Progress in Pain Research and Management
Volume 2

Proceedings of the 7th World Congress on Pain

Progress in Pain Research and Management
Volume 2

Proceedings of the 7th World Congress on Pain

Editors

Gerald F. Gebhart, PhD

Department of Pharmacology
University of Iowa
Iowa City, Iowa, USA

Donna L. Hammond, PhD

Department of Anesthesia and Critical Care
The University of Chicago
Chicago, Illinois, USA

Troels S. Jensen, MD, PhD

Department of Neurology
Aarhus University Hospital
Aarhus, Denmark

IASP PRESS • SEATTLE

Timely topics in pain research and treatment have been selected for publication, but the information provided and opinions expressed have not involved any verification of the findings, conclusions, and opinions by IASP. Thus, opinions expressed in *Proceedings of the 7th World Congress on Pain* do not necessarily reflect those of IASP or of the Officers and Councillors.

No responsibility is assumed by IASP for any injury and/or damage to persons or property as a matter of product liability, negligence, or from any use of any methods, products, instruction, or ideas contained in the material herein. Because of the rapid advances in the medical sciences, the publisher recommends that there should be independent verification of diagnoses and drug dosages.

Library of Congress Cataloging-in-Publication Data

World Congress on Pain (7th : 1993 : Paris, France)
Proceedings of the 7th World Congress on Pain / editors, Gerald F. Gebhart, Donna L. Hammond, Troels S. Jensen.
p. cm. — (Progress in pain research and management ; v. 2)
Includes bibliographical references and index.
ISBN 0-931092-07-8
1. Pain—Congresses. I. Gebhart, Gerald F. II. Hammond, Donna L., 1953- . III. Jensen, Troels Staehelin. IV. Title. V. Series.
[DNLM: 1. Pain—physiopathology—congresses. 2. Pain—drug therapy—congresses. 3. Neuronal Plasticity—physiology—congresses. 4. Central Nervous System—physiology—congresses. WL 704 W927p 1994]
RB127. W67 1993a
616'.0472—dc20
DNLM/DLC
for Library of Congress 94-12699

Published by:

IASP Press
International Association for the Study of Pain
909 NE 43rd St., Suite 306
Seattle, WA 98105 USA
Fax: 206-547-1703

Printed in the United States of America

Contents

Contributors

Preface

If one word were to characterize the 7th World Congress on Pain, it would be *dynamic*. Nearly 4000 participants gathered in an exceptional setting in Paris to make this Congress the largest and most successful meeting to date of the International Association for the Study of Pain. The more than 1500 free communications that were presented in daily poster and slide sessions document the vitality of the IASP membership and the growth in pain research and pain management worldwide. The Congress was unsurpassed as a forum for interdisciplinary interchange of basic and clinical science. In the twenty years since John Bonica convened in Issaquah, Washington, the forerunner of what is now the IASP, this unique international association has continued to grow and mature. The triennial World Congresses that the IASP sponsors and organizes remain the centerpiece of its scientific, educational, and administrative objectives.

The dynamic character of this Congress was reflected in all components of the scientific program. The central theme of the Congress was plasticity of the nervous system in response to insult. From the nociceptor to the cortex, the function and clinical implications of a nervous system changed by injury were incorporated into many parts of the program. In this volume, Schmidt emphasizes the dynamic properties of nociceptors and describes how their function changes when the tissue they innervate is inflamed. Willis describes how plasticity induced as a consequence of peripheral tissue damage influences the excitability of spinal neurons. Free communications included by the editors amplify and complement this important concept, which is changing the way we think about pain and its control, including the circumstance when the injury is intentional (e.g., surgery). As McQuay shows in his review, however, at present only opioids have been documented in appropriately controlled clinical trials to produce a preemptive effect that reduces postoperative hyperalgesia and postoperative opioid requirement for pain control. The chapter by Tohyama, and a number of free communications selected by the editors, provide hope that novel strategies aimed at blocking excitatory amino acid receptors in the spinal cord will be useful in attenuating the increased central excitability that follows peripheral tissue injury. These plastic responses of the nervous system contribute to many pain states, including various chronic pain conditions, as attested to by contributions in several sections of this book.

Above the level of the spinal cord, the nature of pain is more complex and, accordingly, less well understood. Flor discusses the importance of applying careful analysis to pain and pain behaviors in her chapter on the psychobiology of pain, an expanding area of investigation. Keefe and Linton address complementary issues related to pain behaviors and the challenge health care providers face in preventing chronic pain. The importance of these topics to the membership of IASP is attested to by the number of free communications at the Congress that addressed these issues, some of which are included in this volume. Somerville addresses another important dimension of pain management with her well-tempered discussion of pain, suffering, and ethics, presenting rational argument that pain control and the prevention of suffering are not only medical but ethical imperatives. How pain management is changing, including what patients and health care providers expect and require, is discussed by Miaskowsky and VonKorff.

Opioids remain the most efficacious analgesic drugs available, but they clearly are not without undesirable features. Dickenson reviews what is new about opioids and opioid receptors, and Kayser, the recipient of the Patrick D. Wall Young Investigator Award, reviews the role of the endogenous opioid system in the modulation of pain. Max discusses optimization of opioid use for pain control by combining opioids with other drugs and evaluating the effectiveness of the combination in appropriately designed clinical trials. The issue of development of tolerance to the analgesic effects of opioids is reviewed by Portenoy, who presents evidence that analgesic tolerance is not the limiting component to adequate pain control that it has long been considered to be. The pharmacology of pain control continues to be a central focus in pain research, which Besson discusses from his perspective. Recounting the excitement generated when stimulation-produced analgesia was first described, followed soon by documentation of opiate receptors and the discovery of endogenous opioid peptides, he reviews the disappointment of the basic and clinical science community when it became apparent that this new knowledge would not immediately lead to new and better drugs for pain control. The newest developments he describes, many of which are articulated in this volume, give us ample reason to expect that novel pharmacological entities and new strategies will improve our ability to control pain.

This volume, which is the seventh to summarize the important developments in basic and clinical pain research and pain management reported at a World Congress of the IASP, represents only a small sample of the many excellent presentations at the Congress. It is the first Proceedings of an IASP World Congress to be published by the IASP Press. The IASP has succeeded in attracting new and enthusiastic investigators and practitioners to the field of pain research and pain management, and it is the hope of the editors that the vitality of the IASP and of the 7th World Congress on Pain is reflected in these pages.

Acknowledgments

The editors of this volume and the officers and members of the Council of the International Association for the Study of Pain express their appreciation to the many individuals whose efforts were so important to the success of the 7th World Congress on Pain and of this book.

We first thank our colleagues on the Scientific Program Committee, Allan I. Basbaum, Pedro F. Bejarano, Nikolai Bogduk, J. Edmond Charlton, Kenjiro Dan, Gisele Guilbaud, Mitchell B. Max, Bjorn A. Meyerson, Evelyne Pichard-Leandri, Robert F. Schmidt, Barry J. Sessle, and Judith S. Turner, upon whom the editorial group depended for the outline planning of the scientific program, which was so well received.

We thank the Local Arrangements Committee in Paris, led by Jean-Marie Besson, and his colleagues Yves Lazorthes, Daniel H. Le Bars, François Boureau, Henri Dehen, Gisele Guilbaud, Evelyne Pichard-Leandri, Philippe A. Scherpereel, and Jean-Claude Willer, who helped provide an unrivaled setting for the Congress and who worked hard to ensure that the myriad of small organizational details at the Congress were looked after. Special thanks are due to the Congress Secretariat in Paris, SOCFI, especially to staff members Isabel Bardinet, Patrice Lamot, Inez Burger, and Cécile Briot, who took such great care in overseeing registration and all the on-site meeting details. We are grateful for their hard work on our behalf. We extend special gratitude to Louisa Jones, IASP Executive Officer, for her invaluable efforts in organizing the Congress. Thanks also to IASP staff members Andrew Whipple, Frances Butler, and Bryan Urakawa, whose hard work before and during the congress was an important contribution to the overall success of the meeting.

The editors express appreciation to the staff of the publications department of IASP and IASP Press, Leslie Nelson Bond and Dale Schmidt, for their dedicated work in preparing this book for publication.

On behalf of the Council and members of IASP, the editors acknowledge and express their special appreciation for the financial support given to the 7th World Congress on Pain and related IASP programs by the following persons and groups.

The Mayor of Paris, Jacques Chirac
Rhône-Poulenc Rorer (France)

UPSA Laboratoires (France)
Syntex International (USA)
Institut de Recherches Internationales Servier (France)
Theraplix (France)
The Purdue Frederick Company (USA)
Sanofi Recherche (France)
Janssen Pharmaceutica (Belgium)
Grünenthal GMBH (Germany)
Laboratories Houdé (France)
Sarget (France)
Institut de Recherche Jouveinal (France)
Fondation Ipsen (France)
Kabi Pharmacia (Sweden)
Air France
Celsa (France)
Upjohn (France)
Laboratoires Bard (France)
LPI (Laboratoire Pérouse Implant)(France)

Faulding Pharma Group (Australia)
Infusaid, Inc. (USA)
SmithKline Beecham Pharmaceuticals (Beecham Group PLC) (UK)
Volvo Research Foundation (Sweden)

Astra Farmajoytiske A/S (Norway)
Astra Pharma Inc. (Canada)
Curaflex Infusion Services Inc. (USA)
Cygnus Research Corporation (USA)
Danmeter I/S (Denmark)
Elsevier Science Publishers (The Netherlands)
Fondazione Floriani (Italy)
Fondazione Livia Benini (Italy)
The Haworth Press (USA)
H. Lundbeck A/S Ltd. (Norway)
Medtronic of Canada (Canada)
VZV Research Foundation Inc. (USA)
Whitehall Robbins, Inc. (USA)

Part I

Introductory Remarks

Proceedings of the 7th World Congress on Pain, Progress in Pain Research and Management, Vol. 2, edited by G.F. Gebhart, D.L. Hammond, and T.S. Jensen, IASP Press, Seattle, © 1994.

1

President's Address at the 7th World Congress on Pain: Twenty Years with IASP

Ulf Lindblom

Department of Neurology, Karolinska Sjukhuset, Stockholm, Sweden

Dear IASP members, congress participants, and guests! Let me first address the committee for local arrangements and the French chapter, and express our appreciation and thanks for the enthusiastic and generous support and for all your efforts with sponsors and special preparations for the congress. On behalf of IASP, I ask Professor Jean-Marie Besson to accept our sincerest thanks for welcoming the association to Paris with its 7th World Congress, which I now declare officially opened.

It is a solemn moment when a huge congress like this is launched. The work of literally thousands of basic scientists and clinical investigators is comprised in the congress.With the plenary sessions and the seminars, the ambition is to strike the forefront of research, and yet allude enough to basic concepts in the field to enable the multidisciplinary audience to follow and learn from the presentations. The multidisciplinary character of the IASP puts special demands on the Scientific Program Committee, which arranged 1600 abstracts into sensible sessions with the least possible overlap in topic and time. The committee, chaired by Professor Gerald Gebhart, did an excellent job with that task and with the choice of topics and speakers.

There are special aspects of almost every big congress. One such aspect of this congress is its location in the historical capital of Paris, with its exceptional display and variety of facilities. Another special aspect, which could not have been planned beforehand, is the recent great political change in eastern Europe, which in principle enabled participation here from several additional countries. IASP has recognized the economic restraints in these and several other countries and allocated $70,000 for travel support of our members for this congress. Several applicants from Eastern Europe have been supported this time, and further support has come from European chapters and from companies. The general condition for being eligible for IASP travel support has been that the applicant should submit an abstract of reasonable quality. It is our hope that all participants, especially from countries or regions with few representatives, will disseminate knowledge from the congress in their respective regions.

A third aspect of this congress to which I wish to call attention is the following bizarre contrast: Here are representatives of the international scientific community from many universities and clinics assembled under excellent conditions to discuss the study of pain and improvements of pain control. At the same time, other human beings in other places are actively *producing* incomprehensible amounts of pain and suffering, which we cannot control at all, in terrorist actions, civil war, and other destructive violence. It is despairing to see this going on even in parts of Europe where cultural traditions should have worked to prevent repeated barbarism. However, a historical perspective may yield consolation and inspiration to continue our work. One hundred years ago there was another gathering of the international scientific community in Paris. The topic was not pain but celebration of Louis Pasteur on the occasion of his 70th birthday. As the great scientist of the time, Pasteur was also a humanistic authority. At the jubilee, which was held in the grand auditorium at Sorbonne, Pasteur summarized his life thoughts in a closing speech of thanks that included these words: "You give me the greatest joy possible to be experienced by a human being whose unfaltering conviction is that peace and scientific research will gain victory over war and ignorance, that the peoples of this world will arrive at a mutual understanding not to destroy but to build up, and that the future will belong to those who have accomplished most for our suffering mankind. I place my hope in all the brilliant representatives of Science, Medicine, and Surgery whom I see here around me." It is a grim fact that Pasteur's conviction is still a vision rather than a prophecy, and that it may take another century to come true. But the decreased prevalence of suffering today, and political conditions much better than those 100 years ago, should make it easier for us to maintain the same vision.

The twentieth anniversary of the IASP is a further special facet of this congress. A look in the rear-view mirror tells us that the first international and interdisciplinary pain meeting was called together by our Founding President John Bonica in May 1973. Neither the idea to arrange the meeting nor the proposal to form IASP were sudden ideas of Professor Bonica, but rather the result of almost 30 years of systematic study of pain problems, including the publication of his classic monograph in 1953 and his sustained advocacy for recognition of pain as an important but neglected field, requiring a forum of its own, a multidisciplinary approach, and research about pain mechanisms and improved clinical management.

The first meeting took place in Issaquah, Washington, USA, and attracted 350 registrants. Several prominent pain clinicians and researchers gave scientific papers and took part in the discussion leading to the enthusiastic decision to organize IASP and to arrange triennial multidisciplinary world congresses. The first scientific program committee was chaired by Professor Denise Albe-Fessard, who was also the first President of IASP. Another decision made was to start the journal *Pain,* with Professor Patrick Wall as Editor in Chief. Many senior members I have asked agree that *Pain* was the most important and fundamental endeavor of IASP. The long, devoted contribution by Professor Wall has no doubt been crucial for the journal's establishment as the leading scholarly journal in the pain field. As a token of the appreciation of generations of members and their student fellows who have absorbed wisdom from the pages of *Pain*, IASP has decided to rename the Young Investigator Award to become the Patrick D. Wall Young Investigator Award.

The twentieth anniversary is a natural time to ask what IASP has contributed to the pain field. It is unique to start and build an international and multidisciplinary society from scratch, and it is noteworthy that the original bylaws that define the aims of IASP still monitor our business, with few amendments. Regarding the achievements and impact of IASP on the field of pain, we can identify five target areas: research, education, clinical management, public awareness, and civic adjustments.

The most important contribution of IASP is the implementation of multidisciplinary interaction among research, education, and clinical management. To start with the last, there is little doubt that the formation of multidisciplinary pain groups, which have proliferated like mushrooms in country after country, has advanced clinical management so widely that we can speak of worldwide establishment of the multidisciplinary principle of pain management. IASP has played a significant role toward awareness of the undertreatment of acute pain, toward the acceptance of opioid regimens, and toward the initiation of the WHO cancer pain programs. The hospice movement and pain programs of palliative care medicine have conceivably benefited as well from the interface with IASP.

Among educational achievements, the publications will naturally have the widest and most sustained impact. In addition to *Pain,* IASP has published its Newsletter with a Technical Corner, refresher course material, congress abstracts, proceedings, and a new clinical update in newsletter format. Further, the positive role for undergraduate and postgraduate training of the pain curricula for medicine, pharmacology, dentistry, and nursing, the *Core Curriculum,* and the *Management of Acute Pain* book has been witnessed from all parts of the world. The recent decision to enter the publishing field as IASP Press was taken in order to expand the production of educational material and to publish such material at lower cost, primarily for the benefit of our members. Both the abstract book and the Proceedings of this congress will appear as IASP publications.

In addition to the World Congresses, IASP has endorsed many multidisciplinary and international meetings and refresher courses that have worked indirectly to improve patient care.

It is thus possible to list many IASP contributions to education in the pain field . But what about research? What has IASP meant to the study of pain mechanisms, pathophysiology, and new treatments? There should be no doubt about the general benefit of the multidisciplinary meetings, especially the World Congresses, as inspiring sources of ideas and cross-fertilization between disciplines. When Professor Bonica reviewed the first period of IASP in his presidential address at the Edinburgh Congress in 1981, he pointed out that there had been a significant increase in pain research during the 1970s compared to the long previous "silent period." It was believed that this increase was much due to the appearance of IASP. Today's perspective adds another decade of further and, I must say, astounding increase in interest and awareness of pain as an important field of medicine, and also as a worthwhile target for dedicated research resources. We have witnessed how several pioneers in basic research, from molecular biologists to psychologists, have become actively engaged in pain research and stimulated a generation of students to enter the field. I feel safe to claim that the amount of pain research currently produced would not have reached this level without the nurturing effects of IASP.

Regarding public awareness and civic adjustment in the form of changes of public policies, laws, and regulations, a few examples may be mentioned. IASP's existence and prestige have cleared the way for allocation of federal funds to pain research in at least the United States and Germany. Pain foundations have been established in some countries. The IASP chapters have pursuaded authorities to change the regulations of opioid prescription in at least Germany and Austria. The Dutch chapter has successfully generated substantial support and active sponsorship by the Ministry of Health for pain education of general practitioners and others.

In addition to IASP's general catalytic influence on pain research, I was interested to find out if there were discoveries or other specific scientific advancements that could be ascribed to IASP. An inquiry among senior IASP members yielded a largely negative result: it is difficult to make such assignments. This is not surprising from the point of view that IASP has no funds for direct support of research projects. There is, however, one example where I dare to claim that IASP has initiated a specific scientific advancement, with implications for both basic and clinical research that can hardly be overestimated. That is the work on pain taxonomy, in which I personally have been involved as a member of the committee, persistently and skillfully chaired by Professor Harold Merskey. The *Classification of Chronic Pain: Descriptions of Chronic Pain Syndromes and Definitions of Pain Terms* has provided a basis for improved communication which was badly needed. The taxonomy has further, albeit with a latency of years, spurred interest of basic scientists to investigate some clinical phenomena, as witnessed by recent publications on hyperalgesia and allodynia (W.D. Willis, ed., *Hyperalgesia and Allodynia*, Raven Press, New York, 1992; W.D. Willis, *Mechanical allodynia*, APS Journal, 2,1 [1993] 23–33; G.L. Wilcox, *Spinal mediators of nociceptive neurotransmission and hyperalgesia*, APS Journal, 2,4, [1993] 265–275). From personal experience, I know that the clinical phenomenon that mild mechanical or thermal stimuli may evoke pain in apparently normal skin in patients with neuropathic pain raised no specific interest among neurophysiologists before IASP gave the new term *allodynia* to this condition.

It should be pointed out that there have been significant advancements in the pain field by means of non-IASP initiatives, and these should be given due credit. One is the delineation and description of the fibromyalgia syndrome, which was achieved through exemplary multicenter studies in United States and Canada and the support of the American College of Rheumatology, as well as through recently published monographs on the subject. Another example is headache, which has its own regional and international forum, the International Headache Society. The alignment of the IHS World Congress to overlap with the IASP Congress here in Paris is intended to facilitate cross-fertilization between the two organizations.

An important IASP perspective is in the development of its regional chapters. The first four IASP chapters were founded in 1976 in the German-speaking countries of Austria, Germany, and Switzerland; in Italy; in Scandinavia; and in the United States. After IASP's first 10 years there were 13 chapters. Today, after another 10 years, there are 46 chapters comprising 55 nations. This shows an accelerated development and means that IASP is now truly international, even if some chapters are young and have relatively few members. The total membership worldwide, including both IASP members and other chapter members, is close to13,000.

As incoming President in Adelaide, I called for or anticipated a number of things that might happen during my presidency, which are listed below. Issues in bold are those that definitely have advanced, those in regular type showed some or partial development, and those in italic showed no advancement that I am aware of, at the clinical level.

- **Improved taxonomy**
- Differential diagnosis of chronic pain with pathophysiological testing
- *New specific drugs for chronic pain syndromes*
- *"Hands on" with psychologically enforced pain*
- Studies on pain-related sensory abnormalities
- *Studies on predictors of chronic pain*
- *Studies on pain provocation in painless disease*
- *Recruitment of neurologists, orthopedists, rheumatologists, etc.*
- Fund-raising: **Publications**
  J.J. Bonica Fellowship Fund
  Other capital funds

Some of these points I have already addressed. With regard to new specific drugs for chronic pain syndromes, a lot of research is ongoing, but we are still waiting for clinically useful NMDA-antagonists and analogs of peptides or other endogenous pain-transmission modulators. I had hoped for a breakthrough for chronic pain syndromes with a receptor-targeted drug, as has occurred with sumatriptan for migraine. Fund-raising was certainly one of my priority issues. It has been successful, as during previous periods, with specific projects such as publications, congress activities, and a few prizes, but the only capital fund that has grown, thanks to many donations by members, is the John J. Bonica Fellowship Fund.

Thus, there will be many challenges left in the future for IASP and its incoming Council when I leave office as President by the completion of this Congress. I shall be looking back at several years of exciting work as Councillor, thanks to the spirit of uniquely professional, inspiring, and productive colleagues and collaborators dedicated to contributing toward the important goals of IASP.

Proceedings of the 7th World Congress on Pain,
Progress in Pain Research and Management, Vol. 2,
edited by G.F. Gebhart, D.L. Hammond, and T.S.
Jensen, IASP Press, Seattle, © 1994.

2

Quo Vadis Dolore

John D. Loeser

Professor, Neurological Surgery and Anesthesiology,
Director, Multidisciplinary Pain Center, University of
Washington, Seattle, Washington, USA

The first twenty years of our association have been a spectacular success. We have had stable leadership and administrative support. To no small degree, this is due to the unflaggingly devoted efforts of Louisa Jones, our Executive Director, and her fine administrative staff. It is also due to the selfless efforts by the members of committees and task forces and, in particular, to the hard work of committee chairpersons, Council members and your elected officers.

We have made a difference in four areas of endeavor, as characterized in Ulf Lindblom's Presidential Address to this congress. Research, education, communication, and patient care have all been favorably influenced by our association and the activities of our members.

I would like to review our educational and communications activities first; they are, in my opinion our most important contribution. We have established the largest and most productive congresses for the presentation of research and clinical information. Our journal, *Pain*, under the careful leadership of Patrick Wall since its inception, and now Ronald Dubner and Patrick Wall, is the premier scientific publication focused upon pain. Our other publications provide members and the public with valuable and timely new information—scientific, clinical, and administrative.

We have developed a series of public information resources, but much remains to be done in this area. Our administrative office is bombarded with requests from both the professional and the lay public for all types of information about pain, its treatment, educational opportunities, and referral requests. We have laid the groundwork for a communications network about all aspects of pain, and now we need to put some muscle on the skeleton.

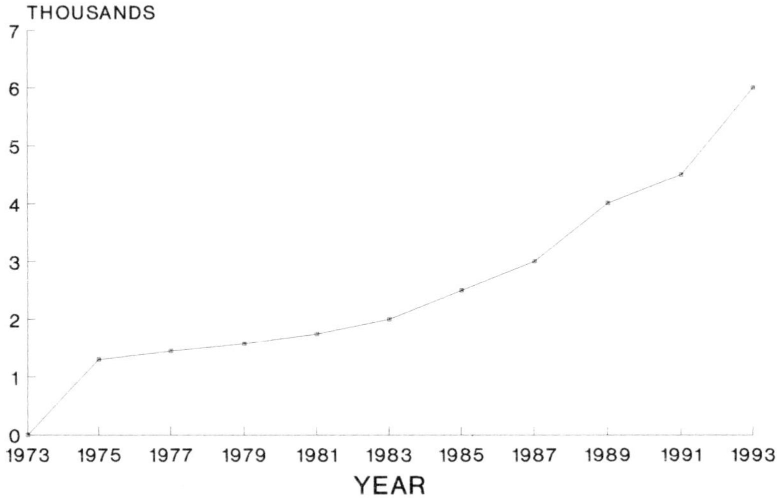

Fig. 1. Number of IASP members.

Another great success has been the development of national and regional chapters that have adopted and implemented the goals of IASP in their own territory. Those of us who have been privileged to travel to countries when chapters are in the process of formation feel great pride, almost like a new grandparent, as the new chapter grows in size and activity.

We have succeeded in making pain a legitimate subject of education, research and patient care in the brief span of twenty years. The explosion of scientific and clinical papers addressing aspects of pain is well known to all in this audience. The pioneers are only one generation ahead of us; some are even present at this meeting.

The growth and development of IASP can be reflected in some of the numbers, but they are dry compared to the knowledge of the people involved in this process. We can look at membership, geographic representation, finances, and attendance at World Congresses to see how we are growing.

Our paid membership is growing geometrically and now is over 6000. In addition, there are about 6000 chapter members in currency-restricted or developing countries who do not pay dues to IASP directly. Our family is, therefore, 12,000 strong (Fig. 1). By the end of this Congress, we will have 30 approved chapters. In addition, there are at least 10 more in the process of formation. I expect that this representation of countries throughout the globe will continue to grow in the several years (Fig. 2). The budget of IASP is heavily influenced by the Congress; I have chosen to present the association's budget data for the years of the Congresses (Fig. 3). As you can see, this

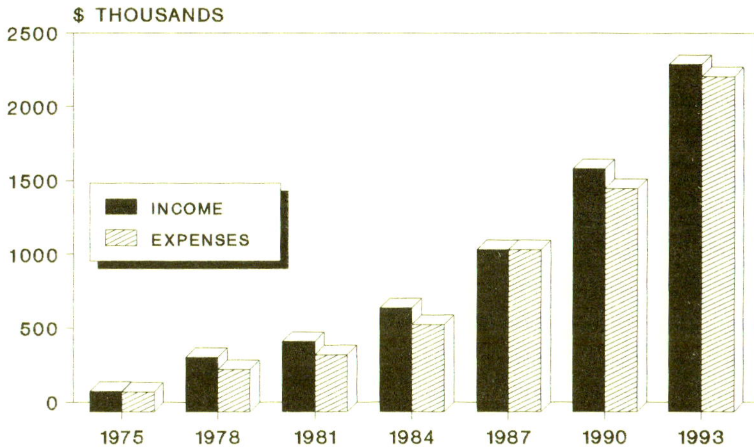

Fig. 2. Number of IASP chapters.

association has been led by fiscally responsible officers and we actually have a reserve fund of several hundred thousand dollars. Finally, the number of delegates at our triennial Congress is a good reflection of the strength of our association (Fig. 4). We expect that all of you present at this Congress, plus an addition thousand or so, will be present in Chicago three years from now.

I would like to talk a moment about the dues policy of IASP. We have struggled to develop an equitable policy that supports our members in developing or currency-controlled countries but does not deplete the resources required to implement other programs. The essential points, as they have now been approved by Council, are:

- Dues will be kept as low as possible.
- Dues will increase for the first time in four years.
- All regular members will pay dues sufficient to cover the basic costs of *Pain* and operations in the central office.
- Dues will be graduated on the basis of income.
- A special membership category exists for individuals in developing or currency-restricted countries. Dues will be $40 US, but the individual will not receive *Pain*.
- We have reaffirmed the policy that a regular chapter must have a minimum of 25 dues-paying members.

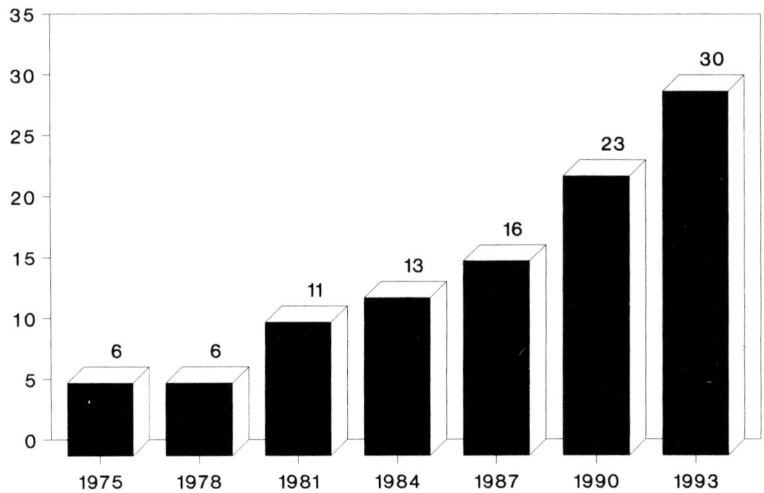

Fig. 3. IASP budget in years of World Congresses.

- Affiliate chapters in currency-controlled or developing countries do not have a minimum number of dues paying members. The members of an affiliate chapter do not pay dues to IASP and do not receive individual mailings or journals. IASP does subsidize affiliate chapters by sending printed resources and journals to a central address for subsequent circulation by the chapter. We have also tried to help fund visiting lecturers.

Our greatest accomplishment is that we have become a community with both soul and purpose: the relief of needless pain and suffering in all of the countries of this world.

There have also been scientific achievements by our members that have been supported by IASP. One of the most important has been the Taxonomy of Pain. Harold Merskey will be known as the Linnaeus of the twentieth century for his efforts.

We have carried on the vision of John J. Bonica, who convened the world's first pain symposium in Issaquah, Washington, USA, in 1973. From that came IASP, and everything that we can accomplish is the fulfillment of his vision and his unceasing efforts for the cause.

Finally, nous sommes montes à Paris; or if it must be in English, one of our great accomplishments has been to hold this Congress in Paris. We need to thank Jean Marie Besson and the Local Arrangements Committee for their fund raising and total support of this Congress.

I would like to set forth my goals for next several years. The first set relate to financial matters that are critical to our association. We must continue the prudent fiscal policies that have been implemented by our treasurer,

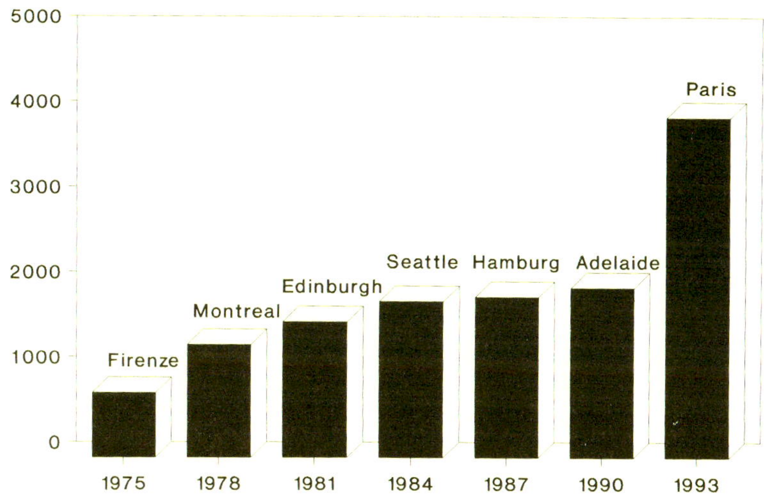

Fig. 4. Number of delegates to World Congresses.

Ron Dubner. Additional money must be set aside in a reserve fund to provide for unforeseen contingencies and generate income. Our dues must be kept as low as possible, but they must cover the true cost of maintaining the central office and services to members. We must develop external funding for specific projects from private sources, be they commercial or charitable. This has been a difficult task for an international organization, but we must redouble our efforts.

The most exciting new development is the program to be undertaken under the leadership of Howard Fields to develop IASP Press. We believe that we can offer our members first-class texts written by the world's experts at a cost far below the commercial publishers. We also hope to develop extensive translation services to expand the readership of our publications.

We must continue to attract and maintain dues-paying members and broaden our geographic representation by facilitating the development of chapters in the developing countries. This will require new programs to send out experts who can serve as the focal points for meetings throughout the world.

The time has come to encourage the development of regional associations of chapters, based upon common geography or common languages. This will provide an opportunity for scientific exchanges that cannot be met in our large, triennial Congress.

Finally, special interest groups can provide another mechanism for the exchange of scientific and clinical information beyond that can occur in a journal or at a large meeting. The development of the Pediatric Special Interest Group has been a source of real pleasure for all; I hope that other groups will continue to develop to meet the needs of our members.

The second president of IASP, my colleague and friend John J. Bonica, delivered an important address at the time of the Third World Congress on Pain of IASP in Edinburgh in August 1981. His review of the developments in research, education, and patient care that had occurred in the first eight years of the existence of our association also charted a course for us to follow. Bonica said, "It is my firm conviction that IASP can and should provide vigorous leadership in helping the biomedical scientific community, the health professions, and society as a whole to effectively meet these challenges."

As you have heard from my predecessor, Ulf Lindblom, we have traveled some distance on the journey first envisioned by John Bonica. Our association has grown in numbers and in geographic representation. We have preserved and even strengthened our unique multidisciplinary membership. The association has directly supported educational activities and has established committees and task forces that have produced useful reports for clinicians, researchers, and educators. We have, in conjunction with the World Health Organization and other political groups, influenced governmental policies. Our publications are widely recognized as being of the finest quality. The triennial Congresses have all been scientific and financial successes; this great Congress that is soon to be concluded has clearly met the needs and goals of its attendees.

I believe that the primary mission of the International Association for the Study of Pain is education: of our members, of scientists in general, of health care practitioners, of governmental officials, and of the public. Associations such as ours can facilitate, through education, organization, and public recognition, the intellectual activities of our members. Although the members of your Council and the Executive Committee can provide the leadership to accomplish some of the tasks that lie ahead, the actual work will, of necessity, be carried out by individual members who are willing to serve on committees and task forces and to undertake the research, patient care, and educational and political activities so vital to our association.

As I have the great honor to be your president for the next three years, I would like to commence my term of office by asking what I believe to be the critical question for the International Association for the Study of Pain: What are you willing to do to keep us moving forward?

Proceedings of the 7th World Congress on Pain, Progress in Pain Research and Management, Vol. 2, edited by G.F. Gebhart, D.L. Hammond, and T.S. Jensen, IASP Press, Seattle, © 1994.

3

Address to the 7th World Congress on Pain

Philippe Douste-Blazy

Minister of Health, Paris, France

I would first like to thank the organizers of the 7th Congress of the International Association for the Study of Pain for their invitation, in particular Professor Lindblom, president of IASP, and Professor Besson, president of the local arrangements committee.

I also greet Professor Yves Lazorthes, whom I know personally, a renowned surgeon known for his skills and his humanity, and I wish to congratulate him on his latest work, *Les Douleurs Rebelles*. The presence today of so many of you is proof of your interest in the fight against pain, a priority for the public health authorities in France, and in which I am personally very interested, both as Minister and as a doctor.

Over the decades, pain has been looked upon as a tragic misfortune. As has been put forward by Professor Jean Bernard of the French Academy, "Medicine has changed more in the last 50 years than in the preceding 50 centuries." However, despite this progress, he added, "pain has attracted less attention. Pain has been looked upon as a symptom and has not been the center of attention for clinicians or researchers." I agree with this famous academician that it should no longer be like this, since scientific progress has given us better means to understand pain. It is no longer possible to give in; we must give all patients access to all possible treatments for pain.

Pain accompanies all pathologies, whether medical or surgical. Each year in France 4 million operations are carried out and 200,000 new cases of cancer are diagnosed, together with the more than 24,000 cases of AIDS that have arisen since the start of the epidemic. Pain is the primary reason for 67% medical consultations in France.

With regard to international cooperation, the exemplary campaign of the World Health Organization should be pointed out. Their efforts over many years to urge every country to develop a program for the relief of cancer pain are starting to bear fruit. I do not forget to acknowledge the International Association for the Study of Pain (IASP), the organizing body for this congress, which by merit of its many activities in the field of pain, and particularly by means of the journal *Pain,* has contributed to doctors' awareness of this important public health issue.

The situation in France is paradoxical: although the nation actively participates in the progress that has been made in neurobiological research such as the pharmacology of analgesics, it must be said that for a long time, the treatment of pain has often been neglected. Many studies have shown that the lack of care and treatment of pain is a common complaint by patients and their relatives but is generally underestimated by health professionals. It has been estimated that as a result of cancer, whatever the stage, 56% of patients suffer pain, and half of those do not receive any analgesic. Only 30% of such pain is correctly treated, although it should be possible to completely eliminate it in 90% of cases.

The lack of treatment or insufficient treatment of pain in children has been recognized only in the past 10 years and arises from misconceptions and prejudices that still determine the majority of therapeutic attitudes of health teams coping with pain in children. In the late 1980s, numerous studies showed that such conceptions of pain in children were not supported by scientific bases. There are effective means of treating pain, in children, but these studies remain dispersed in the literature and among different medical and paramedical specialties. The slowness of France in the area of pain relief (only in 40th place in the world for the consumption of opiates, well behind the Anglo-Saxon and Scandinavian countries) has become a public issue, because people are, with good cause, very aware of these matters.

It is unacceptable, and I say this as a doctor as well as the head of public health in this country, that a significant number of general practitioners do not always have the required forms for the prescription of strong analgesics. It is equally unacceptable that during the initial stages of medical training, half of French medical schools dedicate less than two hours to instruction on pain, and it is not covered except as a symptom within the teaching programs of particular organs and illnesses. What is there in the teaching of the use analgesics that still causes reticence in doctors and pharmacists with regard to the use of opiates, which have such an important role in the fight against pain? Some of this reticence is based on an understandable desire to avoid the problems of side effects and dependence, but there are techniques and therapeutic approaches (based on WHO recommendations) that can control these problems. Can one justify the insupportable and unrelieved suffering of patients at the end of their lives by a poor knowledge of these techniques and approaches? It seems to me that it is essential to organize in medical faculties a balanced and specific teaching program on pain. Every clinician is a doctor of pain.

Over several years, the public health authorities in France, in collaboration with professionals and associations, have fought this situation by means of information and education and by relaxing prescription rules. Furthermore, a working group has been formed for the care of the terminally ill. Their recommendations led to the publication of a bill on 26 August 1986 organizing the health care structures (Palliative Care Units) and encouraging their development. Action has been taken to spread of information: a brochure for doctors, entitled *Soigner et accompagner jusqu'au bout: soulager la souffrance* (Treatment and care until the end of life: the relief of suffering), with details on the techniques of pain relief, has been sent out by the Ministry of Health, and will be revised on the occasion of this congress. In the same way, a report on chronic pain was published in 1991 which listed the specialized treatment units and put forward guidelines on education; my advisors inform me that this publication was exactly what was needed by the groups confronted with this problem.

To take account of the fact that pain in children can and must be treated, the Ministry of Health, together with the Association for the Treatment of Pain in Children, organizes an annual colloquium on this subject. This association, with the aid of the Ministry of Health, has set up a data base on pain in children (PEDIADOL), accessible by Minitel, the national computer network. The Ministry of Health has furthermore placed a campaign against pain among its stated priorities.

The establishment of university and inter-university degree programs in pain education has been encouraged since 1985, and eight faculties now have such a program. The campaign against pain is also one of the most frequent subject areas covered in continuing medical education.

Finally, and most important, since September 1992, doctors have been able to prescribe morphine by the oral route and for a longer period (14 days) than previously allowed. This will ease the problems of doctors and undoubtedly allow better use of this drug.

These actions all have helped to raise the consciousness of both the public and health professionals with regard to pain. There is still much to do, in particular to improve the organization of the specialized treatment of chronic pain and to further the educational aspects. Despite the economic restrictions on health-care expenditure in France, I hope that the campaign against pain will become a priority for the ministry of which I am in charge.

I can now make you part of my wish to know exactly, with the agreement of the involved professionals, the structures needed to overcome pain.

The recommendations of the working group on Intractable Pain will soon lead to the production of a circular establishing a network of multidisciplinary centers with a triple approach: *care* (evaluation, therapy, and follow-up of patients with a doctor), *research,* and *education.* With regard to education, I hope that eventually the subject of pain will be a part of medical studies (second and third levels) and that all doctors will be equipped with the means to relieve suffering in their patients. Education continues, and will do so until the reticence still seen is eliminated.

Finally, I wish to encourage research, and in that regard I must encourage and offer my best wishes to all researchers who are making new contributions to this field and to the clinical application of this research. It is my role as Minister of Health to assure you my support.

Discours, 7ème Congès Mondial sur la Douleur

Philippe Douste-Blazy

Ministre Délégué à la Santé, Paris, France

Je tiens tout d'abord à remercier pour leur invitation les organisateurs de ce 7ème congrès de la Société Internationale pour l'Etude de la Douleur, et plus particulièrement le Professeur Lindblom, président de la Société Internationale pour l'étude de la Douleur et le Dr Besson, président du comité local d'organisation. Je salue également le Professeur Yves Lazorthes que je connais personnellement, grand chirurgien reconnu pour sa compétence et son humanisme et que je tiens à féliciter pour son dernier ouvrage «Les douleurs rebelles.» Votre présence en si grand nombre aujourd'hui, témoigne de votre intérêt pour la lutte contre la douleur, qui est une priorité des autorités de santé publique françaises et à laquelle je suis personnellement très attaché, en tant que Ministre et en tant que médecin.

Pendant des millénaires, la douleur a été vécue comme une tragique fatalité. Comme le souligne le Professeur Jean Bernard de l'Académie Française, "la médecine a plus changé pendant ces 50 dernières années que pendant les 50 siècles précédents (...). Cependant que s'accomplissaient ces progrès, ajoute-t-il, la douleur ne retenait guère l'attention. Elle était tenue pour un symptôme et ne se trouvait pas au centre des préoccupations des médecins, des chercheurs...." En accord avec ce célèbre académicien, il ne devrait plus en être de même aujourd'hui, car les progrès de la science nous ont donné de meilleurs moyens de la maîtriser. Il n'est plus possible de se résigner; il faut absolument donner aux malades toutes les possibilités d'accès au traitement de la douleur.

La douleur se rencontre dans toutes les pathologies aussi bien médicales que chirurgicales: chaque année en France 4 millions d'actes chirurgicaux sont pratiqués, et 20 0000 nouveaux cas de cancers sont diagnostiqués, plus de 24 000 cas de SIDA ont été recensés depuis le début de l'épidémie: sait-on que la douleur représente 67% des premiers motifs de consultation médicale des français?

En matière de coopération internationale, il faut particulièrement souligner l'action exemplaire de l'Organisation Mondiale de la Santé, engagée depuis plusieurs années pour inciter chaque pays à mettre en place un programme de soulagement de la douleur cancéreuse, qui commence à porter ses fruits. Je n'oublierai pas d'associer à cet hommage l'Association Internationale d'Etude de la Douleur (IASP), organisatrice de ce colloque, qui par ses nombreux travaux sur la douleur, et particulièrement par l'intermédiaire de sa revue Pain, a contribué à sensibiliser les médecins sur ce dossier important de santé publique.

La situation de la France est paradoxale: si elle participe activement aux progrès réalisés dans le domaine de la recherche neurobiologique comme dans celui de la pharmacologie des antalgiques, force est de constater que pendant longtemps, le traitement de la douleur a été trop souvent négligé. De nombreux travaux témoignent de l'insuffisance de la prise en charge et du traitement des douleurs dont se plaignent les malades et leurs proches, sous-estimée en général par les professionnels de santé. On estime qu'au cours du cancer, tous stades confondus, 56% des patients présentent des douleurs, pour lesquelles la moitié d'entre eux ne reçoivent aucun antalgique, et que seules 30% des douleurs sont correctement prises en charge, alors qu'il serait possible dans 90% des cas de les soulager entièrement.

Chez l'enfant, l'absence ou l'insuffisance de traitement de la douleur a été mise en évidence depuis moins de 10 ans et tient à des conceptions erronées et des préjugés qui déterminent encore la majorité des attitudes thérapeutiques des équipes soignantes face à la douleur de l'enfant. Dans les toutes dernières années 80, de nombreuses études ont montré que ces conceptions de la douleur chez l'enfant n'étaient étayées par aucun argument scientifique. Des moyens efficaces existent pour lutter contre la douleur, mais ces données restent dispersées dans les publications et entre différentes spécialités médicales et para-médicales. Le retard de la France dans le domaine du soulagement de la douleur (elle se situe seulement au 40ème rang mondial quant à la consommation des morphiniques, ce qui la place loin derrière les pays anglosaxons et scandinaves) est d'autant plus sensible que l'opinion publique est, à juste titre, très attentive à ces questions.

Il n'est pas acceptable, et je m'exprime ici en tant que médecin comme au titre de mes fonctions à la tête de la santé publique dans ce pays, qu'un nombre important de médecins généralistes ne possède toujours pas de carnet à souche, alors qu'il est, vous le savez, nécessaire à la prescription des stupéfiants. Il n'est plus acceptable non plus qu'au cours de la formation initiale des médecins, la moitié des facultés françaises consacre moins de deux heures à l'enseignement sur la douleur en tant que telle, celle-ci n'étant abordée que comme symptôme au cours des enseignements propres à chaque organe et à chaque maladie. Enfin qu'en est-il de l'enseignement sur les antalgiques, qui contribue plus à entretenir les réticences des médecins et pharmaciens face à l'utilisation des morphiniques qu'à une véritable formation à la lutte contre la douleur. Certes ces réticences sont fondées sur un louable souci d'éviter les risques d'accoutumance, comme par la crainte de leurs effets secondaires, mais des techniques et des protocoles thérapeutiques (sur la base des recommandations de l'OMS en la matière) existent actuellement qui permettent de contrôler ces dérives. Et peut-on justifier les souffrances insupportables et non soulagées de certains malades en fin de vie par la méconnaissance de ces techniques et de ces protocoles? L'organisation dans les facultés de médecine d'un enseignement spécifique et équilibré de la douleur m'apparaît indispensable. Tout médecin est, pour beaucoup, médecin de la douleur.

Depuis plusieurs années, les autorités publiques de la Santé en France, en liaison avec les professionnels et les associations ont tenté de lutter contre cette situation en favorisant l'information et la formation, et en assouplissant les règles de prescription. Ainsi un groupe de travail a été constitué sur l'organisation des soins et l'accompagnement des malades en phase terminale. Ses conclusions ont permis la rédaction d'une circulaire du 26 août 1986, organisant les structures de soins (Unités de Soins Palliatifs) et encourageant le développement de ces soins. Des actions d'information ont été entreprises: une brochure, intitulée «Soigner et Accompagner jusqu'au bout: soulager la souffrance,» destinée aux médecins et détaillant les techniques de traitement des douleurs a été diffusée par le Ministère de la Santé, et fait l'objet d'une réédition à l'occasion de ce congrès. De la même manière un rapport a été publié en 1991 sur la douleur chronique, qui définit les structures spécialisées dans son traitement et formule des recommandations sur la formation: mes services constatent que cette publication correspond vraiment à une demande des équipes confrontées à ce problème.

Afin de faire prendre conscience que la douleur de l'enfant peut et doit être traitée, le Ministère de la Santé en liaison avec l'Association pour le Traitement de la Douleur de l'Enfant organisent annuellement un colloque sur ce thème. De même cette association, aidée par les services du Ministère, a mis en place une banque de données sur la douleur de l'enfant, accessible par minitel (PEDIADOL). Le Ministère de la Santé a également inscrit la formation sur la lutte contre la douleur parmi ses priorités.

Ainsi la création de diplômes médicaux universitaires puis interuniversitaires d'enseignement sur la douleur a été encouragée depuis 1985, et à ce jour 8 facultés les ont mis en place. La lutte contre la douleur est également un des thèmes les plus fréquemment abordés lors des sessions de formation médicale continue.

Enfin, et surtout, les médecins peuvent désormais, depuis septembre 1992 prescrire la morphine par voie orale pour une durée plus longue qu'auparavant (14 jours), ce qui devrait faciliter la tâche des médecins et permettre sans doute une meilleure utilisation.

Toutes ces actions ont favorisé une évolution des mentalités, tant du grand public que des professionnels de la santé, à l'égard de la douleur. Beaucoup reste à faire, en particulier améliorer l'organisation des structures spécialisées dans le traitement de la douleur chronique, et poursuivre les efforts entrepris en matière de formation. Malgré les impératifs d'économie de la santé auxquels nous sommes confrontés en France, je souhaite que la lutte contre la douleur soit un thème prioritaire du Ministère dont je suis en charge.

D'ores et déja je peux vous faire part de mon souhait de voir définies précisément, avec l'accord des professionnels concernés, les structures nécessaires à la prise en charge de la douleur.

Les recommandations du groupe de travail sur les douleurs rebelles devraient aboutir prochainement à l'élaboration d'une circulaire organisant leur prise en charge au sein de structures pluridisciplinaires à triple vocation de soins (évaluation, orientations thérapeutiques et suivi des patients en collaboration avec le médecin traitant), de recherches et d'enseignement. En matière de formation, je souhaite qu'à terme, elle soit intégrée au cursus existant des études médicales (2ème et 3ème cycle), afin que tout médecin soit armé pour s'efforcer d'apaiser les souffrances de ses patients. La formation continue doit elle aussi poursuivre ses efforts pour que les réticences encore observées disparaissent.

Enfin je souhaite que la recherche soit encouragée, et à cet égard il me paraît nécessaire de féliciter et d'encourager tous les chercheurs, et parmi eux vous-mêmes, qui êtes à la pointe des acquisitions modernes dans ce domaine, et de leur application clinique. C'est mon rôle comme Ministre Délégué à la Santé de vous assurer de mon soutien.

Part II

Special Lectures

Proceedings of the 7th World Congress on Pain,
Progress in Pain Research and Management, Vol. 2,
edited by G.F. Gebhart, D.L. Hammond, and T.S.
Jensen, IASP Press, Seattle, © 1994.

4

The Pharmacology of Pain: Twenty-five Years of Hope, Despair, and Hope

Jean-Marie Besson

Unité de Recherches de Physiopharmacologie du Système Nerveux de l'INSERM (U 161) and E.P.H.E., Laboratoire de Physiopharmacologie de la Douleur, Paris, France

When I entered into the field of pain research more than twenty-five years ago, studies devoted to the pharmacology of pain were scarce and difficult to interpret. At that time the number of chemicals thought to be involved in pain processes could be counted on the fingers of one hand, and most of the investigations were essentially devoted to the site of actions of morphine and aspirin. Lim and coworkers (1964), using original and very sophisticated experiments on cross-circulation in the dog, had already established that the main site of action of non-opioid analgesics was the periphery, and the main sites of action of opioids were in the central nervous system. As one can see in this volume, today the problem is much more complex because some recent data suggest an additional action of morphine at peripheral sites and an action at central sites for nonsteroidal anti-inflammatory drugs (NSAIDs).

Research in the field of pain has expanded considerably over the past twenty-five years. This is mainly due to formulation of the gate control theory, discovery of the various sites of action of morphine, and discovery of opioid receptors and endogenous opioids. In parallel, the involvement of numerous endogenous substances including monoamines, various peptides, and excitatory amino acids in the transmission and modulation of pain has been established.

Thus today there are many strategic approaches to the development of new analgesic compounds. During the past twenty-five years, I have been lucky to be actively involved in this field of research. This chapter does not claim to be exhaustive or to delve deeply into a specific area of pain research. I would like instead to recount the main experimental steps I have experienced since the mid-1960s, including our hopes, our wavering, our disillusionments, and finally our confidence in present and future research for the design of new analgesic compounds.

This chapter consists of three parts:

1. *A start like a trumpet fanfare.* The early progress in neurophysiology led to more functional pharmacological research. Those were the glory years of the direct spinal depressive effects of morphine, of the descending monoaminergic systems, and of endogenous opioids.

2. *Complexities, difficulties, and doubts.*

3. *The reasons for hope.*

This survey reflects my own point of view, but I feel that it is reasonably optimistic. Indeed, we all know how very time-consuming and difficult it is to design an analgesic drug for clinical use. We should avoid being too enthusiastic and giving false hope to patients suffering from intractable pain.

A START LIKE A TRUMPET FANFARE

The gate control theory of pain played a major role in the development of both experimental and clinical pain research. This theory gave rise to lively discussions with the supporters of the specificity theory of pain. I realized immediately that if the trigger cells of the gate control theory so nicely described by Wall (1967) and coworkers had something to do with pain, their responses to noxious stimuli should be depressed by morphine. At the end of the 1960s, I went to University College London to watch an experiment, and back in Paris we started to record the activity of dorsal horn neurons. In 1971 we clearly demonstrated in spinalized animals that a morphine-like drug named phenoperidine depressed the responses of deep dorsal horn neurons to noxious stimulation (Besson et al. 1973).

That same year I was invited to Ulm, Germany, to participate in a satellite symposium of the International Congress of Physiology. I presented several aspects of our work on the pharmacology of dorsal horn neurons. Present were Ainley Iggo, Ed Perl, Robert Schmidt, Manfred Zimmermann, and others. I was severely criticized for using intra-arterial injections of bradykinin (largely used today), and to my great despair the audience was totally unresponsive to the part of my presentation related to phenoperidine. We were not defeated by this apparent lack of interest, however, for we quickly demonstrated a direct depressive effect of morphine itself at the spinal level. In the extensive studies performed in our group by Daniel Le Bars and coworkers, we showed that these effects are dose-dependent, stereospecific, and reversed by naloxone (Conseiller et al. 1972; Le Bars et al. 1974, 1975, 1976; Le Bars and Besson 1981). These results were confirmed by other groups: J. Henry in Montreal (Calvillo et al. 1974), L. Kitihata in New Haven (Kitahata et al. 1974), and W. Zieglgänsberger in Munich (Zieglgansberger and Bayerl 1976). Then, by using local administration of morphine by microiontophoresis, Duggan and colleagues (1976) demonstrated that the main site of action of morphine was the superficial dorsal horn.

Despite the fact that the results obtained by these electrophysiological investigations were homogenous and extremely convincing, most of the pharmacologists, physiologists, and clinicians remained very skeptical about their functional significance. People started to believe in the spinal cord when a high density of opioid receptors and endogenous opioids were found in the superficial dorsal horn (LaMotte et al. 1976). At the same time, Yaksh and colleagues demonstrated that intrathecal injection of few micrograms of morphine in a variety of species induced a potent and long-lasting analgesia (Yaksh and Rudy 1976).

As shown in Fig. 1, this triggered a rush to study the spinal cord. The figure shows a rough MEDLINE analysis of the number of papers devoted to the effect of opioids at the spinal cord level each year from 1966 to 1993, and one can observe that the interest in this question continues.

In this volume, Anthony H. Dickenson discusses in detail the various mechanisms of action of morphine. The data obtained with intrathecal morphine led to a wave of enthusiasm for intrathecal injections. In 1976, the basic discoveries produced immediate clinical applications, and it was rational to jump from animals to humans. In my opinion, the other side of the coin is that during the past 15 years intrathecal injections of various drugs have been used, not always with enough caution, in animals and also unfortunately in humans. More than 100 different drugs have been injected, sometimes with a lack of rationality, and not always following the criteria defined by Yaksh (1989). Those criteria refer to the classical principles of pharmacology, to the necessity of clearly differentiating the sensory and motor effects of the injected drugs, and finally to checking possible toxic effects. The intrathecal administration of drugs is an elegant technique extremely useful for the study of the pharmacology of pain at the spinal level. Intrathecal injections are not, however, a universal panacea, and clinicians must be extremely prudent in selecting drugs for such a purpose—the spinal cord is not a trash can.

Other very exciting and promising approaches to the pharmacology of pain started in the early 1970s. They related to the supraspinal modulation of the segmental transmission of pain studied initially by the group of Anders Lundberg in Sweden (Engberg et al. 1968) and by Patrick Wall (1967). The subsequent demonstration of stimulation produced analgesia (SPA) in animals and humans provided powerful evidence for a behaviorally relevant, highly

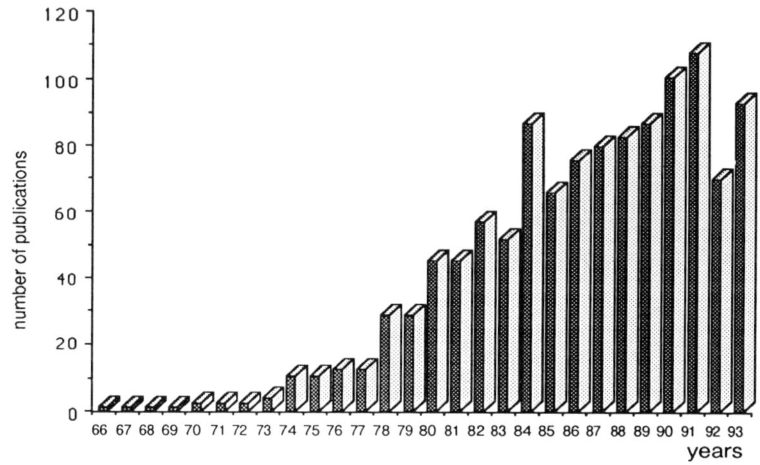

Fig. 1. Rough MEDLINE analysis of the number of papers devoted to the effects of opioids at the spinal cord level each year from 1966 to 1993.

selective brain stem control of nociceptive transmission. These initial discoveries were at the origin of an explosion of research in this field; my coverage is limited to the beginning of the story, showing how, in the mid-1970s, the first outlines of a nociceptive modulation network emerged. Reynolds (1969) first reported on three rats the antinociceptive effects induced by electrical stimulation in the periaqueductal gray matter (PAG). Dave Mayer, Huda Akil, John Liebeskind, and colleagues (1971) in Los Angeles further characterized this phenomenon, demonstrating that stimulation at sites throughout the PAG inhibited nociception. In 1972, Liebeskind came to Paris for a sabbatical year. At first, the project was to study the effects of PAG stimulation on the activities of dorsal horn neurons to establish directly the involvement of descending systems in SPA. I was still doubtful, because from my own experience with deep brain or cortical stimulation I was well aware that it was relatively easy to inhibit the activities of dorsal horn neurons using high intensities of current. At that time, electrophysiological investigations were performed exclusively in the cat. To set the scene before starting electrophysiological experiments, we first decided, with Liebeskind, Gisèle Guilbaud, and Jean-Louis Oliveras, to evaluate the effects of PAG stimulation in freely moving cats.

In the first stage of our experiments we demonstrated in these animals that electrical stimulation within the ventral PAG induced powerful analgesia. Then we anesthetized the same animals, and using the same parameters of central stimulation, we reported a strong depressive effect induced by PAG stimulation on the responses of dorsal horn neurons to noxious stimulation.

These experiments, run in parallel, led us to conclude that the antinociceptive effects induced by deep brain stimulation were due, at least in part, to the activation of descending inhibitory systems (Guilbaud et al. 1972; Liebeskind et al. 1973; Oliveras et al. 1974). The involvement of descending inhibition in SPA was then behaviorally and electrophysiologically confirmed by Basbaum, Clanton, and Fields (1976), who described a suppression of the effects of deep brain stimulation after lesion of the dorsolateral funiculus of the spinal cord in the rat.

The promising results we published in 1972–74 led Oliveras to perform an extensive behavioral mapping study of more than 300 stimulation sites in the brain stem of the freely moving cat (Oliveras et al. 1979; Besson et al. 1981). At the PAG level in the cat, the effective stimulation sites for the induction of analgesia without aversive side effects were essentially located in its ventral and ventrolateral sites. Thus our results strongly differed from those of the UCLA group, who obtained in the rat analgesia from stimulation sites located throughout the PAG (Mayer et al. 1971). Interestingly, a closer examination of effective sites in the cat ventral PAG revealed that the main target for SPA was in fact the dorsal raphe nucleus (DRN), rich in serotonin-containing neurons. That is why we immediately investigated the effects of the stimulation of other raphe nuclei. We found that extremely powerful analgesia was obtained by stimulation of the nucleus raphe magnus located at the bulbo-pontine level (Redjemi et al. 1974; Oliveras et al. 1975). In certain cases, these antinociceptive effects were as powerful as those obtained after administration of several tens of milligrams of morphine. Thus in 1975 we clearly identified in the cat the areas involved in SPA. They correspond to the DRN, the dorsal part of the central superior nucleus of the raphe, and the nucleus raphe magnus. Electrophysiological investigations performed by the groups of Howard Fields in San Francisco and of John Wolstencroft in the United Kingdom suggested that the effects of PAG were mediated through the raphe magnus (Fields and Anderson 1978; Lovick et al. 1978).

The interest in analgesia induced by deep brain stimulation was enhanced by analogies with some of the mechanisms of action of morphine. Several groups showed that powerful analgesic effects could be obtained by micro-injection of several micrograms of morphine into the PAG (see references in Yaksh and Rudy 1978) and nucleus raphe magnus (Dickenson et al. 1979; Levy and Proudfit 1979). Furthermore, the UCLA group (working on the PAG) and our group (nucleus raphe magnus) demonstrated cross-tolerance between SPA and morphine analgesia (Mayer and Hayes 1975; Oliveras et al. 1978). In addition, the analgesic effects of central stimulation of these regions could be reduced or diminished by naloxone, suggesting that stimulation elicited a release of endogenous opioids (Akil et al. 1976; Oliveras et al. 1977).

These experiments gave rise to a torrent of written words and many criticisms, but now, almost twenty years later, we stand by our results with the nucleus raphe magnus, and Liebeskind's group has localized the key regions within the PAG.

Over the past twenty years, an enormous number of articles have been devoted to the influence of descending inhibitory systems. Numerous techniques have been used, including anatomy, physiology, pharmacology, neurochemistry, and behavior. The main groups interested in pain research publish very sophisticated papers. I know perfectly well that the literature on the subject is highly controversial, but even if at the start a few groups oversimplified the story, I emphasize the fact that these initial investigations led these groups to suggest as early as the mid-1970s that opioids and serotonin strongly influence the activity of descending systems. I confess that over many years I strongly supported the 5-hydroxytryptamine (5-HT) story, but in the light of more recent investigations, especially those of Herbert Proudfit (1992) and Susan Fleetwood-Walker (1992), we have much evidence strongly supporting the involvement of descending noradrenergic systems in the modulation of pain via alpha-2 noradrenergic receptors.

The few examples I have selected clearly indicate that 5-HT agonists, alpha-2 noradrenergic agonists, and of course more selective opioid agonists could lead to new analgesic compounds devoid of side effects. Accurate and time-saving research techniques have been developed, great hopes have begun to emerge. Several tens of thousands of molecules have been synthesized as possible analgesics. Unfortunately, as one of our colleagues in pharmacology, the director of a major pharmaceutical laboratory, recently pointed out, the pharmaceutical industry cannot be proud of its recent activity in the discovery of original analgesic substances. Indeed, as you know, the bark of the willow tree, which contains salicin, and the poppy were used before Christ, and today there are only a small number of new molecules in use, mostly NSAIDs. To give another example, some anticonvulsants and antidepressants are now used to try to suppress particular types of pain, notably those arising from lesions of the peripheral and central nervous systems. Here again, the use of these substances does not result from rational research but simply from accidental observations by some particularly attentive clinicians.

COMPLEXITIES, DIFFICULTIES, AND DOUBTS

Today, I must admit that for my part I feel quite disappointed, because we were expecting more rapid and striking progress in the field. In fact we are facing not only methodological difficulties but also the complexities of the nervous system, which has led to doubts and despair.

One could discuss for hours the methodological difficulties and the complexities inherent in the pharmacology of pain. We must recognize that very often we have a tendency to interpret our results according to our own conceptual inclinations and to focus more on differences of interpretation than on contradictory data. To illustrate this point, I have arbitrarily selected two examples: the tests used in evaluating the antinociceptive effects of drugs and the coexistence and corelease of neurotransmitters. I discuss below some problems relevant to the multiplicity of receptor types and subtypes; however, other major pharmacological aspects such as pharmacodynamics, route of administration, intermittent versus chronic exposure, tolerance, cross-tolerance, and physical dependence will not be covered.

The relevance or even the lack of relevance of the main pharmacological acute screening tests to clinical pain states has been repeatedly discussed. The tests used to evaluate antinociceptive activity include noxious heat, pressure to the tail or paw pinch, colorectal distension, intraperitoneal chemical irritants, and subcutaneous administration of formalin. In most cases these stimuli are applied to normal animals in the absence of hyperalgesia, allodynia, and hyperesthesia. Some of these tests depend on spinal mechanisms, while others also involve supraspinal structures. Some of them are extraordinarily sensitive to a particular class of analgesics; others are too optimistic and lead to false positive interpretations. In addition, in numerous behavioral experiments only one nociceptive test is used, and the exact method can vary from author to author. These few remarks indicate why, with the exception of morphine, there are often controversies in the literature relevant to the pharmacology of pain. There is a need for the standardization of behavioral models in nociception.

More important, these models are limited, and most of them do not mimic chronic pain states. Chronic pain states differ markedly from acute pain by nature of their persistence and by the adaptive changes well illustrated by the phenomenon of plasticity, which has been described at various levels of the nervous system. Such limitations led to the use and development of more appropriate chronic pain models, which mainly represent inflammatory pain and neuropathic pain. The development of these new experimental models is essential not only for the detection of new analgesics but also for better understanding of pain syndromes that are poorly managed clinically. In this volume, Gary Bennett discusses peripheral neuropathies, so I would like here to focus a little bit on chronic arthritis.

Adjuvant induced arthritis in the rat was essentially used by the pharmaceutical industry to detect the analgesic effects of NSAIDs. In 1978, Colpaert proposed and used for the first time the arthritic rat as an animal model of chronic pain (Colpaert et al. 1982). Numerous behavioral studies have shown that these animals clearly displayed hyperalgesia and certain clinical signs that resemble chronic pain. With Guilbaud and Daniel Menétrey, our laboratory introduced at the beginning of the 1980s a model for electrophysiological investigations in the rat at both spinal cord and thalamic levels (Gautron and Guilbaud 1982; Menétrey and Besson 1982). At both levels we observed dramatic changes in the responsiveness of neurons implicated in nociceptive processes. At the dorsal horn level, for example, these modifications consisted of: (1) an increase in the size of their cutaneous receptive field; (2) a high level of background discharge in the absence of any intentional stimulation (sustained or sporadic); and (3) some neurons (in the superficial and deep dorsal horn) receiving A-delta and/or C inputs were maximally driven by light mechanical stimulation with no subsequent increase in their discharge in response to noxious stimuli.

These modifications could reflect hyperalgesia and spontaneous nociceptive reactions observed in the arthritic rat. They are in keeping with the well-known clinical observations that in rheumatism disease in humans, flashes of pain can appear spontaneously or be caused just by touch of the inflamed area.

Without excluding central mechanisms, we attributed the observed modifications to the activation and sensitization of thin primary afferent fibers due to the release of various chemicals into the microenvironment of the nociceptors. Subsequent studies performed in our laboratory by Guilbaud and Iggo confirmed this hypothesis. Recording thin peripheral fibers innervating the inflamed ankle in the polyarthritic rat, they described the appearance of a spontaneous background discharge, a decrease in the threshold of these fibers to mechanical stimulation, and an exacerbated response to subthreshold stimulation. They further showed that in normal rat these fibers were extremely difficult to excite. In the same year, 1985, using another model of arthritis, Hans-Georg Schaible and Robert Schmidt reported at the level of the cat knee joint the presence of receptors normally silent but active in acute inflammation, for which they have coined the expression "sleeping nociceptors." The German group (see Schmidt, this volume) performed careful, convincing, and extensive studies over several years on these subjects. It is now well established that a certain number of nociceptors present in other tissues are silent and unexcitable under healthy conditions.

These electrophysiological findings speak for themselves, and they strongly emphasize that inflammatory models are an absolute necessity for pharmacological pain research.

Over the past five years, several models of inflammation have been developed, and an enormous amount of information has been published. These studies concern the modalities of activation of peripheral nociceptors, the peripheral or central release of neurotransmitters, the gene expression of various peptides, the plasticity of the nervous system, and of course the pharmacology of analgesics or putative analgesics, including not only those acting at the periphery but also those acting centrally (see several chapters in this volume).

A question that remains to be answered, however, is the validity of animal models in predicting an analgesic effect in humans. This is particularly true for the design of peptide agonists and antagonists. For instance, large differences have been seen in the amino acid sequences of substance P (SP) receptors in humans and rats. Consequently, it is not surprising that among the various SP antagonists designed by the pharmaceutical industry, some of them have more affinity in humans than in rats, and vice versa. As mentioned by Ray Hill (1991), this raises a particular problem for the industry, because it may mean that a direct jump must be made from a mechanistic in vitro screening program to evaluation of analgesic efficacy in humans. This may be the way in which major progress can be made, but it requires courage and willingness to invest large sums of money for safety evaluation.

Another methodological problem I discuss briefly is the microinjection techniques that have been used to precisely locate the sites of action of various drugs. These techniques require consideration of the diffusion of the injected substance and the high local concentration attained, which could be much greater than that following systemic injection or the concentration in the synaptic cleft under physiological conditions. No doubt these techniques are essential, but we must remember that in more than 99% of cases in humans, the relief of pain is based mainly on oral administration of analgesics. So why not return more frequently to systemic administration of drugs?

Another difficulty encountered in the design of safe analgesics is the fact that some chemicals possibly involved in the transmission or in the modulation of pain and their receptors are widely distributed throughout the nervous system. This is especially the case for peptides and excitatory or inhibitory amino acids. Most of them are involved in multiple physiological functions. This could lead to unexpected undesirable side effects, as reported, for instance, for kappa-opioid receptor agonists or for N-methyl-D-aspartate (NMDA) receptor antagonists.

I now wish to consider the complexity of the nervous system, considering particularly the "jungle" of neurochemical anatomy and the colocalization and corelease of neurotransmitters. The complexity of the neurochemical neuroanatomy is well illustrated by the spinal cord. Indeed, most of the classical neurotransmitters and a considerable number of neuropeptides are present in the dorsal horn. Thus, theoretically, they could be released at this level and intervene in the transmission of nociceptive processes.

As shown in Fig. 2, some of these substances are contained in primary

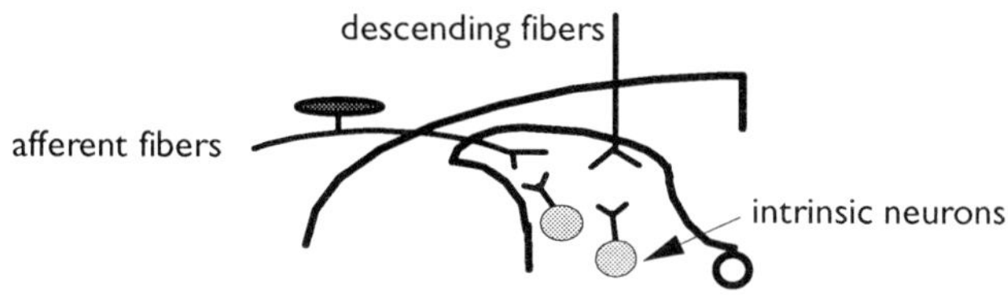

primary afferent fibers		intrinsic neurons		descending fibers	
SP	GLU	enkephalin	GABA	5-HT	NE
CGRP	ASP	dynorphin	GLU	SP	enkephalin
CCK	ATP	GAL	ACh	TRH	CCK
SOM	VIP	SP	5HT	SOM	GAL
ocytocin	NKA	neurotensin	NKA	β-endorphin	DA
vasopressine	NPK	SOM	NKB	F-8F-NH2	glycine
gastrin	NPY	CCK	NPY	EAA	ACh
angiotensin	GRF	DA		adenosine	
dynorphin A 1-17	ANP				
dynorphin B	PHI				
leu-enkephalin	PHM				
alpha-MSH	F-8-F-NH2				

Fig. 2. The jungle of chemical neuroanatomy in the spinal cord. Some of these data are controversial and must be considered with caution for many reasons, especially those obtained with immunohistochemistry.

afferent fibers or intrinsic neurons, others are located in terminals of supraspinal origin. These data must be considered with caution for many reasons, especially those obtained with immunohistochemistry. The role of some of these substances remains obscure. However, the involvement of others in pain processes has been relatively well established. This is the case for SP, glutamate, and calcitonin gene-related peptide (CGRP) in primary fibers; enkephalin and gamma-aminobutyric acid (GABA) in intrinsic neurons; and norepinephrine (NE) and 5-HT in descending fibers.

Another complexity of the network is further complicated by the fact that some of the peptides, for instance SP, cholecystokinin (CCK), and somatostatin (SOM), are localized not only in primary afferent neurons but also in intrinsic neurons and descending fibers. Interestingly others, like CGRP, seem to be located exclusively in primary afferent fibers. Here again we must be extremely careful in considering the data and not fall into temptation, as we all have in becoming infatuated with the molecule of the moment. For instance, fifteen years ago, SP was considered to be *the* pain neurotransmitter; now glutamate has many supporters, and in 1992 nitric oxide was the molecule of the year.

Additional complexity is provided by the coexistence of several peptides and classical neurotransmitters in the same neuron. For instance, SP and glutamate coexist in some primary afferent fibers. Since several compounds are coreleased from the same central terminals, the problem is extraordinarily complex. If two compounds such as SP and glutamate are capable of producing excitation alone, for example, then the action of both may need to be blocked to produce transmission failure. Thus in this condition it is difficult to predict the effects of antagonists. This is probably why the effects of systemic administration of NMDA or SP antagonists are weaker than expected. One can speculate that the use of drug cocktails to target multiple transmitters would be a highly interesting strategy. This is illustrated in a theoretical diagram in Fig. 3, where it is also indicated that morphine remains the analgesic of choice.

I would like to mention that we cannot entirely explain the effects of morphine only by direct and indirect action at the spinal level. Indeed, several series of experiments performed in our laboratory have shown that neuronal responses recorded at the level of various supraspinal structures are depressed by lower doses of intravenous morphine than those required to depress the activity of dorsal horn neurons. For instance, in our laboratory, Jean-François Bernard and coworkers have described a new pain pathway, the spino-ponto-amygdaloid pathway: some neurons located in the superficial dorsal horn and exclusively driven by noxious inputs densely project to the lateral parabrachial (PB) nucleus at the pontine level, and then there is direct projection to the central nucleus of the amygdala. We have shown that the doses of morphine needed to depress the responses to noxious stimulation in the PB and amygdala are lower than those required to act at the spinal level. This is not surprising, since opioid receptors are located in both the superficial dorsal horn and the lateral parabrachial area. It must be stressed that this pathway, which we believe to be implicated in the affective emotional aspects of pain, is highly sensitive to morphine.

Until now I may have sounded quite skeptical. I think it was necessary, in order to moderate our enthusiasm a bit. In fact I am optimistic, and I briefly describe below reasons for this hope.

THE REASONS FOR HOPE

The reasons for hope are multiple. They are based on the development of new technologies and new strategies for pharmacological approaches.

With the various biochemical techniques, it is possible to specify rapidly the number of receptor sites for a newly synthesized substance and the affinity

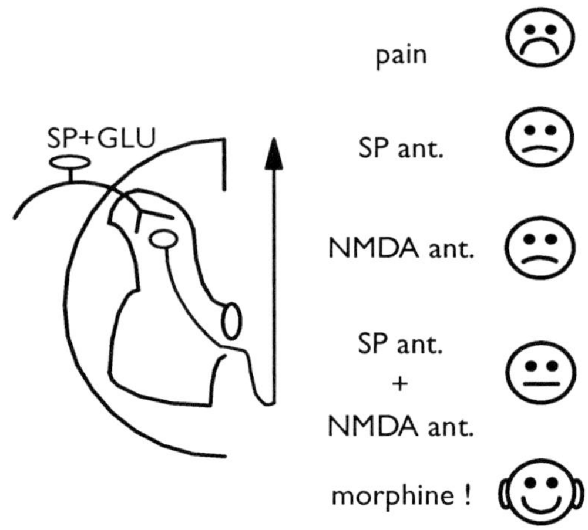

Fig. 3. Theoretical aspects of the colocalization of peptides and excitatory amino acids in primary afferent fibers and of their corelease in the dorsal horn of the spinal cord (for further information see text).

of the substance for a given receptor type. These techniques can be used on brain slices, allowing selection of substances according to the strength of their action. One can therefore quickly analyze the effects of certain molecules in a very small number of animals, and only after this first screening are the most promising molecules studied in vivo in different animal species, particularly rodents. In other words, we have moved from empiricism to rationalism.

The considerable progress achieved during the past few years in the field of molecular biology and in the definition of chemical studies has also led to significant advances. The primary sequence of numerous receptors, that is, their amino acid sequence, has been obtained through molecular biology. We have been waiting for many years for the cloning of opioid receptors, and suddenly during the past eight months, mu, delta, and kappa receptors have been cloned. The delta receptor was cloned in the mouse by Brigitte Kieffer in Strasbourg and Chris Evans in Los Angeles in December 1992. In July 1993, during the international narcotic research conference held in Sweden, we learned that both kappa and mu receptors had also been cloned.

Even more exciting is that we can now gauge the structure of the natural molecule by using nuclear magnetic resonance. A precise representation of the molecule is obtained, which can be visualized on a television screen. Because the receptors are at least one hundred times larger than their messengers, few of them have yet been analyzed. Computer models can be developed, however, to simulate the manner in which the chemically synthesized agonists or antagonists interact with the receptor. These experiments, known as docking, are used more and more as a guide for chemical synthesis.

Understanding the pharmacology of pain is first of all trying to comprehend its pathophysiological mechanisms. I have already discussed what we are expecting from the use of pain models. Now I briefly consider the interest of a relatively recent technique of visualization of activity using immediate early gene expression. The demonstration by Steve Hunt and coworkers (1987) that sensory stimulation rapidly induced c-*fos* expression in dorsal horn neurons gave rise to many investigations. Evidence is accumulating that the dorsal horn neurons expressing c-*fos* are those receiving noxious inputs. Recently, with Catherine Abbadie, we demonstrated that the number of *fos*-like immunoreactive neurons in lumbar spinal cord correlates with the development of adjuvant-induced arthritis (Fig. 4; Abbadie and Besson 1992). This c-*fos* expression, appearing in the absence of any intentional stimulus, was significantly reduced by a chronic treatment with aspirin or acetaminophen. In parallel, these two compounds strongly reduced the clinical signs of the disease. This technique using the expression of immediate early genes is highly promising for study of both physiological and pharmacological pain processes.

Of course, another source of hope for future pharmacological advances lies in the enormous number of strategies for the development of novel analgesics. Some of these strategies are based on classical approaches, whereas others are totally original.

Despite the importance of supraspinal mechanisms in nociceptive processes, it appears that the primary afferent neuron constitutes a favored target for the development of novel efficacious agents for the relief of pain. Indeed, drugs acting at the supraspinal level could produce marked psychoactive side effects.

Numerous strategies are being developed at the peripheral level. They include the design of bradykinin receptor antagonists (B2-B1), cyclo-oxygenase inhibitors, neurokinin 1 (NK1) receptor antagonists, 5-HT antagonists, noradrenergic antagonists, ion channel blockers, blockade of interleukin 1-β, capsaicin derivatives, kainate receptor antagonists, antagonists of growth factors, and inhibitors of nitric oxide synthase. One can observe that sometimes these approaches are based on rational targets but, to me, others seem to be highly speculative.

It is not necessary to insist on the strategies developed at the spinal level; here again, they are numerous and include the design of antagonists for the transmitters released by primary afferent fibers and the design of agonists at the inhibitory neurotransmitter receptors.

Reinforcing or mimicking the actions of monoaminergic descending systems is another direction. Interestingly, tricyclic antidepressants, which block the reuptake of norepinephrine and/or serotonin, are largely used for the treatment of neuropathic pain. Noradrenergic alpha-2 agonists are very popular, but they can produce side effects, especially hypotension and sedation. I previously mentioned that we were disappointed when manipulating the activity of

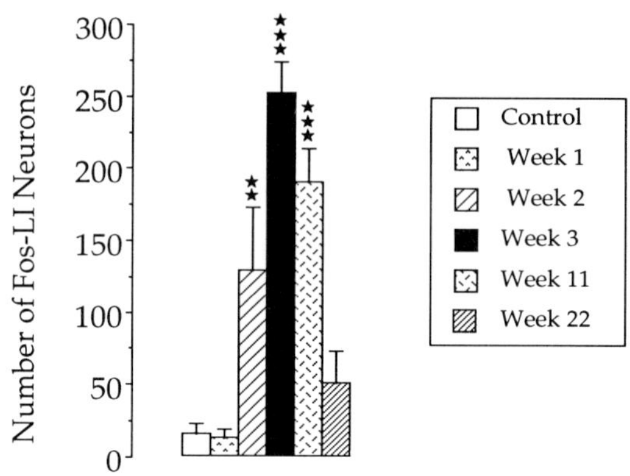

Fig 4. Fos-LI during the development of adjuvant-induced arthritis. Histogram presenting the number of *fos*-like immunoreactive (*fos*-LI) neurons in the lumbar spinal enlargement, from L2 to L6, following injection of Freund's adjuvant. Six groups of rats are considered: control animals and animals at 1, 2, 3, 11, and 22 weeks postinjection (n = 7 in each group). Results are expressed as mean (± S.E.M.) number of *fos*-LI neurons per 3 × 40 mm section for 5 lumbar segments. Significance is expressed using PLSD Fisher's test, taking the control group as reference (** $P < 0.01$, *** $P < 0.001$). Note that the number of *fos*-LI neurons increases at week 2 and at week 3, when hyperalgesia signs are maximal, decreases slightly at week 11, and decreases greatly at week 22. (Adapted from Abbadie and Besson 1992)

the bulbospinal serotonergic system. In Chapter 45 of this volume, Michel Hamon and coworkers describe the multiplicity of 5-HT receptors, and we await the introduction of highly selective, well-characterized, and potent agonists of serotonin receptor subtypes to mimic the activity of bulbospinal 5-HT systems.

In the field of opioid research, we can expect novel agonists devoid of side effects, but there is another rational approach that has the advantage of being more physiological. It is based on the fact that endogenous opioids are quickly destroyed by two enzymes. Bernard Roques and colleagues (1993) in Paris have produced mixed inhibition of enkephalin-degrading enzymes. An increase in the concentration of enkephalin followed and pain threshold was elevated in freely moving animals. More recently we found that pretreatment with those mixed inhibitors produced a dose-dependent decrease in c-*fos* expression in the neurons located in the superficial dorsal horn. We must recognize that the antinociceptive effects of these molecules are less potent than those of morphine, but they do seem to have the advantage of producing only minor side effects.

Arriving at the end of this trip through the puzzle of the pharmacology of pain, I repeat that we are faced with multifactorial interactions and that the use of cocktails to address cooperative interactions between drugs or between several modalities of action of the same drug could be highly promising.

In conclusion, it is difficult to compete with morphine for its analgesic efficacy, but theoretically this is a challenge that can be met. The most important thing is to fill some of the gaps in the treatment of pain using substances that have no side effects, even after long-term treatment. In addition, there are multiple pains due to various pathophysiological mechanisms, and one could speculate that some specific new chemicals would be selectively effective against certain types of pain. This is another reason for great hope in our battle against pain.

ACKNOWLEDGMENTS

To John Bonica: John, we are indebted to you for founding the IASP. We have a great admiration for your work, for your energy, and for your tenacious fight to relieve pain. Please be sure of my warmest gratitude.

I express here my deep gratitude to my coworkers old and young, some of whom have been supporting and tolerating me over many years. I also thank Professor Denise Albe-Fessard, from whom I first learned neurophysiology.

REFERENCES

Abbadie, C. and Besson, J.-M., C-fos expression in rat lumbar spinal cord during the development of adjuvant-induced arthritis, Neuroscience, 48 (1992) 985–993.

Akil, H., Mayer, D.J. and Liebeskind, J.C., Antagonism of stimulation produced analgesia by naloxone, a narcotic antagonist, Science, 191 (1976) 961–962.

Basbaum, A.I., Clanton, C.H. and Fields, H.L., Opiate and stimulus produced analgesia: functional anatomy of a medullo-spinal pathways, Proc. Natl. Acad. Sci. USA, 73 (1976) 4685–4688.

Besson, J.M., Wyon-Maillard, M.C., Benoist, J.M., Conseiller, C. and Hamann, K.F., Effects of phenoperidine on lamina V cells in the cat dorsal horn, J. Pharmacol. Exp. Ther., 187 (1973) 239–245.

Besson, J.M., Oliveras, J.L, Chaouch, A. and Rivot, J.P., Role of the raphe nuclei in stimulation produced analgesia. In: B. Haber, S. Gabay, T. Issidorides and S.G.A. Alivisatos (Eds.), Serotonin, Neurochemistry and Function. Advances in Experimental Biology and Medicine, Vol. 33. Plenum Press, New York, 1981, pp 153–176.

Calvillo, O., Henry, J.L. and Neuman, R.S., Effects of morphine and naloxone on dorsal horn neurones in the cat, Can. J. Physiol. Pharmacol., 52 (1974) 1207–1211.

Colpaert, F.C., Meert, T.H., De Witte, P.H. and Schmidt, P., Further evidence validating adjuvant arthritis as an experimental model of chronic pain in the rat, Life Sci., 31 (1982), 67–75.

Conseiller, C., Menétrey. D., Le Bars, D. and Besson, J.M., Effets de la morphine sur les activitiés des interneurones de la couche V de Rexed de la corne dorsale chez le rat spinal, J. Physiol. (Paris), 65 (1972) 220–221A.

Dickenson, A.H., Oliveras, J.L. and Besson, J.M., Role of the nucleus raphe magnus in opiate analgesia as studied by the microinjection technique in the rat, Brain Res., 170 (1979) 95–111.

Duggan, A.W., Hall, J.G. and Headley, P.M., Morphine, enkephalin and the substantia gelatinosa, Nature, 264 (1976) 456–458.

Engberg, I., Lundberg, A. and Ryall, R.W., Reticulospinal inhibition of interneurones, J. Physiol.

(Lond.), 194 (1968) 225–236.
Evans, C.J., Keith, D.E., Morrison, H., Magendzo, K. and Edwards, R.H., Cloning of a delta opioid receptor by functional expression, Science, 258 (1992) 1952–1955.
Fields, H.L. and Anderson, S.D., Evidence that raphe spinal neurons mediate opiate and midbrain stimulation produced analgesia, Pain, 5 (1978) 333–349.
Fleetwood-Walter, S.M., The antinociceptive effects of noradrenerigic agonists on the activity of spinal dorsal horn neurones. In: J.M. Besson and G. Guilbaud (Eds.), Towards the Use of Noradrenergic Agonists for the Treatment of Pain, Elsevier, Excertpa Medica, ICS 1006 (1992) 181–195.
Gautron, M. and Guilbaud, G., Somatic responses of ventrobasal thalamic neurons in polyarthritic rats, Brain Res., 237 (1982) 459–471.
Guilbaud, G., Besson, J.M., Liebeskind, J.C. and Oliveras, J.L., Analgésie induite par stimulation de la substance grise périaqueducale chez le chat: données conportementales et modifications de l'activité des interneurones de la corne dorsale de la moelle, C.R. Acad. Sci. (Paris), 275 (1972) 1055–1057.
Hill, R.G., Criteria for the development of analgesic drugs: a personal view from the perspective of the pharmaceutical industry. In: A.I. Basbaum and J.M. Besson (Eds.), Towards a New Pharmacotherapy of Pain, John Wiley and Sons, Chichester, 1991, pp. 293–329.
Hunt, S.P., Pini, A. and Evan, G., Induction of c-fos-like protein in spinal cord neurons following sensory stimulation, Nature, 328 (1987) 632–634.
Kieffer, B., Befort, C., Gaveriaux-Ruff, C. and Hirth, C.G., The δ opioid receptor: isolation of a cDNA by expression cloning and pharmacological characterization, Proc. Natl. Acad. Sci. USA, 89 (1992), 12048–12052.
Kitahata, L.M., Kosaka, Y., Taub, A., Bonikos, K. and Hoffert, M., Lamina specific suppression of dorsal-horn unit activity by morphine sulfate, Anesthesiology, 41 (1974) 39–48.
Lamotte, C., Pert, C. and Snyder, S., Opiate receptor binding in primate spinal cord: distribution and changes after dorsal root section, Brain Res., 112 (1976) 407–412.
Le Bars, D. and Besson, J.M., The spinal site of action of morphine in pain relief: from basic research to clinical applications, Trends Pharmacol. Sci, 2 (1981) 323–325.
Le Bars, D., Menétrey, D., Conseiller, C. and Besson, J.M., Comparaison chez le chat spinal et le chat décérébré, des effets de la morphine sur les activités des interneurones de type V de la corne dorsale de la moelle, C.R. Acad. Sci., 279 (1974) 1369–1371.
Le Bars, D., Menétrey, D., Conseiller, C. and Besson, J.M., Depressive effects of morphine upon lamina V cells activities in the dorsal horn of the cat, Brain Res., 98 (1975) 261–277.
Le Bars, D., Guilbaud, G., Jurna, I. and Besson, J.M., Differential effects of morphine on response of dorsal horn lamina V type cells elicited by A and C fibre stimulation in the spinal cat, Brain Res., 115 (1976) 518–524.
Levy, R.A. and Proudfit, H.K., Analgesia produced by microinjection of baclofen and morphine at brain stem sites, Eur. J. Pharmacol., 57 (1979) 43–55.
Liebeskind, J.C., Guilbaud, G., Besson, J.M. and Oliveras, J.L., Analgesia from electrical stimulation of the periaqueductal gray matter in the cat: bahavioral observations and inhibitory effects on spinal cord interneurons, Brain Res., 50 (1973) 441–446.
Lim, R.K.S., Guzman, F., Rogers, D.W., Goto, K., Braun, C., Diskerson, G.D. and Enge, R.J., Site of action of narcotic and non-narcotic analgesics determined by blocking bradykinin-evoked visceral pain, Arch. Int. Pharmacodyn., 152 (1964) 25–58.
Lovick, T.A., West, D.C. and Wolstencroft, H.H., Response of raphe spinal and other bulbar raphe neurones to stimulation of the periaqueductal gray in the cat, Neurosci. Lett., 8 (1978) 45–49.
Mayer, D.J. and Hayes, R.L., Stimulation produced analgesia: development of tolerance and cross-tolerance to morphine, Science, 188 (1975) 941–943.
Mayer, D.J., Wolfe, T.L., Akil, H., Carder, B. and Liebeskind, J.C., Analgesia from electrical stimulation in the midbrain of the rat, Science, 174 (1971) 1351–1354.
Menétrey, D. and Besson, J.M., Electrophysiological characteristics of dorsal horn cells in rats with cutaneous inflammation resulting from chronic arthritis, Pain, 13 (1982) 343–364.

Oliveras, J.L., Besson, J.M., Guilbaud, G. and Liebeskind, J.C., Behavioral and electrophysiological evidence of pain inhibition from midbrain stimulation in the cat, Exp. Brain Res., 20 (1974) 32–44.

Oliveras, J.L., Redjemi, F. Guilbaud, G. and Besson, J.M., Analgesia induced by electrical stimulation of the inferior centralis nucleus of the raphe in the cat, Pain, 1 (1975) 139–145.

Oliveras, J.L., Hosobuchi, Y., Redjemi, F. Guilbaud, G. and Besson, J.M., Opiate antagonist naloxone strongly reduces analgesia induced by stimulation of a raphe nucleus (centralis inferior), Brain Res., 120 (1977) 221-229.

Oliveras, J.L., Hosobuchi, Y., Bruxelle, J., Passot, C. and Besson, J.M., Analgesic effects induced by electrical stimulation of the nucleus raphé magnus in the rat: interaction with morphine analgesia. In: Abstracts: 7th International Congress of Pharmacology, Paris, Vol. 1, 1978, p. 119.

Oliveras, J.L., Guilbaud, G. and Besson, J.M., A map of serotoningeric structures involved in stimulation producing analgesia in unrestrained, freely moving cats, Brain Res., 164 (1979) 317–322.

Proudfit, H.K., The behavioural pharmacology of the noradrenergic descending system. In: J.M. Besson and G. Guilbaud (Eds.), Towards the Use of Noradrenergic Agonists for the Treatment of Pain, Elsevier, Excerpta Medica, ICS 1006 (1992) 119–136.

Redjemi, F., Oliveras, J.L., Guilbaud, G. and Besson, J.M., Analgésie induite par la stimulation du noyau central inférieur du raphé chez le chat, C.R. Acad. Sci. (Paris), 279 (1974) 1105–1107.

Reynolds, D.V., Surgery in the rat during electrical analgesia by focal brain stimulation, Science, 164 (1969) 444–445.

Roques, B.P., Noble, F., Daugé, V., Fournié-Zaluski, F. and Beaumont, A., Neutral endopeptidase 24.11: structure, inhibition, and experimental and clinical pharmacology, Pharmacol. Rev., 45 (1993) 87–146.

Wall, P.D., The laminar organization of dorsal horn and effects of descending impulses, J. Physiol. (Lond.), 188 (1967) 403–423.

Yaksh, T.L., Studies in animals should precede human use of spinally administered drugs, Anesthesiology, 70 (1989) 4–6.

Yaksh, T.L. and Rudy, T.A., Analgesia mediated by a direct spinal action of narcotics, Science, 192 (1976) 1357–1358.

Yaksh, T.L. and Rudy, T.A., Narcotic analgetics: C.N.S. sites and mechanisms of action as revealed by intracerebral injection techniques, Pain, 4 (1978) 299–360.

Zieglgansberger, W. and Bayerl, H., The mechanisms of inhibition of neuronal activity by opiates in the spinal cord of cat, Brain Res., 115 (1976) 111–128.

Correspondence to: Jean-Marie Besson, DSc, INSERM U161, 2 rue d'Alesia, 75014 Paris, France. Tel: 33-1-4589-3662; Fax: 33-1-4588-1304.

Proceedings of the 7th World Congress on Pain, Progress in Pain Research and Management, Vol. 2, edited by G.F. Gebhart, D.L. Hammond, and T.S. Jensen, IASP Press, Seattle, © 1994.

5

Death of Pain: Pain, Suffering, and Ethics

Margaret A. Somerville

McGill Centre for Medicine, Ethics and Law, McGill University, Montreal, Quebec, Canada

INTRODUCTION

The title *Death of Pain* can be interpreted in two ways: either the person dies of pain, or the pain dies but not the person, or at least does not die of pain.

It is possible that a person could die of pain directly, because being in pain could conceivably shorten life. All of the person's physical and psychological resources are focused on dealing with the pain and are exhausted sooner than would otherwise have occurred. A person also can die of pain indirectly; for instance, by committing suicide because of pain. In one case that came to my attention, an elderly man, who had been in chronic pain for a long time was refused pain relief treatment by a locum tenens physician on the grounds that the man was addicted to the pain relief drugs prescribed by his regular physician. This old man returned home and committed suicide by hanging himself. His elderly wife found him dead in their woodshed. Physicians are often concerned that pain relief treatment might shorten the life of a person for whom it is prescribed. But perhaps it never occurred to this physician that the opposite could happen, that the refusal to prescribe pain relief treatment could shorten this man's life.

A person also can die of pain indirectly in another sense. Fear of being left in pain is one of the major forces giving rise to calls for euthanasia. We need to compare killing the person suffering the pain with killing the pain but not the person who suffers. In other words, in some cases euthanasia may be proposed or used (for instance, possibly in some cases in the Netherlands; Somerville 1993) as a substitute for compassionate and adequate pain relief treatment.

If failure to relieve pain can have deathly consequences, why might anyone be left in pain? A response to this question first requires facts. We can sometimes overlook the importance of having good facts in dealing with ethical issues. This is a serious mistake. Good facts (including, if necessary, research to establish these) are essential to good ethics, which, in turn, is essential to good law.

Second, we need to consider our obligations with respect to provision of pain relief treatment. What ought we do (that is, we have an ethical, and I will suggest legal, duty to do)? And, what ought not we do (that is, we have an ethical and legal duty not to do)? And, what not ought we do (that is, we may or may not do, because there is no duty either to act or not to act)?

Having determined our obligations, how should we promote honoring them? One way is through the formulation of concepts that will encourage the fulfillment of these obligations. We need to keep in mind that concepts, and the language in which we choose to articulate them, are neither neutral nor just descriptive. The concepts that we use to deal with important issues such as provision of pain relief treatment, both reflect and form us as individuals, institutions, and society, and determine our attitudes, values, beliefs, responses, and actions. This is particularly true in relation to issues such as pain relief treatment or euthanasia, in which powerful emotional and value-based factors are at play.

Concepts relevant to establishing values, attitudes, and beliefs that relate to provision of pain relief treatment are discussed in the second section of this chapter. The third section briefly discusses the relationship between pain relief treatment and euthanasia.

WHY IS A PERSON LEFT IN PAIN?

It is important to ask, "Why is a person left in pain?" Such a question is the necessary first step toward sensitizing ourselves to the ethical issues that are raised and to eliciting an appropriate ethical response. We also should keep in mind that the questions we are now asking are often more indicative of the ways in which we will act in the future than the responses we are giving in the present, which tend to reflect the past. As with many apparently simple questions, the answers to the question, "Why is a person left in pain?" reflect a complex reality that is not possible to explore comprehensively here.

Factors relevant to our nonsensitivity to the pain of others range from cultural to personal, from historical to self-protective, from psychological (for example, that we lose pain memory) to social. They include attitudes of health care professionals to pain relief treatment, to pain itself, and the influence of culture on these attitudes. They also include problems with communication of the fact of being in pain; eliciting what can be called a pain relief reaction in a health care professional; the inability of persons in pain to verbalize their pain, for instance, in the case of young children; distancing from the person in pain by the person who could provide pain relief treatment; and simply indifference to pain on the part of the person who has an obligation to relieve the pain.

HEALTH CARE PROFESSIONALS' ATTITUDES

Health Care Professionals' Attitudes to Pain Relief Treatment

Sadly, it is still not uncommon to hear health care professionals state that a person in pain is "just a complainer" or that "I do not want my patients to become addicted." Recently, I was consulted by a physician who told me the following story: She was on night call at a major hospital that treated many old and chronically ill patients. She was called to see a man who was in severe pain with advanced metastatic carcinoma of the prostate. When she examined his chart, she found that the only pain relief treatment that had been ordered was Tylenol. She changed the order to morphine, brought his pain under control, and gave instructions that morphine was to be used in a way that would keep the pain under control. She did not work at the hospital the following night, but was there again the night after and was called to see this same man because he was in pain. On her way into the room, she commented to the nurse that obviously they needed to increase the dose of morphine. The nurse replied that the man was not on morphine, he was on Tylenol. The attending physician, during the day, had changed the order, noting in the patient's record that he would not have his patients becoming drug addicts. The physician on night call made a formal complaint to the director of professional services at the hospital. He said that he was aware of this attending physician's attitude, but he was having great difficulty in convincing this particular physician to provide adequate pain relief treatment. The physician had argued he was exercising his right to professional autonomy in deciding what pain relief treatment should be given.

The case just described is shocking as an isolated incident. It is even more shocking to learn of another, similar case, involving a different attending physician in the same hospital, that occurred a few weeks later. A man dying of cancer of the larynx who was suffering from severe abdominal cramps and had barely slept for three days, was likewise given only Tylenol by his attending physician. This raises the issue of the "tone" of an institution with respect to provision of adequate pain relief treatment. The tone in this institution, if these examples are typical of conduct in relation to pain relief treatment, is highly unacceptable. We need to be aware that a few persons at the highest level of authority in an institution are usually the role models who set the "tone" that governs such matters (Barber et al. 1973). They have serious and important obligations in this regard and must recognize and fulfill them.

Health Care Professionals' Attitudes to Pain

Tradition can still exercise an influence on attitudes to pain, particularly those of practitioners in tradition-based and tradition-sensitive professions such as medicine. Historically, prior to anesthetics, physicians needed to be able to inflict pain to have any chance of curing or helping patients and, in many instances, of saving lives. In American medicine prior to 1850, there was a tradition that relief of suffering was at most a secondary concern in comparison to saving life, and only acceptable when it imposed no danger to life. Such historical antecedents may still have some strong subliminal effects (Somerville 1986).

Moreover, some physicians may be indifferent to pain or at least to pain suffered by persons categorized in certain ways. For instance, it is often noted that terminally ill persons are in effect abandoned by some health care professionals, resulting in what Dr. Jay Katz has called "intense premortem loneliness" (Katz 1984). Many persons would rather be dead than unloved, abandoned and, too often, left in pain (Somerville 1993). As I will discuss shortly, asking for euthanasia may be one response of those who find themselves in such a situation.

We also need to keep in mind that physicians' attitudes are not formed in isolation; they reflect the larger culture. In this regard, it is interesting that:

> mid-century America witnessed the growth of a masculine cult of toughness and callousness. This antisentimental glorification of insensitivity took two very different forms: one a reaffirmation of the traditional manly ability to endure pain; and the second, a newer more mechanical form of indifference to suffering. [Unless we are aware of such factors,] it may be

> hard to imagine the extent to which the calculus of suffering constituted a major revolution in the techniques of decision-making in medicine. (Pernick 1983)

In short, health care professionals have *not* always seen it as their role to be concerned about pain and suffering or, even, have seen it as *not their role*. These attitudes of physicians reflected wider cultural attitudes. This raises a further related question concerning how closely contemporary health care professionals' attitudes to pain and suffering reflect those of the community. This in turn leads to consideration of the nature of these latter attitudes. One way to examine this issue is to identify the factors in a given community or culture that elicit a reaction to relieve pain or suffering.

COMMUNICATION

A response to relieve pain and suffering requires that the presence of pain and suffering be communicated to the person who can act to relieve it. The form of the communication can determine whether it is effective in eliciting such a response.

Some unpublished work by Dr. Ellen Corin is interesting in this regard (Corin, personal communication). She found that in North America health care professionals often did not respond to persons who claimed to be in serious pain and suffering until they articulated their claim in terms of rights—"I have a right to treatment" (for example, pain relief treatment). In contrast, in France (and some other French-speaking countries) "rights talk" did not elicit any such response and tended to be ignored; however, if persons claimed to be in pain and suffering, health care professionals responded to them. This shows that there is a cultural basis to a communication that will influence whether it is effective in eliciting a response of providing treatment to relieve the pain.

We also need to be aware of other aspects of communication of pain and suffering if we are to respond to such a communication appropriately. For example, those who are unable to verbalize their pain, and therefore to communicate it by describing it in words, are often regarded as not suffering pain. Research on our failure to treat or prevent pain in children has demonstrated this phenomenon. For instance, we carry out medical interventions on children with little or no pain relief treatment, that we would never undertake on adults without such treatment (Anand and Hickey 1987; Rogers 1992). Or, historically, persons of low intelligence or even of low socioeconomic status (e.g., slaves) were regarded as not having the same sensitivity to pain (Pernick 1983).

It is also easier to detach from those who cannot communicate with us, or those whose status or position we do not identify with. In short, it is easier to disidentify from persons who cannot communicate with us, either through words or by virtue of what we recognize as their obvious similarities to us. This, in turn, results in our depersonalizing them. Sometimes, we even deliberately avoid communication with others in order to take advantage of this reaction. For example, researchers who were forced personally to seek informed consent had difficulty carrying out risky or painful experiments on the persons with whom they communicated. They did not have this same difficulty if they did not personally communicate with them (Lally and Barber 1974; Barber et al. 1973; Gray 1975). One function of ethical and legal requirements relating to health care (for example, those relating to informed consent), is to act as a countermeasure to such reactions, which place others at risk as well as dehumanizing them. To summarize, disidentification from and depersonalization of others can be seen as a method of blocking communication. Such methods may be consciously or unconsciously used, especially in situations in which the content of the communication we receive is frightening or painful to us, which is often true of the communication of pain.

Communication of pain may also be blocked because, when we are in serious pain, it possesses us: we are the pain. Other persons may then act to disidentify from the pain that is seen as us, rather than identifying with us as a person, albeit one who happens to be in pain. They may do this as a protective mechanism, almost as though the pain could be contagious and from fear that they might find themselves in similar pain. Even health care professionals can have such reactions. Instead of empathy (feeling what it feels like for the other), when we see another in pain we may seek disidentification (this is not me and could not be me), and often, as a result, we depersonalize the other (the person in pain is not a person like me and even not a person), which is a way of protecting ourselves.

The ultimate, most horrible example of this phenomenon of disidentification and depersonalization, that necessarily results in dehumanization, is torture. The torturer dehumanizes his or her victim and, in the process, himself or herself as well (Scarry 1985). Although torture might seem far removed from many of the realities in which we live and work in a health care context, we need to be aware of the terrible fact that in many and possibly the majority of cases of torture today, physicians are involved (in some contexts the number of such cases has been alleged to be as high as 90%; Editorial 1990; Grodin 1993). The involvement of physicians in administering the death penalty, for instance, in some U.S. states (Truog and Brennan 1993), is a related issue.

Both the infliction of pain and the infliction of death isolate the other person. At one level, they are "isolation rituals" (Schulmann 1980) that function to reassure those carrying out the rituals that the situation of the other person could not happen to them. They also have the effect of bonding those carrying out the ritual through shared guilt for what they have done to the other person over whom they exercise power.

Recognizing how horrible these situations are, and that they are far removed from any personal experience of the vast majority of health care professionals, could we nevertheless learn from them? For instance, could the actions of health care professionals in ignoring pain have some of the same causes and display some of the same characteristics as infliction of torture? These are tough questions to face, but they need to be asked if we are to remedy the situation of persons being left in pain. Moreover, these questions are not fanciful or simply theoretical. The Supreme Court of Canada recently was required to determine whether a Canadian Criminal Code provision (R.S.C. 1980 c.C-46 [as amended], sec. 241[b]) that made assisted suicide (and therefore physician-assisted suicide) an offense was unconstitutional (Rodriguez vs. British Columbia [Attorney General] [1993] 107 D.L.R. [4th] 342). The Court considered, among other issues, whether this prohibition constituted cruel and unusual treatment or punishment, which is prohibited by the Canadian Constitution, through its effect of prohibiting physicians from helping persons in severe pain to terminate their lives (Supreme Court of Canada 1993). The Court split five to four, the majority holding that the provision prohibiting assisted suicide was constitutional. The prohibition on cruel and unusual treatment or punishment was held not to be contravened by the prohibition on assisting suicide, because this did not constitute any "treatment" of the plaintiff by the state, as is required for unconstitutional action under the Canadian Charter of Rights. This aspect of the case is of interest in the context of the current discussion because it was argued that leaving persons in unbearable pain and suffering could contravene the prohibition on cruel and unusual treatment or punishment, that is, the prohibition of torture.

Yet another barrier to communication in relation to pain is the issue of truth telling in a situation of terminal illness. If a person is not told the truth about a condition, then, particularly in a community or culture in which the use of opioids to relieve pain is entirely or predominantly associated with fatal illness, adequate pain relief treatment may not be provided because doing so would itself reveal the truth about the person's condition.

THE LAW AND PAIN AND SUFFERING

The Law's Response to Pain and Suffering

The law's response to pain and suffering reflects some of the same reticence that we find in medicine. For instance, there have long been fears of both fraudulent claims and opening the "flood-gates of litigation" through recognizing claims and awarding damages for so-called pure mental injury, that is, psychological harm that does not arise directly from physical injury (Somerville 1986).

Courts also speak of not awarding compensation for the "normal vicissitudes of life." These are almost always defined to include injury in the form of pure mental pain, for example, grief or bereavement in situations where the person for whom one grieves was wrongfully killed. Even when damages for pain and suffering can be recovered through a legal action, courts have limited the amount of such damages. For instance, large jury awards in the United States for damages for pain and suffering, including in some medical malpractice cases, were probably a major cause of the Supreme Court of Canada placing a limit of $(C)100,000 (adjusted for inflation since the ruling in 1978) on the total amount of such damages (Teno v. Arnold [1978] 2 S.C.R. 287).

Fear of Legal Liability

Fear of legal liability on the part of health care professionals also can inhibit the provision of adequate pain relief treatment. This is especially likely if the treatment necessary to relieve pain could, or even is likely to, shorten life. Such situations are, however, in practice becoming less likely, as more sophisticated pain relief treatments emerge.

Although there are no cases in which legal liability has been imposed for the provision of reasonably necessary pain relief treatment, and authoritative bodies such as the U.S. President's Commission for the Study of Ethical Problems in Medicine (1983), the Law Reform Commission of Canada (1982), and, most recently, the House of Lords in England (Airedale NHS Trust v. Bland [1993] 1 ALL E.R. 821; [1993]1 H.L.J. 7) have stated that the provision of necessary pain relief treatment is not a matter of potential legal liability, physicians still seem to believe that it is. We need to ask why: Is the fact that sometimes what we know and what we feel are different, relevant to explaining this belief?

Some recent work on physicians' attitudes about withholding treatment, as compared with withdrawal of treatment, is interesting in this respect (Solomon 1992). One group of researchers in the United States found that although physicians understood that withholding and withdrawing treatment were governed by the same ethical and legal principles, many of them did not feel that this was true. They were much less comfortable with withdrawing treatment than withholding it. The former was seen as a more difficult decision to justify than the latter, which could translate to a feeling of being at greater risk of legal liability for making an unacceptable decision regarding withdrawal of treatment, as compared with withholding it.

In any case, one radical response to preventing situations of unreasonable failure on the part of physicians to relieve pain would be to threaten to sue physicians for gross medical malpractice for such conduct. (I have focused on physicians here because they are the least complicated category of health care professionals from a legal point of view, with respect to imposing liability, because they have full authority to order and administer pain relief treatment. Other health care professionals will have correlative obligations and liability.) If it is not possible to get across the message that physicians do not need to be frightened of legal liability for giving reasonably necessary pain relief treatment, one remedy might be to bring home the message that they need to be concerned about legal liability for not doing so. I do not as a general principle advocate suing physicians, but leaving a person in pain is such a serious matter that if there is no other way to ensure the provision of adequate pain relief treatment, such an approach is merited.

In short, leaving persons in pain can be regarded not only as unethical, but also as negligence (I am tempted to say criminal negligence). It also should be regarded as unprofessional conduct; that is, it should constitute a basis for disciplinary action by the relevant professional licensing body. This approach is not out of line, indeed it is consistent, with that taken in relation to legal liability of physicians and other health care professionals in general and disciplinary action involving them. Leaving a person in pain can be regarded as equivalent to other culpable omissions by physicians in relation to treatment, for example, failure to remove an acutely inflamed appendix in a situation in which no reasonably competent physician would fail to act. Moreover, not only the acts of individuals can be regarded as negligent, but also *systems*, within which professionals with obligations to provide pain-relief treatment work, can be "guilty" of negligence.

Negligent Systems

A negligent system is yet another reason that pain may not be adequately treated. An example can be seen in the film *Terms of Endearment*. The young woman dying of breast cancer is in terrible pain, and her mother begs the nurse for help. The nurse replies that there are still 30 minutes to wait until she will give the next morphine injection on schedule. This is a horrifying, but too common event in many hospitals—the rules and system are treated as being more important than the patient; the health care professional's feeling of comfort, calm, and security (he or she need not make any decisions, but simply follow orders) takes priority over the agony of the patient.

A recent event reported in the press in Montreal well illustrates yet another negligent system for the delivery of pain relief treatment. It involved a young physician attending a young man dying of AIDS who was in terrible pain; at midnight there was no more morphine available in the hospital ward, and the physician was told that "the pharmacy does not open again until tomorrow morning at 9 o'clock." In desperation, the young doctor thought of giving a lethal injection of potassium chloride, which, unlike morphine, was available on the ward.

Unreasonable failure to consult a specialist or to seek a second opinion can constitute medical malpractice. I propose that this legal rule also should be applied in relation to unreasonable failure to consult on the treatment of pain. Likewise, unreasonable failure to establish a system of access to pain specialists, which is reasonably available to physicians or patients, could constitute "systems negligence."

We also need to consider whether our approaches in trying to stop drug (ab)use could constitute an ethically and legally unacceptable system at a macro level, in particular because of the effects of these efforts on the provision of pain relief treatment to residents of developing countries. Thirty percent of such persons die with no pain relief treatment (Lancet 1984) because narcotics are not available. The reason is that developed countries have attached demands to aid packages that these developing countries join "the war on drugs." This probably does little to reduce illegitimate use of these drugs, but it does seriously inhibit their legitimate, indeed required, use.

CONCEPTS

BASES OF OBLIGATIONS TO RELIEVE PAIN

Substantive concepts that could support claims of access to pain relief treatment include those of trust, human rights, respect for persons, respect for human dignity, relief of suffering, healing (which can be contrasted with curing), and covenant.

Trust. Trust is essential to the formation and maintenance of all good human relationships. But not all forms of trust are the same. For example, we can compare paternalistically based trust—"blind trust"—with trust based on an egalitarian relationship—"earned trust" (Katz 1984). Blind trust is founded on role, status, position, and power, and operates on the basis of a principle that can be summarized as: "You should (query: must) trust me because I know what is best for you and will act only in your best interests." In contrast, earned trust is not based on role, status, position, or power, but on a principle that can be stated as: "You can trust me because I will show that you can trust me."

The theory of trust that we espouse and use will affect the approaches that we take in practice. For example, in a health care professional-patient relationship based on blind trust, the health care professional is likely to control the giving of treatment for the relief of pain. If the same type of relationship is based on earned trust, control is shared with or given to the patient. Suffering occurs when we lose control over what happens to us, accompanied by a sense of our own disintegration (Cassel 1982). Having control reduces pain and suffering; therefore, the earned trust approach can be regarded as a pain and suffering relief mechanism.

Another difference in effect between the two theories is that while we can demand the blind trust of those we leave in pain, we cannot earn their trust. In other words, failure to relieve pain is antithetical to establishing earned trust, which is the essential base of contemporary health care professional-patient relationships.

Human rights. To leave a person in avoidable pain and suffering should be regarded as a serious breach of fundamental human rights. There have been recent challenges to the universality of concepts of human rights, often along the lines that these concepts are a creation of modern Western democracies and are related to their political ideology and social culture, in particular, their emphasis on individualism (Somerville 1992). At least in a narrow sense, there may be some truth to these criticisms. These difficulties may be overcome, however, if we focus on the spirit of what we seek to achieve by promoting human rights and look for ways in which this can be developed and enhanced in all societies. One way, it is suggested, is to focus on promoting respect for all persons.

Respect for all persons. We should recognize that:

- the informing principle of human rights is one of *respect for all persons*;
- such respect *is* a universal requirement which, in some of our societies, we implement through concepts of legal rights;
- the concept of respect for all persons is inextricably linked to a concept of human ethics, as well as, ideally, to one of legally enforceable human rights (Somerville 1992); and

- that to leave a person in avoidable pain and suffering is to show great disrespect and to breach fundamental requirements of human ethics and human rights.

According to the *Oxford English Dictionary*, the word respect means to "look back"; to regard; to consider; a relationship of one person or thing *to* another; heed, care, attention; to treat with consideration. We can compare looking back and looking down. We need to look back on (respect) and relate to others in pain in all of the senses denoted and connoted by the word respect. And we need to avoid looking down on them, which connotes and denotes the opposite. Such an attitude and approach would do much to remedy the situation of leaving a person in pain. As an aside, but of crucial importance, we also need to look back on and not to abandon those in a form of pain that has its source at a more macro level, for example, those who are caught in devastating wars or civil conflict. We also have obligations to do whatever we can to relieve their suffering.

Human dignity. The term human dignity can operate as another expression of respect for persons and for their human rights, but it also can be misused. The latter can occur if human dignity is regarded as an extrinsic (attributed) characteristic of some persons, rather than an intrinsic (essential) feature of all persons by virtue of their being human. When human dignity is used as an extrinsic or attributed characteristic, it can be argued that some persons do not have dignity and, therefore, there are no requirements to respect them.

Relief of suffering. No more worthy goal can be promoted than the relief of suffering. It is a goal that gives a common aim to each of the disciplines of medicine, ethics, and law. In the exercise of our various professions, we all are or should be seeking relief of suffering, although we may do so in different ways.

The aim of relief of suffering is also a basis of consensus for "right thinking" persons. Starting from consensus, rather than disagreement, can be important in setting a constructive tone for, and therefore in determining the outcomes of, our analyses and discussions. We feel differently about others with whom we disagree, when we start from consensus as compared with disagreement. In short, the starting point that we choose to use in analyzing an issue, including that of provision of pain relief treatment, is not neutral with respect to the decisions we make concerning such matters. While, however, relief of suffering is an important starting point for analysis, this principle is not absolute in its operation. For instance, euthanasia in the form of the administration of lethal injections, even though intended to relieve suffering, would not be justified (Somerville 1993).

Finally, placing emphasis on an aim of relief of suffering has important impact on values, attitudes, and beliefs of individuals and society, and on symbolism. As a shared value, in particular, it has an important impact in terms of establishing a "high" ethical tone and an appropriate legal tone of a society.

Healing (as compared with curing). Too strong an emphasis only on an aim of curing can cause us to ignore or to abandon those who cannot be cured. We need to emphasize that such persons can still be healed; for example, their pain can be healed. Further, we need to recognize that this is an immensely important task and of the utmost value.

Covenant. The relationship between patients and health care professionals can be characterized as a covenant or fiduciary relationship, concepts that are both also related to trust. Part of the covenant between, for instance, a physician and a patient is that the physician has an obligation to provide access to treatment that the patient needs for the relief of pain.

Covenant is related to the legal concept of contract, but has a less materialistic aura and often involves the notion of the sacred, especially in terms of the nature of the obligations engendered through use of the concept. Consequently, within the context of covenant, one could speak of sacred duties to relieve suffering by providing pain relief treatment.

ANALYZING FROM ETHICS TO LAW

Another concept relevant to obligations to relieve pain can seem to constitute an unimportant change at first. But, in fact, it has far-reaching implications. In contrast to the substantive concepts discussed above, this is more a process or procedural concept. It needs to be kept in mind, however, that "form is no mere formality;" procedural concepts can have profound impact on substance. This concept involves a change in our order of analysis, namely, moving from ethics to law rather than from law to ethics.

Take, for example, the question of whether we should provide pain relief treatment that could shorten life, but which is necessary to relieve pain. Analyzing from law to ethics seems, in many instances, to have indicated to physicians that provision of such treatment is *not allowed.* In contrast, analyzing from ethics to law indicates the *opposite*; ethics would require that we act to relieve pain and that the law would accommodate, and certainly not prohibit, such action. This shows another important point, which has been mentioned already: our starting points, or initial or basic presumptions, are not neutral in their effect on the outcomes of our analyses and, therefore, on our decisions. Nowhere is this more true than in relation to treatment decisions at the end of life, including decisions relating to so-called physician-assisted suicide and euthanasia.

DECISIONS AT THE END OF LIFE AND EUTHANASIA

FEARS

The issues raised by euthanasia are complex and diverse (Somerville, 1993) and it is not possible to discuss them in any depth here. However, some points regarding the interrelationship of relief of pain and euthanasia are particularly relevant with respect to the ethics of providing or failure to provide pain relief treatment.

Almost everyone fears pain and being left in pain. Paradoxically, the power of modern medicine to prolong life raises fears, including of suffering and pain experienced as a result of such prolongation. These fears are sometimes summed up in statements that have a certain dramatic impact, for instance, that a person would rather be dead than "left to the mercy of doctors and their machines" (Fenigsen 1989). Some persons argue that the way to avoid these dangers, and the fear that they engender, is by making euthanasia available.

DEFINITION OF EUTHANASIA

First, we need to be careful to define what we mean by euthanasia. There is a range of medical interventions or noninterventions at the end of life that includes the right to refuse treatment; withdrawal of "life support" including artificial hydration and nutrition; provision of pain relief treatment, even that which could shorten life, if this is reasonably necessary to relieve pain; suicide; assisted suicide; and, finally, euthanasia.

Euthanasia *is not* refusal of treatment by a competent person or through either "advance directives" or a validly appointed substitute decision-maker. Euthanasia *is not* the failure to treat or withdrawal of treatment when treatment is futile. And euthanasia *is not* the provision of necessary treatment for the relief of pain or other symptoms of serious physical distress, even though this treatment could shorten life.

Euthanasia *is* an intervention undertaken with the primary intention of killing the person subject to it, including what can be described as physician-assisted suicide. To define euthanasia comprehensively and accurately requires a somewhat technical and legalistic description. Euthanasia can be defined as "an intervention or nonintervention by one person, to end the life of another person, who is terminally ill, for the purpose of relieving suffering, with the intent of causing the death of the other person, except where the primary intent is either to provide treatment necessary for the relief of pain or other symptoms of serious physical distress, or nonprovision or withdrawal of treatment is justified, in particular, because there is a valid refusal of treatment or the treatment is futile" (Somerville 1993).

Euthanasia is an enormously complex topic that needs the most careful and in-depth consideration and analysis. The issues raised range from those of personal morality and autonomy, to setting the "legal and ethical tone" of society itself, because the position that we take on euthanasia, both as individuals and as a society, will affect important values, attitudes, and beliefs.

Even if at an individual level we regard euthanasia as morally acceptable in some circumstances, the impact that institutionalizing and even more so legalizing it would necessarily have at a societal level makes it highly unacceptable. This would change one of the most fundamental principles on which our society is founded—namely, *that we do not kill each other*—to one that we do in certain circumstances.

There are four basic presumptions from which to choose as a starting point for analysis undertaken to establish a position on euthanasia. These are:

1. "no euthanasia," which is the position taken by most jurisdictions;
2. "no euthanasia unless . . . ," which is the position taken, for example, in theory in the Netherlands;
3. "yes euthanasia is allowed, but . . . ," which is the position taken in practice in the Netherlands; and
4. "yes euthanasia is allowed," which is not a position taken by any jurisdiction.

Currently, most societies maintain a "no euthanasia" basic presumption, but there is increasing pressure to change to a "no euthanasia unless . . ." position (with the conditions for the exception being articulated), or even, a "yes euthanasia is allowed but . . ." presumption (with, likewise, the conditions for the exception being stated).

To the extent that fears of pain and being left in pain are a contributing factor in eliciting calls to legalize euthanasia, it is imperative to change any reality that provides a basis for such fear. We should regard ourselves as having the strongest of ethical obligations to achieve such change. This change is of the utmost importance to the persons whose pain will consequently be relieved; to the reality and image of health care professions and professionals as *caring* professions and professionals (and correlatively avoiding their being and being seen as *not caring* ones if they fail to act to relieve pain); and to society, itself, particularly if we are to maintain some of our most important symbolism and values.

CONCLUSION

We must ensure that we seek ways to relieve suffering and to kill pain, not persons with pain and suffering. As professionals with the greatest accumulated expertise and experience in the world on how to achieve the former and avoid the latter, physicians and nurses have an extraordinarily heavy responsibility to those fellow humans who seek their care when they are in pain, and to society, itself.

In closing, I would like to tell you how my interest in the topic of pain and suffering at interfaces of medicine and law arose. My father was in Australia and dying of widely disseminated prostatic carcinoma. I was telephoned in Canada and told that he had developed brain metastases and would die within a few days. I flew to Australia to find him largely mentally incoherent and in great pain. I insisted on calling in a pain specialist. To cut short the story, we discovered that he had aspirin poisoning—he was being given an aspirin and morphine mixture in increasing doses to try to control his pain. His treatment was immediately changed, the pain brought under control, and he became entirely lucid. He lived almost pain-free for another nine months. He said two things to me: that he wanted to live as long as he could, but not if he had to endure such terrible pain; and that I must do something to help others who were in the same situation as he had been—as he put it, probably not many of them had daughters who, as we say in Australia, "would go berserk" as I had done, to obtain essential pain-relief treatment for him.

Our decisions on how to deal with pain and suffering will depend, in part, on what we *can* do. This in turn depends on research; appropriate clinical systems; education of health care professionals about pain relief treatment; provision of access to health care, including pain relief treatment; and so forth. Our decisions and actions in relation to pain relief treatment will be among the most important that we will engage in, in terms of both humane and compassionate care of those who come to us in pain and establishing "the ethical and legal tones" of the societies of the twenty-first century. It is no small challenge to be charged with both making those decisions and acting on them.

ACKNOWLEDGMENTS

This research has been supported in part by Grant No. 806-92-0024, Social Sciences and Humanities Research Council of Canada.

REFERENCES

Anand, K.J. and Hickey, P.R., Pain and its effects in the human neonate and fetus, N. Engl. J. Med. 317 (1987) 1321–1329

Barber, B., Lally, J.J., Makarushka, J.L. and Sullivan, D., Problems of Social Control in Medical Experimentation, New York, Russell Sage Foundation, 1973, pp. 113, 133–143.

Cassel, E., The nature of suffering and the goals of medicine, N. Engl. J. Med., 306 (1982) 639–644.

Editorial, Conscience and complicity, Lancet, 336 (1990) 720.

Fenigsen, R., A case against dutch euthanasia, Hastings Cent. Rep., 19, 1 (Spec. Suppl.) (1989) 24.

Gray B.H., Human Subjects in Medical Experimentation, John Wiley & Sons, New York, 1975.

Grodin, M., Review of Medicine Betrayed: The Participation of Doctors in Human Rights Abuse, Report of a Working Party, British Medical Association, Soc. Sci. Med., 37 (1993) 277–278.

Katz, J., Silent World of Doctor and Patient, Free Press, New York, 1984, pp. 207 and ff.

Lally, J. and Barber, B., The compassionate physician: frequency and social determinants of physician-investigator concern for human subjects, Social Forces, 53, 2 (1974) 289–296

Lancet, Cancer and the Third World (note), Lancet, i (1984) 1136.

Law Reform Commission of Canada, Euthanasia, aiding suicide and cessation of treatment, Working Paper 28, Protection of Life Series, Minister of Supply and Services, Ottawa, 1982, p. 71.

Pernick, M.S., The calculus of suffering in nineteenth century surgery, Hastings Cent. Rep., 13 (1983) 26.

President's Commission for the Study of Ethical Problems in Medicine and Biomedical and Behavioral Research, Deciding to Forgo Life Sustaining Treatment, U.S. Government Printing Office, Washington, D.C., 1983, pp. 77–82.

Rogers, M.C., Do the right thing: pain relief in infants and children, N. Engl. J. Med., 326 (1992) 55–56.

Scarry, E., The Body in Pain: The Making and Unmaking of the World, Oxford University Press, New York, 1985.

Schulmann, D., Remembering who we are: AIDS and law in a time of madness, AIDS and Public Policy, 3 (1988) 75–76.

Solomon, M., Health care professionals and treatment at the end of life, Presentation at annual meeting of American Society of Law and Medicine, October 30–31, 1992, Cambridge, Mass., USA.

Somerville, M.A., Pain and suffering at the interfaces of medicine and law, University of Toronto Law Journal, 36 (1986) 286–317.

Somerville, M.A., Human rights and medicine: the relief of suffering. In: I. Cotler and P.P. Eliadis, (Eds.), International Human Rights Law: Theory and Practice, Canadian Human Rights Foundation, Montreal, 1992, pp. 505–522.

Somerville, M.A., The song of death: the lyrics of euthanasia, Journal of Contemporary Health Law and Policy 9 (1993) 1–76 and references cited therein.

Supreme Court of Canada, Rodriguez vs. British Columbia (Attorney General) (1993) 107 D.L.R. (4th) 342.

Truog, R.D. and Brennan, T.A., Participation of physicians in capital punishment, N. Engl. J. Med., 329 (1993) 1346–1349.

Working Party, British Medical Association, Medicine Betrayed: The Participation of Doctors in Human Rights Abuse, Zed Books, London, 1993, 234 pp.

Correspondence to: Margaret A. Somerville, AM, FRSC, McGill Centre for Medicine, Ethics, and Law, 3690 Peel St., Montreal, Quebec, Canada H3A 1W9. Tel: 514-398-7401; Fax: 514-398-4668.

Proceedings of the 7th World Congress on Pain,
Progress in Pain Research and Management, Vol. 2,
edited by G.F. Gebhart, D.L. Hammond, and T.S.
Jensen, IASP Press, Seattle, © 1994.

6

The World Health Organization Program in Cancer Pain Relief and Palliative Care

Kathleen M. Foley

Department of Neurology, Memorial Sloan-Kettering Cancer Center, New York, New York, USA

HISTORICAL PERSPECTIVE: WORLD HEALTH ORGANIZATION AND INTERNATIONAL ASSOCIATION FOR THE STUDY OF PAIN COLLABORATIVE EFFORTS

The international program in cancer pain sponsored by the International Association for the Study of Pain (IASP) had its origins at the association's First World Congress on Pain in Florence, Italy, in 1975 with a one-day meeting organized by Dr. John Bonica. This meeting served as a focal point for the creation of an informal group of international pain specialists who would meet and debate the current approaches to cancer pain treatment. In 1978, the First International Symposium on Pain of Advanced Cancer was held in Venice, Italy, under the organizational direction of Drs. John Bonica and Vittorio Ventafridda (1979). This meeting served as a unifying impetus to the development of international collaborative efforts in defining treatment strategies for patients with pain and cancer. The published proceedings served as a useful compendium of papers on the scope of cancer pain and the current diagnostic and therapeutic approaches available (Bonica and Ventafridda 1979). Many members of the IASP participated in this meeting and urged a more organized focus on cancer pain treatment at an international level.

In 1980, Dr. Bonica met with World Health Organization (WHO) leaders to discuss the importance of pain as an international health care problem. Dr. Jan Stjernsward, head of the WHO Cancer Unit, responded to Dr. Bonica's call for action. Following several preliminary discussions and through the efforts of Drs. Bonica, Ventafridda, and Mark Swerdlow, a WHO consultation meeting was held in Pomerio, Italy, in October of 1982. At this historic meeting the participants prepared draft guidelines on which the "Method for Relief of Cancer Pain" was based. This method emphasized the need for comprehensive evaluation of cancer patients with pain and provided a simple outline for the use of analgesic drugs. It represented the consensus of a group of experts on cancer pain management and was based on the concept that pharmacotherapy should be the mainstay of treatment for this symptom.

Field testing of the method and numerous related studies worldwide have demonstrated the safety and efficacy of this approach for the management of patients with pain (Cleeland 1990; Ventafridda et al. 1990).

In 1986, as a result of a WHO Expert Panel on the Comprehensive Management of Cancer Pain, a summary report was published as *Cancer Pain Relief.* This monograph has now been translated into 22 languages and has had wide distribution (Fig. 1; World Health Organization 1986). Its guidelines identified cancer pain as an important and neglected public health issue in developed and developing countries. It emphasized analgesic drug therapy as the essential component of the treatment approach and it recommended that every WHO member country develop a national cancer control program that would include pain relief as one of its major facets.

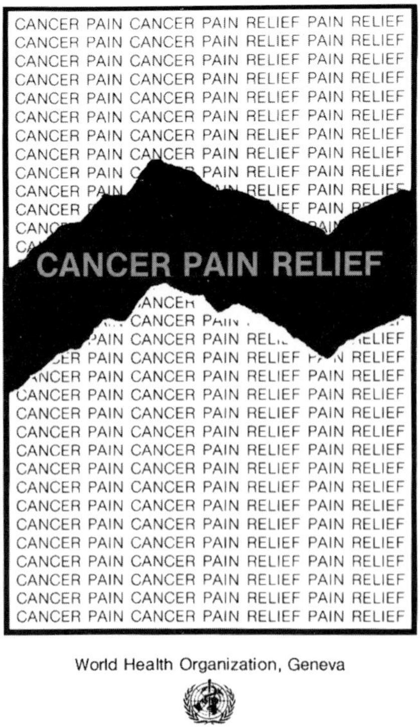

Fig. 1.

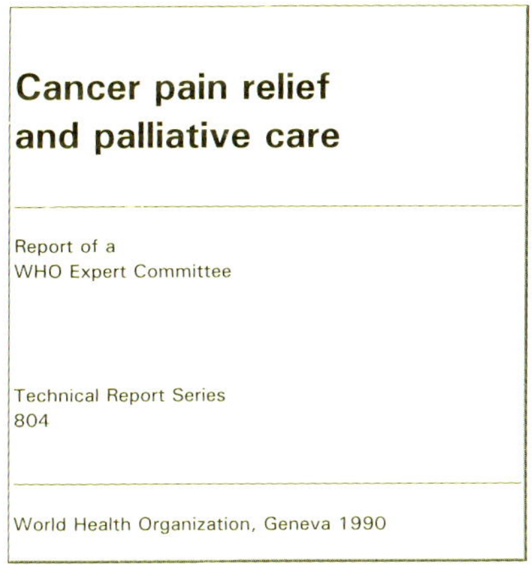
Cancer pain relief and palliative care

Report of a
WHO Expert Committee

Technical Report Series
804

World Health Organization, Geneva 1990

Fig. 2.

In 1988, the Second International Congress on Cancer Pain was held in Rye, New York; its proceedings detailed the efforts of the WHO Cancer Pain Relief Program in advocating for a broader perspective of symptom control and pain to encompass palliative care (Foley et al. 1990).

By 1989, the WHO Expert Panel on Cancer Pain Relief had reviewed and officially endorsed guidelines on teaching and training of health care professionals in cancer pain relief. Most important, it extended the focus of the WHO program in cancer pain to include palliative care. It published a second monograph, *Cancer Pain Relief and Palliative Care,* which has now been translated into seven languages (Fig. 2; World Health Organization 1990). The WHO Cancer Unit subsequently was renamed the WHO Cancer and Palliative Care Unit to identify its broader scope. At each step along the way, many participants in the development of the WHO program have been members of the IASP (Foley and Portenoy 1993).

The IASP responded rapidly to the development of the WHO program and created a subcommittee of the Education Committee focused on Cancer Pain Relief in Developing Countries (Foley and Portenoy 1993). This subcommittee functioned from 1984 to 1990 as a network devoted to the improvement of cancer pain treatment throughout the world. IASP supported in various ways the activities of WHO. To further facilitate its goal to improve cancer pain treatment internationally, the IASP became a nongovernmental organization (NGO) member of the WHO. In this capacity, the IASP has provided consultation and comment on WHO activities that may impact on the evaluation and treatment of patients with cancer and pain. This mechanism allows IASP to have representation at the WHO Assembly and provides a forum for discussion and debate on important common topics. Moreover, the IASP has created an official position of Liaison to WHO, which is currently filled by Drs. Kathleen M. Foley and Charles Cleeland.

At IASP World Congresses on Pain, the topic of cancer pain relief has been given an important place in the program, including plenary lectures, topical seminars, and special sessions (Takeda 1991). Moreover, in 1991 the IASP Council officially established a Task Force on Cancer Pain. The task force established working groups to address three important aspects of cancer pain and palliative care: the Working Group on Opioid Regulation, the Working Group on Education, and the Working Group on Multicenter Studies (Foley and Portenoy 1993).

IASP members now also work closely with WHO through a series of collaborating centers, of which there are currently seven, that serve as an interinstitutional network to support WHO programs at national and international levels (Table I). These centers are important channels for the global exchange of information, experience, and expertise consistent with the objectives and priorities of the WHO Program in Cancer Pain Relief and Palliative Care. All seven centers are associated with internationally recognized institutions that assign high priority to the promotion of the WHO Cancer and Palliative Care Unit, and all seven are directed by persons who are also members of IASP. Through collaborating centers, information about new initiatives in the WHO Program in Cancer Pain Relief and Palliative Care is well integrated.

CURRENT STATUS OF THE WHO PROGRAM IN CANCER PAIN RELIEF AND PALLIATIVE CARE

The principal objective of the WHO Program in Cancer Pain Relief and Palliative Care is to advocate for adequate pain relief and palliative care to all cancer patients in the world through existing health care systems. This program is one of the four priorities of WHO's Comprehensive Cancer Control activities. The other three are prevention, early detection linked with curative treatment, and the establishment of national cancer control programs in member states.

Estimates predict rapid increases in the incidence of cancer worldwide (Stjernsward 1993). Of an estimated 9 million new cancer cases in 1985, 4 million occurred in developed countries and 5 million in developing countries. It is predicted that by the year 2015, two-thirds of all cancers—an estimated 10 million of 15 million new cases—will occur in the developing countries

Table I
World Health Organiation collaborating centers in cancer pain relief and palliative care

WHO Collaborating Center for Quality of Life in Cancer Care St. Boniface General Hospital Research Center 351 Tache Avenue Winnipeg, Manitoba, Canada R2H 2A6	Dr Harvey Schipper, Director Telephone: 204-235-3850 Fax: 204-235-1231
WHO Collaborating Center for Palliative Cancer Care Churchill Hospital Oxford OX3 7LJ, England	Dr, Robert Twycross, Director Telephone: 44-865-751156 Fax: 44-865-741862
WHO Collaborating Center for Cancer Pain Relief National Cancer Institute Via Venezia 1 20133 Milan, Italy	Dr. Vittorio Ventafridda, Director Telephone: 39-2-877240 Fax: 39-2-720 22493
WHO Collaborating Center for Cancer Pain Relief and Quality of Life Saitama Cancer Center 818 Komuro Ina, Saitama 362, Japan	Dr. Fumikazu Takeda, Director Telephone: 81-48-722-1111 Fax: 81-48-832-1664
WHO Collaborating Center for Research and Training in Methods of Assessment of Quality of Life in Relation to Health Care The Netherlands Cancer Institute Plesmanlaan 121 1066 CX Amsterdam, The Netherlands	Dr. Frits Van Dam, Director Telephone: 31-20-616-2527 Fax: 31-20-616-2527
WHO Collaborating Center for Cancer Pain Research and Education Memorial Sloan-Kettering Cancer Center 1275 York Avenue New York, NY 10021, USA	Dr. Kathleen M. Foley, Director Telephone: 212-639-6594 Fax: 212-717-3081
WHO Collaborating Center for Symptom Evaluation in Cancer Care University of Wisconsin Medical School 1900 University Avenue Madison, WI 53705, USA	Dr. Charles Cleeland, Director Telephone: 608-263-7662 Fax: 608-263-0259

(Stjernsward 1993). At present, less than 5% of the resources committed to cancer control internationally are available to the developing countries where more than half of the world's cancer patients live.

According to the current available data on cancer treatment, one-third of cancers are preventable and another one-third are potentially curable if they are diagnosed early in their course (Stjernsward 1993). There is sufficient scientific knowledge to put into practice national cancer control programs encompassing cancer pain relief and palliative care. It has become most apparent, however, that in most developing countries, facilities and human resources to prevent, detect, diagnose, and treat cancer are in short supply. Large amounts of financial and human resources are often expended on curative treatment at a relatively high cost, but with a limited effect for a small, select population (Stjernsward and Teoh 1993). From WHO projections, 80–90% of cancer patients in developing countries will continue to be diagnosed with far-advanced and incurable cancer, if they are diagnosed at all. It is for this population especially that active treatment of pain and provision of palliative care should be the realistic options.

The WHO recommends that countries developing public health programs in cancer pain relief and palliative care first establish three process measures to monitor and evaluate programs (see Fig. 3): (1) the development of national policies, such as cancer control policies, that assure patients access to cancer pain and palliative care treatment; (2) broad educational programs for health care professionals and the public, such as medical and nursing curricula and media coverage about pain management; and (3) analgesic drug availability, including recommendations to governments on ways to facilitate opioid availability for severe cancer pain. These proposed methods are economically feasible and can have far reaching effects. They are closely linked, requiring achievements in all three areas to facilitate the development of such programs. Some of the impressive results of implementing these measures internationally are briefly summarized in the next section. It is beyond the scope of this presentation to give credit to all individuals who have made the WHO program a reality. The dramatic progress to date serves as a hopeful sign of the possibility of far-reaching changes to improve the care of patients with pain worldwide.

WHO PROCESS MEASURES

NATIONAL POLICIES

The World Health Organization's guiding principle for health care policy is to develop technologies that can be easily applied in a variety of existing health care systems for broad populations of patients. To date, many countries have developed national guidelines on cancer pain and palliative or terminal care. In some of these countries, true national policies have been developed; in others, guidelines for care have been developed but have not been institutionalized as national policy. As of 1993, Canada, Finland, Mexico, The Nether-

Cancer

RELIEVING CANCER PAIN

PROCESS MEASURES: (Foundation)

Costs little, but big effects
Necessary before outcome measures
All three should be done, namely:

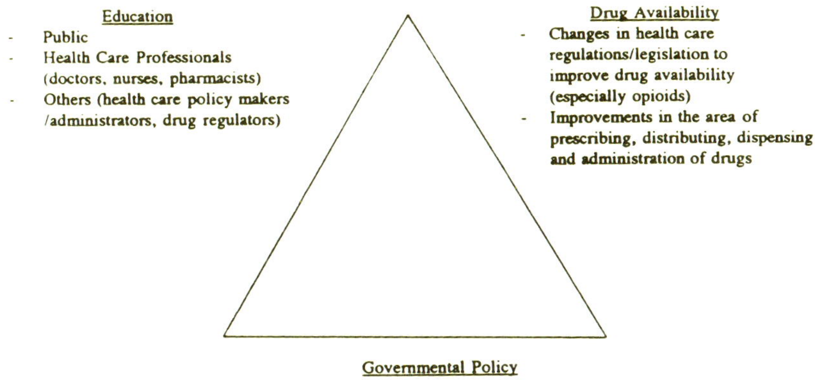

- National or state policy emphasizing the need to alleviate chronic cancer pain through education, drug availability and governmental support/endorsement.
- The policy can stand alone, be part of an overall national/state cancer control programme, be part of an overall policy on care of the terminally ill, or be part of a policy on chronic intractable pain, etc.

Fig. 3. WHO process measures to monitor and evaluate programs in cancer pain relief and palliative care.

lands, the Philippines, Sweden, and Vietnam had official policies. Australia, the United States, France, Italy, Thailand, and Japan had guidelines that addressed cancer pain and terminal care (Stjernsward and Teoh 1993).

The Philippines serves as an example of a developing country that has formulated a national cancer control program and has developed the basic infrastructure necessary to develop an program in cancer pain relief and palliative care (Laudico 1993). Similarly, Indonesia has developed recommendations that are in the process of being implemented (Lickiss 1993). Models other than the WHO model have been used to create programs in cancer pain relief and palliative care in some countries. For example, in Singapore, cancer pain treatment and palliative care has developed from the hospice movement and a broad-based volunteer effort (Goh 1993). In contrast to the Philippines, government funding has not yet identified palliative care as a priority in health care provision and planning, and philanthropy continues to support the major efforts of this program. Similarly, in Argentina, a strong grass-roots effort relies on volunteer support without governmental input (Wenk 1990, 1993). From 1985 to 1993, there has been an increase in official clinical programs in cancer pain and palliative care from only 1 to now over 20 teams in 14 cities throughout Argentina.

One model that has been successful is development of cancer pain and palliative care programs that originated in cancer centers, including the National Cancer Institute in Milan, Italy, the Saitama Cancer Center in Saitama, Japan, and Memorial Sloan-Kettering Cancer Center in New York City, USA (Foley and Portenoy 1993; Takeda 1990, 1993). These centers also serve as WHO Collaborating Centers. In developing countries, national cancer centers also have taken a leadership position, for example, the National Cancer Institute in Vietnam and China (Cai 1991; Chen 1992; Duc 1991; Sun 1993). In Colombia, a grass-roots hospice program combined efforts with the National Cancer Institute to develop a national program (Bruera 1993; DeLima 1993). These models demonstrate different approaches that eventually will develop into national programs and public health policy.

As discussed above, in some instances national policies have created the programs, whereas in others, national programs have aided in governmental development and institutionalization of such care as a basic right. There appears to be no single best way for countries to develop palliative care programs. Each country must rely on its own organizational system and make health care for patients with advanced disease a priority. Ideally, national policies facilitate and legislate not only a patient's right to care, but also the necessary components of education and drug availability which are so critical for the appropriate achievement of public health programs. The World Health Organization and the International Association for the Study of Pain are involved in ongoing joint efforts to foster national policies. There is, however, a strong impetus to endorse the need and provide support to national programs where governmental policies are not or have not been a possible solution.

If one uses policy as an outcome measure, the dramatic explosion of policy regarding cancer pain and palliative care internationally indicates increasing recognition of the need for health care programs to care for this patient population.

EDUCATION

Publication

Since *Cancer Pain Relief* was published in 1986, more than 250,000 copies have been distributed in 22 different languages (World Health Organization 1986), making it the second most translated publication in WHO history. It was recently selected as one of seven WHO clinical manuals considered indispensable to hospitals at a first referral level. *Cancer Pain Relief and Palliative Care,* now available in seven languages, establishes clear policies and priorities for public health approaches in palliative care (World Health Organization 1990). Currently in the works are two new monographs, the first of which, *Guidelines for Opioid Availability,* revises the guidelines in *Cancer Pain Relief* to broaden the number of drugs involved and to include a guide for opioid availability (World Health Organization, in press; Joranson 1993). The second, entitled *Cancer Pain Relief and Palliative Care in Children with Cancer,* should be available by the end of 1994. Two other monographs are pending: a *Symptom Manual* that addresses the issues of symptoms other than pain and the current approaches for treatment, and a *Family Manual* that addresses the role and activities of the family in the care of advanced cancer patients with pain and other symptoms. The two published works and the five pending will provide useful texts for the educational efforts for the WHO Program in Cancer Pain Relief and Palliative Care.

A short video tape describing the WHO program also is currently available from the WHO office. Several other publications have served to promote the WHO program at both national and international levels. Major textbooks including *The Oxford Textbook of Palliative Medicine,* edited by Drs. Doyle, Hanks, and MacDonald, and textbooks in oncology and medicine include chapters describing the WHO Program in Cancer Pain Relief and Palliative Care (Doyle et al. 1993). Proceedings from IASP World Congresses include chapters discussing this effort, as do the proceedings from the Second International Congress on Cancer Pain (Foley et al. 1990).

Cancer Pain Release, a newsletter edited by Dr. Sophie Colleau, distributes reports on the progress of the national and international programs to alleviate cancer pain. This publication is available in English and Spanish and is sent to IASP chapters, where it can be reproduced for distribution to local members. It serves as an important document that reports on changes in national policies, professional education, regulatory issues, and analgesic availability. The *Journal of Pain and Symptom Management* has published overviews of the major efforts in the WHO program worldwide and has included several reports on individual country programs.

Curriculum and Position Papers

Various organizations have developed core curricula for instruction on issues in cancer pain. The IASP *Core Curriculum* serves as a useful model of the broad educational needs for health care professionals (Fields 1991). Several countries, including Canada and Australia, have also developed specific palliative care curricula. A specific cancer pain curriculum has been developed by the American Society of Clinical Oncology (ASCO). This organization, which represents the largest group of clinical oncologists nationally and internationally, based its core curriculum for professional education on the IASP core curriculum. ASCO has recommended that this cancer pain curriculum be integrated into oncology training programs (American Society of Clinical Oncology Ad Hoc Committee on Cancer Pain 1992).

The Oncology Nursing Society, the largest association of oncology health professionals in the world, has published a position paper on cancer pain and has advocated a variety of national, regional, and local educational activities to facilitate the broad education of nurses in cancer pain management (Spross and Moore 1993; Spross et al. 1993).

The Agency for Health Care Policy and Research has published guidelines for health care professionals in cancer pain as well as a family educational booklet (Jacox 1994a,b).

Professional and Public Education

Another important advance in education, which encompasses health care professionals as well as the public, is the development of a model program referred to as the Cancer Pain Initiatives (Dahl 1993; Dahl and Joranson 1990; Greene 1993; Grossman 1993). These volunteer, interdisciplinary organizations, developed in the United States at a statewide level, include physicians, nurses, pharmacists, social workers, psychologists, and medical educators, as well as representatives of clinical care facilities, professional organizations, and government. They work together to enhance their own and their colleagues' awareness of the cancer pain problem and the advantages of appropriate pain management. Their current challenge is to maintain efforts at professional education and patient and family education, and to focus at the federal and state level on restrictions placed on drug availability for patients with pain and cancer. The Wisconsin Cancer Pain Initiative has led the development of these programs and has been a major force in statewide development. More than 33 of the 50 U.S. states have such programs in place or in development (Greene 1993).

The Wisconsin model serves as a useful approach for nationwide efforts. Many countries have taken surveys comparable to those done at a statewide level to address knowledge and attitudes of health care professionals and the public on issues of cancer pain and palliative care. Surveys in France and Germany helped to determine some of the important barriers to effective pain relief (Brasseur and Larue 1993; Zenz 1993). Both studies demonstrated the undertreatment of cancer pain and identified barriers including lack of professional education, excessive regulation of opioid analgesics, and a low priority given to this approach. Such surveys provide a useful way for each country or local area to assess barriers to effective pain relief.

Comparable to the state initiatives has been the development of large organizations such as the European Association for Palliative Care (EAPC), which has over 1400 members, publishes its own journal, and has developed guidelines for cancer pain relief and palliative care (Ventafridda et al. 1993). This organization brings together professionals working in the field of palliative care by promoting an exchange of experience. The EAPC regards the education and training of health care providers as one of its major priorities. It is currently working with the Commission of the European Community to elaborate recommendations for member countries for the inclusion of courses on palliative care in physicians' education. Particularly important is that many countries—Germany, Denmark, Sweden, Greece, Poland, Spain, and Switzerland, to name only a few—have actively participated in the EAPC.

DRUG AVAILABILITY

In the WHO strategy for cancer pain relief programs, availability of analgesics, including opioids, is a critical factor (World Health Organization 1986, 1990). Although the drugs included in the *Cancer Pain Relief* guidelines are on the Essential Drug List of the WHO, it rapidly became apparent that there is little or no use of one of the most important, morphine, in half of the countries in the world. Almost all morphine is consumed in developed countries. Joranson and others have reviewed the availability of opioids for cancer pain and have examined the trends in morphine consumption, the barriers to opioid availability, and the potential approaches to improving drug availability worldwide (Angarola 1990; Cai 1991; Chen 1992; Joranson 1993; Kishida 1991).

The WHO considers a country's morphine consumption to be an important indicator of progress toward improved cancer pain relief. Of interest, since 1984, when the WHO Program in Cancer Pain Relief and Palliative

Care began, the global consumption of morphine has increased by 272% (Joranson 1993; United Nations International Narcotics Control Board 1992). However, 57% of all morphine was consumed by the 10 countries that have ranked highest in per capita consumption for a number of years (United Nations International Narcotics Control Board 1992). These are developed countries and include Australia, Canada, Denmark, Iceland, Ireland, New Zealand, Norway, Sweden, the United Kingdom, and the United States. In fact, the 20 countries with the highest per capita consumption of morphine are developed countries. These 20 countries account for 86% of the morphine consumed in the world. The remaining 14% was consumed in approximately 100 other countries, which have the majority of the world's population. There definitely was an increase in morphine consumption in less developed countries, including China, Uruguay, Argentina, Zimbabwe, Venezuela, Romania, and Malta. Moreover, morphine has become available for the first time in Mexico, Vietnam, and India as a result of these countries' efforts to make cancer pain relief a priority (Ba Duc 1993; Romo et al. 1990; Vijayaram 1993).

It has been well recognized by international health and drug regulatory authorities that opioid analgesics are not sufficiently available for the treatment of cancer pain in many places throughout the world. The International Narcotics Control Board (INCB), which regulates global production and distribution of opioids, has requested that all countries take steps to assure that opioids are available for pain management, particularly for cancer pain (United Nations International Narcotics Control Board 1989). Demonstrated barriers to opioid availability are numerous and vary from country to country. Some countries do not have the resources and health care infrastructure to produce and distribute medicines. Others have not given a high priority to the treatment of pain. In some countries, specific drug laws prohibit or restrict the availability and medical use of opioids. For each of these barriers, specific approaches need to be developed. Both Japan and the Philippines, for example, need to change drug laws to facilitate physician prescription of opioid analgesics for cancer pain (Kishida 1991; Laudico 1993). The WHO Expert Panel and other experts have advocated that each country develop an action plan that defines existing barriers within the country to opioid availability and create an action plan to deal with these barriers.

The WHO Expert Committee on Cancer Pain Relief and Active Supportive Care prepared a *Guideline for Opioid Availability* (World Health Organization, in press) to assist health care workers and national regulators in their efforts to improve the availability of essential drugs, including opioid analgesics. The guidelines provide information about the requirements for opioid production and distribution that must be observed to make morphine and other opioids available for patients and to prevent drug diversion to illicit uses. They address issues of communication and cooperation among regulators, health care professionals, and pharmaceutical manufacturers. Not well recognized is the fact that national governments determine the amount of opioid analgesics that can be imported or manufactured by their country. National drug regulatory authorities prepare and submit to the INCB annual estimates of the quantity that their country will need for medical and scientific purposes during the next year. Although the INCB must confirm all national estimates, it is the responsibility of the national governments to determine medical need for opioids. If a country's annual estimates prove to be inadequate, the national authority may submit an amended estimate to the INCB, which can rapidly confirm revised estimates. Continually challenging the program of opioid availability are the risk of diversion and the reality of drug abuse throughout the world. These barriers, however, need to be carefully assessed on a country by country basis. National and international cooperation with drug enforcement agencies is critical to facilitate the WHO Program in Cancer Pain Relief and Palliative Care.

FUTURE DIRECTIONS

Significant progress characterized by international cooperation, national and community leadership, and extraordinary volunteerism has been made. Through the independent as well as as the collaborative efforts of the IASP and the WHO, improved pain management and palliative care are a reality for a large number of cancer patients worldwide. Continued expansion of this clinical program, a broad clinical and basic research agenda to address the scientific basis of symptom control, and strong advocacy programs to ensure institutionalization of care for this population of patients are the next steps to ensure integration of a standard of care that respects the needs of the patient with pain.

REFERENCES

American Society of Clinical Oncology Ad Hoc Committee on Cancer Pain, Cancer pain assessment and treatment curriculum guidelines, J. Clin. Oncol., 101 (1992) 1976–1982.

Angarola, R.T., Availability and regulation of opioid analgesics. In: K.M. Foley, J.J. Bonica, V. Ventafridda, and M.V. Callaway (Eds.), Second International Congress on Cancer Pain. Advances in Pain Research and Therapy, Vol. 16. Raven Press, New York, 1990, pp. 513–524.

Ba Duc, N., Vietnam: status of cancer pain relief and palliative care. J. Pain Symptom Manage., 8 (1993) 440–442.

Bonica, J.J. and Ventafridda, V. (Eds.), International Symposium on Pain of Advanced Cancer. Advances in Pain Research and Therapy, Vol. 2. Raven Press, New York 1979, 734 pp.

Brasseur, L. and Larue, F., France: status of cancer pain relief and palliative care. J. Pain Symptom Manage., 8 (1993) 412–415.

Bruera, E., Palliative care in Latin America. J. Pain Symptom Manage., 8 (1993) 365–368.

Cai, Z., The international control of narcotic drugs for licit requirements. Cancer Pain Relief and Quality of Life. Proceedings of the Workshop on Cancer Pain Relief and Quality of Life. Saitama, 16–17 December 1990. WHO Collaborating Center for Cancer Pain Relief and Quality of Life at Saitama Cancer Center, Saitama, 1991, pp. 60–63.

Chen, Y.Q., The policy and measures for narcotics control in China (monograph)., International Workshop on Cancer Pain Relief and Research, 17 June 1992, Beijing, China. Beijing International Medical Exchange Center, Beijing, 1992.

Cleeland, C.S., Demonstration projects for cancer pain relief. In: K.M. Foley, J.J. Bonica, V. Ventafridda, and M.V. Callaway (Eds.), Second International Congress on Cancer Pain. Advances in Pain Research and Therapy. Raven Press, Vol. 16. New York, 1990, pp. 465–473.

Dahl, J.L., State cancer pain initiatives. J. Pain Symptom Manage., 8 (1993) 372–375.

Dahl, J.L., and Joranson, D.E., The Wisconsin cancer pain initiative. In: K.M. Foley, J.J. Bonica, V. Ventafridda, M.V. Callaway (Eds.), Second International Congress on Cancer Pain. Advances in Pain Research and Therapy, Vol. 16. Raven Press, New York 1990, pp. 499–504.

DeLima, L., Colombia: status of cancer pain relief and palliative care, J. Pain Symptom Manage., 8 (1993) 404–406.

Doyle, D., Hanks, G.W.C., and MacDonald, N. (Eds.), Oxford Textbook of Palliative Medicine, Oxford University Press, New York, 1993.

Duc, N.B., The problems in cancer pain relief in Viet Nam. Cancer Pain Relief and Quality of Life. Proceedings of the Workshop on Cancer Pain Relief and Quality of Life. Saitama, 16–17 December 1990. WHO Collaborating Center for Cancer Pain Relief and Quality of Life at Saitama Cancer Center, Saitama, 1991, p. 56

Fields, H.L. (Ed.), Core Curriculum for Professional Education in Pain, IASP Publications, Seattle, 1991.

Foley, K.M. and Portenoy, R.K., World Health Organization–International Association for the Study of Pain: joint initiatives in cancer pain relief, J Pain Symptom Manage., 8 (1993) 335–339.

Foley, K.M., Bonica, J.J., Ventafridda, V., Callaway, M.V. (Eds), Second International Congress on Cancer Pain. Advances in Pain Research and Therapy, Vol. 16. Raven Press, New York, 1990.

Goh, C., Singapore: status of cancer pain relief and palliative care, J. Pain Symptom Manage., 8 (1993) 431–433.

Greene, P.E., America responds to cancer pain: a survey of state cancer pain initiatives, Cancer Practice, 1 (1993) 65–71.

Grossman, S.A., United States: status of cancer pain relief and palliative care, J. Pain Symptom Manage., 8 (1993) 437–439.

Jacox, A., Carr, D.B., Payne, R., et al., Management of Cancer Pain. Clinical Practice Guideline no. 9. AHCPR Publication no. 94-0592. Agency for Health Care Policy and Research, U.S. Department of Health and Human Services, Public Health Service, Rockville, Md. 1994a.

Jacox, A., Carr, D.B., Payne, R., et al., Managing Cancer Pain. Consumer Version, Clinical Practice Guideline no. 9. AHCPR Publication no. 94-0595. Patient Guide. Agency for Health Care Policy and Research, U.S. Department of Health and Human Services, Public Health Service, Rockville, Md., 1994b.

Joranson, D.E., Availability of opioids for cancer pain relief: recent trends, assessment of system barriers, New York health organization guidelines, and the risk of diversion, J. Pain Symptom Manage., 8 (1993) 353–360.

Kishida, S., Narcotics control in cancer pain management and improvement in legislative factors in

Japan. Cancer Pain Relief and Quality of Life. Proceedings of the Workshop on Cancer Pain Relief and Quality of Life, Saitama, 16–17 December 1990. WHO Collaborating Center for Cancer Pain Relief and Quality of Life at Saitama Cancer Center, Saitama, 1991, pp. 57–59.

Laudico, A.L., The Philippines: status of cancer pain relief and palliative care, J. Pain Symptom Manage., 8 (1993) 429–430.

Lickiss, J.N., Indonesia: status of cancer pain relief and palliative care, J. Pain Symptom Manage., 8 (1993) 423–424.

Romo, J.I.R., Sanchez, R.P., Garcia, C.A., and Lujan, M., Mexico's WHO Cancer Pain Relief Program. In: K.M. Foley, J.J. Bonica, V. Ventafridda, and M.V. Callaway (Eds.), Second International Congress on Cancer Pain. Advances in Pain Research and Therapy, Vol. 16. Raven Press, New York, 1990, pp. 489–498.

Spross, J.A. and Moore, P., The Oncology Nursing Society: commitment and activities promoting cancer pain relief, J. Pain Symptom Manage., 8 (1993) 376–380.

Spross, J.A., McGuire, D.B. and Schmitt, R.M., Oncology Nursing Society position paper on cancer pain, Oncol. Nurs. Forum, 17 (1993) 595–614.

Stjernsward, J., Palliative medicine: a global perspective. In: D. Doyle, G.W.C. Hanks and N. MacDonald (Eds.), Oxford Textbook of Palliative Medicine, Oxford University Press, New York, 1993, pp. 803–816.

Stjernsward, J. and Teoh, N., Current status of the global cancer control program of the World Health Organization, J. Pain Symptom Manage., 8 (1993) 340–347.

Sun, Y., China: status of cancer pain and palliative care, J. Pain Symptom Manage., 8 (1993) 399–403.

Takeda, F., Japan's WHO Cancer Pain Relief Program. In: K.M. Foley, J.J. Bonica, V. Ventafridda, and M.V. Callaway (Eds.), Second International Congress on Cancer Pain. Advances in Pain Research and Therapy, Vol. 16. Raven Press, New York, 1990, pp. 475–484.

Takeda, F., WHO Cancer Pain Relief Programme. In: M.R. Bond, J.E. Charlton and C.J. Woolf (Eds.), Proceedings of the VIth World Congress on Pain, Pain Research and Clinical Management, Vol. 4. Elsevier, Amsterdam, 1991, p. 467–474.

Takeda, F., Japan: status of cancer pain relief and palliative care, J. Pain Symptom Manage., 8 (1993) 425–426.

United Nations International Narcotics Control Board, Demand for and Supply of Opiates for Medical and Scientific Needs, United Nations, New York, 1989.

United Nations International Narcotics Control Board, Narcotic Drugs: Estimated World Requirements for 1993, Statistics for 1991, United Nations, Vienna, 1992.

Ventafridda, V., Caraceni, A., and Gamba, A., Field-testing of the WHO Guidelines for Cancer Pain Relief: summary report of demonstration projects. In: K.M. Foley, J.J. Bonica, V. Ventafridda and M.V. Callaway (Eds.), Second International Congress on Cancer Pain. Advances in Pain Research and Therapy, Vol. 16. Raven Press, New York, 1990, pp. 451–464.

Ventafridda, V., DeConno, F. and Blumhuber, H., Palliative care in Europe, J. Pain Symptom Manage., 8 (1993) 369–371.

Vijayaram, S., India: status of cancer pain relief and palliative care, J. Pain Symptom Manage., 8 (1993) 421–422.

Wenk, R., Argentina's WHO Cancer Pain Relief Program. In: K.M. Foley, J.J. Bonica, V. Ventafridda and M.V. Callaway (Eds.), Second International Congress on Cancer Pain. Advances in Pain Research and Therapy, Vol. 16. Raven Press, New York, 1990, pp. 485–488.

Wenk R., Argentina: status of cancer pain relief and palliative care, J. Pain Symptom Manage., 8 (1993) 385–387.

World Health Organization, Cancer Pain Relief, World Health Organization, Geneva, 1986.

World Health Organization, Cancer Pain Relief and Palliative Care: Report of the WHO Expert Committee, World Health Organization, Geneva, 1990.

World Health Organization, Guidelines for Opioid Availability: Annex 1 to the Report of the Expert

Committee on Cancer Pain Relief and Active Supportive Care, World Health Organization, Geneva, in press.
Zenz, M., Germany: status of cancer pain relief and palliative care, J. Pain Symptom Manage., 8 (1993) 416–418.

Correspondence to: Kathleen Foley, MD, Department of Neurology, Memorial Sloan-Kettering Cancer Center, 1275 York Ave., New York, NY 10021, USA. Tel: 212-639-7050; 212-717-3081.

Proceedings of the 7th World Congress on Pain,
Progress in Pain Research and Management, Vol. 2,
edited by G.F. Gebhart, D.L. Hammond, and T.S.
Jensen, IASP Press, Seattle, © 1994.

7

Pain Management: Quality Assurance and Changing Practice

Christine Miaskowski

Department of Physiological Nursing, University of California, San Francisco, California, USA

INTRODUCTION

The need to evaluate the quality of patient care, as well as other variables in pain management, is becoming extremely important in light of the world-wide crisis in health care. The debates around health care reform center on balancing cost issues with issues of access and quality. Fundamental to finding solutions to the health care crisis and evaluating the outcomes of health care reform will be the ability to *measure* cost, access, and quality.

Previously published clinical surveys (Marks and Sachar 1973; Sriwatanakul et al. 1983; Donovan et al. 1987; Oden 1989), as well as abstracts from this meeting (Boureau and Sahmoud 1993; Galichon et al. 1993), continue to demonstrate that routine management of postoperative pain results in undertreatment of the patient. Similar documentation exists on the undertreatment of cancer-related pain (Bonica 1985; Daut et al. 1982; Twycross and Fairfield 1982).

These studies have provided the impetus for several professional organizations, including the International Association for the Study of Pain (IASP) and the American Pain Society (APS), as well as several government and regulatory agencies including the Canadian Council on Health Facilities Accreditation and the Agency for Health Care Policy and Research (AHCPR), to develop and publish standards or guidelines on the management of acute or cancer-related pain. Implicit or explicit in each of the standards and guidelines published to date is the call for a systematic evaluation of the scope of pain management services provided by an organization, as well as the quality and cost of these activities. In addition, these standards and guidelines recommend that organizations conduct patient satisfaction surveys as part of an evaluation of the quality of pain management services provided.

This chapter focuses on the issues surrounding the evaluation of the quality of pain management, particularly in the areas of acute and cancer-related pain. The main reasons for limiting discussion to these two pain problems are as follows:

- Extensive research on the undertreatment of pain in these patient populations is available.
- Standards/guidelines for evaluation are published.
- Pain problems are of relatively short duration.
- Pain problems are associated with fewer psychological implications.

As mentioned previously, abundant research has documented that patients experiencing acute and cancer-related pain are not receiving quality pain management. In addition, several professional organizations and government agencies have issued guidelines for the management of acute and cancer-related pain that can be used as the basis for developing a quality improvement (QI) program.

In addition, recent QI data suggest that an evaluation of a specific episode of care is preferable to an evaluation of care in general. Acute pain and most cases of cancer-related pain are time-limited as compared to chronic pain of nonmalignant origin; thus, the issues related to quality evaluation of pain management for these complaints may be simpler and more easily managed by a health care organization than a detailed evaluation of chronic pain of nonmalignant origin. Data and experience obtained from measuring quality of acute and cancer-related pain management should provide direction for future research on the evaluation of the quality of pain management of patients experiencing chronic pain of nonmalignant origin. Finally, in respect to use of patient satisfaction surveys as a measure of the quality of pain management, acute and cancer-related pain are associated with fewer psychological issues (e.g., issues of secondary gain) as compared to chronic pain of nonmalignant origin, factors that might influence patients' responses to satisfaction surveys.

This chapter begins with a discussion of the current concepts underlying the measurement of quality of care. It will review the specific guidelines/standards for the management of acute and cancer-related pain that have been published by professional organizations and government and regulatory agencies. Emphasis is placed on the issues surrounding the use of patient satisfaction surveys to evaluate the quality of pain management. Specifically, the chapter summarizes data on the pros and cons of patient satisfaction surveys in general and reviews the limited amount of available data on the use of patient satisfaction surveys to evaluate the quality of pain management. The chapter concludes with a series of recommendations that can guide future quality of care studies in pain management.

QUALITY ASSURANCE VERSUS QUALITY IMPROVEMENT

Continuing a tradition established by Florence Nightingale, Donabedian began writing, in the mid-1960s, about evaluating the quality of medical care (Donabedian 1966). Since then, the concepts fundamental to evaluating the quality of health care have evolved. In the late 1980s, new terms appeared in the literature to replace *quality assurance* (QA). The new language includes such terms as *quality improvement* (QI), *continuous quality improvement* (CQI), and *total quality management* (TQM). Some may consider this a kind of alphabet soup approach to the evaluation of quality of care. However, the question is whether or not there are fundamental differences in the assumptions or approaches used with QA versus QI techniques or strategies.

Table I contrasts the fundamental assumptions underlying a QI approach to quality measurement as opposed to the way the process of QA has been conceptualized. The process of QA recommends that standards of care be established as yardsticks or measurement criteria. The QA approach believes

Table I
Comparison of quality improvement versus quality assurance

Quality Improvement	Quality Assurance
Improve continuously	Meet standards
Rely on process control and design improvement	Rely on inspection to improve
Leaders enable and support	Leaders exhort and enforce
Workers try hard	Workers don't try hard enough
Quality saves	Quality costs
Customers are partners	Customers are problems
Learn from data	"Gut fact" understanding

Source: Adapted from McEachern et al. 1991.

that external authorities, not those persons directly involved in the process of care, can define the attributes of good care. The QA approach is somewhat punitive in that it recommends that once an authority establishes a standard, some authority also evaluates compliance with the standard. The QA approach suggests that one of the main reasons a standard is not met is usually because workers don't try hard enough or work hard enough. To rectify the deficit in the quality of care, authority figures enforce sanctions and impose rules. The QA process of evaluation is usually viewed as a costly venture to perform and maintain. Customers, in this case patients, are seen as problems or outsiders, irrelevant to the process of QA. The QA process seeks to identify "bad apples" in an organization and either improve their performance or punish them in some way.

However, Donabedian (1990) suggests that "system design and performance monitoring are two inseparable, mutually supportive components of quality." He makes the distinction between production efficiency and clinical efficiency. Donabedian states that "optimal care is optimal production and clinical efficiency assessed jointly by the health care practitioner and the fully informed patient, guided by the patient's own values and interests." These ideas, as well as concepts from the manufacturing industry espoused by Deming (1986) and tested in Japan, suggest that a paradigm shift in evaluating quality of care is in order, namely a QI approach.

The QI approach recommends that a process of care be examined from a systems perspective. The QI view espouses that problems with achieving high-quality care are not the result of problems with people but with the processes and systems of care delivery. This approach suggests that processes of care occur on a continuum and that the goal of quality management is to improve continuously. To improve the quality of care provided to patients, the *processes* of care must be understood. Understanding any process of care, for example the administration of pain medications, requires input and participation from those involved in the process, namely workers and customers. The QI process is a data-driven approach that requires participation from *all* the participants (i.e., workers and customers). The QI process improves the quality of the product or the output, in this case some aspect of health care delivery/services, and saves money. It destroys the bad apple approach and puts control of quality in the hands of the providers.

One of the major issues with the QI approach, which has worked so successfully in the manufacturing industry is whether it is applicable to a largely service industry such as health care. Fig. 1 illustrates McEachern's concept (1991) of how Deming's model of continuous QI can be applied to health care. The model suggests that health care professionals (HCPs) are charged with designing the best value health care services. The model is

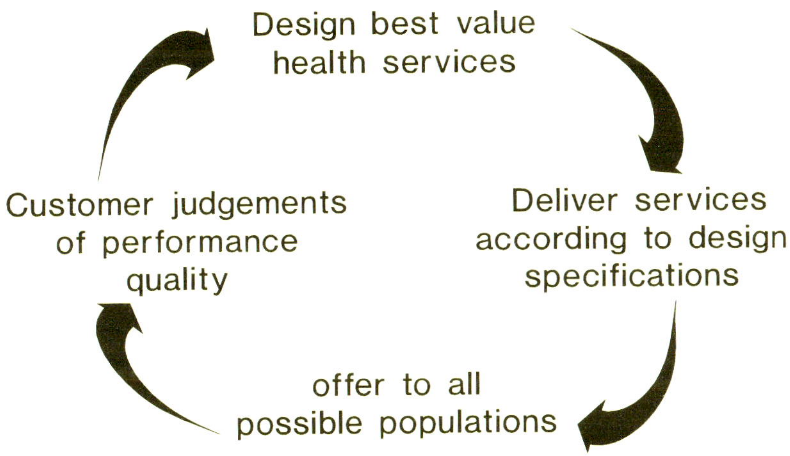

Fig. 1. The Deming model of continuous quality improvement applied to health care. (McEachern et al. 1991)

driven by the new age of consumerism that exists, at least, in the industrialized world. Customers drive this new model in which health care organizations will succeed or fail based on their ability to produce services that meet customer needs, desires, and expectations. Not only do HCPs need to design the services, they must then deliver them according to advertised specifications. Inherent in the model is an exquisite marketing plan and ongoing evaluation from customers about the quality of the services provided (McEachern et al. 1991).

The model has two basic assumptions that HCPs need to grapple with, and pain practitioners in particular need to discern, before progress can be made. The first assumption is that HCPs understand who the customer is. In this QI model, a customer is defined as any person or product receiving an output of the process. Customers in health care include patients, payers, regulators, providers, and the government. All of these customers need to be considered when designing any health care service. The second assumption of the QI model is that HCPs have sufficient knowledge about their customers expectations and needs. However, in today's health care system, HCPs lack not only the customers' input but also a systematic way of incorporating that input into improving the system. Health care professionals need to consider ways of obtaining information from consumers and incorporating these data into the processes of care. This chapter will consider in more detail the need for a customer focus in planning and evaluating health care services in the section that discuss the use of patient satisfaction surveys to evaluate the quality of care.

Table II
Summary of published pain-related Quality Assurance/Quality Improvement standards or guidelines

I. Canadian Council of Health Facilities Accreditation—QA-Related Palliative Care Program Standards

A. The Palliative Care Program has planned and conducted systematic activities for monitoring and evaluating the quality of patient care, including a plan for action(s) and follow-up to ensure that the action(s) is effective in continually improving the quality of care.

II. American Pain Society's QA Standards on Acute and Cancer-related Pain

A. Acute pain and chronic cancer pain are recognized and effectively treated.
B. Information about analgesics is readily available.
C. Patients are promised attentive analgesic care.
D. Explicit policies for the use of advanced technologies are defined
E. Adherence to standards is monitored.

III. Agency for Health Care Policy and Research QA Guidelines

A. General Considerations

1. Institutional process of acute pain management begins with the affirmation that patients should have access to the best level of pain relief that may safely be provided.
2. Each institution should develop the resources necessary to provide the best and the most modern pain relief appropriate to its patients and should designate who and/or which departments are responsible for the required activities.
3. Formal means must be developed and used within each institution to assess pain management practices and to obtain patient feedback to gauge the adequacy of pain control.

B. Key Items to be Included in an Institutional QA Program

1. Patient comfort and satisfaction with pain management.
2. How those options are best applied.
3. The range and appropriateness of options available within a particular institution.
4. Minimizing side effects and complications related to pain control.

PAIN-RELATED QA/QI ACTIVITIES—HOW DO WE MEASURE UP?

The process of QA/QI in pain management is still in its infancy. In relationship to the entire quality measurement field, some of the pain-related quality of care activities are more QA-focused, while others are more QI-focused. Most of the published work to date on pain-related QA/QI activities focuses on an evaluation of acute pain and cancer-related pain. This work has emphasized assessment of the quality, or more accurately the poor quality, of pain management of these two types of pain within acute care hospitals or terminal care/palliative care organizations.

Two organizations and one governmental agency have published standards/guidelines on quality pain management, which are summarized in Table II. In 1992, the Canadian Council of Health Care Facilities published palliative care program (PCP) Standards to be used by a palliative care service, a program, a unit, or a consultation team (Canadian Council of Health Facilities Accreditation 1992). These standards address the purpose, organizational structure, policies and procedures, human and physical resources, orientation programs, staff development and continuing education requirements, and patient care activities that are necessary for a PCP to provide quality care to the terminally ill. A separate QA standard calls for a systematic evaluation of patient care that ensures continuous improvement in the quality of care. The document's patient care standard requires that the plan of care is based, in part, on the patient's choice of care and/or treatment and the expressed desires and preferences of the patient and the family. In the United States, the Joint Commission on the Accreditation of Health Care Organizations has published similar standards for the care of the terminally ill.

The American Pain Society (APS) in 1991 published QA standards for the relief of acute and cancer pain (Committee on Quality Assurance Standards 1991). Doctors Max and Donovan, cochairs of the APS committee, charged pain professionals as well as all HCPs to implement several basic standards. A fundamental approach that needs to be promoted as part of the process of quality pain management in every organization is that acute pain and cancer pain must be recognized and effectively treated. The APS standards recommend that pain assessments be done regularly and that pain intensity measures be documented in a visible place on the patients' charts. The APS QA Committee believes that knowledge will change practice and thus recommended that information about analgesics be made readily available to all HCPs. Inherent in the information standard is the need to educate all HCPs about pain assessment and management.

The APS QA Standard II speaks to empowering patients by letting them know that pain management is an important part of their care. The committee also recommended the development of policies and procedures for advanced technologies and that these policies delineate role accountability of all HCPs. Finally, the committee recommended that an interdisciplinary committee monitor adherence to these standards. The APS standards indicate that patient satisfaction survey data should be used as part of the quality monitoring process. Miaskowski and Donovan have described strategies for implementing the APS QA Standards in acute care settings (Donovan and Miaskowski 1992) and on oncology units (Miaskowski and Donovan 1992).

Most recently, a new federal agency, the Agency for Health Care Policy and Research (AHCPR), was established in the United States to enhance the quality, appropriateness, and effectiveness of health care services and access to such services. To achieve its mission, AHCPR supports broad-based scientific research as well as the development of clinical practice guidelines (CPG). In 1992 AHCPR published the first CPG on the management of acute pain. The goals of this guideline are to: (1) reduce the incidence and severity of postoperative and posttraumatic pain; (2) educate patients about the need to communicate unrelieved pain so that they can receive prompt evaluation and effective treatment; (3) enhance patient comfort and satisfaction; and (4) contribute to fewer postoperative complications and in some instances shorter stays after surgical procedures (Acute Pain Management Guideline Panel 1992).

A key component of the Acute Pain Guideline is the recommendation that an organization must establish responsibility for effective pain relief. The guideline recommends that organizations develop the resources necessary to provide effective pain relief and determine which HCPs are responsible for which aspects of pain management. In addition, the guideline calls for the establishment of an formal means to assess the process of pain management within an organization. The AHCPR Acute Pain Guideline incorporated many of the recommendations from the APS QA Standards (Committee on Quality Assurance Standards 1991) in recommending the key items to be included in the development of a QA plan. These items include an evaluation of patient comfort and satisfaction with pain management as well as an evaluation of patient outcomes including side effects and complications associated with pain management. Several authors have described how HCPs may implement the Acute Pain Guideline with adult and pediatric patients (Hester et al. 1992; Miaskowski et al. 1992b).

All these standards and guidelines recommend a process of pain management that requires involvement of the patient in evaluating the quality of care they received. As discussed previously, most of the work on evaluating the quality of both acute and cancer pain management has focused on identifying the bad apples in pain management, namely HCPs undertreatment of these common pain problems. Very little work has been done on obtaining information from consumers on the quality of pain management. In addition, very little work has been done defining the processes of care surrounding pain management. The next portion of this chapter will focus on what is known about patient satisfaction with health care in general and then will review the limited work summarizing patient satisfaction data on pain management.

PATIENT SATISFACTION—TO ASK OR NOT TO ASK?

Patient satisfaction is defined as a health care recipient's reaction to salient aspects of the service experience (Cleary et al. 1988). Several factors have stimulated research in evaluating the quality of health care using patient satisfaction surveys. The first reason for the increase in patient satisfaction research is the increase in consumer sophistication. The age of consumerism is upon us and the popular press is not reticent to release consumer reports on health care organizations (*U.S. News and World Report* 1993). As consumers are becoming more sophisticated about care and services, providers are becoming more attentive to patients' concerns and desires. In some ways this increased attentiveness may be motivated by a climate of increased competition for patients. However, social scientists are becoming more interested in health services research, and governmental agencies, at least in the United States, are providing some financial support for this type of research (Cleary et al. 1988).

Again, Donabedian (1980) has set the stage by discussing the use of patient satisfaction surveys to assess the quality of care. Donabedian (1980) defines quality of care as "the worth or excellence of various attributes of health care." He suggests that three aspects of care must form the basis of quality care measurement: the technical process of care, interpersonal features of the provider-patient relationship, and amenities. The attributes of the technical process of care refer to the various procedures involved in making a diagnosis or managing a patient's problem. The interpersonal features refer to interpersonal communication skills of HCPs. Finally, amenities refer to the physical facilities and resources available to provide health care services.

It is important to realize that patients can provide two different types of satisfaction data, namely ratings and reports. Ratings capture the *personal* evaluations of attributes of providers and services. Ratings are more *subjective* because they reflect both personal experiences and the standards consumers apply when evaluating care (Davies et al. 1988).

In contrast, consumer reports deal with what did or did not occur in a given health care encounter. Consumer reports are more *objective* and can potentially be confirmed by an outside observer (Davies et al. 1988). Table III provides an example of how this type of rating system versus reporting system might be applied to gathering patient satisfaction about pain management.

While these measurement distinctions seem to be relatively straightforward, major controversies exist among HCPs about the validity and reliability of patient satisfaction data to be used to evaluate the quality of health care,

Table III
Distinction between patient ratings and reports of technical and interpersonal aspects of pain management

	Technical	Interpersonal
Rating	Evaluation (excellent to poor) of the thoroughness of the pain history by the health care professional	Evaluation (excellent to poor) of staffs' responses to reports of pain
Report	Indication (yes–no) of whether the health care professional determined the following: description, location, and severity of the pain	Indication (yes–no) of whether staff told the patient that pain management was an important part of care

Table IV summarizes the key arguments for and against the use of patient satisfaction data.

Arguments that question the validity of patient satisfaction data suggest that the information reflects something other than the processes involved in health care. The first argument against the validity of patient satisfaction data states that because consumer ratings of health care correlate with a person's attitudes toward the community, satisfaction with life, health status, and selected demographic variables (i.e., age, educational level, income, and ethnicity) that these ratings tell us more about the consumers than about the quality of care. For example, one correlation that has been found across numerous surveys is that older patients are more satisfied with their health care than are younger patients.

However, as Davies and Ware from the Rand Corporation point out, these correlations are difficult to interpret because we know little about the relationship among these factors and what should be the exact magnitude of the correlations between them. In addition, while opponents of consumer involvement in rating health care suggest that these relationships may indicate a consumer bias, they fail to recognize the real probability that features of health care and individual characteristics are probably related in the real world (Davies et al. 1988).

The second argument "holds that consumers can be 'seduced' by the number of tests and procedures received, into believing that the services provided were appropriate and well-performed" (Davies et al. 1988). In other words, does quantity equate with quality in the eyes of the patient and are patient satisfaction surveys really quantity reports as opposed to quality reports or ratings? The results of two experimental studies (Davies et al. 1986; Sox et al. 1981) suggest that consumers' ratings of care do reflect, at least in part, how many services they received. However, more research is needed in this area, and pain researchers could examine the relationships between pa-

Table IV
Arguments against and for the use of patient satisfaction data

Against	For
Data reveal more about the consumers that about the quality of care.	Consumers' assessments of quality predict their behaviors in the marketplace.
Data reflect how much was done, not how well it was done.	Consumers need not necessarily be qualified judges to provide accurate information about quality.
Consumers disagree with HCPs' judgments about quality.	Data from consumers may be less expensive than other QI sources of data.
Data simply reflect whether the provider was nice to patients.	Data from consumers provide information not otherwise available.

tient satisfaction and the use of technology versus no technology in the management of acute pain and cancer-related pain.

Some persons who challenge consumer ratings of health care suggest that the judgments of HPCs are the only criteria that can be used to judge the quality of patient care. These persons claim that consumers lack the technical knowledge and appropriate standards for judging the science and technology of health care (Davies et al. 1988). As Davies and Ware (1988) point out, "this argument encounters its first difficulty in holding consumers to a standard that is far from uniform." Brook's (1973) and Eddy's (1984) work suggest that HCPs do not always agree with their own or each other's judgments of technical quality. Therefore, why should we expect consumers' ratings to agree perfectly with HCPs? In addition, we should not expect consumers' ratings to agree perfectly with HCPs because the two groups have different perspectives on the process of health care. However, two studies (Chang et al. 1984; Erlich et al. 1961) have examined the congruence between consumers' and HCPs' judgments of quality care. In general, consumers tend to rate care more favorably than do HCPs. However, there appears to be better agreement between the two groups on judgments of poor care.

The final argument against the validity of patient satisfaction data states that consumers' ratings simply reflect whether HCPs were nice to the patient. The real issue underlying this argument is whether the providers' interpersonal communication skills interfere with patients' accurate assessments of the technical processes of care. Davies and Ware (1988) point out that relatively strong correlations (on the order of 0.60 to 0.70) have been found between consumers' ratings of the interpersonal aspects of care and the technical quality of care. However, additional studies by DiMatteo and colleagues (1980), Korsch and coworkers (1968), and Stiles and colleagues (1979) have demonstrated in a variety of clinical and experimental situations that patients are able to distinguish between high and low technical quality encounters coupled with high or low interpersonal encounters.

The arguments favoring the use of consumers' ratings of care are compelling. First, the literature suggests that consumers' assessments of quality predict their behaviors in the marketplace. Specific behaviors that have been linked to consumers' ratings of quality-related features of care include: doctor-shopping, complaints and disenrollment from group health-care plans, compliance with the therapeutic regimen, recommending a source of care to others, and use of health care services (Davies and Ware 1988).

Consumers who are positive about the technical and interpersonal aspects of care they receive are significantly less likely to change physicians (Kosteller et al. 1976; Marquis, et al. 1983). Additional studies have shown that patients who were more satisfied with the quality of their health care were more likely to recommend a certain HCP to a friend or relative (Ware 1981), were more likely to follow a therapeutic regimen (Ware et al. 1976), and were more likely to use health care services (Kravitz 1975; Mirowsky and Ross 1983).

Arguments against the use of consumer data question the accuracy of patients' ratings or judgments about the quality of care. Data from an experiment conducted by Ware and coworkers (1978) suggest that consumers can provide accurate reports of the technical aspects of care. Consumers and physicians watched videotaped simulations and, using a checklist, reported whether specific history and physical exam items were performed or not performed. Consumers were as accurate as physicians in scoring the history and physical exam items that were done.

An additional advantage to using patient satisfaction data is that it may be less expensive data to obtain compared with other QI approaches, including medical record abstraction. Recent estimates suggest that medical record abstraction and data entry can cost anywhere from \$15 to \$45 per record. However, before a definitive conclusion can be made, comparative cost analyses for obtaining patient satisfaction data need to be performed.

Perhaps the most compelling argument for using consumer data to evaluate the quality of care is that these data provide unique information that is not available from any other data source. In addition, Vuori (1987) has suggested that when HCPs are trying to determine the patient's role in the evaluation of the quality of care, they need to consider the differences in the roles that HCPs and patients play relative to the QA process. According to Vuori (1987), the difference between the role of the health care provider and the role of the patient in QA resembles that between the hen and the pig in the preparation of eggs and bacon: the hen is involved in the process, but the pig is committed. Vuori's analogy provides a compelling argument for involving patients in evaluating the quality of the pain management.

METHODS OF MEASURING PATIENT SATISFACTION

Fitzpatrick (1991) provides a review of the important general considerations in conducting patient satisfaction surveys. The various dimensions of patient satisfaction that can be surveyed include humaneness, informativeness, overall quality, competence, bureaucracy, access, cost, facilities, outcome, continuity, and attention to psychosocial problems. Investigators must determine what aspects they want to measure and whether they are more interested in obtaining patient ratings or reports of the quality of care. In addition, investigators must choose a specific method for obtaining the patient satisfaction data (i.e., an interview, a self-report questionnaire prior to a patient's discharge, a mailed questionnaire, or a telephone survey). Table V summarizes the advantages of an interview versus a self-report approach to data collection.

Parker and Kroboth (1991) summarize the practical problems that can be encountered when conducting patient satisfaction surveys. Some problems include: (1) access to patients (issues related to ease of recruiting participation from inpatients versus outpatients); (2) the establishment of appropriate patient selection criteria to obtain the specific data needed to answer the study questions; (3) validity and reliability of the survey instrument; (4) problems with consent and ensuring the patient's confidentiality; (5) consideration to specific patient characteristics including age, severity of illness, literacy level, and language; and (6) procedural issues including when to conduct the survey in relationship to the episode of care that is being evaluated, cost, training of

Table V
A comparison of the use of interviews versus questionnaires to obtain data on patient satisfaction

Interview	Self-Report Questionnaire
Sensitivity to patient concerns	Standardization of items
Flexibility in covering topics	No interviewer bias
Rapport	Anonymity is maintained
Clarification of ambiguous items or reasons for the items	Low cost of data gathering
Respondent adherence	Less need for trained staff
More scope to follow up nonrespondents	

interviewers to ensure inter-rater reliability, and plans for data management and analysis. All these aspects of survey design and preparation need to be planned in advance to promote the collection of valid patient satisfaction data.

PATIENT SATISFACTION WITH PAIN MANAGEMENT

As mentioned previously, the QA Committee of the APS and the AHCPR Acute Pain Guideline Panel recommended that patient satisfaction surveys of pain management be conducted. The APS QA Committee (Committee on Quality Assurance Standards 1991) published a model patient satisfaction survey and charged HCPs with the task of testing the instrument and providing feedback. Table VI summarizes the key dimensions of the APS patient satisfaction survey and whether the key items require a consumer rating or a report.

To date, only two studies have been conducted using the APS Patient Satisfaction Survey to assess the quality of acute and cancer-related pain management (Miaskowski et al. 1994, Ward and Gordon 1994). One additional study conducted by Miaskowski and Nye (unpublished data) also will be presented as part of this discussion.

The patient satisfaction studies were done in three different acute care hospitals. All three studies included patients experiencing acute and/or cancer-related pain. A total of 404 patients were assessed. The Ward and Gordon study (1994) included 31 children. The two studies conducted by Miaskowski and colleagues (Miaskowski et al. 1994; Miaskowski, unpublished data) were conducted using patient interviews, while the Ward and Gordon study used a patient self-report questionnaire.

Table VII compares data from three of the key items on the survey (pain intensity, pain relief, and waiting time for pain medications), as well as the patients' satisfaction ratings. Patients were asked to report, on a 0 to 10 numeric rating scale (with 0 being no pain and 10 being the worst possible pain), their pain intensity at the time of the survey and the worst pain they had experienced in the past 24 hours. The three studies show marked similarities in both intensity measures. At two of the study sites, pain relief scores also were assessed using a 0 to 10 scale. Ratings of pain at its least ranged from 1.93 to 3.07. The final common parameter that was evaluated was waiting time for medications. In all three studies, more than 40% of the patients had to wait longer than 15 minutes for pain medications. Taken together, these data suggest that hospitalized patients suffer moderate to severe pain that is not well relieved. In addition, patients need to wait long periods of time to receive pain medications.

Table VI
Dimensions of the American Pain Society's patient satisfaction survey

Dimension	APS Survey
Outcome	Measure of pain relief following treatment (rating)
Overall quality	Satisfaction with pain relief (rating)
Humaneness	Satisfaction with staff response (rating)
Competence	Health professional who was helpful with pain management (report)
Bureaucracy	Waiting time for pain medications (report)
Informativeness	MD/RN instruct patient to report pain (report)

However, when patients were asked (through a Likert scale) how satisfied they were with the staffs' responses to their pain management needs, 84–99% stated that they were either satisfied or very satisfied with the staffs' responses. However, all three studies showed a statistically significant negative correlation between pain intensity scores and patient satisfaction scores. That is, patients with lower pain intensity scores were more satisfied with their overall pain management while patients with higher pain intensity scores were more dissatisfied.

The data from these three studies suggest that while patients reported experiencing moderate to severe pain and had to wait relatively long periods of time for pain medications, in most cases they were satisfied with their pain management. Miaskowski's and Ward's data are supported by data and conclusions from several abstracts presented at the 7th World Congress on Pain by investigators in Denmark (Skadborg et al. 1993), Spain (Bosch et al. 1993), and the United States (Dauber et al. 1993; LaPerriere et al. 1993). These investigators found similar results and drew similar conclusions, namely that patients were undermedicated and experienced severe pain, but were satisfied with the quality of their pain management.

Both Miaskowski and Ward and their colleagues came to similar conclusions about the use of patient satisfaction surveys to assess the quality of pain management. One critical dimension that needs to be evaluated, and may help interpret these types of satisfaction data, is a careful evaluation of patients' expectations of pain and pain relief. One published study (Carr 1990) and one study reported as an abstract at the Congress (Miralles et al. 1993) have evaluated surgical patients' expectations of postoperative pain and found that patients, when asked preoperatively, underestimated the amount of pain they would experience postoperatively. However, neither study reported evaluating

Table VII
Comparison of patient satisfaction data from three pain studies

	Miaskowski et al. 1994	Miaskowski and Nye, unpublished	Ward and Gordon 1994
Pain intensity scores (mean ± SD)			
Now	4.32 (2.9)	4.2 (3.0)	3.6 (2.4)
Worst	7.6 (2.2)	7.3 (2.5)	6.6 (2.8)
Pain relief score (mean ± SD)			
Pain at its least	3.1 (2.6)	—	1.9 (1.9)
Waiting time for pain medications (% of patients responding)			
0–15 minutes	52.1	59.7	60.0
16–30 minutes	22.5	3.6	16.0
> 30 minutes	24.0	14.0	8.0
Satisfaction with staff response (% of patients responding)			
Very satisfied	72.5 (RN + MD)	49 (RN + MD)	57/48 (RN/MD)
Satisfied	26.4 (RN + MD)	36 (RN + MD)	33/36 (RN/MD)

the relationship between expectations of pain, or perhaps more importantly, expectations of pain relief, and patients' ratings of satisfaction with pain management. Ratings of patients' expectations of pain and pain relief need to be incorporated into future studies that attempt to evaluate the quality of pain management.

ISSUES IN ASSESSING PATIENT SATISFACTION WITH PAIN MANAGEMENT AND PRACTICE RECOMMENDATIONS

Table VIII enumerates several recommendations for design of studies to evaluate the quality of acute and cancer-related pain management. Based on the current information available in the QI literature, quality of care evaluations should focus on a discrete or specific episode of care rather than a survey of patients' general assessments of the quality of care they received. Pain studies need to focus on a specific portion of the pain experience (e.g., for a specific surgical procedure or for a specific period during the cancer pain experience).

Pain practitioners need to develop well-designed QI studies that evaluate specific patient populations. Consideration must be given to patient inclusion and exclusion criteria to ensure that certain groups of patients are not systematically ignored while other groups are overstudied. Now that some general survey information on patient satisfaction with pain management is available, studies of vulnerable patient populations (e.g., intensive care unit patients who cannot self-report pain, patients with language barriers, children, the elderly) must be purposefully designed and data compared with previously published reports.

Based on the data from the Miaskowski group (1994) and Ward and Gordon (1994) studies, patient evaluations of their satisfaction with pain management should be done using a descriptive numeric rating scale rather than a Likert scale to obtain a greater range of possible responses. In addition, if the satisfaction survey is conducted using an interview format, the interviewer should explore with the patient, in a nonthreatening manner, any incongruities between pain intensity ratings and level of satisfaction with pain relief.

Another recommendation related to conducting patient satisfaction surveys of pain management is that *all* survey responses need to be triangulated to obtain an overall assessment of the quality of care provided by a health care organization. In other words, HCPs must consider the responses to all survey items, not just the satisfaction questions when evaluating the overall quality of a pain management program. Failure to consider all of the survey data may lead to erroneous conclusions and a failure to identify critical factors that require modification and improvement.

As stated previously, several questions need to be added to pain satisfaction surveys that evaluate patients' expectations about the amount of pain they will experience and the amount of relief that will be provided. The relationship between patients' expectations and satisfaction with pain management needs to be determined.

Pain practitioners dealing with acute and cancer-related pain management need to broaden their approach and conduct both inpatient and outpatient pain satisfaction surveys. Most of the work on patient satisfaction with pain management has been done with hospitalized patients. This contrasts with the general work on patient satisfaction with health care that primarily focuses on outpatients. In the area of acute pain, a critical population that is growing exponentially is the ambulatory surgery population. Assessments of the quality of their pain management in the ambulatory surgery setting extending into the home is an important area for future research. In addition, oncology patients are receiving more of their care on an outpatient basis. The quality of pain management in ambulatory care settings must be assessed.

Not only does patient satisfaction with pain management need to be as-

Table VIII
Recommendations for assessing patient satisfaction with pain management

1.	Evaluate an episode of pain.
2.	Develop specific patient inclusion/exclusion criteria.
3.	Evaluate patient satisfaction with pain management and care providers using a descriptive numeric rating scale (i.e., not a Likert type scale).
4.	Explore with patients incongruities in pain intensity ratings and their ratings of their level of satisfaction with pain management.
5.	Triangulate survey responses to determine the overall quality of pain management within an organization.
6.	Evaluate patients' expectations for pain and pain relief.
7.	Conduct inpatient and outpatient patient satisfaction surveys.
8.	Evaluate patient satisfaction with pain management across health care settings (e.g., inpatient, ambulatory care, hospice, nursing home, home, private physician offices).
9.	Evaluate caregiver satisfaction with pain management.
10.	Link patient satisfaction data with patient outcomes (e.g. quality of life, mood, side effects and complications, functional status).
11.	Evaluate the cost of patient satisfaction surveys of pain management.
12.	Conduct qualitative analyses of patient satisfaction with pain management and patients' opinions of factors that would improve the quality of pain management.

sessed in inpatient and outpatient settings, assessments of quality need to be done *across* settings, particularly at points of transition in care. For example, the question arises, "Is the quality of pain management maintained when an oncology patient is transferred from a hospice or home setting to an acute care hospital for an emergency procedure?"

Work by Ferrell and colleagues (1991) demonstrates that caregivers of oncology patients are intimately involved in the pain experience of the patient. Surveys need to be conducted on caregivers' satisfaction with the quality of pain management that a patient receives. Caregiver data may provide different insights into the processes of care governing pain management and may assist HCPs to develop more effective QI strategies.

Patient satisfaction data on pain management must begin to be linked to patient outcomes. Previous work (Davies and Ware 1988) has shown that patients who were more satisfied with their care were more compliant with the therapeutic regimen. Does a similar relationship hold for patients who are satisfied with their pain management? Would patients increase the use of pharmacologic and nonpharmacologic interventions that might result in subsequent improvements in quality of life, mood, and/or functional status if they

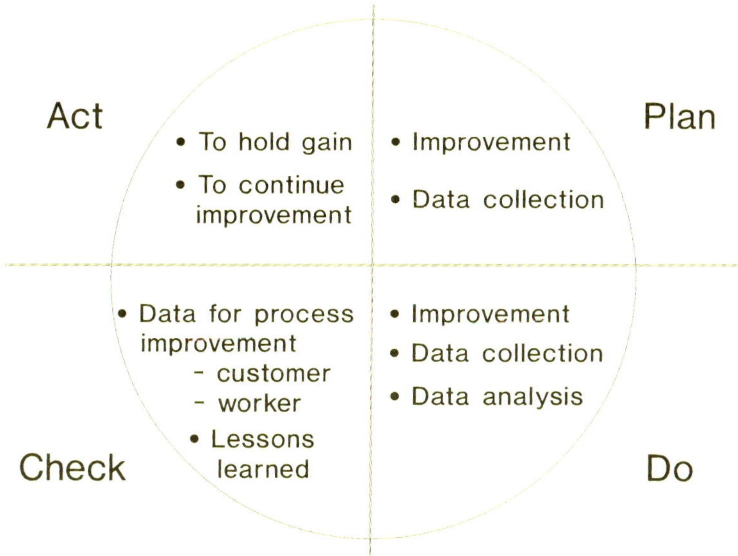

Fig. 2. Key aspects of the quality improvement action plan. (McEachern et al. 1991)

were satisfied with the quality of their pain management? Further research on the relationship between patient satisfaction and patient outcomes is warranted.

The costs of patient satisfaction surveys conducted using interviews or self-report questionnaires need to be determined. Is the yield, in terms of information obtained that can be used to continuously improve the process of pain management, worth the expense of obtaining it? Are there cheaper and more effective ways to obtain the same type of information?

Finally, the use of qualitative approaches to obtaining patient satisfaction data need to be evaluated. In-depth patient interviews that are then subjected to content analysis for recurrent themes may provide useful information for HCPs to use when redesigning the processes of pain management. These in-depth interviews could focus on patients' opinions about key factors that could be implemented or modified to improve the quality of pain management.

CONCLUSION—A CALL TO ACTION!

The QI improvement process is a call to action! Fig. 2 illustrates the key aspects of the action plan. Once the process of care that requires improvement is identified, HCPs must *Plan* the data collection process and procedures. If pain management is the process to be evaluated, the plan may involve a patient satisfaction survey. The *Do* portion of the process involves data collection and analysis. The next step involves validating the data (i.e., *Check*) with those involved in the process of care (e.g., in the case of pain management, both HCPs and patients). Once the data are validated an action plan is designed and implemented, HCPs would use the *Act* step to implement the process of improvement, sustain the improvement, and begin the process again to evaluate the gains that have been made in the process of delivering quality pain management. Coyle and colleagues at the Memorial Sloan-Kettering Cancer Center reported one example of using the QI process to implement the APS QA Standards (Coyle et al. 1993). The ongoing QI process applied to pain management, which includes the patient as part of the process, should improve the quality of pain care. Additional studies are needed to determine the effectiveness of such QI activities in changing both patients' and HCPs' behaviors, specifically related to pain management.

REFERENCES

Acute Pain Management Guideline Panel., Acute Pain Management: Operative or Medical Procedures and Trauma: Clinical Practice Guideline, AHCPR Pub. no. 92-0032, Agency for Health Care Policy and Research, Public Health Service, U.S. Department of Health and Human Services, Rockville, Md., 1992, 145pp.

Bonica, J.J., Treatment of cancer pain: current status and future needs. In H.L. Fields, R. Dubner, and F. Cervero (Eds.), Proceedings of the IVth World Congress on Pain. Advances in Pain Research and Therapy, Vol. 9. Raven Press, New York, 1985, pp. 589–616.

Bosch, F., Bassols, A., Zavala, S., Moral, M.V. and Bansos, J.E., Prevalence, characteristics, and treatment of pain in a Spanish hospital. In: Abstracts: 7th World Congress on Pain, IASP Publications, Seattle, 1993, p. 90.

Boureau, E. and Sahmoud, T., The prevalence of acute and chronic pain in the French general medical practice. In: Abstracts: 7th World Congress on Pain, IASP Publications, Seattle, 1993, p. 90.

Brook, R.H., Quality of Care Assessment: A Comparison of Five Methods of Peer Review, DHEW Pub. no. HRA 74-3100, Department of Health, Education, and Welfare, Washington, D.C., 1973, 301 pp.

Canadian Council of Health Facilities Accreditation., Palliative Care Program Standards, Ottawa, Ontario, 12pp.

Carr, E.C.J., Postoperative pain: patients' expectations and experiences, J. Adv. Nurs., 15 (1990) 89–100.

Chang, B.C., Uman, G.C., Linn, L.S., Ware, J.E. and Kane, R.L., The effect of systematically varying components of nursing care on satisfaction in elderly ambulatory women, West. J. Nurs. Res., 6 (1984) 367–379.

Cleary, P.D. and McNeil, B.J., Patient satisfaction as an indicator of quality care, Inquiry, 25 (1988) 25–36.

Committee on Quality Assurance Standards, American Pain Society, American Pain Society quality assurance standards for relief of acute pain and cancer pain. In: M.R. Bond, J.E. Charlton and C.J. Woolf (Eds.), Proceedings of the VIth World Congress on Pain. Pain Research and Clinical Management, Vol. 4. Elsevier, Amsterdam, 1991, pp. 185–189.

Coyle, N., Thaler, H., Bookbinder, M., Brown, M., Kiss, M., Layman, M., Derby, S., Gianella, A., Foley, K. and Portenoy, R., Implementing the American Pain Society (APS) standards for cancer pain management: program development and pilot study. In: Abstracts: 7th World

Congress on Pain, IASP Publications, Seattle, 1993, p. 166.
Dauber, A., Carr, D.B. and Breslau, A. Burn survivors' pain experiences: a questionnaire-based study. In: Abstracts: 7th World Congress on Pain, IASP Publications, Seattle, 1993, p. 281.
Daut, R.L. and Cleeland, C.S., The prevalence and severity of pain in cancer, Cancer, 50 (1982) 1913–1916.
Davies, A.R. and Ware, J.E., Jr., Involving consumers in quality of care assessment, Health Aff., 7 (1988) 33–48.
Davies, A.R., Ware, J.E., Brook, R.K., Peterson, J.R. and Newhouse, J.P., Consumer acceptance of prepaid and fee-for-service care: results from a randomized trial, Health Serv. Res., 21 (1986) 429–452.
Deming, W.E., Out of Crisis, Center for Advanced Engineering Study, Massachusetts Institute of Technology, Cambridge, Mass., 1986, 201 pp.
DiMatteo, M.R., Taranta, A., Freedman, H.S. and Prince, L.M., Predicting patient satisfaction from physician's nonverbal communication skills, Med. Care, 18 (1980) 376–387.
Donabedian, A., Evaluating the quality of medical care, Millbank Q., 44 (1966) 166–171.
Donabedian, A., Explorations in Quality Assessment and Monitoring. Vol. 1: The Definition of Quality: Approaches to Its Assessment. Health Administration Press, Ann Arbor, Michigan, 1980, 163 pp.
Donabedian, A., Quality and cost: choices and responsibilities, J. Occup. Med., 32 (1990) 1167–1172.
Donovan, M. and Miaskowski, C., Striving for a standard of pain relief, Am. J. Nurs., 92 (1992) 106–107.
Donovan, M., Dillon, P. and McGuire, L. Incidence and characteristics of pain in a sample of medical-surgical inpatients, Pain, 30 (1987) 69–78.
Eddy, D.M., Variations in physician practice: the role of uncertainty, Health Aff., 19 (1984) 74–89.
Erlick, J., Morehead, M.A. and Trussell, R.E., The Quantity, Quality, and Costs of Medical and Hospital Care Secured by a Sample of Teamster Families in the New York Area, Columbia University School of Public Health and Administrative Medicine, New York, 1961, 209 pp.
Ferrell, B.R., Rhiner, M., Cohen, M.S. and Grant, M., Pain as a metaphor for illness. Part I: Impact of cancer pain on family caregivers. Oncol. Nurs. Forum, 18 (1991) 1303–1309.
Fitzpatrick, R., Surveys of patient satisfaction: I. Important general considerations, BMJ, 302 (1991) 887–889.
Galichon, B., Pages, D. and Boccard, E., Acute pain in ambulatory children. In: Abstracts: 7th World Congress on Pain, IASP Publications, Seattle, 1993, p. 145.
Hester, N.O., Jacox, A., Miaskowski, C. and Ferrell, B., Development of guidelines for the management of pain in infants, children, and adolescents undergoing operative and medical procedures, MCN, 17 (1992) 146–152.
Korsch, B.M., Gozzi, E.K. and Francis, V., Gaps in doctor-patient communication, Pediatrics, 42 (1968) 855–869.
Kosteller, J., Kane, R.L. and Olsen, D., Issues underlying prevalence of "doctor-shopping" behavior, J. Health Soc. Behav., 17 (1976) 328–339.
Kravitz, J., The relationship of attitudes to discretionary physician and dentist use by race and income. In: R. Andersen, J. Kravitz and O. Anderson (Eds.), Equity in Health Care Services, Ballinger Publishing, Cambridge, 1975, 295 pp.
LaPerriere, J.A., Sienon, L.O. and Milo, K.M., Monitoring the quality of analgesic treatment of acute and chronic cancer related pain using patient outcome measures. In: Abstracts: 7th World Congress on Pain, IASP Publications, Seattle, 1993, p. 280.
Marks, R.M. and Sachar, E.J., Undertreatment of medical inpatients with narcotic analgesics, Ann. Intern. Med., 78 (1973) 173–181.
Marquis, M.S., Davies, A.R. and Ware, J.E., Patient satisfaction and change in medical care provider: a longitudinal study, Med. Care, 21 (1983) 821–829.
McEachern, J.E., Makens, P.K., Buchanan, E.D. and Schiff, L., Quality improvement: an imperative for medical care, J. Occup. Med., 33 (1991) 364–375.
Miaskowski, C. and Donovan, M., Implementation of the American Pain Society Quality Assur-

ance Standards for Relief of Acute Pain and Cancer Pain in oncology in nursing practice, Oncol. Nurs. Forum, 19 (1992) 411–415.
Miaskowski, C., Jacox, A., Hester, N.O. and Ferrell, B., Interdisciplinary guidelines for the management of acute pain: implications for quality improvement, J. Nurs. Care Qual., 7 (1992) 1–6.
Miaskowski, C., Nichols, R., Brody, R. and Synold, T., Assessment of patient satisfaction utilizing the American Pain Society's quality assurance standards on acute and cancer-related pain, J. Pain Sympt. Manage., 9 (1994) 5–11.
Miralles, F.S., Galan, A.G, Robles, E., Ortuno, P., Crespo, J., Lopez, A.G. and Iranzo, J., The assessment of patients expectations and experiences about postoperative pain. In: Abstracts: 7th World Congress on Pain, IASP Publications, Seattle, 1993, p. 577.
Mirowsky, J. and Ross, C.E., Patient satisfaction and visiting the doctor: a self-regulating system, Soc. Sci. Med., 17 (1983) 1353–1361.
Oden, R., Acute postoperative pain: incidence, severity, and the etiology of inadequate treatment, Anesthesiology Clinics North America, 7 (1989) 1–15.
Parker, S.C. and Kroboth, F.J., Practical problems of conducting patient satisfaction surveys, J. Gen. Intern. Med., 6 (1991) 430–435.
Skadborg, M.K., Behrens, J.K., Anker-Moller, E., Ahlburg, P., Skadborg, J. and Christiansen, J.H., Quality assurance of postoperative pain treatment II. Evaluation by patient questionnaire. In: Abstracts: 7th World Congress on Pain, IASP Publications, Seattle, 1993, p. 396.
Sriwatanakul, K., Kelvie, W., Lasagna, L., Calimlim, J., Weis, O. and Mehta, G., Analysis of narcotic usage in the treatment of postoperative pain, JAMA, 250 (1983) 926–929.
Sox, H.C., Jr., Margulies, I. and Sox, C.H., Psychologically mediated effects of diagnostic tests, Ann. Intern. Med., 95 (1981) 680–685.
Stiles, W.B., Putnam, S.M., James, S.A. and Wolf, M.H., Dimensions of patients' and physicians' roles in medical screening interviews, Soc. Sci. Med., 13a (1979) 335–341.
Twycross, R. and Fairfield, S., Pain in far-advanced cancer, Pain, 2 (1982) 77–79.
U.S. News and World Report, America's best hospitals, 115 (1993) 66–74.
Vuori, H., Patient satisfaction—an attribute or indicator of the quality of care? QRB, March (1987) 106–108.
Ward, S. and Gordon, D., Application of the American Pain Society quality assurance standards, Pain, 56 (1994) 299–306.
Ware, J.E., Medical Satisfaction Surveys, 1977–1980: A Report of the Prepaid Health Research, Evaluation, and Development Project, California State Department of Health Services, Sacramento, California, 1981, 289pp.
Ware, J.E., Snyder, M.K. and Wright, W.R., Development and Validation of Scales to Measure Patient Satisfaction with Health Care Services, Vol I, Part B: Results Regarding Scales Constructed from the Patient Satisfaction Questionnaire and Measures of Other Health Perceptions, National Technical Information Service, Springfield, Va., 1976, 305 pp.
Ware, J.E., Kane, R.L. and Davies-Avery, A., Effects of differences in quality of care on patient satisfaction and other variables: an experimental simulation. In: Proceedings of the Seventeenth Annual Conference on Research in Medical Education, Association of Medical Colleges, Washington, D.C., 1978, 102 pp.

Correspondence to: Christine Miaskowski, RN, PhD, FAAN, Associate Professor, Department of Physiological Nursing, University of California, Box 0610-N611Y, San Francisco, CA 94143, USA. Tel: 415-476-9407; Fax: 415-476-8899.

Proceedings of the 7th World Congress on Pain,
Progress in Pain Research and Management, Vol. 2,
edited by G.F. Gebhart, D.L. Hammond, and T.S.
Jensen, IASP Press, Seattle, © 1994.

8

Perspectives on Management of Back Pain in Primary Care

Michael VonKorff

Center for Health Studies, Group Health Cooperative of Puget Sound, Seattle, Washington, USA

This chapter considers the promise and the problems of pain management in primary care settings. Based on a series of studies we have conducted concerning the epidemiology of common pain conditions and how they are managed in a large health care delivery system (Dworkin et al. 1992), as well as relevant studies of pain management in primary care settings carried out by other investigators, critical issues will be identified. The focus is back pain, because its care is widely acknowledged to be one of the most vexing problems in the organization and delivery of primary health care services.

PRIMARY CARE: WHERE MOST PAIN PATIENTS ARE TREATED

Primary medical care, as defined by Starfield (1992), is "the point of entry into the health care system and the locus of responsibility for organizing care for patients and for populations over time." Pain is one of the most frequent reasons for visiting a doctor. Patients seeking medical care for common pain conditions are most likely to be seen in primary care settings (Fig. 1). For example, back pain, headache, abdominal pain, chest pain, and neck pain are among the 20 most common reasons for visiting primary care physicians in the United States (American Academy of Family Physicians 1987). Primary care physicians are asked to manage large numbers of pain patients in less time and with fewer resources than are available to specialists. They are sometimes frustrated by the difficulties of caring for chronic pain patients, and are eager for new approaches to managing pain.

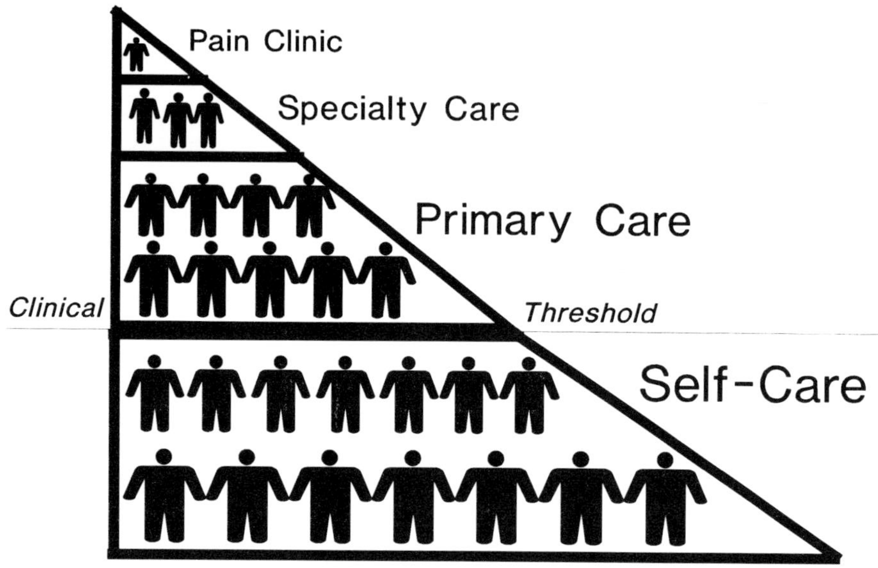

Fig. 1. Most common sites of care for back pain.

THE INTERFACE BETWEEN SELF-CARE AND SPECIALTY CARE

In any given year, about half the adult population experiences an episode of back pain (Sternbach 1986). Most persons with back pain employ self-care, while one in four seeks health care (VonKorff et al. 1988). Among those seeking medical care, about 70% of the physician visits for back pain in the United States take place in primary care settings (Cypress 1983). Primary care is the interface between self-care and specialty care. An important role of primary care is to support and enhance self-care for the large majority of back pain patients not requiring specialty services.

A SETTING FOR COST-EFFECTIVE MANAGEMENT

For many reasons, primary care is a critical setting for ensuring cost-effective management of back pain (see Starfield 1992).

1. Primary care is *population-based.* It is the only part of the health care system that aspires to serve the entire population and their most common health care needs.

2. Primary care is the *setting of first contact.* It is an accessible setting where early intervention is possible.
3. It provides *continuity of care* and is *comprehensive.* The physician knows the patient, assumes continuing responsibility for the patient and, in addition to diagnosing and treating disease, attends to psychological and social factors in illness.
4. Primary care physicians are the *gate-keepers to specialty care.* They triage patients requiring specialized services, while controlling access to costly or potentially harmful specialty services not warranted by medical need.
5. Primary care aspires to be *cost-effective.* Primary care seeks to provide essential services to the many persons seeking care at a cost that society can afford.

At the same time, primary care of back pain is beset with problems including:

1. *Stigmatization of chronic pain patients.* Primary care physicians often stereotype chronic pain patients as difficult, dependent, and poorly motivated (Klein et al. 1982; Cherkin et al. 1988).
2. *Inadequate pain control.* General practitioners have been criticized for suboptimal use of pain medications and for failure to use nonpharmacologic methods of pain control (Portenoy 1989; Melzack 1990; Turk, Holzman and Kerns 1986).
3. *Overmedicalization of pain management.* Primary care physicians may sanction disability, provide a gateway to misuse of pain medications, and discourage self-care by implicitly promising a medical solution to chronic pain (Fordyce 1976; Osterweis et al. 1987).
4. *Discordant expectations of doctors and patients.* Many patients expect their doctor to be able to explain the cause of the back pain, cure back pain, and restore functioning. Primary care physicians tend to view their role as providing palliative care until back pain resolves on its own (Cherkin et al. 1988). Given these discordant expectations, it is not surprising that the care of back pain is regarded by both patients and physicians as fraught with difficulties, frustrations, and misunderstandings.

With these perspectives as background, this chapter is organized around three observations about back pain in primary care that challenge us to reexamine and rethink assumptions about how back pain should be managed in primary care.

1. The course of back pain in primary care is typically recurrent or chronic, *not* acute.

2. Primary care of back pain patients often does not follow behavioral guidelines for preservation of function or fostering self-care of patients with chronic or recurrent pain.

3. Evidence that management of back pain patients in primary care can either cause chronic disability or prevent it through early intervention is, as yet, inconclusive.

I will review research supporting these three assertions, and consider implications of this research for patient care.

BACK PAIN IN PRIMARY CARE IS TYPICALLY CHRONIC-RECURRENT, NOT ACUTE

It is often assumed that back pain usually runs an acute course. This statement is typical: "Of those seeking care . . . almost half improve in a week and almost 90% are better within a month, regardless of treatment" (Kelsey 1982). Only a small percentage, perhaps 10–15% of back pain patients in primary care, are expected to develop chronic pain that persists beyond four to six weeks (Deyo 1993). Primary care physicians routinely tell patients that their back pain will go away within a few weeks (Cherkin et al. 1991). The assumption that in primary care back pain typically runs an acute course is the basis for emphasizing acute palliative care.

An important study recently challenged the belief that back pain is typically an acute condition. Philips and Grant (1991) reported that the number of acute onset back pain patients still reporting pain at six months was considerably higher than expected (40%) and concluded that, "If expectations for improvement provided by a general practitioner are based on [only 10–15% reporting pain at six weeks], many individuals will feel frustrated and concerned." Patients led to expect rapid recovery may be unprepared to adapt to an ongoing back pain problem.

We recently completed a longitudinal study of back pain patients in primary care that assessed long-term course (VonKorff et al. 1992; VonKorff et al. 1993). Over one year, we enrolled 1213 back pain patients, interviewing them about one month after their index visit. We then reinterviewed more than 85% of these patients at one- and two-year follow-ups. At the one-year follow-up, one-third (34%) reported chronic back pain, defined as pain present on at least half the days in the prior six months, while twenty-one percent reported back pain every day for six months. When results from the one- and two-year follow-ups were combined, 44% were experiencing chronic back

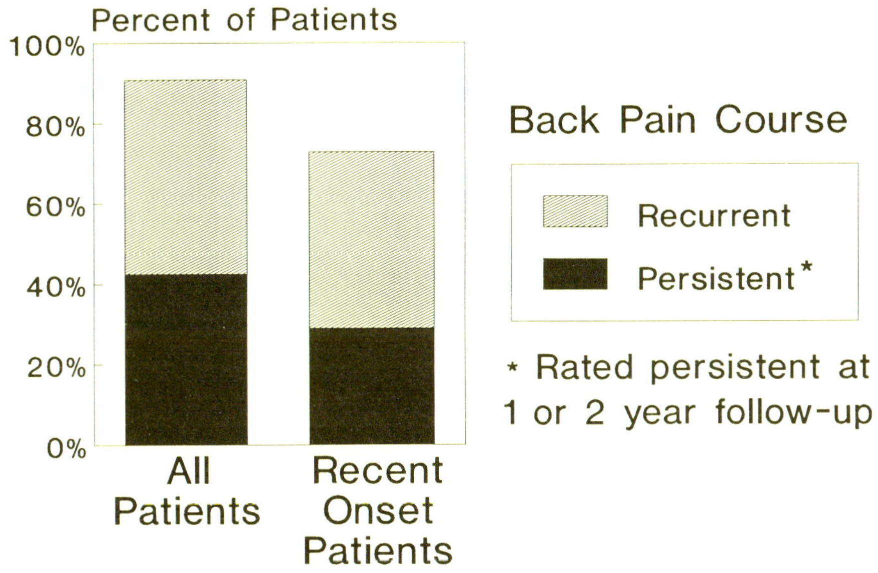

Fig. 2. Assessment of the course of back pain over one or two years by patients receiving primary care.

pain at either the one- year or the two-year follow-up.

At each follow-up, we had patients assess their back pain as a one-time problem, a recurrent problem, or a persistent problem (Fig. 2). On at least one of the follow-up interviews, 43% of the patients described their back pain as a persistent problem. When this analysis was restricted to cases who reported recent first onset of back pain at baseline (that is, the first episode of back pain had occurred within six months of the baseline interview), 29% described their back pain as a persistent problem at one or both of the follow-up interviews. Among those not reporting persistent back pain, the large majority characterized their back pain as a recurrent problem.

Confusion about whether back pain is typically an acute or a chronic condition in primary care is not surprising. Over time, the same back pain patient may experience recurrent episodes of back pain, periods when back pain has entered a chronic phase, and acute, severe flare-ups that usually last less than a week. To date, only limited epidemiologic research has focused on these phases in the natural history of back pain or on factors controlling transitions from one phase to the next.

Recurrent back pain is typical in primary care, while chronic phases of back pain are common. Given its natural history, back pain management in primary care should be appropriate for patients with chronic-recurrent pain. Does primary care of back pain patients conform to behavioral principles for preserving function, fostering successful adaptation to chronic pain, and preventing over-reliance on medical care?

MANAGEMENT CONSIDERATIONS

BEHAVIORAL GUIDELINES FOR PRESERVING FUNCTION

Behavioral principles for preservation of function and preventing maladaptive pain behaviors among chronic pain patients have been articulated by Fordyce (1976), Turk (Turk et al. 1983, 1986), and others. These principles suggest that routine medical care for back pain patients should:

1. *Emphasize patient education* to provide patients information and skills necessary for successful adaptation to chronic pain;
2. *Limit expectations of medical cure*, so that patients adopt an active rather than a passive stance toward their illness;
3. *Prescribe bed rest and pain medications on a time-limited rather than a pain contingent basis;* and
4. *Encourage patients to progressively increase their activity levels.*

We have assessed whether management of back pain patients in primary care follows these general guidelines in the health maintenance organization where our longitudinal study of back pain patients was conducted.

INADEQUATE PATIENT EDUCATION

We asked patients to rate the quality of medical care and patient education for back pain provided by their primary care physician. Seventy-five percent of the study patients gave favorable ratings on a scale measuring global satisfaction with medical care. Typical items on this scale included: The doctor was very thorough in the physical examination of your back; You were treated like your back pain was an important problem and not all in your head. In contrast, less than half of the patients (49%) gave favorable ratings on items assessing the quality of patient education about back pain. Typical items on this scale included: Your visit to the doctor helped you feel you could control your back pain; After your visit to the doctor, you fully understood how to take care of your back problem. Similar results indicating inadequate patient education about back pain have been reported by Deyo (Deyo and Diehl 1986) and Cherkin (Cherkin and MacCornack 1989).

PALLIATIVE INTERVENTIONS GUIDED BY DYSFUNCTION, NOT PAIN

In primary care, patients are usually instructed to take medications as needed for pain. They may be advised to rest without clear instructions for when to resume activities, or to let pain guide resumption of activities. Fordyce (1976) has hypothesized that pain contingent palliative care reinforces activity limitations and other maladaptive pain behaviors. We have examined how the severity of chronic pain dysfunction influences prescribing of acute palliative interventions, often on a pain-contingent basis. Dysfunctional chronic pain, as empirically defined by Turk and Rudy (1987, 1988), refers to a constellation of severe pain, interference with activities, suffering, and maladaptive pain behaviors. Patients with chronic pain dysfunction may be most vulnerable to deleterious effects of pain-contingent acute care.

To examine differences in management of back pain patients across the severity spectrum, we developed a brief method to assess chronic pain dysfunction suitable for use in primary care practice (VonKorff et al. 1992). Severity of chronic pain dysfunction was graded using seven questions: three pain intensity ratings, three interference ratings, and an item asking about activity limitation days due to pain. Persons at Chronic Pain Grade I have mild back pain while those at Grade II report high pain intensity but low levels of interference with activities. Chronic Pain Grades III and IV include persons with moderate to severe pain dysfunction. Dysfunctional pain patients at Grades III and IV are more likely to be depressed, to be chronic users of medical care, and to have less favorable long-term outcomes than are patients at Grades I and II.

At baseline, about one-third of the back pain patients in our research reported mild back pain, a slightly smaller proportion reported high-intensity back pain without dysfunction, while somewhat more than one-third were graded as having moderate to severe pain dysfunction (VonKorff et al. 1993). The following results indicate how acute palliative care of back pain patients differed by grade of dysfunctional chronic pain.

The likelihood of back pain patients receiving opioid medications increased with the severity of pain dysfunction. Grade III and IV patients limiting their activities were much more likely to be managed with opioids than were Grade II patients with intense back pain but without significant dysfunction (Fig. 3). A similar pattern was observed for sedative-hypnotic medications and for polypharmacy. In multivariate analyses, pain-related disability

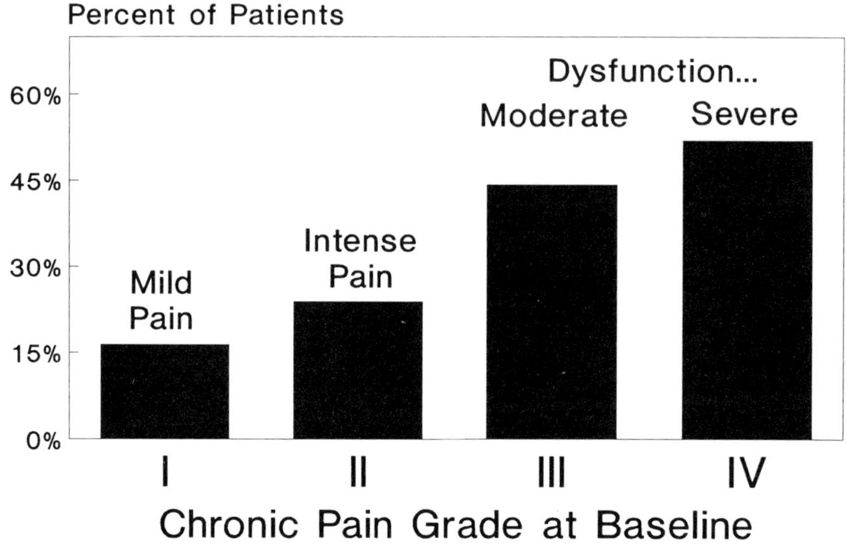

Fig. 3. Percentage of patients receiving primary care for different grades of back pain who were managed with opioid medications (n = 1185).

was a stronger predictor of whether a patient was managed with opioids, sedative-hypnotics, and polypharmacy than were pain intensity ratings, chronicity, or the physician's diagnosis.

Bed rest and extended bed rest recommendations were also markedly increased among dysfunctional patients. Physicians were most likely to recommend bed rest to the dysfunctional patients at Grades III and IV (Fig. 4). In multivariate analyses, bed rest recommendations were more strongly associated with pain-related disability than with pain intensity, chronicity or the physician's diagnosis.

In contrast, physicians were not more likely to tell dysfunctional back pain patients to resume activities even if they caused some pain. Only one in five dysfunctional back pain patients reported being advised to resume activities even if they caused some pain.

DOES PAIN-CONTINGENT MANAGEMENT CAUSE CHRONIC DISABILITY?

In summary, patients often viewed education as inadequate. Pain medications and bed rest were most likely to be prescribed to dysfunctional patients

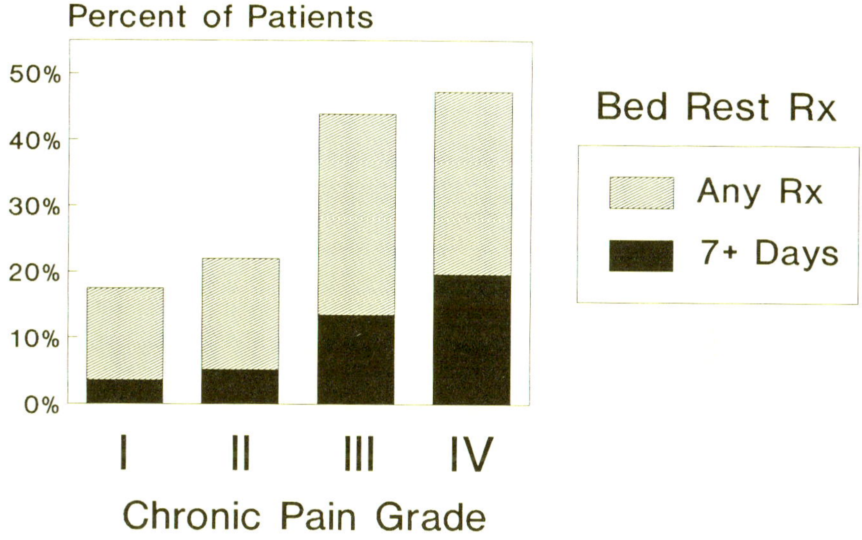

Fig. 4. Percentage of patients receiving primary care for different grades of back pain for whom bed rest was recommended (n = 1180).

who may be the most vulnerable to reinforcement of maladaptive pain behaviors. But, few dysfunctional patients received advice to resume activities even if they caused some pain. These results suggest that management of back pain patients in primary care often does not conform to behavioral guidelines for management of patients with chronic or recurrent pain. This raises the question: Does pain contingent management of back pain in primary care cause chronic disability? If it does, then early intervention according to behavioral principles might be expected to prevent chronic disability.

Fordyce conducted the first study relevant to this question (Fordyce et al. 1986). He randomized back pain patients in primary care to either a pain contingent or a behavioral pain management program. The primary care physician implemented both programs. In the pain contingent management program, patients were advised to use pain medications as needed for pain and were permitted to refill their prescriptions. They also were told to let pain guide resumption of activities. In the behavioral care program, patients were prescribed time-scheduled pain medication without provision for refill. Time-scheduled increases in activity levels were recommended. There were no differences in outcomes between the two groups at six weeks. However, at a

9- to 12-month follow-up, patients assigned to the behavioral care program reported significantly lower levels of impairment on a scale assessing such activities as lifting and walking. Philips conducted a randomized trial to assess a graded activation program for acute onset back pain patients (Philips et al. 1991). Patients were randomly assigned to either counseling that pain should guide return to function or to a program of graded activation. There were no differences in pain status or in frequency of exercise at three- or six-month follow-up. While pain outcomes were not changed, a difference in coping strategies between the two groups was observed. Patients assigned to the graded activation program more often reported that they exercised even when they were experiencing back pain. But, to reiterate, this difference was not accompanied by reported differences in the frequency of exercise.

Deyo carried out a third experimental study (Deyo et al. 1986). Back pain patients in primary care were randomly assigned to a prescription of either two days or seven days of bed rest. Patients prescribed seven days of bed rest reported significantly more days off work at the three-week follow-up. Interestingly, the large majority of patients prescribed seven days of bed rest did not fully comply with the recommendation. At the three-month follow-up, there were no differences in days off work or other measures of disability between the two groups. The initial difference in days off work, resulting directly from the physician's orders, did not extend to longer term effects in days off work or to more generalized effects on disability status.

In our own observational research, we obtained results similar in some respects to those reported by Deyo. We classified 44 primary care physicians as having a practice style characterized by a low, medium, or high frequency of prescribing acute palliative interventions including opioid medications, sedative-hypnotic medications, polypharmacy, and bed rest. Patients treated by physicians with a low, medium, and high frequency of prescribing acute palliative interventions did not differ in pain intensity, chronicity, diagnosis, or in other patient characteristics.

At the one-month assessment, patients treated by physicians who infrequently prescribed acute palliative care were less likely to be dysfunctional (Fig. 5). This difference was highly significant after controlling for pain intensity, chronicity, diagnosis, and other patient variables. However, despite the initial differences in disability across the practice style groups, the differences in disability did not persist at long-term follow-up. The patient groups that were initially more dysfunctional, treated by physicians who tended to rely more heavily on acute palliative care, did not show higher levels of disability at long-term follow-up. These results are not consistent with naturally occurring differences in pain management practice style having a strong effect on

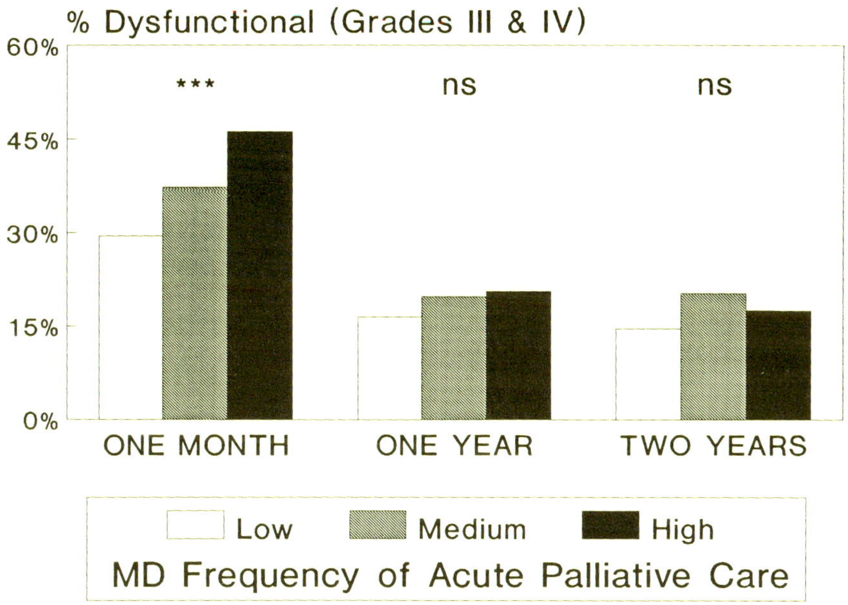

Fig. 5. Percentage with moderate to severe pain dysfunction among patients treated by a physician with a low, medium, or high frequency of prescribing bed rest and pain medications.

the long-term risks of chronic disability.

However, patients cared for by frequent prescribers of pain medications and bed rest did have substantially higher costs of back pain care over the following year. The total costs of back care were 80% higher among patients treated by physicians who frequently prescribed acute palliative care relative to the patients of infrequent prescribers. The mean total costs of care were: $426 for patients treated by physicians who infrequently prescribed acute palliative interventions, $506 for the intermediate physicians, and $767 for physicians who most frequently prescribed acute palliative interventions (F = 4.9, df = 2,879, *P* = .008). Cost differences were primarily due to inpatient and specialty care. Cost differences due to primary care visits, pain medications, and radiographic studies were negligible. The higher cost physicians, those who frequently prescribed bed rest and pain medications, also received less favorable ratings from their patients on items assessing the quality of patient education about back pain.

A possible interpretation of these results is that the physicians who relied more heavily on acute palliative care, and who provided less adequate patient education about back pain and self-care, may have fostered greater reliance on medical care, resulting in increased costs of back pain care. These results suggest the possibility that pain-contingent palliative care may be guided by the patient's initial severity of chronic pain dysfunction and may subsequently induce increased use of health care services (and presumably greater dependence on health care providers), but without necessarily causing chronic disability. Future research will need to differentiate the effects of different strategies of caring for back pain patients on pain-related disability and on health care-related pain behaviors such as doctor visits and use of pain medications. It also remains to be determined if more substantial cognitive-behavioral interventions delivered early to dysfunctional back pain patients in primary care could improve long-term patient outcomes.

Taken together, the results of these four studies suggest that pain-contingent, acute palliative care among back pain patients in primary care may reduce short-term activity levels, increase use of services and costs of care long-term, and influence patient pain coping strategies. I make these statements cautiously because results of existing studies have been inconsistent and have not been replicated. At present, evidence that differences in the management of back pain patients in primary care can either cause or prevent long-term disability is inconclusive.

CLINICAL AND RESEARCH EFFORTS NEEDED

The research I have reviewed raises more questions than answers. Clinical and research efforts to understand and to improve pain management in primary care are clearly needed. Research on methods of preventing disability and increasing the cost-effectiveness of care would be of particular significance. Unfortunately, many pain patients, but few pain clinicians or researchers, are found in primary care. On the clinical side, one need is for primary care clinics to provide consultation-liaison services on pain management that assist physicians in managing selected chronic pain patients while providing continuing medical education in pain management in the practice setting of the primary care physician.

Primary care research is urgently needed to produce more reliable knowledge about how to reduce the suffering, disability and health care costs of pain patients in primary care. The increasing emphasis on primary care in the United States and elsewhere makes this an opportune time for new efforts to address critical issues of how to manage pain patients. Increased clinical and research efforts by members of the IASP in this important area of patient care would be a welcome development.

ACKNOWLEDGMENTS

This work was supported by research grants from the National Institute of Dental Research (P01 DE08773), Samuel F. Dworkin, Principal Investigator; and from the Agency for Health Care Policy and Research (R01 HS06168).

REFERENCES

American Academy of Family Physicians, Facts About: Family Practice, American Academy of Family Physicians, Kansas City, Mo., 1987.

Cherkin, D.C. and MacCornack, F.A., Patient evaluations of low back pain care from family physicians and from chiropractors, West. J. Med., 150 (1989) 351–355.

Cherkin, D.C., MacCornack, F.A. and Berg, A.O., The management of low back pain: a comparison of the beliefs and behaviors of family physicians and chiropractors, West. J. Med., 149 (1988) 475–480.

Cherkin, D., Deyo, R.A., Berg, A.O., Bergman, J.J. and Lishner, D.M., Evaluation of a physician education intervention to improve primary care for low-back pain I: impact on physicians, Spine, 16 (1991) 1168–1172.

Cypress, B.K., Characteristics of physician visits for back symptoms: a national perspective, Am. J. Public Health, 73 (1983) 389–395.

Deyo, R.A., Back pain revisited: newer thinking on diagnosis and therapy, Consultant, 33 (1993) 88–100.

Deyo, R.A. and Diehl, A.K., Patient satisfaction with medical care for low-back pain, Spine, 11 (1986) 28–30.

Deyo, R.A., Diehl, A.K. and Rosenthal, M., How many days of bed rest for acute low back pain? A randomized clinical trial, N. Engl. J. Med., 315 (1986) 1064–1070.

Dworkin, S.F., VonKorff, M. and LeResche, L., Epidemiologic studies of chronic pain: a dynamic-ecologic perspective, Annals Behavioral Medicine, 14 (1992) 3–11.

Fordyce, W.E., Behavioral Methods in Chronic Pain and Illness, C. V. Mosby, St. Louis, 1976.

Fordyce, W.E., Brockway, J.A., Bergman, J.A. and Spengler, D., Acute back pain: a control group comparison of behavioral vs. traditional management methods, J. Behav. Med., 5 (1986) 127–140.

Kelsey, J.L., Epidemiology of Musculoskeletal Disorders, Oxford University Press, New York, 1982.

Klein, D., Najman, J., Kohrman, A.F. and Munro, C., Patient characteristics that elicit negative responses from family physicians, J. Family Practice, 5 (1982) 881–888.

Melzack, R., The tragedy of needless pain, Sci. Am., 262 (1990) 27–33.

Osterweis, M., Kleinman, A. and Mechanic, D., Pain and disability: clinical, behavioral and public policy perspectives, National Academy Press, Washington D.C., 1987.

Philips, H.C. and Grant, L., The evolution of chronic back pain problems: a longitudinal study, Behav. Res. Ther., 29 (1991) 435–441.

Philips, H.C., Grant, L. and Berkowitz, J., The prevention of chronic pain and disability: a preliminary analysis, Behav. Res. Ther., 29 (1991) 443–450.

Portenoy, R.K., Opioid therapy in the management of chronic back pain. In: C.D. Tollison (Ed.), Interdisciplinary rehabilitation of low back pain, Williams and Wilkins, Baltimore, 1989, pp

137–157.
Starfield, B., Primary Care: Concept, Evaluation, Policy. Oxford University Press, New York, 1992.
Sternbach, R.A., Survey of pain in the United States: the Nuprin Pain Report, Clin. J. Pain, 2 (1986) 49–53.
Turk, D.C. and Rudy, T.E., Towards a comprehensive assessment of chronic pain patients: a multiaxial approach, Behav. Res. Ther., 25 (1987) 237–249.
Turk, D.C. and Rudy, T.E., Toward an empirically derived taxonomy of chronic pain patients: integration of psychological assessment data, J. Consult. Clin. Psychol., 56 (1988) 1–6.
Turk, D.C., Meichenbaum, D. and Genest, M., Pain and Behavioral Medicine: A Cognitive Behavioral Perspective, Guilford Press, New York, 1983.
Turk, D.C., Holzman, A.D. and Kerns, R.D., Chronic pain. In: K.A. Holroyd and T.L. Creer (Eds.), Self Management of Chronic Disease: Handbook of Clinical Interventions and Research, Academic Press, Orlando, 1986, pp. 441–471.
VonKorff, M., Dworkin, S.F., LeResche, L. and Kluger, A., An epidemiologic comparison of pain complaints, Pain, 32 (1988) 173–183.
VonKorff, M., Ormel, J., Keefe, F. and Dworkin, S.F., Grading the severity of chronic pain, Pain, 50 (1992) 133–149.
VonKorff, M., Deyo, R.A., Cherkin, D. and Barlow, W., Back pain in primary care: outcomes at one year, Spine, 18 (1993) 855–862.

Correspondence to: Michael VonKorff ScD, Center for Health Studies, Group Health Cooperative of Puget Sound, 1730 Minor Avenue, Suite 1600, Seattle, WA 98101, USA. Tel: 206-287-2874; Fax: 206-287-2871.

Part III

Psychologic Factors Related to Chronic Pain

Proceedings of the 7th World Congress on Pain,
Progress in Pain Research and Management, Vol. 2,
edited by G.F. Gebhart, D.L. Hammond, and T.S.
Jensen, IASP Press, Seattle, © 1994.

9

Basic Issues in the Psychobiology of Pain

Herta Flor[a] and Niels Birbaumer[b,c]

[a]*Department of Psychology, Humboldt-University, Berlin, Germany;* [b]*Institute for Medical Psychology and Behavioral Neurobiology, University of Tübingen, Germany; and* [c]*Department of General Psychology, University of Padova, Italy*

INTRODUCTION

Several animal studies have demonstrated that peripheral lesions such as the laceration of a nerve, the amputation of a digit, or the deafferentation of a limb, lead to extensive reorganization of the areas in the somatosensory cortex that represent the respective body region (Jenkins et al. 1990b; Pons et al. 1991). For example, the amputation of the third digit in an owl monkey led to an invasion by the adjacent digits of the space that represented the third digit in the somatosensory cortex. Stimulation of digits adjacent to the amputation site elicited activity in the area formerly occupied by the amputated digit (Merzenich et al. 1984).

These studies point toward an astonishing plasticity of the primary sensory areas of the adult cortex, which previously was thought to be firmly wired and unmodifiable after an early developmental stage (Hubel and Wiesel 1970). In addition to physical variables, behavioral changes such as operant learning also continuously influence the structure of cortical representation zones. For example, Jenkins et al. (1990a) trained a monkey to use only the three middle digits of one hand to reach for food that was presented on a rotating disk. This learning process led to an expansion of the region in the somatosensory cortex that represents the digits involved in the training. This finding implies that the often used distinction of somatogenic and psychogenic processes in general and the differentiation of psychogenic and somatogenic pain syndromes in particular is irrelevant. Behavioral changes affect physiological processes and physiological processes are routinely modified by environmental influences and learning.

Kandel (1991, pp. 1027–1028) succinctly states: "There is a tendency in medicine and psychiatry to think that biological and social determinants of behavior act on separate levels of the mind... this distinction is unwarranted. Everyday events—sensory stimulation, deprivation, and learning—can cause an effective disruption of synaptic connections under some circumstances and reactivation of connections under others. It is therefore incorrect to imply that certain diseases (organic diseases) affect mentation by producing biological changes in the brain, whereas other diseases (functional diseases) do not." He proposes to give up the biological/not biological distinction and to ask instead: "To what degree is a biological process determined by genetic and developmental factors, to what degree is it determined by a toxic or infectious agent and to what degree is it environmentally or socially determined?"

The main task of the psychobiological approach to chronic pain is thus to identify the psychological—specifically, the learning processes—that influence pain and to examine their physiological and neurochemical basis and the brain mechanisms underlying their action. This chapter will focus on operant and respondent learning mechanisms (for a review of the role of observational learning see Craig 1987).

INSTRUMENTAL (OPERANT) CONDITIONING OF CHRONIC PAIN

Fordyce (1976) was the first to propose the important role of operant learning in chronic pain. His assumption was that once the acute pain phase is over pain behaviors, that is, observable expressions of pain, may be maintained by environmental contingencies. Linton et al. (1985) further extended this operant view to the development of passive behaviors. Recent experimental evidence demonstrates that not only pain behaviors, but also the subjective experience of pain as well as physiological correlates of pain, are subject to operant learning mechanisms. For example, in an experiment in our laboratory we compared patients whose spouses frequently positively reinforced pain behaviors (solicitous spouses) to patients whose spouses ignored or punished their partners' pain behaviors (nonsolicitous spouses) (Flor, Breitenstein, et al., in press). The patients participated in a cold pressor test (CPT) while their spouses were either present or absent. Patients with nonreinforcing, nonsolicitous spouses indicated pain thresholds that were comparable to those of patients with reinforcing, solicitous spouses when they were alone during the CPT. However, when the spouses were present the group with a reinforcing

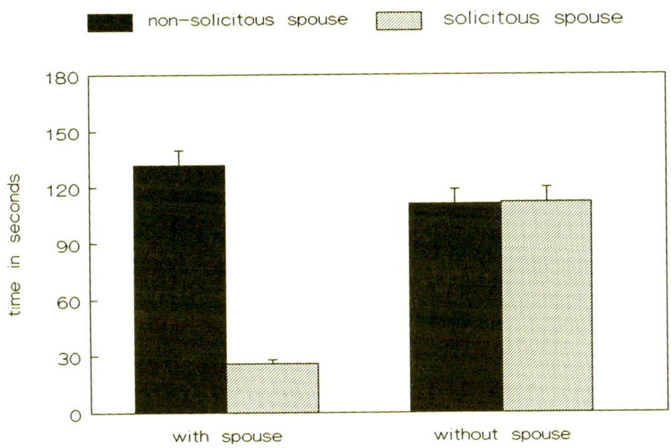

Fig. 1. Pain thresholds determined in the cold pressor test with or without the spouse present. Spouse solicitousness was assessed by the West Haven–Yale Multidimensional Pain Inventory

spouse had significantly lower pain thresholds (i.e., indicated pain much sooner) compared to the group with a nonreinforcing spouse (Fig. 1).

The patients with solicitous spouses thus reported the identical stimulus as much more painful when the spouse observed them. Lousberg et al. (1992) reported similar data for chronic pain patients in a treadmill test; patients with solicitous spouses showed elevated pain levels compared to patients with nonsolicitous spouses.

Not only subjective pain reports or observable pain behaviors, but also physiological correlates of pain, are subject to operant learning. Miltner et al. (1988) reported that the N150/P260 component of the evoked cortical potential, which is a good correlate of subjectively experienced pain (Bromm 1984), is modifiable by operant learning. The increase or decrease of this component was systematically reinforced by a biofeedback paradigm; subjects were rewarded for the correct increase or decrease of the brain response. This learned change in amplitude of the pain-related potential was highly significant and was accompanied by a change in pain perception. Subjects who learned to decrease the N150-P260 amplitude experienced less pain, while subjects who learned to increase this amplitude experienced more pain. Thus, operant learning influences all levels of the pain experience and may establish powerful memories for pain-related responses.

PAVLOVIAN (RESPONDENT) CONDITIONING OF CHRONIC PAIN

Linton et al. (1985) proposed a respondent or Pavlovian conditioning model of chronic pain. They assumed that pain as an unconditioned stimulus may lead to numerous physiological reactions that will then be conditioned to all stimuli that are present along with the painful stimulation. If these learned associations occur often and with great intensity, pain may develop that is now maintained by the respondent learning process. This learned pain response is no longer related to the initial cause of the acute pain, although it may be localized at the same site and may have comparable qualities.

We first became aware of this possibility when we examined the peripheral psychophysiological characteristics of chronic back pain (CBP) patients. In a laboratory situation, the patients were asked to simply remember and report stressful or painful episodes they had previously experienced. A general stressor (mental arithmetic) and a neutral situation (recital of the alphabet) were used as control conditions. Only the *personally relevant* stress and pain conditions elicited marked increases in muscle tension at the site of pain, not the control conditions (Flor et al. 1985). Muscles distal to the site of pain, heart rate, or skin conductance were not differentially affected by the presence of pain (Fig. 2).

This site-specificity as well as the specificity of the response to the muscular system was confirmed in a second and a third study that included an additional group of temporomandibular pain and dysfunction patients (TMPD) and used imagery of stressful life events (Flor et al. 1991, 1992). Whereas the TMPD patients displayed the maximum response in the masseter muscles, the CBP patients responded most with the lumbar muscles, and the healthy controls showed their maximum response in the cardiovascular system. Similar results have been reported by Arntz et al. (1991).

In addition, a slower return to baseline after the termination of the stressor was observed at the site of pain in the pain patient groups. This result also has been replicated by Moulton and Spence (1991), who examined musicians with upper limb pain. This extended maintenance of high levels of muscle tension is pain-inducing (Christensen et al. 1986a,b). Dickson-Parnell and Zeichner (1988) also observed muscular hyperreactivity in patients with pain-related premenstrual syndrome.

The increased muscle tension can, if it persists over sufficient time, cause pain via ischemia, hypoxia, and an increase in receptor sensitivity. These muscular reactivities are most likely classically conditioned because they are evoked by personally relevant pain and stress situations but not by general (unconditioned) stressors (Flor et al. 1990).

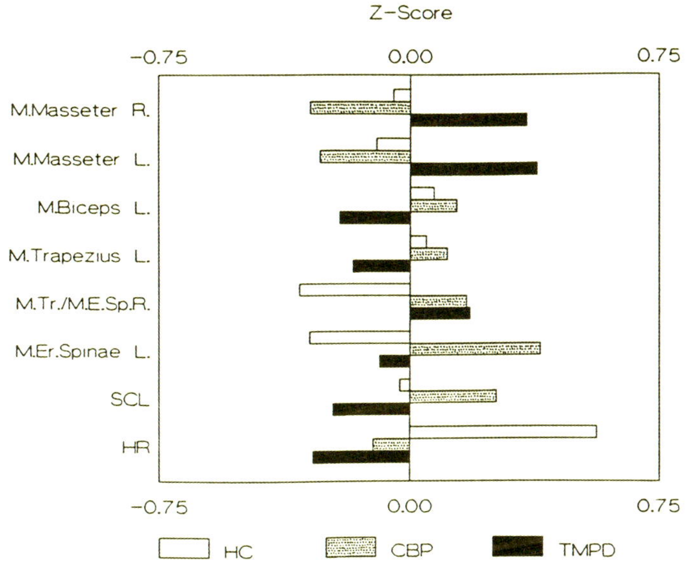

Fig. 2. Reactivity to the imagery of a personally relevant stressor of various muscle groups (m. masseter right and left; m. biceps left; m. trapezius left; m. trapezius or m. erector spinae right; m. erector spinae left), skin conductance level (SCL), and heart rate (HR) in a group of healthy controls (HC), a group of back pain patients (CBP), and a group of temporomandibular pain and dysfunction patients (TMPD). The reactivity was converted to standardized z-scores to achieve comparable values for the various physiological measures.

We have recently begun to test the conditioning of pain behavior hypothesis in healthy subjects. We subjected students to moderately aversive electric shock, at the same time using simple tones or slides of different emotional valence as neutral (conditioned) stimuli. Intracutaneous shock to the finger leads to an increase in muscle tension in the flexor communis digitorum muscle. After several pairings of the shock and the tone, the tone itself elicits a marked muscular response. Even more effective are conditioned stimuli that are associated with genetically "prewired" negative emotions such as an angry face. These signals of impending pain may themselves acquire the ability to elicit pain-inducing responses. We found that students who frequently complain about neck and shoulder pain acquire these conditioned muscular responses faster and that these responses are more resistant to extinction (Flor and Birbaumer 1994). Thus, many stimuli that were once associated with pain (such as certain body positions, movements, emotions, or external situations) may gain a pain-inducing function through respondent conditioning.

CLASSICAL CONDITIONING OF NEUROCHEMICAL MECHANISMS RELATED TO PAIN

Learning mechanisms are not limited to muscular reflexes. The activation of pain-inhibiting and pain-inducing transmitter systems (e.g., of the endogenous opioid system) is also subject to conditioning. For example, in animal research the phenomenon of stress-induced analgesia (SIA), which is partially opioid-mediated, has been described extensively (Amit and Galina 1986). If rats are exposed to shock they show an increase in pain threshold, usually measured by the tail-flick response. Certain forms of this SIA are reversible with naloxone. Stress analgesia is also subject to Pavlovian conditioning (e.g., Maier 1989). Wiertelak et al. (1992a,b) recently showed that there is also a conditioned anti-analgesia; safety signals (e.g., a light always given after the shock) effectively abolish conditioned stress analgesia involving the release of cholecystokinin. Maier et al. (1992) also reported the existence of conditioned hyperalgesia. Lithium chloride induces feelings of sickness and nausea that are accompanied by heightened pain sensitivity. If this substance is paired with saccharin, saccharin alone can also induce this now learned hyperalgesia. Maier, Watkins, and their colleagues are currently studying the brain circuits as well as the transmitters responsible for these learned pain modulatory effects (Watkins et al. 1992).

In humans, Willer and his colleagues (1981) have shown the existence of opioid-mediated stress analgesia by using a nociceptive reflex as a dependent variable. We recently began a study to show that stress analgesia also can be classically conditioned in humans; in a second study we showed that it is opioid-mediated. Students were exposed to noise plus mental arithmetic stress for five days (the UCS), which was paired with green light as the CS in the conditioning groups. On the seventh day we tested whether pain thresholds and pain tolerance had changed. The students who had participated in the conditioning sessions responded with a marked increase in pain threshold and tolerance on day seven to the green light alone (CS+). The control group, which did not receive a green light on the test day, did not change its pain perception, nor did a second control group that had only received the stress trials and was now exposed to the green light (Flor et al., unpublished data).

In a second experiment we used a differential conditioning design; the tick tock of a clock was always followed by shock (CS+), whereas a beeping noise was never followed by shock (CS–). On two test days either naloxone or placebo was given in the presence of either the CS+ or the CS–. Naloxone clearly reversed the conditioned stress analgesia whereas placebo did not affect it (Flor et al., unpublished data; see Fig. 3).

Thus, learning modifies not only autonomic and muscular but also neurochemical pain-related processes.

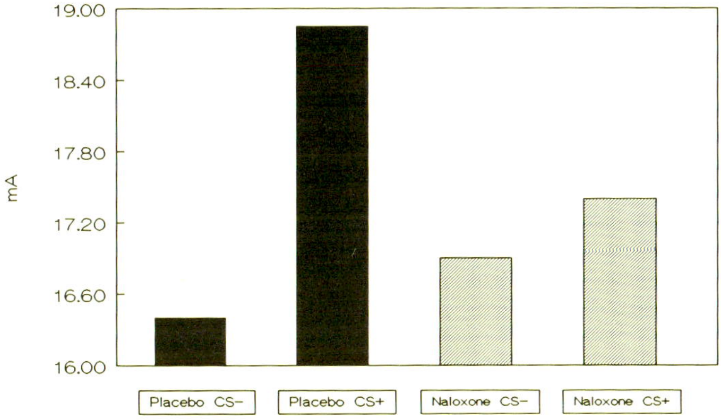

Fig. 3. Conditioned stress analgesia: pain tolerance to conditioned stimuli (CS+) and control stimuli (CS–) during test sessions for the placebo and Naloxone group. Naloxone eliminates the conditioned stress analgesia.

PAIN-EVOKED BRAIN RESPONSES AND CORTICAL PLASTICITY

The described learning processes not only affect the respective physiological and neurochemical processes but also have profound effects on the brain in the form of pain memories. Modern theories of memory and learning differentiate declarative or explicit from nondeclarative or implicit memory systems (Squire 1987). Operant and respondent learning processes form both explicit and especially implicit memories that the person is not aware of but that have important influences on perception and motor action. Chronic pain patients' memories differ from those of persons unaffected by pain and these memories influence their pain perception and pain behaviors (Erskine et al. 1990). For example, we found that pain patients remember more negative or unpleasant events from their lives and fewer positive or pleasant events irrespective of their current pain state (Flor et al. 1993b).

Moreover, previous experience with pain seems to sensitize chronic pain patients to new pains. Using intracutaneous electric shock we could show that chronic back pain patients have lower perception and pain thresholds as well as lower tolerance levels than do healthy controls or patients with episodic pain (Flor et al. 1993b).

The cortical mechanisms of these pain memories are currently being investigated. We believe that conditioning leads to the formation of both local and global (Hebbian) neural cell assemblies that underlie these memories.

Local cell assemblies in the somatosensory cortex may expand through pain-related learning and damage their receptive field site. Global cell assemblies involve thalamo-cortical and cortico-limbic as well as cortico-cortical associations, which are newly established or modified during learning. Melzack (1991) has described comparable changes as the neuromatrix that might underlie phantom limb pain. Surface-negative slow cortical potentials develop during conditioning and prime cortical areas involved in response execution lower their firing thresholds and thus form the basis of these associative processes (Birbaumer et al. 1990). Even long after conditioning has ended, these cell assemblies may easily be activated (ignited) by conditioned stimuli and give rise to conditioned pain responses.

Results from nonlinear analyses of the spontaneous EEG substantiate the assumption of more activated cell assemblies during retrieval of pain memories in chronic pain patients. The memory of a painful event elicits a much higher dimensional complexity of the EEG in chronic pain patients than in healthy controls (Lutzenberger et al. 1993). We have previously suggested that the dimensional complexity measure of the spontaneous EEG might be an indicator of the number of simultaneously active cell assemblies (Lutzenberger et al. 1992). Evoked potential studies showed that although chronic back pain patients receive much lower levels of stimulation, they produce comparably high amplitudes of the evoked response (similar to healthy controls), indicating a central sensitization for noxious stimulation (Flor et al. 1993b).

We further investigated these findings with a magnetoencephalographic study (Flor et al. 1993a), which confirmed our evoked potential findings. Moreover, we found a high correlation between chronicity and the magnitude of the pain-evoked magnetic field. Using stimulation at both the pain site (the lower back) and a site unaffected by the pain (finger), we showed that the magnitude of the response to back stimulation in the 100-msec range was clearly elevated in a highly chronic patient group. Pain-evoked magnetic fields were significantly lower in less chronic pain patients and in healthy controls. Source analyses using a single equivalent current dipole model suggested that this activity comes from the primary somatosensory cortex (Fig. 4).

Earlier primary subcortical and cortical components of the evoked magnetic field around 50 msec did not differentiate between the groups, suggesting a cortical origin for this heightened response. Later components (150 msec, 250 msec) did not show a back/finger differentiation, but showed a generally elevated response in the very chronic patients. These data strongly suggest both expansion of the representation of the body part affected by pain in the primary somatosensory cortex and an activation of more cell assembles by noxious stimulation in chronic pain patients.

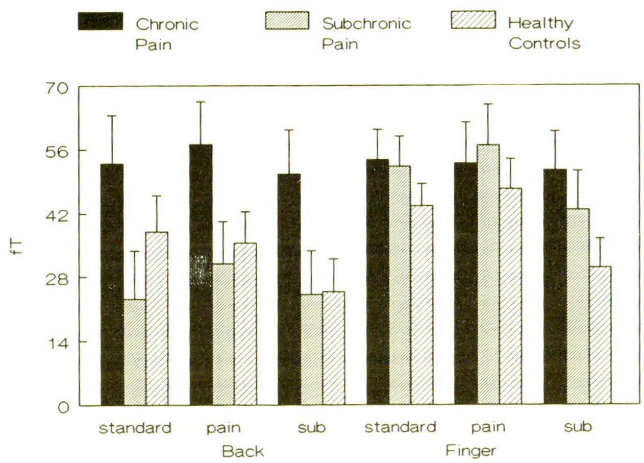

Fig. 4. Root mean square (RMS) values of the magnetically evoked fields at 100 msec poststimulus in the chronic back pain group (average duration of pain 18 years), the subchronic pain group (average duration 7 years), and a healthy control group.

We have extended these studies to patients who suffer from phantom limb pain. Ramachandran et al. (1992) reported that they could elicit painful and nonpainful sensations in the phantom limb by stimulation of the face or the proximal stump in upper limb amputees. The authors suggested that this phenomenon, which they called remapping, might be a perceptual correlate of changes in the cortical representation of the amputated limb and neighboring areas. They hypothesized that the face and the stump area invaded the region of the primary somatosensory cortex that was formerly occupied by the amputated limb and that this cortical plasticity might be a neurophysiological basis for phantom limb sensation and phantom pains.

This hypothesis was tested in five phantom limb patients (Elbert et al., unpublished data). Light vibratory stimuli were applied to the fifth and first digit of the intact arm, and bilaterally to the upper arm and face regions. A 37-channel biomagnetometer was used to assess the cortical response to stimulation. In healthy subjects the evoked magnetic responses of each of the hemispheres contralateral to the site of stimulation were comparable in size and location. In the five phantom pain patients the evoked magnetic fields of the upper arm and chin contralateral to the phantom side were substantially greater than those from the hemisphere contralateral to the intact side. Both their size and location resembled the magnetic fields evoked by the finger stimulation.

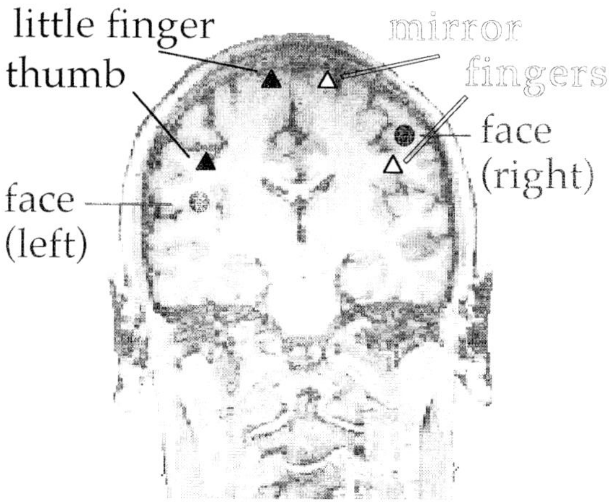

Fig. 5. Localization of the dipoles of the chin and finger representation on the magnetic resonance image of one upper limb amputee with phantom limb pain and sensations. In this patient the left arm was amputated. "Mirror fingers" denotes the assumed location of the finger representation of the amputated hand based on the measured locations of the representation of the intact hand.

Fig. 5 shows the location of the cortical representation of the fingers and the chin of the intact side and the chin of the amputated side of one patient on a magnetic resonance image. The region of the somatosensory cortex that represents the chin has moved closer to the region where the amputated finger used to be represented.

A statistical analysis of the Euclidean distances of the chin and the first and fifth digit representations of the intact side and the mirror images of the fingers and the chin of the phantom side yielded a highly significant effect. The chin-finger distance was 1–2 cm shorter in the somatosensory cortex representing the amputated side as compared to the intact side. These results confirm our hypothesis that plastic changes of the cortex may play an important role in the processing and the learned acquisition of increased sensitivity to somatosensory and painful stimulation.

The psychobiological view of chronic pain has important assessment and treatment implications. Thorough behavioral and psychophysiological assessments (cf. Turk and Melzack 1992) of the chronic pain patient are essential if we take these findings seriously. Both operant and respondent conditioning, which are instrumental in creating psychophysiological dysfunction, can be used therapeutically. For example, enhanced peripheral and central psychophysiological reactivity can be modified by biofeedback to reduce muscular reactivity (Flor and Birbaumer 1993) or operant conditioning of evoked cortical responses (Miltner et al. 1988). Further research should focus on demonstrating how these behavioral and psychophysiological methods change the biological substrate of response to pain. Kandel (1991, p. 1028) wrote: "It is intriguing to think, then, that insofar as psychotherapy is successful in bringing about substantive changes in behavior, it does so by producing alterations in gene expression. Treatment...by psychotherapeutic intervention should, if successful, also produce structural changes." The same should be true for behavioral treatments of chronic pain.

ACKNOWLEDGMENTS

Supported by the Deutsche Forschungsgemeinschaft (Forschergruppe "Klinische Psychophysiologie des Schmerzes" / Research Group "Clinical Psychophysiology of Pain" Bi 195/24-1 and grants Fl 156/1-6 and Fl 156/3).

REFERENCES

Amit, Z. and Galina, Z.H., Stress-induced analgesia: adaptive pain suppression, Physiol. Rev., 66 (1986) 1091–1120.

Arntz A., Merckelbach H., Peters M. and Schmidt A.J.M., Chronic low back pain, response specificity, and habituation to painful stimuli, J. Psychophysiology, 5 (1991) 177–188.

Birbaumer, N., Elbert, T., Canavan, A., and Rockstroh, B., Slow potentials of the cerebral cortex and behavior, Physiol. Rev., 70 (1990), 1–41.

Bromm, B., Pain-related components of the cerebral potential. Experimental and multivariate statistical approaches. In: B. Bromm (Ed.), Pain Measurement in Man. Neurophysiological Correlates of Pain. Elsevier, Amsterdam, 1984, pp. 257–290.

Christensen, L.V., Physiology and pathophysiology of skeletal muscle contraction: Part I. Dynamic activity, J. Oral Rehabil., 13 (1986a) 451–461.

Christensen, L.V., Physiology and pathophysiology of skeletal muscle contraction: Part II. Static activity, J. Oral Rehabil., 13 (1986b) 463–477.

Craig, K.D., Consequences of caring: pain in the human context, Can. J. Psychol./Psychol. Canad., 28 (1987) 311–321.

Dickson-Parnell, B. and Zeichner, A., The premenstrual syndrome: psychophysiological concomitants of perceived stress and chronic back pain, Pain, 34 (1988) 61–69.

Elbert, T., Ray, W.J., Kowalik, Z.J., Skinner, J.E., Graf, K.E. and Birbaumer, N., Chaos and physiology: deterministic chaos in excitable cell assemblies. Physiol. Rev., 74 (1994) 1–47.

Erskine, A., Morley, S. and Pearce, S., Memory for pain, Pain, 41 (1990) 255–265.

Flor, H. and Birbaumer, N., Comparison of the efficacy of EMG biofeedback, cognitive behavior therapy, and conservative medical interventions in the treatment of chronic musculoskeletal pain, J. Consult Clin. Psychol., 61 (1993) 653–658.

Flor, H. and Birbaumer, N., Psychophysiological methods in the assessment and treatment of chronic pain. In: J. Carlson and R. Seifert (Eds.), Biobehavioral Self-Regulation and Health, Vol. 2. Plenum, New York, 1994, 171–184.

Flor, H., Turk, D.C. and Birbaumer. N., Assessment of stress-related psychophysiological reac-

tions in chronic back pain patients, J. Consult. Clin. Psychol., 53 (1985) 354–364.
Flor, H., Birbaumer, N. and Turk, D.C., The psychobiology of chronic pain, Adv. Behav. Res. Ther., 12 (1990) 47–84.
Flor, H., Birbaumer, N., Schulte, W. and Roos, R., Stress-related EMG responses in patients with chronic temporomandibular pain, Pain, 46 (1991) 145–152.
Flor, H., Birbaumer, N., Schugens, M.M. and Lutzenberger, W., Symptom-specific responding in chronic pain patients and healthy controls, Psychophysiology, 29 (1992) 452–460.
Flor, H., Birbaumer, N., Braun, C., Elbert, T., Ross, M. and Hoke, M., Chronic pain enhances the magnitude of the magnetic field evoked by painful stimulation. In: L. Deecke, C. Baumgartner, G. Stroink and S.J. Williamson (Eds.), Recent Advances in Biomagnetism. 9th International Conference on Biomagnetism. Elsevier, Amsterdam, in press.
Flor, H., Birbaumer, N., Fürst, M., Lutzenberger, W., Elbert, T. and Braun, C., Evidence of enhanced peripheral and central responses to painful stimulation in states of chronic pain, Psychophysiology, 30 (1993) 9.
Flor, H., Breitenstein, C. and Birbaumer, N., Operant reinforcement, spouse interaction, and pain perception: a psychophysiological analysis, Behavior Therapy, in press.
Fordyce, W.E., Behavioral methods in chronic pain and illness, Mosby, St. Louis, 1976.
Hubel, D.H. and Wiesel, T.N., The period of susceptibility to the physiological effects of unilateral eye closure in kittens, J. Physiol. (Lond.), 206 (1979) 419–436.
Jenkins, W.M., Merzenich, M.M., Ochs, M.T., Allard, T. and Guic, E.C., Functional reorganization of somatosensory representations within area 3b of adult owl monkey after behaviorally controlled stimulation, J. Neurophysiol., 63 (1990a) 82–104.
Jenkins, W.M., Merzenich, M.M. and Recanzone, G., Neocortical representational dynamics in adult primates: implications for neuropsychology, Neuropsychologia, 28 (1990b) 573–584.
Kandel, E.R., Cellular mechanisms of learning and the basis of individuality. In: E.R. Kandel, J.H. Schwarz and T.M. Jessell (Eds.), Principles of Neural Science, 3rd ed., Elsevier, Amsterdam, 1991, pp. 1009–1031.
Linton, S.J., Melin, L. and Götestam, K.G., Behavioral analysis of chronic pain and its management. In: M. Hersen, A. Bellack and H. Eisler (Eds.), Progress in Behavior Modification, Vol. 18. Academic Press, New York, 1985.
Lousberg, R., Schmidt. A.J.M. and Groenman, N., The relationship between spouse solicitousness and pain behaviour: searching for more experimental evidence, Pain, 51 (1992) 75–80.
Lutzenberger, W., Birbaumer, N., Flor, H., Rockstroh, B. and Elbert T, Dynamic analysis of the human EEG and intelligence. Neurosc. Lett., 143 (1992) 10–14.
Lutzenberger, W., Flor, H., Birbaumer, N. and Fürst, M., Chronic pain enhances electro-cortical responses to painful stimulation, Soc. Neurosci. Abstr., 19 (1993) 233.
Maier, S., Determinants of the nature of environmentally induced hypoalgesia, Behav. Neurosci. 103 (1989) 131–143.
Maier, S.F., Wiertelak, E.P. and Watkins, L.R., Endogenous pain facilitatory systems: anti-analgesia and hyperalgisia, American Pain Society Journal, 1 (1992) 191–198.
Melzack, R.A., The gate control theory 25 years later: new perspectives on phantom limb pain. In: M.R. Bond, J.E. Charlton and C.J. Woolf (Eds.), Proceedings of the VIth World Congress on Pain. Pain Research and Clinical Management, Vol. 4. Elsevier, Amsterdam, 1991, pp.9–21.
Merzenich, M.M., Nelson, R.J., Stryker, M.P., Cynader, M.S., Schoppman, A. and Zook, J.M., Somatosensory cortical map changes following digit amputation in man, J. Comp. Neurol., 224 (1984) 591–605.
Miltner, W., Larbig, W. and Braun, C., Biofeedback of somatosensory event-related potentials: can individual pain sensations be modified by self-control of event-related potentials? Pain, 35 (1988) 205–213.
Moulton, B. and Spence, S.H., Site-specific muscle hyper-activity in musicians with occupational upper limb pain, Behav. Res. Ther., 30 (1991) 375–386.

Pons, T., Garraghty, P.E., Ommaya, A.K., Kaas, J.H., Taub, E. and Mishkin, M., Massive cortical reorganization after sensory deafferentation in adult macaques, Science, 252 (1991) 1857–1860.

Ramachandran, V.S., Stewart, M., Rogers-Ramachandran, D.C., Perceptual correlates of massive cortical reorganization, Neuroreport, 3 (1992) 583–586.

Squire, L.R., Memory and Brain. Oxford University Press, New York and Oxford, 1987.

Turk, D.C. and Melzack, R., Trends and future directions in human pain assessment. In: D.C. Turk and R. Melzack (Eds.), Handbook of Pain Assessment, Guilford Press, New York, 1992, pp. 473–479.

Watkins, L.R., Maier, S.F. and Wiertelak, E.P., The amygdala is necessary for the expression of conditioned but not unconditioned analgesia, Behav. Neurosci., 107 (1993) 402–405.

Wiertelak, E.P., Maier, S.F. and Watkins, L.R., Cholecystokinin antianalgesia: safety cues abolish morphine analgesia, Science, 256 (1992a) 830–833.

Wiertelak, E.P., Watkins, L.R. and Maier, S.F., Conditioned inhibition of analgesia, Animal Learning and Behavior, 20 (1992b) 339–349.

Willer, J.C., Dehen, H. and Cambier, J., Stress-induced analgesia in humans: endogenous opioids and naloxone-reversible depression of pain reflexes, Science, 212 (1981) 689–690.

Correspondence to: Prof. Dr. Herta Flor, Fachbereich Psychologie der Humboldt-Universität zu Berlin, Oranienburger Straße 18, D-10178 Berlin, Germany, Tel: 49-30-2805115, Fax: 49-30-2824046, e-mail: hflor@rz.hu-berlin.de

Proceedings of the 7th World Congress on Pain,
Progress in Pain Research and Management, Vol. 2,
edited by G.F. Gebhart, D.L. Hammond, and T.S.
Jensen, IASP Press, Seattle, © 1994.

10

Pain Behavior Concepts: Controversies, Current Status, and Future Directions

Francis J. Keefe[a,b] and John Lefebvre[b]

[a]Department of Psychiatry, Pain Management Program, Duke University Medical Center, and [b]Deparment of Psychology: Social and Health Sciences, Duke University, Durham, North Carolina, USA

To watch someone in pain, particularly someone we know or love, can be a compelling experience. The look of pain on the person's face, the altered body position, and descriptions of pain tell us much about the pain experience. Such signals are important in communicating pain to others and have been called pain behaviors (Fordyce 1976). Pain clinicians and pain theorists consider pain behaviors to be extremely important in understanding chronic pain (Keefe 1989). Clinicians attend to pain behaviors and try to interpret their meaning in light of information about the tissue pathology basis of pain. Pain behaviors are an important component in each of the major theories of chronic pain (Keefe 1989).

Over the past 20 years, a behavioral perspective on pain has emerged that views pain behavior as central to the development and maintenance of chronic pain. This chapter provides an overview of the behavioral perspective. The first section reviews behavioral concepts used to understand pain behavior. The second section describes the current status of major methods used to assess pain behavior. The third section presents controversial issues in pain behavior assessment and treatment. The chapter concludes with a discussion of several new directions for research on pain behavior.

THE CONCEPT OF PAIN BEHAVIOR

The theoretical foundations of behavioral approaches to pain are based on behavioral and cognitive-behavioral models of human behavior. These models have two major hallmarks. First, they emphasize the importance of behavior

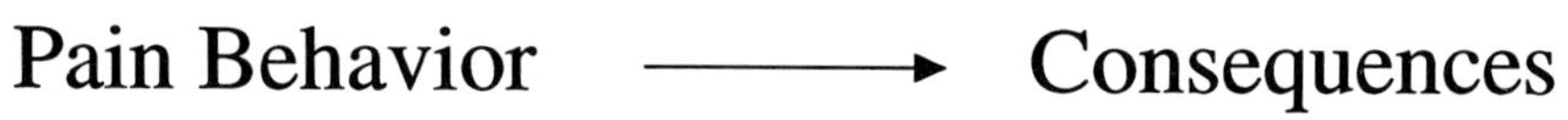

Fig. 1. Basic elements of the operant behavioral model of pain behavior.

in understanding pain. What patients say or do when they have pain are viewed as important factors influencing chronic pain. Second, these models underscore the need to directly sample and carefully measure pain behavior in the settings in which pain is likely to be a problem, using both reliable and valid measurement methods.

The behavioral concepts used to analyze pain behavior have evolved over the years. The earliest behavioral model was based on operant conditioning principles (Fordyce 1976). Fig. 1 illustrates the basic elements of the operant model, which draws attention to the relationship between pain behavior and its consequences. Chronic pain patients, for example, might learn to associate pain behavior with reinforcing consequences such as attention from a solicitous spouse, access to pain medication, or avoidance of unpleasant activities. These consequences, in some chronic pain patients, are highly reinforcing and can serve to maintain pain behavior patterns long after the normal healing time. Research has shown that pain behavior patterns can be altered by manipulating their consequences (Keefe and Gil 1986). Reinforcing well behaviors while simultaneously reducing reinforcement for pain behaviors can produce significant changes in the activity level and medication intake of chronic pain patients (Fordyce et al. 1973).

In the late 1970s and early 1980s, behavioral research and clinical practice began to raise questions about the adequacy of the operant model in explaining pain behavior (Keefe and Gil 1986). Other variables in addition to response consequences were seen as important to the development and maintenance of pain behavior. In 1979, Fordyce presented a revised behavioral model of pain behavior that went beyond the operant model and attempted to take into account the influence of biological and psychological variables (Fordyce 1979). This model, presented in Fig. 2, incorporates four basic classes of variables: (1) nociception—nervous system responses to aversive input, (2) pain—the conscious perception of nociceptive input, (3) suffering—which reflects the negative emotional responses to nociception and pain, and (4) pain behavior—overt behaviors communicating that pain is experienced. This model was important in the development of behavioral theories of pain because it highlighted the multiple factors influencing pain behavior. The model not only

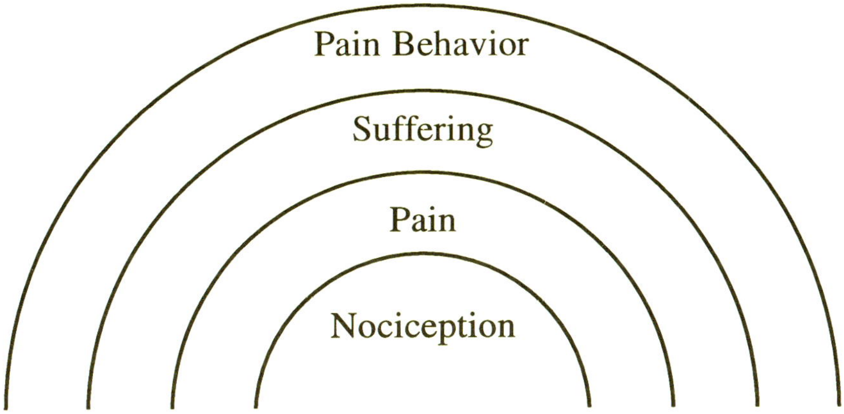

Fig. 2. Fordyce's (1979) revised behavioral model of pain.

views pain behavior as a product of behavioral and social factors, it also emphasizes the role of psychological and somatic variables in determining such behavior. Recent research based on this model has attempted to determine the relative importance of somatic, behavioral, and psychological factors in explaining pain behavior in different chronic pain populations (e.g., Keefe et al. 1984; Keefe et al. 1986; Keefe et al. 1987).

Recently, behavior theorists have developed even more comprehensive models based on systems theory (Kanfer and Schefft 1988; Schefft and Lehr 1985). The systems model differs from earlier models of pain behavior in three important ways. First, as depicted in Fig. 3, the systems model maintains that pain behavior can be controlled by multiple and interactive factors. Some pain behaviors, such as motor and verbal operants, may be classified as primarily controlled by environmental factors (alpha variables). Other pain behaviors may be characterized as biological responses to physical nociceptive stimuli (gamma variables). Still other pain behaviors may be under psychological control (beta variables). Pain behavior, for example, may reflect psychological self-control efforts in which patients are attempting to cognitively or behaviorally regulate their pain.

A second characteristic of the systems model, depicted in Fig. 4, is that it places pain behaviors in a broader context. This context not only views the consequences of pain behavior as important, it also highlights the role that stimulus events (e.g., environmental cues—an alpha variable) and organismic variables (e.g., biological factors—a gamma variable, or psychological events—a beta variable) can play in determining pain behavior.

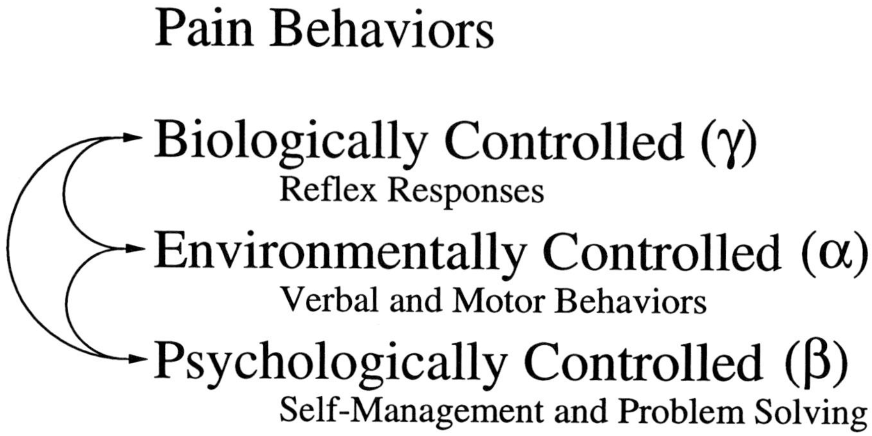

Fig. 3. The systems model views pain behavior as controlled by multiple and interactive factors: (1) alpha variables—environmental factors, (2) beta variables—psychological factors, and (3) gamma variables—biological factors.

A third important feature of this model is that it includes feedback and feedforward loops to emphasize that changes in one part of the system can influence and alter other parts. For example, a patient who has been socially reinforced (a consequence variable) for engaging in well behaviors may become much more confident in the ability to engage in demanding physical activities (a psychological variable) and may show much lower levels of emotional arousal (a biological variable) when attempting such activities.

Systems models provide the conceptual basis for new cognitive-behavioral approaches to pain management (Turk et al. 1983). These approaches help patients reconceptualize their pain and provide them with training in skills such as self-monitoring, relaxation training, activity pacing, and cognitive coping methods. These skills are important because they enable patients to directly regulate their own pain behavior.

PAIN BEHAVIOR ASSESSMENT METHODS

A variety of methods have been developed for recording and analyzing pain behavior. These methods can be grouped into three basic categories: (1) self-monitoring techniques, (2) automated recorders, and (3) observation methods.

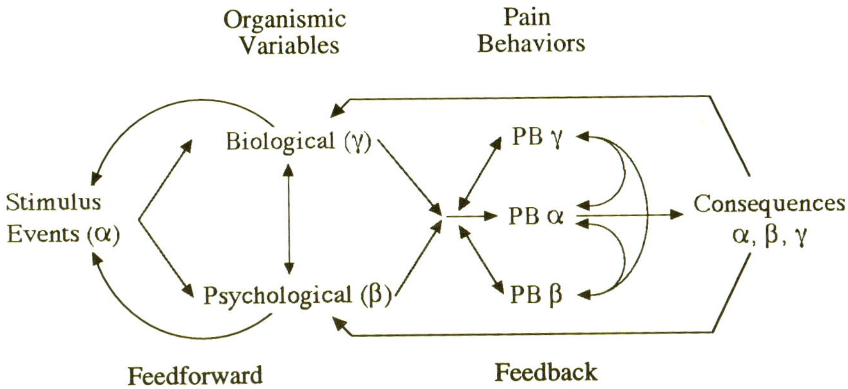

Fig. 4. A systems model of pain behavior based on the General Systems Model presented by Kanfer and Schefft. (Adpated by permission from Kanfer and Schefft 1988, p. 53, © 1988 by the authors).

SELF-MONITORING

In self-monitoring the patient keeps a behavior record. The daily activity diary developed by Fordyce (1976) is a good example of self-monitoring methods. The diary requires patients to make hourly entries of the amount of time spent in three positions: sitting, standing or walking, and reclining. The diary also includes a column for recording medication intake. Using this diary, the clinician can calculate two pain behavior indices: (1) downtime—the amount of time spent reclining, and (2) pain medication intake—the amount of analgesic and opioid medication taken daily.

In analyzing diary data it is important to try identify pain behavior patterns that may be maladaptive and that could serve as potential targets for behavioral intervention. For example, patients who spend an inordinate amount of time reclining each day may benefit from a graded activation program that encourages a gradual increase in the amount of time spent standing or walking. Patients who take extra pain medication may benefit from a behavioral program that delivers these medications on a specific schedule (e.g., every four hours) and with gradually tapered doses.

Self-monitoring is a practical approach to assessing pain behavior. Concerns, however, have been raised about the reliability and validity of diary data provided by patients (Sanders 1983). Recent studies, however, suggest that high-quality data can be obtained if patients receive systematic training in self-monitoring methods. Follick et al. (1984), for example, found that when they provided such training, their patients' diary records of activity correlated highly with data recorded using an objective activity monitor.

Recently, researchers in health psychology and behavioral medicine have shown increased interest in the use of daily diary methods (Affleck et al. 1991). Two factors have contributed to this interest. First, diary records provide more timely measures of behavior than do retrospective questionnaire methods. Second, diary methods provide repeated measures of behavior and allow a study of processes that change over time. This factor is especially important in pain behavior assessment where the level of pain behavior may change as patients undergo treatment. Finally, newly developed statistical methods permit sophisticated analyses of daily diary data (Affleck et al. 1991). These analyses can control for potential confounding effects (e.g., autocorrelation) and provide quantitative information on the temporal relationships between pain and subsequent pain behavior.

Affleck and his colleagues have used innovative daily study methods to analyze self-monitoring data recorded from arthritis patients (Affleck et al. 1991; Affleck et al. 1992). They found that patients who reported a higher frequency of daily coping had a pronounced linear decline in daily pain ratings over a 75-day recording period.

AUTOMATED RECORDING

A second method for assessing pain behavior is to use electrical or mechanical devices that automatically record the behavior of interest. Several monitors have been developed to record downtime or uptime in chronic pain patients. One of the earliest uptime recorders consisted of a clock placed on the patient's bed that was activated by a switch each time the patient got out of bed (Cairns et al. 1976). Later variations of this approach (Sanders 1980; Follick et al. 1985) used a microswitch placed on the patient's leg to automatically record standing or walking time on the timing unit of an electronic calculator.

In our own lab we have evaluated several electromechanical devices for recording pain-related behaviors. In one set of studies we tested an electromechanical monitor for assessing gait patterns in patients with chronic low-back pain (Keefe and Hill 1985). The monitor used a transducer placed in the subject's shoes that produced an electrical signal proportional to the amount of force placed on it. The transducer was connected to a polygraph that directly recorded several gait parameters. Using the monitor, we recorded measures of gait from a sample of 18 patients with chronic low-back pain and 18 pain-free normal controls. Comparisons of these two subject groups revealed that the chronic pain patients walked much more slowly, took shorter steps, and showed more gait asymmetries than did the control subjects. In the patients with low-back pain, disability/financial compensation status correlated with gait patterns. Patients receiving disability or financial compensation payments had longer stride lengths and swing time than did patients not receiving compensation.

In a second set of studies we tested the utility of an actometer in assessing activity level in chronic pain patients (Morrell and Keefe 1988). An actometer is a self-winding watch that is sensitive to accelerative forces that occur during daily activities. The second hand on the face of the watch advances when the subject moves. The amount of activity can be measured by setting the watch to a standard time (e.g., 1:00 P.M.) and then at standard intervals recording the time elapsed. Research by Tryon (1985) using pain-free subjects provided strong support for the reliability and validity of the actometer.

Our research was designed to assess the applicability of the actometer to patients with a common chronic pain condition—low-back pain. We first tested the instrument's internal reliability having patients wear two actometers while walking a standard distance. The reliability was quite high; both actometers showed almost identical readings. We then examined the test-retest reliability by having patients walk the same course on three different days. We found a high level of inconsistency in actometer readings over the three days of recording. The only factor that appeared to explain this inconsistency was that the patients with low-back pain may have engaged in more limping and altered gait patterns when walking on one day versus another.

Recent developments in portable accelerometer technology are important because they potentially can provide more objective and reliable measures of activity in chronic pain patients. A newly developed accelerometer, the Actigraph ambulatory activity monitor (Ambulatory Monitoring Inc., Ardsley, NY, USA), has several features that increase its utility in pain assessment. First, the sensitivity of this device can be adjusted to reduce the confounding effects of movement artifacts such as limping. Second, the Actigraph not only detects the quantity of movements but also their intensity. This feature is particularly important in gauging the clinical significance of a physical conditioning program designed to increase activity and reduce pain behavior. Finally, the Actigraph has a microprocessor that periodically samples movement and stores the information gathered for subsequent downloading on a microcomputer. Continuous data on activity thus can be collected over periods ranging to 11 days. Patterson et al. (1993) recently conducted a study validating the Actigraph in pain-free subjects. The instrument showed excellent test-retest reliability and correlated well with physiological and self-report measures of activity.

The Actigraph appears to be one of the most promising electromechanical methods for assessing pain-related behavior patterns. However, our experience with the actometer strongly suggests that the reliability and validity of this device should not be judged solely on the basis of data gathered from pain-free populations (e.g., Patterson et al. 1993). The best way to test the utility of electromechanical devices such as the Actigraph is to examine their applicability to populations of patients suffering from persistent pain.

OBSERVATION METHODS

Pain behaviors occur with sufficient frequency to allow direct observation and recording in clinical settings. In the early 1980s we developed and validated a structured pain behavior observation protocol for recording pain behaviors in patients with chronic low-back pain (Keefe and Block 1982). To elicit pain behavior, the protocol requires that patients engage in a series of simple daily activities (sitting, standing, walking, and reclining) for periods of one to two minutes. Patients were videotaped for 10 minutes while engaging in these activities and the videotapes were subsequently scored by trained observers. The observers recorded the occurrence/nonoccurrence of five pain behaviors using ongoing 20-second observe and 10-second record intervals. The definitions of the five pain behaviors were: (1) guarding—abnormally stiff, interrupted, or rigid movement, (2) bracing—a stationary pain avoidant posture in which one limb supports and maintains an abnormal distribution of weight, (3) rubbing—touching, rubbing, or holding the affected area of pain for three or more seconds, (4) grimacing—an obvious facial expression of pain, and (5) sighing—an obvious exaggerated exhalation of air.

We conducted a series of four experiments to evaluate the observation protocol (Keefe and Block 1982). Experiment I showed that observers were highly reliable in coding the pain behaviors (interobserver percentage agreement = 80–96%) and that the level of pain behavior was highly correlated with the patients' own ratings of pain (r = .71, P < .01). Experiment II indicated the observation protocol was sensitive enough to detect changes in pain behavior occurring over the course of an inpatient pain management treatment program. Experiment III supported the construct validity of the observation protocol in that the level of pain behavior correlated with naive observers' ratings of the patients' pain. Experiment IV revealed that the observation protocol was able to discriminate patients having low-back pain from pain-free normal and depressed subjects.

Taken together, the findings of our initial four experiments provided strong evidence for the reliability and validity of the observation protocol. The observation protocol subsequently has been widely applied as a measure of treatment outcome in studies evaluating behavioral treatments for chronic low-back pain (e.g., Turner 1982). This protocol also has been used in several studies examining the relation of pain behavior to measures of depression, psychological distress, and coping (Keefe et al. 1984; Keefe et al. 1987). Several investigators have adapted this protocol for use with other chronic pain populations. Evidence for the reliability and validity of this observation method has been gathered in studies of patients with rheumatoid arthritis (Anderson et al. 1987), osteoarthritis (Keefe et al. 1987), and cancer (Ahles et al. 1990).

Although videotaped protocols are useful in sampling pain behavior, research has shown that direct observations of pain behavior can be reliably gathered in naturalistic settings without using videotape (Keefe and Williams 1992). In our own research we have found that observers watching physical examinations can reliably record pain behavior in patients with low-back pain (Keefe et al. 1984). Richards et al. (1982) have provided strong support for the reliability of an observation method for recording pain behavior during bedside rounds. Cinciripini and Floreen (1982) also have documented the reliability of a pain behavior observation system for collecting hourly records of pain and well behaviors from patients hospitalized for pain management.

CONTROVERSIAL ISSUES IN PAIN BEHAVIOR ASSESSMENT AND TREATMENT

The pain behavior concept is controversial. Consideration of these controversies is important to understanding the pain behavior construct and its applications. The controversial issues can be grouped into two basic categories: (1) those related to pain behavior assessment, and (2) those related to behavioral interventions designed to treat pain behavior.

CONTROVERSIES IN PAIN BEHAVIOR ASSESSMENT

In two recent papers (Keefe and Dunsmore 1992a, 1992b) we identified and discussed five criticisms that arise from using pain behavior observation methods to assess chronic pain patients. These criticisms include: the pain behavior construct is too simplistic, the focus on pain behavior denies the existence of pain, the question of whether pain behavior is an expression of pain or a coping response, the measures of pain behavior may not be useful in clinical settings, and the notion that pain behavior has been oversold. Table I summarizes our response to each of these criticisms, which we do not consider to be valid. Many arise from a lack of understanding of the current status of behavior assessment research on pain.

CONTROVERSIES IN PAIN BEHAVIOR TREATMENT

Several criticisms have been raised about applications of behavioral therapy and cognitive-behavioral therapy techniques to the modification of pain behavior. These criticisms have centered around four common themes: behavioral therapies dehumanize the patient, behavioral therapies ignore historical variables affecting pain behavior, improvements following behavioral therapy are temporary, and behavioral therapies are expensive. We will address each criticism in turn.

Behavioral Treatments Dehumanize the Patient

Critics of behavioral treatments for pain contend that these treatments, through their emphasis on changing behavior, invariably devalue the patient's wants and needs. According to this view, behavioral therapies indirectly manipulate pain behavior by controlling the environment. The environment is programmed to determine when the patient is active or rests and what others will say or do when around them. The main concern is that the patient has little control over the process of treatment and individual wishes and goals are ignored.

This criticism demonstrates a basic misunderstanding of the therapy process in behavioral pain management. Informed consent has always been a basic part of behavioral treatment. Fordyce (1976), one of the pioneers of behavioral treatment, emphasized the importance of obtaining fully informed consent. He recommended that the treatment objectives, target behaviors, therapy techniques, and likely outcomes be fully discussed with both the patient and spouse before starting treatment. Sternbach (1978), another early advocate of behavioral treatment, recommended using written contracts as part of the informed consent process. A behavioral contract can be negotiated with patients that specifies the treatments that will be offered and likely treatment outcomes. The contract also can indicate expectations of both the patient (e.g., that pain will be reevaluated at regular intervals) and the therapist (e.g., that the patient will not make unnecessary late-night calls). By signing the written contract, both patient and therapist indicate their commitment to a common set of goals and methods of treatment.

The process of obtaining informed consent is often therapeutic (Keefe et al. 1978). Many chronic pain patients are uncertain about what behavioral treatment is and find that the information provided in the informed consent process is helpful and reassuring. When patients are involved in setting their own treatment goals, and clear about the objectives and methods of treatment, cooperation and compliance with treatment is greatly enhanced (Keefe et al. 1978).

Table I
Controversies in pain behavior assessment

Controversy	Description	Response
Pain behavior is too simplistic.	Behavioral clinicians and researchers tend to view pain behaviors solely as operant behaviors maintained by the environment.	Behavioral theorists emphasize that pain behavior is influenced not only by the environment but by nociception, constitutional factors, and personality.
Pain behavior denies the existence of pain.	Measures of pain behavior ignore the conscious experience of pain. Pain cannot be reduced to a set of pain behaviors.	Pain and pain behavior are separate but related. Behavioral researchers do not ignore this issue, but rather frequently study the relation of pain perception to overt pain behavior.
Pain behavior is not an objective index of pain.	Pain behaviors are supposed to be objective indexes of pain, but fail to meet this goal.	It is the methodlogy that is objective. Pain behavior measures provide objective measures of behavior, not pain. Behavioral observation is one of the most objective and reliable means of recording pain behavior.
Is pain behavior a coping response or a means of expressing pain?	Certain pain behaviors may communicate to others the experience of pain, but they also may serve to control pain (e.g., rubbing a sore joint).	Any behavior that reliably communicates pain to others is a pain behavior regardless of intent.
Pain behavior measures need further development.	People change their behavior when being observed (reactivity). Behavioral data collected in one place and one time can not be generalized to other places or occasions.	Reactivity is a problem for all assessment methods. However, steps can be taken to minimize the effects of reactivity. There are several ways to enhance the generalizability of pain behavior measures.
Pain behavior has been oversold.	Behavioral clinicians and researchers have exaggerated the importance of pain behaviors.	The problem may not be that the concept has been oversold, but that others are too eager to reduce the complexity of chronic pain by applying the pain behavior concept in an overly simplistic fashion.

Source: Modified from Keefe and Dunsmore (1992a,b)

In summary, criticism of behavioral treatment programs as dehumanizing ignores the fact that pain behaviors are not modified without the active and ongoing consent of the patient. Although the environment might be structured to reinforce well behaviors and reduce pain behaviors (e.g., through training of the spouse in reinforcement techniques), this is done with the patient's approval. Furthermore, behavioral programs train patients in self-control techniques such as relaxation training and activity-pacing methods to provide them with a way to directly control and reduce their own pain behavior.

Behavioral Treatments Ignores Historical Information

Another criticism of behavioral treatment is that it ignores background or historical information that may be important in understanding pain behavior. According to this view, behavioral therapists focus solely on current behavior and its controlling variables and consider irrelevant earlier determinants of pain behavior, such as childhood or early adult experiences with pain or illness.

This criticism that behavioral treatment ignores historical variables is surprising given the emphasis on learning and conditioning inherent in behavioral theories of pain. Pain behaviors are seen as learned patterns that have their origins in early experiences with pain. In discussing the acquisition of pain behavior, Fordyce (1976) identified a number of early learning experiences that can influence how patients subsequently cope with chronic pain. For example, he discussed the role that parental responses play in the learning of pain behavior patterns. Children whose parents are relatively nonresponsive to pain may be prone as adults to be stoic in displaying pain behavior. On the other hand, children whose parents show an excessive amount of concern about pain and who are prone to overrespond to illness or pain may be much more prone to exhibit pain as adults. Fordyce maintained that children may learn maladaptive pain behaviors through modeling or imitation of their parents. Many patients having chronic pain grew up with parents who themselves suffered from chronic pain or illness. Children also may learn that the display of pain behavior enables them to avoid unpleasant situations. The child who develops abdominal pain when anxious about an upcoming test may learn that this pain provides an excuse to avoid going to school.

An emphasis on the history of pain behavior also is evident in the assessment strategies used in analyzing pain behavior. An important component in behavioral interviewing of pain patients is the identification of historical variables influencing pain behavior (Fordyce 1976). Diary data help the clinician analyze patterns of pain behavior occurring over the weeks and months prior to treatment. Data from psychological tests such as the Minnesota Multiphasic

Personality Inventory (MMPI) also help to place pain behavior in the context of longstanding personality traits. Many of the cognitive-behavioral questionnaires used in pain assessment such as the Pain Beliefs and Perceptions Inventory (Williams and Thorn 1989) identify enduring trait-like patterns of attitudes that can exert a strong historical influence on the development and maintenance of pain behavior.

In summary, behavioral treatment specialists recognize that pain behavior patterns are learned. Understanding the history of these behaviors, both for early childhood and more recent experiences, is crucial to attempts to change pain behavior. If behavioral treatment is to be effective, a careful analysis of historical influences on pain behavior is essential (Fordyce 1976).

Improvements Following Behavioral Therapy Are Temporary

A third criticism of behavioral treatment is that reductions in pain behavior achieved through behavioral intervention are only temporary at best. With an overreliance on achieving behavior change by controlling the patient's environment, the initial gains produced in the therapeutic environment are lost once the patient returns home.

Behavioral theorists (Fordyce 1976; Turk et al. 1983) recognize that successful outcomes can only be achieved when steps are taken to ensure that patients maintain long-term improvements in pain behavior. Two methods are typically incorporated into behavioral programs to enhance the maintenance of changes in pain behavior (Keefe and Van Horn 1993). The first method is behavioral spouse training. As Fordyce (1976) noted, spouses can be systematically taught to discriminate pain from well behaviors, to avoid reinforcing pain behavior, and to prompt more functionally effective well behaviors. Training of spouses can help them understand the goals of behavioral treatment and prevent them from unwittingly reinforcing maladaptive pain behaviors.

Although spouse training is widely used in behavioral treatment, the literature on its effectiveness is limited. We are conducting a study to test whether behavioral spouse training can enhance the efficacy of a cognitive-behavioral treatment program for osteoarthritis patients with persistent knee pain. Preliminary results are promising and suggest that spouse training does lead to better treatment outcomes.

A second approach to enhancing the maintenance of changes in pain behavior is to provide patients with training in relapse prevention methods (Marlatt and Gordon 1985), which have been helpful in enhancing the long-term maintenance of behavioral interventions for smoking (Hall et al. 1984), obesity (Perri 1984), and alcoholism (Chaney 1978). Relapse prevention training uses methods derived from cognitive therapy to help patients identify high-risk situations that might lead to relapse, pinpoint early warning signs of relapse, and cognitively rehearse different relapse situations. This training also uses behavioral rehearsal to provide therapist modeling of coping skills for handling setbacks, patient rehearsal, and therapist feedback. Training in self-monitoring (e.g., daily diary recording) and self-reinforcement also can help patients enhance their own abilities to regulate pain behavior.

In summary, behavioral theory recognizes that a person must plan for maintenance of behavior change, not expect that it will occur. Spouse training and relapse prevention efforts can provide effective means of enhancing long-term improvements in pain behavior.

Behavioral Treatments Are Expensive

Critics also raised concerns that the costs of behavioral treatments for managing pain are much higher than those of other treatment alternatives, such as medication. This view stems from the belief that behavioral treatment requires an extended stay in a highly structured in-patient program followed by intensive outpatient treatment. Given the growing emphasis on decreasing medical costs, such a treatment course may simply be impractical.

In their early days, behavioral treatment programs primarily occurred in inpatient settings (Fordyce et al. 1973) where the patient's behavior could be monitored closely and staff could provide consistent reinforcement for well behaviors. Although some tertiary care treatment centers still maintain an inpatient behavioral unit for treating chronic pain, most behavioral treatment programs are now delivered in outpatient settings. These outpatient treatment programs are much less costly and appear to be quite effective.

One of the main arguments for implementing behavioral treatment is that it may reduce medical costs. Caudill et al. (1991) conducted a cost-benefit analysis of an outpatient behavioral pain management program. The program involved group sessions held weekly for 10 weeks. The patients treated were members of a health maintenance organization (HMO) that provided all their medical care. To study the impact of the behavioral treatment program, the investigators assessed patient visits for pain and other medical problems at 12 and 24 months post-intervention. The results indicated that patients treated in the behavioral program showed a 36% reduction in total clinic visits over the course of treatment. This reduction in clinic visits was maintained at the two-year follow-up assessment. Patients who had the highest frequency of health care use prior to behavioral treatment showed the greatest reduction in post-treatment clinic visits. The authors estimated that the intervention saved about $12,000 in the first year and $23,000 in the second year. These figures did not include the cost savings for potential reduction in diagnostic assessment and prescription drug use.

Another argument for the cost-effectiveness of behavioral treatments is that they can be used to prevent the development of pain behavior patterns. Fordyce et al. (1986) compared the efficacy of a behavioral program for recent-onset low-back pain to more traditional medical management. Subjects in this study were workers who had injured their back on the job. These subjects were randomly assigned to either a medical management or behavioral treatment condition. Subjects in the medical management condition followed a traditional back pain regimen of exercise, medications, and bedrest. These subjects were instructed to let pain be their guide in determining when to take medications, rest, and exercise. Subjects in the behavioral treatment condition received the same medical treatments delivered on a time-contingent rather than pain-contingent basis. Thus, patients receiving behavioral treatment took their medications, rest breaks, and exercise according to a predetermined schedule. Over the course of behavioral treatment the amount of medication and rest was gradually decreased and the amount of exercise increased. Results of the study indicated no difference in outcome between the two treatment regimens six weeks after treatment, but at one-year follow-up the group of patients receiving behavioral treatment were doing much better than patients receiving medical management. Patients in the behavioral treatment condition had significantly lower levels of impairment, less body area affected by pain, and lower levels of health care use than did patients receiving the traditional medical management protocol.

NEW DIRECTIONS IN PAIN BEHAVIOR RESEARCH

Research on pain behavior has grown dramatically over the past five years. Several exciting and important new directions have emerged. This section highlights three: (1) analysis of pain-related behaviors during functional tasks, (2) sequential analysis of pain behaviors and spouse responses, and (3) studies of observer judgments of pain behavior displays.

PAIN BEHAVIOR DURING FUNCTIONAL TASKS

Studies of pain behavior usually sample these behaviors during relatively nondemanding tasks such as sitting, walking, or reclining. Many patients, however, experience pain primarily when they engage in more complex, physically demanding tasks at work or home. Pain behavior researchers are beginning to extend behavior sampling methods to these more natural tasks. This approach to task analysis has important implications for both pain assessment and treatment.

An excellent example of this new emphasis on task analysis is research by Feuerstein (Feuerstein and Fitzgerald 1992) on sign language interpreters who were experiencing persistent pain. The subjects in this research worked as interpreters for deaf students attending the Rochester Institute of Technology. The task of interpreting is a demanding one that involves repeated and forceful movements of the fingers, hands, forearms, and shoulders. In the college classrooms in which these subjects worked, interpreting sessions could last up to 50 minutes. Interpreters had few formal breaks and little control over the pace of interpreting, which was mainly determined by the lecturer. More than half of the interpreters had persistent pain due to problems such as tendinitis in the wrist or shoulder. Work absenteeism was a significant problem with 45% of the full-time interpreters out of work or on a reduced workload because of pain.

Feuerstein and Fitzgerald (1992) sought to analyze the task of interpreting to identify behavior patterns that discriminated interpreters having pain from those who were pain free. They studied two groups: one that had pain during interpreting (n = 16) and a group without pain during interpreting (n = 13). All subjects were videotaped during an experimental session that involved a 5-minute baseline rest period, 20-minute interpreting session, and 5-minute recovery period. The material chosen for the interpreting session, a selection from *The Merchant of Venice,* was rated as demanding in content, pace, and style of delivery. Trained observers scored each videotape to measure specific behaviors that might be related to the development or exacerbation of pain. The results indicated that interpreters having pain took significantly fewer rest breaks per minute, showed a much higher level of hand/wrist deviations from neutral, more frequent excursions outside a reasonable work envelope, and a much more rapid pace of interpreting. In addition, subjects' ratings of pain were highly correlated with the frequency of hand/wrist deviations and pace of interpreting. Taken together, these findings indicated that sign language interpreters having pain showed a pattern of behaviors related to work style that clearly discriminated them from interpreters without pain.

Based on these findings, Feuerstein and his colleagues developed a behavioral intervention designed to alter the pain-related behaviors they had identified (Feuerstein and Fitzgerald 1992). This program had two basic components. First, the interpreters were encouraged to try to reduce the length of interpreting sessions to 25 minutes and to increase the number of rest breaks. To provide the interpreters with more control over their work, they were asked to work more closely with lecturing faculty. Second, the interpreters were taught to limit their effort during work sessions. Interpreters learned to avoid the use of excessive force or abnormal postures. The behavioral treatment program led to a marked reduction in the frequency of pain and pain-related absences. Importantly, interpreters were able to change their maladaptive pain behavior patterns without compromising the quality of their interpreting.

Analyzing pain behavior during work tasks appears to be a promising approach. This method may be particularly helpful in pinpointing behavior patterns that may be important in the development and maintenance of pain. By identifying these target behaviors, clinicians can better tailor behavioral interventions to the particular demands of an injured worker. Early identification of such problem behaviors also can help to implement behavioral interventions in a timely fashion and thereby prevent persistent pain.

ANALYSIS OF PAIN BEHAVIORS AND SPOUSE RESPONSES

Pain behaviors can be viewed as part of a continuing stream of behaviors that involve not only the patient having pain, but the responses of others to that behavior. Recent research by Joan Romano and her colleagues at the University of Washington (Romano 1991, 1992) has attempted to provide a sequential analysis of pain behavior by studying not only the behavior exhibited by a patient having pain but the spouse's response. This research involved direct observations of 50 chronic pain patients and 33 control couples. Couples were videotaped as they performed routine household activities such as sweeping the floor, bundling newspapers, or carrying small artificial logs across the room. The couples were asked to perform the tasks together, with the only demand being that the patient stay involved in the task in some way. Trained observers scored the videotapes and coded sequences of patient-spouse interaction using the Living in Family Environments coding system (Hops et al. 1990). This system coded not only verbal and nonverbal pain behaviors exhibited by patients, but also spousal responses that were solicitous (e.g., physical assistance, taking over the task), aggressive (e.g., expressions of disapproval or criticism), or facilitative (e.g., praise or encouragement).

Romano and her colleagues have published two studies summarizing their findings. The first study (Romano et al. 1991) identified several behavior patterns that differentiated the pain and control couples. Spouses of pain patients showed a much higher level of solicitous behavior and a much lower level of facilitative behavior than did spouses of pain-free control subjects. The second study (Romano et al. 1992) systematically examined the timing of spousal responses in relationship to pain behavior. Specifically, this study sought to determine whether solicitous or aggressive spouse behaviors regularly occurred just before or just after pain behaviors. The results obtained indicated that spouses of patients having pain were significantly more likely to engage in solicitous behavior before or after nonverbal pain behaviors than were spouses of control patients.

Taken together, these findings provide strong support for operant theories that hypothesize that spouses may maintain maladaptive responses to pain by prompting or positively reinforcing pain behaviors. These results have important implications for pain management efforts. They suggest that spouses need to be involved in treatment to become more aware of how they are responding to pain behavior and to help them learn to prompt and reinforce more adaptive, well behaviors.

The methods of sequential analysis potentially could be used to study how patients interact with other important persons in their environment. For example, studies of patient-child interactions may provide insights into the effects of pain on the family and the degree to which parental pain behaviors influence children's responses to pain. Studies of patient and health care provider interactions also could help identify responses that serve to reinforce pain behaviors or encourage more adaptive coping efforts.

OBSERVER JUDGMENTS OF PAIN BEHAVIOR

Pain behaviors communicate the experience of pain, and so are subject to interpretation by others. Studies in our lab have demonstrated that some behaviors, such as guarded movement or facial expressions of pain, are more salient indicators of pain than are other behaviors (Keefe and Block 1982). Researchers are beginning to systematically investigate the variables that influence observer judgments about pain. An interesting recent study by Prkachin (1992) examined the effects of genuine and faked facial displays of pain on observers' ratings of pain. The videotaped stimuli for this study consisted of facial expressions gathered under two conditions: (1) during exposure to a series of shocks ranging from painless to severe pain, and (2) during instructions to simulate facial expressions to these shock stimuli. Ten observers who were naive with respect to the genuine/faked status of the subject's facial expressions watched videotapes of these facial expressions and rated both the pain experienced by the subject and their confidence in whether the subject viewed was feigning the response.

Prkachin found that faked pain expressions appeared to observers to be stronger than genuine pain expressions at the mild level of pain, but equal at the higher levels of pain intensity. Interestingly, even though the expressions of pain were equivalent in terms of intensity at high levels of pain, the naive observers were able to discriminate the genuine from faked expressions across the entire range of pain stimuli. The naive observers ratings of subjects' pain also correlated more highly with the actual intensity of genuine than faked pain expressions. Taken together, these findings suggest that observers may be particularly sensitive to genuine expressions of pain behavior. As Prkachin suggests, observers do not make judgments about the genuineness of pain-related facial expressions solely on the basis of intensity, but appear to attend to other factors, perhaps temporal or configural, in arriving at judgments about the aversiveness of the experience.

More research is needed to understand how observers make judgments about pain behavior. An observer's level of experience with persons having persistent pain may play an important role in the judgment process. Naive observers may use different criteria in making judgments about pain behavior than do spouses or clinicians who work with chronic pain patients. Studying these judgment processes in different groups of observers may help us better understand how they respond to patients having persistent pain.

CONCLUSIONS

The pain behavior concept has had a major impact on chronic pain management. This concept has led to the development of new behavioral treatment methods and new approaches to behavioral assessment. The theoretical formulations of pain behavior have evolved substantially over the past 20 years. While pain behavior concepts have been criticized, many of the criticisms are based on early theoretical models that have since been revised. Research has underscored the role that biological, social, and psychological variables can play in controlling pain behavior. Further advances in research and treatment can be expected in the coming years. These advances are likely to foster an even greater appreciation of the complexity and richness of the pain behavior concept.

REFERENCES

Affleck, G., Tennen, H., Urrows, S. and Higgins, P., Individual differences in the day-to-day experience of chronic pain: a prospective daily study of rheumatoid arthritis patients, Health Psychol., 10 (1991) 419–426.

Affleck, G., Tennen, H., Urrows, S. and Higgins, P., Neuroticism and the pain-mood relation in rheumatoid arthritis: insights from a prospective daily study, J. Consul. Clin. Psychol., 60 (1992) 119–126.

Ahles, T.A., Coombs, D.W., Jensen, L., Stukel, T., Maurer, L.H. and Keefe, F.J., Development of a behavior observation technique for the assessment of pain behaviors in cancer patients, Behav. Ther., 21 (1990) 449–460.

Anderson, K.O., Bradley, L.A., McDaniel, L.K., Young, L.D., Turner, R.A., Agudelo, C.A., Keefe, F.J., Pisko, E.J., Snyder, R.M. and Semble, E.L., The assessment of pain in rheumatoid arthritis: validity of a behavioral observation method, Arthritis Rheum., 30 (1987) 36–43.

Cairns, D., Thomas, L., Mooney, V. and Pace, J.B., A comprehensive treatment approach to

chronic low back pain, Pain, 2 (1976) 301–308.
Caudill, M., Schnable, R., Zuttermeister, P., Benson, H. and Friedman, R., Decreased clinic use by chronic pain patients: response to behavioral medicine intervention, Clin. J. Pain, 7 (1991) 305–310.
Chaney, E.F., O'Leary, M.R. and Marlatt, G.A., Skill training with alcoholics, J. Consul. Clin. Psychol., 46 (1978) 1092–1104.
Cinciripini, P.M. and Floreen, A., An evaluation of a behavioral program for chronic pain, J. Behav. Med., 5 (1982) 375–389.
Feuerstein, M. and Fitzgerald, T.E., Biomechanical factors affecting upper extremity cumulative trauma disorders in sign language interpreters, J. Occup. Med., 34 (1992) 257–263.
Follick, M.J., Ahern, D.K. and Laser-Wolston, N., Evaluation of a daily activity dairy for chronic pain patients, Pain, 19 (1984) 373–382.
Follick, M.J., Ahern, D.K., Laser-Wolston, N., Adams, A.E. and Molloy, A.J., An electromechanical recording device for the measurement of "uptime" or "downtime' in chronic pain patients, Arch. Phys. Med. Rehab., 66 (1985) 75–79.
Fordyce, W.E., Behavioral Methods for Chronic Pain and Illness, C.V. Mosby, Saint Louis, 1976.
Fordyce, W.E., Environmental factors in the genesis of low back pain. In: J.J. Bonica, J.E. Liebeskind and D.G. Albe-Fessard (Eds.), Proceedings of the Second World Congress on Pain. Advances in Pain Research and Therapy, Vol. 3. Raven Press, New York, 1979, pp 659–666.
Fordyce, W.E., Brockaway, J.A., Bergman, J.A. and Spengler, D., Acute back pain: a control-group comparison of behavioral vs traditional management methods, J. Behav. Med., 9 (1986) 127–140.
Fordyce, W.E., Fowler, R.S., Lehmann, J.R., DeLateur, B.J., Sand, P.L. and Trieschmann, R.B., Operant conditioning in the treatment of chronic pain, Arch. Phys. Med. Rehab., 54 (1973) 399–408.
Hall, S.M., Rugg, D., Tunstall, C. and Jones, R.T., Preventing relapse to cigarette smoking by behavioral skills training, J. Consul. Clin. Psychol., 52 (1984) 372–382.
Hops, H., Biglan, A., Tolman, A., Arthur, J., Sherman, L., Warner, P., Romano, J., Turner, J., Friedman, L., Bulcroft, R., Holcomb, C., Oosternink, N. and Osteen, V., Living in Family Environments (LIFE) Coding System, rev. ed., Oregon Research Institute, Eugene, Ore., 1990.
Kanfer, F.H. and Schefft, B.K., Guiding the Process of Therapeutic Change, Research Press, Champaign, Ill., 1988.
Keefe, F.J, Behavioral measurement of pain. In: C.R. Chapman and J.D. Loeser (Eds.), Issues in Pain Measurement, Raven Press, New York, 1989, pp. 405–424.
Keefe, F.J. and Block, A.R., Development of an observation method for assessing behaviors in chronic low back pain patients, Behav. Ther., 13 (1982) 363–375.
Keefe, F.J. and Dunsmore, J., Pain behavior: concepts and controversies, Am. Pain. Soc. J., 1 (1992a) 92–100.
Keefe, F.J. and Dunsmore, J., The multifaceted nature of pain behavior, Am. Pain. Soc. J., 1 (1992b) 112–114.
Keefe, F.J. and Gil, K.M., Behavioral concepts in the analysis of chronic pain syndromes, J. Consul. Clin. Psychol., 54 (1986) 776–783.
Keefe, F.J. and Hill, R.W., An objective approach to quantifying pain behavior and gait pattern in low back pain patients, Pain, 21 (1985) 153–161.
Keefe, F.J. and Van Horn, Y., Cognitive-behavioral treatment of rheumatoid arthritis pain: understanding and enhancing maintenance of treatment gains, Arthritis Care Res., 6 (1993) 213–222.
Keefe, F.J. and Williams, D.A., Pain behavior assessment. In: D.C. Turk and R. Melzack (Eds.), Handbook of Pain Assessment, Guilford Press, New York, 1992, pp. 275–294.

Keefe, F.J., Kopel, S.A. and Gordon, S.B., A practical guide to behavioral assessment, Springer, New York, 1978.

Keefe, F.J., Wilkins, R.H. and Cook, W.A., Direct observation of pain behavior in low back pain patients during physical examination, Pain, 20 (1984) 59–68.

Keefe, F.J., Wilkins, R.H., Cook, W.A., Crisson, J.E. and Mulbhaier, L.H., Depression, pain, and pain behavior, J. Consul. Clin. Psychol., 54 (1986) 665–669.

Keefe, F.J., Caldwell, D.S., Queen, K.T., Gil, K.M., Martinez, S., Crisson, J.E., Ogden, W. and Nunley, J., Osteoarthritic knee pain: a behavioral analysis, Pain, 28 (1987) 309–321.

Marlatt, G.A. and Gordon, J.R., Relapse prevention: maintenance strategies in the treatment of addictive behaviors, Guilford Press, New York, 1985.

Morell, E.M. and Keefe, F.J., The actometer: an evaluation of instrument applicability for chronic pain patients, Pain, 32 (1988) 265–270.

Patterson, S.M., Krantz, D.S., Montgomery, L.C., Deuster, P.A., Hedges, S.M. and Nebel, L.E., Automated physical activity monitoring: validation and comparison with physiological and self-report measures, Psychophysiology, 30 (1993) 296–305.

Perri, M.G., Shapiro, R.M., Ludwig, W.W., Twentyman, C.T. and McAdoo, W.G., Maintenance strategies for the treatment of obesity: an evaluation of relapse prevention training and posttreatment contact by mail and telephone, J. Consul. Clin. Psychol., 52 (1984) 404–413.

Prkachin, K.M., Dissociating spontaneous and deliberate expressions of pain: Signal detection analyses, Pain, 51 (1992) 57–65.

Richards, R., Nepomuneco, C., Riles, M. and Suer, A., Assessing pain behavior: the UAB pain behavior scale, Pain, 14 (1982) 393–398.

Romano, J.M., Turner, J.A., Friedman, L.S., Bulcroft, R.A., Jensen, M.P. and Hops, H., Observational assessment of chronic pain patient-spouse behavioral interactions, Behav. Ther., 22 (1991) 549–567.

Romano, J.M., Turner, J.A., Friedman, L.S., Bulcroft, R.A., Jensen, M.P., Hops, H. and Wright, S.F., Sequential analysis of chronic pain behaviors and spouse responses, J. Consul. Clin. Psychol., 60 (1992) 777–782.

Sanders, S., Toward a practical instrument system for the automatic measurement of "uptime" in chronic pain patients, Pain, 9 (1980) 103–109.

Sanders, S.H., Automated versus self-monitoring of "up-time" in chronic low back pain patients: a comparative study, Pain, 15 (1983) 399–406.

Schefft, B.K. and Lehr, B.K., A self-regulatory model of adjunctive behavior change, Behav. Modif., 9 (1985) 458–476.

Sternbach, R.A., Treatment of the chronic pain patient, J. Hum. Stress, 4 (1978) 11–15.

Tryon, W.W., Measurement of human activity. In: W.W. Tryon (Ed.), Behavioral Assessment in Behavioral Medicine, Springer, New York, 1985, pp. 200–206.

Turk, D.C., Meichenbaum, D. and Genest, M., Pain and behavioral medicine: a cognitive behavioral perspective, Guilford Press, New York, 1983.

Turner, J.A., Comparison of group progressive-relaxation training and cognitive-behavioral therapy for chronic low back pain, J. Consul. Clin. Psychol., 50 (1982) 757–765.

Williams, D.A. and Thorn, B.E., An empirical assessment of pain beliefs, Pain, 36 (1989) 351–358.

Correspondence to: Francis J. Keefe, PhD, Department of Psychiatry, Pain Management Program, Box 3159, Duke University Medical Center, Durham, NC 27710, USA. Tel: 919-684-6212; Fax: 919-684-8629.

Proceedings of the 7th World Congress on Pain,
Progress in Pain Research and Management, Vol. 2,
edited by G.F. Gebhart, D.L. Hammond, and T.S.
Jensen, IASP Press, Seattle, © 1994.

11

The Challenge of Preventing Chronic Musculoskeletal Pain

Steven J. Linton

Department of Occupational and Environmental Medicine,
Örebro Medical Center, Örebro, Sweden

INTRODUCTION

The challenge of preventing chronic musculoskeletal pain (MSP) is an enticing aim that appears to be essential if we are to come to grips with this escalating problem. In spite of a lack of detailed knowledge about the complexities of MSP, there is nevertheless information relevant to prevention that presents a challenge in two areas. The first is to develop screening procedures that would help us efficiently identify persons at risk. The second challenge is to implement early interventions to prevent chronic problems.

Mastering these two areas would provide the ideal framework for effective secondary prevention from the health care provider's perspective. In this chapter I define secondary prevention as interventions taken between the first treatment for acute pain until a full chronic problem has developed (Fig. 1). I will focus on secondary forms of prevention because they are most relevant for health care professionals. This chapter provides an overview, rather than detailed review, of the latest trends in preventive strategies for MSP problems and risk factors relevant for screening and preventive interventions.

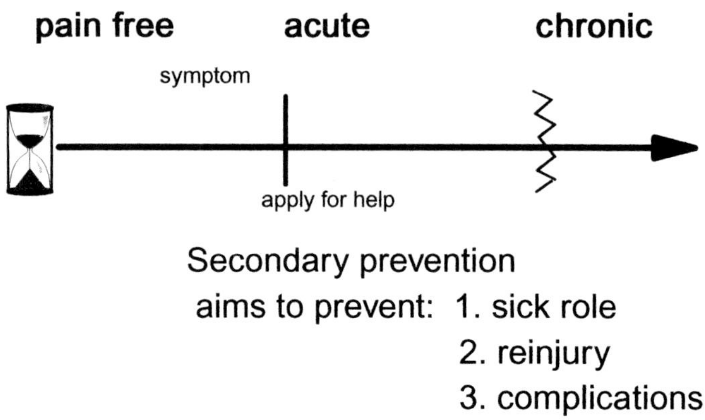

Fig. 1. The temporal aspect of the development of chronic pain stressing secondary prevention possibilities.

BACKGROUND

THE NEED FOR PREVENTION

It would be difficult to overstate the well-documented need for prevention, as MSP problems consume stupendous amounts of health care and compensation resources. Suffice it to say that MSP accounts for more than 25% of all sick absenteeism and is a leading consumer of health care and disability compensation resources (Bigos and Battié 1992; Linton 1992; Pope et al. 1991). Back pain alone amounts to about 20 million sick days per year in the United States and 28 million in Sweden (Nachemson 1992). The total cost has been estimated at $20–50 billion in the United States and some $10 billion in Sweden (Nachemson 1992). Coupled with the vast amount of suffering for the patient, his or her family, and friends, the malady takes on unmeasurable proportions.

However, not all patients develop chronic problems and, in fact, about 85% recover undramatically within six weeks (Frymoyer 1992). A relatively small number of patients nevertheless become chronic cases and these estimated 2–10% of the sufferers devour roughly 75–85% of the resources (Nachemson 1992). Although rehabilitation efforts are certainly of considerable value, there is little reason to believe they may be a substitute for prevention since many patients will continue to have problems or relapse (Linton 1992; Flor et al. 1992; Turk and Rudy 1991). Thus, there is a real need for the effective prevention of chronic MSP.

MODEL OF CHRONIC PAIN DEVELOPMENT

Fordyce (1976) was among the first to describe how learning factors may influence the development of chronic problems. A key concept is what happens between acute injury and a fully developed chronic problem. It has become increasingly clear that for MSP, progressive diseases are the rare exception rather than the rule (Frymoyer 1992; Nachemson 1992). Instead, Fordyce (1976) suggested that as healing occurs over time, cognitive-behavioral processes may nevertheless support pain behaviors so that the problem persists or is actually exacerbated. Indeed, in Western society pain complaints may be reinforced with attention, medication, relief of responsibility, and treatments according to the principle that the greater the number and intensity of pain behaviors the more attention and treatment. A central process may be the reinforcement of passive behaviors, i.e., that behaviors such as resting, reading, and watching television, which may be pleasant and associated with little or no pain, become predominant. Moreover, patients may learn to avoid many taxing everyday activities, leading to a new and comparatively passive lifestyle. In addition, social (e.g., decreased contact) and cognitive (e.g., seeing oneself as handicapped) changes constitute a full-fledged sick role in which one might say that the patient makes a career out of his or her problem. Vital to this process is a substantial period of time to allow these factors an opportunity to operate.

THE PROBLEM OF PREVENTION

If prevention is so badly needed, why then haven't prevention programs been put forward more aggressively? At least three intricate problems appear to have impeded their development. The first is the matter of definitions. In the usual medical situation there is a fairly strictly defined biological state that is to be prevented. However, this is not the case with MSP. Consequently, we may ask what we should be preventing: tissue damage, a disease process, dysfunction, or the experience of pain itself. Chronic pain is not a single disease, but a collection of several problems mostly defined by symptoms. Using the theoretical model outlined above, researchers have often pragmatically defined what is to be prevented as: reinjury, development of the sick role, and complications due to insufficient self-care skills. Thus, the aim is most often to prevent dysfunction rather than a biological disease process.

The coordination of services is a second stumbling block retarding development because preventive action usually requires contributions from several clinics and agencies, as well as the family, friends, and workplace. Practitioners then, may not have the authority or feel that it is their responsibility to attempt prevention, and the enormity of the undertaking in itself may hinder initiation. Economic issues also may be involved in that those institutions incurring the costs may not be those reaping the benefits.

Another obstacle in preventive work is the logistics of doing methodologically proper preventive research. This type of research requires prospective studies with rather large, representative populations that need to be followed with a well-defined protocol over periods of one to five years.

RISK FACTORS AND SCREENING

The first challenge in preventing chronic MSP is identifying patients at risk. The usual course of prevention is to identify risk factors and subsequently to initiate an intervention to modify these factors. The public health approach, which has stressed primary prevention and manipulation of the environment, has not yet proved effective for MSP (Spitzer 1993; Wickström 1992). Most health-care providers are attuned to the clinical approach where observed signs in a patient represent risk appraisal and early treatment the prevention strategy. The search for risk factors has been conducted from various perspectives. It is important to recognize that investigations may study risks for different results such as poor treatment outcome, poor compliance, development of chronic problems (for acute patients), or reinjury. These studies also may involve diverse populations, including patients whose problems are chronic, prechronic, or acute, and the general population.

Risk factors used for screening patients should fulfill several requirements. These include the usual psychometric qualities of reliability, validity, and sensitivity/specificity. Moreover, the method should be relatively inexpensive and easy to administer and interpret. At best, a screening procedure based on demonstrated risk factors would identify patients likely to develop chronic problems or relapse and would provide valuable information concerning successful intervention.

RISK FACTORS

Several risk factors primarily for back pain have emerged during the past decade. Table I summarizes the variables in the categories of medical, demographic, psychosocial, and work and family. Unfortunately, most medical (e.g., duration of pain, surgeries) and demographic factors (e.g., age, gender, education level) are difficult or impossible to alter. Thus, while they may predict disability, they do not provide a route for intervention. A common observation, moreover, is that medical and demographic factors tend to be of lesser

Table I
An overview of risk factors for the development of chronic musculoskeletal pain

Area	Example
Medical	pain duration treatment history
Demographic	age gender employability
Psychosocial	psychopathology pain perception/beliefs pain behaviors/dysfunction
Work and Family	support for return

importance than previously believed and that psychosocial factors including work and the family may be central (Bigos and Battié 1992; Frymoyer 1992; Linton 1992; Nachemson 1992). This chapter examines the various risk areas, stressing those that may be most relevant for screening.

MEDICAL FACTORS

Several physical and diagnostic variables associated with MSP problems might be used to predict disability (Burton and Tollotson 1991), including the number of previous surgeries, duration of the pain problem, and history of disability (absenteeism) (Frymoyer 1992; Nachemson 1992). In fact, the report of back pain is often the best predictor of future back injury reports (e.g., Biering-Sörensen 1984; Bigos and Battié 1992; Deyo and Diehl 1988). However, the medical diagnosis has had relatively little impact. Most patients are given a nonspecific diagnosis and only about 1% have what might be termed serious, medically treatable maladies such as tumors, infections, or fractures (Frymoyer 1992). Other factors that may be important are spinal range of motion, straight leg raising impairments, absence of neurologic abnormalities, and reduced muscle strength. Indeed, the role of muscle strength has been heatedly debated. While many chronic sufferers undoubtably have reduced strength, only a few prospective studies have examined strength as a potential risk factor. Although Cady et al. (1979) report a connection between strength and back pain, the Boeing study that prospectively followed more than 3000 employees showed no significant association between back injury and strength, flexibility, or aerobic capacity (Battié et al. 1989). The most singular aspect of the few prospective studies to date has been the absence or low degree of a relationship between physical variables and the incidence of MSP (Bigos and Battié 1992).

Demographic Variables

Age, education, and gender have been repeatedly reported to be associated with disability and pain. However, the mechanism as well as the potency of the relationship is unclear (Biering-Sörensen 1984; Deyo and Diehl 1988; Frymoyer 1992; Heliövaara 1989; Vällfors 1985). Low education and income also have been regarded as risk factors, although they are confounded by occupation as less educated people tend to have greater physical demands at work.

PSYCHOLOGICAL VARIABLES

Psychopathology, pain behaviors, and cognitions have been suggested as fundamental variables in the development of chronic MSP. Psychopathology historically has been assessed most often by the Minnesota Multiphasic Personality Inventory (MMPI). Although the MMPI reliably indicates the "neurotic triad" of elevated hypochondriasis, depression, and hysteria in chronic patients, it lacks discriminant validity and therefore is of questionable use in risk assessment (McCreary et al. 1977). Depression, anxiety, and elevated somatic awareness, termed distress, also are related to MSP problems. Main and coworkers (1992) for instance, have shown that scores on the Modified Somatic Perception Questionnaire and the Modified Zung Depression Index may be used to classify patients seeking orthopedic help into four groups based on the level of risk involved for poor outcome. The mechanism is not clear, but these patients may not be as prepared as others to deal with a pain problem.

The level of pain behavior and function a patient exhibits seems to be tied directly to the development of a chronic MSP problem. A system of pain behavior measurement is an excellent way to assess current pain status and treatment outcome (Dworkin and Whitney 1992) and studies of pain behavior suggest a relationship with MSP problems (Keefe and Williams 1992; Talo et al. 1992; Turner, et al. 1983). Theoretically, pain behaviors are believed to be instrumental in the development of avoidance (Fordyce 1976; Waddell and Turk 1992) and consequently may be potent indicators of risk for chronic MSP development. In some studies, scores on the nonorganic signs test that evaluates some specific "inappropriate" pain behaviors in the clinic (Main et al. 1992; Waddell and Turk 1992) increased with the amount of failed treatment (LaCroix et al. 1990; Waddell et al. 1984). However, Bradish et al. (1988) in a clinical trial found no correlation between the nonorganic signs and activity levels one year later.

Several lines of recent research suggest that a patient's perceptions, attributions, beliefs, and coping style (i.e., cognitions) may serve as key screening factors. Pain cognitions apparently set the stage for actual behavior and consequently appear to be important predictors of future behavior. A patient's beliefs about the relationship between pain and activity provide a relevant illustration. Jensen and Karoly (1992) have found that patients' perceptions of themselves as disabled are inversely related to activity level for chronic sufferers. They reported that a belief that activity exacerbates pain predicted activity level, psychological functioning, and health care utilization. Riley et al. (1988) found that scores on the Pain and Impairment Relationship Scale, which consists of 15 statements about one's ability to function despite pain, demonstrated a significant correlation to functional impairment, and were replicated by Slater et al. (1991).

A more specific assessment of fear and avoidance of activities focuses on the patient's belief about how physical activity and work would affect back pain (Waddell et al. 1993). These authors demonstrated that fear-avoidance beliefs concerning work were strongly related to absenteeism due to back pain. Moreover, this fear-avoidance was identified with a questionnaire containing just 16 items.

Negative cognitions also have been reported to be related to developing pain problems. Reesor and Craig (1988), for instance, found that maladaptive thoughts were the major difference between chronic pain patients with and without maladaptive signs. Williams and Thorn (1989) demonstrated that with chronic pain patients the negative factors of self-blame, pain as a mystery, and enduring pain predicted treatment outcome. Pain-elicited affective responses also have been found to predict future headaches (LaCroix and Barbaree 1992). Moreover, Gil et al. (1990) have shown that patients with chronic pain actually have more frequent negative thoughts than do patients with intermittent pain, while Partridge and Johnston (1989) found that perceived control of recovery is associated with actual recovery rates. Finally, Boston et al. (1990) found a clear correlation between negative cognitions and measures of pain intensity, distress and disruption.

The above data on negative cognitions agree with results concerning coping strategies in which patients who do not catastrophize, believe they can control their pain, and do not define themselves as disabled function substantially better than do those who do not (Jensen et al. 1991). However, to date no studies in the pain coping literature have prospectively followed subjects to determine who develops persistent pain (Keefe et al. 1992).

Work and Family

Support from family and work associates may be an important aspect of recovery. Job satisfaction, work demands, and above all relations with co-workers and supervisors are fairly strongly related to injuries and problems in returning to work (Bigos et al. 1991, 1992; Linton 1990; Nachemson 1992). Bigos et al. (1991) found job satisfaction to be a strong predictor of acute injury while Linton and Bradley (1992), as well as Feuerstein and Thebarge (1991), found supervisor support to be a central factor related to return to work. Keep in mind that Waddell et al.'s (1993) findings above concerning fear of return to work also are relevant. Thus, the work environment including social relations, work demands, and content may hinder or assist patients in their efforts to return to a normal life. Similarly, the family may provide a source of support for the patient's recovery, or vice versa, and may be related to the actual development of the problem (Bradley et al. 1992; Romano et al. 1991).

SCREENING

Despite the isolation of several risk factors, there have been problems in developing a successful screening methodology. This situation is illustrated by the attempt of Lehmann and colleagues (1993) to prospectively predict return to work among 55 patients with occupationally related low back pain of two to six weeks' duration. Using physical examinations and an extensive battery of questionnaires, they found few correlations with chronicity, but nevertheless concluded that patients who perceive their pain as being work-related and who have been off work for more than two weeks are at high risk. One problem in developing screening techniques is the diversity of patient populations in relation to the large number of risk variables, which may result in poor sensitivity or specificity. While several risk factors are undoubtably correlated, to date it has been difficult to reduce the number of factors and maintain accuracy. Although a set of factors may successfully classify 75% of a research population with regard to risk for chronic development, the "misses" nevertheless represent a significant number of people. Moreover, one might expect the accuracy to decrease when the technique is applied clinically where patient populations may be more heterogenous. However, Iezzi et al. (1992) maintain, based on their results from a cross-sectional study, that it should be possible to screen for problem patients shortly after injury. These researchers found that psychological variables could be used to discriminate between healthy controls, dysfunctional, and functional chronic low back pain patients.

Unfortunately, current practice often means that no systematic screening is conducted at all, or that only the duration of disability is employed in a risk analysis. This is paradoxical because waiting until a patient has been off work, for example, three to six months may signify that the development of a chronic condition is already well underway. Moreover, basing screening only on the time factor would seem to be an ineffective use of resources. Not in the least, many patients have relapses with increasing amounts of sick leave (Biering-Sörensen 1984; Rossignol et al. 1992), and screening based on such a time factor obviously would not detect these patients at an early point.

With the knowledge available today, more efficient methods of screening should be possible. A suitable method probably will provide a graded evaluation, just as cardiovascular risk is assessed, rather than an all or none statement. Psychosocial variables, in addition, would seem to be relevant and most likely central to the screening, thus underscoring the need for patients and health care workers alike to understand that:

1. risk factors are not necessarily causal factors, but may be factors that maintain or catalyze chronic problems, and
2. identification of risk factors ought to be used to help the patient, i.e., to provide better care.

To date there is no accepted, standard screening device. As noted, many risk factors have been reported and some bold attempts have been made to develop screening methods. Thus, while the challenge of developing an efficient screening method remains, its resolution appears to be within reach.

PREVENTIVE INTERVENTIONS

The second challenge we face in preventing chronic MSP is providing effective interventions. In spite of the lack of standardized risk appraisal, several attempts have been made to prevent the development of MSP. These studies have keyed on the time factor (i.e., the amount of time off work or since injury). Consequently, we shall begin with those programs designed for "prechronics" and work our way toward those meant for acute pain problems.

FUNCTIONAL RESTORATION

Work hardening or functional restoration programs might be considered as a preventive strategy since they usually are oriented toward patients having pain at least three to four months (i.e., on the borderline of being a chronic pain patient). The functional restoration approach stresses reconditioning and is designed to maximize the person's ability to return to work.

An outcome evaluation of this type of program for upper extremity disorders illustrates this type of treatment. Feuerstein et al. (1993) compared two similar groups of patients with one group receiving multidisciplinary restoration while the other group received care as usual. A comprehensive work reentry program, designed to facilitate a transition from disability to work, emphasized attitudes and health behaviors. Over a four to six week period, patients participated in physical conditioning, work simulation/conditioning, work-related pain and stress management, and ergonomic consultation. Subjects in the usual care group were managed by their primary care physician. At a 17-month follow-up, 74% of the restoration group had returned to work compared to 40% for the treatment as usual reference group. The authors noted the need for modifications in the workplace to maximize long-term results for the restoration group.

The above data are fairly typical of work hardening programs, which report that 55–85% of their patients return to work (Hazard et al. 1991). However, patients are typically off work several months before entering these programs (Feuerstein et al. averaged eight months off work), and thus they are probably not preventive in nature. Nevertheless, the application of work restoration programs at the minimum disability criteria of three months, which several programs use, may prove to be of interest as a preventive measure.

SUBACUTE PAIN PATIENTS

Several attempts have been made to identify patients with subacute pain and to provide subsequent interventions that, in addition to treating the pain, might prevent the problem from becoming chronic. Occupational health care services have been used to identify nurses at risk for developing chronic back pain because these nurses had been taking increasing amounts of sick leave for the pain (Linton et al. 1989). Then, participants were randomly assigned to either a waiting-list control or a group receiving a five-week program of physical and behavioral therapy aimed at preventing reinjury and minor pains from becoming medical problems. Results at a six-month follow-up demonstrated that the treatment group had significantly greater improvements than did the control group on virtually every variable (e.g., pain intensity, sleep, observed pain behaviors, mood, activities, and helplessness). Moreover, the intervention broke an upward trend in pain-related sick leave, suggesting that secondary prevention may be effective.

Lindström et al. (1992) have shown that a behavioral approach to reconditioning patients with subacute low back pain is quite effective. A considerable proportion of those off work for more than eight weeks develop chronic problems, so Lindström et al. (1992) randomly assigned such patients to an "as usual" treatment group or an "early" activation group. The activation group received measurement of functional capacity, a workplace visit, participation in a back school, and an individualized exercise program based on operant learning principles. Results indicated that the activation group returned to work earlier and had significantly less sick leave during follow-up than did the controls as illustrated in Fig. 2. Although sick leave for back pain still occurred, this study clearly indicates that a broad-based intervention at the subacute stage emphasizing an operant-based exercise program produces less sick leave relative to usual treatment methods.

A similar result was found in a 12-center trial of early activation and education started an average of 41 days after injury. These patients returned to work earlier and accumulated less costs than did matched controls (Mitchell et al. 1990).

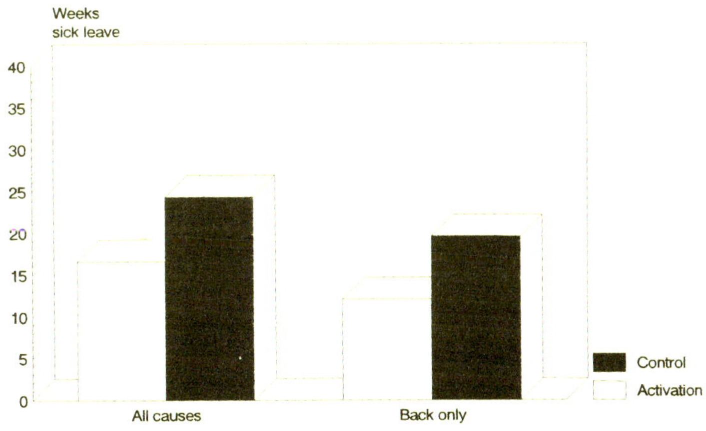

Fig. 2. Sick absenteeism (all causes and back pain related), for patients with subacute pain, during the second year of follow-up for the treatment as usual control group and the early activation group in the study by Lindström et al. (1992).

ACUTE PAIN PATIENTS

Rather than waiting to see which patients relapse or continue to have problems, another approach is to attempt to prevent chronic pain by providing proper care the first time the patient seeks help. Fordyce and colleagues (1986) reported on the effects of behaviorally oriented management of acute back pain. They randomly assigned 107 patients with pain onset during the preceding 10 days to one of two groups. The control group received treatment as usual with analgesics and activity recommendations on an as needed, pain-contingent basis. The behavioral group, however, made use of time-contingencies so as to avoid reinforcing pain behaviors and the sick role. Analgesics, if used at all, were to be taken on a fixed-time schedule, and the prescription was limited. Similarly, activity limits, if any, were based on a physician-specified time interval, and exercises were to be done at fixed times. Results at the 9 to 12-month follow-up showed that while the traditional treatment group had increased levels of claimed impairment, the behavioral group had returned to pre-onset levels. Certainly, this study demonstrates that the method of caring for patients with acute back pain has an effect on the development of impairment and consequently may be used to promote (back) health.

Another approach to acute management for the prevention of chronic problems was based at the workplace. Haig et al. (1990) compared results of previous treatment methods at a tertiary care hospital with a new program for employees off work two days or more for MSP. The treatment attempted to establish good communication with the patient, identified factors delaying return, and maintained regular communication with the workplace to enhance a modified return to work. Overall, the new program, as compared to earlier care, resulted in a 33% improvement in return to work. Although this report suggests that a workplace-based early intervention that primarily addresses communication and return-to-work issues may be an effective preventive measure, the study is restricted by its uncontrolled design and limited outcome measures.

In our own work (Linton et al. 1993) we have investigated the effects of an early, active, behavioral intervention designed to prevent first-time acute pain from developing into a chronic problem. We randomly assigned 198 patients seeking health care for acute MSP to either a treatment as usual control group or an early, active behavioral treatment group. The early treatment reinforced functional and other "well" behaviors and underscored the importance of maintaining everyday activities and a return to work. Usual treatment consisted of a prescription for analgesics and advice to rest, both on an as needed basis. Records indicated that about half the patients had a history of previous sick leave for pain (Study I), while half were first-time

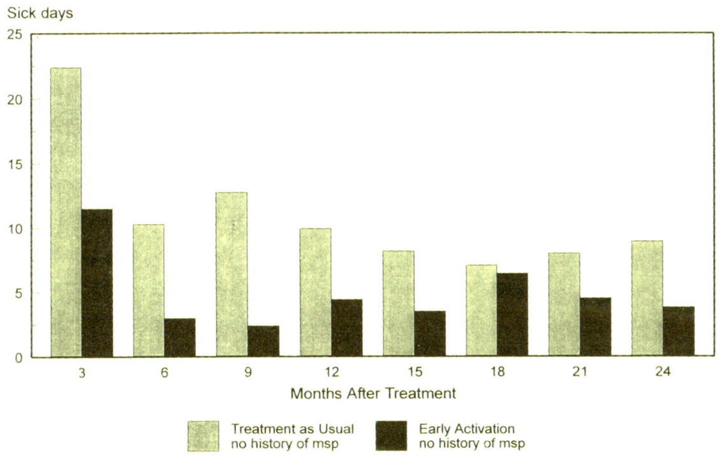

Fig. 3. Mean number of sick absenteeism days for MSP per quarter during a two-year follow-up for "first-time" sufferers of acute MSP showing the difference between usual treatment and early activation. (Data for the first year are from Linton et al. 1993; data from the second year have not been previously published.)

sufferers (Study II). For those with a previous history of pain (Study I), both groups improved greatly at the one-year follow-up as compared to pretest, but there were virtually no differences between the groups.

However while both groups of first-timers (Study II) also made great improvements, the early, active behavioral group had significantly less sick leave relative to the control group as shown in Fig. 3. The risk of developing chronic pain, moreover, was reduced by more than eight-fold. This finding suggests that relatively small changes in acute pain treatment routines may prevent the development of chronic problems. Also, the results suggest that the content and timing of the treatment apparently are critical because those with previous pain problems did not benefit in the same way was did first-timers.

Even though several studies have shown that early interventions can be effective, not all results have been positive. For example, Cherkin et al. (1991) provided an educational program for physicians meant to improve the primary care of back pain. Despite the course's perceived benefit to doctors, there was no actual improvement in patient outcome, possibly indicating that information alone is not sufficient in changing routine care.

Likewise, Greenwood et al. (1990) found that an early program of claims management provided by the Worker's Compensation Fund actually resulted in increased costs. This finding shows, once again, that the mere fact that an intervention is provided early is not sufficient for improving outcome.

Finally, the use of an early exercise program was found to be no better than an ultrasound placebo treatment (Faas et al. 1993). Acute back pain patients received ultrasound, treatment by a physician, or an exercise program, but no substantial differences were found between the groups. Contrary to much current thinking, Faas et al. concluded that exercise therapy should not be recommended. This study may indicate that exercise, in itself, is not a sufficient ingredient in prevention.

SUMMARY OF INTERVENTION RESULTS

Several studies have shown positive results, and overall a pattern emerges where the application of learning factors from the cognitive-behavioral conception of the development of chronic pain seems to be a decisive element in successful programs. Examples have been presented that show the timing itself (i.e., an early intervention) was not sufficient. Moreover, some programs using singular approaches (e.g., exercise or case management) did not produce significantly better improvements than did control conditions. Thus, while the timing of the intervention seems to be important, the content of the program relative to the type of patient also appears to be significant.

One plausible explanation for the diversity of results may be that some programs, although initiated early, actually inadvertently reinforce pain behavior. The attention, for instance, a patient receives in the acute or subacute programs may not be provided on a well-behavior contingency. These early treatment programs, in addition, may provide more contact with health-care providers and thus more opportunities to be sick listed. Patients may cognitively interpret the "new, sudden, and thorough" interest in their MSP problem as confirmation of a significant illness, if the attention is provided noncontingently or pain-contingent. Even exercise therapy may inadvertently reinforce pain behavior if proper contingency management is not practiced. Fordyce et al. (1989), for example, were careful in stressing fixed-time contingencies for medication and exercise rather than as needed, pain-based contingencies. Thus, the details of the method of administration may be central to the results obtained. If this speculation holds true, it not only might explain differences in reported results, but provide an avenue to enhance current programs.

Another common denominator of successful programs may be their emphasis on good communication, workplace contacts, and follow-up. Most of the programs reporting significant gains included information/communication with the patient and most often some sort of contact with the workplace. The latter often was used to enhance an early return to work and alter any barriers that might exist at work. The need for follow-up is obvious and requires little articulation. Put directly, almost all patients who develop chronic MSP have a considerable previous history of health care seeking and absenteeism, and consequently proper follow-up might be an excellent tool in prevention programs. Furthermore, relapse may often be related to poor adherence. Thus follow-up would provide an extraordinary opportunity to detect patients at risk and maintain effective intervention. Ultimately, follow-up may oil the wheels of the patient's readjustment to a normal lifestyle.

RECAPITULATION

The humanitarian as well as socioeconomic and medical need for the prevention of chronic MSP is urgent. Effective secondary prevention seems to be within our grasp if we can meet the challenge of screening, providing very early interventions matched to patients' needs, and finally follow-up each case sufficiently to enhance maintenance and prevent relapse. Substantial gains have been made in identifying potent risk factors that are relevant for clinical risk appraisal. Yet, to date there is no accepted methodology for screening. Therefore, preventive treatment has keyed on the time factor only, stressing early, active treatments to counter the development of the sick role. Promising results have been reported for prechronic, subacute, and acute pain problems, indicating that changes in the delivery of care may result in distinct improvements. Proper treatment of acute MSP patients seeking help for the first time, for example, may reduce the risk of becoming a chronic sufferer by eight-fold as compared to usual treatment.

Negative findings, however, also have been reported, and an analysis suggests that the content and timing of care in relation to the type of patient is crucial. Moreover, programs that are broad-based and conducted according to cognitive-behavioral principles seem to obtain the best results. Finally, the need for thorough follow-up was underscored as a method of preventing relapse, maintaining adherence and detecting problem patients early on.

We must continue to make bold attempts to meet the challenge of preventing chronic MSP. Knowledge to date has laid a good foundation, but the house is yet to be built.

REFERENCES

Battié, M.C., Bigos, S.J., Fisher, L.D., Hansson, T.H., Jones M.E. and Wortley, M., Isometric lifting strength as a predictor of industrial back pain reports, Spine, 4 (1989) 851–856.

Biering-Sörensen, F., A One-Year Prospective Study of Low Back Trouble in a General Population, Danish Medical Association, Copenhagen, 1984.

Bigos, S.J. and Battié, M.C., Risk factors for industrial back problems, Seminars in Spine Surgery, 4 (1992) 2–11.

Bigos, S.J., Battié, M.C., Spengler, D.M., Fisher, L.D., Fordyce, W.E., Hansson, T.H., Nachemson, A.L. and Wortley, M.D., A prospective study of work perceptions and psychosocial factors affecting the report of back injury, Spine, 16 (1991) 1–6.

Boston, K, Pearce, S.A. and Richardson, P.H., The pain cognitions questionnaire, J. Psychosom. Res., 34 (1990) 103–109.

Bradish, C.F., Lloyd, G.J., Aldam, C.H., Albert, J., Dyson, P., Doxey, N.C.S. and Mitson, G.L., Do nonorganic signs help to predict the return to activity of patients with low-back pain? Spine, 13 (1988) 557–560.

Bradley, L.A., Haile, J.M. and Jaworski, T.M., Assessment of psychological status using interviews and self-report instruments. In: D.C. Turk and R. Melzack (Eds.), Handbook of Pain Assessment, Guilford, New York, 1992, pp. 193–213.

Burton, A.K. and Tillotson, K.M., Prediction of the clinical course of low-back trouble using multivariable models, Spine, 16 (1991) 7–14.

Cady, L.D., Bischoff, D.P. and O'Connell, E.R., Strength and fitness and subsequent back injuries of firefighters, J. Occup. Med., 21 (1979) 269–272.

Cherkin, E., Deyo, R.A. and Berg, A.O., Evaluation of a physician education intervention to improve primary care for low-back pain. II. Impact on patients, Spine, 16 (1991) 1173–1178.

Deyo, R.A. and Diehl, A.K., Psychosocial predictors of disability in patients with low back pain, J. Rheumatol., 15 (1988) 1557–1564.

Dworkin, S.F. and Whitney, C.W., Relying on objective and subjective measures of chronic pain: guidelines for use and interpretation. In: D.C. Turk and R. Melzack (Eds.), Handbook of Pain Assessment, Guilford, New York, 1992, pp. 429–446.

Faas, A., Chavannes, A.W., van Eijk, J.T.M. and Gubbels, J.W., A randomized, placebo-controlled trial of exercise therapy in patients with acute low back pain, Spine, 18 (1993) 1388–1395.

Feuerstein, M. and Thebarge, R.W., Perceptions of disability and occupational stress as discriminators of work disability in patients with chronic pain, J. Occup. Rehab., 1 (1991) 185–195.

Feuerstein, M., Callan-Harris, S., Hickey, P., Dyer, D., Armbruster, W. and Carosella, A.M., Multidisciplinary rehabilitation of chronic work-related upper extremity disorders, J. Occup. Med., 35 (1993) 396–403.

Flor, H., Fydrick, T. and Turk, D.C., Efficacy of multidisciplinary pain treatment centers: a meta-analytic review, Pain, 49 (1992) 221–230.

Fordyce, W.E., Behavioral Methods for Chronic Pain and Illness, Mosby, St. Louis, 1976.

Fordyce, W.E., Brockway, J.A., Bergman, Ja.A. and Spengler, D., Acute back pain: a control-group comparison of behavioral vs traditional management methods, J. Behav. Med., 9 (1986) 127–140.

Frymoyer, J.W., Predicting disability from low back pain, Clin. Orthop., 279 (1992) 101–109.

Gil, K.M., Williams, D.A., Keefe, F.J. and Beckham, J.C., The relationship of negative thoughts to pain and psychological distress, Behav. Ther., 21 (1990) 349–362.

Greenwood, J.G., Wolf, H.J., Pearson, J.C., Woon,C.L., Posey, P. and Main, C., Early intervention in low back disability among coal miners in West Virginia: negative findings, J. Occup. Med., 32 (1990) 1047–1052.

Haig, A.J., Linton, P., McIntosh, M., Moneta, L and Mead, P.B., Aggressive early medical management by a specialist in physical medicine and rehabilitation, J. Occup. Med., 32 (1990) 241–244.

Hazard, R.G., Matheson, L.N., Lehmann, T.R. and Frymoyer, J.W., Rehabilitation of the patient with chronic low back pain. In: M.H. Pope, G.B. Andersson, J. Frymoyer and D.B. Chaffin (Eds.), Occupational Low Back Pain: Assessment,Treatment, and Prevention, Mosby-Year Book, St. Louis, 1991, pp.194–208.

Heliövaara, M., Risk factors for low back pain and sciatica, Ann. Med., 21 (1989) 257–264.

Iezzi, A., Adams, H.E., Stokes, G.S., Pilon,R.N, and Ault, L.C., An identification of low back pain groups using biobehavioral variables, J. Occup. Rehab., 2 (1992) 19–33.

Jensen, M.P. and Karoly, P., Pain-specific beliefs, perceived symptom severity, and adjustment to chronic pain, Clin. J. Pain, 8 (1992) 123–130.

Jensen, M.P., Turner, J.A., Romano, J.M. and Karoly, P., Coping with chronic pain: a critical review of the literature, Pain, 47 (1991) 249–283.

Keefe, F.J. and Williams, D.A., Assessment of pain behaviors. In: D.C. Turk and R. Melzack (Eds.), Handbook of Pain Assessment, Guilford, New York, 1992, pp. 275–294.

Keefe, F.J., Salley, A.N. and Befebvre, J.C., Coping with pain: conceptual concerns and future directions, Pain, 51 (1992) 131–134.

LaCroix, R. and Barbaree, H.E., Pain-elicited responses and their role in predicting future pain duration and severity, Behav. Res. Ther., 30 (1992) 471–478.

Lacroix, J.M., Powell, J., Lloyd, G.J., Doxey, M.C.S., Mitson, G.L. and Aldam, C.F., Low-back pain: factors of value in predicting outcome, Spine, 15 (1990) 495–499.

Lehmann, T.R., Spratt, K.F. and Lehmann, K.K., Predicting long-term disability in low back injured workers presenting to a spine consultant, Spine, 18 (1993) 1103–1112.

Lindström, I., Öhlund, C., Eek, C., Wallin, L., Peterson, L.E., Fordyce, W.E. and Nachemson, A.L., The effect of graded activity on patients with subacute low back pain: a randomized prospective clinical study with an operant-conditioning behavioral approach, Phys. Ther., 72 (1992) 279–290.

Linton, S.J., Risk factors for neck and back pain in a working population in Sweden, Work and Stress, 4 (1990) 41–49.

Linton, S.J., The behavioral management and prevention of chronic pain. In: G.R. Caddy and D.G. Byrne (Eds.), Behavioral Medicine: International Perspectives, Vol 2, Ablex Publishing, Norwood, N.J., 1992, pp.253–294.

Linton, S.J. and Bradley, L.A., An 18-month follow-up of a secondary prevention program for back pain: help and hindrance factors related to outcome maintenance, Clin. J. Pain, 8 (1992) 227–236.

Linton, S.J., Bradley, L.A., Jensen, I., Spangfort, E. and Sundell, L., The secondary prevention of low back pain: a controlled study with follow-up, Pain, 36 (1989) 197–207.

Linton, S.J., Hellsing, A.L. and Andersson, D., A controlled study of the effects of an early intervention on acute musculoskeletal pain problems, Pain, 54 (1993) 353–359.

Main, C.J., Wood, P.L.R., Hollis, S., Spanswick, C.C. and Waddell, G., The distress and risk assessment method: a simple patient classification to identify distress and evaluate the risk of poor outcome, Spine, 17 (1992) 42–52.

McCreary, C., Turner, J. and Dawson, C., Differences between functional versus organic pain patients, Pain, 4 (1977) 73–78.

Mitchell, R.I. and Carmen, G.M., Results of a multicenter trial using an intensive active exercise program for the treatment of acute soft tissue and back injuries, Spine, 15 (1990) 514–521.

Nachemson, A.L., Newest knowledge of low back pain, Clin. Orthop., 279 (1992) 8–20.

Partridge, C. and Johnston, M., Perceived control of recovery from physical disability: measurement and prediction, Br. J. Clin. Psychol., 28 (1989) 53–59.

Pope, M.H., Andersson, G.B., Frymoyer, J. and Chaffin, D.B., Occupational low back pain: assessment, treatment, and prevention, Mosby-Year Book, St. Louis, 1991.

Reesor, K.A. and Craig, K., Medically incongruent chronic back pain: physical limitations, suffering and ineffective coping, Pain, 32 (1988) 35–45.

Riley, J.F., Ahern, D.K. and Follick, M.J., Chronic pain and functional impairment: assessing beliefs about their relationship, Arch. Phys. Med. Rehab., 59 (1988) 579–582.

Romano, J.M., Turner, J.A., Friedman, L.S., Bulcroft, R.A., Jensen, M.P. and Hops,H., Observable assessment of chronic pain patient-spouse behavioral interactions, Behav. Ther., 22 (1991) 549–567.

Rossignol, M, Suissa,S. and Abenhaim, L., The evolution of compensated occupational spinal injuries, Spine, 17 (1992) 1043–1047.

Slater, M.A., Itall, H.F. Atkinson, J.H. and Garfin, S.R., Pain and impairment beliefs in chronic low back pain: validation of the Pain and Impairment Relationship Scale (PAIRS), Pain, 44 (1991) 51–56.

Spitzer, W.O. Low back pain in the workplace: attainable benefits not attained, Br. J. Ind. Med., 50 (1993) 385–388.

Talo, S., Rytökoski, U. and Puukka, P., Patient classification, a key to evaluate pain treatment: a psychological study in chronic low back pain patients, Spine, 17 (1992) 998–1011.

Turk, D.C. and Rudy, T.E., Neglected topics in the treatment of chronic pain patients: relapse, non-compliance, and adherence enhancement, Pain, 44 (1991) 5–28.

Turner, J.A., Robinson, J. and McCreary, C.P., Chronic low back pain: predicting response to nonsurgical treatment, Arch. Phys. Med. Rehab., 64 (1983) 560–563.

Vällfors, B., Acute, subacute and chronic low back pain: clinical symptoms, absenteeism and working environment, Scand. J. Rehab. Med., Suppl. 11 (1985) 1–85.

Waddell, G. and Turk, D.C., Clinical assessment of low back pain. In: D.C. Turk and R. Melzack (Eds.), Handbook of Pain Assessment, Guilford, New York, 1992, pp. 15–36.

Waddell, G., Bircher, M., Finlaysson, D. and Main, C.J., Symptoms and signs: physical disease or illness behaviour? Br. Med. J., 289 (1984) 739–741.

Waddell, G., Newton, M., Henderson, I., Somerville, D. and Main, C.J., A Fear-Avoidance Beliefs Questionnaire (FABQ) and the role of fear-avoidance beliefs in chronic low back pain and disability, Pain, 52 (1993) 157–168.

Wickström, G., Evaluation of work-related intervention studies to prevent chronification of back disorders, Publication of Health Risks and Prevention Policy group, Wissenschaftszentrum Berlin fur Sozialforschung, 1992.

Williams, D.A. and Thorn, B.E., An empirical assessment of pain beliefs, Pain, 36 (1989) 351–358.

Correspondence to: Steven J. Linton, PhD, Department of Occupational and Environmental Medicine, Örebro Medical Center Hospital, S-70185 Örebro, Sweden. Tel: 46-19-152456; Fax: 46-19-120404.

Proceedings of the 7th World Congress on Pain,
Progress in Pain Research and Management, Vol. 2,
edited by G.F. Gebhart, D.L. Hammond, and T.S.
Jensen, IASP Press, Seattle, © 1994.

12

Pain Thresholds, Symptom Severity, Coping Strategies, and Pain Beliefs as Predictors of Health Care Seeking in Fibromyalgia Patients

Laurence A. Bradley, Graciela S. Alarcón,
Ronald W. Alexander, Mireya Triana,
Leslie A. Aaron, and Katharine E. Stewart

Division of Clinical Immunology and Rheumatology and the Multipurpose Arthritis and Musculoskeletal Diseases Center, University of Alabama at Birmingham, Birmingham, Alabama, USA

Fibromyalgia (FM) is a disorder that is defined by chronic diffuse muscular pain and low pain thresholds ($\leq$ 4 kg) at 11 or more of 18 specific anatomic sites that are termed *tender points* (Wolfe et al. 1990). Recent investigations have demonstrated that patients with FM, relative to controls, also display significantly lower pain thresholds at several *control points* (Granges and Littlejohn 1993). These findings suggest that FM may represent a generalized pain perception disorder associated with alterations in central nervous system processes such as sleep patterns, psychological states, or neuropeptides involved in pain transmission (see Boissevain and McCain 1991 for a complete review).

Efforts to study FM have greatly increased since the publication of the American College of Rheumatology (ACR) classification criteria for this disorder (Wolfe et al. 1990). However, our understanding of pain perception in FM has been limited by the fact that nearly all patient samples studied to date have consisted of persons who have sought treatment from specialists at tertiary care medical centers or practices. These patient samples may not be representative of the population of persons with FM, many of whom may not seek medical care for their symptoms. Indeed, studies of tertiary care patients are likely to be biased because these persons tend to have more severe physical and psychological symptoms (Wolfe 1990).

The present study is the first attempt to identify the factors that differentiate persons with FM who seek medical treatment for their symptoms at a tertiary care center from those who do not attempt to obtain health care. To accomplish this aim, we examined pain thresholds as well as self-reports of subjective pain, disability, fatigue, pain coping strategies, and pain-related beliefs among three groups of subjects. These groups included: (a) patients drawn from a university-based rheumatology practice who had sought treatment for FM; (b) persons recruited from the local community who met the ACR criteria for FM, but who had not sought medical care for their pain in the past 10 years (i.e., nonpatients); and (c) control subjects without FM who were recruited from the local community.

We hypothesized that patients with FM would display significantly lower pain thresholds at tender points and control points and report significantly higher levels of fatigue and disability than would nonpatients and controls. We also hypothesized that the nonpatients would show significantly lower pain thresholds and report significantly higher fatigue and disability levels than would the control subjects. Finally, we hypothesized that the patients, relative to the nonpatients, would report significantly higher pain levels as well as greater use of negative pain coping strategies and pain-related beliefs.

METHOD

This investigation was approved by the Institutional Review Board of the University of Alabama at Birmingham (UAB) on March 1, 1991.

SUBJECTS

All subjects were volunteers who were paid $25 to participate in this study.

Patients

This sample included 33 patients (30 women, 3 men) with FM recruited from the 1992 rheumatology clinic database at UAB as well as current referrals to the clinic. A board-certified rheumatologist validated the diagnosis of FM using the ACR criteria and ruled out other rheumatologic diagnoses on clinical grounds.

Nonpatients

This sample consisted of 23 residents (22 women, 1 man) of the Birmingham community who met the ACR criteria for FM but who had not sought medical care for their pain in the past 10 years. Potential subjects had responded to advertisements in local newspapers asking volunteers with widespread pain or aching to telephone a central number at UAB. We conducted a telephone screening interview for FM (Wolfe et al. 1985) and asked the volunteers several questions regarding their health care history. If they met the interview criteria for nonpatients with FM, they were asked to come to the rheumatology clinic for a physical examination that was performed by one of the investigators (GSA). Those who met the ACR criteria for FM and who did not meet criteria for any other rheumatologic diagnoses were asked to participate in the study.

Controls

This sample consisted of 20 residents (18 women, 2 men) of the Birmingham community who did not suffer from pain and who did not meet the ACR criteria for FM or other rheumatologic diagnoses. Potential controls had responded to advertisements in local newspapers asking for volunteers without muscular aches and pains. We evaluated volunteers with the same procedure used to evaluate the nonpatients. However, these persons were asked to participate in the study only if they failed to meet the interview criteria for FM and if physical examination showed they did not suffer from FM or other rheumatologic disorders.

MATERIALS

Pain Threshold Stimulus

A standard dolorimeter (Chatillon Instruments, Kew Gardens, NY) was used to assess pain threshold at five paired (left, right) tender points included in the ACR criteria for FM and five paired control points. The tender points (TPs) included: the knee at the medial fat pad; the second rib at the second costochondral junctions; the gluteal at the upper outer quadrant of the buttocks; the trapezius at the midpoint of the upper border; and the low cervical at the anterior aspect of the intertransverse spaces at C5–C7. These were chosen to obtain a representative sample of TPs above and below the waist. The control points (CPs) consisted of: the midfoot at the midpoint of the dorsal third metatarsal; the midtibia (anteromedial surface); the tensor fascia latae, 5 cm inferior to the anterior superior iliac spine; the ulna midshaft; and the frontal, 5 cm superior to the orbit. These were chosen from CPs used in previous pain threshold studies of patients with FM and allowed us to sample from the upper and lower body segments (e.g., Wolfe et al. 1990).

Self-Report Questionnaires

Subjects were administered several self-report measures of symptoms associated with FM and pain coping strategies and beliefs. The symptom measures included the McGill Pain Questionnaire (MPQ; Melzack 1975), Sickness Impact Profile (SIP; Bergner et al. 1980), and the Fatigue Severity Scale (FSS; Krupp et al. 1989). These measures evaluated subjects' perceptions of their pain, disability, and fatigue, respectively. The remaining measures included the Coping Strategies Questionnaire (CSQ; Rosenstiel and Keefe 1983), Pain Beliefs and Perceptions Inventory (PBPI; Williams and Thorn 1989), and the Self-Efficacy Scales (SES; Lorig et al. 1989). The CSQ assesses the frequency with which subjects use eight strategies for coping with pain (e.g., reinterpreting pain sensations, catastrophizing, praying and hoping). The PBPI measures three dimensions of beliefs about pain: stability of pain, self-blame, and perceptions of pain as mysterious. The SES assesses the extent to which persons believe they can perform specific behaviors to control their pain and other disease-related symptoms.

PROCEDURE

After giving informed consent, each subject received an appointment for an assessment at the UAB General Clinical Research Center and was asked to discontinue all analgesic, anti-inflammatory, and psychotropic medication for four days prior to the assessment. One week before the assessment, each subject received by mail the FSS; patients and nonpatients also received the PBPI and the SES. The subject received written instructions and a subsequent telephone call with a reminder to complete these measures and to bring them to the assessment as well as to discontinue medication as previously requested.

One of four graduate research associates (ReAs) administered a pain threshold assessment to each subject. The ReA began the assessment by collecting demographic information regarding age and education level. The ReA also asked patients and nonpatients to report the length of time since onset of their pain. Next, the ReA identified the subject's TP and CP locations by surface landmarks and marked them with a colored pen. The ReA then instructed the patient in the use of a seven-category rating scale to report perceptions of dolorimeter stimulation. The scale was printed on a 21.5-cm by 28-cm card and included the following categories: 0 = no sensation, 1 = faint pressure, 2 = moderate pressure, 3 = severe pressure, 4 = faint pain, 5 = moderate pain, and 6 = severe pain.

The ReA used a computer-generated random order to determine whether to first assess pain threshold for all TPs or CPs. Regardless of the order of the assessments, the ReA evaluated pain threshold at each TP and CP in a predetermined order for all subjects. The ReA assessed pain threshold by applying steady and increasing pressure with the dolorimeter at a rate of 1 kg/1.54 cm^2 each second in a direction perpendicular to the skin. The patient viewed the rating scale during the assessment and indicated the moment that she or he perceived that the dolorimeter stimulation matched the category of faint pain. The ReA then withdrew the dolorimeter and repeated the procedure at the next TP or CP. The dolorimeter pressures that evoked faint pain at each of the TPs were averaged to produce a mean pain threshold level. The same procedure was performed to produce a mean pain threshold for the CPs.

Following the pain threshold assessment, the ReA administered at least one self-report measure to each subject. Controls completed only the SIP, whereas patients and nonpatients completed this measure as well as the MPQ and CSQ.

STATISTICAL ANALYSIS

The first set of analyses consisted of a series of one-way analyses of variance (ANOVAs) that compared the three subject groups on age and education. An ANOVA also was used to compare the patients and nonpatients with respect to time since pain onset.

The second set of analyses consisted of a series of ANOVAs that compared the three subject groups with regard to pain thresholds at TPs and CPs and responses to the SIP and FSS. *T*-tests for nonorthogonal comparisons were used to test the hypotheses regarding group differences on these variables.

Finally, *t*-tests were used to test hypotheses regarding differences between patients and nonpatients on the MPQ, CSQ, PBPI, and SES. The Bonferroni correction for multiple comparisons was used to adjust the alpha levels for analyses of the eight CSQ scales ($P = .006$), three PBPI scales ($P = .017$), and two SES ($P = .025$).

RESULTS

Table I shows that there were no differences among the subject groups with regard to age, education, and time since pain onset. Thus, it was not necessary to control for these variables in the subsequent analyses.

Fig. 1 shows the mean pain thresholds at the TPs and CPs as a function of subject group. Consistent with the hypotheses, we found significant differences among the subject groups at the TPs (F = 89.67, P = .0001) and CPs (F = 101.13, P = .0001); patients with FM displayed significantly lower pain thresholds than did both the nonpatients and the controls (Ps = .001). The nonpatients also showed significantly lower pain thresholds than did the controls at the TPs and CPs (Ps = .001).

Subjects' reports of pain, disability, and fatigue produced similar results. Table II shows that consistent with the hypotheses, there were significant differences among the subject groups in scores on the MPQ (t = 2.81, P = .01), SIP (F = 32.67, P = .0001), and the FSS (F = 46.68, P = .0001). Patients with FM reported significantly higher levels of pain, disability, and fatigue than did nonpatients (Ps < .01). In addition, both patients and nonpatients reported significantly higher levels of disability (Ps < .04) and fatigue (Ps = .001) than did controls.

The findings regarding reports of pain coping strategies and beliefs also were consistent with the hypotheses. Table III shows that patients with FM produced significantly higher scores than did nonpatients on two of the CSQ scales, praying and hoping (t = 3.29, P = .001) and catastrophizing (t = 3.44, P = .001), as well as on the pain stability scale of the PBPI (t = 3.71, P < .001). The patients also displayed significantly lower scores than did nonpatients on the SES for pain (t = 4.30, P = .001) and other symptoms (t = 5.33, P < .001).

Table I
Mean (± S.E.M.) demographic variables as a function of subject group

	Subject Group		
Demographic Variable	Patients	Nonpatients	Controls
Age (years)	44.88 ± 1.90	49.96 ± 2.35	42.65 ± 3.60
Education (years)	12.94 ± 0.38	13.52 ± 0.49	14.05 ± 0.40
Time since onset of pain (months)	69.48 ± 13.60	96.96 ± 25.17	—

Note: There are no significant differences among the subject groups on any of the demographic variables.

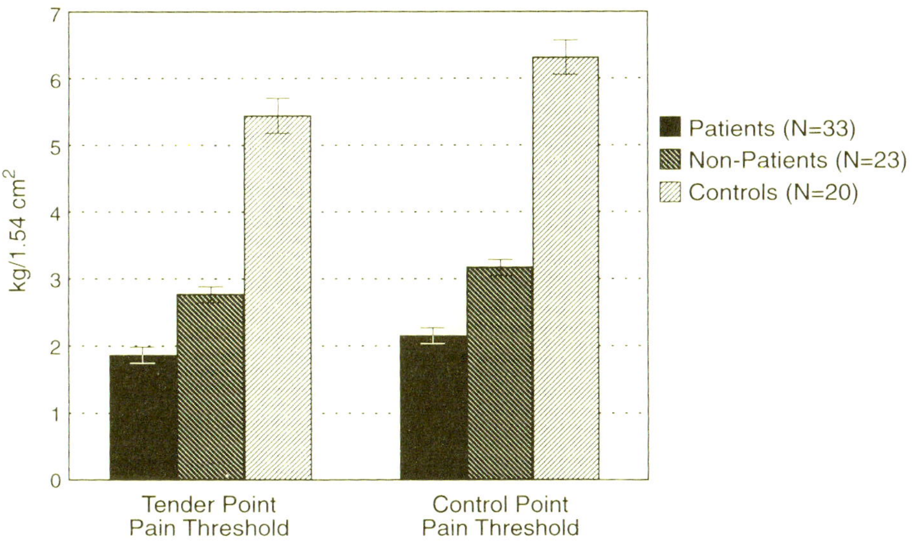

Fig. 1. Mean (± S.E.M.) pain threshold levels at tender points and control points as a function of subject group. Patients with FM show significantly lower pain thresholds than non-patients and controls at both tender and control points (*P*s = .001). Nonpatients also show significantly lower pain thresholds than controls at tender and control points (*P*s =.001).

DISCUSSION

We have demonstrated that both patients and nonpatients with FM, relative to control subjects, exhibit low pain thresholds in response to dolorimeter stimulation at TPs and CPs. Similarly, patients and nonpatients also report significantly higher levels of fatigue and disability than do controls. These findings indicate that persons with FM, regardless of whether or not they seek medical treatment, display generalized low pain thresholds for pressure stimulation that are accompanied by high levels of fatigue and disability. This suggests that central nervous system factors, such as altered sleep patterns, psychological states, and neuropeptide levels, contribute to the symptoms of FM. Indeed, we recently found that patients with FM show reduced levels of regional cerebral blood flow (rCBF) to the caudate nucleus and that rCBF to this structure is strongly associated with pain thresholds at TPs and CPs (Mountz et al. 1993).

Our results also provide important information regarding the factors that are associated with health care seeking behavior among persons with FM. We found that patients, relative to nonpatients, show significantly lower pain

Table II
Mean (± S.E.M.) reports of pain, disability, and fatigue as a function of subject group

Variable	Subject Group Patients	Nonpatients	Controls
McGill Pain Questionnaire (MPQ)*	30.89 ± 2.19	22.89 ± 2.57	—
Sickness Impact Profile (SIP)†	18.29 ± 2.04	5.70 ± 1.20	0.22 ± 0.10
Fatigue Severity Scale (FSS)†	5.96 ± 0.20	4.35 ± 0.33	2.56 ± 0.21

*Patients > nonpatients, P = .01
†Patients > nonpatients > controls, Ps = .036–.001

threshold levels at TPs and CPs and report significantly higher levels of pain, disability, and fatigue. Thus, similar to studies of patients with irritable bowel syndrome, symptom severity is associated with seeking medical treatment for FM (Drossman et al. 1988). Importantly, we also produced the first evidence that several cognitive variables differentiate patients with FM from nonpatients. For example, patients report significantly greater usage of two pain coping strategies, praying and hoping as well as catastrophizing, that are significantly associated with disability among patients with chronic pain (Jensen et al. 1992). In addition, patients report significantly lower levels of self-efficacy for reducing pain and related symptoms and display a significantly greater belief that their pain will remain stable. These results are similar to those found in a recent population-based study of health care seeking for medical

Table III
Mean (± S.E.M.) reports of pain coping strategies and beliefs as a function of subject group

Variable	Subject Group Patients	Nonpatients	P value
CSQ praying and hoping	3.27 ± 0.28	1.89 ± 0.29	0.001
CSQ catastrophizing	2.22 ± 0.27	0.94 ± 0.23	0.001
PBPI pain stability	3.01 ± 0.13	2.20 ± 0.18	0.001
SES pain	33.03 ± 3.63	57.39 ± 4.36	0.001
SES other symptoms	38.73 ± 3.44	65.00 ± 3.23	0.001

CSQ = Coping Strategies Questionnaire
PBPI = Pain Beliefs and Perceptions Inventory
SES = Self-Efficacy Scales

symptoms (Cameron et al. 1993). This investigation revealed that, among 366 members of a health maintenance organization (HMO), persons who sought medical treatment for new symptoms reported significantly higher levels of pain as well as more frequent usage of passive coping strategies (similar to praying and hoping) than did persons who did not seek treatment. Health care seekers also rated their coping efforts as significantly less effective in reducing symptoms (i.e., low self-efficacy) than did persons who did not obtain medical care.

In summary, we have provided evidence that central nervous system factors are associated with the pain and other symptoms of FM among patients who seek treatment at a tertiary care medical center as well as among persons who do not seek medical treatment. We also have demonstrated that patients with FM, relative to nonpatients, display lower pain thresholds and report higher levels of pain, more frequent usage of negative coping strategies and pain-related beliefs, and lower levels of self-efficacy for controlling pain and other symptoms. However, our data are cross-sectional and require replication in a longitudinal, prospective investigation. We will therefore continue to follow our subjects for two years and will record health care seeking for FM among the nonpatients. This follow-up will allow us to determine if the same factors that are associated with health care seeking in the present analysis also differentiate patients from nonpatients during the longitudinal portion of the study.

ACKNOWLEDGEMENTS

This investigation was supported by the National Institute of Arthritis, Musculoskeletal and Skin Diseases (2P60 AR 20641-15) and the National Center for Research Resources (5 M010032).

REFERENCES

Bergner, M., Bobbitt, R.A., Carter, W.B., et al., The Sickness Impact Profile: development and final revision of a health status measure, Med. Care, 19 (1981) 787–805.

Boissevain, M.D. and McCain, G.A., Toward an integrated understanding of fibromyalgia syndrome. I. Medical and pathophysiological aspects, Pain, 45 (1991) 227–238.

Cameron, L., Leventhal, E.A. and Leventhal, H., Symptom representations and affect as determinants of care seeking in a community-dwelling, adult sample population, Health Psychol., 12 (1993) 171–179.

Drossman, D.A., McKee, D.C., Sandler, R.S., et al., Psychosocial factors in the irritable bowel syndrome: a multivariate study of patients and non-patients with irritable bowel syndrome, Gastroenterology, 95 (1988) 701–708.

Granges, G. and Littlejohn, G., Pressure pain threshold in pain-free subjects, in patients with chronic regional pain syndromes, and in patients with fibromyalgia syndrome, Arthritis Rheum., 36 (1993) 642–646.

Jensen, M.P., Turner, J.A. and Romano, J.M., Chronic pain coping measures: individual vs. composite scores, Pain, 51 (1992) 273–280.

Krupp, L.B., La Rocca, N.G., Muir-Nash, J., et al., The fatigue severity scale: application to patients with multiple sclerosis and systemic lupus erythematosus, Arch. Neurol., 46 (1989) 1121–1123.

Lorig, K., Chastain, R.L., Ung, E., et al., Development and evaluation of a scale to measure perceived self-efficacy in people with arthritis, Arthritis Rheum., 32 (1989) 37–44.

Melzack, R., The McGill Pain Questionnaire: major properties and scoring methods, Pain, 1 (1975) 277–299.

Mountz, J.M., Alexander, R.W., Bradley, L.A., et al., Regional cerebral blood flow (rCBF) in caudate nuclei is associated with pain thresholds in patients with fibromyalgia (FM), Arthritis Rheum., 36 (1993) S221.

Rosentiel, A.K. and Keefe, F.J., The use of coping strategies in chronic low back pain patients: relationship to patient characteristics and current adjustment, Pain, 17 (1983) 33–44.

Williams, D.A. and Thorn, B.E., An empirical assessment of pain beliefs, Pain, 36 (1989) 351–358.

Wolfe, F., Methodological and statistical problems in the epidemiology of fibromyalgia. In: J.R. Fricton and E. Awad (Eds.), Myofascial Pain and Fibromyalgia. Advances in Pain Research and Therapy, Vol. 17. Raven Press, New York, 1990, pp. 147–163.

Wolfe, F., Hawley, D.J., Cathy, M.A., et al., Fibrositis: symptom frequency and criteria for diagnosis: an evaluation of 291 rheumatic disease patients and 58 normal individuals, J. Rheumatol., 12 (1985) 1159–1163.

Wolfe, F., Smythe, H.A., Yunus, M.B., et al., The American College of Rheumatology 1990 criteria for the classification of fibromyalgia: report of the multicenter criteria committee, Arthritis Rheum., 33 (1990) 160–172.

Correspondence to: Laurence A. Bradley, PhD, Division of Clinical Immunology and Rheumatology, UAB Station / MEB 615, 1813 6th Avenue South, Birmingham, AL 35294, USA. Tel: 205-934-9614; Fax: 205-934-8493.

Proceedings of the 7th World Congress on Pain,
Progress in Pain Research and Management, Vol. 2,
edited by G.F. Gebhart, D.L. Hammond, and T.S.
Jensen, IASP Press, Seattle, © 1994.

13

Comparative Sensory Evaluation of Parietal Tissues in Painful and Nonpainful Areas in Fibromyalgia and Myofascial Pain Syndrome

Leonardo Vecchiet, Maria Adele Giamberardino, Paolo de Bigontina, and Luca Dragani

Institute of Medical Pathophysiology, "G. D'Annunzio" University of Chieti, Chieti, Italy

INTRODUCTION

In spite of the theoretical recognition of fibromyalgia (FS) and myofascial pain syndrome (MPS) as independent forms of chronic musculoskeletal pain with distinct diagnostic criteria (Simons 1990; Boissevain and McCain 1991), the differentiation of the two remains difficult in many cases in routine medical practice. The sensory characterization of parietal tissues in both syndromes is a crucial element. Most studies to date have evaluated pain thresholds to pressure stimulation in painful sites (i.e., tender spots [TePs] and trigger points [TrPs]) and nonpainful areas. Although all report an increased sensitivity to pain at both TePs and TrPs, controversial results have been obtained regarding the sensitivity outside the typical painful spots of the two disorders, with some authors claiming a decreased pain threshold in fibromyalgic patients (Lautenschlager et al. 1988; Tunks et al. 1988, 1991, 1993; Scudds et al. 1989; Wolfe et al. 1990) and others a sensory normality (Campbell et al. 1983). No attempt has been made, moreover, to differentiate between the sensitivity of superficial and deep parietal tissues in painful and nonpainful sites (Wall 1993), because the pressure pain threshold test, although practical in routine examination, stimulates superficial as well as deep receptors, making it difficult to attribute any hypersensitivity to a specific parietal structure. Our study attempted to better characterize the sensory disorder of both syndromes by evaluating pain thresholds, measured by means of electrical stimulation, individually in the three parietal tissues (skin, subcutaneous tissue, and muscle), of painful and nonpainful areas in patients diagnosed as having FS or MPS in comparison with those recorded in corresponding sites of normal subjects.

MATERIALS AND METHODS

PATIENT SELECTION CRITERIA

We screened fibromyalgia patients and those with myofascial pain syndrome of the trapezius muscle of one side who were seeking medical care for musculoskeletal pain at the Institute of Medical Pathophysiology of the "G. D'Annunzio" University.

We used the FS diagnostic criteria of the American College of Rheumatology (Wolfe et al. 1990), with the further condition that the TeP be present in the upper border of the trapezius muscle; criteria for MPS of the trapezius were those described by Simons (1990) for an active TrP (TrP1) located in the upper border of the muscle.

Patients were examined by two clinicians separately and were admitted to the study when diagnosed by both as falling into the FM or MPS categories. To identify FS and MPS groups with a comparable extent of spontaneous symptomatology, patients were asked during examination to indicate on a VAS scale the usual intensity of the pain experienced (Rollman and Lautenbacher 1993).

FS Patients

Thirteen patients were selected (12 women and 1 man, aged 31–57 years, mean age 42.15 ± 7.11) who complained of bilateral pain posteriorly in the neck, in the upper trapezius and lumbar regions, and anteriorly in the quadriceps regions. Seven of them also reported cephalalgic crises with pain mainly in the fronto-orbital area of one side. The diffuse pain had started two to five years before (mean 45.23 ± 13.98 months), with a subcontinuous pattern and a mean intensity of 58.69 ± 14.29 mm of VAS. All patients had 13–18 TePs in the typical locations (Wolfe et al. 1990)

MPS Patients

Twenty-two patients were selected (13 women and 9 men, aged 30–55 years, mean age 40.77 ± 8.91). All had a typical trigger point included in a taut palpable band located in the upper aspect of the trapezius muscle (TrP1) (Travell and Simons 1983) and pain referred both spontaneously and on compression of the TrP unilaterally, upward along the posterolateral aspect of the neck to the mastoid region. In three cases, the pain also extended to the side of the head, to the temporal region and behind the orbit. The painful symptoms had begun one to four years previously (mean 31.72 ± 11.23 months), with pain of usual intensity of 63.59 ± 14.37 mm of VAS experienced on an intermittent basis.

In all patients, we measured pain threshold to electrical stimulation of the cutaneous, subcutaneous, and muscular tissue of: (1) tender spot (TeP) and trigger point (TrP) areas, respectively, at trapezius level on one side and (2) nonpainful areas (deltoid region, on one side).

We compared the results with those recorded in 30 normal subjects (15 women and 15 men, aged 27–50 years, mean age 38.26 ± 7.31) in corresponding areas. The fibromyalgic group consisted almost entirely of women, so we also compared thresholds recorded only in female subjects of the different groups (12 FS, 13 MPS patients, 15 normals).

TECHNIQUE OF MEASUREMENT OF PAIN THRESHOLDS TO ELECTRICAL STIMULATION

We used a Lace Electronics three-channel (ES-3) square-wave stimulator and constant-current isolator (CCI-2) with a digital display showing current intensity in mA (range 0–30). A double-trace Goldstar oscilloscope (model 05-7020) verified the shape of the stimulation wave by measuring the fall in voltage via a 5KΩ resistance placed in series with the tissues tested. Stimulation consisted of 18-msec trains of single 0.5-msec square waves, frequency 310 Hz, delivered automatically every 2 sec.

Surface electrodes were used for the skin, a 10-mm circular plate in Ag/AgCl (reference electrode) and a cylinder in Ag/AgCl with a 0.3-mm diameter base (stimulating electrode). They were stuck to the skin with conductor paste, 1 cm apart with the stimulating one placed in the middle of the TeP or TrP at trapezius level and in the median portion of the deltoid region. An adjustable parallelogram was connected to the stimulating electrode through a spring device, allowing the pressure exerted on the skin to remain constant throughout measurement. Two needle electrodes were employed for subcutaneous and muscular tissues (25 mm long, isolated with Teflon except for 2 mm at the tip), inserted vertically into the respective layers, 1.5 cm apart, with the TeP or TrP halfway between them.

In each tissue, the pain threshold (pricking pain for the skin, prickling pain for the subcutaneous tissue, and cramplike pain for the muscle) was measured by the method of the limits (Vecchiet et al. 1988,1990,1993). Measurements were performed: (1) in the pain-free interval for MPS patients and in the phase of minor pain (below the usual VAS score) in FS patients, (2) always at the same time of day (10–12 A.M.) in patients and normals, (3) in the same period of the menstrual cycle in fertile women (early follicular phase, 2nd–6th day). They were carried out in a quiet, comfortable environment always by the same experimenter, who was different from the clinicians selecting the patients and unaware of the diagnosis.

Before starting measurement in the chosen sites in both patients and normal subjects, the experimenter performed preliminary test measurements in a control area (usually the dorsal aspect of the forearm) to familiarize them with the procedure. Neither patients nor controls had taken any drug for the 72 hours preceding all tests.

STATISTICAL ANALYSIS

We calculated means ± S.E.M. of thresholds for each tissue for patients and normal subjects. Student's *t* test for paired samples was used to compare painful and nonpainful areas within each group of subjects (FM patients, MPS patients, and normal subjects). Comparison between corresponding areas in different groups was made by Student's *t* test for unpaired samples. Significance level was assessed at $P < 0.05$.

RESULTS

FIBROMYALGIC PATIENTS

In the tender point (TeP) area, pain thresholds to electrical stimulation were significantly lower than normal in the cutaneous, subcutaneous, and muscular tissue. Outside the TeP area, thresholds were higher than in the TeP, with a significant difference for the muscle, but were still significantly lower than normal in the three tissues (Fig. 1; Table I).

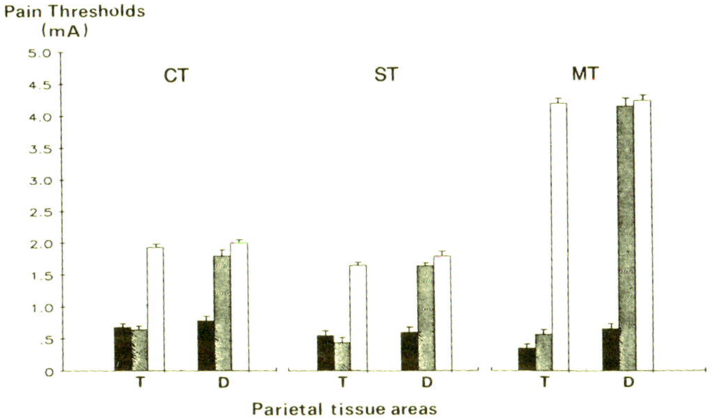

Fig. 1. Pain thresholds to electrical stimulation (mA; means ± S.E.M.) of cutaneous (CT), subcutaneous (ST), and muscular (MT) tissues in the trapezius (T) and deltoid (D) areas in fibromyalgic patients (solid bars; n = 13), myofascial pain syndrome patients (striped bars; n = 22), and normal subjects (open bars; n = 30). Trapezius area in patients: painful site (TeP for FS, TrP for MPS); deltoid area in patients: nonpainful site.

MYOFASCIAL PAIN SYNDROME PATIENTS

In the trigger point (TrP) area, pain thresholds were significantly lower than normal in the cutaneous, subcutaneous, and muscular tissues. Outside the TrP area, thresholds were significantly higher than in the TrP in the three tissues and not significantly different from normal (Fig. 1; Table I).

FIBROMYALGIC PATIENTS VERSUS MYOFASCIAL PAIN SYNDROME PATIENTS

FS with respect to MPS patients showed: (1) in the painful area (TeP vs. TrP), similar thresholds in skin and subcutaneous tissue (no significant difference) and significantly lower thresholds in muscle; (2) in the nonpainful area, a significantly lower threshold in all three tissues (Table I).

COMPARISON BETWEEN FEMALE SUBJECTS OF PATIENT AND NORMAL GROUPS

Table II reports thresholds in women of FS, MPS, and normal groups. All comparisons gave results identical to those performed with mixed male-female groups, except for the comparison between muscular thresholds of TePs and TrPs, which showed no statistically significant difference.

Table I
Statistical comparison of pain thresholds in patients and normal subjects

	Skin		Subcutaneous Tissue		Muscle	
FS (painful vs. nonpainful sites)	n.s.		n.s.		P < 0.003	
MPS (painful vs. nonpainful sites)	P < 0.0001		P < 0.0001		P < 0.0001	
	Trapezius	Deltoid	Trapezius	Deltoid	Trapezius	Deltoid
FS vs. normals	P < 0.0001	P < 0.0001	P < 0.0001	P < 0.0001	p < 0.0001	P < 0.0001
MPS vs. normals	P < 0.0001	n.s.	P < 0.0001	n.s.	P < 0.0001	n.s.
FS vs. MPS	n.s.	P < 0.0001	n.s.	P < 0.0001	P < 0.04	P < 0.0001

Note: Comparison of painful and nonpainful areas in FS and MPS patients: Student's t test for paired samples.
Comparison between corresponding areas of FS, MPS, and normal subjects: Student's t test for unpaired samples.
Trapezius: painful site in patients (TeP for FS, TrP for MPS): deltoid: non-painful site in patients
n.s. = not significant

DISCUSSION

The results of this study on the sensory evaluation in fibromyalgic and myofascial pain syndrome patients versus normals suggest several considerations. First, the tenderness commonly found at both TePs and TrPs is not exclusively attributable to the muscular structure but appears to be distributed in all three parietal tissues, as shown by the pain threshold decrease to electrical stimulation in the skin, subcutaneous tissue, and muscle. Second, provided that the extent of the spontaneous painful symptoms are comparable in FS and MPS, tender and trigger points do not appear to differ much from a sensory standpoint in spite of the different characteristics emerging at physical examination (TrPs located in taut, palpable bands, eliciting local twitch responses on pincer palpation and referred pain on compression with TePs exhibiting only local tenderness) (Travell and Simons 1983, Simons 1990). A third and most important consideration is the finding of hyperalgesia of all three parietal tissues outside the painful sites in FS, in contrast to the sensory normality seen in MPS at the same level.

On the whole, the results of the study indicate that, regarding sensory examination, the comparison between TePs and TrPs alone does not allow us to distinguish FS from MPS. The crucial element for the differential diagnosis

Table II
Pain thresholds to electrical stimulation of parietal tissues in female patients and normals (mA; mean ± S.E.M.)

	Fibromyalgia		Myofascial Pain Syndrome		Normals	
	Trapezius	Deltoid	Trapezius	Deltoid	Trapezius	Deltoid
Skin	0.71 ± 0.01	0.78 ± 0.08	0.65 ± 0.11	1.80 ± 0.13	1.93 ± 0.08	1.97 ± 0.06
Subcutaneous tissue	0.54 ± 0.06	0.61 ± 0.08	0.47 ± 0.11	1.59 ± 0.06	1.63 ± 0.06	1.71 ± 0.09
Muscle	0.36 ± 0.05	0.67 ± 0.07	0.53 ± 0.12	4.02 ± 0.16	4.11 ± 0.09	4.23 ± 0.11

Note: FS, n = 12; MPS, n = 13; normals, n = 15.

of the two disorders would instead be a systematic study and comparison of painful with nonpainful areas. This is certainly valid for cases such as those described in this study, which are paradigmatic of the two syndromes, with MPS patients complaining of strictly regional pain in contrast to FS patients who have diffuse aching. It is also true, however, for more intricate situations such as that of MPS patients with diffuse pain from multiple trigger points in different muscles. In our experience in patients of exactly this type, we find normal sensitivity in areas outside latent or active TrPs and their respective targets (unpublished observations).

The results of our study also lead us to formulate some pathophysiological considerations. In the case of myofascial pain syndrome, the strict localization of tenderness in painful areas is consistent with the claimed regional nature of the disorder, whose starting point would lie in the formation of TrPs in muscles or their fascia mainly as a consequence of traumatic-microtraumatic events (Travell and Simons 1983; Simons 1990; Vecchiet et al. 1991).

The hypersensitivity also found at trigger level in the superficial parietal tissues could be accounted for on the basis of a *superficialization* process of pain from the muscular focus, similar to what is observed for many clinical conditions involving algogenic foci in other deep somatic structures or viscera (Vecchiet et al. 1989; Giamberardino et al. 1994).

In the case of fibromyalgia, the finding of a diffuse hyperalgesic state, involving not only the muscular structure but also the more superficial tissues in painful as well as nonpainful areas, would seem to provide further support to the hypothesis of the intervention of central pathogenetic mechanisms (Smythe 1976; Wall 1993). This would affirm the idea of "fibromyalgia reflecting an aberration of normal central mechanisms of pain, with abnormality that could arise from a deficiency in the inhibitory system, accentuation of the facilitatory system, or both" (Yunus et al. 1992a,b).

ACKNOWLEDGMENTS

This work was supported by the Italian National Research Council (CNR). C.n.: 9300756PF41, Targeted Project "Prevention and Control of Disease Factors," Subproject "Stress," "Neurophysiological and Psychological Aspects of Fibromyalgic Syndromes."

REFERENCES

Boissevain, M.D. and McCain, G.A., Toward an integrated understanding of fibromyalgia syndrome. I. Medical and pathophysiological aspects, Pain, 45 (1991) 227–238.

Campbell, S.M., Clark, S., Tindell, E.A., Forehand, M.E. and Bennett, R.M., Clinical characteristics of fibrositis (I): a "blinded" controlled study of symptoms and tender points, Arthritis Rheum., 26 (1983) 817–824.

Giamberardino, M.A., de Bigontina, P., Martegiani, C. and Vecchiet, L., Effects of extracorporeal shock-wave lithotripsy on referred hyperalgesia from renal/ureteral calculosis, Pain, 56 (1994) 77–83.

Lautenschlager, J., Bruckle, W., Schnorrenberger, C.C. and Muller, W., Die Messung von Druckschmerzen im Bereich von Sehnen und Muskeln bei Gesunden und Patienten mit generalisierter Tendomyopathie (Fibromyalgie-Syndrom), Z. Rheumatol., 47 (1988) 397–404.

Rollman, G.B. and Lautenbacher, S., Hypervigilance effects in fibromyalgia: pain experience and pain perception. In: H. Vaeroy and H. Merskey (Eds.), Progress in Fibromyalgia and Myofascial Pain. Pain Research and Clinical Management, Vol. 6. Elsevier, Amsterdam, 1993, pp. 149–159.

Scudds, R.A., Trachsel, L.C.E., Luckhurst, B.J. and Percy, J.S., A comparative study of pain, sleep quality and pain responsiveness in fibrositis and myofascial pain syndrome, J. Rheumatol., 16, Suppl. 19 (1989) 120–126.

Simons, D.G., Muscular pain syndromes. In: J.R. Fricton and E. Awad (Eds.), Myofascial Pain and Fibromyalgia. Advances in Pain Research and Therapy, Vol. 17. Raven Press, New York, 1990, pp. 1–41.

Smythe, H.A., "Fibrositis" as a disorder of pain modulation, Clin. Rheum. Dis., 5 (1976) 823–832.

Travell, J.G. and Simons, D.G., Myofascial Pain and Dysfunction: The Trigger Point Manual. William and Wilkins, Baltimore, London, 1983.

Tunks, E., Clinical experimental investigations in fibromyalgia and myofascial pain. In: H. Vaeroy and H. Merskey (Eds.), Progress in Fibromyalgia and Myofascial Pain. Pain Research and Clinical Management, Vol. 6. Elsevier, Amsterdam, 1993, pp. 161–172.

Tunks, E., Crook, J., Norman, G. and Kalaher, S., Tender points in fibromyalgia, Pain, 34 (1988) 11–19.

Tunks, E., McCain, G.A., Hart, L.E., Teasell, R.W., Rollman, G.B., DeShane, P.J., McDermid, A.J. and Goldsmith, C.H., The reliability of physical findings in patients with fibromyalgia and myofascial pain syndromes, Arthritis Rheum., 34, Suppl. (1991) 190.

Vecchiet, L., Galletti, R., Giamberardino, M.A., Dragani, L. and Marini, F., Modifications of cutaneous, subcutaneous and muscular sensory and pain thresholds after the induction of an experimental algogenic focus in the skeletal muscle, Clin. J. Pain, 4 (1988) 55–59.

Vecchiet, L., Giamberardino, M.A., Dragani, L. and Albe-Fessard, D., Pain from renal/ureteral calculosis: evaluation of sensory thresholds in the lumbar area, Pain, 36 (1989) 289–295.

Vecchiet, L., Giamberardino, M.A., Dragani, L., de Bigontina, P. and Albe-Fessard, D., Latent myofascial trigger points: changes in muscular and subcutaneous pain thresholds at trigger point and target level, Journal of Manual Medicine, 5 (1990) 151–154.

Vecchiet, L., Giamberardino, M.A. and Saggini, R., Myofascial pain syndromes: clinical and

pathophysiological aspects, Clin. J. Pain, 7, Suppl. (1991) S16–S22.
Vecchiet, L., Giamberardino, M.A. and de Bigontina, P., Referred pain from viscera: when the symptom persists despite the extinction of the visceral focus. In: F. Sicuteri et al. (Eds.), Pain versus Man. Advances in Pain Research and Therapy, Vol. 20. Raven Press, New York, 1992, pp. 101–110.
Vecchiet, L., Dragani, L., de Bigontina, P., Obletter, G. and Giamberardino, M.A:, Experimental referred pain and hyperalgesia from muscles in humans. In: L. Vecchiet, D. Albe-Fessard, U. Lindblom (Eds.), and M.A. Giamberardino (Assoc. Ed.), New Trends in Referred Pain and Hyperalgesia. Pain Research and Clinical Management, Vol. 7. Elsevier, Amsterdam, 1993, pp. 239–249.
Wall, P.D., The mechanisms of fibromyalgia: a critical essay. In: H. Vaeroy and H. Merskey (Eds.), Progress in Fibromyalgia and Myofascial Pain. Pain Research and Clinical Management, Vol. 6. Elsevier, Amsterdam, 1993, pp. 53–59.
Wolfe, F., Smythe, H.A., Yunus, M.B., et al., The American College of Rheumatology 1990: criteria for the classification of fibromyalgia, Arthritis Rheum., 33 (1990) 160–172.
Yunus, M.B., Fibromyalgia: a dysfunctional syndrome with chronic pain. In: F. Sicuteri, L. Terenius, L. Vecchiet and C.A. Maggi (Eds.), Pain versus Man. Advances in Pain Research and Therapy, Vol. 20. Raven Press, New York, 1992a, pp. 133–140.
Yunus, M.B., Towards a model of pathophysiology of fibromyalgia: aberrant central pain mechanisms with peripheral modulation, J. Rheumatol., 19 (1992b) 846–850.

Correspondence to: Prof. Leonardo Vecchiet, Semeiotica Medica, Ospedale "SS. Annunziata," via P.A. Valignani, 66100 Chieti, Italy. Tel: 39-871-345460; Fax: 39-871-349108.

Proceedings of the 7th World Congress on Pain,
Progress in Pain Research and Management, Vol. 2,
edited by G.F. Gebhart, D.L. Hammond, and T.S.
Jensen, IASP Press, Seattle, © 1994.

14

Patient Explanatory Models for Temporomandibular Disorders

Donna L. Massoth,[a] Samuel F. Dworkin,[a,b] Coralyn W. Whitney,[a] Robert G. Harrison,[a] Leanne Wilson,[a] and Judy Turner[b]

[a]*School of Dentistry, Department of Oral Medicine, and* [b]*School of Medicine, Department of Psychiatry and Behavioral Sciences, University of Washington, Seattle, Washington, USA*

INTRODUCTION

When a person seeks medical care, the provider's primary objective is to diagnose the problem and render appropriate treatment so that the patient is protected from significant and/or progressive disease. Patients seeking relief from chronic pain often have symptoms that are difficult to diagnose, including those which are vague and diffuse as well as those which appear disproportionate to the degree of measurable organic pathology. These challenging diagnostic dilemmas can be further complicated by the social and emotional sequelae of chronic pain, represented as a complex web of personal and interpersonal variables, which over time are intricately woven into the patient's pain experience. The clinician may experience difficulty in assigning a definitive diagnosis to explain the patient's experience of pain. Such difficulty may be attributed to lack of sensitivity of current diagnostic instruments and techniques; alternatively, the clinician may conclude that the symptoms are psychogenic, that the patient is exaggerating symptoms, or even that the patient is malingering.

Dworkin and colleagues (1992) have described a model that characterizes chronic pain, including Temporomandibular Disorders (TMD) pain, as arising from multiple and interrelated biologic, psychologic, and social factors. According to this model, the chronic pain experience arises from a complex interaction of nociception, pain perception, cognitive appraisal, behavioral responses to pain, and socioculturally defined roles for persons in pain. The subjective experience of pain thus depends not only on the sensory stimulation of pain receptors (nociception), but also on what the person attends to, how the experience is cognitively appraised, what coping mechanisms are activated in response to the stimulus, and the social and cultural contexts that shape the patient's perceptions and responses of illness.

The management of chronic pain has expanded beyond treating biomedical factors alone and now incorporates a broader array of treatment strategies, consistent with the current biopsychosocial understanding of chronic pain. The current reliance on and extensive use of cognitive behavioral treatment approaches in the multidisciplinary management of chronic pain reflects this shift in paradigms from a biomedical to a biopsychosocial understanding of chronic pain. Cognitive behavioral (CB) therapies aim to modify patients' beliefs, attitudes, and expectancies about pain (e.g., explanatory models of pain; Turk et al. 1983), and to extinguish pain behaviors and facilitate return to adaptive levels of activity and social function (Fordyce et al. 1985). Thus, CB therapies aim to help patients manage and cope with chronic pain so they can regain productive lives, whether or not pain is completely and permanently resolved.

Kleinman (1980) has promulgated the concept of explanatory models as an organizing construct for understanding illness from a biopsychosocial perspective. Explanatory models of illness are defined as the views, notions, beliefs, and expectancies about an illness episode (Kleinman 1988). Explanatory models are specific to the person, shaped by the culture, and representative of the person's attempt to make sense of the illness experience—that is, how the person perceives, experiences, and copes with disease. Each person carries a set of beliefs about the cause of his or her illness, time and mode of onset of symptoms, what maintains or aggravates symptoms, expected course of the illness, and appropriate treatments. These beliefs and expectancies are shaped by past illness episodes as they are personally experienced or observed in others (Chrisman 1977). Within each medical encounter, patients and their families and practitioners will have discrete and possibly quite independent explanatory models of illness.

The elucidation of TMD explanatory models should enhance understanding of TMD-related illness behavior and subsequent therapeutic strategies. Yet, there are few concise measures for assessing patients' explanatory models for TMD that are useful in both clinical and research settings. We developed and pilot-tested measures to assess patients' explanatory models of TMD and to determine if the measures developed were related to relevant clinical examination and psychosocial measures.

METHODS

SUBJECTS

Study participants included 71 patient volunteers experiencing pain and related symptoms of TMD and enrolled in an ongoing, brief cognitive-behavioral (CB) intervention study (Dworkin et al., in press). These patients were predominantly Caucasian women (81.7%) with a mean age of 38 years. More than 82% of patients reported full-time employment, and more than 84% reported formal education and/or technical training beyond high school.

PROCEDURES

For six-months, dental hygienist examiners recruited consecutive patients from the CB intervention study during the three-month follow-up interview. Within 10 days after signing informed consent to participate in this pilot study, patients were contacted by telephone and asked questions concerning their explanatory models for TMD.

Patients recruited from the intervention study received a baseline evaluation by a TMD specialist from the TMD Clinic of Group Health Cooperative of Puget Sound or the Faculty Oral Medicine Clinic at the University of Washington School of Dentistry. Following baseline evaluation, patients were randomized to receive either usual dental treatment (UT) or usual dental treatment plus a brief cognitive-behavioral (CB) intervention. Of 71 participants in the explanatory models study, 34 received usual dental treatment and 37 received the intervention. The brief CB intervention emphasized a biopsychosocial explanatory model of TMD and focused on patient-management strategies for the relief of chronic pain.

MEASURES

1. Explanatory Model (EM) scores were derived from a measure (Fig. 1) designed to assess patients' global explanations of the relative roles played by physical factors, behavior and/or stress in each of three TMD dimensions—cause, exacerbation, and treatment efficacy. Each of the three TMD

People who have TMD often say that it was **originally caused** by some combination of (1) physical factors, (2) harmful habits to the jaws/head/neck, and/or (3) stress and emotional upset. What combination would seem appropriate for your particular TMD problem?

Please distribute 100 percentage points among these three categories to describe how they may have **originally caused** your TMD problem. For example, one could assign 34% to physical factors, 33% to harmful habits, and 33% to stress to indicate that all three categories were equally important in originally causing his or her TMD. Any combination that adds up to 100% is fine.

What percentage of your TMD problem was ***originally caused*** by:

- Physical Factors ______
- Harmful Habits to Jaws/Head/Neck ______
- Stress or Emotional Upset ______

100%

What percentage of your TMD problem is ***aggravated*** by:

- Physical Factors ______
- Harmful Habits to Jaws/Head/Neck ______
- Stress or Emotional Upset ______

100%

What percentage of ***TMD treatments*** should be directed toward eliminating or lessening the impact of:

- Physical Factors (such as) ______
- Harmful Habits to Jaws/Head/Neck ______
- Stress or Emotional Upset ______

100%

Fig. 1. The Explanatory Models Questionnaire for TMD assesses patients' global perceptions of the relative importance of physical factors, behavior, and/or stress in each of three TMD dimensions—cause, exacerbation, and treatment efficacy.

dimensions is assigned three scores depicting patients' global perceptions of the relative importance (from 0 to 100%) played by physical factors, behavior (e.g., bruxism), and stress along that one dimension. Together, the physical, behavior, and stress scores total 100% for each TMD dimension of cause, exacerbate, and treatment efficacy. Nine EM scores, with potential ranges of 0–100%, were thus developed for each subject.

We also developed composite measures to represent patients' global beliefs about factors that influence the *course* of TMD—that is, what makes their TMD worse, and concomitantly, what makes it better. The person has little opportunity to change the initial causes of TMD. Yet, the course of TMD may be modified following the recognition of TMD-exacerbating agents and the initiation of effective strategies to ameliorate symptoms. The composite scores that integrate the TMD exacerbation and treatment efficacy dimensions are summed across physical, behavior, and stress domains. Thus, three composite scores, with potential ranges from 0 to 200%, are developed for each subject.

2. Clinical measures included *mandibular range of motion (unassisted)* and *muscle palpation score*. Unassisted mandibular range of motion, measured in millimeters between the edges of the maxillary and mandibular central incisors, assessed the patient's ability to open the jaw without pain and without assistance by an examiner (Dworkin and LeResche 1992). Muscle palpation score was assessed by patient report of pain elicited in response to palpation of 20 predetermined extraoral sites on the muscles of mastication. One point is assigned to each of 10 bilateral palpation sites for which pain is elicited, leading to a score ranging from 0 to 20 (Dworkin et al. 1990a).

3. Self-report measures were collected for sociodemographic and pain history variables. Specific pain measures included *characteristic pain* and *pain interference*. Characteristic pain, representing the average of scores for present, average, and worst pain intensity in the past two months, was assessed using a 0–10 point scale anchored by 0 as "no pain" and 10 as "worst possible pain." The measure of characteristic pain is somewhat more reliable than a single measure of average pain (Dworkin et al. 1990b). Pain interference with daily, work, and social/recreational activities in the previous two months was measured by a 0–10 point scale anchored by 0 as "no interference" and 10 as "unable to carry on any activities."

4. Somatization was assessed by items from the Symptom Checklist 90-Revised (SCL 90-R) (Derogatis 1983) somatization scale. Items that specifically refer to pain (e.g., presence of back pain, headaches) were excluded to eliminate confounding between TMD pain symptomatology and nonpain-related somatization. Age- and sex-adjusted and standardized scale scores were computed for all subjects based on norms derived for the study population from which more than half of the present study sample was drawn (Dworkin et al. 1990c; Von Korff et al. 1988).

5. Graded Cronic Pain Status was assessed using a 0–IV scale for Graded Chronic Pain (GCP) Severity (Von Korff et al. 1992) that incorporates characteristic pain level, degree of interference due to pain, and number of days of activity lost due to pain. The reliability and validity of this graded chronic pain scale have been established with separate primary care samples of headache, back pain, and TMD patients. The scale has demonstrated utility for associating pain-related dysfunction to psychological, psychosocial, and clinical variables (Von Korff et al. 1992; Graff-Radford et al. 1991). Chronic

Table I
Sample characteristics at baseline

	UT (N = 34)	CB (N = 37)	Combined (N = 71)
Gender (% female)	76.5	86.5	81.7
Mean age (years)	36.7	39.2	38
% with TMD Pain for:			
< 6 months	14.7	29.7	22.5
6–24 months	17.7	13.5	15.5
2–5 years	32.3	21.6	26.8
> 5 years	35.3	35.2	35.2
Mean pain ratings (past 2 months):			
Characteristic pain (0–10)	4.46	4.96	4.72
Interference with daily activities (0–10)	3.65	3.41	3.52
Days with facial pain	40.21	46.68	43.58
Activity limitation days	6.29	4.11	5.15
Clinical measures:			
Unassisted mandibular opening (mm)	33.1	33.8	33.5
Muscle palpation score (0–20)	7.62	4.92	6.21

UT = Patients in Usual Treatment group
CB = Patients in Cognitive-Behavioral Intervention group

pain severity is graded into four hierarchical classes: Grade I—low disability, low pain intensity; Grade II—low disability, high pain intensity; Grade III—high disability, moderately limiting; and Grade IV—high disability, severely limiting. Persons qualifying as Grade III or IV almost exclusively reported high-intensity pain (e.g., pain greater than 5 on a 10-point scale). For present purposes, Grades I and II TMD patients were defined as psychosocially functional while Grades III and IV were defined as dysfunctional.

6. Coping variables assessed the nature and efficacy of *pain coping style* using the Vanderbilt Pain Management Inventory (VPMI) (Brown and Nicassio 1987). The VPMI is an 18-item self-report questionnaire that incorporates two scales, Active Coping and Passive Coping, which reflect groups of strategies employed by chronic pain patients to deal with their pain. Items of the Active Coping scale reflect efforts by the patient to function despite the pain, or to distract oneself from the pain. The Passive Coping scale assesses tendencies such as depending on others for help in pain control, engaging in wish-fulfilling thoughts, and restricting functioning due to pain. A measure of pain coping efficacy also was assessed using an item from the Coping Strategies Questionnaire (CSQ) (Rosenstiel and Keefe 1983), which asks patients to rate their ability to control pain on a 0–6 scale.

Table II
Explanatory model scores:
distributions for combined sample (N = 71)

	Sample Mean (%)	(SD)	Sample Median (%)
EXPLANATORY MODEL SCORE*			
TMD causes			
% attributed to Physical	52.5	(34.6)	50
% attributed to Behavioral	25.8	(21.0)	25
% attributed to Stress	21.7	(22.9)	15
	100.0		
TMD exacerbation			
% attributed to Physical	27.4	(29.2)	20
% attributed to Behavioral	42.6	(23.8)	50
% attributed to Stress	30.0	(22.1)	25
	100.0		
TMD treatment efficacy			
% attributed to Physical	33.2	(33.5)	25
% attributed to Behavioral	35.9	(25.3)	33
% attributed to Stress	31.0	(25.3)	33
	100.0		
COMPOSITE EXPLANATORY MODEL SCORE†			
Physical Score	60.6	(56.0)	50
Behavior Score	78.5	(43.7)	85
Stress Score	60.9	(44.3)	53

*Range = 0–100%
†Range = 0–200%

RESULTS

Patients assigned to the UT and CB conditions were comparable at baseline on demographic and pain history variables (Table I). Overall, 35% of patients reported TMD pain of greater than five years duration. The sample mean for characteristic pain rating was 4.72 (0–10 scale), with patients reporting an average of five activity limitation days in the two months prior to baseline evaluation. The mean for unassisted mandibular opening was 33.5 mm.

Explanatory Model (EM) scores were developed, using 0–100% rating scales, to measure patients' global perceptions of the relative roles played by physical factors, behavior, and stress in influencing TMD cause, exacerba-

Table III
Composite explanatory model scores: correlations (r) with 3-month examination and interview measures (combined sample, N = 71)

	Composite Explanatory Model Score		
	Physical (r)	Behavior (r)	Stress (r)
Clinical measures			
Unassisted mandibular opening	–0.30*	0.06	0.33**
Muscle palpation score	0.19	–0.16	–0.08
Characteristic pain (0-10)	0.18	–0.21	–0.02
Psychosocial variables			
SCL-90 somatization†	0.25*	–0.23*	–0.09
VPMI passive coping	0.32**	–0.31**	0.10
VPMI active coping	–0.08	0.09	0.01
Ability to control pain	–0.25*	0.23*	–0.10

* $P < .05$
** $P < .01$
† Somatization subscale with pain items removed

tion, and treatment efficacy. Sample mean and median values, as shown in Table II, indicate that EM scores are not skewed, and show variability between subjects. On average, patients rated physical factors as most important in initially causing TMD ($\bar{x}$ = 52.5 ± 34.6), followed by behavioral factors ($\bar{x}$ = 25.8 ± 21.0), and stress ($\bar{x}$ = 21.7 ± 22.9). Patients' ratings of the importance of physical factors, behaviors, and stress in exacerbating TMD were more evenly distributed (means of 27.4, 42.6, and 30.0, respectively), as were their ratings of expected efficacy of physically, behaviorally, and psychosocially-oriented TMD treatments (means of 33.2, 35.9, and 30.9, respectively).

Consistency was often observed among EM scores for the TMD exacerbate and treatment efficacy dimensions. The correlations (*r*) between EM scores of exacerbate and treatment efficacy, across the physical, behavioral, and psychosocial domains were .67, .58, and .75, respectively, explaining 33–56% of the variance between relevant variables. Composite explanatory model (CEM) scores were derived by summing the physical, behavior, and stress EM scores across TMD exacerbation and treatment efficacy dimensions, yielding three CEM scores (0–200%) per subject. Table II also shows descriptive data for CEM scores.

Physical, behavioral, and stress explanatory models for TMD were examined for their association with clinical indices, characteristic pain, and

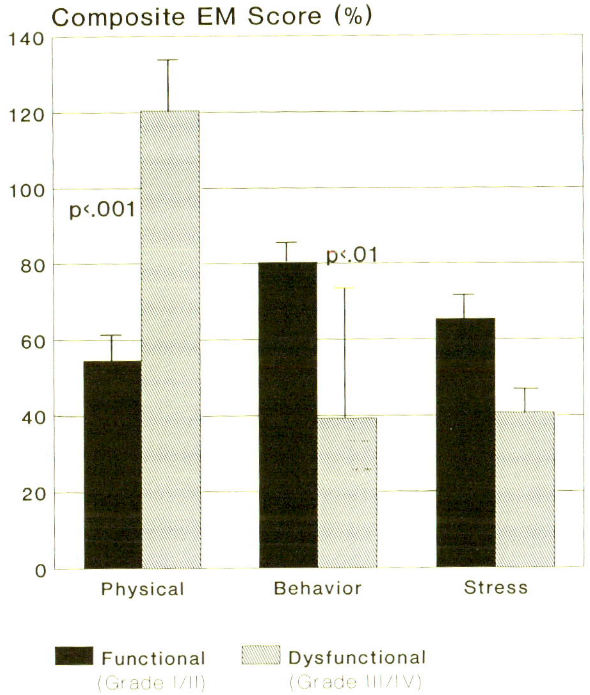

Fig. 2. Composite Explanatory Model (EM) scores for low (Chronic Pain Grades I/II) versus high (Chronic Pain Grades III/IV) pain-related disability.

psychosocial variables, as measured by Pearson product-moment correlations (Table III). Unassisted mandibular opening was correlated with lower CEM physical scores ($r = -0.30$; $P < .05$) and higher CEM stress scores ($r = 0.33$; $P < .01$). Muscle palpation tenderness and self-report ratings of characteristic pain experienced in the past two months were not significantly related to CEM score.

Table III also shows correlations among CEM scores, somatization, and coping style. CEM physical score was positively correlated with mean somatization score ($r = 0.25$; $P < .05$) and VPMI Passive Coping score ($r = 0.32$; $P < .01$), and negatively correlated with ability to control pain ($r = -0.25$; $P < .05$). By comparison, CEM behavior score was negatively correlated with mean somatization score ($r = -0.23$; $P < .05$) and VPMI Passive Coping ($r = -0.31$; $P < .01$), and tended toward a positive association with ability to control pain ($r = 0.23$; $P < .05$). No significant relationships were observed between CEM scores and VPMI Active Coping.

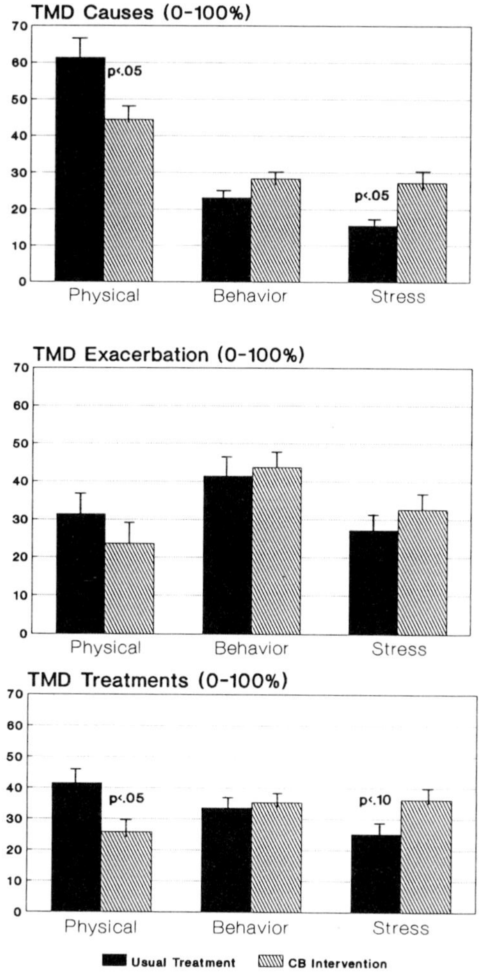

Fig. 3. TMD Explanatory Model Scores for patients receiving usual dental treatment versus a brief cognitive-behavioral intervention.

Fig. 2 shows the association between pain-related disability, assessed by chronic pain grade (0–IV), and CEM scores. Functional (Grades I/II) patients had significantly lower CEM physical scores than did dysfunctional (Grades III/IV) patients ($t = 3.29$; $df = 64$; $P < .001$). By contrast, functional patients had significantly higher CEM behavior scores than did dysfunctional patients ($t = -2.64$; $df = 64$; $P < .01$).

Finally, TMD explanatory models were compared between patients receiving usual dental treatment and patients receiving usual treatment plus the brief CB intervention. Fig. 3 shows that patients exposed to the CB intervention, compared with UT patients, rated physical factors as less important in TMD causes ($t = 2.11$; $df = 69$; $P < .05$) and in TMD treatment efficacy ($t = 2.09$; $df = 69$; $P < .05$), and stress and psychosocial factors as more important in

TMD causes ($t = -2.22$; $df = 69$; $P < .05$) and in TMD treatment efficacy ($t = -1.85$; $df = 69$; $P < .10$).

DISCUSSION

A primary objective of this pilot study was to examine the utility of global explanatory model measures for research with TMD patients. First, it is apparent that patients with TMD are capable of responding to questions about the relative roles that physical factors, behaviors, and psychosocial stressors play in explaining TMD cause, exacerbation, and treatment efficacy. The EM scores showed adequate variability in subject response, indicating that TMD explanatory models differ among persons and can be measured. In general, many of the patients in this study had a biologically-oriented explanation for TMD causes, but shifted their focus to a mixed, or biopsychosocial perspective with respect to TMD exacerbation and types of treatment viewed as efficacious. CEM scores, which are a linear combination of EM exacerbate and EM treatment efficacy scores, indicated that on average, patients had a biopsychosocial view of the factors that influence the *course* of their TMD. The TMD specialists participating in this study typically advocate a biopsychosocial explanatory model of TMD and emphasize conservative dental therapies. Thus, patient explanatory models seem to mirror the explanatory models of their clinicians.

A series of analyses examined the associations among CEM scores and relevant clinical examination variables. Self-reported pain and muscle palpation tenderness were not significantly related to subject's global beliefs about the influence of physical, behavior, or stress factors on the course of TMD. By contrast, unassisted jaw opening was significantly correlated with CEM scores. Patients showing limited mandibular opening rated physical factors as more influential in the course of their TMD, while patients with maximal mandibular opening rated stress factors as more important. Unassisted mandibular opening requires that the patient open the mouth until pain, a subjective symptom, is experienced. Perhaps patients who endorse more physically-oriented explanations of TMD are more guarded during mandibular movement as a function of perceived structural damage to the temporomandibular joint apparatus.

Other analyses examined the associations among CEM scores and relevant psychosocial variables. Somatization scores (excluding pain items) were observed to be highest in patients reporting primarily physical explanations of TMD and lowest in those reporting behavioral explanations of TMD. Similarly, dysfunctional TMD patients (high pain-related disability) gave physical factors more than twice the weight given by functional TMD patients (low pain-related disability) when explaining their TMD. Conversely, functional patients gave twice as much weight to behavioral factors.

High-somatization patients, typically characterized by the tendency to report numerous physical symptoms and to seek health care frequently (Dworkin et al. 1993), have demonstrated poorer response to multidisciplinary treatment for TMD (McCreary et al. 1992). Dysfunctional TMD patients seek TMD treatment from more health care providers than do their nondysfunctional counterparts, even though clinical signs appear to be comparable between these two groups (Dworkin and Massoth, in press). Thus, it is plausible that highly somatizing and/or dysfunctional TMD patients, who endorse a more biologic explanatory model for their condition, more frequently pursue physical treatments for their illness and may be less receptive to broad-based treatment approaches that include modifying behaviors that cause or exacerbate their pain condition.

Comparisons among CEM scores and various coping measures were also provocative. Those attributing physical factors as most influential in the course of TMD endorsed both passive pain coping strategies and lower self-ratings of pain coping efficacy. By contrast, these same coping strategies were inversely related to the strength of belief that behaviors most strongly influenced the course of TMD. Prior research has demonstrated the relationship of passive pain coping strategies to patients' reports of increased pain, greater functional impairment, and greater affective disturbance (Brown and Nicassio 1987; Keefe and Dolan 1986; Rosenstiel and Keefe 1983). In addition, pain coping efficacy has been correlated with current pain status (Bandura 1986; O'Leary 1985) and continued presence of pain after one year (Massoth et al. 1990). It is possible that patients who endorse a physical explanatory model of TMD tend to wait and see how their perceived structural aberrations will respond to treatment, while patients who endorse behavioral explanatory models feel better able to influence TMD symptomatology through modification of their behavior.

Patients exposed to the brief CB intervention in addition to usual treatment, compared with patients receiving usual treatment alone, rated stress and psychosocial factors as more important in their TMD. This finding seems consistent with the intervention's emphasis on the potential role of stress in TMD pain and its focus on patient self-management strategies for the relief of chronic pain. This investigation was not designed to evaluate pre- to postintervention changes in TMD explanatory models; however, this will be an important and exciting line of research for future study.

CONCLUSIONS

This pilot investigation has demonstrated that patient explanatory models for TMD can be measured and show adequate variability between persons. In addition, these measures were meaningfully associated with clinical examination and relevant psychosocial measures such that patients who endorsed physical explanatory models of TMD reported more subjectively-influenced clinical TMD signs, higher somatization, more pain-related disability, and endorsed more passive pain coping strategies. By contrast, patients who endorsed behavioral explanatory models of TMD reported fewer subjectively-influenced clinical TMD signs, less somatization, less pain-related disability, and endorsed fewer passive pain coping strategies.

While these findings are provocative, they are certainly preliminary. Specifically, correlations were low to moderate, which could reflect the imperfect nature of this early measuring instrument. Potential interactions among treatment group, chronic pain grade, and explanatory model scores require further exploration. In addition, further examination of health care use among patients with behavioral versus physical TMD explanatory models will help delineate patterns of self-care for chronic pain and pain-related disability within these populations.

ACKNOWLEDGMENTS

This research was supported by grants PO1 DE08773 and 5P30 DE09743 from the National Institute of Dental Research. The contributions of Muneera Merchant, Kimberly Huggins, and Linda LeResche to this research are gratefully acknowledged.

REFERENCES

Bandura, A., Self-efficacy mechanism in physiological activation and health-promoting behavior. In: J. Madden IV, S. Matthysse and J. Barchas (Eds.), Adaptation, Learning and Affect, Raven Press, New York, 1986.

Brown, G.K. and Nicassio, P.M., Development of a questionnaire for the assessment of active and passive coping strategies in chronic pain patients, Pain, 31 (1987) 53–64.

Chrisman, N., The health seeking process: an approach to the natural history of illness, Cult. Med. Psychiatry, 1 (1977) 351–377.

Derogatis, L.R., SCL-90-R: administration, scoring and procedures manual—II for the revised version, Clinical Psychometric Research, Towson, Md., 1983.

Dworkin, S.F. and Massoth, D.L., Temporomandibular disorders and chronic pain: disease or illness? J. Pros. Dent., in press.

Dworkin, S.F. and LeResche, L., Research diagnostic criteria for temporomandibular disorders, J.

Craniomandib. Disord. Facial Oral Pain, 6 (1992) 301–355.
Dworkin, S.F., Huggins, K.H., LeResche, L., Von Korff, M., Howard, J., Truelove, E. and Sommers, E., Epidemiology of signs and symptoms in temporomandibular disorders: clinical signs in cases and controls, J. Am. Dent. Assoc., 120 (1990a) 273–281.
Dworkin, S.F., Von Korff, M., Whitney, C.W., LeResche, L., Dicker, B.G. and Barlow, W., Measurement of characteristic pain in field research, Pain, 55 (1990b) 290.
Dworkin, S.F., Von Korff, M.R. and LeResche, L., Multiple pains and psychiatric disturbance: an epidemiologic investigation, Arch. Gen. Psychiatry, 47 (1990c) 239–244.
Dworkin, S.F., Von Korff, M.R. and LeResche, L., Epidemiologic studies of chronic pain: a dynamic-ecologic perspective, Ann. Behav. Med., 14 (1992) 3–11.
Dworkin, S.F., Wilson, L. and Massoth, D.L., Somatizing as a risk factor for chronic pain. In: R.C. Grzesiak and D.S. Ciccone (Eds.), Psychologic Vulnerability to Chronic Pain, 1993, in press.
Dworkin, S.F., Turner, J.A., Wilson, L., Massoth, D.L., Whitney, C., Huggins, K.H., Burgess, J., Sommers, E. and Truelove, E., Brief group cognitive-behavioral intervention for TMD, Pain, in press.
Fordyce, W.E., Roberts, A.H. and Sternbach, R.A., The behavioral management of chronic pain: a response to critics, Pain, 22 (1985) 113–125.
Graff-Radford, S.B., Reeves, J.L. and Janetta, P.J., Evaluation and management of the difficult facial pain patient. Presentation at the 10th Annual Scientific Meeting of the American Pain Society, New Orleans, Nov. 7–10, 1991.
Keefe, F.J. and Dolan, E., Pain behavior and pain coping strategies in low back pain and myofascial pain dysfunction syndrome patients, Pain, 24 (1986) 49–56.
Kleinman, A., Patients and Healers in the Context of Culture: An Exploration of the Borderland between Anthropology, Medicine, and Psychiatry, University of California Press, Berkeley, 1980.
Kleinman, A., The Illness Narratives: Suffering, Healing and the Human Condition, Basic Books, New York, 1988.
Massoth, D.L., Barlow, W., LeResche, L., Dicker, B.G., Whitney, C.W., Dworkin, S.F. and Von Korff, M., Perceived ability to control pain and continued TMD pain (abstract), Pain, Suppl. 5 (1990) 531.
McCreary, C.P., Clark, G.T., Oakley, M.E. and Flack, V., Predicting response to treatment for temporomandibular disorders, J. Craniomandib. Disord. Facial Oral Pain, 6 (1992) 161–170.
O'Leary, A., Self-efficacy and health, Behav. Res. Ther., 23 (1985) 437–451.
Rosenstiel, A.K. and Keefe, F.J., The use of coping strategies in chronic low back pain patients: relationship to patient characteristics and current adjustment, Pain, 17 (1983) 33–44.
Turk, D.C., Meichenbaum, D. and Genest, M., Pain and Behavioral Medicine: A Cognitive Behavioral Perspective, Guilford Press, New York, 1983.
Von Korff, M., Dworkin, S.F., LeResche, L. and Kruger, A., An epidemiologic comparison of pain complaints, Pain, 32 (1988) 173–183.
Von Korff, M., Ormel, J., Keefe, F.J. and Dworkin, S.F., Grading the severity of chronic pain, Pain, 50 (1992) 133–149.

Correspondence to: Donna L. Massoth, DDS, PhD, University of Washington, Department of Oral Medicine SC-63, Seattle, WA 98195, USA. Tel: 206-543-5912, Fax: 206-685-8412.

Proceedings of the 7th World Congress on Pain,
Progress in Pain Research and Management, Vol. 2,
edited by G.F. Gebhart, D.L. Hammond, and T.S.
Jensen, IASP Press, Seattle, © 1994.

15

The Relationship Between Pain and Depression: A Longitudinal Study of Early Synovitis

Suzanne M. Skevington

School of Social Sciences, University of Bath, Avon, UK

INTRODUCTION

Considerable controversy surrounds the debate about the incidence and intensity of depression in chronic pain patients. The link between the two is widely reported but difficult to explain. Perhaps more puzzling is not that some people in pain become depressed, but why so many do not appear to be depressed. In a comprehensive review of the epidemiological, methodological, and theoretical factors that influence the relationship between pain and depression, Romano and Turner (1985) concluded that there was little consistent evidence to support the view that syndromal depression is more common in chronic pain patients. The presence of depressive symptoms was much more likely than a major syndrome of clinical depression. Other estimates put the figure for clinical depression at around 30% (DeVellis 1993).

From the extensive literature on depression, three main hypotheses have been identified that concern the timing and relationship of depressive thoughts or cognitions to the onset of depression itself, and these may be relevant to the understanding of how the relationship between pain and depression works and why it only affects some of those in pain. Looking at vulnerability to depression, Abramson et al. (1978) proposed that when faced with a negative, uncontrollable, and aversive event, those who were more inclined to interpret that event using a certain cluster of explanatory beliefs would be more likely to develop learned helplessness and therefore become depressed. If they believed the event to be uncontrollable (beyond control), stable (persisting in time), global (pertaining to many other areas of life), and internal (bearing personal responsibility), rather than controllable, unstable, specific, and external (the responsibility of others), collectively this explanatory style would predispose that person to be helpless. If self-blame was an integral part of this pattern, then it was expected that self-esteem would be lowered.

This antecedent model describes the way depressive cognitions precede the onset of helplessness depression; pain as a particularly aversive occurrence provides a good test of these ideas. It seems a plausible that those who become helpless and depressed following the onset of a painful illness are more inclined to have explained previous unpleasant events in this particular way, but this model of depression has not been directly tested for those in pain (Romano and Turner 1985). A revised model of hopelessness now places much more emphasis on the contributions of stable and global attributions (Abramson et al. 1989).

One alternative to the antecedent model is the consequence hypothesis, where depressive cognitions would be expected to occur at the same time as the depression rather than precede or cause it. A third scar hypothesis predicts that any episode of depression that occurred in the period before the onset of pain is liable to have left psychological scars or residues, which will then predispose those who are later exposed to an aversive event to become helpless and depressed. These three models have been compared by looking at the incidence of psychiatric depression in communities in the United States (Lewinsohn et al. 1981) and United Kingdom (Dent and Teasdale 1988) using prospective longitudinal designs. Both studies gave greatest support to the consequence hypothesis, found little evidence for an antecedent model, and none for the scar hypothesis. Do any of these models explain the relationship between pain and depression?

Surveying chronically ill patients with rheumatoid arthritis (RA), Brown et al. (1989) reported that depression at the beginning of their study strongly predicted depression six months later (55% of the variance), but pain did not predict changes in depression. Brown (1990) reported that episodes of pain and depression were distinct and correlated syndromes and found that this weak relationship persisted even when confounding somatic symptoms common to the two conditions were removed.

Pain is a symptom of greatest concern to patients with rheumatoid arthritis, and reducing pain is a primary goal of seeking medical treatment (Skevington 1986). Pain and the serious functional difficulties that develop as the disease progresses make the concept of helplessness seem particularly appropriate to this disease group. The Arthritis Helplessness Index (AHI), designed to examine perceptions of controllability in this group, has had widespread use. For instance, Fitzpatrick et al. (1990) gave the AHI to chronic RA outpatients and found that the sickest patients (as shown in clinical tests) also were the most helpless on this measure. This cross-sectional study showed that those who said they had most helplessness also believed they had less personal control, had lower self-esteem, and more depressive symptoms. However, it is debatable whether the aspects of controllability investigated within the AHI constitute an adequate test of the learned helplessness hypothesis, because there is no direct operational means of evaluating the four separate attributional styles described by Abramson et al. (1978).

As these models have not been directly tested for those at the early stages of potentially chronically painful illness, our study reported a prospective longitudinal design to examine evidence for the three hypotheses, looking at the relationship between depression and depressive cognitions in outpatients with early synovitis (commonly associated with the onset of rheumatoid arthritis).

METHODS

Patients admitted to a specialist outpatient clinic with the symptoms of early synovitis were interviewed on the day of admission, immediately before their first consultation with a senior rheumatologist, so that beliefs and expectations could be assessed before outpatient treatment began. General practitioners refer patients to this clinic sited in the Royal National Hospital for Rheumatic Diseases, Bath, at a much earlier stage of the disease than is common in rheumatology clinics in the United Kingdom. Interviews and assessments were carried out on three occasions over two years (mean 22.2 months) from the time of admission (Fig. 1).

Of the 74 patients approached, 69 volunteered to take part at stage I, of which 30 were men, and 98% Caucasian. The mean age was 45.5 years (SD = 16), the mean duration of illness was 2.7 years (median six months), mean school-leaving age was 15 (SD = 1.4), and mean occupational grading was middle class. By stage III, 43% were still outpatients, 35% had confirmed RA, and 27% were seropositive. Of those who left the study, 17 were discharged (most within two consultations), 6 refused, 1 died and 1 was untraceable. Thus, 44 of the original 69 patients (64%) were available at stage III.

Five scales measuring 13 variables were used to assess participants at each stage of the study. Self-reports of depressive symptoms were obtained using the 12-item Wakefield Self-Assessment Depression Inventory (WSADI) (Snaith et al. 1971). Scores from two items on sleep were removed because sleep problems are common to both pain and depression. A modified version

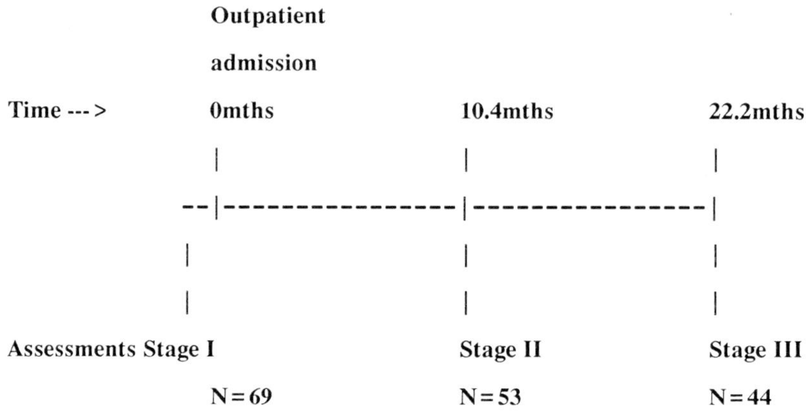

Fig. 1. Prospective longitudinal design of the study.

of the Carlson Adjective Checklist assessed levels of social and personal self-esteem (Skevington et al. 1987). The Beliefs in Pain Control Questionnaire (BPCQ; Skevington 1990) was used to evaluate three types of beliefs about controlling pain. Three subscales evaluate beliefs in the personal responsibility for pain control (Internal Scale), beliefs that the doctors control pain (Powerful Doctors scale) and beliefs that pain occurs by chance or from misfortune (Chance Happenings scale). It has been standardized for use with arthritis patients. Depressive attributions about painful symptoms were investigated using the four attributional dimensions proposed by Abramson et al. (1978). The four seven-point ratings were completed for each of the painful joints or sites recorded by that patient and so were tailored to the condition of each patient. Means for each person's joints and sites were calculated separately for internal-external, stable-unstable, global-specific, and controllable-uncontrollable dimensions (Skevington 1993). A modified version of the McGill Pain Questionnaire (MPQ) adapted for arthritis and low-back pain patients assessed the qualities of sensory, affective, and evaluative pain, and total pain weightings were calculated for each subscale (Skevington 1979).

RESULTS AND DISCUSSION

The levels of depressive symptoms recorded throughout this study were fairly low. Ranging from 0 to 36, the mean score at stage I was 12.6 (SD = 5.8), at stage II 12.0 (SD = 7.0), and at stage III = 11.7 (SD = 6.8). Only five patients obtained or exceeded a score of 24 throughout the study, a level that provides tentative evidence of primary clinical depression. These findings support Romano and Turner's (1985) observation that few pain patients are severely depressed.

SCAR HYPOTHESIS

The 44 patients who completed all three stages were divided into two groups, and the five with high depression scores were removed. Those who reported an episode of depression prior to the onset of their pain (N=19) were compared with those who believed they had not been depressed (N=20). Univariate F-tests of all stage I variables showed no significant differences, so there was no evidence to support a scar hypothesis.

ANTECEDENT HYPOTHESIS

Hierarchical multiple regressions were performed to find out whether cognitions before treatment began had any power to predict depression at either of the two later stages. Blocks of variables were entered into the analysis as follows: first, the four depressive attributions and two self-esteem variables, which had been identified as important by the learned helplessness model, followed by pain then pain control.

The best predictor of whether patients would be depressed at either of the two later stages was their level of depressive symptoms at the time of admission. The more depression they reported on their first visit, the more depressed they were likely to be one and two years later. In each analysis, 34% of the variance in later depression was explained by the level of depressive symptoms expressed at the time of admission.

When the 12 cognitive variables were added, they increased the amount of depression explained to 54% at stage II, and 60.4% at stage III, but at neither stage did this increase significantly improve the prediction of future depression. More specifically, expectations that the pain would continue (stable) ($t = 2.03$, $P = 0.049$), and poor personal self-esteem ($t = 2.17$, $P = 0.036$) at the start, contributed to explaining depression a year later, but only weakly. Those who believed from the outset that their pain would be uncontrollable ($t = 2.41$, $P = 0.021$) and that it was beyond their personal control ($t = 2.13$, $P = 0.040$) were more likely to be depressed after two years of treatment.

But does the presence of depression mask the expression of other cognitions? Do the features above remain significant if depression scores at the time of admission are removed from the analysis? Repeating these regressions, we found that stable attributions remained important in explaining depressive symptoms after a year ($t = 2.48$, $P = 0.017$) and so did not appear to be affected by the presence of depression. But affective pain ($t = 2.33$, $P = 0.025$) and beliefs in the powers of doctors to control pain ($t = 2.26$, $P = 0.029$) emerged as cognitive features (F change = 2.12, $P < 0.038$) that appeared to have been masked by the presence of depression. Affective pain also was important in explaining depression after two years of treatment ($t = 2.23$, $P = 0.034$), together with social self-esteem ($t = 2.17$, $P = 0.038$) (F change = 3.02, $P < 0.007$). So the presence of depressive symptoms throughout the first two years of treatment may mask the expression of affective pain, which could be a consistent predictor of depressive symptoms later in the illness. These results provide insights into the complex and elusive interaction between pain and depression.

In an additional test of the antecedent hypothesis, we compared those who were most depressed at the end of the study (scored 15+) with those who had few depressive symptoms (10 or less), using each of the variables obtained at stage I. Those who were most depressed at stage III were more likely to have believed from the start that their pain would be stable ($t = 2.64$, $P <.01$) and uncontrollable ($t =2.22$, $P < .03$).

CONSEQUENCE HYPOTHESIS

To test the consequence hypothesis, cognitive variables were regressed against depression scores obtained at the same stage. The consequence hypothesis was supported at stage I and stage III; the results failed to reach significance at stage II. Depressive cognitions explained 42% of the variance in depression at stage I (F change = 3.18, $P < 0.002$), but at stage III, a sizable 72% was explained (F change = 5.73, $P <.001$). It is worth noting that at both these stages, together the three pain measures (F = 5.77, $P = 0.002$ at stage I; F = 7.55, $P = 0.001$ at stage III) and four attributional dimensions (F = 3.43, $P = 0.015$ at stage I; F = 3.06, $P = 0.033$ at stage III) combined to substantially improve the prediction of depression. However, the specific type of pain and style of attribution involved proved to be quite different for the two time periods, so that at admission, affective pain ($t = 3.81$, $P = 0.001$) and attributions that the pain would be uncontrollable ($t = 2.12$, $P = 0.039$) and stable ($t = 2.12$, $P = 0.49$), best predicted depression at that time. But after two years treatment, sensory pain ($t = 2.16$, $P = 0.40$) combined with affective pain ($t = 2.30$, $P = 0.029$) and global attributions ($t = 2.33$, $P = 0.027$), provided the best predictors.

COMPARING ANTECEDENT AND CONSEQUENCE HYPOTHESES

It was important to compare the results from the antecedent hypothesis with those for the consequence hypothesis because if the cognitive variables predict depression within the same time period, they cannot then be viewed as true antecedents of depression at a later date. In this case, some of the above results that appear to support an antecedent hypothesis would be negated. The following conclusions may be drawn:

1. Two depressive attributions appeared to be antecedents to depression, but these results were compromised by significant contributions to the consequence model. Beliefs that the pain is uncontrollable and stable turn out not to be antecedents but a consequence of depression at the time of admission. Global attributions are an important consequence of depression after two years of treatment. Internal-external attributions are not significant in any model. These results, which constitute a direct test of the theory, lead to the rejection of the antecedent learned helplessness model as an explanation for the incidence and onset of depression in these pain patients.

2. While two true antecedents of depression helped to explain it, neither made a significant contribution to its later prediction. These were personal self-esteem at admission and initial beliefs in a lack of personal responsibility for pain control. They provide only minor and indirect support for the learned helplessness concept.

3. Affective and sensory pain are prime consequences of depression in RA. While chronic pain sufferers commonly report affective pain, this prospective longitudinal design shows that affective pain is an important consequence of depression much earlier in the disease process than has been formerly acknowledged: as early as the first visit to outpatient clinics.

4. Furthermore, sensory and affective pain better predict depression when the illness is chronic than do depressive attributions alone, but when pain is assessed along with depressive attributions, together they have major predictive power. Two years after the start of treatment, affective and sensory pain together with global attributions predicted a major part of depression at this chronic stage.

5. Affective pain was found to be both an antecedent and a consequence of pain at most stages, but its antecedent properties were largely masked by the presence of depression throughout this two-year period. These results suggest that the contribution of affective pain to the pain-depression cycle may hitherto have been underestimated in those at the early stages of painful disease.

CONCLUSION

The results from this study showed no evidence for a scar hypothesis, weak evidence for an antecedent hypothesis, and the strongest evidence for the consequence hypothesis. It shows that, for those faced with the negative and aversive onset of painful early synovitis symptoms, important depressive cognitions accompany depressive symptoms rather than precede or cause it. This concurs with the findings from previous prospective longitudinal community studies of psychiatric morbidity by Lewinsohn et al. (1981) and Dent and Teasdale (1988).

The best predictor of depression later in the disease is how much patients are depressed at the time they are admitted to an early synovitis clinic. While Brown et al. (1989) reported this feature for chronic RAs, our study shows that it occurs much earlier in the development of this painful disease.

The main limitations to this study are first that the retrospective data used to test the scar hypothesis may not be entirely reliable due to inaccuracies in the prior reporting of depression. Second, the sample size is small and has low statistic power. Third, while the attrition rate was quite high, this was largely due to the withdrawal of patients after stage I who had been suffering from inflammatory conditions, e.g., trauma, which were only temporary and without serious implications.

IMPLICATIONS FOR PRACTICE

Three main implications can be drawn from this work. First, even subclinical levels of depression should be treated much more seriously at the earliest stages of the development of a painful disease and its treatment. Second, as it progresses, rheumatoid arthritis can spread to more and more joints, but these stable and uncontrollable attributions may represent an overly pessimistic view of the future. Is it realistic for patients with the early symptoms of rheumatoid arthritis to believe that their pain will continue and be beyond their control? Jayson and Dixon (1980) reported that of those who attend for treatment, a quarter recover completely, a quarter heal but have slight residual joint damage that does not interfere with their ability to work, 40% have continual disease activity, but only 10% are severely crippled with the chronically painful and disabling condition that represents the widespread image of this disease. Furthermore, the development of better NSAIDs have improved the treatment of pain and inflammation in RA by providing a long-term means of pain control for many patients. So for some patients with early synovitis, stable and uncontrollable attributions may represent inappropriate pessimism.

Psychological therapies in the form of attributional retraining (Forsterling 1985) and social support groups, specially convened for those who are at an early stage of the disease, could provide preemptive counseling and good role models. Better public education by national institutions such as the Arthritis and Rheumatism Council, and Arthritis Care in Britain already go some way to providing this service. But action against these beliefs, which increase personal vulnerability to depression, need to be targeted systematically.

Third, from a pragmatic viewpoint it seems unlikely that newly admitted outpatients will readily disclose any expectations that their pain will continue and be uncontrollable for fear of affronting the rheumatologist and appearing to challenge clinical competence at the point that they most wish to engage the physician's help. For social desirability reasons, many rheumatologists may be unable to access those depressive cognitions that are central to predictions about whether patients will become depressed. Consequently, the health care team needs to be involved in screening patients' beliefs at the outset, and to be trained to take prophylactic action where necessary by offering psychosocial care right from the start to those who appear to be most vulnerable to future depression.

REFERENCES

Abramson, LY, Seligman, M.E.P. and Teasdale, J.D., Learned helplessness in humans: critique and reformulation, J. Abnorm. Psychol., 87 (1978) 49–74.

Abramson, L.Y., Metalsky, G.I. and Alloy, L.A., Hopelessness depression: a theory based subtype of depression, Psychol. Rev., 96, 2 (1989) 358–372.

Brown, G.K., A causal analysis of chronic pain and depression, J. Abnorm. Psychol., 99, 2 (1990) 127–137.

Brown, G.K., Nicassio P.M. and Wallston, K.A., Pain coping strategies and depression in rheumatoid arthritis, J. Consult. Clin. Psychol., 57, 5 (1989) 652–657.

Dent, J. and Teasdale, J.D., Negative cognitions and the persistence of depression, J. Abnorm. Psychol., 97, 1 (1988) 29–34.

De Vellis, B.M.E., Depression in rheumatological diseases. In: S. Newman and M. Shipley (Eds.), Psychological Aspects of Rheumatoid Disease, Ballières Clinical Rheumatology, Vol. 7:2, London, 1993, pp. 241–257.

Fitzpatrick, R., Newman, S., Lamb, R. and Shipley, M., Helplessness and control in rheumatoid arthritis, Int. J. Health Sci., 1, 1 (1990) 17–23.

Forsterling, F., Attributional retraining: a review, Psychol. Bull., 98, 3 (1985) 495–512.

Jayson, M.I.V. and Dixon, A.StJ., Rheumatism and Arthritis: What You Should Know about the Problems and Treatment, Pan, London, 1980.

Lewinsohn, P.M., Steinmetz, J.L., Larson, D.W. and Franklin, J., Depression-related cognitions: antecedent or consequence, J. Abnorm. Psychol., 90 (1981) 213–219.

Romano, J.M. and Turner, J.A., Chronic pain and depression: does the evidence support the relationship? Psychol. Bull., 97 (1985) 18–34.

Skevington, S.M., Pain and locus of control: a social approach. In: D.J. Oborne, M.M. Gruneberg and J.R. Eiser (Eds), Research in Psychology and Medicine, Vol. 1, Academic Press, London, 1979, pp. 61–69.

Skevington, S.M., Psychological aspects of pain in rheumatoid arthritis: a review, Soc. Sci. Med., 23, 6 (1986) 567–575.

Skevington, S.M., A standardised scale to measure beliefs about controlling pain (BPCQ): a preliminary study, Psychol. Health, 4 (1990) 221–232.

Skevington, S.M., Depression and causal attributions in the early stages of a chronic painful

disease: a longitudinal study of early synovitis, Psychol. Health, 8 (1993) 51–64.
Skevington, S.M., Blackwell, F. and Britton, N.F.B., Self-esteem and perception of attractiveness: an investigation of early rheumatoid arthritis, Br. J. Med. Psychol., 60 (1987) 45–52.
Snaith, R.P., Ahmed, S.N., Mehta, S. and Hamilton, M., Assessment of the severity of primary depressive illness: Wakefield Self-Assessment Depression Inventory, Psychol. Med., 2 (1971) 143–149.

Correspondence to: Suzanne M. Skevington, PhD, School of Social Sciences, University of Bath, Claverton Down, Bath, BA2 7AY, Avon, UK. Tel: 44-225-826826; Fax: 44-225-826381 (group 3); E-mail: S.M.Skevington@bath.ac.uk

Part IV

The Nociceptor as a Dynamic Entity

Proceedings of the 7th World Congress on Pain,
Progress in Pain Research and Management, Vol. 2,
edited by G.F. Gebhart, D.L. Hammond, and T.S.
Jensen, IASP Press, Seattle, © 1994.

16

Silent and Active Nociceptors: Structure, Functions, and Clinical Implications

Robert F. Schmidt, Hans-Georg Schaible,
Karl Meßlinger, Bernd Heppelmann,
Ulrike Hanesch, and Matthias Pawlak

Physiologisches Institut der Universität Würzburg, Würzburg, Germany

This brief outline on the structure and function of nociceptors in mammals, including humans, emphasizes three "take-home messages":

1. Basic research has revealed that nociceptors are not a homogeneous population of sensory receptors with high thresholds. Rather, nociceptors are extremely diverse in nature.

2. All widely held simple concepts regarding the structural and functional properties of nociceptors have crumbled under the weight of ever increasing evidence to the contrary. Such concepts included, for instance, that all fine (unmyelinated and thinly myelinated) somatovisceral primary afferents have high thresholds, or that all nociceptive units either contain substance P (SP) or at least another of the more common peptides, or that all nociceptors and only nociceptors are excited by capsaicin.

3. A nociceptor is not born to be and to remain that kind of fellow for the rest of his life. It is a dynamic entity, shifting its properties under the influence and according to the necessities of its environment.

Data to support these statements will be taken mainly from our own work on the knee joint of the rat and cat. They will be supplemented by reviewing the considerable and fundamental contributions of many other laboratories around the world.

CAN WE RECOGNIZE NOCICEPTORS FROM THEIR STRUCTURE?

INNERVATION OF THE KNEE JOINT

The medial articular nerve (MAN) and the posterior articular nerve (PAN) form the major innervation of the cat's knee joint (Freeman and Wyke 1967). Their afferent and efferent fiber content is shown in Table I. Each nerve contains approximately 650 afferent fibers, mainly of groups III and IV, and another 500 unmyelinated sympathetic efferents (Langford and Schmidt 1983). In the group IV fiber range the maximum of the diameter distribution is between 0.3 and 0.4 μm for the afferent fibers, whereas that maximum is around 0.8 to 0.9 μm for the sympathetic efferent ones (Heppelmann et al. 1988). The latter study and that of Langford and Schmidt (1983) also determined the respective numbers of the group I–III fibers (Table I). The small contribution of the group I fibers in the PAN is presumably due to stray fibers joining in from muscle spindles of the popliteus muscle (McIntyre et al. 1978). Thus, the majority of afferent fibers in both nerves belongs to the fine afferent category consisting of groups III and IV (MAN 91%, PAN 74%).

Little in general is known about the ultrastructure of the sensory endings of fine afferent nerve fibers in visceral, superficial cutaneous, or deep tissues. In particular, the structure of nocisensors and their eventual specializations in tissue, relative to other "free nerve endings," is unknown. Therefore, using methods described in detail elsewhere (Heppelmann et al. 1989), we conducted several studies devoted to these questions. We inspected serial sections of the terminal parts of group III and group IV articular afferents at distances up to 300 μm under the electron microscope and produced three-dimensional computer-assisted reconstructions. The specimen section of Fig. 1 shows sensory endings of a group III and a group IV unit innervating the knee joint capsule.

TERMINALS OF GROUP III AFFERENTS

The final part of any group III afferent fiber consists of three major segments (Fig. 2A) (Heppelmann et al. 1990a): (1) The proximal part of the afferent fiber is myelinated and runs within a perineural sheath. Most likely, action potentials are conducted from Ranvier node to Ranvier node in this area. (2) More distally, an intermediate part has lost its myelin at the last half of the Ranvier node, but is still within the perineural sheath. However, its ultrastructure is already comparable to that of the distal portion described next. The length of the intermediate part is 7–98 μm. (3) The distal portion,

Table I
Composition of the nerves inntervating the knee joint of the cat

	Medial Articular Nerve	Posterior Articular Nerve
Afferents	630 (100%)	680 (100%)
Group I (A-alpha) Fibers	0 (0%)	27 (4%)
Group II (A-beta) Fibers	59 (9%)	149 (22%)
Group III (A-delta) Fibers	131 (21%)	94 (14%)
Group IV (C) Fibers	440 (70%)	410 (60%)
Sympathetic Fibers	500	515

also free of myelin, starts at the end of the perineural sheath. It runs into the tissue, splits into several branches, and forms the sensory terminal tree. This terminal tree usually consists of 2–4 larger branches with an overall length of about 80–200 µm. In addition, there are short side branches with 10–20 µm length. The branches innervate a predominantly two-dimensional area of tissue of about 150 × 200 µm (Heppelmann et al. 1990b).

The intermediate and final fiber parts of group III fibers display regular axonal thickenings; in three-dimensional reconstructions they appear to be lined up like pearls on a string. These axonal beads, as we like to call them, contain numerous mitochondria, glycogen granules, and vesicles (Figs. 1 and 3) (Heppelmann et al. 1990b). A count indicates about 7 beads per 100 µm of fiber length. The terminal branches of group III afferents show end bulbs similar in size and content to the axonal beads. Within these end bulbs the mitochondria loose their regular orientation. Also, the neurofilament core described in the next paragraph is no longer visible.

A further important feature of the group III fiber terminals is that a neurofilament core consisting of numerous microfilaments runs in the center of their axoplasma (Figs. 1 and 3 [left]). In this area no organelles and barely any microtubules can be seen. This finding is so specific for group III fibers that they can be identified by it. We may speculate that this neurofilament core serves as a "backbone" for the quite extended unmyelinated terminal parts of the group III afferents, because relative to the group IV fibers, they have a much worse relation of surface area to volume.

TERMINALS OF GROUP IV AFFERENTS

The unmyelinated afferent group IV fibers have a proximal and a distal terminal part. The proximal one is defined as that still within the perineural sheath, the distal one as that outside (Fig. 2B; there is no intermediate portion because there is no myelin sheath). The major branches of the distal portion

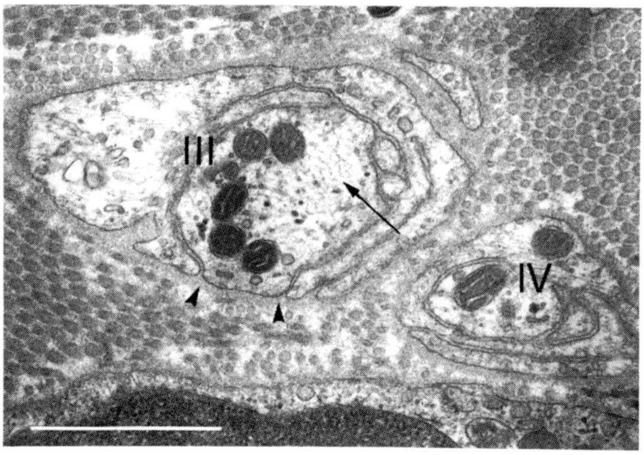

Fig. 1. Electron micrograph of a cross-section of a group III and a group IV sensory ending in the articular capsule of the cat's knee joint. The sensory axon of the group III fiber contains mitochondria, some glycogen particles (black), and different vesicles. Centrally arranged neurofilaments form a "neurofilament core" (arrow), which is characteristic for group III fibers and has never been observed in sensory axons of group IV. The group III axon is partly devoid of Schwann cell covering (between arrowheads). The axoplasm underlying this bare area is darker, indicating a specific (receptive?) function. Scale bar 1 µm.

are quite long, sometimes more than 300 µm. They frequently have short side branches less than 10 µm in length (Heppelmann et al. 1990b). The fibers usually run parallel to vessels, but the distances to the vessel walls may vary considerably. As in the group III units, the final fiber sections display regular axonal beads containing an above average number of mitochondria, glycogen granules, and vesicles (Heppelmann et al. 1990b). Counting these beads showed that in group IV units there are 9–10 per 100 µm (as compared to 7 in group III units).

TRANSDUCTION SITES OF SENSORY ENDINGS

The distal portions of group III and IV units are incompletely covered by Schwann cells; about one-third of the axonal membrane surface is separated only by a basal lamina from its immediate environment (Fig. 1). These areas not covered by Schwann cells show below the fiber membrane a fine filamentous plasma that is somewhat more electron dense than is the common axoplasma. These areas look similar to the receptor matrix described by Andres and von Düring (1973). Most likely they represent transduction sites of these units.

To return to the initial question, it is obviously not possible to recognize nociceptors solely by looking at their "coarse" ultrastructure as displayed in Figs. 1–3, at least not yet. But if our notion materializes, namely that nociceptors may be recognized by their cytoplasmic contents (see below), hitherto unrec-

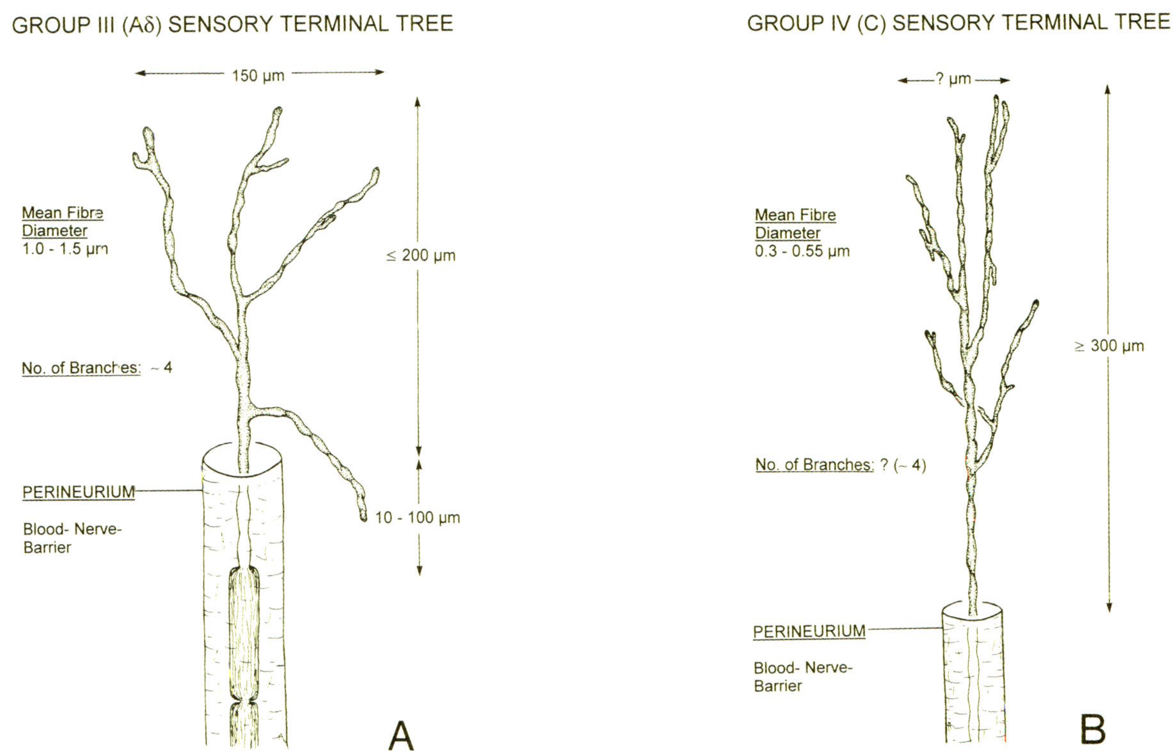

Fig. 2. Schematic drawings of group III (**A**) and IV (**B**) sensory endings in the knee joint capsule of the cat. The terminal trees are formed by several branches of various orientations. Group III sensory terminal trees innervate an area of about 200 × 150 µm. Their mean fiber diameter is within 1.0–1.5 µm. Group IV sensory terminal trees are up to 300 µm long. Their extension, however, is not known in detail. The mean fiber diameter is about 0.3–0.55 µm.

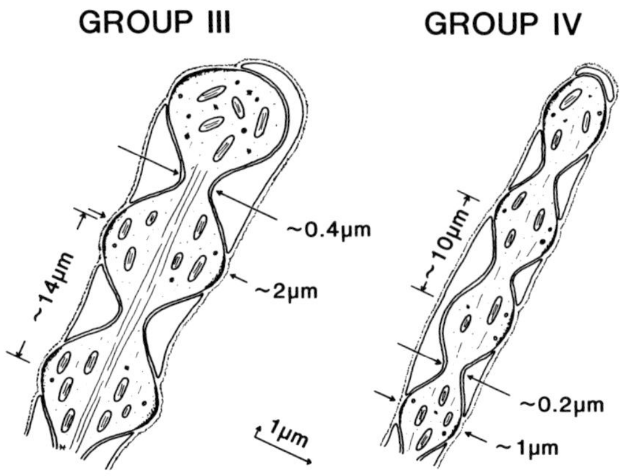

Fig. 3. Schematic drawing of the terminal portion of a group III (**left**) and group IV (**right**) nerve fiber with approximate dimensions obtained by three-dimensional reconstructions. The sensory axons consist of periodically arranged thick and thin segments forming spindle-shaped beads. The axolemma is not completely ensheathed by its accompanying Schwann cells; the bare areas presumably are receptive sites. A central axis of neurofilaments ("neurofilament core") exists only in sensory axons of group III fibers.

ognized features of the terminal branches and their relation to their environment may provide new clues to allow their differentiation from terminals sensitive to non-noxious stimuli.

CAN WE RECOGNIZE NOCICEPTORS FROM THEIR FUNCTIONAL CHARACTERISTICS—AND IF SO, HOW MANY ARE THERE IN A KNEE JOINT?

Single-fiber studies have been carried out on the afferent innervation of the knee joint of cats and rats anesthetized with alpha-chloralose and immobilized with pancuronium. In cats, both units in the posterior articular nerve (PAN) and in the medial articular nerve (MAN) have been studied, but most of the investigations were done on MAN units. This nerve innervates the medial and anteromedial regions of the articular capsule of the knee joint, the medial collateral ligament, the medial part of the annular ligament, the patellar ligament, the infrapatellar fat pad, and the medial part of the patellar periosteum (Freeman and Wyke 1967). The techniques used in these experiments (i.e., the dissection of the right leg, the setting-up of the animal on the mounting table, and the performance of passive limb movements) have previously been described in detail (Schaible and Schmidt 1983a,b; 1985).

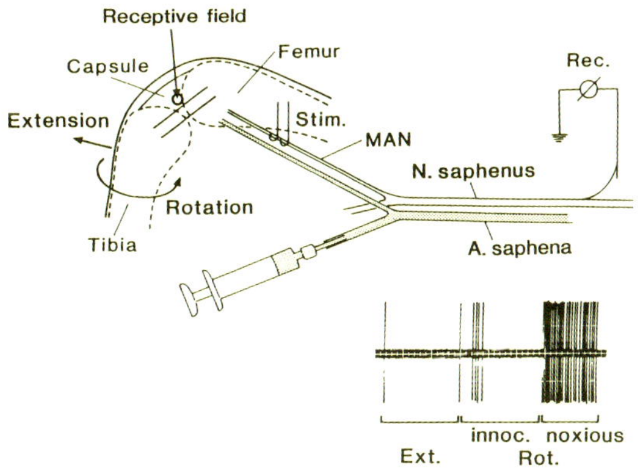

Fig. 4. Schematic representation of the cat knee joint preparation for electrophysiological recordings of articular afferents. Single units are characterized by their conduction velocity measured between the stimulation electrode *(Stim.)* placed under the medial articular nerve *(MAN)* and the recording electrode *(Rec.)* and by their responses to mechanical (movements, pressure onto the receptive field) and chemical stimuli (agents injected close to the joint). The specimen shown with a von Frey threshold of 12.5 g was weakly activated by innocuous inner rotation, but responded vigorously to noxious rotations of the lower leg.

A schematic view of the experimental situation is shown in Fig. 4. To enable close intra-arterial injection of inflammatory mediators and other chemical agents, a fine plastic catheter is fitted in the saphenous artery. The fine afferent fibers are searched in filaments of the saphenous nerve dissected in the inguinal region. Whether such a filament contains MAN nerve fibers is tested by single-pulse electric stimulation of the MAN close to the joint. If several units appear, the filament is progressively split until only one fiber can be activated. The fibers are identified by their conduction velocities, calculated from the time required for an action potential to cover the distance between the stimulating and recording electrodes. Articular afferent units conducting at less than 2.5 m/s were classified as group IV (or C) fibers, those with conduction velocities from 2.5 to 20 m/s as group III (or A-delta) units. Group II units have conduction velocities greater than 20 m/s.

RESPONSE PROPERTIES OF GROUP II UNITS

Group II articular afferents (conduction velocity 21–65 m/s) usually have no resting discharges and low mechanical thresholds (Fig. 6). Most are excited by gentle local stimuli and by movements in the working range of the knee joint. Although they encode pressure and particularly movement stimuli up to the noxious range, their responses are more closely related to the particular type of stimulus (e.g., movement in a specific direction) than to intensity (innoxious vs. noxious). These results suggest that they presumably subserve proprioceptive functions such as deep pressure sensation and kinesthesia (Dorn et al. 1991; Proske et al. 1988; Schaible and Grubb 1993), and that they probably are not involved in joint nociception and pain.

RESPONSE PROPERTIES OF GROUP III AND IV UNITS

In articular group III and group IV afferent units resting discharges occur in no more than one-third of all fibers (Fig. 6). The frequency of these irregular discharges is low, usually below 0.5 Hz (Schaible and Schmidt 1983a,b). Fig. 5 and the upper right panel of Fig. 6 show that the units with fine afferent nerve fibers can be grouped together according to their movement sensitivity, ranging from units that are readily or only marginally activated by non-noxious events, through units that are only activated by noxious movements, to units that are not activated by any movements, even extremely noxious ones (movement-insensitive units; they are excited by *local* mechanical stimulation, i.e., they have circumscribed receptive fields). Approximately 55% of the group III and 70% of the group IV units either respond only to (potentially) noxious movements or completely fail to respond to movements (Schaible and Schmidt 1983b). Units in the PAN also can be grouped into different categories, but the vast majority of the group IV fibers in this nerve do not respond to mechanical stimulation at all (Grigg et al. 1986). Therefore, at least 60% of all fine afferent fibers innervating the knee joint of the cat have nociceptive properties when classified by mechanical stimuli (Table II).

Those afferent units which in the normal joint are not excited by any movements may lack significant function except under pathological conditions (Schaible and Schmidt 1983b; Schaible and Grubb 1993). Kruger supposed that in normal tissue those afferents may subserve an efferent rather than an afferent function (Kruger 1987). Fibers that are only activated by noxious mechanical stimuli can be referred to as nocisensors as defined by the specificity theory. The units that are readily excited while the joint is being moved through its normal working range cannot be considered nociceptive (for further discussion on movement-insensitive and completely silent units see below).

STRUCTURE-FUNCTION RELATIONSHIPS: FIRST INSIGHTS

As outlined here, many new findings in the fields of electrophysiology, cytochemistry, and ultrastructure allow us to characterize and identify slowly conducting fine afferent fibers, but there are some "missing links" that prevent us from being able to finally characterize a nociceptor and to distinguish it from other fine afferents. A particularly difficult gap to bridge concerns the

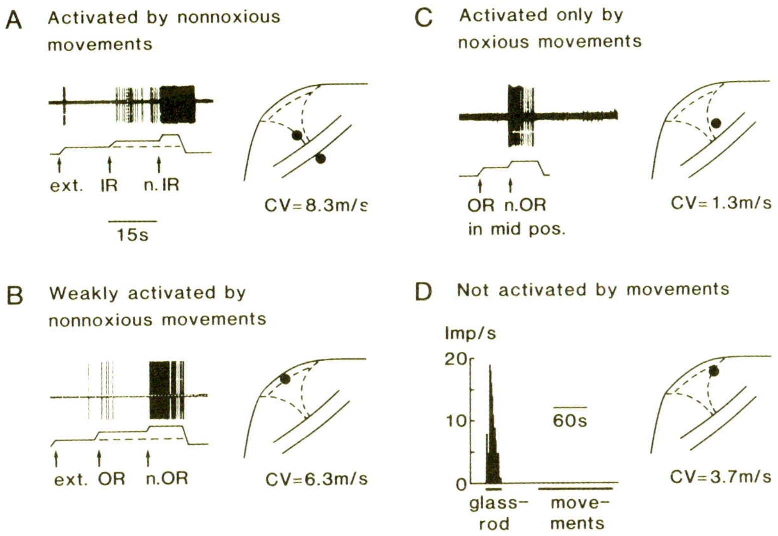

Fig. 5. Classification of fine articular afferents from the MAN according to their response during passive movements of the knee joint. The insets on the right of each record display the receptive fields on the medial aspect of the joint capsule and the conduction velocity *(CV)* of each unit. The time scale in **A** also applies to **B** and **C**. *Ext.*, extension; *IR* and *OR*, innocuous inward and outward rotations, respectively (pronation and supination, respectively); *n.IR* and *n.OR*, noxious inward and outward rotations, respectively; *mid pos.*, mid position (normal resting position of the joint between flexion and extension). The activity in **D** is displayed as a peristimulus-time histogram; the movement program included noxious flexions, extensions, and rotations.

relationship between structure and function. For instance, afferent fibers of groups II to IV, which are defined by their axon diameter and conduction velocity (Boyd and Davey 1968; Freeman and Wyke 1967; Boyd 1954; Novotny 1973), supposedly terminate in the knee joint either in corpuscular receptors (group II units) or in so-called free nerve endings (Figs. 1–3). But apart from some types of corpuscular receptors, this correlation is poorly confirmed and the borders between these groups are shaky. Furthermore, the primary processes of signal transduction and transformation of the generator potential to action potentials are probably independent and spatially separated, but we do not know where these processes take place. As described above, we can discriminate three (group III) or two (group IV fibers) segments of peripheral nerve fiber terminals, but their relative role in the electrophysiological processes remains open. Thirdly, slowly conducting afferents show a variety of responses and response characteristics to mechanical, chemical, and thermal stimuli, and these properties are rather independent of their

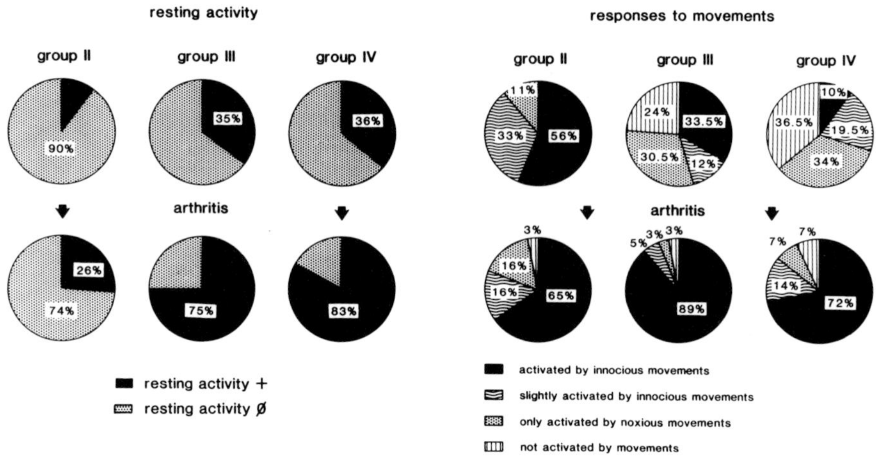

Fig 6. Relative distributions (percentages) of the various afferent units in the knee joint of the cat as classified in regard to their conduction velocities (groups II, III, IV), their resting activity (**left**), and their responsiveness to passive joint movements (**right**). The upper row shows the results obtained from normal joints, the lower row those obtained during an experimental arthritis. Note the rather small changes induced by the inflammation in the group II afferents. The figure does not show an increase in the frequency of the spontaneous and evoked discharges induced by inflammation.

conduction velocity. However, the sensory endings of thinly myelinated and unmyelinated fibers can be found in different layers and associated to different histological structures of the knee joint capsule, which again may be a structural finding related to their functional properties. Finally, the ultrastructure of the sensory endings, as already outlined above, is also variable in respect to shape, free area (not covered by Schwann cells), and organelle content of the sensory axon, which may or may not be related to the physiological properties.

Our attempt to make some progress in relating physiological, cytochemical, and morphological data to answer some of these questions led to experiments involving different techniques.

First we tried to determine whether the various types of articular afferents show some differences in the location of their receptive fields on the joint capsule and the ligaments. For instance, we examined the distribution of receptive fields of polymodal sensors (those having mechano- and chemosensitivity) vs. specific mechanosensitive units (no excitation to close intra-arterial injection of 2.6 µg bradykinin), but could not discern any significant difference. However, there may be some differential in the distribution of the receptive fields of movement-sensitive vs. movement-insensitive articular units, the latter being almost entirely restricted to the triangle between the borders of the condyli of the femur and tibia and the patellar ligament. This finding raises the question as to whether some movement-insensitive or completely silent nocisensors may be located in menisci, cruciate ligaments, or in the infrapatellar fat body, all close to the joint cavity where they are primarily exposed to an inflammation of the knee joint.

Second, we have started to mark receptive fields of functionally characterized group II–IV afferents for a subsequent histological study (both by light and electron microscopy). To date, only Kruger et al. (1988), in a study of testicular afferents, have attempted morphological identification of sensory endings of physiologically pre-examined slowly conducting afferents. Our study examining the structure and function of identified sensory endings produced these preliminary results: (1) At the "preparative level" the microdissection of functionally mapped receptive fields showed that endings of high-threshold group III and IV afferents (nocisensor units) are more frequently related to ligaments (medial collateral and patellar) than are low-threshold units. (2) At the "microscopic level" (histotopography of sensory endings) we have so far analyzed four group III units. Of these, two were high threshold (HT-units or nocisensors) and two were low threshold (LT). The HT units were located in dense connective tissue (stratum fibrosum of capsule or ligament structure), and the LT units were located in soft connective tissue related to delicate

Table II
Number of nociceptive units and distribution of neuropeptides in primary afferents of the medial articular nerve (MAN)

ELECTROPHYSIOLOGYAND MORPHOMETRY	
MAN afferent fibers	630 (100%)
Nociceptive afferents	
Group II	6 (1%)
Group III	71 (11%)
Group IV	310 (49%)
	387 (~60%)
Non-nociceptive afferents	243 (~40%)
IMMUNOHISTOCHEMISTRY	
Substance P	18%
Neurokinin A	8%
CGRP	35%
Somatostatin	18%

collagen fibers. It will be interesting to see whether these findings can be confirmed and a general principle be evolved from such measurements. (3) At the "ultrastructural level" we have measured the mean axon diameter of two group III units with different conduction velocity. We found that the rapidly conducting group III unit (conduction velocity 12.8 m/s) had indeed a thicker sensory axon within its terminal (mean diameter 1.6 μm) than did the slowly conducting unit (conduction velocity 6.4 m/s; axon diameter 1.1 μm). Morphometrical measurements of the volume density of the mitochondria within the sensory axon may elucidate the relationship between the content of organelles and the activity of distinct group III fibers (see discussion below).

It is immediately obvious from this brief sketch of our recent findings that many methodological difficulties make progress slow in our attempt to relate structure, particularly ultrastructure, to function. Nevertheless, we consider these experiments a valuable tool in the study of structure-dependent characteristics of nociceptors.

TOTAL SENSORY OUTFLOW AT REST AND DURING MOVEMENT FROM NORMAL JOINTS

Using the histological data and the results of recording the discharges of individual fine afferents, Heppelmann (1990) estimated the number of afferent impulses reaching the spinal cord when the knee joint is at rest and in response to a single flexion movement from the mid-position of the joint. Sufficient data were only available for the MAN, so the estimate has been restricted to that particular input (Table II). In the normal joint 35% of the group III and 36% of the group IV afferents have a mean resting activity of 10 and 19 impulses per minute, respectively. Group II fibers are barely active at rest. Altogether this totals some 1800 impulses per 30 seconds entering the spinal cord from a knee joint resting in mid-position (Dorn et al. 1991; Schaible and Schmidt 1985; Heppelmann 1990). A flexion, extension, or rotatory movement in the working range of a normal joint excites 89% of group II afferents, 45.5% of group III, and 29.5% of group IV afferents, i.e., they are of low threshold (Heppelmann et al. 1987). In the MAN these percentages amount to 240 afferent fibers with low thresholds and 390 fibers with high thresholds. Again, it is not absolutely settled which type of information is signaled to the nervous system by these discharges. Most units respond to more than one type of joint movement, i.e. only in an imprecise way may these discharges contribute to measuring joint movement and direction. During a simple flexion movement the afferent volley consists of approximately 4400 impulses per 30 seconds (including the resting discharges).

CAN WE RECOGNIZE NOCICEPTORS FROM THEIR CYTOPLASMIC, PARTICULARLY THEIR PEPTIDE CONTENT?

DISTRIBUTION OF MITOCHONDRIA

The cytoplasmic content of the fine afferents may offer special hints about their sensory properties. Certainly the mitochondria are not regularly distributed in the terminal axons. They accumulate in the axonal beads of both group III and group IV fibers (and in the end bulbs of the group III afferents), whereas barely any mitochondria can be seen in the thin fiber segments between the axonal beads. In addition, their volume density increases considerably in the intermediate and, particularly, the distal portions of group III fibers relative to the proximal ones.

Moreover, the volume density of mitochondria varies considerably from fiber to fiber. Therefore, in a population of 21 group III and 41 group IV afferents the average volume of mitochondria per surface area of the fiber has been determined over a length of 15–108 μm in steps of 1 μm. Calculating the relationship "volume per surface area" is somewhat unusual, but it is used here to highlight eventual differences in the relation between the ATP-producing organelles, namely the mitochondria, and the energy-using structures, in particular the membranes of the afferent units. In the proximal areas of group III afferents we found an average volume-to-surface ratio of 0.004 to 0.030 μm^3 per μm^2. In contrast, in the distal areas we found both a considerable increase of these values and, secondly, a much wider fluctuation of the measured volume-to-surface ratios (0.016–0.080 μm^3 per μm^2) (Heppelmann et al. 1994).

The group IV terminals contain much less mitochondria than do the group III terminals. Within any individual fiber profile we never saw more than 4–7 cross-cut mitochondria at once. Because the fiber surface is so much smaller, the volume-to-surface ratio in the proximal part is comparable with that of the group III units (0.001–0.025 μm^3 per μm^2). In contrast to the group III units, however, we did not see a significant increase in the density of mitochondria between the proximal and the distal portion of the group IV fibers. Also, no increase in the fluctuation of the values could be seen (0.003–0.019 μm^3 per μm^2).

If it is agreed that the total volume of mitochondria is proportional to the production and storage of ATP as a readily available pool of energy, then the results presented here point to considerable differences in the energy requirements between individual units of group III and group IV fibers, particularly in the group III range. Actually, for skeletal muscle a linear relation exists

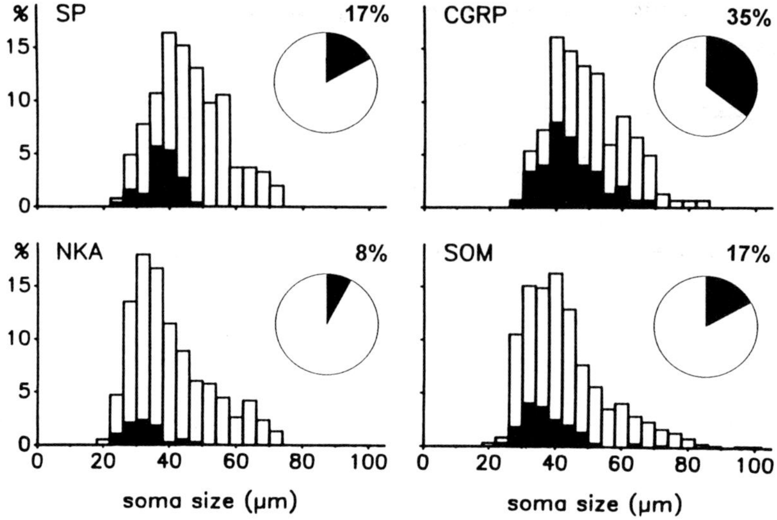

Fig. 7. Proportion and soma size distribution of knee joint afferents with a positive immunoreaction for substance P *(SP)*, calcitonin gene-related peptide *(CGRP)*, neurokinin A *(NKA)*, and somatostatin *(SOM)* (black bars and segments) in relation to all retrogradely labelled dorsal root ganglion cells innervating the knee via the medial articular nerve (white bars and segments). SP-, NKA-, and SOM-like immunoreactivity are only found in small- or intermediate-sized perikarya (< 50 μm), whereas CGRP-like immunoreactivity is also present in some large-sized dorsal root ganglion cells.

between the oxidative capacity of this tissue and the total volume of mitochondria (Schwerzmann et al. 1988). In lobster muscle receptor organs a positive correlation has been found between the concentration of mitochondria and the electrophysiological responses of these cells (Mayes and Govind 1989); neurons with a low mechanical threshold and a long adaptation time showed a high density of mitochondria, whereas neurons with high mechanical thresholds and a short adaptation time contained significantly less mitochondria. As both cell types contain nearly the same amount of electrogenic pumps in their membranes (Edman et al. 1986), the functional character of these cells seems to be determined by their oxidative capacity (Mayes and Govind 1989).

In analogy to these findings, we propose the following suggestions for the fine articular afferent fibers: (1) Because the saltatory conduction of action potentials in the proximal portions of group III afferents requires only a small amount of energy, the density of mitochondria is low in these portions whereas in the distal portions a much higher energy consumption requires the presence of more mitochondria. (2) In the group IV fibers the differences in mitochon-

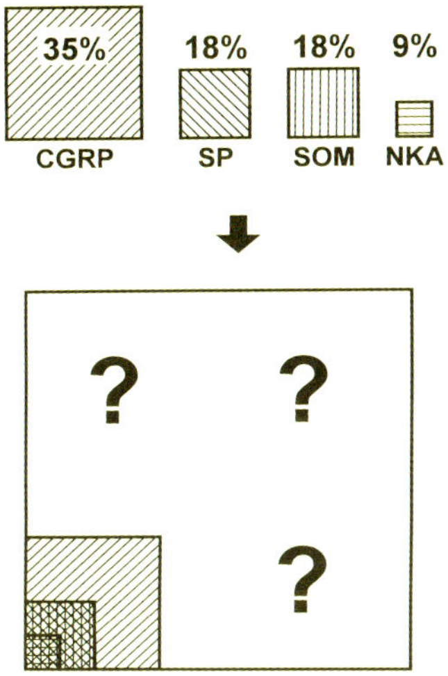

Fig. 8. Proportions of cat's articular afferents synthetizing CGRP, SP, SOM, and NKA. The four neuropeptides are co-localized to a great extent. NKA-positive perikarya contain SP, SOM, and CGRP as well. SP and SOM are nearly completely co-localized and additionally contain CGRP. The peptidergic content of about 65% of articular afferents is unknown (?).

drial content between the proximal and distal portions are small because both areas use approximately the same amount of energy (mainly because of the lack of a myelin sheath). (3) The large variations in mitochondrial content of the terminal portions of various individual units may be related to differences in their sensory function, namely the high-threshold (nociceptive) fine afferents containing less mitochondria per surface area than do low-threshold mechanosensitive units because high-threshold units are activated much more rarely than low-threshold units, and vice versa.

NEUROPEPTIDE CONTENT OF FINE ARTICULAR AFFERENT TERMINALS

Neuropeptides are found in all sensory ganglia of all species, especially in small-diameter neurons (for review see Hökfelt et al. 1986). There is some agreement that they modulate the transmission of (nociceptive?) information and have local effector functions (Ferrell and Russell 1985; Holzer 1988; Inagaki and Kito 1986; Kupfermann 1991). Of particular interest are the tachykinins substance P (SP) and neurokinin A (NKA), calcitonin gene-related peptide (CGRP), and somatostatin (SOM), which have been demonstrated in various dorsal root ganglia. There is good evidence that these neuropeptides play a key role in nociception. For example, various types of noxious stimulation lead to the release of these peptides in the spinal cord (Duggan et al. 1987, 1988, 1990; Hope et al. 1990; Morton et al. 1988; Schaible et al. 1990, 1992; Morton and Hutchison 1989).

Experiments with retrograde labeling of MAN afferents with the fluorescent dye Fast Blue and with subsequent immunocytochemical staining (PAP-method) of the dorsal root ganglia cells for the neuropeptides SP, NKA, SOM and CGRP (Hanesch et al. 1991, 1992) produced these major results: (1) SP-, NKA- and SOM-like immunoreactivities (SP-, NKA-, SOM-li) were evenly distributed throughout the cytoplasm; CGRP-like immunoreactivity (CGRP-li) occurred either as an even or as a punctate granule-like staining across the cytoplasm, or as a combination of both; (2) CGRP-li was found within 35%, SP-li and SOM-li in 17% and 18%, respectively, of the MAN afferents; only 8% of the afferents were NKA positive (Fig. 7); (3) The examined neuropeptides were nearly exclusively localized in small to intermediate-sized cell bodies (< 50 µm; Fig. 7), which are known to give rise predominantly to group IV and some group III fibers; and (4) CGRP was found additionally in some large perikarya (> 50 µm; Fig. 7), which probably give rise to myelinated nerve fibers of groups I and II, and to some group III fibers (75% of CGRP-li is localized in small and intermediate-sized perikarya, 25% is found in large perikarya).

Roughly 60% of the MAN afferents have high mechanical thresholds, which make them candidates for nociceptors (see above and Table II). Obviously not all contain the peptides just discussed. Even if it is assumed that only nociceptive afferents contain such peptides, only about 30% could contain SP or SOM, and no more than 10% of the nociceptors could contain NKA. These percentages would have to be further reduced given that considerable co-localization exists (Fig. 8), and that low-threshold mechanosensitive neurons also may contain these peptides (Leah et al. 1985). Thus, one of the major conclusions of our investigation (emphasized in Table II) is that no simple correlation between a peptide in an afferent fiber and the sensory function of that fiber (e.g., nociception) seems to exist in articular afferents, and most likely in afferents from other tissues, such as viscera.

WHY ARE WE SPEAKING OF NOCICEPTORS AS DYNAMIC ENTITIES?

EFFECTS OF INFLAMMATION

An acute experimental arthritis is induced in two steps. First, a 4% solution of kaolin suspended in distilled water is injected into the knee joint cavity. Thereafter, the knee joint is rhythmically bent and extended for 15 minutes. Second, 0.15–0.3 ml of a 2% solution of carrageenan is injected into the joint cavity, and the joint is again flexed and extended for another 5 minutes. This procedure leads to a long-lasting inflammation with behavioral changes in the awake cat and histological signs of acute severe inflammation with cellular infiltration (Coggeshall et al. 1983; Schaible and Schmidt 1988a; Grigg et al. 1986). As a consequence, profound changes occur in the resting and evoked discharge characteristics of fine articular afferents (Coggeshall et al. 1983; Guilbaud et al. 1985; Schaible and Schmidt 1985, 1988b; Grigg et al. 1986; Schaible and Grubb 1993).

During inflammation, resting activity is observed in 75% of group III and 83% of group IV units of the MAN (Fig. 6, lower left panel). The discharges are irregular and sometimes of high frequency. Both the percentages of units with resting activity and the frequencies of their discharges are more than twice as high as in the control sample. Their resting activity might represent the neural correlate of spontaneous pain, and the large number of fibers exhibiting resting activity under inflammatory conditions also implies (and has been confirmed by direct observation, see below) that in any case there are numerous nociceptors (usually silent in the normal joint) that exhibit resting activity under these conditions.

Nearly all fine afferent units from inflamed joints have low thresholds to movement, and most respond well to flexion and extension (Fig. 6, lower right panel). The increase in the number of easily excitable afferents corresponds to the clear decrease in the number of units belonging to the other classes. Specifically, the number of units in the normal joint that respond only to noxious movements or respond not at all becomes very small as soon as the joint is inflamed.

DIRECT OBSERVATION OF THE SENSITIZATION OF ARTICULAR AFFERENTS DURING AN EXPERIMENTAL ARTHRITIS

The results discussed so far led us to conclude that an inflammatory lesion of the joint causes sensitization of high-threshold (nociceptive) afferents, sensitization of low-threshold (non-nociceptive) afferents, and induction of mechanosensitivity in units without movement-induced sensitivity or without any mechanosensitivity. As, however, the comparison of samples of afferent units from normal and inflamed joints leaves some uncertainty about inflammation-induced changes of the discharge behavior of individual articular units, we studied the effects of inflammation on these afferents directly by recording from them prior to inflammation and then during a developing arthritis. This approach allowed us, in addition, to determine the time course of sensitization that could not be analyzed previously (Schaible and Schmidt 1988a,c).

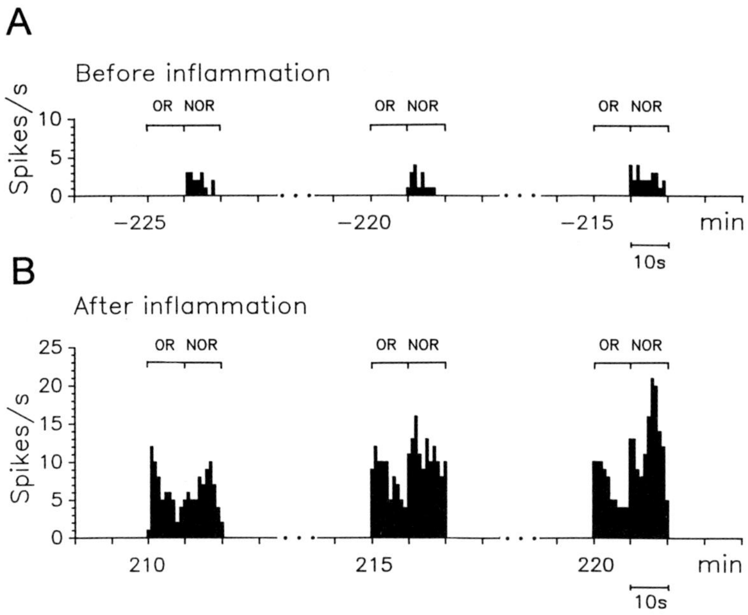

Fig. 9. Peristimulus time histogram of a group II fiber (c.v. 22.4 m/s) that was examined before and after an experimental arthritis. Before induction of the inflammation (**A**) the unit responded only to noxious outer rotation *(NOR)*. After the onset of inflammation (**B**) the afferent was sensitized to movement and responded vigorously to noxious as well as nonnoxious outer rotation *(OR)*.

The results show that remarkable differences exist in the time course of sensitization of the various types of articular afferents (Schaible and Schmidt 1988a). In high-threshold afferents, including originally silent ones ("sleeping" nocisensors), the sensitization becomes evident within the second to third hour after induction of inflammation with a later increase that persists for many hours (Fig. 9). In contrast, low-threshold units in the group II and III fiber ranges develop increased activity principally in the first hour after the injection of the inflammatory compounds, sometimes starting immediately after the injection (usually low-threshold group II units); these increased responses vanish more or less completely in the later stages of the inflammation.

It is necessary to discriminate three categories of units with different "levels of unresponsiveness": (1) units that do not respond to movements but have a receptive field and a response to KCl (cf. Fig. 5D, Fig. 6); (2) units that respond neither to movements nor to local mechanical stimulation (no detectable receptive field), but show a typical response to KCl; and (3) units

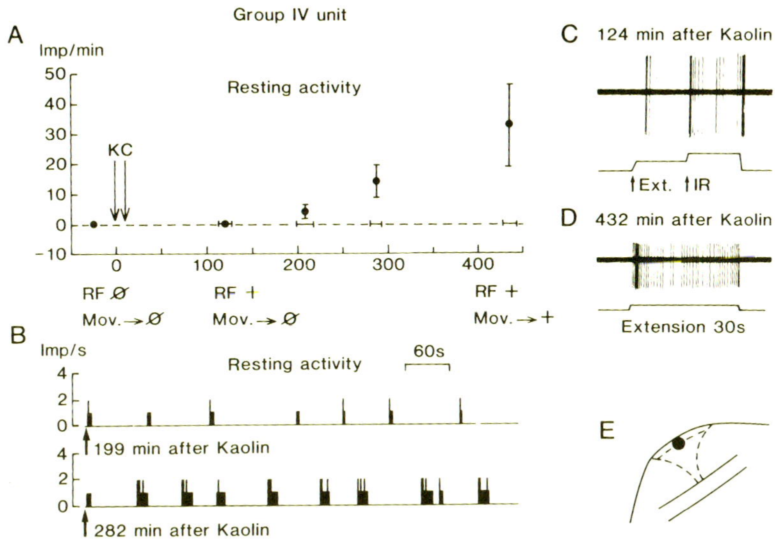

Fig. 10. Effect of an experimental arthritis on a silent afferent, group IV unit. **A:** Mean and standard deviation of resting discharges quantified during the indicated times (bars). **B:** Peristimulus time histograms. **C** and **D:** Responses to movements in the inflamed state; *Ext.*, extension; *IR*, pronation. **E:** receptive field *(dot)*.

having no mechanosensitivity and no clear response to KCl. Resting activity is practically always absent in all three types of units. Units in all three categories became sensitized in the course of inflammation, some to the point that they developed activity at rest and vigorous responses to movements in the working range of the joint. Fig. 10 gives a striking example of a category 2 unit becoming sensitized in the course of inflammation.

Actually, the existence of mechanoinsensitive (i.e., silent) primary afferents in the articular nerves of the cat's knee joint slowly but steadily emerged over the years 1983 to 1988 (Schaible and Schmidt 1983a,b, 1984, 1985, 1988a,c; Grigg et al. 1986). In addition, it became obvious that under both physiological and pathophysiological conditions, there is most likely a continuity of mechanical thresholds for articular fine afferents, ranging from very low to deep into the range of silent units. Under physiological conditions the spectrum of thresholds is rather evenly distributed over this range, whereas under pathophysiological conditions, such as an experimental arthritis, all units become sensitized and the spectrum of thresholds is skewed, i.e., most units can now be activated by stimuli that under normal conditions are completely innocuous.

SILENT NOCICEPTORS IN OTHER TISSUES AND IN OTHER SPECIES INCLUDING HUMANS

Since their original description in articular nerves of the cat, silent primary afferent units have been described in various tissues; they seem to be widespread if not universal in the mammalian somatoafferent systems. A first brief review on this topic published in 1990 by McMahon and Koltzenburg summarizes reports on the existence of silent primary afferents in the urinary bladder of the cat (Häbler et al. 1990, 1988), and preliminary evidence on silent units in the skin of the rat and monkey, which was substantiated by more extensive publications in the following year (rat: Handwerker et al. 1991; monkey: Meyer et al. 1991). In the same year silent afferent units were described in the colon of the cat (Jänig and Koltzenburg 1991).

More recently, additional support for the existence of silent afferent units has come from in vivo studies on the skin of the monkey (Davis et al. 1993) and recordings from afferent units of the cat's and rat's veins and perineurium (W. Jänig, personal communication, 1993). In humans, Torebjörk and Handwerker (personal communication, 1994; see also Magerl et al., this volume; Torebjörk, this volume), using microneurographic recordings from skin nerves, have detected a considerable percentage of fine afferent units that could not be activated by mechanical stimuli until the skin was irritated by mustard oil or comparable procedures.

Thus, in summary, silent primary afferent units may be a universal feature of the somatoafferent system of mammals, and, presumably, of other vertebrates. Many details of their functional characteristics and their possible afferent and efferent functions have still to be elucidated. For instance, many of the mechanoinsensitive units can be activated by chemical stimulation, particularly by close ia. injection of algesic substances such as bradykinin, but whether such stimuli have any physiological significance is open for discussion. Furthermore, no evidence is available yet whether silent afferents have more prominent efferent functions than other fine afferent units (Kruger 1987). There is, however, little doubt that they form a special population of fine afferent units that only comes into play under pathophysiological conditions, thus providing a special alarm system to inform the organism on particularly threatening noxious situations.

TOTAL SENSORY OUTFLOW AT REST AND DURING MOVEMENT FROM INFLAMED JOINTS

The percentage of fibers having resting activity and their mean discharge frequency increase considerably in the course of inflammation (Fig. 6). As already mentioned, 75% of group III and 83% of group IV afferents become

Table III
Outflow from a normal and an inflamed knee joint of the cat based on data from the medial articular nerve

	Normal Joint	Inflamed Joint	Change
Resting activity*	1,800	11,100	x 6.2
Low threshold units	245 fibers	550 fibers	x 2.3
Movement*	4,400	30,900	x 7.0

* Action potentials per 30 seconds.

spontaneously active with a mean resting activity of 54 and 46 impulses per minute, respectively. Also, some of the group II afferents develop resting activity. Both factors contribute to the increase of afferent activity from 1,800 to 11,100 impulses reaching the spinal cord within 30 seconds with the joint in resting position (Table III; Dorn et al. 1991; Schaible and Schmidt 1985). The peripheral neurobiological correlate for pain at rest from an inflamed joint seems to consist of these impulses conducted through the MAN together with those in the PAN, which most likely undergo a similar sensitization. It appears not too far fetched to assume that similar mechanisms of sensitization operate not only in acute inflammatory, but possibly also in chronic pain processes. Inflammation of the joint reduces the mechanical thresholds of most of the afferent fibers regardless of their threshold found under normal conditions (see above). A movement in the normal working range of the joint, such as the test flexion used here, will now excite approximately 550 units in the MAN, and, in addition, the discharge rates of those low-threshold units is now much higher than previously. All in all, in the MAN the afferent volley in response to the test movement now consists of some 30,900 impulses per 30 seconds, i.e., about seven times more than under normal conditions (Table III; in individual afferents that have been studied consecutively both under normal and inflamed conditions, the afferent discharges sometimes increased more than 100-fold). This huge volley, together with the corresponding one in the PAN, obviously transmits those messages responsible for the noxious reflexes and the pain perception when moving an inflamed joint.

WHICH FACTORS ARE RESPONSIBLE FOR THE SENSITIVITY CHANGES OF NOCICEPTORS?

Which of the many changes induced by inflammation are responsible for the sensitization and excitation of nocisensors is still an open question. Mechanical factors (increase of the tissue turgor by cellular and interstitial edema) and thermal factors (increase in local temperature as a consequence of vasodi-

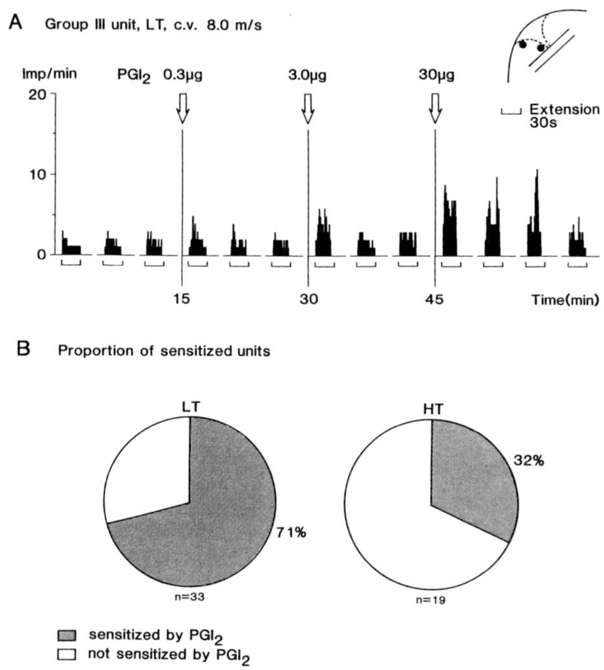

Fig. 11. Sensitization of articular afferents by PGI_2 to movement. **A:** Low-threshold *(LT)*, group III unit with a conduction velocity *(c.v.)* of 8.0 m/s; responses to extension (expressed as PSTH) were gradually increased by increasing doses of PGI_2. *Inset:* position of receptive fields of this unit. **B:** proportion of low-threshold *(LT)* and high-threshold *(HT)* afferents sensitized by PGI_2

latation, not the vasodilatation itself) could in part be responsible for the sensitization, but we do not know of any clinical or experimental findings supporting such an assumption.

On the other hand, there are several good reasons to believe that chemical factors are the decisive component in the sensitization caused by inflammatory processes. Many inflammatory mediators accumulate in the inflamed tissue, for instance bradykinin, serotonin, and eicosanoids such as prostaglandins and leukotrienes (Barlas et al. 1985; Hargreaves et al. 1988; Atik 1990; Egg 1984; Larsson et al. 1989; Melli 1988). These are either locally released or synthesized. In several tissues such inflammatory mediators could either excite the nocisensors directly or could sensitize them for other stimuli (Lang et al. 1990; Beck and Handwerker 1974; Birrell et al. 1990a; Kanaka et al. 1985; Mense and Meyer 1988; Raja et al. 1988; Schaible and Schmidt 1988b; Martin 1990; Mizumura et al. 1987; Neugebauer and Schaible 1988). For instance, close arterial injection of prostaglandins into the joint tissue led to an increase of the afferent responses to joint movements (Fig. 11) but also to the subsequent injection of bradykinin (Grubb et al. 1991; Birrell et al. 1990a; Schaible and Schmidt 1988b; Schepelmann et al. 1992).

Many, if not all, knee joint afferents differ in their responsiveness to distinct inflammatory mediators, leading to a pronounced diversity of their chemical sensitivity. As an example, most of the articular afferents tested are sensitive to prostaglandin I_2 . However, we found that a larger proportion of low-threshold compared to high-threshold fibers was sensitized to mechanical stimuli following the application of prostaglandin I_2 (Fig. 11), whereas a smaller proportion of low-threshold compared to high-threshold fibers was sensitized to bradykinin.

In respect to the mode of action of the various inflammatory mediators on fine afferents (percentage of fibers being excited and/or sensitized, time course of the effect, etc.) it has to be assumed that several mediators act together to produce the changes in the receptive properties observed during inflammation. Several other substances also could participate in the sensitization processes, including potassium ions, serotonin, histamine, and eventually also H^+ ions (pH) and catecholamines (Birrell et al. 1990b; Herbert and Schmidt 1992; Heyer et al. 1989; Moncada et al. 1978; Neugebauer and Schaible 1988; Neugebauer et al. 1989; Sicuteri 1967).

The neuropeptides do not seem to have a major role in the sensitization process. Perhaps some induce the production of prostaglandin E_2 in synovial tissue (Lotz et al. 1987) and these prostaglandins in turn act on joint afferents in an excitatory or sensitizing manner (Schaible and Schmidt 1988b; Schepelmann et al. 1992). On the other hand at least some of the neuropeptides, particularly CGRP and substance P (but not somatostatin), are substantially up-regulated in the course of acute and chronic inflammation (Fig. 12; Hanesch et al. 1993a,b). This up-regulation probably leads to a substantial increase in spinal release and a consequent modulation of the synaptic transmission in the nociceptive pathways (Schaible et al. 1992).

The manifold changes occurring in the course of inflammation in the population of articular afferents are summarized in Fig. 13. In normal joints the majority of afferent units have high thresholds (upper panel, white units), and only few of them contain peptides (dots). Under inflammatory conditions (lower panel) the number of low-threshold units (black) is greatly increased (see also Fig. 6), and there is also a substantial increase of the number of fine afferents containing peptides (for details see legend).

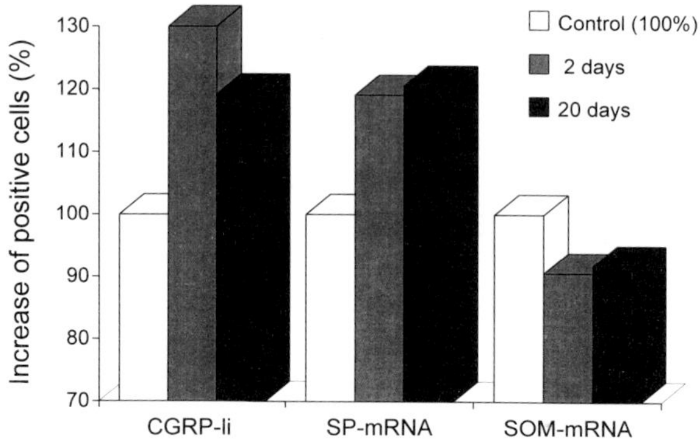

Fig. 12. Increase of the proportion of CGRP-like immunoreactive perikarya and of perikarya with a positive in situ hybridization signal for SP-mRNA and SOM-mRNA. Ipsilateral dorsal root ganglia L4–L6 of rats with a unilateral inflammation in the ankle region at day 2 (light gray bars) and day 20 (dark gray bars) post inoculation. The proportion of stained neurons on the control sides was set at 100% (white bars). The values obtained for each side at days 2 and 20 were expressed as percent of control.

CLINICAL IMPLICATIONS: IS THE NOCICEPTOR STILL A WORTHWHILE TARGET FOR ANALGESIC DRUGS?

NONSTEROIDAL ANTI-INFLAMMATORY DRUGS (NSAIDs)

Drugs such as acetylsalicylic acid (ASA) and indomethacin are used for the analgesic and antiphlogistic treatment of inflammation in joints. For a long time it has been assumed that not only the antiphlogistic but also the analgesic effect of these drugs is mediated by an action at the inflammation site. This assumption was based on the results of different experimental approaches, but not on the recording of single-unit activity originating in the inflamed tissue (for a review of the literature see Heppelmann et al. 1986). Therefore, we performed experiments to test whether the systemic application of two common NSAIDs, namely ASA and indomethacin, reverses the effects of an acute experimental arthritis on fine articular afferents. According to the assumption about the peripheral site of action of these drugs, depressant effects on the activity in units from inflamed joints should be seen as an indicator for the peripheral analgesic action.

An example of the results obtained is shown in Fig. 14. Resting discharges and movement-evoked activity originating in the inflamed tissue were reduced following the application of these drugs. This depression presumably

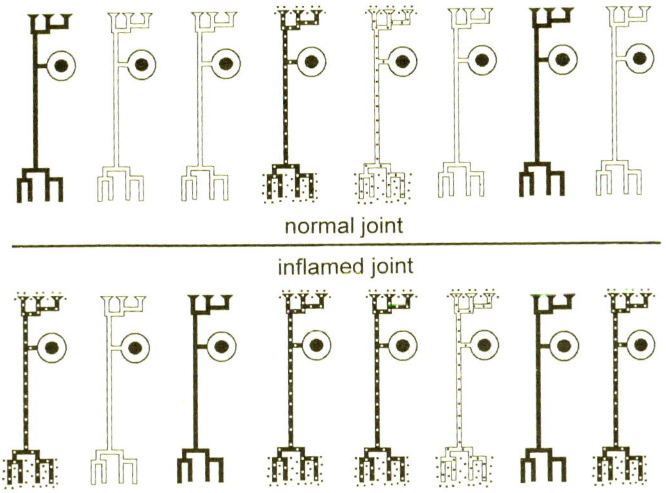

Fig. 13. Schematic representation of the afferent innervation of a normal and an inflamed joint. According to electrophysiological studies, the majority of the primary afferents of a normal joint seem to be nociceptors (white neurons); other units are low-threshold (black neurons). Immunohistochemical studies revealed that only a small proportion contain the neuropeptides SP, NKA, CGRP, and/or SOM (black and white dots). In an inflamed joint most of the nociceptive afferents are sensitized, becoming low-threshold in character. In addition, a higher number of afferents synthesize the neuropeptides SP and CGRP, whereas the proportion of SOM-synthezising neurons seems to be unaffected.

reflects the analgesic action of these anti-inflammatory substances at the peripheral nerve fiber (Guilbaud and Iggo 1985; Heppelmann et al. 1986). The time course of these effects concurs with clinical experience. In patients the analgesic effect of aspirin starts within the first hour after the application, and it may be maximal after one hour and lasts two to several hours. Depressive effects on the resting activity in single units from inflamed knee were found within the first hour after intravenous injection, starting in most units within the first 10 or 20 minutes. Thus the onset of the depression and the continuous decline of ongoing discharges fit well to the clinical manifestation of pain relief after treatment with anti-inflammatory drugs. In yet another respect our results fit well to the clinical experience; even after long observation times the resting activity and the movement-evoked discharges were never completely blocked. The extent of sensitization was reduced, but sensitization was never abolished within the recording time. This may correspond to the weak analgesic potency of NSAIDs.

EXCITATORY AND DESENSITIZING EFFECTS OF CAPSAICIN

Capsaicin is well known as a toxic agent that selectively impairs and/or destroys slowly conducting afferent fibers. Low doses of capsaicin can be used to activate such afferents and to elicit acute painful sensations. In cutaneous nerves this drug seems to preferentially excite thin myelinated and unmyelinated nociceptive afferents, whereas non-nociceptive afferents are rarely activated by the compound (for a review of the literature see He et al. 1990). Joint afferents show a similar selectivity for high-threshold afferents (He et al. 1988). But it has to be appreciated, as shown in the summing up of many experiments in Fig. 15, that this selective action is by far not an absolute one. It is best, although only in a negative sense, for group III fibers with conduction velocities greater than 11 m/s which were never excited even by high

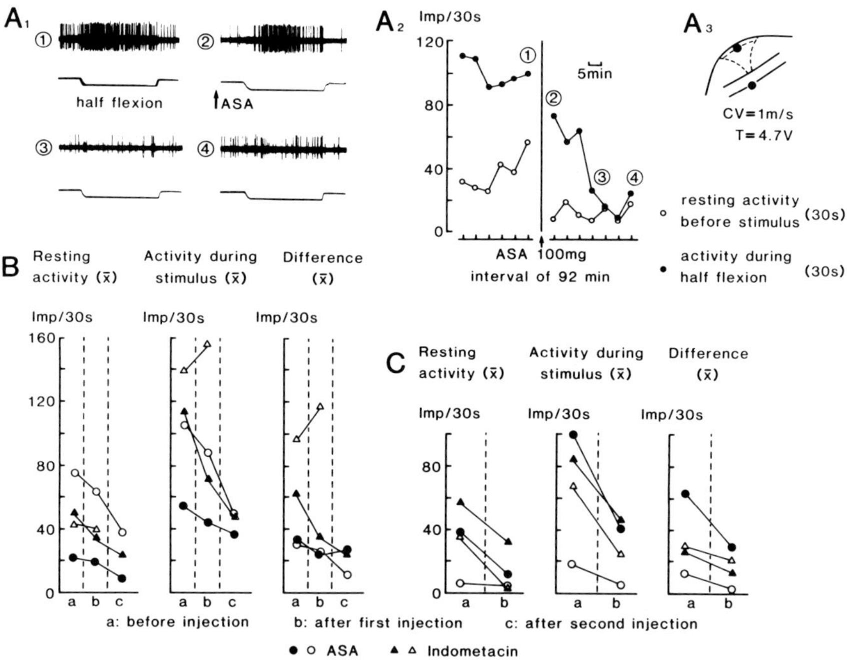

Fig. 14. A: The effect of aspirin (*ASA*) on motion-induced responses in a group IV unit from an inflamed joint. **A$_1$:** Half flexion before and at various times after aspirin administration as indicated in **A$_2$**. **A$_2$:** Quantitative evaluation of all responses to movements. **A$_3$:** Receptive fields of the afferent unit. **B, C:** Quantitative evaluation of group III (B) and group IV (C) units. The means are given for the resting activity 30 seconds prior to movement, the activity during movement, and the differences between movement-induced and resting activity.

doses of capsaicin regardless of their mechanical threshold (left panel in Fig. 15). For the slow group III fibers (middle panel) as well as the group IV fibers (right panel), we noted many exceptions in both directions; units with low mechanical threshold were excited by capsaicin and high-threshold units were unaffected. Nevertheless, it seems worth mentioning that capsaicin is "better" in discriminating between high-threshold and low-threshold fine afferent units than any other substance (e.g., bradykinin, various prostaglandins, serotonin) tested so far in this respect.

The excitation induced by capsaicin in fine articular afferent units is closely coupled to a suppression of the responses to subsequent mechanical and chemical stimuli (He et al. 1990). Such a "desensitizing" effect of capsaicin on afferents confirms other studies that used different preparations and different types of recording (He et al. 1990). Our study and others suggest that these effects are largely independent of the target tissue of the afferents and also of the species. Our experiments on single, identified afferents showed in addition that the desensitizing effect is evoked in myelinated as well as in unmyelinated afferents, and that this desensitization predominantly occurs in nociceptive units. It also became evident that the suppression of the responses

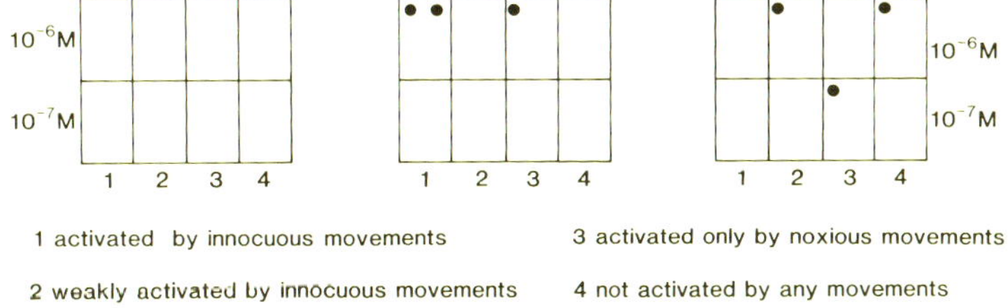

Fig. 15. Sensitivity to capsaicin of a population of 84 fine afferents recorded from the knee joints of 24 cats. The units were classified in three panels in regard to their conduction velocity and to their responses to passive movements of the knee joint (left to right in each panel according to the key given at the bottom of the figure; cf. also Fig. 5). The study included only units that were readily excited by a close ia. bolus injection of 0.3 ml twice isotonic KCl solution. Units that did not respond to a 0.3 ml bolus injection of 10^{-4} M capsaicin were classified as unresponsive (Ø; uppermost row in each panel).

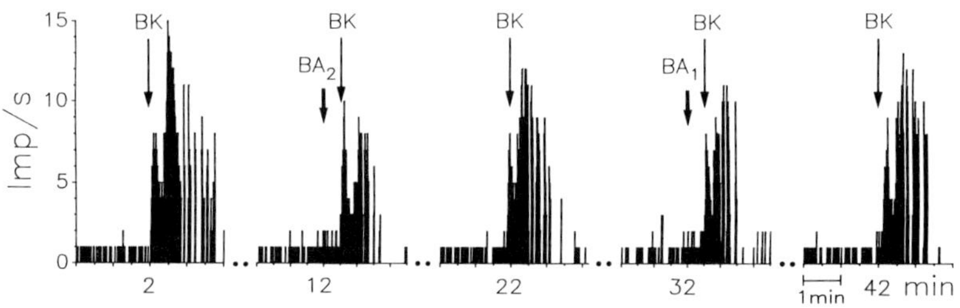

Fig. 16. Continuous recording (PSTH) of a high-threshold group IV fiber (conduction velocity 0.5 m/s) that was repetitively stimulated by 0.26 μg of bradykinin *(BK)*. Both the B_1 antagonist des-Arg^9-Leu^8-BK *(BA_1)* and the B_2 antagonist Thi^{5,8},D-Phe^7-BK *(BA_2)* administered 30 seconds prior to BK (at doses of 26 μg per bolus at 12 and 32 minutes, respectively) slightly inhibited the response to BK.

is closely related to an excitatory effect of capsaicin, as responses were not inhibited in units that were not excited by capsaicin or only by high doses. The mechanism of this inhibitory action of capsaicin is not known, but there are good reasons to believe that capsaicin triggers an intraneuronal process that subsequently inhibits the transduction process (He et al. 1990).

BRADYKININ ANTAGONISTS

Bradykinin (BK) is an important mediator of inflammation and a potent algesic substance that is found in inflammatory exudates of humans suffering from arthritis as well as in experimentally inflamed tissues of animals (Barlas et al. 1985; Hargreaves et al. 1988). As previously described, it excites a high proportion of fine articular afferents, both from normal and inflamed joints (Meßlinger et al. 1994, also for a recent summary of the literature). Since pharmacological evidence became available that the nociceptive actions of BK are mainly due to stimulation of the B_2 receptor, this receptor has become a target for the design of specific competitive antagonists (Hargreaves et al. 1988). Electrophysiological recordings from nociceptive afferents as well as pain rating tests showed an antinociceptive effect of those B_2 receptor antagonists (Dray et al. 1988; Mizumura et al. 1990; Whalley et al. 1987). In other preparations, however, antagonistic effects of these agents were short-lasting, and rather prominent agonistic effects make them doubtful candidates for peripherally acting analgetics (Khan et al. 1992).

In agreement with these findings, our own studies of the action of B_2 antagonists (and also a B_1 antagonist) on fine articular units have revealed that both show partly inhibitory and partly excitatory and/or sensitizing effects (Fig. 16). The inhibitory effects were short-lasting and did not depend on

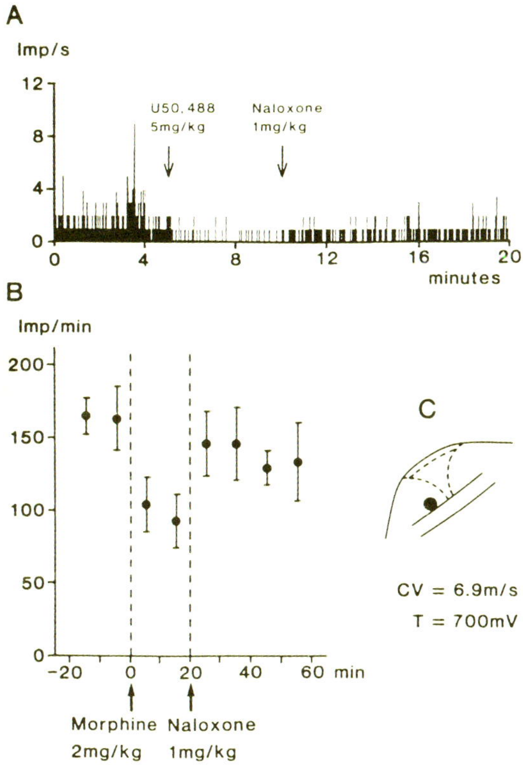

Fig. 17. Effects of intra-arterial injection of U50488 (**A**) and morphine (**B**) on the spontaneous discharge of a single group III afferent in the MAN. Naloxone reversed the actions of both drugs. **C**: The location of the receptive field of this unit on the medial aspect of the knee joint. *T*, electrical threshold of the fiber under observation; *CV*, conduction velocity.

functional characteristics such as mechanical sensitivity or ongoing activity of the afferents. Although inhibitory effects of both antagonists dominated, the average response to BK of all units tested with the B_1 or B_2 antagonist was not significantly weaker than that of the control units due to the partial agonist effects just mentioned (this laboratory, unpublished). Recently, however, a new long-acting and potent B_2 antagonist, HOE 140, was developed that provides new hope that BK antagonists may become useful antinociceptive drugs (Correa and Calixto 1993; Ferreira et al. 1993; Lembeck et al. 1991).

PERIPHERAL OPIOID ANTINOCICEPTION

In recent years evidence has accumulated to suggest that opiates can act at neuronal sites in afferent fibers. Opiate receptors were identified on small-diameter afferent terminals in the spinal cord and on cell soma in dorsal root ganglia (Stein et al. 1990). An inhibitory effect on the calcium-dependent component of the action potential in dorsal root ganglion neurons in culture was described for a range of opiate agonists. The vasodilatation and extravasation in the skin induced by antidromic nerve stimulation were inhibited by various opiates, which may result from inhibition of neuropeptide release from sensory terminals during electrical stimulation. Under various experimental and clinical conditions, a series of opiates and their antagonists showed peripheral analgesic and algesic effects, respectively (for literature see Stein et al. 1991; Stein 1993; Czlonkowski et al. 1993; Russell et al. 1987).

We have contributed to the unfolding story of peripheral opiate receptors and their potential analgesic action by studying the peripheral effects of a range of mu- and kappa-opiate agonists on the spontaneous impulse traffic in small-diameter afferents from the acutely inflamed joint (Russell et al. 1987). At the time the model was chosen, the symptoms of inflammation could clearly be reduced by cyclo-oxygenase inhibitors (Heppelmann et al. 1986) or partly mimicked by prostaglandins E_1 and E_2 (Heppelmann et al. 1985; Schaible and

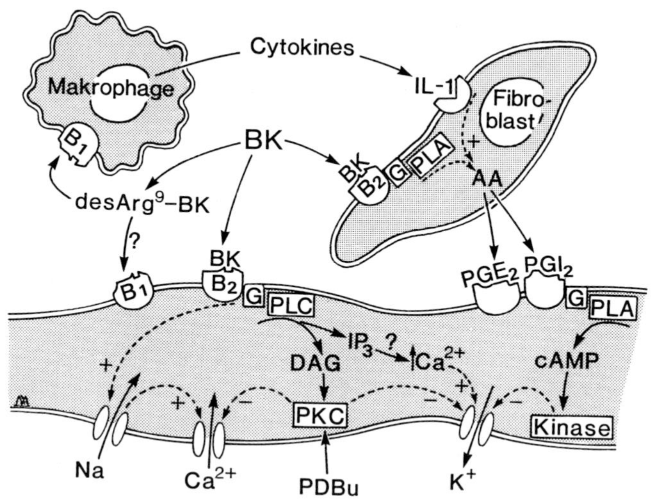

Fig. 18. Potential intracellular mechanisms and interactions between makrophages, fibroblasts, and sensory endings after activation of B_1 and B_2 receptors by bradykinin *(BK)* and desArg⁹-BK, respectively. Apart from direct stimulation of sensory endings involving the second messengers DAG and IP_3, an important action of BK seems to be the stimulation of the arachidonic acid *(AA)* metabolism in fibroblasts (and other cells) and the production of prostaglandins *(PGE_2, PGI_2)*, which in turn activate the sensory endings using the adenyl cyclase-cAMP system. Protein kinase C *(PKC)* can experimentally be activated by phorbol esters such as phorbol dibutyrate *(PDBu)* instead of DAG. In the inflamed state an important sidepath may be the production of cytokines such as interleukin 1 *(IL-1)* by makrophages activated through stimulation of B_1 receptors.

Schmidt 1988b). In this model we expected an antinociceptive effect of opiates to be reflected in a depression of the spontaneous discharges of individual fine primary afferent fibers. As Fig. 17 shows, these expectations were fully justified. The spontaneous discharges of nearly all of the tested fine afferent units from inflamed joints were significantly inhibited by one or several opiates in a naloxone-reversible manner. These data provided the first electrophysiological demonstration that opiates may act on opiate receptors located at peripheral sites of primary afferent fibers and hence exert a peripheral analgesic effect. Most of the subsequent evidence on the peripheral analgesic action of opiates is still indirect (Stein et al. 1990, 1991; Stein 1993; Czlonkowski et al. 1993).

SUMMARY

After summing up the recent data on the peripheral processes of nociception—as this chapter intended by using articular nociception as an example—we must admit that the physical and chemical processes involved

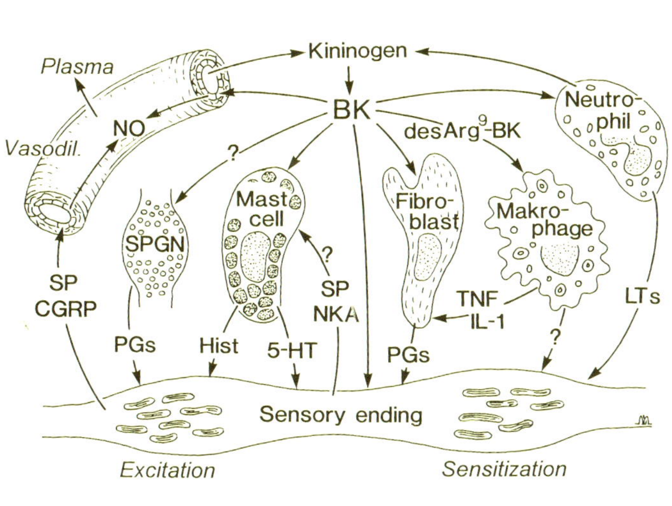

Fig. 19. Direct and indirect excitatory and sensitizing pathways of bradykinin *(BK)* involving different cell types in the normal (**left side**) and additional cells in the inflamed articular tissue (**right side**). BK may indirectly act by production of inflammatory mediators such as prostaglandins *(PGs)*, histamine *(His)*, serotonin *(5-HT)*, leukotrienes *(LTs)*, and cytokines *(TNF, IL-1)*. Neuropeptides such as substance P *(SP)*, neurokinin A *(NKA)*, and calcitonin gene-related peptide *(CGRP)* released from small-diameter sensory endings may cause a neurogenic inflammation, thereby increasing the production of inflammatory mediators.

are much more complicated than predicted 10 years ago, and this complexity seems to increase further with any factor that is carefully analyzed. When we are looking, for instance, at the bradykinin system mentioned in the previous section, we learn from recent studies that at least two different receptors mediate various aspects of nociception (Fig. 18). In contrast to the former opinion that only B_2 receptors mediate the excitatory action of bradykinin (Dray et al. 1988; Mizumura et al. 1990; Whalley et al. 1987), recent studies seem to confirm a decisive role of B_1 receptors in specific inflammatory states (Correa and Calixto 1993; Perkins et al. 1993), a finding that was first proposed on the basis of pharmacological experiments (Burch et al. 1989). It is still a matter of discussion whether B_1 receptors already exist and are simply activated under inflammatory conditions or whether they are synthesized de novo (Mantione and Rodriguez 1990; Marceau et al. 1980); their importance seems to depend on the type of inflammation and/or the preparation used (Correa and Calixto 1993; Perkins et al. 1993). Moreover, both bradykinin receptors mentioned seem to be located on various cell systems.

A direct action of bradykinin on sensory endings seems likely (Steranka et al. 1988), although there is also good evidence for indirect actions via endothelial cells, fibroblasts, synoviocytes, mast cells, sympathetic postganglionic terminals, and (in inflamed tissue) macrophages and neutrophils, all causing various chains of intracellular events, some of which are outlined in Fig. 18 (for a recent review see Dray and Perkins 1993). Most important seems to be the production of cytokines such as interleukins and tumor necrosis factor, and the consecutive production of other inflammatory mediators such as prostaglandins when the cell's various systems are switching from the normal to the inflamed state (Burch et al. 1989; Ferreira et al. 1993). This means that, in addition to nociceptive cascades following acute noxious events (Fig. 19, left hand side), under pathological conditions, such as an arthritis, other pathways may involve cells that produce additional algesic and/or inflammatory mediators (right-hand side in Fig. 19).

Similar to the bradykinin system representatively worked out in more detail in this paragraph, all these mediators are likely to form a complex framework of actions and reactions that finally affect the nociceptive terminals, eliciting excitatory and sensitizing effects, and these processes may again depend on the pathological conditions of the tissue. Consequently, all attempts to treat painful states by agents that block peripheral receptors involved in nociception would critically depend on the pathological condition of the lesioned tissue. It seems unlikely that there is one drug that would serve as a universal analgesic for treatment of all inflammatory pains. On the other hand, the better we understand these specific systems, the better our chances to design specific drugs targeted on specific peripheral sites for a selective inhibition of nociceptive processes.

ACKNOWLEDGMENTS

Work reported from this laboratory has been supported by the Deutsche Forschungsgemeinschaft, the Wilhelm-Sander-Stiftung, and the Volkswagenstiftung, and by a Max-Planck-Forschungspreis.

REFERENCES

Andres, K.H. and von Düring, M., Morphology of cutaneous receptors. In: Iggo, A. (Ed.), Handbook of Sensory Physiology, Vol. 2., Springer, Berlin, 1973, pp. 3–28.

Atik, O.A., Leukotriene B4 and prostaglandin E2-like activity in synovial fluid in osteoarthritis, Prostaglandins Leukot. Essent. Fatty Acids, 34 (1990) 253–254.

Barlas, A., Sugio, K. and Greenbaum, L.M., Release of T-kinin and bradykinin in carrageenin induced inflammation in the rat, FEBS Lett., 190 (1985) 268–270.

Beck, P.W. and Handwerker, H.O., Bradykinin and serotonin effects on various types of cutaneous nerve fibers, Pflügers Arch., 347 (1974) 209–222.

Birrell, G.J., Grubb, B.D., Iggo, A. and McQueen, D.S., Actions of PGE2 and cicaprost on the sensitivity of high-threshold mechanoreceptors in normal and inflamed ankle joints of the anaesthetized rat, J. Physiol., 420 (1990a) 33.

Birrell, G.J., McQueen, D.S., Iggo, A. and Grubb, B.D., The effects of 5-HT on articular sensory receptors in normal and arthritic rats, Br. J. Pharmacol., 101 (1990b) 715–721.

Boyd, I.A., The histological structure of the receptors in the knee joint of the cat correlated with their physiological response, J. Physiol., 124 (1954) 476–488.

Boyd, I.A. and Davey, M.R., Composition of Peripheral Nerves, E&S Livingstone, Edinburgh, 1968.

Burch, R.M., Connor, J.R. and Tiffany, C.W., The kallikrein-kininogen-kinin system in chronic inflammation, Agents Actions, 27 (1989) 258–260.

Coggeshall, R.E., Hong, K.A., Langford, L.A., Schaible, H.-G. and Schmidt, R.F., Discharge characteristics of fine medial articular afferents at rest and during passive movements of inflamed knee joints, Brain Res., 272 (1983) 185–188.

Correa, C.R. and Calixto, J.B., Evidence for participation of B1 and B2 kinin receptors in formalin-induced nociceptive response in the mouse, Br. J. Pharmacol., 110 (1993) 193–198.

Czlonkowski, A., Stein, C. and Herz, A., Peripheral mechanisms of opioid antinociception in inflammation: involvement of cytokines, Eur. J. Pharmacol., 242 (1993) 229–235.

Davis, K.D., Meyer, R.A. and Campbell, J.N., Chemosensitivity and sensitization of nociceptive afferents that innervate the hairy skin of monkey, J. Neurophysiol., 69 (1993) 1071–1081.

Dorn, T., Schaible, H.-G. and Schmidt, R.F., Response properties of thick myelinated group II afferents in the medial articular nerve of normal and inflamed knee joints of the cat, Somatosens. Mot. Res., 8 (1991) 127–136.

Dray, A. and Perkins, M., Bradykinin and inflammatory pain, Trends Neurosci., 16 (1993) 99–104.

Dray, A., Bettaney, J., Forster, P. and Perkins, M.N., Activation of a bradykinin receptor in peripheral nerve and spinal cord in the neonatal rat in vitro, Br. J. Pharmacol., 95 (1988)

1008–1010.

Duggan, A.W., Morton, C.R., Zhao, Z.Q. and Hendry, I.A., Noxious heating of the skin releases immunoreactive substance P in the substantia gelatinosa of the cat: a study with antibody microprobes, Brain Res., 403 (1987) 345–349.

Duggan, A.W., Hendry, I.A., Morton, C.R., Hutchinson, W.D. and Zhao, Z.Q., Cutaneous stimuli releasing immunoreactive substance P in the dorsal horn of the cat, Brain Res., 451 (1988) 261–273.

Duggan, A.W., Hope, P.J., Jarrott, B., Schaible, H.-G. and Fleetwood-Walker, S.M., Release, spread and persistence of immunoreactive neurokinin A in the dorsal horn of the cat following noxious cutaneous stimulation: studies with antibody microprobes, Neuroscience, 35 (1990) 195–202.

Edman, A., Gastrelius, S. and Grampp, W., Transmembrane ion balance in slowly and rapidly adapting lobster stretch receptor neurons, J. Physiol., 377 (1986) 171–191.

Egg, D., Concentrations of prostaglandins D2, E2, F2, 6-keto-F1a and thromboxane B2 in synovial fluid from patients with inflammatory joint disorders and osteoarthritis, Z. Rheumatol., (1984) 89–96.

Ferreira, S.H., Lorenzetti, B.B. and Poole, S., Bradykinin initiates cytokine-mediated inflammatory hyperalgesia, Br. J. Pharmacol., 110 (1993) 1227–1231.

Ferrell, W.R. and Russell, N.J.W., Plasma extravasation in the cat knee joint induced by antidromic articular nerve stimulation, Pflügers Arch., 404 (1985) 91–93.

Freeman, M.A.R. and Wyke, B., The innervation of the knee joint: an anatomical and histological study in the cat, J. Anat., 101 (1967) 502–532.

Grigg, P., Schaible, H.-G. and Schmidt, R.F., Mechanical sensitivity of group III and IV afferents from PAN in normal and inflamed cat knee, J. Neurophysiol., 55 (1986) 635–643.

Grubb, B.D., Birrel, G.J., McQueen, D.S. and Iggo, A., The role of PGE2 in the sensitization of mechanoreceptors in normal and inflamed ankle joints of the rat, Exp. Brain Res., 84 (1991) 383–392.

Guilbaud, G. and Iggo, A., The effect of lysine acetylsalicylate on joint capsule mechanoreceptors in rats with polyarthritis, Exp. Brain Res., 61 (1985) 164–168.

Guilbaud, G., Iggo, A. and Tegner, R., Sensory receptors in ankle joint capsules of normal and arthritic rats, Exp. Brain Res., 58 (1985) 29–40.

Handwerker, H.O., Kilo, S. and Reeh, P.W., Unresponsive afferent nerve fibers in the sural nerve of the rat, J. Physiol., 435 (1991) 229–242.

Hanesch, U., Heppelmann, B. and Schmidt, R.F., Substance P- and calcitonin gene-related peptide immunoreactivity in primary afferent neurons of the cat's knee joint, Neuroscience, 45 (1991) 185–193.

Hanesch, U., Heppelmann, B. and Schmidt, R.F., Neurokinin A-like immunoreactivity in articular afferents of the cat, Brain Res., 586 (1992) 332–335.

Hanesch, U., Pfrommer, U., Grubb, B.D., Heppelmann, B. and Schaible, H.-G., The proportion of CGRP-immunoreactive and SP-mRNA containing dorsal root ganglion cells is increased by a unilateral inflammation of the ankle joint of the rat, Regul. Pept., 46 (1993a) 202–203.

Hanesch, U., Pfrommer, U., Grubb, B.D. and Schaible, H.-G., Acute and chronic phases of unilateral inflammation in rat's ankle are associated with an increase in the proportion of calcitonin gene-related peptide-immunoreactive dorsal root ganglion cells, Eur. J. Neurosci., 5 (1993b) 154–161.

Häbler, H.-J., Jänig, W. and Koltzenburg, M., A novel type of unmyelinated chemosensitive nociceptor in the acutely inflamed bladder, Agents Actions, 25 (1988) 219–221.

Häbler, H.J., Jänig, W. and Koltzenburg, M., Activation of unmyelinated afferent fibers by mechanical stimuli and inflammation of the urinary bladder in the cat. J. Physiol., 425 (1990) 545–562.

Hargreaves, K.M., Troullos, E., Dionne, R.A., Schmidt, E.A., Schafer, S. and Joris, J.L., Bradykinin is increased during acute and chronic inflammation: therapeutic implications, Clin. Pharmacol. Ther., 6 (1988) 613–621.

He, X., Schmidt, R.F. and Schmittner, H., Effects of capsaicin on articular afferents of the cat's knee joint, Agents Actions, 25 (1988) 221–224.

He, X., Schepelmann, K., Schaible, H.-G. and Schmidt, R.F., Capsaicin inhibits responses of fine afferents from the knee joint of the cat to mechanical and chemical stimuli, Brain Res., 530 (1990) 147–150.

Heppelmann, B., Morphologisiche Grundlagen periphere und spinaler Prozess beim Gelenkschmerz, Habilitationsschrift, Medizinische Fakultät der Universität Würzburg, Würzburg, Germany, 1990.

Heppelmann, B., Schaible, H.-G. and Schmidt, R.F., Effects of prostaglandins E1 and E2 on the mechanosensitivity of group III afferents from normal and inflamed cat knee joints. In: H. L. Fields, R. Dubner and F. Cervero (Eds.), Proceedings of the Fourth World Congress on Pain. Advances in Pain Research and Therapy, Vol. 9. Raven Press, New York, 1985, p. 91–101.

Heppelmann, B., Pfeffer, A., Schaible, H.-G. and Schmidt, R.F., Effects of acetylsalicylic acid and indomethacin on single goups III and IV sensory units from acutely inflamed joints, Pain, 26 (1986) 337–351.

Heppelmann, B., Herbert, M.K. and Schaible, H.-G., Morphological and physiological characteristics of the innervation of cat's normal and arthritic knee joint. In: L.M. Pubols and B. Sessle (Eds.), Effects of Injury on Trigeminal and Spinal Somatosensory Systems, A.R.Liss, New York , 1987, p. 19–27.

Heppelmann, B., Heuß, C. and Schmidt, R.F. Fibre size distribution of myelinated and unmyelinated axons in the medial and posterior articular nerves of the cat's knee joint, Somatosens. Mot. Res., 5 (1988) 273–281.

Heppelmann, B., Meßlinger, K. and Schmidt, R.F., Three-dimensional reconstruction of fine afferent nerve fibres in the knee joint capsule, Eur. J. Cell Biol., 48, Suppl. 25 (1989) 115–118.

Heppelmann, B., Meßlinger, K., Neiss, W.F. and Schmidt, R.F., The sensory terminal tree of "free nerve endings" in the articular capsule of the knee. In: W. Zenker and W. L. Neuhuber (Eds.), The Primary Afferent Neuron: A Survey of Recent Morpho-Functional Aspects, Plenum Press, New York, 1990a, p. 73–85.

Heppelmann, B., Meßlinger, K., Neiss, W.F. and Schmidt, R.F., Ultrastructural three-dimensional reconstruction of group III and group IV sensory nerve endings ("free nerve endings") in the knee joint capsule of the cat: evidence for multiple receptive sites, J. Comp. Neurol., 292 (1990b) 103–116.

Heppelmann, B., Meßlinger, K., Neiss, W.F. and Schmidt, R.F., Mitochondria in fine afferent nerve fibres of the knee joint in the cat: a quantitative electron-microscopical examination, Cell Tissue Res., 275 (1994) 493–501.

Herbert, M.K. and Schmidt, R.F., Activation of normal and inflamed fine articular afferent units by serotonin, Pain, 50 (1992) 79–88.

Heyer, G., Hornstein, O.P. and Handwerker, H.O., Skin reactions and itch sensations induced by epicutaneus histamine application in atopic dermatitis and controls, J. Invest. Dermatol., 93 (1989) 492–496.

Hökfelt, T., Holets, V.R., Staines, W., Meister, B., Melander, T., Schalling, M., Schultzberg, M., et al., Coexistence of neuronal Messengers: an overview. In: T. Hökfelt, K. Fuxe and B. Pernow (Eds.), Coexistence of Neuronal Messengers: A New Principle in Chemical Transmission. Progress in Brain Research. Elsevier, Amsterdam, 1986, pp. 33–70.

Holzer, P., Local effector functions of capsaicin-sensitive sensory nerve endings: nvolvement of tachykinins, calcitonin gene-related peptide and other neuropeptides, Neuroscience, 24 (1988) 739–768.

Hope, P.J., Jarrot, B., Schaible, H.-G., Clarke, R.W. and Duggan, A.W., Release and spread of immunoreaktive neurokinin A in the cat spinal cord in a model of acute arthritis, Brain Res., 533 (1990) 292–299.

Inagaki, S. and Kito, S., Peptides in the peripheral nervous system. In: P. C. Emson, M.N. Rossor and M.Tohyama (Eds.), Progress in Brain Research, Vol. 66, Elsevier, Amsterdam, 1986, pp. 269–316.

Jänig, W. and Koltzenburg, M., Receptive properties of sacral primary afferent neurons supplying the colon, J. Neurophysiol., 65 (1991) 1067–1077.

Kanaka, R., Schaible, H.-G. and Schmidt, R.F., Activation of fine articular afferent units by bradykinin, Brain Res., 327 (1985) 81–90.

Khan, A.A., Raja, S.N., Manning, D.C., Campbell, J.N. and Meyer, R.A., The effects of bradykinin and sequence-related analogs on the response properties of cutaneous nociceptors in monkeys, Somatosens. Mot. Res., 9 (1992) 97–106.

Kruger, L., Morphological correlates of "free" nerve endings: a reappraisal of thin sensory axon classification. In: R.F. Schmidt, H.-G. Schaible and C.Vahle-Hinz. (Ed.), Fine Afferent Nerve Fibres and Pain, VCH, Weinheim, 1987.

Kruger, L., Kumazawa, T., Mizumura, K., Sato, J. and Yeh, Y., Observations on electrophysiologically characterized receptive fields of thin testicular afferent axons: a preliminary note on the analysis of fine structural specializations of polymodal receptors, Somatosens. Mot. Res., 5 (1988) 373–380.

Kupfermann, I., Functional studies of cotransmission, Physiol. Rev., 71 (1991) 683–732.

Lang, E., Novak, A., Reeh, P.W. and Handwerker, H.O., Chemosensitivity of fine afferents from rat skin in vitro, J. Neurophysiol., 63 (1990) 887–901.

Langford, L.A. and Schmidt, R.F., Afferent and efferent axons in the medial and posterior articular nerves of the cat, Anat. Rec., 206 (1983) 71–78.

Larsson, J., Ekblom, A., Henriksson, K., Lundeberg, T. and Theodorsson, E., Immunoreactive tachykinins, calcitonin gene-related peptide and neuropeptide Y in human synovial fluid from inflamed knee joints, Neurosci. Lett., 100 (1989) 326–330.

Leah, J.D., Cameron, A.A. and Snow, P.J., Neuropeptides in physiologically identified mammalian sensory neurones, Neurosci. Lett., 56 (1985) 257–263.

Lembeck, F., Griesbacher, T., Eckhardt, M., Henke, S., Breipohl, G. and Knolle, J., New, long-lasting, potent bradykinin antagonists, Br. J. Pharmacol., 102 (1991) 297–304.

Lotz, M., Carson, D.A. and Vaughan, J.H., Substance P activation of rheumatoid synoviocytes: neural pathway in pathogenesis of arthritis, Science, 235 (1987) 893–895.

Mantione, C.R. and Rodriguez, R., A bradykinin (BK)1 receptor antagonist blocks capsaicin-induced ear inflammation in mice, Br. J. Pharmacol., 99 (1990) 516–518.

Marceau, F., Barabé, J., St.-Pierre, S. and Regoli, D., Kinin receptors in experimental inflammation, Can. J. Physiol. Pharmacol., 58 (1980) 536–542.

Martin, H.A., Leukotriene B4 induced decrease in mechanical and thermal thresholds of C-fiber mechanonociceptors in rat hairy skin, Brain Res., 509 (1990) 273–279.

Mayes, J.J. and Govind, C.K., Higher mitochondrial density in slow versus fast lobster sensory neurons, Neurosci. Lett., 102 (1989) 87–90.

McIntyre, A.K., Proske, U. and Tracey, D.J., afferent fibres form muscle receptors in the posterior nerve of the cat's knee joint, Exp. Brain Res., 33 (1978) 415–424.

McMahon, S. and Koltzenburg, M., Novel classes of nociceptors: beyond Sherrington, Trends Neurosci., 13 (1990) 199–201.

Melli, M., Assessment of plasma leukotriene and prostaglandin levels during adjuvant arthritis and kaolin-induced paw oedema in rats, Prostaglandins Leucot. Essent. Fatty Acids, 33 (1988) 173–178.

Mense, S. and Meyer, H., Bradykinin-induced modulation of the response behaviour of different types of feline group III and IV muscle receptors, J. Physiol., 398 (1988) 49–63.

Meßlinger, K., Pawlak, M., Schepelmann, K. and Schmidt, R.F., Responsiveness of slowly conducting articular afferents to bradykinin: effects of an experimental arthritis, Pain, in press.

Meyer, R.A., Davis, K.D., Cohen, R.H., Treede, R.-D. and Campbell, J.N., Mechanically insensitive afferents (MIAs) in cutaneous nerves of monkey, Brain Res., 561 (1991) 252–261.

Mizumura, K., Sato, J. and Kumazawa, T., Effects of prostaglandins and other putative chemical intermediaries of the activity of canine testicular polymodal receptors studied in vitro, Eur. J. Physiol., 408 (1987) 565–572.

Mizumura, K. , Minagawa, M. , Tsujii, Y. and Kumazawa, T., The effects of bradykinin agonists

and antagonists on visceral polymodal receptor activities, Pain, 40 (1990) 221–227.
Moncada, S., Ferreira, S.H. and Vane, J.R., Pain and inflammatory mediators. In: J. R. Vane and S. H. Ferreira (Eds.), Handbook of Experimental Pharmacology, Vol. 50, Springer, Berlin, 1978, pp. 588–616.
Morton, C.R. and Hutchison, W.D., Release of sensory neuropeptides in the spinal cord: studies with calcitonin gene-related peptide and galanin, Neuroscience, 31 (1989) 807–815.
Morton, C.R., Hutchison, W.D. and Hendry, I.A., Release of immunoreactive somatostatin in the spinal dorsal horn of the cat, Neuropeptides, 12 (1988) 189–198.
Neugebauer, V. and Schaible, H.-G., Peripheral and spinal components of the sensitization of spinal neurons during an acute experimental arthritis, Agents Actions, 25 (1988) 234–236.
Neugebauer, V., Schaible, H.-G. and Schmidt, R.F., Sensitization of articular afferents to mechanical stimuli by bradykinin, Pflügers Arch., 415 (1989) 330–335.
Novotny, V., Relation between receptor kind and afferent fibre diameter in the knee-joint capsule of the cat, Acta Anat., 86 (1973) 436–450.
Perkins, M.N., Campbell, E. and Dray, A., Antinociceptive activity of the bradykinin B_1 and B_2 receptor antagonists, des-Arg^9, [Leu^8]-BK and HOE 140, in two models of persistent hyperalgesia in the rat, Pain, 53 (1993) 191–197.
Proske, U., Schaible, H.-G. and Schmidt, R.F., Joint receptors and kinaesthesia, Exp. Brain Res., 72 (1988) 219–224.
Raja, S.N., Meyer, R.A. and Campbell, J.N., Peripheral mechanisms of somatic pain, Anesthesiology, 68 (1988) 571–590.
Russell, N.J.W., Schaible, H.-G. and Schmidt, R.F., Opiates inhibit the discharges of fine afferent units from inflamed knee joint of the cat, Neurosci. Lett., 76 (1987) 107–112.
Schaible, H.-G. and Grubb, B.D., Afferent and spinal mechanisms of joint pain, Pain, 55 (1993) 5–54.
Schaible, H.-G. and Schmidt, R.F., Activation of groups III and IV sensory units in medial articular nerve by local mechanical stimulation of knee joint, J. Neurophysiol., 49 (1983a) 35–44.
Schaible, H.-G. and Schmidt, R.F., Responses of fine medial articular nerve afferents to passive movements of knee joint (abstract), J. Neurophysiol., 49 (1983b) 1118–1126.
Schaible, H.-G. and Schmidt, R.F., Mechanosensibility of joint receptors with fine afferent fibres, Exp. Brain Res., Suppl. 9 (1984) 284–297.
Schaible, H.-G. and Schmidt, R.F., Effects of an experimental arthritis on the sensory properties of fine articular afferent units, J. Neurophysiol., 54 (1985) 1109–1122.
Schaible, H.-G. and Schmidt, R.F., Time course of mechanosensitivity changes in articular afferents during a developing experimental arthritis, J. Neurophysiol., 60 (1988a) 2180–2195.
Schaible, H.-G. and Schmidt, R.F., Exitation and sensitization of fine articular afferent units from cat's knee joint by prostaglandin E_2 (PG E_2), J. Physiol., 403 (1988b) 91–104.
Schaible, H.-G. and Schmidt, R.F., Direct observation of the sensitization of articular afferents during an experimental arthritis. In: R. Dubner, G.F. Gebhardt and M.R. Bond (Eds.), Proceedings of the Vth World Congress on Pain. Pain Research and Clinical Management, Vol. 3. Elsevier, Amsterdam, 1988c, pp. 44–50.
Schaible, H.-G., Jarrott, B., Hope, P.J. and Duggan, A.W., Release of immunoreactive substance P in the spinal cord during development of acute arthritis in the knee joint of the cat: a study with antibody microprobes, Brain Res., 529 (1990) 214–223.
Schaible, H.-G., Hope, P.J., Lang, C.W. and Duggan, A.W., Calcitonin gene-related peptide causes intraspinal spreading of substance P released by peripheral stimulation, Eur. J. Neurosci., 4 (1992) 750–757.
Schepelmann, K., Meßlinger, K., Schaible, H.-G. and Schmidt, R.F., Inflammatory mediators and nociception in the joint: excitation and sensitization of slowly conducting afferent fibers of the cat's knee by prostaglandin I2, Neuroscience, 50 (1992) 237–247.
Schwerzmann, K., Hoppler, H., Kayar, S.R. and Weibel, E.R., Oxidative capacity of muscle and mitochondria: correlation of physiological, biochemical and morphometric characteristics, Proc. Natl. Acad. Sci. USA, 86 (1988) 1583–1587.

Sicuteri, F., Vasoneuroactive substances and their implication in vascular pain. In: A.P. Friedmann (Ed.), Res. Clin. Stud. Headache, Karger, Basel, 1967, p. 6–45.
Stein, C., Periphere Opioidrezeptoren und ihre Bedeutung für die postoperative Schmerztherapie, Der Schmerz, 7 (1993) 4–7.
Stein, C., Hassan, A.H.S., Przewlocki, R., Gramsch, C., Peter, K. and Herz, A., Opioids from immunocytes interact with receptors on sensory nerves to inhibit nociception in inflammation, Proc. Natl. Acad. Sci. USA, 87 (1990) 5935–5939.
Stein, C., Comisel, K., Haimerl, E., Yassouridis, A., Lehrberger, K., Herz, A. and Peter, K., Analgesic effect of intraarticular morphine after arthroscopic knee surgery, N. Engl. J. Med., 325 (1991) 1123–1126.
Steranka, L.R., Manning, D. C., DeHaas, C.J., Ferkany, J.W., Borosky, S.A., Connor, J.R., Vavrek, R.J. and Stewart, J.M., Bradykinin as a pain mediator: receptors are localized to sensory neurons and antagonists have analgesic actions, Proc. Natl. Acad. Sci. USA, 85 (1988) 3245–3249.
Whalley, E.T., Clegg, S., Stewart, J.M. and Vavrek, R.J., The effect of kinin agonists and antagonists on the pain response of the human blister base. Naunyn-Schmiedebergs Arch. Pharmacol., 336 (1987) 652–655.

Correspondence to: Prof. Dr. med. Robert F. Schmidt, PhD, Physiologisches Institut der Universität Würzburg, Röntgenring 9, D-97070 Würzburg, Germany. Tel.: 49-931-31-730, Fax: 49-931-54-553.

Proceedings of the 7th World Congress on Pain,
Progress in Pain Research and Management, Vol. 2,
edited by G.F. Gebhart, D.L. Hammond, and T.S.
Jensen, IASP Press, Seattle, © 1994.

17

Changes in the Functional Organization of the Dorsal Horn During Acute Myositis and Following Muscle Nerve Axotomy

Götz Beylich, Ulrich Hoheisel, Klaus Koch,
and Siegfried Mense

*Institut für Anatomie und Zellbiologie, Universität Heidelberg,
Heidelberg, Germany*

INTRODUCTION

Recent data from animal experiments suggest that pathological alterations in peripheral tissues induce neuroplastic changes at the spinal cord level that may be related to such clinical symptoms as spread of pain or transition from acute to chronic pain. Other workers have shown that following peripheral lesions, the response behavior of dorsal horn neurons changes. The experimental lesions used were inflammation of joints (Calvino et al. 1986; Schaible et al. 1987) or of subcutaneous tissues of the paw (Hylden et al. 1989), as well as section of peripheral nerves (Wall et al. 1981; Brown et al. 1984) or dorsal roots (Basbaum and Wall 1976). Data on the spinal effects of myositis or an acute muscle nerve axotomy are lacking.

METHODS

We performed experiments on adult Sprague Dawly rats. We deeply anesthetized the animals initially with thiopental-sodium (Trapanal, BYK) 100 mg/kg intraperitoneally, followed by small doses of the same anesthetic intravenously

(10–20 mg/kg per hour) to maintain a deep level of anesthesia. The anesthesia was considered to be deep if no gross changes in blood pressure (exceeding 10 mm Hg) and no flexor reflexes occurred upon noxious stimulation of the hindlimb or tail. Muscular relaxation was induced with pancuronium bromide (Pancuronium, Organon) and maintained by subsequent doses as required. We repeatedly tested for the presence of flexor reflexes during recovery from muscular relaxation. The animals were artificially ventilated with a gas mixture of 47.5% O_2, 2.5% CO_2, and 50% N_2. The spinal cord was exposed by a laminectomy at the thoracolumbar level.

We recorded the activity of single dorsal horn neurons in the spinal segments L3–L6 in a randomized mapping procedure. Extracellular recordings were made using glass micropipettes filled with 5% NaCl (DC resistance 7–15 MOhm). As a search stimulus during microelectrode tracking, we used electrical stimulation of dorsal roots L3–L6 (square wave pulses of 5 V amplitude, 0.3 ms duration, repetition rate 0.33 Hz).

We studied the excitability of the neurons with electrical stimulation of the common peroneal (PER), sural (SU), and gastrocnemius-soleus (GS) nerves. The maximal stimulus intensity for testing for A-fiber input from a given nerve was 2.5 V at a stimulus duration of 0.3 ms. This stimulus strength corresponded to 20–25 times threshold of the A-fiber volley in the dorsal roots. We detected no stimulus spread among the large nerves at this strength. With stimuli to the GS nerves exceeding 1.2 V, however, A-fibers in the tibial nerve (TIB n.) were also excited. Thus, the 2.5 V stimulus elicited effects via both the GS nerves and TIB n. (GS/TIB input). To study the effects of input from the GS alone, we used only dorsal horn neurons having a maximal GS n. threshold of 1 V and/or a mechanosensitive receptive field (RF) in the GS muscle. For supramaximal stimulation of C-fibers, we applied single pulses or trains of 3 pulses at 20 ms interval and of up to 50 V amplitude. At this strength, no stimulus spread to adjacent nerves sufficient for activating C-fibers occurred.

We induced inflammation of the GS muscle by injecting it with a 2% solution of carrageenan in Tyrode. Animals with normal, non-injected, muscles were used as a control. In the experiments employing axotomy, we ligated and cut the GS nerves close to the muscle during a reversible cold block of the section site. A stimulating electrode was placed proximal to the ligature. Neither inflammation nor axotomy had a detectable influence on the electrical threshold of the A-fibers in the GS nerves. The activity of single dorsal horn neurons was recorded 2–8 hours after inducing the lesions.

For superfusion of the spinal cord with antagonists to transmitter/modulator substances, a pool was formed around the L3 segment. Via a strip of filter paper, the segment was continuously superfused with artificial cerebrospinal fluid to which antagonists at a concentration of 100 μM were added. We tested the following compounds: spantide (Sigma), a relatively unspecific tachykinin antagonist; MK-801 (Research Biochemical Incorporated), an open channel antagonist at the N-methyl-D-aspartate (NMDA) receptor; and N^G-monomethyl-L-arginine (NMMA; Sigma), a nitric oxide (NO) synthase blocker. The superfusion with antagonists started 30 minutes before the experimental myositis was induced and was continued for the rest of the experiment.

RESULTS

AXOTOMY

The background activity of the neurons was not significantly altered by axotomy. The proportion of cells having background activity remained almost constant, and there was only a small trend to a higher mean discharge frequency.

Under control conditions, stimulation of A-fibers in the GS nerves (1 V stimulus) had the largest effects in the medial dorsal horn of the L4 and L5 segments. There, 20–30% of the neurons responding to dorsal root stimulation could be activated by A-fiber input from the GS, whereas in the lateral dorsal horn and in the L6 and L3 segments the proportion varied around 10% (Fig. 1). The main effect of GS axotomy was a reduction in the number of cells responding to GS A-fiber input; in the lateral L4–L6 segments the responses vanished completely. The decrease in responsiveness to GS A-fiber input became significant only five or more hours after axotomy.

The effects of the GS/TIB input (2.5 V stimulus) showed the same change, namely a highly significant decrease in the proportion of responding neurons. In contrast, the proportion of neurons responding to A-fiber input from the SU and PER n. at the same stimulus strength increased. For the SU n., the increase was significant in the lateral horn only, that is, in that region of the dorsal horn that showed the most marked decrease in response to stimulating the GS/TIB nerves.

Responses of dorsal horn neurons to C-fiber input from the GS/TIB nerves (50 V stimulus) were almost completely missing in animals with intact GS nerves, and no change could be detected following axotomy (Fig. 2B). There was, however, a significant increase in responsiveness to C-fiber input from the SU n. in the lateral dorsal horn in axotomized animals (Fig. 2D).

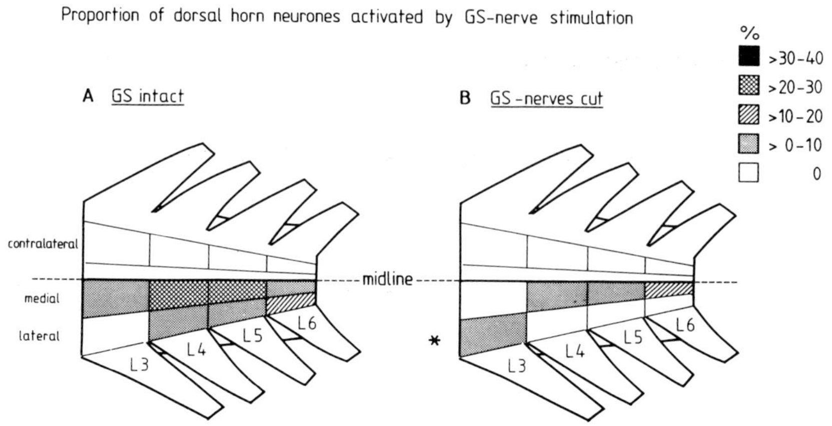

Fig. 1. Dorsal view of the rat lumbar spinal cord showing the effect of GS axotomy on the proportion of neurons activated by electrical stimulation of A-fibers in the GS nerves (1 V stimulus). In the left half of the cord (ipsilateral to the axotomy), each segment is divided in a medial and lateral portion; the percentage of neurons responding to GS input is indicated by different grades of shading. A, data from animals with intact GS muscle. B, data from animals with cut GS nerves. The asterisk marks a statistically significant decrease in the number of responding neurons in the lateral dorsal horn of the L3–L6 segments (* $P < 0.05$; *U* test, two-tailed).

MYOSITIS

Background Activity and Changes in Responsiveness

The proportion of neurons exhibiting background activity increased significantly from approximately 10% to 20% during myositis; the mean discharge frequency, however, showed only an insignificant trend to higher values.

In animals with a myositis of the GS muscle, the population of neurons responding to A-fiber input (1 V stimulus) from that muscle increased in size. The effect was most marked in the lateral dorsal horn, where more than 30% of the cells responded in myositis animals, whereas under control conditions the proportion was less than 10% ($P < 0.001$; Fig. 3). In the lateral L3 segment there was a qualitative change, in that responses to stimulation of the GS nerves appeared which were completely missing in control animals. These effects were strongly restricted to input from the inflamed muscle, since additional activation of A-fibers in the TIB n. (2.5 V stimulus, GS/TIB input) abolished the significance. The proportion of neurons responding to A-fiber

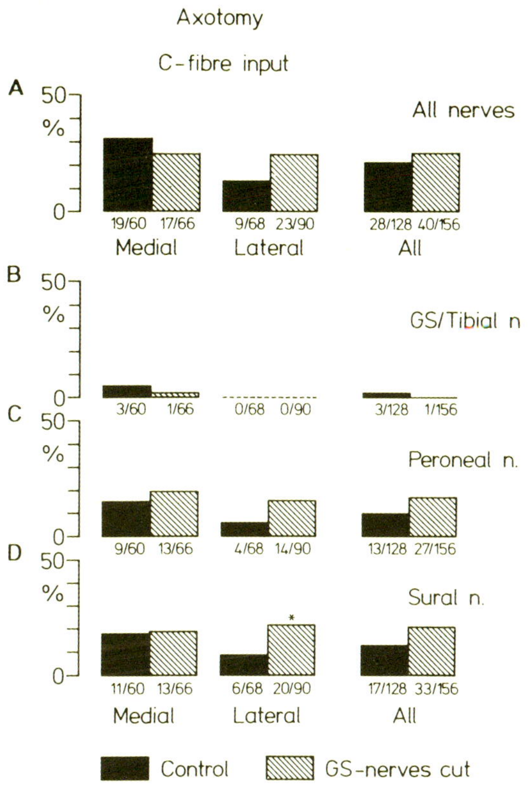

Fig. 2. Effects of GS axotomy on the stimulating efficacy of C-fiber input from the nerves GS/TIB, PER, and SU. The ordinates scale gives the proportion of neurons activated by C-fiber input. Filled bars show data from control rats with intact GS nerves, hatched bars data from axotomized rats. Results obtained from neurons in the medial and lateral halves, respectively, of the L3–L6 segments are evaluated separately; "all" indicates pooled data from the medial and lateral dorsal horn). A, stimulating effects of all nerves evaluated together. **B–D**, effects of stimulation of the nerves GS/TIB. (**B**), PER (**C**), and SU n. (**D**). The effects of SU C-fiber stimulation showed a significant increase in the lateral dorsal horn (*D*; *, $P < 0.05$).

input from the other hindlimb nerves likewise was not significantly altered at a stimulus strengths of 1 and 2.5 V.

The effect of the myositis on the responses to C-fiber input had the same direction as that of GS axotomy, namely an increase in responsiveness in the lateral dorsal horn. However, there were quantitative differences: during myositis, the responses to C-fiber input from both PER and SU n. showed highly significant increases (Fig. 4), whereas following axotomy the increase just reached significance and was restricted to the SU n.

Spinal Cord Superfusion with Antagonists

In this series of experiments, we made recordings in the L3 segment only—that is, in that segment which showed the most marked changes during myositis. Superfusion of the spinal cord with spantide resulted in a significant reduction of the proportion of neurons responding to A-fiber input from the GS (1 V stimulus; Fig. 5). The proportion of neurons responding to C-fiber input from the tested nerves (GS/TIB, SU, PER) was likewise significantly reduced by spantide. The NMDA antagonist MK-801 led to an insignificant reduction of the number of cells responding to GS A-fiber input (1 V stimulus) and had no significant influence on the responses to C-fiber input from the three nerves. Superfusion with the NO synthase blocker NMMA had almost no effect on the excitability of the dorsal horn neurons by A- and C-fiber input, but caused a highly significant increase in the proportion of neurons having background activity ($P < 0.001$).

Immunohistochemical Examination of the Dorsal Horn

The results of the superfusion experiments indicated that the release of substance P (SP) may be important for the excitability changes in the dorsal horn. Therefore, SP-immunoreactivity and calcitonin gene-related peptide (CGRP)-immunoreactivity (SP- and CGRP-IR) were visualized in the dorsal horn of the L3 segment 7–8 hours after induction of the myositis and were morphometrically evaluated. The area of SP-IR showed no detectable side-to-side differences and no differences between control and inflamed animals. There was, however, a broadening of the CGRP-immunoreactive (ir) band in the myositis animals, in the medial half of the dorsal horn, in a region that

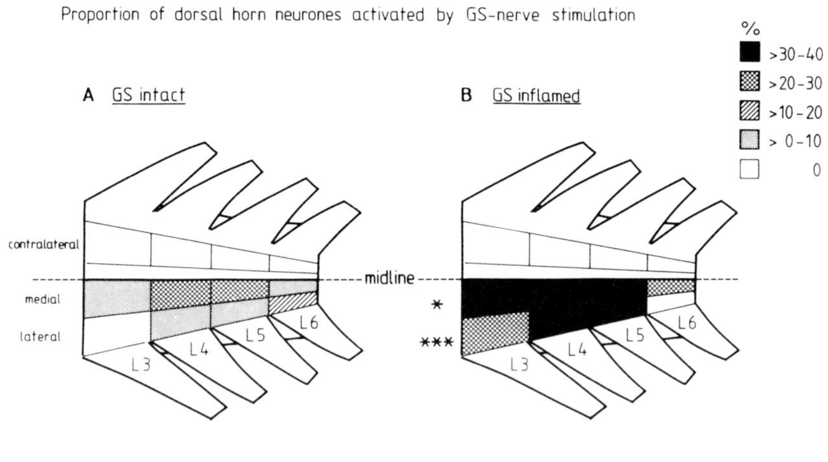

Fig. 3. Dorsal view of the rat lumbar spinal cord showing the effect of an experimental myositis of the GS muscle on the proportion of neurons activated by electrical stimulation of A-fibers in the GS nerves (1 V stimulus). Presentation of data as in Fig. 1. The increase in the proportion of neurons responding to GS input was significant in both the medial (*, $P < 0.05$) and the lateral (***, $P < 0.001$) dorsal horn in the L3–L6 segments.

somatotopically corresponds to the site of the myositis in the lower hindlimb. In axotomized animals, the ir band showed a reduction in width in the same location in the superficial dorsal horn.

DISCUSSION

The results show that an acute lesion of a peripheral nerve or skeletal muscle leads to marked changes in the functional organization of dorsal horn neurons within a few hours. Because of the short interval between lesion and data sampling, morphological changes in the dorsal horn are unlikely to be involved in these effects. Such changes can not be excluded, however, because the formation of new active zones of synapses has been reported to occur within 2 hours in the adult rat (Sperry and Goshgarian 1993).

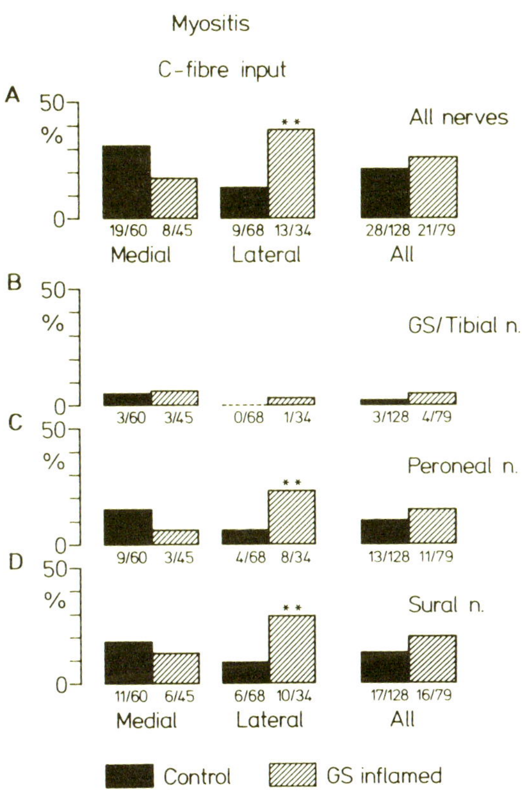

Fig. 4. Effects of a myositis of the GS muscle on the stimulating efficacy of C-fiber input from the nerves GS/TIB, PER, and SU. Presentation of data as in Fig. 2. Note that the C-fiber input from both the PER (**C**) and SU (**D**) nerves was more effective in the myositis animals (**, $P < 0.01$), whereas the responsiveness to C-fiber input from the inflamed muscle (GS/TIB n.) was largely unaffected (**B**).

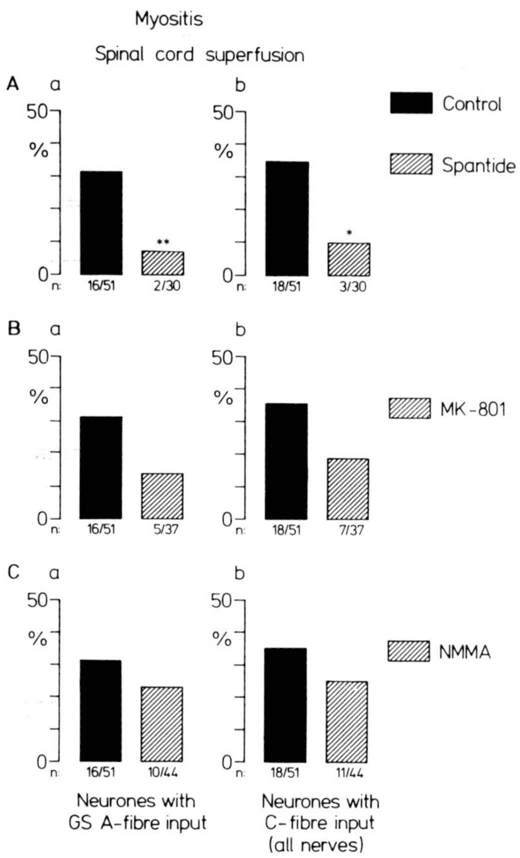

Fig. 5. Effects of spinal cord superfusion with antagonists on the responsiveness of dorsal horn neurons in the L3 segment to A- and C-fiber input in myositis animals. The left column of data (**A a, B a, C a**) shows the proportion of neurons responding to A-fiber input from the GS nerves (1 V stimulus); the right column (**A b, B b, C b**) the proportion of neurons activated by C-fibers in at least one of the nerves tested (50 V stimulus). Filled bars (control) show data from myositis animals whose spinal cord was superfused with artificial cerebrospinal fluid; hatched colums show data from myositis animals whose spinal cord was superfused with the antagonists spantide (**A**), MK-801 (**B**), and NMMA (**C**).

As to the responsiveness of dorsal horn neurons to A-fiber input from the GS, axotomy and myositis had opposite effects: following axotomy, the excitability by input from the cut GS nerves decreased, whereas during myositis it increased. However, as far as the stimulating effect of C-fiber input from PER and SU n. is concerned, the results obtained with the two experimental lesions were qualitatively similar. This suggests that the changes in responsiveness to A-fiber input may be caused by factors different from those controlling the effects of C-fiber input.

The changes in dorsal horn excitability after acute axotomy may be the first step in the long-term functional reorganization of the dorsal horn that has been reported to occur days after cutting of peripheral nerves (Devor and Wall 1981) or dorsal roots (Basbaum and Wall 1976). The simplest interpretation of the reduced excitability to GS A-fiber input in axotomized animals is that it reflects a hyperpolarization of dorsal horn neurons caused by a lack of excitatory postsynaptic potentials (EPSPs), which normally maintain the neurons in a depolarized state. This interpretation implies that under normal circumstances the ongoing activity in muscle afferents has a facilitatory action on the excitability of dorsal horn neurons driven by the cut nerves, and simultaneously an inhibitory action on the stimulating effects of the SU and PER n.

In experimental animals with intact GS muscle and nerve, spontaneous afferent activity of low frequency is present in a small proportion of muscle group III and IV fibers (Mense and Meyer 1985) and in almost all muscle spindle primary endings. Following the above line of thinking, the abolition of this activity might lead to a change in polarization (de- or hyperpolarization) of dorsal horn neurons. The data of the present study are not sufficient to answer this question. However, the finding that the electrical threshold and background activity of dorsal horn neurons were largely unchanged following axotomy speaks against the above assumption. Moreover, the decreased efficacy of the GS input became significant only five or more hours after axotomy.

During a carrageenan-induced myositis, activity in slowly conducting muscle afferent units increases (Diehl et al. 1993); the same applies to primary endings of muscle spindles (Yu, Scherotzke, and Mense, unpublished). A possible mechanism for the increased responsiveness of dorsal horn neurons to GS A-fiber input in the myositis animals is that the increased afferent activity leads to a constant depolarization of the second-order neurons. The largely unchanged frequency of background activity and electrical threshold speak against this mechanism, whereas the increase in the proportion of active neurons during myositis is compatible with a postsynaptic depolarization.

Another possible explanation for the observed effects is that the experimental lesions interfered with the turnover (synthesis, transport, release, degradation) of neuropeptides that influence the excitability of dorsal horn neurons. It is well known that section of peripheral nerves leads to reduced levels of SP and CGRP in the nerve proximal to the lesion and in the dorsal horn (Jessell et al. 1979; Barbut et al. 1981; Villar et al. 1991), whereas the levels of galanin (GAL) and vasoactive intestinal polypeptide (VIP) are increased (Shehab and Atkinson 1986; Hökfelt et al. 1987; Villar et al. 1991). Most of these changes have been studied days or weeks following axotomy; no data are available on the effects of an acute axotomy.

Inflammatory lesions of various tissues in the periphery are followed by an increase in SP and CGRP levels in the spinal nerve and the dorsal horn (Holland and Goldstein 1990; Gillardon et al. 1991; Donnerer et al. 1992). CGRP may be indirectly involved in the inflammation-induced hyperexcitability of dorsal horn neurons by increasing the expression of immediate-early genes

(Galeazza et al. 1992). Whether the broadening of the CGRP-ir band in the myositis animals is due to an increase in synthesis or a decrease in release (as has been described for SP [McCarson and Goldstein 1990]) is unknown.

In experiments on acute arthritic monkeys, a decrease in SP-IR and variable effects on the CGRP-IR have been found ipsilateral to the lesion (Sluka et al. 1992). Possible explanations for this difference are that in the present study the animals underwent extensive surgery including laminectomy, and that search stimuli at C-fiber intensity were applied every 3 seconds. These procedures might lead to an increased synthesis of CGRP early in the experiment.

The broadening of the CGRP-ir region is possibly associated with an increased efficacy of SP, because CGRP is known to enhance the action of SP by inhibiting its degradation (Le Greves et al. 1985) and by facilitating its diffusion in the dorsal horn (Schaible et al. 1992). Therefore, CGRP could play an important role for the postulated function of SP as a volume transmitter (Fuxe and Agnati 1991). Other factors that are up-regulated by peripheral inflammatory lesions and may enhance neuronal excitability are dynorphin (DYN; Nahin et al. 1992) and nerve growth factor (NGF; Lewin et al. 1992).

The data obtained with superfusion of the spinal L3 segment with antagonists suggest that SP- and probably also NMDA-receptor activation is involved in the myositis-induced changes in the dorsal horn. SP has been and still is controversely discussed as a pain transmitter in the central nervous system (Nicoll et al. 1980; Frenk et al. 1988). The neuropeptide excites predominantly nociceptive neurons in the dorsal horn (Henry 1976; Randic and Miletic 1977; Davies and Dray 1980), is released from primary afferent fibers during peripheral inflammatory lesions (see above), and has altered levels in chronic pain patients (Almay et al. 1988; Vaeroy et al. 1988). In animal experiments in which the spinal cord was superfused with SP, it caused an increase in the degree of convergence in dorsal horn neurons (Hoheisel and Mense 1992). This action could well lead to the increased responsiveness to GS A-fiber input in the lateral dorsal horn in myositis animals.

Spantide has been reported to have negative side effects such as local anesthetic (Yoshizawa et al. 1987) or neurotoxic actions (Post and Paulsson 1985). In our experiments, spantide did not appear to have toxic actions, because it did not change the background activity of dorsal horn neurons, and it reduced the responses to GS input without affecting the stimulating effects of the PER n.

Iontophoretically applied NMDA has been shown to excite predominantly nociceptive dorsal horn neurons (Aanonsen et al. 1990). For the present study, the excitatory amino acid is of particular interest because NMDA receptors are thought to be involved in processes associated with neuroplastic changes such as wind-up (Dickenson and Sullivan 1990; Coderre 1992), secondary hyperalgesia (Dougherty and Willis 1991), and long-term potentiation (LTP) in the hippocampus (Bliss and Collingridge 1993). In hyperalgesic animals, prophylactic administration of MK-801 has been found to prevent one of the main signs of hyperalgesia in dorsal horn neurons, namely the increase in size of their RFs (Ren et al. 1992).

Besides having vascular actions, NO influences neuronal processes such as synaptic transmission in sympathetic ganglia (Sheng et al. 1992) and induction of LTP. The actions of NO are mediated via activation of cyclic guanosine monophosphate (cGMP; for recent reviews, see Snyder 1992; Meller and Gebhart 1993). L-NMMA and L-NAME block the NO synthase (Belvis et al. 1991; Ialenti et al. 1992). In the present study, NO did not contribute to the observed changes in the functional organization of the dorsal horn. However, a block of NO synthase had a highly significant excitatory effect on the background activity. The physiological relevance of this finding is obscure at present; it may be related to the observation that NO has a tonic inhibitory action on spinal nociceptive transmission (Zhuo et al. 1993).

As to the clinical importance of the findings, the increased proportion of neurons having background discharge in myositis animals might be associated with spontaneous pain in patients if the impulse activity is present in nociceptive neurons, and with dys- or paresthesias if it occurs in non-nociceptive cells. The main myositis-induced change in the functional organization of the dorsal horn was an increase in size of the neuron population responding to A-fiber input from the inflamed muscle. The effect was most marked in the lateral dorsal horn, where cells are situated that normally process information from deep tissues of the proximal hindlimb (Yu and Mense 1990). This means that cells in the lateral dorsal horn acquired additional input from the GS (i.e. from the distal hindlimb). If a similar change also occurs in patients, it may form the basis of proximal referral of pain and dysesthesia, because under the influence of the lesion, an input from the distal leg may cause activity in neurons that mediate sensations from the proximal leg. Proximal (as well as distal) referral of muscle pain occurs in patients with trigger points in skeletal muscle (Travell and Simons 1983), and proximal referral of muscle pain can be elicited in humans by electrical stimulation of muscle nerve fascicles (Torebjörk et al. 1984).

REFERENCES

Aanonsen, L.M., Lei, S. and Wilcox, G.L., Excitatory amino acid receptors and nociceptive neurotransmission in rat spinal cord, Pain, 41 (1990) 309–321.

Almay, B.G.L., Johansson, F., von Knorring, L., LeGreves, P. and Terenius, L., Substance P in CSF of patients with chronic pain syndromes, Pain, 33 (1988) 3–9.

Barbut, D., Polak, J.M. and Wall, P.D., Substance P in spinal cord dorsal horn decreases following peripheral nerve injury, Brain Res., 205 (1981) 289–298.

Basbaum, A.I. and Wall, P.D., Chronic changes in the response of cells in adult cat dorsal horn following partial deafferentation: the appearance of responding cells in a previously non-responsive region, Brain Res., 116 (1976) 181–204.

Belvis, M.G., Stretton, D. and Barnes, P.I., Nitric oxide as an endogenous modulator of cholinergic neurotransmission in guinea-pig airways, Eur. J. Pharmacol., 198 (1991) 219–221.

Bliss, T.V.P. and Collingridge, G.L., A synaptic model of memory: Long-term potentiation in the hippocampus, Nature, 361 (1993) 31–39.

Brown, A.G., Fyffe, R.E.W., Noble, R. and Rowe, M.J., Effects of hind limb nerve section on lumbosacral dorsal horn neurones in the cat, J. Physiol., London, 354 (1984) 375–394.

Calvino, B., Villanueva, L. and Le Bars, D., Dorsal horn (convergent) neurones in the intact anaesthetized arthritic rat. I. Segmental excitatory influences, Pain, 28 (1986) 81–98.

Coderre, T.J., Contribution of protein kinase C to central sensitization and persistent pain following tissue injury, Neurosci. Lett., 2 (1992) 181–184.

Davies, J. and Dray, A., Depression and facilitation of synaptic responses in cat dorsal horn by substance P administered into substantia gelatinosa, Life Sci., 27 (1980) 2037–2042.

Devor, M and Wall, P.D., Plasticity in the spinal cord sensory map following peripheral nerve injury in rats, J. Neurosci., 1 (1981) 679–684.

Dickenson, A.H. and Sullivan, A.F., Differential effects of excitatory amino acid antagonists on dorsal horn nociceptive neurones in the rat, Brain Res., 506 (1990) 31–39.

Diehl, B., Hoheisel, U. and Mense, S., The influence of mechanical stimuli and of acetylsalicylic acid on the discharges of slowly conducting afferent units from normal and inflamed muscle in the rat, Exp. Brain Res., 92 (1993) 431–440.

Donnerer, J., Schuligoi, R. and Stein, C., Increased content and transport of substance P and calcitonin gene-related peptide in sensory nerves innervating inflamed tissue: evidence for a regulatory function of nerve growth factor in vivo, Neuroscience, 49 (1992) 693–698.

Dougherty, P.M. and Willis, W.D., Enhancement of spinothalamic neuron responses to chemical and mechanical stimuli following combined micro-iontophoretic application of N-methyl-D-aspartic acid and substance P, Pain, 47 (1991) 85–93.

Eide, P.K., Effects of intrathecal substance P and a substance P antagonist on a reflex to noxious heat are independent of changes in tail skin temperature, Acta Physiol. Scand., 140 (1990) 539–543.

Frenk, H., Bossut, D. and Mayer. D.J., Is substance P a primary afferent neurotransmitter for nociceptive input? I. Analysis of pain-related behaviors resulting from intrathecal administration of substance P and 6 exitatory compounds, Brain Res., 455 (1988) 223–231.

Fuxe, K. and Agnati, L.F., Two principal modes of electrochemical communication in the brain: volume versus wiring transmission, In: K. Fuxe and L.F. Agnati (Eds.), Volume Transmission in the Brain, Novel Mechanisms for Neural Transmission, Raven Press, New York, 1991.

Galeazza, M.T., Stucky, C.L. and Seybold, V.S., Changes in (^{125}J) hCGRP binding in rat spinal cord in an experimental model of acute, peripheral inflammation, Brain Res., 591 (1992) 198–208.

Gillardon, F. Morano, I. and Zimmermann, M., Time course of altered levels of calcitonin gene-related peptide in rat spinal cord following skin ultraviolet irradiation, Regul. Pept., 34 (1991) 107.

Henry, J.L., Effects of substance P on functionally identified units in cat spinal cord, Brain Res., 114 (1976) 439–451.

Hökfelt, T., Wiesenfeld-Hallin, Z., Villar, M. and Melander, T., Increase of galanin-like immunoreactivity in rat dorsal root ganglion cells after peripheral axotomy, Neurosci. Lett., 83 (1987) 217–220.

Hoheisel, U. and Mense, S., The influence of substance P on the synaptic efficicacy of afferent input to dorsal horn neurones in the rat, Pflügers Arch., 420 (Suppl. 1) (1992) R 22.

Holland, L.N. and Goldstein, B.D., Changes of substance P-like immunoreactivity in the dorsal horn are associated with the "phasic" behavioral response to a formalin stimulus, Brain Res., 537 (1990) 287–292.

Hylden, J.L.K., Nahin, R.L., Traub, R.J. and Dubner, R., Expansion of receptive fields of spinal lamina I projection neurons in rats with unilateral adjuvant-induced inflammation: the contribution of dorsal horn mechanisms, Pain, 37 (1989) 229–243.

Ialenti, A., Ianaro, A., Moncada, S. and DiRosa, M., Modulation of acute inflammation by endogenous nitric oxide, Eur. J. Pharmacol., 211 (1992) 177–182.

Jessell, T., Tsunoo, A., Kanazawa, F. and Otsuka, M., Substance P in the dorsal horn of rat spinal cord after section of the peripheral processes of primary sensory neurons, Brain Res., 168 (1979) 247–259.

Le Greves, P., Nyberg, F., Terenius, L. and Hökfelt, T., Calcitonin gene-related peptide is a potent inhibitor of substance P degradation, Eur. J. Pharmacol., 115 (1985) 309–311.

Lewin, G.R., Winter, J. and McMahon, S.B., Regulation of afferent connectivity in the adult spinal cord by nerve growth factor, Eur. J. Neurosci., 4 (1992) 700–707.

McCarson, K.E. and Goldstein, B.D., Time course of the alteration in dorsal horn substance P levels following formalin: blockade by naloxone, Pain, 41 (1990) 95–100.

Meller, S.T. and Gebhart, G.F., Nitric oxide (NO) and nociceptive processing in the spinal cord, Pain, 52 (1993) 127–136.

Mense, S. and Meyer, H., Different types of slowly conducting afferent units in cat skeletal muscle and tendon, J. Physiol., London, 363 (1985) 403–417.

Nahin, R.L., Hylden, J.L.K. and Humphrey, E., Demonstration of dynorphin A1-8 immunoreactive axons contacting spinal cord projection neurons in a rat model of peripheral inflammation and hyperalgesia, Pain, 51 (1992) 135–143.

Nicoll, R.A., Schenker, C. and Leeman, S.E., Substance P as a transmitter candidate, Ann. Rev. Neurosci., 3 (1980) 227–268.

Post, C. and Paulsson, I., Antinociceptive and neurotoxic actions of substance P analogues in the rat's spinal cord after intrathecal administration, Neurosci. Lett., 57 (1985) 159–164.

Randic, M. and Miletic, V., Effect of substance P in cat dorsal horn neurones activated by noxious stimuli, Brain Res., 128 (1977) 164–169.

Ren, K., Hylden, J.L.K., Williams, G.M., Ruda, M.A. and Dubner, R., The effects of a non-competitive NMDA receptor antagonist, MK-801, on behavioral hyperalgesia and dorsal horn neuronal activity in rats with unilateral inflammation, Pain, 50 (1992) 331–344.

Schaible, H.-G., Schmidt, R.F. and Willis, W.D., Enhancement of the responses of ascending tract cells in the cat spinal cord by acute inflammation of the knee joint, Exp. Brain Res., 66 (1987) 489–499.

Schaible, H.-G., Hope, P.J., Lang, C.W. and Duggan, A.W., Calcitonin gene-related peptide causes intraspinal spreading of substance P released by peripheral stimulation, Eur. J. Neurosci., 4 (1992) 750–757.

Shehab, S.A.S. and Atkinson, M.E., Vasoactive intestinal polypeptide (VIP) increases in the spinal cord after peripheral axotomy of the sciatic nerve originate from primary afferent neurons, Brain Res., 372 (1986) 37–44.

Sheng, H., Hughes, M.L., Murad, F. and Briggs, C.A., Evidence that nitric oxide mediates the cyclic GMP response to synaptic activity in the rat superior cervical ganglion, Brain Res., 597 (1992) 343–345.

Sluka, K.A., Dougherty, P.M., Sorkin, L.S., Willis, W.D. and Westlund, K.N., Neural changes in acute arthritis in monkeys. III. Changes in substance P, calcitonin gene-related peptide and glutamate in the dorsal horn of the spinal cord, Brain Res. Rev., 17 (1992) 29–38.

Snyder, S.H., Nitric oxide and neurons, Curr. Opin. Neurobiol., 2 (1992) 323–327.

Sperry, M.A. and Goshgarian, H.G., Ultrastructural changes in the rat phrenic nucleus developing within 2 h after cervical spinal cord hemisection, Exp. Neurol., 120 (1993) 233–244.

Torebjörk, H.E., Ochoa, J.L. and Schady, W., Referred pain from intraneural stimulation of muscle fascicles in the median nerve, Pain, 18 (1984) 145–156.

Travell, J.G. and Simons, D.G., Myofascial pain and dysfunction. In: The trigger point manual. Williams and Wilkins, Baltimore, London, 1983.

Vaeroy, H., Helle, R., Forre, 0., Kass, E. and Terenius, L., Elevated CSF levels of substance P and high incidence of Raynaud's phenomenon in patients with fibromyalgia: new features for diagnosis, Pain, 33 (1988) 21–26.

Villar, M.J., Cortés, R., Theodorsson, E., Wiesenfeld-Hallin, Z., Schalling, M., Fahrenkrug, J., Emson, P.C. and Hökfelt, T., Neuropeptide expression in rat dorsal root ganglion cells and spinal cord after peripheral nerve injury with special reference to galanin, Neuroscience, 33 (1989) 587–604.

Villar, M.J., Wiesenfeld-Hallin, Z., Xu, X.-J., Theodorsson, E., Emson, P.C. and Hökfeld, T., Further studies on galanin-, substance P-, and CGRP-like immunoreactivities in primary sensory neurons and spinal cord: Effects of dorsal rhizotomies and sciatic nerve lesions, Exp. Neurol., 112 (1991) 29–39.

Wall, P.D., Fitzgerald, M. and Gibson, S.J., The response of rat spinal cord cells to unmyelinated afferents after peripheral nerve section and after changes in substance P levels, Neuroscience, 6 (1981) 2205–2215.

Woolf, C.J., Shortland, P. and Coggeshall, R.E., Peripheral nerve injury triggers central sprouting of myelinated afferents, Nature, 355 (1992) 75–78.

Yoshizawa, T., Kanazawa, I. and Nakanishi, T., Substance P antagonist (spantide) suppresses the compound action potentials of the rat sciatic nerve in vitro, Neuropeptides, 10 (1987) 181–188.

Yu, X.-M. and Mense, S., Somatotopical arrangement of rat spinal dorsal horn cells processing input from deep tissues, Neurosci. Lett, 108 (1990) 43–47.

Zhuo, M., Meller, S.T. and Gebhart, G.F., Endogenous nitric oxide is required for tonic cholinergic inhibition of spinal mechanical transmission, Pain, 54 (1993) 71–78.

Correspondence to: Prof. Dr. med. S. Mense, Institut für Anatomie und Zellbiologie, Im Neuenheimer Feld 307, D-69120 Heidelberg, Germany. Tel: 49-6221-564193; Fax: 49-6221-563071

Proceedings of the 7th World Congress on Pain,
Progress in Pain Research and Management, Vol. 2,
edited by G.F. Gebhart, D.L. Hammond, and T.S.
Jensen, IASP Press, Seattle, © 1994.

18

Different Mechanisms (Receptor Subtypes and Second Messenger Actions) Implicated in PGE_2-Induced Sensitization of the Responses to Bradykinin and to Heat of Polymodal Receptors

Takao Kumazawa, Kazue Mizumura,
and Hisashi Koda

Department of Neural Regulation, Research Institute of Environmental Medicine, Nagoya University, Nagoya, Japan

INTRODUCTION

Prostaglandins (PG) are known to cause hyperalgesia in man and animals (Moncada et al. 1978). A convergent line of evidence has revealed that polymodal receptors play an important role in signaling pain, particularly the types of pain commonly encountered clinically (Bessou and Perl 1969; Grigg et al. 1986; Kumazawa and Mizumura 1980; Kumazawa et al. 1987a,b; Ochoa and Torebjörk 1989). As shown in Fig. 1, PGE_2 enhances the response of polymodal receptors to bradykinin (BK) at a low concentration, which does not evoke discharge of the sensory receptor. However, it enhances heat responses at concentrations 100 times greater than those for BK responses (Kumazawa et al. 1992a; Mizumura et al. 1987, 1991). This marked difference in the effective concentration of PGE_2 for inducing sensitization of the two responses suggests that different types of PGE receptors are involved in these phenomena. Based on pharmacological studies carried out mainly on visceral tissue preparations, PGE receptors are subdivided into three sub-

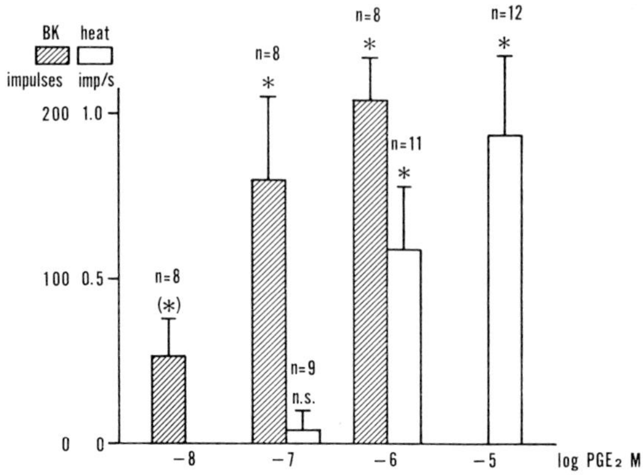

Fig. 1. Comparison of PGE_2-induced augmenting effects on BK and heat responses of polymodal receptors. Hatched columns show net increase in number of impulses evoked by BK (0.1 μM); open columns show net increase in mean discharge rate during heat stimulation. Abscissa: concentrations of PGE_2; * significant change ($P < 0.05$). (From Kumazawa et al. 1992a)

types: EP_1, EP_2, and EP_3 (Coleman et al. 1990) (Table I). Reports implicating the EP receptor subtypes in nociceptor functions apparently have not been published to date.

This study is aimed at clarifying the PGE receptor subtype(s) and the second messenger(s) that are implicated in the PGE_2-induced enhancement on BK and heat responses of polymodal receptors. A preliminary report on portions of our results has been published (Kumazawa et al. 1992b, 1993).

METHODS

We have previously described general experimental procedures (Kumazawa et al. 1987b). Briefly, single- or multi-unit discharges of polymodal receptors, which were identified by the responses to mechanical and heat stimulation as well as to BK, were recorded in testis-spermatic nerve in vitro preparations from deeply anesthetized dogs. stimulus solutions were applied by replacing the Krebs solution bathing the receptive field. In experiments to clarify the EP receptor subtypes, aspirin (550 μM) was applied throughout the experimental period. In these experiments, BK (1 μM BK mixed with 550 μM aspirin and 10 μM captopril) was applied for one minute at intervals of about 10 minutes in the single-dose method and for about 15 minutes at an interval between 50 and 100 minutes in the cumulative method. In the other experiments, BK (0.1 μM,

Table I
EP receptor subtypes, the agonists and antagonist, and the actions of the second messengers. These agonists and antagonist selective for the three subtypes were used in this experiment.

Subtype	Agonist	Antagonist	2nd Messenger
EP_1	17-phenyl trinor PGE_2	AH6809	IP_3, DAG ↑
EP_2	butaprost	none	cAMP ↑
EP_3	M&B28767	none	cAMP ↓

1 min) was tested every 10 minutes. Heat stimulation by preheated Krebs solution (42–48°C) was applied for 30 seconds at intervals of 5 or 10 minutes. AH6809 (donated by Dr. B.M. Bain, Glaxo), 17-phenyl trinor PGE_2 (Cayman Chemical), butaprost (donated by Dr. P.J. Gardiner, Bayer) and M&B28767 (donated by Dr. M.P.L. Caton, Rhone-Poulenc) were used as the EP_1 antagonist, and EP_1-, EP_2-, and EP_3-agonists, respectively (Armstrong et al. 1990; Coleman et al. 1985, 1990; Gardiner 1986). The effects of EP receptor agonists were tested by one or both of the single- and cumulative-dose methods (Fig. 2). After establishing a control group by ascertaining stabilization of the responses, EP receptor agonists were given as pretreatments according to the single-dose method for three minutes before BK- or heat-stimulation. In the cumulative method, EP receptor agonists were cumulatively applied every two minutes with BK at concentrations from 1 nM to 10 μM, when the BK-induced discharge rate reached a quasi-steady state or a slowly declining phase. For quantitative evaluation, the augmenting effect caused by the two-minute application of PGE analogues is expressed by the net increases in mean discharge rates: those at effective concentrations minus those at the ineffective level, as schematically shown in Fig. 2A. Effects of the elevation of intracellular cAMP were tested by either five-minute pretreatment with forskolin (Fo, 5–10 μM) or a mixture of dibutyryl cAMP (dBcAMP, 20–100 μM) and 3-iso-butyl-1-methyl-xanthine (IBMX, 20–100 μM) before BK or heat. Fo, dBcAMP, and IBMX were obtained from Sigma.

MECHANISMS OF PGE_2-INDUCED AUGMENTATION OF BRADYKININ RESPONSES

EFFECTS OF EP RECEPTOR AGONISTS AND ANTAGONIST

M&B28767, an EP_3 receptor agonist, cumulatively applied during the quasi steady or slowly declining phase of BK-induced discharges, augmented the BK response (Fig. 2A). This enhancement is similar to that previously observed with PGE_2 (Mizumura et al. 1991). At 1 nM, M&B28767 was ineffective in all seven cases; at 3 nM, slight augmentation of the BK responses occurred in two of three cases. Above 10 nM, enhancement was observed in all cases. Fig. 3 shows average net increases, which are calculated as shown in Fig. 2A; the effect was concentration-dependent.

In clarifying that the effect of the EP_3 receptor agonist is not limited to the adapted phase of the BK response, the effects of pretreatment with PGE analogues at a single concentration also were tested as shown in Fig. 2B

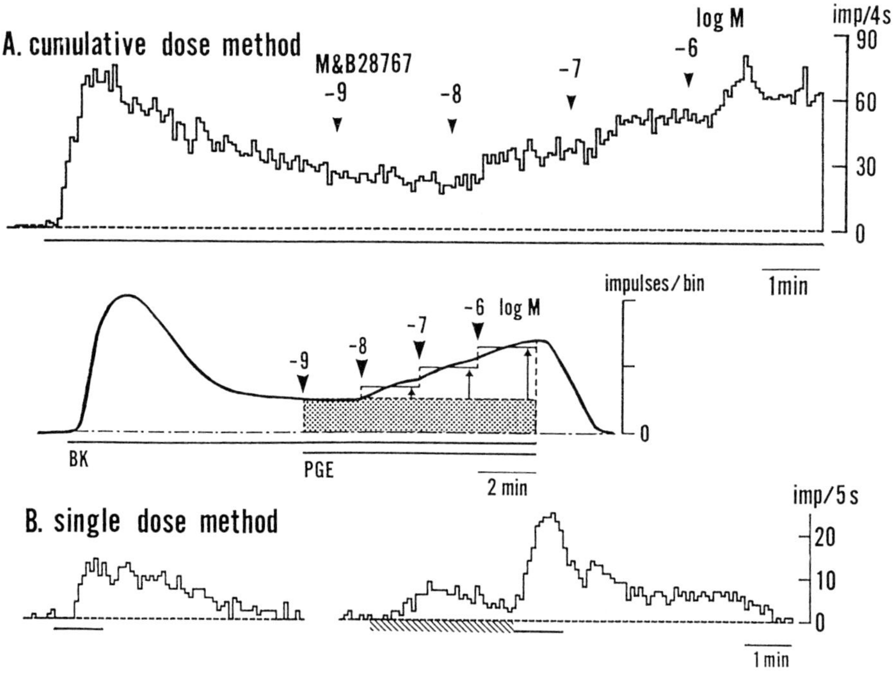

Fig. 2. Examples of enhancement of BK responses induced by the EP_3 receptor agonist (M&B2876). **A:** Cumulative-dose method. The upper trace shows peri-stimulus time histograms of discharges evoked by application of BK (1 μM, horizontal line at the bottom). M&B28767 (1 nM–1 μM) was applied every two minutes during a quasi-steady state of BK-evoked response from low to high concentrations (shown by arrowheads above the trace). Quantitative evaluations are shown schematically in the lower trace. Net increases, as shown by heights of arrows, are expressed as the mean discharge rates during the two-minute application of PGE at effective concentrations, minus the rates of ineffective concentrations (shaded level). **B:** Single-dose method. The response (peri-stimulus time histogram) to BK (1 μM, 1 min, shown by horizontal line at the bottom), following three-minute treatment with M&B28767 (0.1 μM, shown by horizontal hatching) was compared with the control BK response (left).

(single-dose method). Compared with control BK responses, the discharges evoked by BK after treatment with M&B28767 were greater and of longer duration. The total number of BK-evoked impulses after three-minute pretreatment with M&B28767 at 10 nM was significantly greater than control ($P < 0.01$, n = 9).

The effects of butaprost, an EP_2 receptor agonist, on BK responses also were tested by methods similar to those used for M&B28767. Although PGE_2 at 0.1 μM clearly augmented the BK response, butaprost at 0.1–10 μM did not substantially affect it (Fig. 4A). Average net changes in mean discharge rates induced by butaprost in this range of concentrations were negligible. The effects induced by the single-dose method also confirmed this result (Fig. 4B).

PGE_2-induced increases in mean discharge rates of BK responses were compared in the presence and absence of AH6809, an EP_1 receptor antagonist, in the same preparation. The presence of the EP_1 receptor antagonist neither abolished nor substantially suppressed the PGE_2-effect; on the contrary, the PGE_2-effects in the absence of AH6809 were slightly smaller (Fig. 5). These apparently lesser effects are caused by tachyphylaxis, because the effects in the absence of AH6809 were tested in the later period of the experiment.

17-phenyl trinor PGE_2, a relatively selective EP_1 receptor agonist, augmented the BK response, but the necessary concentrations were 100 times greater than those for M&B28767. This enhancement, however, was not suppressed by the EP_1 receptor antagonist AH6809 (10 μM).

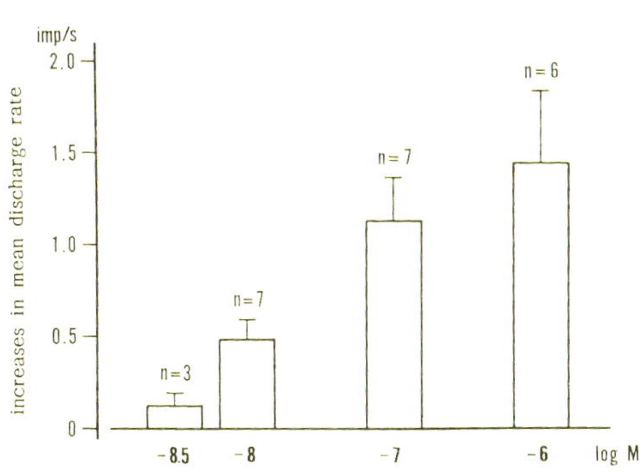

Fig. 3. Average increases in BK responses in the presence of different concentrations of M&B28767 (cumulative-dose method). Ordinate: net increases in mean discharge rates induced by M&B28767 (30 nM–1 μM) compared with those at 1 nM (ineffective concentration). Abscissa: concentration of M&B28767.

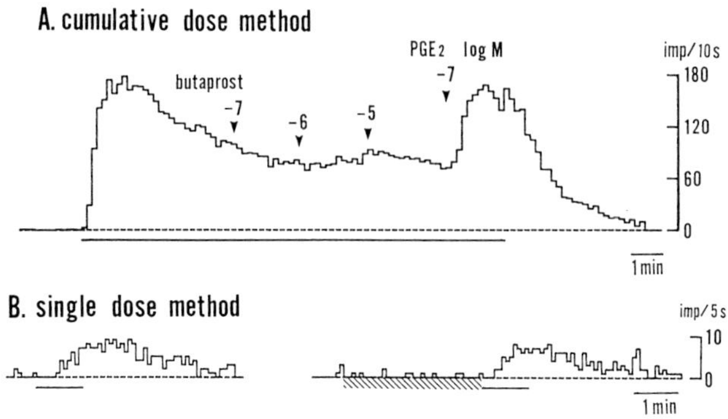

Fig. 4. Effects of the EP_2 receptor agonist (butaprost) on BK responses. Representations are similar to Fig. 2. **A:** Cumulative-dose method. Butaprost (0.1–10 μM) applied every two minutes (shown by arrowheads), did not substantially affect the BK response, although PGE_2 (0.1 μM) augmented the BK response. **B:** Single-dose method. Three-minute pretreatment with butaprost (1 μM, shown by horizontal hatching) did not augment the BK response. Unit of measurement is the same as in Fig. 2B.

These results indicate that the EP_3 receptor is implicated in the PGE_2-induced sensitization of the response to BK.

EFFECTS OF THE ELEVATION OF cAMP

It has been widely thought that the pain-enhancing effects of prostaglandins are mediated by increases in cAMP activity (Ferreira 1981). The results described above are not in accord with this concept because the EP_3 receptor agonist, which causes suppression of cAMP activity (Coleman et al. 1990; Sugimoto et al. 1992), mimics the augmenting effect of PGE_2 on BK responses. The effects of elevations in cAMP on the responses of polymodal receptors to BK (0.1 μM, 1 minute) were investigated by five-minute pretreatment with either Fo (an activator for adenylyl cyclase) or a mixture of dBcAMP (a membrane-permeable analogue of cAMP) and IBMX (an inhibitor of cAMP phosphodiesterase). Because tachyphylaxis is a prominent consequence of initial exposure to BK (Kumazawa et al. 1987b), these substances were tested after ascertaining that responses to BK had stabilized. As shown in Fig. 6, both treatments suppressed the BK responses. Average mean discharge rates evoked by BK were significantly decreased by Fo ($P < 0.005$, n = 8) and by the mixture of dBcAMP and IBMX ($P < 0.025$, n = 13).

These data suggest that a process that lowers intracellular cAMP en-

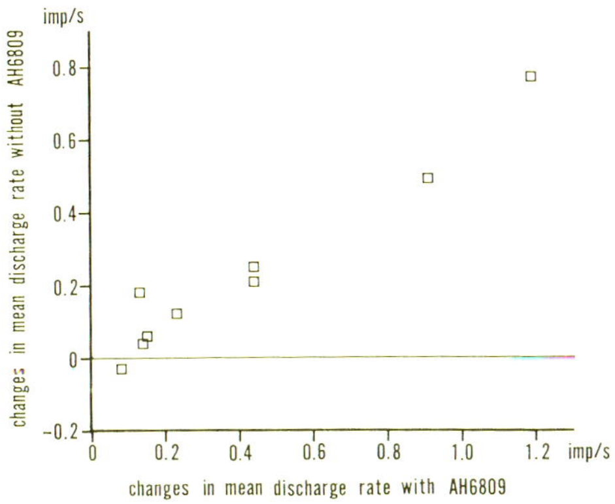

Fig. 5. Effects of the EP$_1$ receptor antagonist (AH6809) on PGE$_2$-induced augmentation of BK responses. Net increases in mean discharge rates induced by each concentration of cumulatively applied PGE$_2$ are plotted in the presence of AH6809 (1 or 10 μM; abscissa) against those in its absence (ordinate). Tested in the same preparation. The presence of the EP$_1$ receptor antagonist did not suppress the PGE$_2$-effect (see text).

hances BK responses, and they further support involvement of the EP$_3$ receptor subtype in sensitization of the response of polymodal receptors to BK.

MECHANISMS OF PGE$_2$-INDUCED AUGMENTATION OF HEAT RESPONSES

EFFECTS OF EP RECEPTOR AGONISTS

PGE$_2$ significantly augmented heat responses at concentrations 100 times greater than required to augment BK responses (Fig. 1). Identification of the EP receptor subtypes implicated in the enhancement of heat responses was performed by using the agonists selective for the three receptor subtypes. As shown in Fig. 7, a three-minute pretreatment with butaprost, at concentrations between 1 nM and 10 μM that did not affect BK responses, concentration-dependently enhanced heat responses of a polymodal receptor unit. Compared with the control heat responses, butaprost in concentrations greater than 10 nM caused significant increases in mean discharge rates ($P < 0.01$, n = 6). Significant increases were observed after pretreatment with M&B28767 and 17-phenyl trinor PGE$_2$, but the necessary concentrations were 1 μM and 10 μM, respectively. The great disparity in the effective concentrations between butaprost and M&B28767 or 17-phenyl trinor PGE_2 suggests that the EP_2 receptor is implicated in the sensitization of heat responses.

EFFECTS OF ELEVATION OF cAMP

Stimulation of the EP_2 receptor subtype is known to increase intracellular cAMP (Coleman et al. 1990); thus, elevation of cAMP levels is expected to augment heat responses. Contrary to BK responses, five-minute pretreatment with Fo or the mixture of dBcAMP and IBMX clearly augmented the heat responses (Fig. 8). Average mean discharge rates evoked by heat stimulation were significantly increased by Fo ($P < 0.01$, n = 9) and by the mixture of dBcAMP and IBMX ($P < 0.005$, n = 13).

DISCUSSION

The subtypes of PGE receptors and the activities of second messengers by these receptors have been shown in various tissues (Coleman et al. 1990).

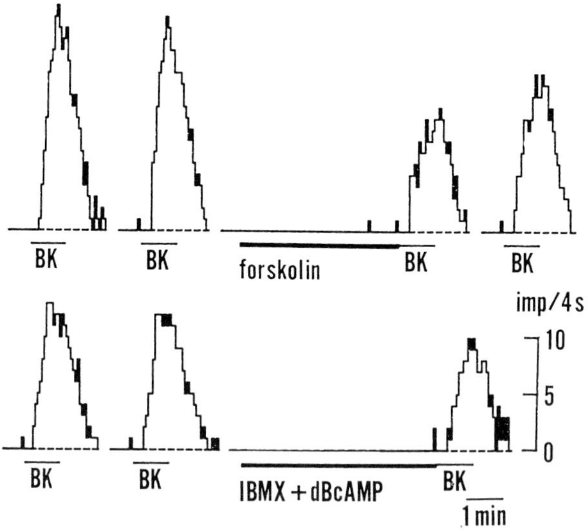

Fig. 6. Increase in adenylyl cyclase activity suppressed BK responses of polymodal receptors. Peri-stimulus time histograms are presented according to the order in which they were recorded. Forskolin (10 μM) or a mixture of a membrane-permeable cAMP (dBcAMP, 20 μM) and an inhibitor of phosphodiesterase (IBMX, 20 μM) was applied during the period marked by the thick horizontal bar. Both treatments suppressed the responses to BK (0.1 μM).

However, no reports have been published to date on the EP receptors and second messengers implicated in PGE-induced sensitization of nociceptor functions. This study, using agonists and an antagonist selective for EP receptor subtypes, revealed that EP_3 and EP_2 receptors are implicated in the PGE_2-induced sensitization of BK and heat responses, respectively, of visceral nociceptors. The validity of this conclusion may be limited, however, because antagonists for the EP_3 and EP_2 receptors are not presently available; moreover, selectivity of the agonists and antagonist for each receptor is not absolute. Nevertheless, our study indicated that among the three receptor agonists, M&B28767, an EP_3 receptor agonist, significantly augmented the BK response, while butaprost, an EP_2 receptor agonist, augmented heat responses. Each substance was effective at concentrations of at least two orders less than those of the other substances. The marked difference in the effective concentrations of the EP receptor agonists appears to support the above conclusion. Furthermore, the experiments using treatments to elevate intracellular cAMP levels strongly support this conclusion.

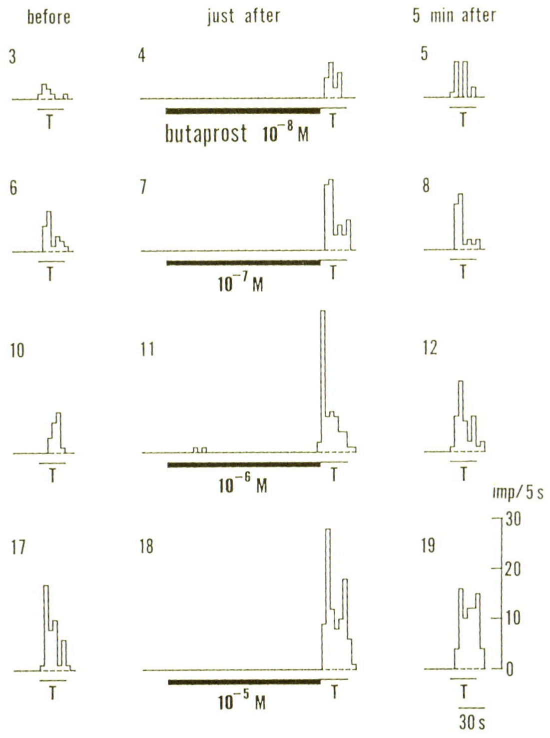

Fig. 7. The EP_2 receptor agonist (butaprost) augmented responses to heat in a concentration-dependent manner. Peri-stimulus time histograms of heat responses of a single unit, repetitively tested at intervals of more than five minutes, are presented according to the order of testing (shown by the number at the left shoulder of each trace). Responses to heat (T, 48°C) following three-minute pretreatment with butaprost (10 nM–10 μM, shown by thick horizontal bars) are compared with those five minutes before and after treatment.

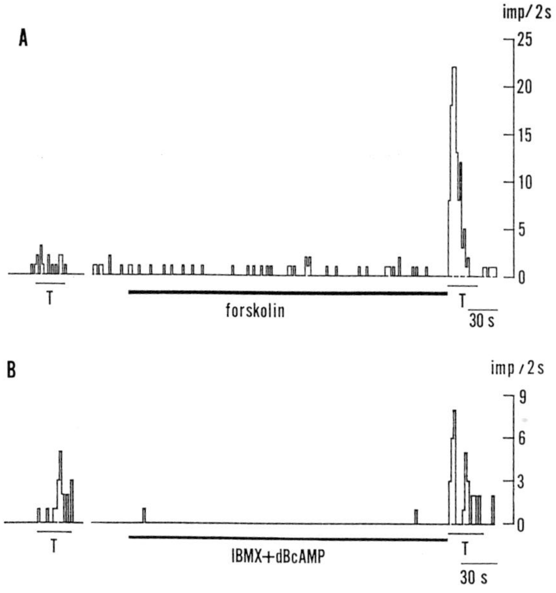

Fig. 8. Increase in adenylyl cyclase activity augmented the heat responses of polymodal receptors. Representations are similar to Fig. 6. T: 48°C; forskolin: 10 μM; dBcAMP: 20 μM; IBMX: 100 μM.

Different subtypes of EP receptors are thought to be associated with different second messenger systems (Coleman et al. 1990). Our study revealed that elevation of cAMP, either by Fo or a mixture of dBcAMP and IBMX, augmented heat responses (Mizumura et al. 1993). In contrast, the same treatment suppressed BK responses. These results are in accord with those obtained using the EP_2 and EP_3 receptor agonist, the activation of which gives rise to increases and decreases in cAMP, respectively (Table I).

Increases in cAMP levels by PGs are widely known (Wellmann and Schwabe 1973) and it long has been thought that the pain-enhancing effects of PGs are mediated by increases of cAMP activity (Ferreira 1981). It was thus unexpected that our study found that two different types of EP receptors that induce opposite changes in cAMP were involved in the PGE_2-induced sensitization of the polymodal receptor. It is especially noteworthy that the EP_3 receptor would be implicated in the sensitization of primary nociceptive neurons. Sugimoto et al. (1992) have succeeded for the first time in isolating a cDNA clone for the EP_3 subtype of PGE receptor from mouse kidneys. They also have reported that forskolin-induced cAMP accumulation is inhibited by

PGE_2 as well as by M&B28767 in the cells in which the cDNA of the EP_3 receptor was transfected.

Ashby (1988) has reported that stimulatory and inhibitory receptors for PGE-induced activation of adenylyl cyclase exist in platelets and that PGE binds to the inhibitory receptor at lower concentrations than to the stimulatory receptor. The difference in effective concentrations for PGE-binding to the stimulatory and inhibitory receptors in platelets is phenomenologically similar to those observed in the PGE_2-induced sensitization of the heat and BK responses of polymodal receptors. Mechanisms of the cAMP-dependent processes involved in these phenomena remain to be clarified.

ACKNOWLEDGMENTS

The authors are grateful to Ms. Yoshiko Yamaguchi for producing the graphics and assisting in the preparation for this manuscript. This work was supported in part by Grants-in-Aid for Scientific Research from the Japanese Ministry of Education, Science, and Culture.

REFERENCES

Armstrong, R.A., Matthews, J.S., Jones, R.L. and Wilson, N.H., Characterization of PGE_2 receptors mediating increased vascular permeability in inflammation. In: B. Sameulsson et al. (Eds.), Advances in Prostaglandin, Thromboxane, and Leukotriene Research, Vol. 21. Raven Press, New York, 1990, pp. 375–378.

Ashby, B., Cyclic AMP turnover in response to prostaglandins in intact platelets: evidence for separate stimulatory and inhibitory prostaglandin receptors, Second Messengers Phosphoproteins, 12 (1988) 45–57.

Bessou, P. and Perl, E.R., Response of cutaneous sensory units with unmyelinated (C) fibers to noxious stimuli, J. Neurophysiol., 32 (1969) 1025–1043.

Coleman, R.A., Kennedy, I. and Sheldrick, R.L.G., AH6809, a prostanoid EP_1 receptor blocking drug, Br. J. Pharmacol., 85 (1985) 273P.

Coleman, R.A., Kennedy, I., Humphrey, P.P.A., Bunce, K. and Lumley, P., Prostanoids and their receptors. In: J.C. Emmett (Ed.), Membranes and Receptors. Comprehensive Medicinal Chemistry, Vol. 3. Pergamon Press, Oxford, 1990, pp. 643–714.

Ferreira, S.H., Inflammatory pain, prostaglandin hyperalgesia and the development of peripheral analgesics, Trends Pharmacol. Sci., 2 (1981) 183–186.

Gardiner, P.J., Characterization of prostanoid relaxant/inhibitory receptors (psi) using a highly selective agonist, TR4979, Br. J. Pharmacol., 87 (1986) 45–56.

Grigg, P., Schaible, H.-G. and Schmidt, R.F., Mechanical sensitivity of group III and IV afferents from posterior articular nerve in normal and inflamed cat knee, J. Neurophysiol., 55 (1986) 635–643.

Kumazawa, T. and Mizumura, K., Mechanical and thermal responses of polymodal receptors recorded from the superior spermatic nerve of dogs, J. Physiol. (Lond.), 299 (1980) 233–245.

Kumazawa, T., Mizumura, K. and Koda, H., Involvement of EP_3 subtype of prostoglandin E receptors in PGE_2-induced enhancement of the bradykinin response of nociceptors, Brain Res.,

632 (1993) 321–324.
Kumazawa, T., Mizumura, K. and Sato, J., Modulations of testicular polymodal receptor activity: implication of receptors in inflammatory pain. In: R.F. Schmidt, H.-G. Schaible and C. Vahle-Hinz (Eds.), Fine Afferent Nerve Fibers and Pain, VCH Verlagsgesellschaft, Weinheim, 1987a, pp. 147–157.
Kumazawa, T., Mizumura, K. and Sato, J., Response properties of polymodal receptors studied using in vitro testis superior spermatic nerve preparations of dogs, J. Neurophysiol., 57 (1987b) 702–711.
Kumazawa, T., Mizumura, K., Minagawa, M., Koda, H., Tujii, Y. and Sato, J., Differences in the response of the polymodal receptor to heat stimulation and to bradykinin. In: R. Inoki, Y. Shigenaga and M. Tohyama (Eds.), Processing and Inhibition of Nociceptive Information, Elsevier, Amsterdam, 1992a, pp. 3–8.
Kumazawa, T., Mizumura, K., Minagawa, M., Narumiya, S. and Namba, T., PGE_2-induced enhancement of bradykinin responses of polymodal receptors is mediated by EP_3 receptors, Soc. Neurosci. Abstr., 18 (1992b) 200.
Mizumura, K., Sato, J. and Kumazawa, T., Effects of prostaglandins and other putative chemical intermediaries on the activity of canine testicular polymodal receptors studied in vitro, Pflugers Arch., 408 (1987) 565–572.
Mizumura, K., Sato, J. and Kumazawa, T., Comparison of the effects of prostaglandins E_2 and I_2 on testicular nociceptor activities studied in vitro, Naunyn Schmiedebergs Arch. Pharmacol., 344 (1991) 368–376.
Mizumura, K., Koda, H. and Kumazawa, T., Augmenting effects of cyclic AMP on the heat response of canine testicular polymodal receptors, Neurosci. Lett., 162 (1993) 75–77.
Moncada, S., Ferreira, S.H. and Vane, J.R., Pain and inflammatory mediators. In: J.R. Vane and S.H. Ferreira (Eds.), Inflammation, Handbook of Experimental Pharmacology, Vol. 50., Springer, Berlin, 1978, pp. 588–616.
Ochoa, J. and Torebjork, E., Sensations evoked by intraneural microstimulation of C nociceptor fibres in human skin nerves, J. Physiol. (Lond.), 415 (1989) 583–599.
Sugimoto, Y., Namba, T., Honda, A., Hayashi, Y., Negishi, M., Ichikawa, A. and Narumiya, S., Cloning and expression of a cDNA for mouse prostaglandin E receptor EP_3 subtype, J. Biol. Chem., 267 (1992) 6463–6466.
Wellmann, W. and Schwabe, U., Effects of prostaglandins E_1, E_2, and F_{2a} on cyclic AMP levels in brain in vivo, Brain Res., 59 (1973) 371–378.

Correspondence to: Dr. Takao Kumazawa, Department of Neural Regulation, Research Institute of Environmental Medicine, Nagoya University, Nagoya 464-01 Japan. Tel: 81-52-789-3861; Fax: 81-52-789-3889; E-mail: e43466a@nucc.cc.nagoya-u.ac.jp

Proceedings of the 7th World Congress on Pain,
Progress in Pain Research and Management, Vol. 2,
edited by G.F. Gebhart, D.L. Hammond, and T.S.
Jensen, IASP Press, Seattle, © 1994.

19

Nociceptor Dynamics in Humans

Erik Torebjörk

Department of Clinical Neurophysiology,
University Hospital, Uppsala, Sweden

INTRODUCTION

This chapter provides a short description of the receptive properties of human nociceptors, based on results obtained through microneurography. The work was done on cutaneous nociceptors, particularly C nociceptors. I describe novel classes of human nociceptors, including C units that are insensitive even to strong mechanical and heat stimuli in normal skin but are excited by chemical agents and become sensitive to mechanical and/or heat stimuli after chemical irritation. Recent observations indicate that the receptive fields of mechanoresponsive C nociceptors are complex, with normally insensitive branches that can be sensitized by chemical irritation and then acquire sensitivity to mechanical stimuli. Thus, human nociceptors are heterogenous and complex, and their receptive properties may change considerably following tissue injury and inflammation. Such peripheral sensitization of nociceptors probably contributes to primary hyperalgesia to heat and to pressure following chemical injury. In addition, the temporal and spatial summation of nociceptor impulses after such injury will affect the signal processing in the central nervous system and lead to various forms of secondary hyperalgesia.

METHODS

Microneurography involves microelectrode recordings of impulses from single myelinated or unmyelinated fibers in peripheral nerves in awake humans (Vallbo and Hagbarth 1968). It allows researchers to obtain information on the physiological response properties of different types of human nociceptive and non-nociceptive nerve endings. Because subjects can report what they feel when their peripheral nerve fibers are stimulated by natural or electrical stimuli, various types of psychophysical studies also can be performed in the same experimental sessions. The experiments reported here were approved by the local ethics committees and were performed after obtaining informed consent from the subjects.

RESULTS AND DISCUSSION

A-DELTA NOCICEPTORS

It is notoriously difficult to record from A-delta fibers in microneurography experiments. A possible explanation is that the electrode tip must be close to a node of Ranvier to detect the signals, and the statistical likelihood of this is fairly low. However, one type of A-delta nociceptor found in both glabrous (Torebjörk 1985, Torebjörk and Ochoa, unpublished data) and hairy skin (Adriaensen et al. 1983) responds to high-intensity mechanical stimuli. Another type, found only in hairy skin, is activated by mechanical, heat, and/or chemical stimuli (Adriaensen et al. 1983). Their response properties are reminiscent of those of type I and II A-delta nociceptors in monkey skin (Meyer et al. 1985). Human A-delta nociceptors, like those in the monkey (Meyer and Campbell 1981), are sensitized by repeatedly heating the skin to noxious (50°C) temperatures; the lowering of their heat thresholds following such treatment correlates with primary heat hyperalgesia at the site of the lesion, as reported by subjects in experiments by Gotoh et al. (1993).

C POLYMODAL OR C MECHANO-HEAT NOCICEPTORS

Most work in humans has focused on cutaneous C-fiber nociceptors. Initially, C polymodal nociceptors responsive to mechanical, heat, and chemical stimuli were recognized (Torebjörk and Hallin 1970; van Hees and Gybels 1972; Torebjörk 1974). These receptors have also been termed C mechano-heat nociceptors (CMH units; LaMotte et al. 1982). Their receptive properties are similar to those of C polymodal nociceptors in the cat (Bessou and Perl 1969) and the monkey (Beitel and Dubner 1976; Kumazawa and Perl 1977; LaMotte et al. 1984). Combined psychophysical and neurophysiological experiments in humans indicate that these nociceptors can provide a peripheral neuronal basis for determination of heat pain threshold, at least in hairy skin (van Hees and Gybels 1981; LaMotte et al. 1982). Furthermore, a nearly linear relation found between the mean suprathreshold response functions in a population of CMH nociceptors and the median ratings of pain suggests that these nociceptors can provide an essential code for magnitude judgments of heat pain (Torebjörk et al. 1984). This is supported by the finding that CMH nociceptors are activated by small increments of 0.1–0.5°C on a base temperature of 48°C, which is matched by the human capacity to detect such increments as increasingly painful (Robinson et al. 1983).

A typical feature of CMH nociceptors is their sensitization after heat injury to their receptive fields. The lowering of thresholds to heat stimuli and the enhanced responses to suprathreshold stimuli correlate with enhanced subjective pain ratings to the same stimuli, indicating that not only A-delta but also CMH nociceptors contribute to primary hyperalgesia to heat in hairy skin (LaMotte et al. 1982, Torebjörk et al. 1984). The situation seems to be different in the glabrous skin of the hand. Neurophysiological studies in monkey have shown that only sensitization of A-delta nociceptors matches the heat hyperalgesia following a burn lesion, whereas CMH nociceptors are desensitized (Meyer and Campbell 1981).

NOVEL CLASSES OF HUMAN C NOCICEPTORS

It has long been recognized that there exist in monkey skin a rich diversity of C nociceptors that respond differentially to mechanical, mechanothermal, or thermal stimuli (Georgopolous 1976). Monkey skin also has very high threshold or insensitive cutaneous nociceptors that may be activated by chemical irritation (Meyer et al. 1991; Davis et al. 1993). Such insensitive nociceptors have also been found in the skin of the rat (Handwerker et al. 1991; Kress et al. 1992), and in the knee joint (Schaible and Schmidt 1985) and the urinary bladder of the cat (Häbler et al. 1988).

To identify these nociceptors in human skin, Handwerker and I and our collaborators have used an electrical transcutaneous search technique to find the innervation territory for C-fibers from which we could record. Steel needles were then inserted 5–10 mm apart within that territory, and the C-fiber responses to regular electrical intracutaneous stimulation every 4 seconds were continuously monitored throughout the ensuing experiment. At such a low stimulation frequency, the C-fiber latencies are fairly constant, but any extra impulse evoked by an additional mechanical, thermal, chemical, or electrical stimulus applied to the skin can be detected as a transient slowing of conduction velocity of the activated unit during the relative refractory period (Torebjörk and Hallin 1974; Torebjörk 1974). Extra impulses elicited in association with sympathetic reflex discharges are detected in the same way (Hallin and

Torebjörk 1974). This technique has proven to be very sensitive and useful to differentiate afferent and sympathetic C-fibers and to classify different types of afferent C units (Torebjörk and Hallin 1976).

We have recently detected several classes of human cutaneous C nociceptors that were not previously described (Schmidt et al. 1994). Apart from the common CMH nociceptor, we found C nociceptors that respond only to mechanical stimuli (CM), others that respond to heat only (CH), and some that are insensitive even to strong mechanical (> 750 mN) and heat (> 50°C) stimuli. The latter are termed CM_iH_i, as suggested by Handwerker and Kobal (1993). In a sample of 76 C units in hairy skin on the foot and lower leg within the innervation territory of the peroneal nerve, we found 45% CMH, 13% CM, 6% CH, 24% CM_iH_i and 12% sympathetic units.

Topical application of mustard oil (100% solution of allyl-iso-thiocyanate) for 5 minutes and/or capsaicin (1% dissolved in ethanol) for 30 minutes excited about 60% of CMH units and about one-third of CM and CM_iH_i units. After this treatment, some CM, CH, and CM_iH_i nociceptors acquired a new sensitivity to a stimulus modality to which they had previously been insensitive. Furthermore, expansion of the mechanoreceptive field size was detected in some CM and CMH units following chemical irritation (Schmelz et al., unpublished data). This finding is consistent with the observation of Thalhammer and LaMotte (1982), who found expansion of the heat-treated parts of the receptive fields of CMH units in hairy skin in monkeys. Detailed mapping of the innervation territory with transcutaneous electrical stimuli revealed that the mechanoreceptive field expansion after chemical irritation occurred only in those parts innervated by electrosensitive but otherwise insensitive branches within the complex receptive fields (Schmelz et al., unpublished data). We conclude that in human skin there are not only insensitive C nociceptor units that can be sensitized by chemical irritation, but also other types of C nociceptors with "silent branches," which can be sensitized by such treatment.

DYNAMICS OF HUMAN NOCICEPTORS AND CENTRAL SENSITIZATION

The data above indicate that human cutaneous nociceptors are heterogenous and their receptive properties may change considerably following tissue injury and inflammation. The lowering of thresholds, the enhanced responses to supraliminal stimuli, and the acquisition of responsiveness to new stimulus modalities as demonstrated here probably contribute to primary hyperalgesia to heat and to mechanical pressure, as seen experimentally following topical application of mustard oil or capsaicin. The temporal and spatial summation of nociceptor impulses will also change the signal processing at central levels in the nervous system and lead to various forms of secondary hyperalgesia.

In their model with intracutaneous injection of capsaicin, LaMotte et al. (1991) showed that after the initial severe pain has subsided, there was secondary hyperalgesia to gentle stroking for an hour or two in a wide area surrounding the injection site. Recordings from nociceptors innervating that area in monkey (Baumann et al. 1991) and human (LaMotte et al. 1992) have not shown any evidence of peripheral sensitization to tactile stimuli. Experiments with selective nerve blocks instead indicate that the tactile hyperalgesia is detectable only in the presence of intact conduction in large myelinated fibers, and can be mimicked by intraneural electrical stimulation of low-threshold mechanoreceptive afferents that normally signal nonpainful touch (Torebjörk et al. 1992). Indeed, nociceptive neurons in the spinal cord in the monkey display increased excitability to A-fiber input following capsaicin injections (Simone et al. 1991).

One form of sensitization of central cells seems to depend on ongoing activity in nociceptive afferents, and quickly disappears when that input is stopped. The magnitude of touch-evoked hyperalgesia after topical application of mustard oil or capsaicin has a linear relation to the degree of background pain, e.g., the amount of nociceptor barrage (Koltzenburg et al. 1992), and the hyperalgesia disappears when the ongoing activity in the sensitized nociceptors is stopped by cooling, as seen in direct microneurographic recordings (LaMotte et al. 1992). The linear relation between background pain and touch-evoked hyperalgesia has been observed also in patients with various forms of neuralgia, regardless of whether or not the pain condition is sympathetically maintained (Koltzenburg et al. 1994). Thus, this particular form of touch-evoked secondary hyperalgesia appears to represent a physiological response of the central nervous system and to be a consequence of an ongoing nociceptor barrage, regardless of its underlying pathophysiological cause (Torebjörk 1992). This nociceptive input need not be very strong; the phenomenon of transient touch-evoked hyperalgesia can be demonstrated after slowly heating the skin without causing detectable pain (Cervero et al. 1993).

It should be emphasized that another form of secondary hyperalgesia to punctate stimuli with von Frey filaments has a much longer time course after capsaicin injection (LaMotte et al. 1991). It probably also represents an example of central sensitization, which is triggered by nociceptor activation but can be maintained for some time in the absence of such input (Kilo et al. 1994).

In their theory to explain the mechanisms of secondary hyperalgesia, LaMotte et al. (1991) postulated the existence in human of chemonociceptors, some of which would have wide branches in the skin, and which were thought to be particularly powerful in their actions to produce central sensitization. Our finding that there are insensitive C units in human skin that are activated and sensitized by chemical irritants is of some interest in this context. We have also seen large and complex receptive fields with mechanoresponsive and silent branches of CM nociceptors on the dorsum of the human foot, extending over skin areas of up to 4.5 cm diameter (Schmelz et al., unpublished data). To what extent such units represent the missing nociceptors in LaMotte's theory remains to be established.

ACKNOWLEDGMENT

Supported by the Swedish Medical Research Council, Grant no 5206.

REFERENCES

Adriaensen, H., Gybels, J., Handwerker, H.O. and van Hees, J., Response properties of thin myelinated (A-delta) fibers in human skin nerves, J. Neurophysiol., 49 (1983) 111–122.

Baumann, T.K., Simone, D.A., Shain, C.N. and LaMotte, R.H., Neurogenic hyperalgesia: the search for the primary cutaneous afferent fibers that contribute to capsaicin-induced pain and hyperalgesia, J. Neurophysiol., 66 (1991) 212–227.

Beitel, R.E. and Dubner, R. , Response of unmyelinated (C) polymodal nociceptors to thermal stimuli applied to monkey's face, J. Neurophysiol. 39 (1976) 1160–1175.

Bessou, P. and Perl, E.R., Responses of cutaneous sensory units with unmyelinated fibers to noxious stimuli, J. Neurophysiol., 32 (1969) 1025–1043.

Cervero, F., Gilbert, R., Hammond, R.G.E. and Tanner, J., Development of secondary hyperalgesia following non-painful thermal stimulation of the skin: a psychophysical study in man, Pain, 54 (1993) 181–189.

Davis, K.D., Meyer, R.A. and Campbell, J.N., Chemosensitivity and sensitization of nociceptive afferents that innervate the hairy skin of monkey, J. Neurophysiol., 69 (1993) 1071–1081.

Georgopoulos, A.P., Functional properties of primary afferent units probably related to pain mechanisms in primate glabrous skin, J.Neurophysiol., 39 (1976) 71–83.

Gotoh, K., Kagosima, Y., Sakurai, K. and Aikawa, S., Marked sensitization of A delta fibers in human skin nerves. In: Abstracts: 7th World Congress on Pain, IASP Publications, Seattle, 1993, p. 24.

Häbler, H.-J., Jänig, W. and Koltzenburg, M., A novel type of unmyelinated chemosensitive nociceptor in the acutely inflamed urinary bladder, Agents Actions, 25 (1988) 219–221.

Handwerker, H.O. and Kobal, G., Psychophysiology of experimentally induced pain, Physiol. Rev., 73 (1993) 639–671.

Handwerker H.O., Kilo, S. and Reeh, P.W., Unresponsive afferent nerve fibres in the sural nerve of the rat, J. Physiol. (Lond)., 435 (1991) 229–242.

Hallin, R.G. and Torebjörk, H.E., Methods to differentiate electrically induced afferent and sympathetic C unit responses in human cutaneous nerves, Acta Physiol. Scand., 92 (1974) 318–331.

Kilo, S., Schmelz, M., Koltzenburg, M. and Handwerker, H.O., Different patterns of hyperalgesia induced by experimental inflammations in human skin, Brain (1994) in press.

Koltzenburg, M., Lundberg, L.E.R. and Torebjörk, H.E., Dynamic and static components of mechanical hyperalgesia in human hairy skin, Pain, 51 (1992) 207–219.

Koltzenburg, M., Torebjörk, H.E, and Wahren, L.K., Nociceptor modulated central sensitization causes mechanical hyperalgesia in acute chemogenic and chronic neuropathic pain, Brain (1994) in press.

Kress, M., Koltzenburg, M., Reeh, P.W. and Handwerker, H.O. Responsiveness and functional attributes of electrically localized terminals of cutaneous C-fibers in vivo and in vitro, J. Neurophysiol., 68 (1992) 581–595.

Kumazawa, T. and Perl, E.R., Primate cutaneous sensory units with unmyelinated (C) afferent fibers, J. Neurophysiol., 40 (1977) 1325–1338.

LaMotte, R.H., Thalhammer, J.G., Torebjörk, H.E. and Robinson, C.J., Peripheral neural mechanisms of cutaneous hyperalgesia following mild injury by heat, J. Neurosci. 2 (1982) 765–781.

LaMotte, R.H., Torebjörk, H.E., Robinson, C.J. and Thalhammer, J.G., Time intensity profiles of cutaneous pain in normal and hyperalgesic skin: a comparison with C-nociceptor activities in monkey and human, J. Neurophysiol., 51 (1984) 1434–1450.

LaMotte, R.H., Shain, C.N., Simone, D.A. and Tsai, E.F., Neurogenic hyperalgesia: psychophysical studies of underlying mechanisms, J. Neurophysiol., 66 (1991) 190–211.

LaMotte, R.H., Lundberg, L.E.R. and Torebjörk. H.E., Pain, hyperalgesia and activity in nociceptive C units in humans after intradermal injection of capsaicin, J. Physiol. (Lond)., 448 (1992) 749–764.

Meyer, R.A. and Campbell, J.N., Myelinated nociceptive afferents account for the hyperalgesia that follows a burn to the hand, Science, 213 (1981) 1527–1529.

Meyer, R.A., Campbell, J.N. and Raja, S.N., Peripheral neural mechanisms of cutaneous hyperalgesia. In: H.L Fields, R.Dubner and F. Cervero (Eds.), Proceedings of the Fourth World Congress on Pain. Advances in Pain Research and Therapy, Vol 9. Raven Press, New York, 1985, pp. 53–71.

Meyer, R.A., Davis, K.D., Cohen, R.H., Treede, R.D. and Campbell, J.N., Mechanically insensitive afferents (MIAs) in cutaneous nerves of monkey, Brain Res., 561 (1991) 252–261.

Robinson, C.J., Torebjörk, H.E. and LaMotte, R.H., Psychophysical detection and pain ratings of incremental thermal stimuli: a comparison with nociceptor responses in humans, Brain Res., 274 (1983) 87–106.

Schaible, H.-G. and Schmidt, R.F., Effects of an experimental arthritis on the sensory properties of fine articular afferent units, J. Neurophysiol., 54 (1985) 1109–1122.

Schmidt, R., Schmelz, M., Forster, C., Ringkamp, M., Torebjörk, H.E. and Handwerker, H.O., Novel classes of responsive and unresponsive C nociceptors in human skin, J. Neurosci. (1994) in press.

Simone, D.A., Sorkin, L.S., Oh, U., Chung, J.M., Owens, C., LaMotte, R.H. and Willis, W.D., Neurogenic hyperalgesia: central neural correlates in responses of spinothalamic tract neurons, J. Neurophysiol., 66 (1991) 228–246.

Thalhammer, J.G. and LaMotte, R.H., Spatial properties of nociceptor sensitization following heat injury of the skin, Brain Res., 231 (1982) 257–265.

Torebjörk, H.E., Afferent C units responding to mechanical, thermal and chemical stimuli in human non-glabrous skin, Acta Physiol. Scand., 92 (1974) 374–390.

Torebjörk, H.E., Nociceptor activation and pain, Philos. Trans. R. Soc. Lond. Biol., 308 (1985) 227–234.

Torebjörk, H.E., Nociceptive and non-nociceptive afferents contributing to pain and hyperalgesia in humans. In: W.D. Willis, Jr. (Ed.), Hyperalgesia and Allodynia, Raven Press, New York, 1992, pp. 135–139.

Torebjörk, H.E. and Hallin, R.G., C-fibre units recorded from human sensory fascicles in situ. Acta

Soc. Med. Ups., 75 (1970) 81–84.

Torebjörk, H.E. and Hallin, R.G., Responses in human A and C fibres to repeated electrical intradermal stimulation, J. Neurol. Neurosurg. Psychiatry, 37 (1974) 653–664.

Torebjörk, H.E. and Hallin, R.G., A new method for classification of C-unit activity in intact human skin nerves. In: J.J. Bonica and D. Albe-Fessard (Eds.), Proceedings of the First World Congress on Pain. Advances in Pain Research and Therapy, Vol 1. Raven Press, New York, 1976, pp. 29–34.

Torebjörk, H.E., LaMotte, R.H. and Robinson, C.J., Peripheral neural correlates of magnitude of cutaneous pain and hyperalgesia: simultaneous recordings in humans of sensory judgments of pain and evoked responses in nociceptors with C-fibers, J. Neurophysiol., 51 (1984) 325–339.

Torebjörk, H.E., Lundberg, L.E.R. and LaMotte, R.H., Central changes in processing of mechanoreceptive input in capsaicin-induced secondary hyperalgesia in humans, J. Physiol. (Lond.), 448 (1992) 765–780.

Vallbo, Å.B. and Hagbarth, K.-E., Activity from skin mechanoreceptors recorded percutaneously in awake human subjects, Exp. Neurol., 21 (1968) 270–289.

van Hees, J. and Gybels, J.M., Pain related to single afferent C fibres from human skin, Brain Res., 48 (1972) 397–400.

van Hees, J. and Gybels, J.M., C nociceptor activity in human nerve during painful and non-painful skin stimulation, J. Neurol. Neurosurg. Psychiatry, 44 (1981) 600–607.

Correspondence to: Erik Torebjörk, MD, PhD, Department of Clinical Neurophysiology, University Hospital, S-751 85 Uppsala, Sweden. Tel: 46-18-663435; Fax: 46-18-556106.

Proceedings of the 7th World Congress on Pain,
Progress in Pain Research and Management, Vol. 2,
edited by G.F. Gebhart, D.L. Hammond, and T.S.
Jensen, IASP Press, Seattle, © 1994.

20

Interaction of Immune-Competent Cells and Nociceptors

Christoph Stein

Department of Anesthesiology and Critical Care Medicine,
Johns Hopkins University, Baltimore, Maryland, USA

INTRODUCTION

Several authors have proposed an interrelation between peripheral sensory nerves and immune cells, based mostly on anatomical findings in inflammatory processes (reviewed in Weihe et al. 1990). Recent neurochemical studies have suggested an interaction of immune-cell derived nerve growth factor with primary afferent neurons innervating inflamed tissue. This interaction apparently results in an upregulation of synthesis, anterograde transport, and release from peripheral terminals of two proinflammatory neuropeptides, substance P and calcitonin gene-related peptide (Donnerer et al. 1992). While these investigations have proposed that such mechanisms sustain pain and inflammation, evidence from more functionally oriented experiments indicates that interactions between the immune system and sensory nerves may well result in the inhibition of pain. Studies concerned with local antinociceptive actions of opioids in peripheral tissues have produced the latter findings.

Peripheral analgesic effects of exogenous opioid agonists are particularly prominent in painful (hyperalgesic) inflammatory conditions (reviewed in Barber and Gottschlich 1992; Stein 1993). Opioid receptors are present on peripheral sensory nerves and are apparently "upregulated" during the development of inflammation. Their endogenous ligands, opioid peptides, are found in resident immune cells within peripheral inflamed tissue. Such opioid peptides mediate local analgesic effects when activated in stressful situations, and suppression of the immune system abolishes these effects (Stein et al. 1990a,b; Przewlocki et al. 1992). These findings have led to our current working hypothesis that endogenous opioid peptides can be secreted from immunocytes, occupy opioid receptors on sensory nerves, and produce analgesia, putatively by inhibiting the excitability of these nerves or by inhibiting the release of excitatory, proinflammatory neuropeptides. This chapter will outline the components of this hypothesis in detail.

PERIPHERAL OPIOID RECEPTORS

Ample biochemical and electrophysiological evidence points to opioid receptors on primary afferent neurons (LaMotte et al. 1976; Fields et al. 1980; Ninkovic et al. 1982). We have demonstrated such receptors immunocytochemically on thinly myelinated and unmyelinated cutaneous nerves, using an anti-idiotypic antibody against mu and delta opioid receptors (Stein et al. 1990b). These findings are in line with functional studies indicating that capsaicin-sensitive, presumably C-fiber neurons mediate the peripheral antinociceptive effect of morphine (Bartho et al. 1990). Following the occupation of neuronal opioid receptors by an opioid agonist, an antinociceptive effect may be brought about by several mechanisms. Firstly, the excitability of the nociceptive input terminal or the propagation of action potentials may be attenuated, possibly via inhibitory G-proteins (Werz and Macdonald 1982; Frank 1985; Russell et al. 1987; Levine and Taiwo 1989; Andreev et al. 1994). Secondly, the release of excitatory compounds (e.g., substance P) from central and/or peripheral endings of primary afferents may be inhibited (Mudge et al. 1979; Yaksh 1988; Yonehara et al. 1992). The latter mechanism also may account for opioid anti-inflammatory actions (Lembeck and Donnerer 1985; Barber and Gottschlich 1992).

Peripheral antinociceptive effects of exogenous opioids are enhanced under inflammatory conditions (for review see Stein 1993). This intriguing phenomenon is yet to be elucidated. It is conceivable that inflammation leads to an increased de novo synthesis and peripherally directed axonal transport of opioid receptors (Young et al. 1980; Laduron 1984). Indeed, using receptor autoradiography with radioactively labeled beta-endorphin (a ligand for mu and delta receptors), we have shown that, within 1–2 days after the induction of peripheral inflammation, the axonal transport of opioid receptors in fibers of the sciatic nerve is greatly enhanced. Saturation and competition experiments indicated that the pharmacological characteristics of these receptors are very similar to those in the brain. Moreover, after 3–4 days, the density of opioid receptors on cutaneous nerve fibers in the inflamed tissue increased profoundly, and this increase was abolished by ligating the sciatic nerve 48 hours beforehand (Hassan et al. 1993). In summary, these findings demonstrate that inflammation enhances the peripherally directed axonal transport of opioid receptors, which leads to an increase in their number ("upregulation") on peripheral nerve terminals.

However, peripheral antinociceptive effects of exogenous opioid agonists have been observed much sooner (within minutes to hours) after the induction of inflammation (Stein 1993; Antonijevic and Stein, unpublished). In contrast to this early occurrence of in vivo antinociceptive effects, the increase in the density of opioid binding sites detected by Hassan et al. (1993) became significant only after three days. Together, these findings suggest that the early antinociceptive actions are not critically dependent upon the number of opioid receptors on cutaneous nerves. Rather, pre-existent, but possibly inactive neuronal opioid receptors may undergo hitherto unidentified changes owing to the specific milieu in inflamed tissue, and thus be rendered active.

The in vitro studies reviewed above have used labels recognizing mu and delta receptors mainly for technical reasons. However, a large body of in vivo data clearly demonstrates that kappa receptors play an equally important role in mediating peripheral opioid antinociception (for review, see Barber and Gottschlich 1992; Stein 1993).

Besides the evidence for opioid receptors on primary afferent neurons, it is important to consider an involvement of sympathetic nerves. Opioid receptors are present on sympathetic postganglionic neurons and can mediate inhibitory effects on vasoconstriction (Illes 1989). Such effects, however, have been ruled out as a mechanism for opioid antinociception (Holland et al. 1987; Stein et al. 1990a). The finding that opioid agonists attenuate bradykinin-induced hyperalgesia and the assumption that such hyperalgesia depends on sympathetic fibers has led to the proposal that opioid receptors on such fibers may contribute to peripheral opioid antinociceptive effects (Taiwo and Levine 1991; but see Koltzenburg et al. 1992).

Studies have found opioid binding sites on immune cells and opioid-mediated modulation of several of their functions (e.g., chemotaxis, superoxide production, mast cell degranulation; Sibinga and Goldstein 1988; Hassan et al. 1993). The significance of such mechanisms for nociception has not been elucidated in detail. There is, however, a body of literature supporting anti-inflammatory actions of opioids (Barber and Gottschlich 1992).

OPIOID PEPTIDES IN CELLS OF THE IMMUNE SYSTEM

Three families of opioid peptides have been well characterized in the central nervous and neuroendocrine systems, each deriving from a distinct gene and precursor protein, namely proopiomelanocortin (POMC), proenkephalin (PENK), and prodynorphin. Appropriate processing yields their respective major representative opioid peptides: beta-endorphin (END), met-enkephalin (ME), and dynorphin (DYN). Each exhibits different affinities for the three opioid receptor types mu, delta, and kappa (Höllt 1986).

The issue whether immune cells are capable of synthesizing opioid peptides, i.e., whether the genes of precursor peptides are expressed and appropriately translated, has been a subject of controversy (Sibinga and Goldstein 1988). Blalock and Smith (1980) were the first to demonstrate POMC-derived peptides in immunocytes. Messenger ribonucleic acid (mRNA) encoding POMC has been found in mouse splenocytes (Westly et al. 1986), lymphocytes (Buzzetti et al. 1989; Smith et al. 1990), and spleen macrophages (Lolait et al. 1986). Lymphocytes and macrophages seem to express POMC mRNA similar to that found in the pituitary and in the hypothalamus, the classical loci for production of POMC-derived peptides (Lolait et al. 1986; Smith et al. 1990). Peripheral blood leukocytes (Buzzetti et al. 1989) and human thymus cells (Lacaze-Masmonteil et al. 1987) appear to contain POMC mRNA molecules about 200 nucleotides shorter than pituitary mRNA, raising doubts about whether this shortened mRNA species is translated into functional POMC protein. PENK mRNA has been demonstrated in normal lymphocytes (Rosen et al. 1989), in activated T-lymphocytes, and in macrophages (Zurawski et al. 1986; Martin et al. 1987). Moreover, this mRNA was highly homologous to rat brain PENK mRNA, abundant and apparently translated, because these cells released immunoreactive ME (Zurawski et al. 1986). Thus, increasing evidence indicates that immune cells produce both POMC- and PENK-derived opioid peptides, but that the specific conditions of stimulation may be crucial (Heijnen et al. 1991; Sacerdote et al. 1991; van Woudenberg et al. 1992; Kilpatrick 1993). Interestingly, in most of these studies, cells were obtained from healthy human subjects or animals and were then stimulated in vitro.

In contrast, we have studied a model which, due to the presence of persistent inflammation (Stein et al. 1988), produces a pathophysiological stimulation of the immune system in vivo. Therefore, it may represent a condition that is closer to the clinical setting than some of the early in vitro studies. We have demonstrated mRNAs encoding POMC and PENK and their respective opioid peptide products END and ME within inflamed tissue. These peptides are found in resident T- and B-lymphocytes as well as monocytes and macrophages (Weihe et al. 1988; Stein et al. 1990b; Przewlocki et al. 1992). Small amounts of DYN also are detectable by immunocytochemistry (Hassan et al. 1992). These findings indicate the presence and synthesis of opioid peptides in different types of inflammatory cells at the site of tissue injury.

RELEASE OF OPIOID PEPTIDES FROM INFLAMMATORY CELLS

The opioid peptides must be released to produce analgesic effects. Although environmental stress is an effective stimulus (Stein et al. 1990a,b; Przewlocki et al. 1992), the exact mechanisms of opioid secretion within inflamed tissue are unknown. Investigations as to whether posttranslational processing in immune cells yields authentic opioid peptides (Lolait et al. 1986; van Woudenberg et al. 1992), and whether such peptides are indeed released, are still scarce (Smith et al. 1986; Zurawski et al. 1986; Heijnen et al. 1991) and were mostly conducted using cells from healthy organisms.

In the pituitary, corticotropin releasing factor (CRF) is a major physiological secretagogue for opioid peptides. Its releasing effects are potentiated by interleukin-1 (IL-1) (Fagarasan et al. 1989), and IL-1 (and other cytokines) can stimulate END release directly (Bernton et al. 1987). Receptors for each of these agents also are present on immune cells (Webster et al. 1990; Dinarello and Thompson 1991). In cultured leukocytes, CRF can stimulate release of END either directly (Smith et al. 1986) or via induction of IL-1, which induces release of END (Kavelaars et al. 1989). Therefore, we hypothesized that CRF and/or cytokines could release opioid peptides from immune cells within inflamed tissue, which then produce antinociception via activation of peripheral opioid receptors. Indeed, the local application of small, systemically inactive doses of CRF, IL-1, and other cytokines produces potent antinociceptive effects in inflamed, but not in noninflamed tissue (Czlonkowski et al. 1993; Schäfer et al. 1994). These effects are reversible by immunosuppression with cyclosporine A, by passive immunization with antibodies against END, and by opioid receptor antagonists. Furthermore, CRF and IL-1 can release END in vitro in immune cell suspensions prepared from lymph nodes (Stein et al. 1994, Schäfer et al. 1994). These findings are consistent with the notion that CRF and cytokines cause secretion of END from immune cells, which subsequently activates opioid receptors on sensory nerves to inhibit nociception.

CLINICAL ANALGESIC EFFECTS OF PERIPHERAL OPIOIDS

The question arises as to whether such peripheral opioid mechanisms are of any significance in the clinical setting. There is a growing body of literature concerning the analgesic efficacy of exogenous opioids outside the central nervous system (Stein 1993). To test opioid actions in the vicinity of peripheral sensory nerve terminals, several controlled studies have examined the intra-articular application of small doses (0.5–6 mg) of morphine during knee surgery (Table I). The effects on postoperative pain were evaluated by various direct (visual analogue scale, numerical rating scale, verbal scales) or indirect parameters (supplemental analgesic consumption, time to first supplemental analgesic requirement).

With the exception of one trial (Raja et al. 1992), all have reported significant analgesic effects demonstrated by at least one of the above measures. These effects were shown to be opioid receptor–specific (Stein et al. 1991), of similar potency to those of conventional local anesthetics, and surprisingly long lasting (up to 48 hours after injection) (Khoury et al. 1992; Joshi et al. 1993b). In addition, one recent study has shown a significantly shortened time to resume normal activities in outpatients receiving 0.5 mg morphine into the mesosalpinx during ligation of the fallopian tubes (Snyder et al. 1993).

None of these papers reported untoward side effects. To confirm a peripheral site of action, equal doses of morphine were administered systemically as a control (Stein et al. 1991) or plasma levels of morphine were measured (Joshi et al. 1992). These levels were much lower than those generally accepted as necessary for central analgesic actions. The reasons for the long duration of these peripheral opioid actions may include a low blood flow to the knee joint, morphine's low lipid solubility and its consequent slow absorption into the circulation, opioid anti-inflammatory actions and/or preemption of central sensitization (Barber and Gottschlich 1992; Woolf and Chong 1993; McQuay, this volume). One trial (Raja et al. 1992) may have failed to detect any effects for several reasons. First, in most studies, the maximum analgesic action of intra-articular morphine occurred between three and eight hours after injection (Table I), a time when half of the subjects in that trial had been discharged from the hospital. Second, these patients had surgery under epidural anesthesia, which may sufficiently block nociceptive inputs to prevent the development of central sensitization and thus result in a generally lower intensity of postoperative pain (Coderre et al. 1993; Woolf and Chong 1993). This may have precluded the detection of any additional analgesic actions, consistent with the finding that intraarticular bupivacaine also had no effect (Raja et al. 1992).

OPIOID PEPTIDES IN HUMAN INFLAMED TISSUE

Findings that intra-articular naloxone antagonizes the effect of locally applied morphine (Stein et al. 1991) and anecdotal evidence for opioid binding in human synovial tissue (Lawrence et al. 1992) indicate that intra-articular opioid receptors are present and capable of mediating analgesia in human

Table I

Clinical studies of the effects of intra-articular morphine on postoperative pain in patients undergoing knee surgery

Pain Assessment Scale	Effect Demonstrated by	Dose (mg)	Peak Effect (hours)	Comments	Authors
VAS, NRS, MPQ, SAC	all	0.5–1	3–6	naloxone reversible central effects excluded	Stein et al. 1991
VAS, SAC	all	1	4–48		Khoury et al. 1992
VAS, TFA, SAC	TFA	6		with epinephrine	Heard et al. 1992
VAS, TFA, SAC	none	3		with epinephrine	Raja et al. 1992
VAS, TFA, SAC	all	5	0–12	plasma levels < 10 ng/ml tourniquet	Joshi et al. 1992
VAS, TFA, SAC	all	5	2–24	drainage, tourniquet	Joshi et al. 1993a
VAS, TFA	all	5	1–24	tourniquet	Joshi et al. 1993b
VAS, NRS, SAC	all	1–2	6–24	with epinephrine	Allen et al. 1993
VAS, SAC	all	5	2–24	tourniquet	McSwiney et al. 1993
VAS, SAC	all	1	8–24		Dalsgaard et al. 1994

Note: VAS, visual analogue scale; NRS, numerical rating scale; MPQ, McGill Pain Questionnaire; SAC, supplemental analgesic comsumption; TFA, time to first analgesic use.

beings. These findings raise the question about the identity and location of the endogenous ligands of such receptors. We used immunochemistry to detect and localize opioid peptides in the synovial tissue from patients who had arthroscopic knee surgery. These patients had acute traumata (several days old) or chronic articular lesions (degenerative arthritis, genetic patellar instability).

We found opioid peptides in all patients studied, regardless of the duration and cause of the articular lesions. Importantly, all synovial tissue samples displayed inflammation, as indicated by leukocytic infiltration. The opioid peptides were localized in synovial lining cells and in immune cells such as lymphocytes, macrophages, and mast cells. The prevailing peptides were END and ME, while only minor amounts of DYN were detected (Stein et al. 1993). These findings are consistent with the animal studies reviewed above and with a recent anecdotal report on the release of opioid peptides from human synovial tissue in vitro (Yoshino et al. 1992).

LOCAL ANALGESIC EFFECT OF ENDOGENOUS OPIOID PEPTIDES IN THE CLINICAL SETTING

Analogous to our previous work in animals (see above), the question arises as to whether the opioids found in synovial tissue are capable of producing a clinically appreciable, local inhibition of pain in a stressful (e.g., postoperative) situation. Therefore, we tested whether blocking of intraarticular opioid receptors by the local administration of the opioid receptor antagonist naloxone would cause increased postoperative pain in patients undergoing arthroscopic knee surgery. To rule out central effects following a potential systemic absorption, the same dose of naloxone was applied intravenously in a control group.

Indeed, postoperative pain was significantly exacerbated in patients receiving naloxone intra-articularly. This pain-enhancing effect was demonstrated by three different subjective measures—the visual analogue scale, a numerical rating scale, and the McGill pain questionnaire—as well as by increased supplemental analgesic requirements (Stein et al. 1993). Taken together, these findings indicate that blocking intraarticular opioid receptors by naloxone prevents their activation by opioid peptides derived from inflamed synovial tissue, and thus exacerbates clinical pain.

CONCLUSIONS

In summary, many experimental and several controlled clinical trials have now demonstrated the analgesic efficacy of small, systemically inactive doses of exogenous opioids administered in the vicinity of peripheral nerve terminals. In addition, endogenous opioid peptides have been detected in inflamed tissue of animals and humans. These peptides are found in cells of the immune system. The opioids apparently activate opioid receptors located on peripheral sensory nerves (nociceptors), thus mediating endogenous inhibition of pain.

These findings have several interesting implications: (1) The local application not only of exogenous opioids but also of enzyme inhibitors preventing the degradation of endogenous opioid peptides (Roques et al. 1993) may provide a new perspective for pain management by producing analgesia without central side effects such as dysphoria, respiratory depression, sedation, nausea, or addiction. (2) In addition to their immunological functions, immunocytes are involved in intrinsic mechanisms of pain inhibition. This finding provides new insights into pain associated with a compromised immune system, such as in the acquired immunodeficiency syndrome or in cancer (O'Neill and Sherrard 1993; Singer et al. 1993). Furthermore, the activation of opioid production and release from immune cells may be a novel approach to the development of peripherally acting analgesics. (3) Finally, these findings fundamentally expand the gate control theory of pain (Melzack and Wall 1965), in that a peripheral gate apparently exists in addition to the well-known central mechanisms of intrinsic pain inhibition.

ACKNOWLEDGMENTS

The author gratefully acknowledges the support and contributions of his colleagues at the Department of Anesthesiology, Ludwig-Maximilians Universität München; the Department of Neuropharmacology, Max-Planck-Institut für Psychiatrie, Martinsried, Germany; the Department of Anesthesiology and Critical Care Medicine, Johns Hopkins University; and the Preclinical Pharmacology Branch, NIH/NIDA, Baltimore, Maryland, USA. All studies were conducted in compliance with the guidelines proposed by the IASP Committee for Research and Ethical Issues (1983) and were approved by the appropriate institutional review boards. Supported by NIH/NINDS grant RO1 NS 32466.

REFERENCES

Allen, G.C., Amand, M.A.S., Lui, A.C.P., Johnson, D.H. and Lindsay, M.P., Postarthroscopy analgesia with intra-articular bupivacaine/morphine: a randomized clinical trial, Anesthesiology, 79 (1993) 475–480.

Andreev, N., Urban, L. and Dray, A., Opioids suppress spontaneous activity of polymodal nociceptors in rat paw skin induced by ultraviolet irradiation, Neuroscience (1994), in press.

Barber, A. and Gottschlich, R., Opioid agonists and antagonists: an evaluation of their peripheral actions in inflammation, Medicinal Res. Rev., 12 (1992) 525–562.

Bartho, L., Stein, C. and Herz, A., Involvement of capsaicin-sensitive neurones in hyperalgesia and enhanced opioid antinociception in inflammation, Naunyn Schmiedeberg's Arch. Pharmacol., 342 (1990) 666–670.

Bernton, E.W., Beach, J.E., Holaday, J.W., Smallridge, R.C. and Fein, H.G., Release of multiple hormones by a direct action of interleukin-1 on pituitary cells, Science, 238 (1987) 519–521.

Blalock, J.E. and Smith, E.M., Human leukocyte interferon: structural and biological relatedness to adrenocortical hormone and endorphins, Proc. Natl. Acad. Sci. USA, 77 (1980) 5972–5974.

Buzzetti, R., McLoughlin, L., Lavender, P.M., Clark, A.J.L. and Rees, L.H., Expression of pro-opiomelanocortin gene and quantification of adrenocorticotropic hormone-like immunoreactivity in human normal peripheral mononuclear cells and lymphoid and myeloid malignancies, J. Clin. Invest., 83 (1989) 733–737.

Coderre, T.J., Katz, J., Vaccarino, A.L. and Melzack, R., Contribution of central neuroplasticity to pathological pain: review of clinical and experimental evidence, Pain, 52 (1993) 259–285.

Czlonkowski, A., Stein, C. and Herz, A., Peripheral mechanisms of opioid antinociception in inflammation: involvement of cytokines, Eur. J. Pharmacol., 242 (1993), 229–235.

Dalsgaard, J., Felsby, S., Juelsgaard, P. and Froekjaer, J., Low-dose intra-articular morphine algesia in day-case knee arthroscopy: a randomized, double-blinded, prospective study, Pain, 56 (1994) 151–154,

Dinarello, C.A. and Thompson, R.C., Blocking IL-1: interleukin 1 receptor antagonist in vivo and in vitro, Immunol. Today, 12 (1991) 404–410.

Donnerer, J., Schuligoi, R. and Stein, C., Increased content and transport of substance P and calcitonin gene-related peptide in sensory nerves innervating inflamed tissue: evidence for a regulatory function of nerve growth factor in vivo, Neuroscience, 49 (1992) 693–698.

Fagarasan, M.O., Eskay, R. and Axelrod, J., Interleukin-1 potentiates the secretion of b-endorphin induced by secretagogues in a mouse pituitary cell line (AtT-20), Proc. Natl. Acad. Sci. USA, 86 (1989) 2070–2075.

Fields, H.L., Emson, P.C., Leigh, B.K., Gilbert, R.F.T. and Iversen, L.L., Multiple opiate receptor sites on primary afferent fibres, Nature, 284 (1980) 351–353.

Frank, G.B., Stereospecific opioid receptors on excitable cell membranes, Can. J. Physiol. Pharmacol., 63 (1985) 1023–1032.

Hassan, A.H.S., Przewlocki, R., Herz, A. and Stein, C., Dynorphin, a preferential ligand for kappa-opioid receptors, is present in nerve fibers and immune cells within inflamed tissue of the rat, Neurosci. Lett., 140 (1992) 85–88.

Hassan, A.H.S., Ableitner, A., Stein, C. and Herz, A., Inflammation of the rat paw enhances axonal transport of opioid receptors in the sciatic nerve and increases their density in the inflamed tissue, Neuroscience, 55 (1993) 185–195.

Heard, S.O., Edwards, W.T., Ferrari, D., Hanna, D., Wong, P.D., Liland, A. and Willock, M.W., Analgesic effect of intraarticular bupivacaine or morphine after arthroscopic knee surgery: a randomized, prospective, double-blind study, Anesth. Analg., 74 (1992) 822–826.

Heijnen, C.J., Kavelaars, A. and Ballieux, R.E., b-endorphin: cytokine and neuropeptide, Immunol. Rev., 119 (1991) 41–63.

Holland, R.L., Harkin, N.E., Coleshaw, S.R.K., Jones, D.A., Peck, A.W. and Telekes, A., Dipipanone and nifedipine in cold induced pain; analgesia not due to skin warming, Br. J. Clin. Pharmacol., 24 (1987) 823–826.

Höllt, V., Opioid peptide processing and receptor selectivity, Annu. Rev. Pharmacol. Toxicol., 26 (1986) 59–77.

Illes, P., Modulation of transmitter and hormone release by multiple neuronal opioid receptors, Rev. Physiol. Biochem. Pharmacol., 112(1989) 169–171.

Joshi, G.P., McCarroll, S.M., Cooney, C.M., Blunnie, W.P., O'Brien, T.M. and Lawrence, A.J., Intra-articular morphine for pain relief after knee arthroscopy, J. Bone Joint Surg., 74-B (1992) 749–751.

Joshi, G.P., McCarroll, S.M., Brady, O.H., Hurson, B.J. and Walsh, G., Intra-articular morphine for pain relief after anterior cruciate ligament repair, Br. J. Anaesth., 70 (1993a) 87–88.

Joshi, G.P., McCarroll, S.M., O'Brien, T.M. and Lenane, P., Intraarticular analgesia following knee arthroscopy, Anesth. Analg., 76 (1993b) 333–336.

Kavelaars, A., Ballieux, R.E. and Heijnen, C.J., The role of IL-1 in the corticotropin-releasing factor and arginine-vasopressin-induced secretion of immunoreactive β-endorphin by human peripheral blood mononuclear cells, J. Immunol., 142 (1989) 2338–2342.

Khoury, G.F., Chen, A.C.N., Garland, D.E. and Stein, C., Intraarticular morphine, bupivacaine and morphine/bupivacaine for pain control after knee videoarthroscopy, Anesthesiology, 77 (1992) 263–266.

Kilpatrick, D.L., Opioid peptide expression in peripheral tissues and its functional implications. In: A. Herz (Ed.), Handbook of Experimental Pharmacology, Vol. 104/II, Opioids II, Springer-Verlag, Berlin, 1993, pp. 551–570.

Koltzenburg, M., Kress, M. and Reeh, P.W., The nociceptor sensitization by bradykinin does not depend on sympathetic neurons, Neuroscience, 46 (1992) 465–473.

Lacaze-Masmonteil, T., De Keyzer, Y., Luton, J.P. and Bertagna, X., Characterization of proopiomelanocortin transcripts in human non-pituitary tissues, Proc. Natl. Acad. Sci. USA, 84 (1987) 7261–7265.

Laduron, P., Axonal transport of opiate receptors in capsaicin sensitive neurones, Brain Res., 294 (1984) 157–160.

LaMotte, C., Pert, C.B. and Snyder, S.H., Opiate receptor binding in primate spinal cord: distribution and changes after dorsal root section, Brain Res., 112 (1976) 407–412.

Lawrence, A.J., Joshi, G.P., Michalkiewicz, A., Blunnie, W.P. and Moriarty, D.C., Evidence for analgesia mediated by peripheral opioid receptors in inflamed synovial tissue, Eur. J. Clin. Pharmacol., 43 (1992) 351–355.

Lembeck, F. and Donnerer, J., Opioid control of the function of primary afferent substance P fibres, Eur. J. Pharmacol., 114 (1985)241–246.

Levine, J.D. and Taiwo, Y.O., Involvement of the mu-opiate receptor in peripheral analgesia, Neuroscience, 32 (1989) 571–575.

Lolait, S.J., Clements, J.A., Markwick, A.J., Cheng, C., McNally, M., Smith, I.A. and Funder, J.W., Pro-opiomelanocortin messenger ribonucleic acid and posttranslational processing of beta-endorphin in spleen macrophages, J. Clin. Invest., 77 (1986) 1776–1779.

Martin, J., Prystowsky, M.B. and Angeletti, R.H., Preproenkephalin mRNA in T-cells, macrophages and mast cells, J. Neurosci. Res., 18(1987) 82–87.

McSwiney, M.M., Joshi, G.P., Kenny, P. and McCarroll, S.M, Analgesia following arthroscopic knee surgery. a controlled study of intra-articular morphine, bupivacaine or both combined, Anaesth. Intens. Care, 21 (1993) 201–203.

Melzack, R. and Wall, P.D., Pain mechanisms: a new theory, Science, 150 (1965) 971–973.

Mudge, A.W., Leeman, S.E. and Fischbach G.D., Enkephalin inhibits release of substance P from sensory neurons in culture and decreases action potential duration, Proc. Natl. Acad. Sci. USA, 76 (1979) 526–530.

Ninkovic, M., Hunt, S.P. and Gleave, J.R.W., Localization of opiate and histamine H1-receptors in the primary sensory ganglia and spinal cord, Brain Res., 241 (1982) 197–206.

O'Neill, W.M. and Sherrard J.S., Pain in human immunodeficiency virus disease: a review, Pain, 54 (1993) 3–14.
Przewlocki, R., Hassan, A.H.S., Lason, W., Epplen, C., Herz, A. and Stein, C., Gene expression and localization of opioid peptides in immune cells of inflamed tissue: functional role in antinociception, Neuroscience, 48 (1992) 491–500.
Raja, S.N., Dickstein, R.E. and Johnson, C.A., Comparison of postoperative analgesic effects of intraarticular bupivacaine and morphine following arthroscopic knee surgery, Anesthesiology, 77 (1992) 1143–1147.
Roques, B.P., Beaumont, A., Dauge, V. and Fournie-Zaluski, M.-C., Peptidase inactivation of enkephalins: design of inhibitors and biochemical, pharmacological and clinical applications. In: A. Herz (Ed.), Handbook of Experimental Pharmacology, Vol. 104/I, Opioids I, Springer-Verlag, Berlin, 1993, pp. 547–584.
Rosen, H., Behar, O., Abramsky, O. and Ovadia, H., Regulated expression of proenkephalin A in normal lymphocytes, J. Immunol., 143 (1989) 3703–3707.
Russell, N.J.W., Schaible, H.G. and Schmidt, R.F., Opiates inhibit the discharges of fine afferent units from inflamed knee joint of the cat, Neurosci. Lett., 76 (1987) 107–112.
Sacerdote, P., Rubboli, F., Locatelli, L., Ciciliato, I., Mantegazza, P. and Panerai, A.E., Pharmacological modulation of neuropeptides in peripheral mononuclear cells, J. Neuroimmunol., 32 (1991) 35–41.
Schäfer, M., Carter, L. and Stein, C., Interleukin-1ß and corticotropin-releasing-factor inhibit pain by releasing opioids from immune cells in inflamed tissue, Proc. Natl. Acad. Sci. USA, 91 (1994) in press.
Sibinga, N.E.S. and Goldstein, A., Opioid peptides and opioid receptors in cells of the immune system, Annu. Rev. Immunol., 6 (1988) 219–249.
Singer, E.J., Zorilla, C., Fahy-Chandon, B., Chi, S., Syndulko, K. and Tourtellotte, W.W., Painful symptoms reported by ambulatory HIV-infected men in a longitudinal study, Pain, 54 (1993) 15–19.
Smith, E.M. and Blalock, J.E., Human lymphocyte production of corticotropin and endorphin-like substances: association with leukocyte interferon, Proc. Natl. Acad. Sci. USA, 78 (1981) 7530–7534.
Smith, E.M., Morril, A.C., Meyer, W.J. and Blalock, J.E., Corticotropin releasing factor induction of leukocyte-derived immunoreactive ACTH and endorphins, Nature, 321 (1986) 881–882.
Smith, E.M., Galin, F.S., Le Boeuf R.D., Coppenhaver, D.H., Harbour D.V. and Blalock, J.E., Nucleotide and amino acid sequence of lymphocyte-derived corticotropin: endotoxin induction of a truncated peptide, Proc. Natl. Acad. Sci. USA, 87 (1990) 1057–1060.
Snyder, D., Dorin, A., van Amerongen, D., Pasternak, R. and Stein, C., Low-dose morphine injected into the mesosalpinx may provide analgesia for outpatient laparoscopic tubal occlusion, Anesthesiology, 79 (1993) A27.
Stein, C., Peripheral mechanisms of opioid analgesia, Anesth. Analg., 76 (1993) 182–191.
Stein, C., Millan, M.J. and Herz, A., Unilateral inflammation of the hindpaw in rats as a model of prolonged noxious stimulation: alterations in behavior and nociceptive thresholds, Pharmacol. Biochem. Behav., 31 (1988) 445–451.
Stein, C., Gramsch, C. and Herz, A., Intrinsic mechanisms of antinociception in inflammation. Local opioid receptors and b-endorphin, J. Neurosci., 10 (1990a) 1292–1298.
Stein, C., Hassan, A.H.S., Przewlocki, R., Gramsch, C., Peter, K. and Herz, A., Opioids from immunocytes interact with receptors on sensory nerves to inhibit nociception in inflammation, Proc. Natl. Acad. Sci. USA, 87 (1990b) 5935–5939.
Stein, C., Comisel, K., Haimerl, E., Lehrberger, K., Yassouridis, A.,Herz, A. and Peter, K., Analgesic effect of intraarticular morphine after arthroscopic knee surgery, N. Engl. J. Med., 325 (1991) 1123–1126. Comment in: N. Engl. J. Med. 325 (1991) 1168–1169.
Stein, C., Hassan, A.H.S., Lehrberger, K., Giefing, J. and Yassouridis, A., Local analgesic effect of endogenous opioid peptides, Lancet, 342 (1993) 321-324. Comment in: Lancet, 342 (1993) 320.

Stein, C., Schäfer, M., Carter, L., Czlonkowski, A., Mousa, S. and Epplen, C., Cytokine-induced antinociception mediated by opioids released from immune cells, Regul. Pept., 50 (1994) S191–S192.

Taiwo, Y.O. and Levine, J.D., Kappa- and delta-opioids block sympathetically dependent hyperalgesia, J. Neurosci., 11 (1991) 928–932.

van Woudenberg, A.D., Hol, E.M. and Wiegant, V.M., Endorphin-like immunoreactivities in uncultured and cultured human peripheral blood mononuclear cells, Life Sci., 50 (1992) 705–714.

Webster, E.L, Tracey, D.E., Jutila, M.A., Wolfe, S.A. and De Souza, E.B., Corticotropin-releasing factor receptors in mouse spleen: identification of receptor-bearing cells as resident macrophages, Endocrinology, 127 (1990) 440–452.

Weihe, E., Nohr, D., Millan, M.J., Stein, C., Müller, S., Gramsch, C. and Herz, A., Peptide neuroanatomy of adjuvant-induced arthritic inflammation in rat, Agents Actions, 25 (1988) 255–259.

Weihe, E., Büchler, M., Müller, S., Friess, H., Zentel, H.J. and Yanaihara, N., Peptidergic innervation in chronic pancreatitis. In: Beger, Büchler, Ditschuneit and Malfertheiner (Eds.), Chronic Pancreatitis, Springer-Verlag, Berlin, 1990, pp. 83–105.

Westly, H.J., Kleiss, A.J., Kelley, K.W., Wong, P.K.Y. and Yuen, P.H., Newcastle disease virus-infected splenocytes express the proopiomelanocortin gene, J. Exp. Med., 163 (1986) 1589–1593.

Werz, M.A. and Macdonald, R.L., Heterogeneous sensitivity of cultured dorsal root ganglion neurones to opioid peptides selective for mu- and delta-opiate receptors, Nature, 299 (1982) 730–733.

Woolf, C.J. and Chong, M.-S., Preemptive analgesia: treating postoperative pain by preventing the establishment of central sensitization, Anesth. Analg., 77 (1993) 362–379.

Yaksh, T.L. Substance P release from knee joint afferent terminals: modulation by opioids, Brain Res., 458 (1988) 319–324.

Yonehara, N., Imai, Y., Chen J.-Q., Takiuchi S. and Inoki, R., Influence of opioids on substance P release evoked by antidromic stimulation of primary afferent fibers in the hind instep of rats, Regul. Pept., 38 (1992) 13–22.

Yoshino, S.I., Koiwa, M., Shiga, H., Nakamura, H., Higaki, M. and Miyasaka, N., Detection of opioid peptides in synovial tissues of patients with rheumatoid arthritis (letter), J. Rheumatol., 19 (1992) 660.

Young, III, W.S., Wamsley, J.K., Zarbin, M.A. and Kuhar, M.J., Opioid receptors undergo axonal flow, Science, 210 (1980) 76–77.

Zurawski, G., Benedik, M., Kamp, B.J., Abrams, J.S., Zurawski, S.M. and Lee, F.D., Activation of mouse T-helper cells induces abundant preproenkephalin mRNA synthesis, Science, 232 (1986) 772–775.

Correspondence to: Christoph Stein, MD, Department of Anesthesiology and Critical Care Medicine, Johns Hopkins Hospital, 600 North Wolfe St., Tower 711, Baltimore, Maryland 21287-8711, USA. Tel: 410-955-5608; Fax: 410-955-0994.

Part V

Central Nervous System Plasticity: Implications for Pain Perception

Proceedings of the 7th World Congress on Pain,
Progress in Pain Research and Management, Vol. 2,
edited by G.F. Gebhart, D.L. Hammond, and T.S.
Jensen, IASP Press, Seattle, © 1994.

21

Central Plastic Responses to Pain

William D. Willis, Jr.

Department of Anatomy and Neurosciences and Marine Biomedical Institute, University of Texas Medical Branch, Galveston, Texas, USA

INTRODUCTION

A dramatic example of a plastic change in somatic sensation is mechanical allodynia. Allodynia (Greek *allo* = other; *odyne* = pain) has been defined by the IASP Subcommittee on Taxonomy as "pain due to a stimulus that does not normally provoke pain" (Merskey 1986; Bonica 1990). In mechanical allodynia, tactile stimuli cause pain or tenderness.

Considerable evidence has been marshaled in recent years that favors the labeled line theory of somatic sensation (Willis and Coggeshall 1991). A labeled-line sensory channel consists of a set of neurons that when activated elicit a sensation of a particular modality. For example, recordings can be made by microneurography from individual myelinated or unmyelinated cutaneous afferent fibers in human peripheral nerves. Such fibers can be classified into mechanoreceptors, thermoreceptors, and nociceptors based on their receptive field properties, exactly as in animal experiments (Vallbo et al. 1979). In human subjects it is possible to elicit sensations when the microelectrode stimulates what are thought to be the same afferent fibers (Vallbo et al. 1984; Torebjörk et al. 1987). For example, repetitive stimulation of the axon of a Pacinian corpuscle often elicits a sensation of vibration, whereas stimulation of the axon of a Merkel cell ending causes a sensation of pressure. Increasing the frequency of stimulation of the Pacinian corpuscle afferent causes an increase in the apparent rate of vibration; increasing the frequency of stimulation of the Merkel cell afferent causes an increase in the intensity of the pressure. The tactile sensations never become painful no matter what the frequency of stimulation. Conversely, stimulation of nociceptors causes pain;

A-delta nociceptors produce sharp pain and C polymodal nociceptors dull or burning pain (Konietzny et al. 1981; Ochoa and Torebjörk 1989).

How then can touch become painful in pathological conditions that result in mechanical allodynia? Several possibilities have been proposed and will be discussed briefly:

1. Nociceptors may become sensitized so that they now respond to normally innocuous stimuli (Ochoa 1992; Price et al. 1989).
2. Central nociceptive neurons become responsive or more responsive to tactile stimuli (Woolf 1992; Willis 1993).
3. Central inhibition is reduced, allowing nociceptive central neurons to respond more to tactile stimuli (Yaksh 1989).
4. There is rewiring of the dorsal horn so that tactile afferent fibers synapse directly onto nociceptive central neurons (Woolf et al. 1992).

MECHANISMS BY WHICH TOUCH CAN BECOME PAINFUL

SENSITIZATION OF NOCICEPTORS

It is well known that cutaneous nociceptors can be sensitized by injury to the skin. For example, mild burns can sensitize either A-delta or C nociceptors, depending on the severity of the burn and its location (Bessou and Perl 1969; Fitzgerald and Lynn 1977; Meyer and Campbell 1981; LaMotte et al. 1983). The sensitization is manifested both by a lowered threshold for activation of nociceptors and by increased responses to normally suprathreshold stimuli. However, if capsaicin causes sensitization of nociceptors, it is more appropriate to denote the resulting sensory changes as hyperalgesia, rather than as allodynia, because hyperalgesia is defined as a lowering of pain threshold and an increase in the intensity of pain associated with a previously painful stimulus at the site of injury (Hardy et al. [1952] 1967; Willis 1992).

ACTIVATION OF CENTRAL NOCICEPTIVE NEURONS BY TACTILE STIMULI

Some nociceptive neurons in the dorsal horn are selectively responsive to noxious stimuli (Christensen and Perl 1979). These nociceptive-specific or high-threshold neurons can easily be conceived to belong to a labeled-line sensory channel for pain. However, it is more difficult to understand their possible role in mechanical allodynia because they do not respond to mechanoreceptors. Other central nociceptive neurons have a convergent input from mechanoreceptors, although their most vigorous responses are to noxious stimuli (Owens et al. 1992; Willis and Coggeshall 1991). These neurons are often called *wide dynamic range* (WDR) or *convergent* neurons. It is not immediately obvious how the responses of these neurons to tactile stimuli fit into the labeled-line concept. However, it is tempting to speculate that such neurons contribute to allodynia (Willis 1993).

An important question to ask about WDR cells is whether their activation causes sensations of touch and pain or just pain. This question has not been answered in a satisfactory fashion, although Mayer, Price, and Becker (1975) made an attempt. They stimulated axons in the anterolateral quadrant of the upper cervical spinal cords of patients having percutaneous cordotomies for pain relief. Pain was always elicited, provided that the stimulus strength and frequency were high enough (Fig. 1). No mention was made of other sensations. By using a double pulse technique, they were able to show that pain could be produced when large myelinated axons were activated. Mayer et al. suggested that these axons were likely to arise from spinothalamic tract (STT) cells of the WDR variety, because in monkeys these cells generally have large myelinated axons (Price and Mayer 1975). However, it could not be shown directly that the axons that evoked pain in the human subjects actually belonged to WDR neurons; furthermore, high-threshold STT cells can have relatively large myelinated axons (Willis et al. 1974).

The study by Mayer et al. (1975) contributes in another way to the argument about the possible function of WDR cells in another way. Stimulation of axons in the anterolateral quadrant using suprathreshold stimuli caused pain in all cases if the stimulus frequency exceeded 25 Hz, but in no case when the frequency was 5 Hz or lower. This suggests that a neural integrator in the central pain system sums activity in the ascending nociceptive pathways. This summated activity must exceed a threshold before pain is sensed at a conscious level. A similar observation has been made for peripheral nociceptors. A low-frequency discharge in nociceptors will not necessarily be accompanied by pain. Furthermore, the time course of discharges in nociceptors and pain may be mismatched, because discharge rates in nociceptors may decrease while pain increases (Van Hees and Gybels 1981; Adriaensen et al. 1984). The frequency of intraneural microstimulation of what are probably small sets of nociceptors must exceed 3 Hz to cause pain (Ochoa and Torebjörk 1989).

Given these observations, it seems reasonable to propose that nociceptive ascending tract neurons in the spinal cord dorsal horn must discharge at some

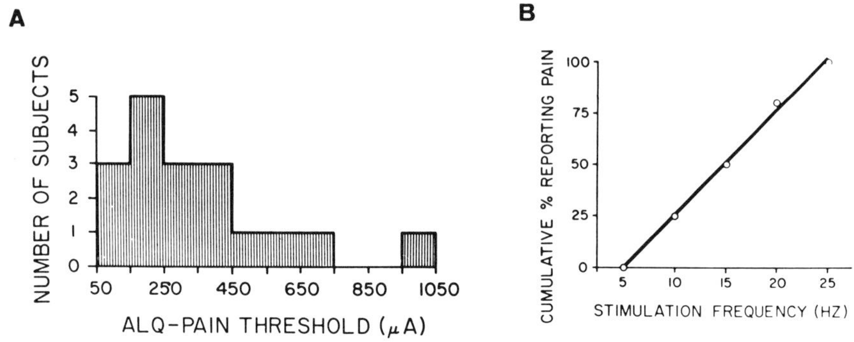

Fig. 1. A: the distribution of pain thresholds in patients in whom axons in the anterolateral quadrant (ALQ) were stimulated during a percutaneous cordotomy (one-second trains of 0.2 ms pulses at 50 Hz were delivered through an electrode in the ALQ). **B:** the proportion of patients who felt pain when the stimulus frequency was varied (stimulus strength was 15% above pain threshold at 50 Hz). (From Mayer et al. 1975)

minimal rate before the signals transmitted to the brain are interpreted as painful. Thus, WDR STT cells that have a minimal input from mechanoreceptors that either do not normally respond overtly with action potentials (Woolf and King 1989), or that respond minimally (Owens et al. 1992), would not signal pain in response to tactile stimuli. Only intense stimuli would cause them to discharge at a sufficiently high rate to signal pain. If this hypothesis is correct, then such convergent STT cells may be regarded as part of a labeled line for pain. In the case of WDR cells, which may have a high background discharge rate and which respond overtly to tactile stimuli, the labeled line is noisy. It can be hypothesized that the brain normally disregards the noise by setting a threshold that must be exceeded by summation of the effects of nerve impulses in the ascending nociceptive pathways. However, if these convergent neurons are sensitized and become hyperresponsive, they may discharge at a high rate when mechanoreceptors are stimulated, and now their activity summates to a level that exceeds threshold for pain and causes allodynia (Willis 1993; Loh and Nathan 1978).

We will discuss evidence for this idea in an experimental model in which allodynia is produced by intradermal injection of capsaicin. Other models being investigated in our laboratory that result in similar plastic changes include mechanical damage of the skin (Owens et al. 1992), neuropathy (Palecek et al. 1992), and arthritis (Dougherty et al. 1992b).

DECREASED INHIBITION

Intrathecal administration of strychnine in rats causes them to become hyperreactive to tactile stimuli (Yaksh 1989). This has been proposed as a model of mechanical allodynia. Strychnine is a selective antagonist of glycine receptors and blocks inhibitory neurotransmission at glycinergic synapses in the spinal cord (Curtis et al. 1971). Clearly, reduced inhibition can result in an increase in the responses of dorsal horn neurons to input from mechanoreceptors. The contribution of a change in the level of central inhibition should be evaluated as a possible explanation for allodynia in particular experimental models.

ANATOMICAL CHANGES

Following transection of the sciatic nerve in rats, several morphological changes occur in the dorsal horn. For example, immunohistochemical staining for the lectins, soybean agglutinin and RL 29, increases in intensity in the superficial dorsal horn (Cameron et al. 1992). Similar changes occur following partial damage to the sciatic nerve by the placement of loose ligatures to produce a mononeuropathy (Cameron et al. 1991). In animals with sciatic nerve transections, myelinated afferent fibers whose endings are normally restricted to the nucleus proprius invade the substantia gelatinosa (Woolf et al. 1992). Sprouting tactile afferent fibers that connect synaptically with nociceptive neurons would provide a mechanism for allodynia. Furthermore, such rewiring could lead to long-lasting sensory changes. However, it is not as yet known if the sprouting tactile afferent fibers establish functional connections or if the postsynaptic neurons are in excitatory or inhibitory pathways.

CAPSAICIN MODEL

Injury to the skin of humans commonly produces pain and several pain-related alterations in sensation, including primary and secondary hyperalgesia and allodynia (Lewis 1942; Hardy et al. [1952] 1967; Willis 1992). Several laboratories have combined efforts to develop an experimental approach to the investigation of the mechanisms underlying these events. The sensory changes produced by intradermal (id.) injections of capsaicin have been examined psychophysically in human subjects by LaMotte, Torebjörk, and their colleagues (Simone et al. 1989a; LaMotte et al. 1991; 1992; Torebjörk et al. 1992). The types of primary afferent nociceptors that are activated by id. capsaicin injections have been surveyed both in human and in animal subjects (Baumann et al. 1991; LaMotte et al. 1992). In parallel animal experiments, recordings have been made from neurons of the spinal cord dorsal horn, including spinothalamic tract (STT) cells, to look for correlations between the human sensory events and single-unit neuronal responses (Simone et al. 1989b; 1991; Dougherty and Willis 1992). Finally, experimental interventions have sought to elucidate the neurochemical mechanisms of the changes in response properties of dorsal horn neurons that presumably underlie the pain, primary and secondary hyperalgesia, and allodynia that result from id. injections of capsaicin (Dougherty and Willis 1991; Dougherty et al. 1992a, 1993; Willis et al. 1992; Palecek et al. 1994a,b).

We performed experiments using anesthetized animals and in accordance with protocols approved by the local Animal Care and Use Committee and with NIH and IASP Guidelines.

SENSORY CHANGES FOLLOWING ID. CAPSAICIN

Capsaicin injected into the skin in human subjects produces immediate, severe burning pain that diminishes to a low level over 10–30 minutes (LaMotte et al. 1991). Within about 15 minutes following the injection, hyperalgesia to heat stimuli occurs in an area extending for 1–2 cm from the injection site (Fig. 2). This is presumably a form of primary hyperalgesia. In addition, the skin becomes tender or painful to stroking with a spring-mounted cotton-tipped applicator (mechanical allodynia), and the weak pain evoked by punctate stimulation with a von Frey filament (bending force of 225 mN) becomes more painful over a broad area of the skin surrounding the injection site

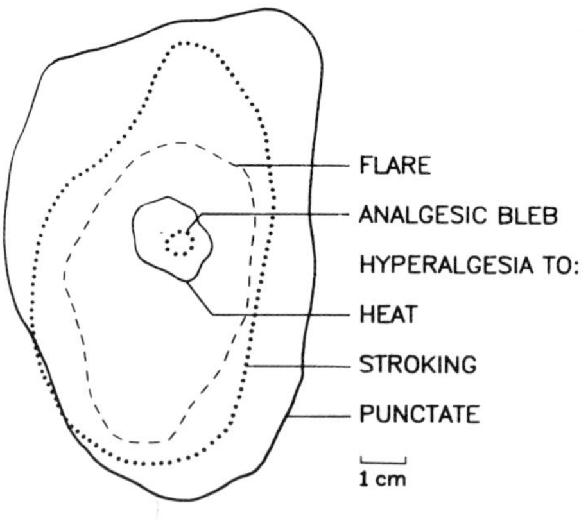

Fig. 2. The concentric lines outline the areas of change that develop following intradermal (id.) injection of capsaicin in human subjects. The areas include: analgesia at the injection site, heat hyperalgesia, flare, mechanical allodynia (hyperalgesia to stroking), and hyperalgesia to punctate stimuli. (LaMotte et al. 1991)

(secondary mechanical hyperalgesia; Fig. 2). A small area of analgesia at the injection site is attributable to an excitotoxic effect of the capsaicin on the terminals of nociceptors that end near the locus of highest concentration of the injected capsaicin (cf., Fitzgerald 1983; Lynn 1990). A noticeable flare extends away from the injection site, but not as far as the maximum extent of the zone of secondary hyperalgesia and mechanical allodynia (Fig. 2).

The mechanical allodynia that results from id. capsaicin injections develops over about 15 minutes and lasts about two hours (Fig. 3; LaMotte et al. 1991). The secondary hyperalgesia that follows id. capsaicin selectively affects mechanical but not thermal responses; there is tenderness to probing the skin with von Frey filaments, but the pain threshold for noxious heat pulses is unchanged. Secondary hyperalgesia to noxious mechanical stimuli develops over 15–30 minutes and lasts for up to 24 hours (Fig. 3).

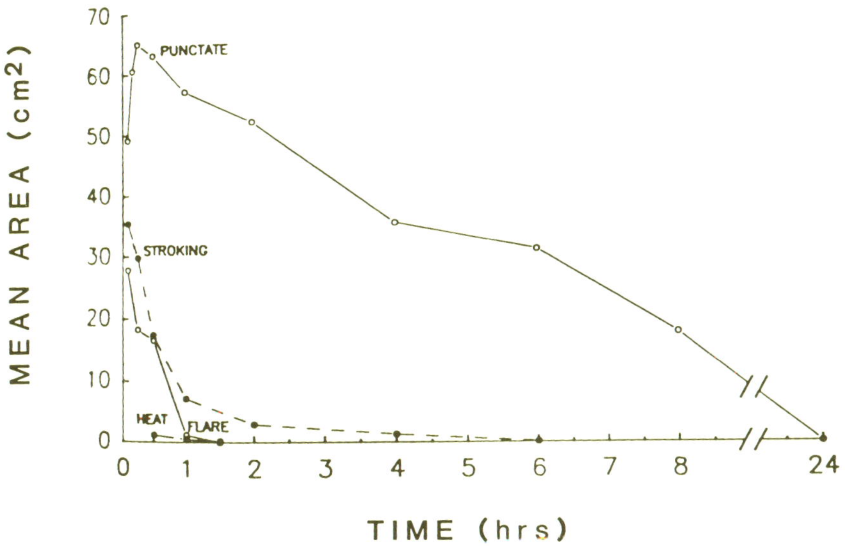

Fig. 3. Time courses of the changes that result from id. capsaicin injection: heat hyperalgesia, flare, mechanical allodynia (stroking), and mechanical hyperalgesia (punctate). (LaMotte et al. 1991)

TYPES OF NERVE FIBERS INVOLVED IN SENSORY CHANGES FOLLOWING INTRADERMAL CAPSAICIN

PAIN

Conduction in C-fibers accounts for the pain that occurs immediately after id. injection of capsaicin. Evidence for this is that the pain is equally intense on both sides of the body when conduction in A-fibers has been blocked by a pressure cuff on one side (Torebjörk et al. 1992). The pain has been attributed largely to the activation of C polymodal nociceptors by the drug (Fitzgerald 1983; Lynn 1990). However, capsaicin also excites several other types of nociceptors (as well as warm receptors), including some that have minimal sensitivity to mechanical stimuli. The latter may be chemosensitive cutaneous nociceptors (Baumann et al. 1991; LaMotte et al. 1992). Nociceptors that are difficult to activate under normal conditions, but that become sensitive to mechanical stimuli under inflammatory conditions, have been recently found in joints (Schaible and Schmidt 1985; 1988), viscera (Häbler et al. 1990), and skin (Handwerker et al. 1991). Experiments that lack sophisticated methodology probably have underestimated the abundance of these so-called sleeping nociceptors.

Although recordings from nociceptors demonstrate their activation by capsaicin, the discharges in monkeys often do not last as long as the pain in humans (Baumann et al. 1991; LaMotte et al. 1992), suggesting that the pain evoked by capsaicin is due only in part to the discharges of nociceptors. The central neural integrator mechanism mentioned above also likely makes a contribution (cf. Price et al. 1977, 1978).

PRIMARY HYPERALGESIA

Primary hyperalgesia following cutaneous damage due to mild burns causes a sensitization of C and A-delta nociceptors (Bessou and Perl 1969; Fitzgerald and Lynn 1977; Meyer and Campbell 1981; LaMotte et al. 1983), so it is generally thought that primary hyperalgesia can be attributed to the sensitization of nociceptors (Willis 1992). Primary hyperalgesia that is produced by id. capsaicin injection in humans occurs despite a conduction block in A-fibers, indicating that the primary hyperalgesia depends on C-fiber input (Torebjörk et al. 1992). Thus, capsaicin presumably has sensitized C-fibers, leading to the primary hyperalgesia. Curiously, nociceptors supplying the skin of monkeys in the area immediately surrounding a capsaicin injection site do not show a change in responsiveness to noxious heat stimuli, making it uncertain if sensitization of nociceptors by capsaicin results in primary hyperalgesia in monkeys (Baumann et al. 1991). However, sensitization of nociceptors to heat by capsaicin is evident when the capsaicin is applied topically to monkey or human skin (Baumann et al. 1991; LaMotte et al. 1992), suggesting that the difficulty in demonstrating a sensitization of nociceptors in monkeys after id. injection of capsaicin may be a sampling problem.

SECONDARY HYPERALGESIA

Nociceptors that supply the skin in the area of secondary hyperalgesia fail to show any changes in responsiveness to mechanical or heat stimuli following id. injection of capsaicin (Baumann et al. 1991; LaMotte et al. 1992). Therefore, there is no direct evidence for the proposal by Lewis (1942) that secondary hyperalgesia depends entirely on a peripheral mechanism involving nocifensive nerve fibers. Instead, it can be concluded that secondary hyperalgesia is due to the sensitization of neurons in the central nervous system caused by the discharges of nociceptors (LaMotte et al. 1991; 1992).

The responsiveness of primary afferent nociceptors supplying the area of secondary hyperalgesia is unchanged, so there is no reason to expect that a change in the threshold for noxious heat stimuli will cause pain. An alternative explanation for the absence of any change in threshold for heat pain in the area of secondary hyperalgesia is that the central pathways for noxious heat and for mechanically-evoked pain involve different interneuronal connections, and only the mechanical nociceptive pathway is sensitized by capsaicin (LaMotte et al. 1991).

MECHANICAL ALLODYNIA

The primary afferent nerve fibers that are responsible for evoking mechanical allodynia appear to be mechanoreceptors supplied by myelinated fibers (Torebjörk et al. 1992). When conduction in A-fibers is interrupted by a pressure block, allodynia cannot be demonstrated following an id. capsaicin injection until the conduction block is relieved (Torebjörk et al. 1992; cf. Loh and Nathan 1978; Dubner et al. 1987; Price et al. 1989; Campbell et al. 1988). Furthermore, using intraneural microstimulation in human subjects, Torebjörk et al. (1992) found a site in a peripheral nerve that, when stimulated electrically, evokes a sensation of touch that is projected to a receptive field in the skin (Fig. 4A). When capsaicin is injected into an area of skin adjacent to the projected receptive field, mechanical allodynia and secondary hyperalgesia develop. At this time, stimulation at the same locus in the nerve now evokes pain as well as touch (Fig. 4B). As the allodynia and secondary

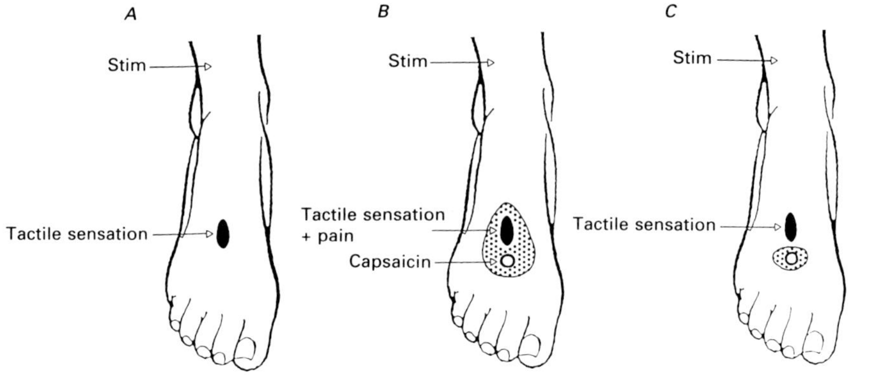

Fig. 4. Sensation evoked by intraneural microstimulation in a human subject. **A:** stimulation caused a tactile sensation that was projected to a receptive field on the dorsum of the foot. **B:** after id. capsaicin injection, an area of secondary hyperalgesia developed that encompassed the projected tactile field; at this time, intraneural stimulation evoked pain as well as touch. **C:** as the secondary hyperalgesia receded to a point distal to the projected field, intraneural stimulation now evoked only a touch sensation. (From Torebjörk et al. 1992.)

hyperalgesia recede from the projected receptive field, stimulation in the nerve no longer produces pain but only touch (Fig. 4C).

ANIMAL MODEL OF CAPSAICIN-INDUCED PAIN, HYPERALGESIA, AND ALLODYNIA

Simone et al. (1989b) have made recordings from dorsal horn neurons in the cat spinal cord before and after id. injections of capsaicin. They found that nociceptive dorsal horn neurons developed an increased responsiveness to innocuous mechanical stimuli following capsaicin. Simone et al. (1991) and Dougherty and Willis (1992) later performed similar experiments in the primate spinal cord, but with recordings from spinothalamic tract (STT) neurons identified by antidromic activation from the ventral posterior lateral nucleus of the contralateral thalamus.

CORRELATE OF PAIN

When capsaicin is injected into the skin, STT cells generally undergo a substantial increase in discharge rate that lasts about 15–20 minutes (Simone et al. 1991; Dougherty and Willis 1992); vehicle injections have little or no effect. The time course of the increased discharges of STT cells parallels that of pain in human subjects (Fig. 5), especially if the STT cells are of the WDR type. High–threshold (HT) STT cells often fail to show a sustained discharge in response to capsaicin, although an initial increase in activity generally occurs.

CORRELATE OF PRIMARY HYPERALGESIA

Capsaicin injected into the receptive field of an STT cell produces increased responses to noxious heat stimuli applied to the injected area and reduces the mean threshold for a response from 48°C to about 32°C (Simone et al. 1991). Responses to noxious mechanical stimuli may be increased or decreased; in the latter case, the reduction can be attributed to the excitotoxic effect of the capsaicin on nociceptor terminals (cf. analgesic effect at the capsaicin injection site in human subjects; LaMotte et al. 1991;1992).

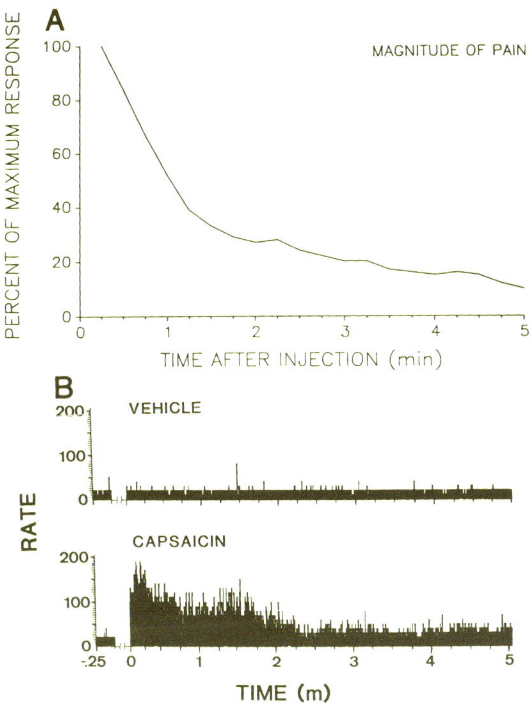

Fig. 5. The curve in **A** shows the normalized mean time course of the magnitude of pain sensation elicited in 17 human subjects by id. injection of capsaicin, expressed as a percentage of maximum. **B** shows the responses of a primate spinothalamic tract (STT) cell to id. injection of vehicle and of capsaicin. (Simone et al. 1991)

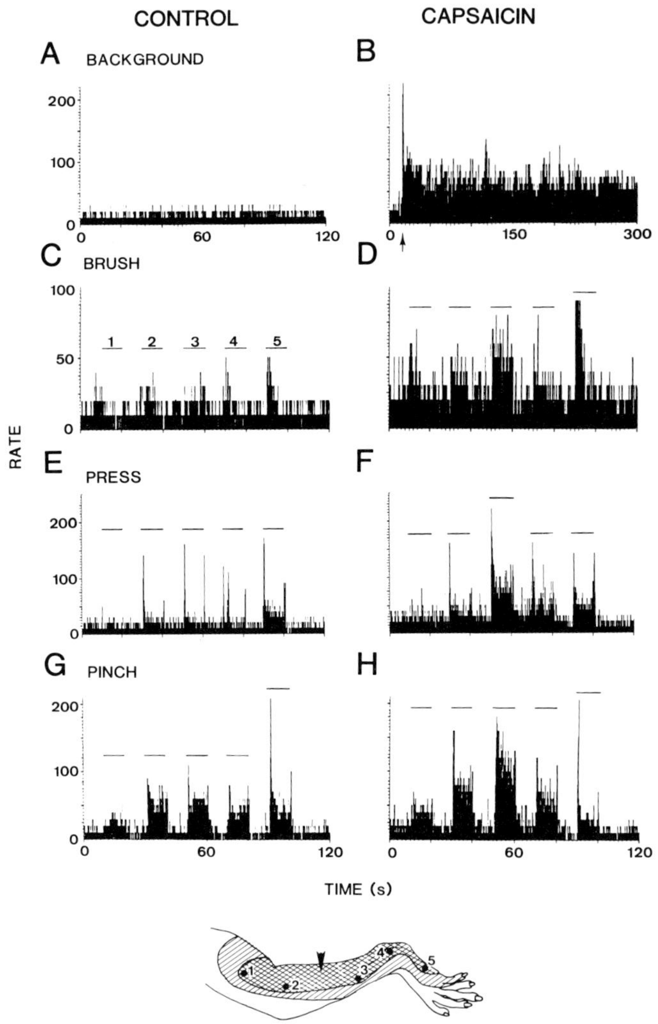

Fig. 6. Responses of an STT cell to mechanical stimuli before and after id. injection of capsaicin. **A** shows the background activity of the cell, and **B** the response to capsaicin. **C, E** and **G** are the responses to stimulation at five sites in the receptive field of the cell (sites indicated in the drawing at the bottom) using innocuous (BRUSH) and noxious (PRESS and PINCH) mechanical stimuli before injection of capsaicin. **D, F** and **H** show the responses to the same stimuli after capsaicin. The enlargement of the receptive field following capsaicin is shown by the singly hatched area in the drawing; the arrow indicates the injection site. (Dougherty and Willis 1992)

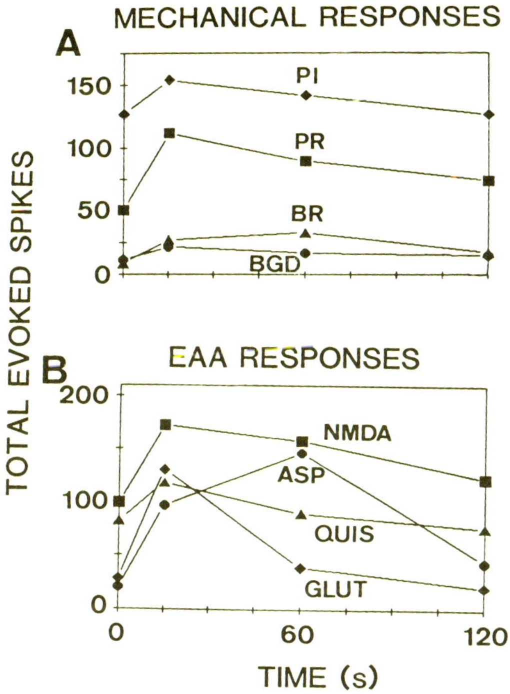

Fig. 7. Time course of the increases in the responses of an STT cell to mechanical stimuli, **A**, and to iontophoretic applications of excitatory amino acids (EAAs), **B**, following an id. injection of capsaicin. Abbreviations: BGD, background; BR, brush; PR, pressure; PI, pinch; ASP, aspartate; GLUT, glutamate; NMDA, N-methyl-D-aspartate; QUIS, quisqualate. (Dougherty and Willis 1992)

CORRELATES OF SECONDARY HYPERALGESIA AND MECHANICAL ALLODYNIA

Responses to innocuous and noxious mechanical stimuli applied to a large area of skin surrounding the injection site increased within 15 minutes after id. injection of capsaicin and remained increased for more than an hour (Figs. 6, 7A; Simone et al. 1991; Dougherty and Willis 1992). The enhanced responses to noxious mechanical stimuli may help explain secondary hyperalgesia, and those to innocuous mechanical stimuli may explain allodynia.

At the time that the responses to innocuous mechanical stimuli are increased, the same STT cells respond more vigorously to iontophoretic application of excitatory amino acids (EAAs; Fig. 7B; Dougherty and Willis 1992) and to electrical stimulation of the largest afferent fibers in the central stump of a cut dorsal root filament (Simone et al. 1991). These observations indicate that the STT cells (1) become more excitable both to locally administered neurotransmitter and also to stimulation of afferent fibers that are unaffected by the capsaicin (because the afferents were disconnected from the periphery by the cut, and (2) are activated more vigorously by A-beta-sized afferent fibers. The first point is consistent with the idea that the capsaicin injection causes central sensitization. Although it is unclear from this experiment whether the sensitization requires continual peripheral input or is strictly a central phenomenon, there is no evidence for a sustained input from the periphery following id. capsaicin injections. The second point is consistent with the observation that the pain of mechanical allodynia can be evoked by activation of A-beta afferent fibers in human subjects (Torebjörk et al. 1992; cf., Loh and Nathan 1978; Dubner et al. 1987; Price et al. 1989; Campbell et al. 1988).

MECHANISMS OF SECONDARY HYPERALGESIA AND MECHANICAL ALLODYNIA

If the neural events observed in recordings from primate STT cells are an adequate model of secondary hyperalgesia and mechanical allodynia, then a study of the mechanisms underlying these events should provide a way to determine the causes of the sensory changes in human subjects.

It is well known that the synaptic terminals of many fine primary afferent fibers in the dorsal horn contain peptides, such as substance P (SP), neurokinin A (NKA), calcitonin gene-related peptide (CGRP), vasoactive intestinal polypeptide (VIP), and others (Willis and Coggeshall 1991). In addition to SP, many afferent terminals in the superficial dorsal horn contain an excitatory amino acid (EAA) neurotransmitter, such as glutamate (GLU) (De Biasi and Rustioni 1988). Electron microscopic immunohistochemical studies of STT cells marked intracellularly by injection of horseradish peroxidase have demonstrated that nearly half of the synaptic profiles in contact with the soma and proximal dendrites contain glutamate (Westlund et al. 1992) and some contain SP (Carlton et al. 1985).

Stimulation of nociceptors by capsaicin causes the release of EAAs and SP in the dorsal horn (Gamse et al. 1979; Sorkin and McAdoo 1993). Therefore, a reasonable hypothesis is that capsaicin sensitizes dorsal horn neurons by activating nociceptors that release EAAs and peptides, such as SP, into the dorsal horn.

ACTION OF EAAs AND SP ON STT CELLS

The most direct way to test the action of EAAs and SP on STT cells is by releasing these substances iontophoretically while recording the discharges of STT neurons (Willcockson et al. 1984a,b; Dougherty and Willis 1991, 1992; Dougherty et al. 1992a, 1993). Iontophoretic application of a number of different EAAs, including glutamate (GLU), aspartate (ASP), N-methyl-

D-aspartate (NMDA), quisqualate (QUIS), α-amino-3-hydroxy-5-methylisoxazole-4-propionic acid (AMPA), and kainate (KAIN), produce an increase in discharge rate (although the responses to different EAAs have different time courses). The excitation of STT cells by these EAAs is produced by actions on non-NMDA or NMDA receptors, as shown by the effects of selective antagonists, such as CNQX and AP-7, applied either iontophoretically or by microdialysis. Alternatively, EAAs can activate metabotropic glutamate receptors and affect neuronal activity by changes in second messenger systems (Palecek et al. 1994b). Applications of SP with relatively small iontophoretic currents often produce little or no change in the

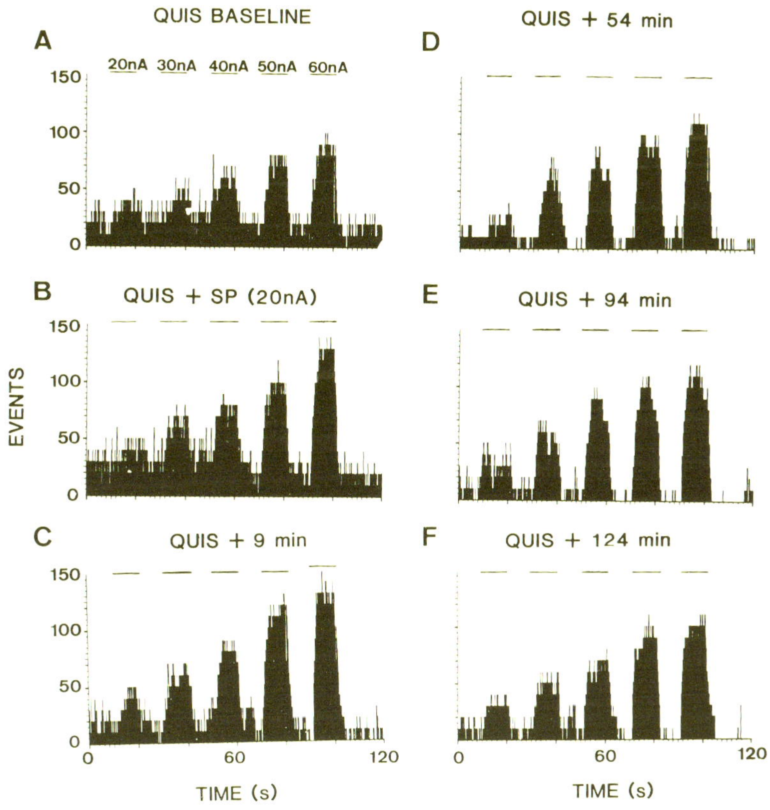

Fig. 8. Responses of an STT cell to iontophoretically applied quisqualate (QUIS) and substance P (SP). **A** shows graded responses to five increasing iontophoretic doses of QUIS. In **B**, the same doses are repeated during coapplication of SP. In C-F, QUIS was repeated at various times after termination of the SP application. The doses (in nA) and times are indicated. (Dougherty et al. 1993)

discharge rates of STT cells. Large iontophoretic doses of SP may excite STT cells or, in some cases, cause an inhibition.

The excitation produced by iontophoretic application of an EAA is quite transient, outlasting by only a short time the iontophoretic current pulse (Dougherty and Willis 1991). Furthermore, repeated applications of the same EAA produce similar or progressively smaller responses. There is no accumulation of excitation as tested with later doses of the same EAA (Dougherty and Willis 1991; Dougherty et al. 1993). However, coapplication of an EAA and SP often causes a long-lasting increase in the responses to later application of the same EAA. For example, Fig. 8A shows the responses of an STT cell to graded iontophoretic doses of QUIS in the absence of SP. The same graded doses of QUIS were released concurrently with SP, and the responses were enhanced (Fig. 8B). The current releasing SP was then turned off, and the responses to QUIS were tested periodically. As seen in Fig. 8C-F, the responses to QUIS were still enhanced at 9, 54, 94, and 124 minutes after the cessation of the SP application.

Similar long-lasting increases in the responses of STT cells to NMDA when coapplied with SP also were observed (Dougherty and Willis 1991). However, coapplication of AMPA and SP produced only short-lasting increases in the responses to AMPA (Dougherty et al. 1993). Interestingly, there were often reciprocal changes in the responses to NMDA and to a non-NMDA agonist (AMPA or QUIS). When the responses to NMDA increased, those to AMPA or QUIS often decreased, and vice versa. Sometimes there was a global decrease in the responses of STT cells to EAAs.

For many of the STT cells studied in these experiments, it was possible to examine periodically the responses of the same neurons to mechanical stimuli applied to their receptive fields. In general, when the responses to an EAA showed a prolonged increase following coapplication of the EAA with SP, the responses to mechanical stimuli also were increased (Dougherty and Willis 1991; Dougherty et al. 1993). AMPA coapplied with SP produced only a short-lasting increase in AMPA responses, and no changes were noted in the responses to mechanical stimuli, perhaps because of the rapid recovery of the excitability of the STT cells. When the responses of STT cells to a variety of EAAs were reduced, there was no change in the responses to mechanical stimulation of the receptive fields (Dougherty et al. 1993).

One weakness of the above experiments is that it is not entirely certain that the effects of iontophoretically released substances are necessarily exerted only on the neuron under observation. However, in vitro experiments using the whole-cell patch-clamp technique show that coapplication of EAAs and SP also enhance responses of isolated neurons to later applications of EAAs (Gu and Huang 1989; Randic et al. 1990).

These experiments were generally consistent with the hypothesis that the release of EAAs and SP from nociceptive afferent fibers activated by capsaicin can cause a long-lasting increase in the excitability of STT cells (and other dorsal horn neurons). Therefore, we tested a second hypothesis: capsaicin produces a long-lasting increase in the excitability of STT cells through the release of EAAs and SP into the dorsal horn.

PREVENTION OF SENSITIZATION OF STT CELLS BY EAA AND SP ANTAGONISTS

We tested this second hypothesis by using microdialysis to administer selective antagonists of non-NMDA, NMDA, and NK1 receptors into the vicinity of STT cells, using microdialysis (Dougherty et al. 1992a; Willis et al. 1992). The experimental paradigm involved two id. injections of capsaicin. The background activity and the responses of the STT cells were tested before and after the first injection of capsaicin; a recovery period of about 90 minutes was allowed, and then similar recordings were made before and after a second injection of capsaicin. As a control procedure, we studied a series of STT cells in the absence of any antagonist to verify that the responses to the two injections of capsaicin are similar. The two capsaicin injections produced similar increases in the initial discharge rate, maintained increases in background discharge, and increases in responses to innocuous and noxious mechanical stimuli.

When the non-NMDA receptor antagonist, CNQX, was introduced into the dorsal horn through a microdialysis fiber, the responses of the STT cells to innocuous and noxious mechanical stimuli and to capsaicin were severely reduced or eliminated (Fig. 9; Dougherty et al. 1992a). We concluded that transmission at the initial synapses in the pathways for mechanoreceptors and nociceptors to STT cells involved activation of non-NMDA EAA receptors. However, when the NMDA antagonist, AP-7, was infused into the dorsal horn, there was no change in the responses of STT cells to innocuous or weakly noxious mechanical stimuli, but the responses to strongly noxious mechanical stimuli and to capsaicin were partially reduced; moreover, the sensitization of the responses of STT cells to mechanical stimuli was eliminated (Fig. 9). We concluded that NMDA receptors are involved in nociceptive transmission to STT cells and that these receptors play an important role in central sensitization.

Administration of the NK1 receptor antagonist, CP 96,345, into the dorsal horn by microdialysis also blocked the sensitization of the responses of STT cells to innocuous and weakly noxious mechanical stimuli (Willis et al. 1992). However, there was no effect on the nociceptive responses themselves.

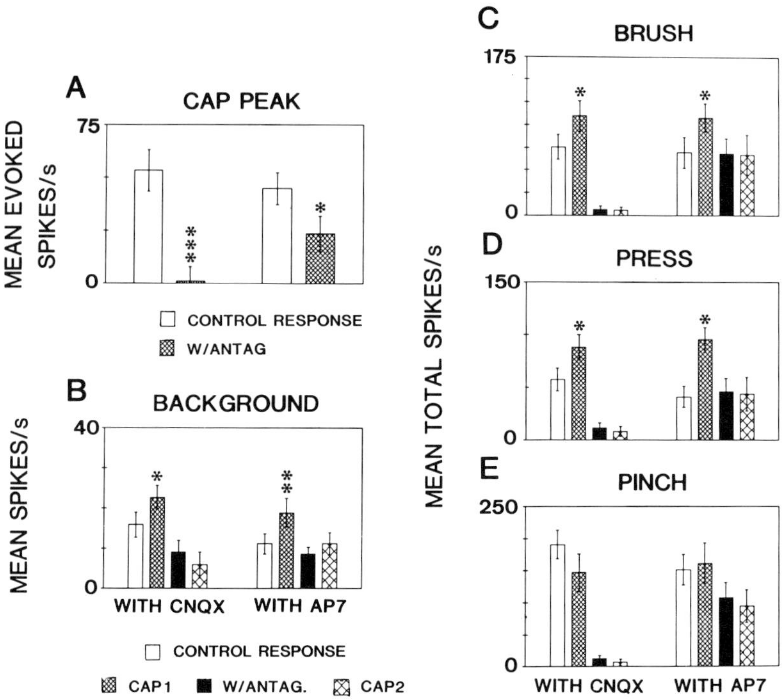

Fig. 9. Effects of EAA antagonists on the enhanced responses of STT cells to mechanical stimuli following id. injection of capsaicin. **A** shows plots of the peak responses to capsaicin without and in the presence of an EAA antagonist (administered by microdialysis). The non-NMDA antagonist, CNQX, nearly eliminated the response to capsaicin, whereas the NMDA antagonist, AP-7, reduced it to about half. **B** shows the effects of capsaicin on the background activity without and with the EAA antagonists. Both CNQX and AP-7 prevented capsaicin from increasing the background activity. **C-E** show the effects of the antagonists on the changes in responses of the cell to mechanical stimuli (sensitization) following capsaicin. CNQX essentially blocked all of the responses, as well as the sensitization. AP-7 did not affect the responses to BRUSH or PRESS, but prevented sensitization of the cell to these stimuli. It did reduce the responses to PINCH. (Dougherty et al. 1992)

Given that CP 96,345 has several effects, including acting as an NK1 receptor antagonist and having an action on calcium channels, we also examined the action of CP 96,344, which has a similar effect on calcium channels but which is not an NK1 receptor antagonist. CP 96,344 did not affect the responses or the sensitization of STT cells. We concluded that the sensitization of STT cells that follows id. capsaicin injections depends on the activation of NK1 receptors, presumably by released SP, as well as on the activation of EAA receptors.

SIGNAL TRANSDUCTION MECHANISMS IN THE SENSITIZATION PROCESS

Several second-messenger systems might play a role in the actions of EAAs and SP. An increase in the concentration of intracellular calcium ions can result from a transmembrane influx through ion channels associated with NMDA receptors (MacDermott et al. 1986) or by release from intracellular stores following activation of NK1 receptors by SP (Helke et al. 1990; Osborne and Ghazi 1989). Later events might include: (1) release of nitric oxide (NO) following activation of nitric oxide synthase and then an action of NO on guanylate cyclase; (2) activation of protein kinase C; or (3) activation of the inositol phosphate system.

Several recent investigations have provided evidence for a role of NO in nociceptive processing (Haley et al. 1992; Kitto et al. 1992; Meller et al. 1992; Babbedge et al. 1993; Radhakrisshnan and Henry 1993; Sorkin 1993). Id. injection of capsaicin also may cause NO release, since the sensitization of STT cells following such injections can be blocked by the NO synthase inhibitor, L-nitroarginine methyl ester(L-NAME), but is unaffected by the inactive isomer (D-NAME) (Palecek et al. 1993).

Evidence that protein kinase C might be involved in the sensitization of STT cells has been provided by experiments that introduced phorbol esters into the dorsal horn by microdialysis (Palecek et al. 1994a). The responses of STT cells to innocuous mechanical stimuli are enhanced by the action of an active phorbol ester but are unchanged by an inactive phorbol ester.

The responses of STT cells to innocuous mechanical stimuli also are increased when trans-ACPD, an agonist of metabotropic glutamate receptors, is introduced into the dorsal horn by microdialysis (Palecek et al. 1994b). Metabotropic glutamate receptors exert their effects by way of second-messenger systems, providing further evidence that second-messenger systems are involved in the sensitization of STT cells. However, studies are needed using selective antagonists of metabotropic glutamate receptors when these become widely available.

CONCLUSIONS

1. Intradermal injections of capsaicin in human subjects produce several sensory effects: pain, primary and secondary hyperalgesia, and mechanical allodynia.

2. All these effects depend upon the activation of nociceptors, particularly C nociceptors, by capsaicin. However, the mechanical allodynia is evoked by activation of large myelinated primary afferent fibers.

3. The time courses of the different sensory events differ. The pain lasts about 15–20 minutes; primary hyperalgesia lasts days; secondary hyperalgesia can last up to 24 hours; mechanical allodynia lasts 1–2 hours.

4. Recordings from primate spinothalamic tract (STT) cells demonstrate neural correlates to the sensory changes observed in humans. Injection of capsaicin into the skin causes a powerful excitation of wide dynamic range STT cells that parallels the time course of pain in human subjects. Noxious stimuli applied in the area of the injection cause enhanced responses of and a lowered threshold for activation of STT cells, changes that resemble the sensory changes of primary hyperalgesia. Responses of the STT cells to noxious and innocuous mechanical stimuli in an area surrounding the injection site also increase for at least 1–2 hours; these changes are similar to the sensory changes in secondary hyperalgesia and mechanical allodynia following id. capsaicin in humans.

5. We propose that STT cells in humans would undergo the same changes as in monkeys and that the changed signaling by STT cells in humans contribute to the pain, primary and secondary hyperalgesia, and mechanical allodynia that subjects report following id. injections of capsaicin.

6. The mechanisms underlying these sensory changes can best be investigated in an animal model. We hypothesized that nociceptive afferent fibers excited by capsaicin release EAAs and peptides, including SP, into the dorsal horn, and that these substances cause a sensitization of dorsal horn neurons, including STT cells.

7. Evidence in favor of this hypothesis includes: demonstrations that noxious stimuli do in fact cause the release of EAAs and SP in the dorsal horn; synaptic terminals on dorsal horn neurons, including STT cells, contain EAAs and SP; iontophoretic coapplication of EAAs and SP can produce long-lasting increases in the excitability of STT as tested by subsequent applications of EAAs and by mechanical stimulation of the receptive field; administration of selective antagonists of EAAs and of SP blocks the sensitization of STT cells by id. injections of capsaicin.

8. Another hypothesis is that the duration of the sensitization of STT cells depends on the activation of any of several second-messenger systems in STT cells. Evidence in favor of this hypothesis includes: blockade of sensitization by an NO synthase antagonist (but not by an inactive isomer); enhancement of the responses of STT cells to innocuous mechanical stimulation by the administration into the dorsal horn of an active phorbol ester (but not by an inactive phorbol ester) and by an agonist of metabotropic glutamate receptors.

9. These studies suggest a variety of potential sites of action for therapeutic interventions for the relief of pain and hyperalgesia.

ACKNOWLEDGMENTS

The author thanks his colleagues for contributions to the work done in Galveston, especially P.M. Dougherty, J.M. Chung, R.H. LaMotte, U.T. Oh, C. Owens, J. Palecek, V. Palecková, D.A. Simone, and L.S. Sorkin. He also thanks Kelli Gondesen and Griselda Gonzales for their expert technical assistance. The experiments were supported by NIH grants NS 09743 and NS 11255 and by an unrestricted grant from the Bristol-Myers Squibb Co.

REFERENCES

Adriaensen, H., Gybels, J., Handwerker, H.O. and Van Hees, J., Nociceptor discharges and sensations due to prolonged noxious mechanical stimulation: a paradox, Hum. Neurobiol., 3 (1984) 53–58.

Babbedge, R.C., Wallace, P., Gaffen, Z.A., Hart, S.L. and Moore, P.K., L-N^G-nitro arginine p-nitroanilide (L-NAPNA) is anti-nociceptive in the mouse, Neuroreport, 4 (1993) 307–310.

Baumann, T.K., Simone, D.A., Shain, C.N. and LaMotte, R.H., Neurogenic hyperalgesia: the search for the primary cutaneous afferent fibers that contribute to capsaicin-induced pain and hyperalgesia, J. Neurophysiol., 66 (1991) 212–227.

Bessou, P. and Perl, E.R., Response of cutaneous sensory units with unmyelinated fibers to noxious stimuli, J. Neurophysiol., 32 (1969) 1025–1043.

Bonica, J.J., The Management of Pain, 2nd ed., Lea & Febiger, Philadelphia, 1990, 2120 pp.

Cameron, A.A., Pover, C.M., Willis, W.D. and Coggeshall, R.E., Evidence that fine primary afferent axons innervate a wider territory in the superficial dorsal horn following peripheral axotomy, Brain Res., 575 (1992) 151–154.

Cameron, A.A., Cliffer, K.D., Dougherty, P.M., Willis, W.D. and Carlton, S.M., Changes in lectin, GAP-43 and neuropeptide staining in the rat superficial dorsal horn following experimental peripheral neuropathy, Neurosci. Lett., 131 (1991) 249–252,

Campbell, J.N., Raja, S.N., Meyer, R.A. and Mackinnon, S.E. Myelinated afferents signal the hyperalgesia associated with nerve injury, Pain, 32 (1988) 89–94.

Carlton, S.M., LaMotte, C.C., Honda, C.N., Surmeier, D.J., DeLanerolle, N.C. and Willis, W.D., Ultrastructural analysis of substance P and other synaptic profiles innervating an identified primate spinothalamic tract neuron, Neurosci. Abstr., 11 (1985) 578.

Christensen, B.N. and Perl, E.R., Spinal neurons specifically excited by noxious or thermal stimuli: marginal zone of the dorsal horn, J. Neurophysiol., 33 (1970) 293–307.

Curtis, D.R., Duggan, A.W. and Johnston, G.A.R., The specificity of strychnine as a glycine antagonist in the mammalian spinal cord, Exp. Brain Res., 12 (1971) 547–565.

De Biasi, S. and Rustioni, A., Glutamate and substance P coexist in primary afferent terminals in the superficial laminae of spinal cord, Proc. Natl. Acad. Sci. USA, 85 (1988) 7820–7824.

Dougherty, P.M. and Willis, W.D., Enhancement of spinothalamic neuron responses to chemical and mechanical stimuli following combined micro-iontophoretic application of N-methyl-D-aspartic acid and substance P, Pain, 47 (1991) 85–93.

Dougherty, P.M. and Willis, W.D., Enhanced responses of spinothalamic tract neurons to excitatory amino acids accompany capsaicin-induced sensitization in the monkey, J. Neurosci., 12 (1992) 883–894.

Dougherty, P.M., Palecek, J., Palecková, V., Sorkin, L.S. and Willis, W.D., The role of NMDA and non-NMDA excitatory amino acid receptors in the excitation of primate spinothalamic tract neurons by mechanical, chemical, thermal, and electrical stimuli, J. Neurosci., 12 (1992**a**) 3025–3041.

Dougherty, P.M., Sluka, K.A., Sorkin, L.S., Westlund, K.N. and Willis, W.D., Neural changes in acute arthritis in monkeys. I. Parallel enhancement of responses of spinothalamic tract neurons to mechanical stimulation and excitatory amino acids, Brain Res. Rev., 17 (1992b) 1–13.

Dougherty, P.M., Palecek, J., Zorn, S. and Willis, W.D., Combined application of excitatory amino acids and substance P produces long-lasting changes in responses of primate spinothalamic tract neurons, Brain Res. Rev., 18 (1993) 227–246.

Dubner, R., Sharav, Y., Gracely, R.H. and Price, D.D., Idiopathic trigeminal neuralgia: sensory features and pain mechanisms, Pain, 31 (1987) 23–33.

Fitzgerald, M., Capsaicin and sensory neurones: a review, Pain, 15 (1983) 109–130.

Fitzgerald, M. and Lynn, B. The sensitization of high threshold mechanoreceptors with myelinated axons by repeated heating, J. Physiol., 265 (1977) 549–563.

Gamse, R., Molnar, A. and Lembeck, F., Substance P release from spinal cord slices by capsaicin, Life Sci., 25 (1979) 629–636.

Gu, Y.P. and Huang, L.Y.M., Effects of excitatory amino acids on neurons isolated from spinal trigeminal nuclei, Neurosci. Abstr., 15 (1989) 947.

Häbler, H.J., Jänig, W. and Koltzenburg, M., Activation of unmyelinated afferent fibres by mechanical stimuli and inflammation of the urinary bladder in the cat, J. Physiol., 425 (1990) 545–562.

Haley, J.E., Dickenson, A.H. and Schachter, M., Electrophysiological evidence for a role of nitric oxide in prolonged chemical nociception in the rat, Neuropharmacol., 31 (1992) 251–258.

Handwerker, H.O., Kilo, S. and Reeh, P.W., Unresponsive afferent nerve fibres in the sural nerve of the rat, J. Physiol., 435 (1991) 229–242.

Hardy, J.D., Wolff, H.G. and Goodell, H., Pain Sensations and Reactions, Williams and Wilkins, New York, 1952. Reprint, Hafner, New York, 1967, 435pp.

Helke, C.J., Krause, J.E., Mantyh, P.W., Couture, R. and Bannon, M.J., Diversity in mammalian tachykinin peptidergic neurons: multiple peptides, receptors and regulatory mechanisms, FASEB J., 4 (1990) 1606–1615.

Kitto, K.F., Haley, J.E. and Wilcox, G.L., Involvement of nitric oxide in spinally mediated hyperalgesia in the mouse, Neurosci. Lett., 148 (1992) 1–5.

Konietzny, F., Perl, E.R., Trevino, D., Light, A. and Hensel, H., Sensory experiences in man evoked by intraneural electrical stimulation of intact cutaneous afferent fibers, Exp. Brain Res., 42 (1981) 219–222.

LaMotte, R.H., Thalhammer, J.G. and Robinson, C.J., Peripheral neural correlates of magnitude of cutaneous pain and hyperalgesia: a comparison of neural events in monkey with sensory judgments in human, J. Neurophysiol., 50 (1983) 1–26.

LaMotte, R.H., Shain, C.N., Simone, D.A. and Tsai, E.F.P., Neurogenic hyperalgesia: psychophysical studies of underlying mechanisms, J. Neurophysiol., 66 (1991) 190–211.

LaMotte, R.H., Lundberg, L.E.R. and Torebjörk, H.E., Pain, hyperalgesia and activity in nociceptive C units in humans after intradermal injection of capsaicin, J. Physiol., 448 (1992) 749–764.

Lewis, T., Pain, Macmillan, London, 1942, 192 pp.

Loh, L. and Nathan, P.W., Painful peripheral states and sympathetic blocks, J. Neurol. Neurosurg. Psychiat., 41 (1978) 664–671.

Lynn, B., Capsaicin: actions on nociceptive C-fibres and therapeutic potential, Pain, 41 (1990) 61–69.

MacDermott, A.B., Mayer, M.L., Westbrook, G.L., Smith, S.J. and Barker, J.L., NMDA-receptor activation increases cytoplasmic calcium concentration in cultured spinal cord neurons, Nature, 321 (1986) 519–522.

Mayer, D.J., Price, D.D. and Becker, D.P., Neurophysiological characterization of the anterolateral spinal cord neurons contributing to pain perception in man, Pain, 1 (1975) 51–58.

Meller, S.T., Pechman, P.S., Gebhart, G.F. and Maves, T.J., Nitric oxide mediates the thermal hyperalgesia produced in a model of neuropathic pain in the rat, Neuroscience, 50 (1992) 7–10.

Merskey, H. (Ed.), Classification of chronic pain: descriptions of chronic pain syndromes and definitions of pain terms, Pain, Suppl. 3 (1986) S217.

Meyer, R.A. and Campbell, J.N., Myelinated nociceptive afferents account for the hyperalgesia that follows a burn to the hand, Science, 213 (1981) 1527–1529.

Ochoa, J., Thermal hyperalgesia as a clinical symptom. In: Willis, W.D. (Ed.), Hyperalgesia and Allodynia, Raven Press, New York, 1992, pp. 151–165.

Ochoa, J. and Torebjörk, E., Sensations evoked by intraneural microstimulation of C nociceptor fibres in human skin nerves, J. Physiol., 415 (1989) 583–599.

Osborne, N.N. and Ghazi, H., The effect of substance P and other tachykinins on inositol phospholipid hydrolysis in rabbit retina, superior colliculus and retinal cultures, Vision Res., 29 (1989) 757–764.

Owens, C.M., Zhang, D. and Willis, W.D., Changes in the response states of primate spinothalamic tract cells caused by mechanical damage of the skin or activation of descending controls, J. Neurophysiol., 67 (1992) 1509–1527.

Palecek, J., Dougherty, P.M., Kim, S.H., Palecková, V., Lekan, H., Chung, J.M, Carlton, S.M. and Willis, W.D., Responses of spinothalamic tract neurons to mechanical and thermal stimuli in an experimental model of peripheral neuropathy in primates, J. Neurophysiol., 68 (1992) 1951–1966.

Palecek, J., Palecková, V. and Willis W.D., The role of nitric oxide in hyperalgesia induced by capsaicin injection in primates. In: Abstracts: 7th World Congress on Pain, IASP Publications, Seattle, 1993, pp. 226–227.

Palecek, J., Palecková, V., Dougherty, P.M. and Willis, W.D., The effect of phorbol esters on the responses of primate spinothalamic neurons to mechanical and thermal stimuli, J. Neurophysiol., 71 (1994a) 529–537.

Palecek, J., Palecková, V., Dougherty, P.M. and Willis, W.D., The effect of trans-ACPD, a metabotropic excitatory amino acid receptor agonist, on the responses of primate spinothalamic tract neurons, Pain, 56 (1994b) 261–269.

Price, D.D. and Mayer, D.J., Neurophysiological characterization of the anterolateral quadrant neurons subserving pain in *M. mulatta*, Pain, 1 (1975) 59–72.

Price, D.D., Hu, J.W., Dubner, R. and Gracely, R.H., Peripheral suppression of first pain and central summation of second pain evoked by noxious heat pulses, Pain, 3 (1977) 57–68.

Price, D.D., Hayes, R.L., Ruda, M. and Dubner, R., Spatial and temporal transformations of input to spinothalamic tract neurons and their relation to somatic sensations, J. Neurophysiol., 41 (1978) 933–947.

Price, D.D., Bennett, G.J. and Rafii, A., Psychophysical observations on patients with neuropathic pain relieved by a sympathetic block, Pain, 36 (1989) 273–288.

Radhakrishnan, V. and Henry, J.L., L-NAME blocks responses to NMDA, substance P and noxious cutaneous stimuli in cat dorsal horn, Neuroreport, 4 (1993) 323–326.

Randic, M., Hecimovic, H. and Ryu, P.D., Substance P modulates glutamate-induced currents in acutely isolated rat dorsal horn neurones, Neurosci. Lett., 117 (1990) 74–80.

Schaible, H.G. and Schmidt, R.F., Effects of an experimental arthritis on the sensory properties of fine articular afferent units, J. Neurophysiol., 54 (1985) 1109–1122.

Schaible, H.G. and Schmidt, R.F., Time course of mechanosensitivity changes in articular afferents during a developing experimental arthritis, J. Neurophysiol., 60 (1988) 2180–2195.

Simone, D.A., Baumann, T.K. and LaMotte, R.H., Dose-dependent pain and mechanical hyperalgesia in humans after intradermal injection of capsaicin, Pain, 38 (1989a) 99–107.

Simone, D.A., Baumann, T.K., Collins, J.G. and LaMotte, R.H. Sensitization of cat dorsal horn neurons to innocuous mechanical stimulation after intradermal injection of capsaicin, Brain Res., 486 (1989b) 185–189.

Simone, D.A., Sorkin, L.S., Oh, U., Chung, J.M., Owens, C., LaMotte, R.H. and Willis, W.D., Neurogenic hyperalgesia: central neural correlates in responses of spinothalamic tract neurons, J. Neurophysiol., 66 (1991) 228–246.

Sorkin, L.S., NMDA evoked an L-NAME sensitive spinal release of glutamate and citrulline, Neuroreport, 4 (1993) 479–482.

Sorkin, L.S. and McAdoo, D.J., Amino acids and serotonin are released into the lumbar spinal cord of the anesthetized cat following intradermal capsaicin injections, Brain Res., 607 (1993) 89–98.

Torebjörk, H.E., Vallbo, A.B. and Ochoa, J.L., Intraneural microstimulation in man: its relation to specificity of tactile sensations, Brain, 110 (1987) 1509–1529.

Torebjörk, H.E., Lundberg, L.E.R. and LaMotte, R.H., Central changes in processing of mechanoreceptive input in capsaicin-induced secondary hyperalgesia in humans, J. Physiol., 448 (1992) 765–780.

Vallbo, A.B., Hagbarth, K.E., Torebjörk, H.E. and Wallin, B.G., Somatosensory, proprioceptive and sympathetic activity in human peripheral nerves, Physiol. Rev., 59 (1979) 919–957.

Vallbo, A.B., Olsson, K.A., Westberg, K.G. and Clark, F.J., Microstimulation of single tactile afferents from the human hand: sensory attributes related to unit type and properties of receptive fields, Brain, 107 (1984) 727–749.

Van Hees, J. and Gybels, J., C nociceptor activity in human nerve during painful and non painful skin stimulation, J. Neurol. Neurosurg. Psychiat., 44 (1981) 600–607.

Westlund, K.N., Carlton, S.M., Zhang, D. and Willis, W.D., Glutamate-immunoreactive terminals synapse on primate spinothalamic tract cells, J. Comp. Neurol., 322 (1992) 519–527.

Willcockson, W.S., Chung, J.M., Hori, Y., Lee, K.H. and Willis, W.D. Effects of iontophoretically released amino acids and amines on primate spinothalamic tract cells, J. Neurosci., 4 (1984a) 732–740.

Willcockson, W.S., Chung, J.M., Hori, Y., Lee, K.H. and Willis, W.D., Effect of iontophoretically released peptides on primate spinothalamic tract cells, J. Neurosci., 4 (1984b) 741–750.

Willis, W.D. (Ed.), Hyperalgesia and Allodynia, Raven Press, New York, 1992, 400 pp.

Willis, W.D. Mechanical allodynia: a role for sensitized nociceptive tract cells with convergent input from mechanoreceptors and nociceptors? APS, 2 (1993) 23–33.

Willis, W.D. and Coggeshall, R.E., Sensory Mechanisms of the Spinal Cord, Plenum Press, New York, 1991, 575 pp.

Willis, W.D., Trevino, D.L., Coulter, J.D. and Maunz, R.A., Responses of primate spinothalamic tract neurons to natural stimulation of hindlimb, J. Neurophysiol., 37 (1974) 358–372.

Willis, W.D., Palecek, J., Palecková, V., Ragland, J. and Dougherty, P.M., Neurokinin receptor antagonists modify the responses of primate STT neurons to cutaneous stimuli, Neurosci. Abstr., 18 (1992) 1023.

Woolf, C.J., Excitability changes in central neurons following peripheral damage: role of central sensitization in the pathogenesis of pain. In: Willis, W.D. (Ed.), Hyperalgesia and Allodynia, Raven Press, New York, 1992, pp. 221–243.

Woolf, C.J. and King, A.E., Subthreshold components of the cutaneous mechanoreceptive fields of dorsal horn neurons in the rat lumbar spinal cord, J. Neurophysiol., 62 (1989) 907–916.

Woolf, C.J., Shortland, P. and Coggeshall, R.E., Peripheral nerve injury triggers central sprouting of myelinated afferents, Nature, 355 (1992) 75–78.

Yaksh, T.L., Behavioral and autonomic correlates of the tactile evoked allodynia produced by spinal glycine inhibition: effects of modulatory receptor systems and excitatory amino acid antagonists, Pain, 37 (1989) 111–123.

Correspondence to: Wm. D. Willis, Jr., MD, PhD, Department of Anatomy and Neurosciences and Marine Biomedical Institute, University of Texas Medical Branch, Galveston, TX 77555-0843, USA. Tel: 409-772-2103; Fax: 409-762-9382.

Proceedings of the 7th World Congress on Pain,
Progress in Pain Research and Management, Vol. 2,
edited by G.F. Gebhart, D.L. Hammond, and T.S.
Jensen, IASP Press, Seattle, © 1994.

22

Electromyographic and Trigeminal Brainstem Neuronal Changes Associated with Inflammatory Irritation of Superficial and Deep Craniofacial Tissues in Rats

James W. Hu, Xian-Min Yu, Mistushiro Sunakawa, Chen Yu Chiang, Daniel A. Haas, Chun L. Kwan, Chih-Mong Tsai, Howard Vernon,[a] and Barry J. Sessle

Faculty of Dentistry, University of Toronto, Ontario, Canada, and
[a]Canadian Memorial Chiropractic College, Toronto, Ontario, Canada

INTRODUCTION

Sensitization of peripheral nociceptors is important in the increased pain sensitivity that develops in the skin immediately surrounding an injury site (so-called primary hyperalgesia, Meyer et al. 1985). However, recent studies also suggest that central as well as peripheral mechanisms are responsible for the hyperalgesia and allodynia that extends beyond the site of cutaneous injury, termed secondary hyperalgesia (LaMotte et al. 1991; Willis 1992). It has been proposed that second-order nociceptive neurons in the spinal dorsal horn are the major sites for this central sensitization in the spinal somatosensory system (Neugebauer and Schaible 1990; Woolf 1992; Cervero et al. 1993; Willis 1993). This central process can be produced by injury or inflammation of deep or visceral tissues and is related to secondary hyperalgesia and manifestations of pain spread and referral associated with deep injury or inflammation (Woolf and Wall 1986; Cook et al. 1987; Hoheisel and Mense

1989; Neugebauer and Schaible 1990). Inflammatory pain may be associated with central opioid changes (Lombard and Besson 1989; Dubner and Ruda 1992), and the initiation and maintenance of the central sensitization process appears to involve N-methyl-D-aspartate (NMDA) receptor mechanisms (Dubner and Ruda 1992; Woolf and Thompson 1992). Recently, nitric oxide (NO) has been suggested as a second messenger for these NMDA receptor mechanisms (Meller and Gebhart 1993).

Our recent studies have sought to determine whether a similar process of central sensitization exists in the trigeminal (V) brainstem sensory nuclear complex and what neurochemical mechanisms may be involved in this process. Our single-unit recording studies have focused on the V subnucleus caudalis because it has been particularly implicated in craniofacial deep pain mechanisms (Sessle and Hu 1991; Hu et al. 1992; Hu 1993; Sessle et al. 1993a,b; Yu et al. 1993b). These studies have been supplemented by studies (Hu et al. 1993; Yu et al. 1993a,c) of possible neuromuscular changes that may accompany neuroplastic changes in the V brainstem complex. We have used mustard oil as a means to produce irritation and inflammation of deep tissues to study the central sensitization process in the V brainstem complex. Mustard oil is an excitant of small-fiber afferents (Reeh et al. 1986; Woolf and Wall 1986; Handwerker et al. 1991) and also acts as an inflammatory irritant (Jancsó et al. 1977; Handwerker and Reeh 1991).

METHODS

Experimentation on all animals conformed to the regulations of the Canadian Council on Animal Care and the Ontario Animals for Research Act and was approved by the University of Toronto Animal Care Committee. Single brainstem units were recorded in the V subnuclei caudalis (1–3 mm behind the obex) or oralis of anesthetized rats paralyzed with a muscle relaxant. Methods and procedures are outlined in detail in our published papers (Hu 1990; Hu et al. 1992; Yu et al. 1993b). A wide range of mechanical, electrical, and thermal stimuli was used to classify each neuron and delineate its mechanoreceptive field (RF) properties. Low-threshold mechanical stimuli included a camel hair brush, and high-threshold mechanical stimuli were applied by watchmaker forceps (pinch). Noxious radiant heat (51–53°C) and bipolar electrical stimulation (2 ms, < 5 mA) were also used for assessment of cutaneous nociceptive properties. A deep RF was documented if no response could be evoked by this wide range of cutaneous stimuli and if a clear response occurred from deep pressure applied by a blunt probe to muscle, bone, tendon, or joint. Furthermore, each neuron functionally classified as a nociceptive skin/mucosa and deep convergent neuron also was classified as either wide dynamic range (WDR) or nociceptive-specific (NS) on the basis of its cutaneous RF properties. In addition, we also tested the excitability of the neuron's responsiveness to electrical stimulation of A-fiber and C-fiber cutaneous afferent inputs. Our aim was to determine whether there are differential neuroplastic effects of cutaneous and deep stimuli on the RF properties of these nociceptive brainstem neurons. Either mineral oil (vehicle for mustard oil) or mustard oil (allyl-isothiocyanate, BDH, Poole) was injected into the deep masseter or tongue (5 mm behind the tongue tip, 3 mm lateral to the tongue midline, and 2 mm below the tongue surface) muscles. Alternatively, either mineral oil or mustard oil also was applied with a cotton swab to the skin 10 mm distal to the cutaneous RF border but overlapping the deep RF of the neuron.

We also conducted a series of electromyographic (EMG) studies in anesthetized, unparalyzed rats to determine if the EMG activity of the jaw and neck muscles can be influenced by mustard oil application to craniofacial tissues. Rats were lightly anesthetized with a mixture of one-third oxygen, two-thirds nitrous oxide, and 0.5–0.8% halothane to achieve a stable plane of anesthesia; noxious pressure applied to the hindpaw could induce a slight flexion reflex response of the hindlimb. EMG activity was recorded by bipolar EMG electrodes (36–40 gauge, single-stranded, Teflon-coated stainless-steel wire; interpolar distance 0.5 cm; exposed tips 0.5 mm) inserted into the ipsilateral digastric and bilateral masseter muscles, and for some experiments, also into the ipsilateral trapezius and bilateral deep neck muscles. Mustard oil (or vehicle) was injected into neck, temporomandibular (TM) joint, or dental tissues. For the neck injection, mustard oil (20%, 20 µl in mineral oil) or mineral oil (20 µl) was injected by a needle into deep paraspinal muscles (Hu et al. 1993). For the TM injection, a preimplanted two-needle assembly with either mustard oil (20%, 20 µl in mineral oil) or mineral oil was placed into the TM region before the EMG recording and injected according to a predetermined schedule (Yu et al. 1992). For the dental injection, mustard oil (98%, 0.25 µl) or mineral oil was applied to a cavity preparation made in the maxillary first molar tooth (Sunakawa et al. 1993a,b).

Inflammation was assessed by the plasma extravasation of Evans' Blue (EB) dye bound to plasma protein (Haas et al. 1992); the EB dye concentration was assessed spectrophotometrically. We also conducted histologic examination and morphometric assessment of the injected tissues to reveal other indicators of inflammation (e.g., congestion and invasion of polymorphonuclear leukocytes; Haas et al. 1992).

The EMG activity of each muscle was amplified (gain: 1000–5000×; bandwidth 30–3000 Hz) and displayed on oscilloscopes, and also recorded on a FM tape recorder, for one minute every 3–5 minutes before the vehicle injection. Immediately after either the vehicle or mustard oil injection, the EMG activity was continuously recorded for 3–5 minutes and thereafter for one minute every 3–5 minutes. The EMG data recorded into the computer was processed off-line with the program Spike2 (CED, Cambridge). The recorded EMG signals were rectified and integrated every second and every 60 seconds to measure the duration of any EMG response induced by mustard oil or vehicle. The integrated EMG area for each 60-second period was used to express EMG activity. The insertion of the injection needle into the deep tissues could itself sometimes induce a small and transient (5–10 second) increase in EMG activity, so we did not begin the injection of the mineral oil or mustard oil until the EMG activity had returned to preinsertion levels. The data analysis did not include the integrated EMG activity associated with any such transient response evoked by insertion of the injection needle.

Before vehicle injection, none of the muscles revealed any variation in EMG activity greater than two standard deviations above the mean EMG amplitude level, so we pooled all preinjection data points for each muscle in each animal to produce a mean value that represented the preinjection level of EMG activity for the muscle in each animal. All postinjection data points were normalized relative to this mean value and expressed as a percentage value of the mean preinjection level of EMG activity. Changes in EMG activity after the injection of either mineral oil or mustard oil were regarded as an increase if one or more EMG data points rose two standard deviations above this mean baseline level.

We also initiated preliminary experiments to test the possible involvement of excitatory amino acid receptor processes in these mustard oil–induced EMG changes: an NMDA noncompetitive inhibitor (MK-801, at a dose of 0.5 mg/kg) and a NO synthase inhibitor (Nω-nitro-L-arginine-methyl-ester [L-NAME], at doses of 10, 30, and 100 mg/kg) were systemically injected 5–10 minutes before mustard oil application. In addition, to test if endogenous opioid receptor mechanisms also might be involved, we administered the opioid antagonist naloxone (1.2–1.3 mg/kg, iv.) 30 minutes after mustard oil application.

RESULTS AND DISCUSSION

CHANGES IN NOCICEPTIVE NEURONS

The injection of mustard oil into the deep masseter muscle enhanced the C-fiber evoked responses of 17 of 39 (44%) nociceptive neurons tested in the rat's subnuclei caudalis and oralis to electrical stimuli applied to their *cutane-*

ous RF (Hu et al. 1992). C-fiber strength electrical stimulation of hypoglossal muscle afferents for about one minute also markedly enhanced the excitability of WDR and NS neurons tested in the subnucleus caudalis (Sessle et al. 1993a). These changes were reversible and were associated with an expansion of the cutaneous RF of the nociceptive neurons, a reduction in their mechanical threshold for activation, and an increase in spontaneous firing. The neuronal changes appeared within 2–5 minutes of the mustard oil injection and lasted for 20–30 minutes; sometimes two phases of mustard oil–induced increased excitability were noted. As we have discussed (Hu et al. 1992; Sessle and Hu 1991; Sessle et al. 1993a), these effects of deep afferent inputs on the cutaneous RF properties of the V nociceptive neurons may relate to neural processes underlying the spread and referral of pain, particularly to cutaneous facial sites. These mechanisms may also contribute to the tenderness and hyperalgesia of superficial tissues that are characteristic of many cases involving injury to deep craniofacial tissues.

The deep application of mustard oil could produce even greater enhancement of the *deep* RF of caudalis nociceptive neurons. A total of 31 caudalis neurons were functionally identified as WDR or NS neurons receiving convergent cutaneous and deep afferent inputs. We tested the effects of mustard oil applied to either tongue muscle or facial skin on their cutaneous and deep RFs (Yu et al. 1993b) and found that the expression of neuroplasticity depended on the site of application of this irritant. Mustard oil injected into the tongue muscle produced a statistically significant and reversible expansion of both the cutaneous and deep RFs (17 of 23 neurons tested). In contrast, application of mustard oil to facial skin resulted in a significant and reversible expansion of the cutaneous RF (7 out of 8 neurons tested), but no deep RF expansion occurred in the 8 neurons tested.

These differential effects of deep and cutaneous afferent inputs may relate to differences in the central sensitization effects between the two types of inputs. While there are differences in neuropeptide content between cutaneous and muscle C-fiber afferents (McMahon et al. 1984), the consequence of these differences on the excitability of central neurons is still unclear. Woolf and Wall (1986), however, have reported that deep (muscle) noxious stimulation at C-fiber strength in spinalized rats produces greater facilitatory effects on the flexion reflex than does cutaneous noxious stimulation at C-fiber strength. Thus, the central effects of activating C-fibers from deep tissue appear to be different from cutaneous C-fiber activation. The time course of the central neuronal changes is much longer than the 3–4 minutes of mustard oil–induced excitation reported with cutaneous primary afferents (Handwerker et al. 1991), thus supporting the view that a central sensitization process contributes to the neuronal changes.

CHANGES IN EMG ACTIVITY

We first conducted a neck EMG study (Hu et al. 1993) to determine if the EMG activity of the jaw and neck muscles could be influenced by the injection of mustard oil into deep paraspinal tissues surrounding the C1 to C3 vertebrae. Vehicle injection (mineral oil, n = 4 rats) did not produce any significant change in EMG activity. In contrast, mustard oil injection (n = 13 rats) induced a statistically significant and reversible increase in EMG activity of the bilateral neck and ipsilateral jaw muscles that was most prominent in the ipsilateral deep neck muscles (Fig. 1A). The increased EMG response evoked by mustard oil was frequently reflected in two phases of enhanced activity. The early phase was initiated immediately (< 20 seconds) following the mustard oil injection and lasted 3 minutes; the second phase occurred 10 to 15 minutes later and lasted 10–15 minutes. The time course of these EMG changes is thus comparable to that (see above) induced by mustard oil in caudalis or oralis neurons (Hu et al. 1992; Yu et al. 1993b), many of which serve as reflex interneurons in jaw and neck motor pathways (Dubner et al. 1978; Sessle and Hu 1991). These findings support the view that the EMG changes are associated with a central sensitization process.

The injection of mustard oil (but not the vehicle, mineral oil) induced an inflammatory reaction in the tissues between the fibers of the rectus capitis posterior muscle that was characterized by congestion and invasion of polymorphonuclear leukocytes (Hu et al. 1993). Plasma extravasation as reflected in increased EB dye content of the tissues also occurred.

We also studied a TM inflammatory model by injecting mustard oil into the periarticular TM tissues of anesthetized rats (Haas et al. 1992; Yu et al. 1992, 1993a). Inflammation was assessed by the plasma extravasation of EB dye, and a spectrophotometric analysis revealed a significantly greater ($P < 0.001$) dye concentration in the injected tissues compared to the contralateral untreated side. A morphometric analysis also revealed a significant increase ($P < 0.001$) in polymorphonuclear leucocyte infiltration compared to the contralateral side (Haas et al. 1992; Yu et al. 1993a). A time-course study of the effect of mustard oil on EB dye extravasation revealed a gradually increasing extravasation of EB dye that was maximal at two hours after administration of mustard oil. In eight anesthetized rats studied to date (Yu et al. 1992), EMG activity was significantly increased above baseline levels in both ipsilateral digastric and masseter muscles after mustard oil injection into the TM region but not after vehicle injection (Fig. 1B). Mustard oil injection into the TM region provoked a strong early phase of EMG increase that gradually subsided. These effects lasted for several minutes, in contrast to the more

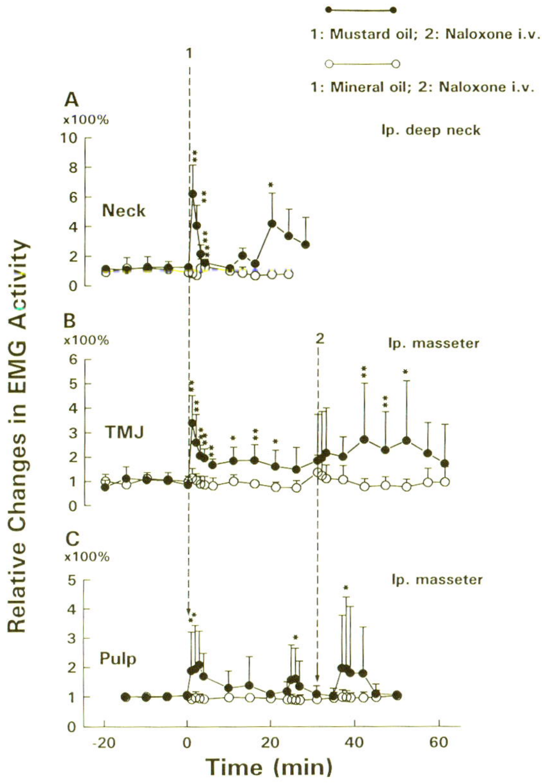

Fig. 1. Changes in EMG activity induced by application of mineral oil or mustard oil to: **A:** the deep paraspinal tissues surrounding the C1–3 vertebrae (mineral oil, n = 4 rats; mustard oil, n = 13 rats); **B:** the temporomandibular (TM) region (mineral oil, n = 6 rats; mustard oil, n = 8 rats); and **C:** the maxillary first molar (mineral oil, n = 6 rats; mustard oil, n = 8 rats). The mean (± SD) data shown are normalized values relative to the mean value of the preinjection level of EMG activity (= 100%) in each rat. Changes in EMG activity of rats receiving mustard oil or mineral oil are indicated by filled or unfilled circles, respectively. * $P < 0.05$ and ** $P < 0.01$ (Wilcoxon test) indicate significant difference between preinjection and postinjection levels of EMG activity. Only one prominent EMG increase induced by mustard oil injected into each tissue has been illustrated. Mineral oil applied to deep paraspinal tissues of the neck, the TM joint region, or the tooth did not induce any significant EMG increase. In contrast, mustard oil induced significant increases in EMG activity of the neck muscles (bilateral deep neck muscles, ipsilateral trapezius) or jaw muscles (ipsilateral digastric and masseter muscles). The opiate antagonist naloxone (1.2–1.3 mg/kg, iv.) was injected in animals receiving mustard oil or mineral oil application to TM region or tooth. When it was administered after the disappearance of the mustard oil–induced EMG response, another significant increase in EMG activity occurred and lasted for 10 minutes. In contrast, administration of naloxone in rats receiving mineral oil did not produce any significant increase in EMG activity (**B** and **C**).

transient EMG effects observed in cats when other algesic compounds such as bradykinin and histamine are applied to TM tissues (Broton and Sessle 1988). The findings suggest that increased EMG activity of jaw muscles may be associated with TM inflammatory conditions and involve a central sensitization process. Moreover, local anesthetic (lidocaine, 1.4 mg/kg) injected into the TM region before the mustard oil injection blocked the EMG activity (but not plasma extravasation) (Yu et al. 1993a). Mustard oil is a small-fiber excitant (see above), so this finding points to the necessity of small-fiber afferent activation in reflexively inducing the central sensitization process after deep injury.

Additional preliminary data also showed that the enhanced EMG activity induced by mustard oil could be blocked by the systemic administration of either the noncompetitive NMDA receptor antagonist, MK-801 (0.5 mg/kg, iv., n = 16 rats), or the NO synthase inhibitor, (L-NAME, 30 and 100 mg/kg but not 10 mg/kg and vehicle injection, iv., n = 24 rats). We have also recently found that MK-801 (0.1 mg/kg, n=5; 0.01 mg/kg, n=5) injected into the third ventricle can also block the evoked EMG activity. These findings suggest that NO and NMDA receptor mechanisms may be involved in the central V neuroplastic changes that we have documented and are consistent with other studies (Dubner and Ruda 1992; Woolf and Thompson 1992; Meller and Gebhart 1993) pointing to their involvement in central sensitization.

The involvement of opioids in the modulation of pain is well known (Basbaum and Fields 1984; Hammond 1986; Sessle 1987; Dubner and Ruda 1992). Lombard and Besson (1989) tested opioid involvement in inflammatory-related pain and showed that the opioid antagonist naloxone (1 mg/kg, iv.) could induce a significant increase in the spontaneous firing as well as enhancement of C-fiber-related responses of dorsal horn nociceptive neurons in polyarthritic rats. We tested the possible involvement of endogenous opioid mechanisms in the increased EMG activities induced by the TM injection of mustard oil by administering naloxone (1.3 mg/kg, iv.) 30 minutes after the mustard oil injection to see if it "rekindled" the EMG activity that had returned to baseline levels by this time (Fig. 1B). The resulting increase of EMG activity suggests that naloxone may have counteracted an opioid suppressive mechanism triggered by the mustard oil–induced inflammatory process or deep afferent input activation. However, naloxone (1.3 mg/kg, iv.), injected 5 minutes before the application of mustard oil did cause significant enhancement of EMG activity induced by the mustard oil injection but had no effect on the extravasation, and did not cause any EMG changes when it was applied either before or after mineral oil injection into the TM region (Yu et al. 1993a).

Another model of the central sensitization process has recently been tested by applying mustard oil directly into the tooth (Sunakawa et al. 1993a,b). The rationale for these experiments is based on the notion that some types of toothache may be associated with activation of pulpal C-fiber afferents, and the possibility that this pain also may reflect a central sensitization process in tooth pulp-related V brainstem sensory and motor neuronal pathways. Mustard oil (n = 8 rats) applied to the first maxillary molar (Sunakawa et al. 1993a,b) evoked a significant increase in EMG activity, often with early and late phases, in the ipsilateral masseter muscle (Fig. 1C). No significant EMG changes occurred following mineral oil application to the tooth (n = 6), or in pulpectomized rats following mustard oil application to the tooth (n = 4). In accordance with our findings outlined above, naloxone (1.2 mg/kg, iv., 30 minutes after mustard oil application to the tooth) also could induce a late enhancement of EMG activity (Fig. 1C).

CONCLUSION

This chapter provides documentation that stimulation of different craniofacial sites as well as cervical paraspinal tissues by an inflammatory irritant results in an inflammatory response in these tissues and in a sustained and reversible activation of jaw or neck muscles. The enhanced EMG activity evoked from the various tissues injected with mustard oil and its abolition by local anesthesia of the injected tissues demonstrate that these enhanced EMG effects can be attributed to reflex responses involving segmental as well as suprasegmental pathways, as opposed to direct effects on muscles by the peripheral spread of mustard oil. In neck injection experiments, activation of neck muscles was more prominent following the mustard oil injection, whereas activation of jaw muscles was more prominent following the mustard oil injection into TM or dental tissues. These results suggest a segmental or somatotopic organization of EMG responses in the head and neck region. The latency and time course of the mustard oil–induced increases in EMG activity are also comparable to the temporal features of the mustard oil–induced increased excitability of sensory neurons in the V spinal tract nucleus, which are the sites of reflex interneurons involved in craniofacial and cervical reflex pathways as well as projection neurons contributing to ascending somatosensory pathways (Dubner et al. 1978; Rossignol et al. 1988; Olsson and Westberg 1989). However, the time courses of both the increased EMG activity and the neuronal hyperexcitability induced by mustard oil (Hu et al. 1992; Yu et al. 1992, 1993a,c) are different from the temporal features of the inflammation process, which may last more than two hours after the application of mustard oil (Reeh et al. 1986; Haas et al. 1992). One factor limiting the duration of the V neuronal and EMG changes may be opioid depressive mechanisms induced by the mustard oil–evoked afferent input. Our data of "rekindling" of EMG activity by the opiate antagonist naloxone demonstrate the involvement of opioid mechanisms in the neuroplastic changes associated with deep tissue injury. Our preliminary EMG data also have raised the possibility that NMDA receptor and NO mechanisms may be involved in the mustard oil–induced changes. These EMG findings are supported by preliminary data obtained from caudalis nociceptive neurons where three of five skin and deep convergent nociceptive caudalis neurons demonstrated a second (i.e., "rekindling") RF expansion following naloxone administration after the initial mustard oil–induced RF expansion had subsided.

In addition to their significance in revealing V central sensitization and possible neurochemical mechanisms involved in the neuroplastic changes, these findings also have clinical significance. They provide insights into how increased cutaneous sensitivity, spread and referral of pain, and associated neuromuscular changes may occur after craniofacial injury or inflammation. The findings also point out the need for therapeutic approaches to reduce nociceptive inputs to the CNS (e.g., with local anesthesia) or their effects (e.g., with opiate drugs) that can potentially prolong posttraumatic craniofacial pain by the central neuroplastic changes that they may induce (e.g., Dubner 1991; Woolf 1992; Mense 1993).

ACKNOWLEDGMENTS

We thank Ken MacLeod for his technical help. This report is supported by U.S. NIH grants DE09559 and DE04786, Canadian MRC grant MT-12286, and funds from the Canadian Memorial Chiropractic College.

REFERENCES

Basbaum, A.I. and Fields, H.L., Endogenous pain control systems; brainstem spinal pathways and endorphin circuitry, Ann. Rev. Neurosci., 7 (1984) 309–338.

Broton, J.G. and Sessle, B.J., Reflex excitation of masticatory muscles induced by algesic chemicals applied to the temporomandibular joint of the cat, Arch. Oral Biol., 33 (1988) 741–747.

Cervero, F., Laird, J.M.A. and Pozo, M.A., Selective changes of receptive field properties of spinal nociceptive neurones induced by visceral noxious stimulation in the cat, Pain, 51 (1992) 335–342.

Cook, A.J., Woolf, C.J., Wall, P.D. and McMahon, S.B., Dynamic receptive field plasticity in rat spinal cord dorsal horn following C-primary afferent input, Nature, 325 (1987) 151–153.

Dubner, R., Pain and hyperalgesia following tissue injury: new mechanisms and new treatment, Pain, 44 (1991) 213–214.

Dubner, R. and Ruda, M.A., Activity-dependent neuronal plasticity following tissue injury and inflammation, Trends in Neurosci., 15 (1992) 96–102.

Dubner, R., Sessle, B.J. and Storey, A.T., The Neural Basis of Oral and Facial Function, Plenum Press, New York, 1978, 483 pp.

Haas, D.A., Nakanishi, O., MacMillan, R.E., Jordan, R.C. and Hu, J.W., Development of an orofacial model of acute inflammation in the rat, Arch. Oral Biol., 37 (1992) 417–422.

Hammond, D.L., Control systems for nociceptive afferent processing: the descending inhibitory pathways. In: Yaksh, T.L. (Ed.), Spinal Afferent Processing, New York, Plenum Press, 1986, pp. 363–390.

Handwerker, H.O., Forster, C. and Kischhoff, C., Discharge patterns of human C-fibers induced by itching and burning stimuli, J. Neurophysiol., 66 (1991) 307–315.

Handwerker, H.O. and Reeh, P.W., Pain and inflammation, In: M.R. Bond, J.E. Charlton and C.J. Woolf (Eds.), Proceedings of the VIth World Congress on Pain. Pain Research and Clinical Management, Vol. 4. Elsevier, Amsterdam, 1991, pp. 59–70.

Hoheisel, U. and Mense, S., Long-term changes in discharge behaviour of cat dorsal horn neurones following noxious stimulation of deep tissues, Pain, 36 (1989) 239–247.

Hu, J.W., Response properties of nociceptive and non-nociceptive neurons in the rat's trigeminal subnucleus caudalis (medullary dorsal horn) related to cutaneous and deep craniofacial afferent stimulation and modulation by diffuse noxious inhibitory controls, Pain, 41 (1990) 331–345.

Hu, J.W., Cephalic myofascial pain pathways. In: J. Olesen and J. Schoenen (Eds.), Tension-Type Headache: Classification, Mechanisms and Treatment, Raven Press, New York, 1993, pp.69–77.

Hu, J.W., Sessle, B.J., Raboisson, P., Dallel, R. and Woda, A., Stimulation of craniofacial muscle afferents induces prolonged facilitatory effects in trigeminal nociceptive brain-stem neurones, Pain, 48 (1992) 53–60.

Hu, J.W., Yu, X.–M., Vernon, H. and Sessle, B.J., Excitatory effects on neck and jaw muscle activity of inflammatory irritant applied to cervical paraspinal tissues, Pain, 55 (1993) 243–250.

Jancsó, G., Kiraly, E. and Jancsó-Gábor, A., Pharmacologically induced selective degeneration of chemosensitive primary sensory neurones, Nature, 270 (1977) 741–743.

LaMotte, R.H., Shain, C.N., Simone, D.A. and Tsai, E.-F. P., Neurogenic hyperalgesia: psychophysical studies of underlying mechanisms, J. Neurophysiol., 66 (1991) 190–211.

Lombard, M.C. and Besson, J.-M., Electrophysiological evidence for a tonic activity of the spinal cord intrinsic opioid systems in a chronic pain model, Brain Res., 477 (1989) 48–56.

McMahon, S.B., Sykova, E., Wall, P.D., Woolf, C.J. and Gibson, S.J., Neurogenic extravasation and substance P levels are low in muscle as compared to skin in the rat hindlimb, Neurosci. Lett., 52 (1984) 235–240.

Meller, S.T. and Gebhart, G.F., Nitric oxide (NO) and nociceptive processing in the spinal cord, Pain, 52 (1993) 127–136.

Mense, S., Nociception from skeletal muscle in relation to clinical muscle pain, Pain, 54, (1993) 241–289.

Meyer, R. A., Campbell, J.N. and Raja, S.N., Peripheral neural mechanisms of cutaneous hyperalgesia, Adv. Pain Res. Ther., 9 (1985) 53–57.

Neugebauer, V. and Schaible, H.-G., Evidence for a central component in the sensitization of spinal neurons with joint input during development of acute arthritis in cat's knee, J. Neurophysiol., 64 (1990) 299–311.

Olsson, K.Å. and Westberg, K.-G., Interneurones in the trigeminal motor system. In: D. van Steenberghe and A. De Laat (Eds.), Electromyography of Jaw Reflexes in Man, Leuven University Press, Leuven, Belgium, 1989, pp. 19–50.

Reeh, P.W., Kocher, L. and Jung, S., Does neurogenic inflammation alter the sensitivity of unmyelinated nociceptors in the rat? Brain Res., 384 (1986) 42–51.

Rossignol, S., Lund, J.P. and Drew. T., The role of sensory inputs in regulating patterns of rhythmical movements in higher vertebrates. In: A.H. Cohen, S. Rossignol and S. Grillner (Eds.), Neural Control of Rhythmic Movements in Vertebrates. John Wiley & Sons, New

York, 1988, pp. 201–283.
Sessle, B.J., The neurobiology of facial and dental pain: present knowledge, future directions, J. Dent. Res. 66 (1987) 962–981.
Sessle, B.J. and Hu, J.W., Mechanisms of pain arising from articular tissues, Can. J. Physiol. Pharmacol., 69 (1991) 617–626.
Sessle, B.J., Hu, J.W. and Yu, X.-M., Brainstem mechanisms of referred pain and hyperalgesia in the orofacial and temporomandibular region. In: L. Vecchiet, D. Albe-Fessard and U. Lindblom (Eds.), New Trends in Referred Pain and Hyperalgesia. Pain Research and Clinical Management, Vol. 7. Elsevier, Amsterdam, 1993a, pp. 59–71.
Sessle, B.J., Yu, X.-M. and Hu, J.W., Trigeminal (V) brainstem neuronal plasticity induced by application of inflammatory irritant to cutaneous and deep tissue. In: Abstracts: 7th World Congress on Pain, IASP Publication, Seattle, 1993b, 131.
Sunakawa, M., Chiang, C.Y., Hu, J.W. and Sessle, B. J., Jaw electromyographic (EMG) activity induced by application of algesic chemicals to the rat tooth pulp, Soc. Neurosci. Abst., 19, 1993a, 1571.
Sunakawa, M., Chiang, C.Y., Kwan, C.L., Hu, J. W. and Sessle, B.J., Increased jaw electromyographic activity induced by application of inflammatory irritant to rat tooth pulp. In: Abstracts: 7th World Congress on Pain, IASP Publications, Seattle, 1993b, 543.
Willis, W. D., Hyperalgesia and allodynia: summary and overview. In: Willis, W.D. (Ed.), Hyperalgesia and Allodynia, Raven Press, New York, 1992, pp. 1–11.
Willis, W.D., Mechanical allodynia: a role for sensitized nociceptive tract cells with convergent input from mechanoreceptors and nociceptors? APS J., 2 (1993) 23–33.
Woolf, C.J., Excitability changes in central neurons following peripheral damage: role of central sensitization in the pathogenesis of pain, In: Willis, W.D. (Ed.), Hyperalgesia and Allodynia. Raven Press, New York, 1992, pp. 221–243.
Woolf, C.J. and Thompson, S.W.N., The induction and maintenance of central sensitization is dependent on N-methyl-D-aspartic acid receptor activation; implications for the treatment of post-injury pain hypersensitivity states, Pain, 44 (1991) 293–299.
Woolf, C.J. and Wall, P.D., Relative effectiveness of C primary afferent fibers of different origins in evoking a prolonged facilitation of the flexor reflex in the rat, J. Neurosci., 6 (1986) 1433–1442.
Yu, X.-M., Hu, J.W., Vernon, H. and Sessle, B.J., Temporomandibular inflammatory irritant induces increased activity of jaw muscles, J. Dent. Res., (Special Issue) 72 (1992) 603.
Yu, X.-M., Hu, J.W., Haas, D. A., Vernon, H. and Sessle, B.J., Opioid involvement in jaw electromyographic (EMG) responses induced by injection of inflammatory irritant into temporomandibular joint (TMJ). In: Abstracts: 7th World Congress on Pain, IASP Publications, Seattle, 1993a, 544.
Yu, X.-M., Sessle, B. J. and Hu, J. W., Differential effects of cutaneous and deep application of inflammatory irritant on the mechanoreceptive field properties of trigeminal brain stem nociceptive neurons, J. Neurophysiol., 70 (1993b) 1704–1707.
Yu, X.-M., Sessle, B. J. and Hu, J.W., Opioid involvement in electromyographic (EMG) and neuronal responses induced by injection of inflammatory irritant into deep tissues, Soc. Neurosci. Abst., 19 (1993c) 108.

Correspondence to: Barry J. Sessle, Faculty of Dentistry, University of Toronto, 142 Edward Street, Toronto, Ontario M5G 1G6, Canada. Tel: 416-979-4921; Fax: 416-979-4936.

Proceedings of the 7th World Congress on Pain,
Progress in Pain Research and Management, Vol. 2,
edited by G.F. Gebhart, D.L. Hammond, and T.S.
Jensen, IASP Press, Seattle, © 1994.

23

Receptor and Cellular Mechanisms Involved in Mustard Oil–Induced Activation of Dorsal Horn Neurons

Fiona E. Munro,[a] Marie R. Young,[a]
Susan M. Fleetwood-Walker,[a]
Rachel M.C. Parker,[a] and Rory Mitchell[b]

[a]Department of Preclinical Veterinary Sciences, Royal (Dick) School of Veterinary Studies, University of Edinburgh, Summerhall, Edinburgh, and [b]MRC Brain Metabolism Unit, Edinburgh, UK

INTRODUCTION

For many years substance P (SP) has been a prominent candidate for the transmitter of primary afferent nociceptive fibers (Henry 1976). Although considerable evidence suggests a role for SP (and NK_1 receptors) in nociceptive transmission (Coderre et al. 1993; Maggi et al. 1993), it is unlikely to be the only relevant transmitter. SP together with neurokinin A (NKA) and excitatory amino acids (EAAs) are released into the dorsal horn by noxious or high-intensity stimulation of afferents (Duggan et al. 1990; Skilling et al. 1988; Petermann et al. 1986). Evidence from both electrophysiological and reflex studies suggests that transmitters such as NKA and EAAs also may be crucial to nociception through their actions at NK_2, NMDA, and non-NMDA receptors (Coderre et al. 1993).

Several lines of evidence point to a role for NKA in nociceptive transmission. Ligand binding (Yashpal et al. 1990) and mRNA hybridization studies (Takeda and Krause 1991) have confirmed that there are NK_2 receptors in the spinal cord. NKA is present in primary sensory neurons (Ogawa et al. 1985) and is released by capsaicin from primary afferent terminals (Saria et al.

1986). In a model of acute nociception, we have previously shown that the responses of dorsal horn neurons to brief thermal (but not mechanical) noxious cutaneous stimuli are inhibited by selective NK_2 but not NK_1 receptor antagonists (Fleetwood-Walker et al. 1990, 1992a). Also in an in vitro spinal cord/dorsal root preparation, neuronal activity evoked by brief application of capsaicin to the dorsal root ganglion is inhibited by a selective NK_2 antagonist (Urban et al. 1992). Following both noxious mechanical and noxious thermal stimuli, release of NKA-immunoreactive material is detected throughout the dorsal horn in a diffuse pattern (Duggan et al. 1990; Hope et al. 1990) and intrathecal administration of NKA gives rise to behavioral responses indicative of pain (Cridland and Henry 1986; Fleetwood-Walker et al. 1990).

The EAA glutamate is present at high levels in local interneurons of the dorsal horn (Rizzoli 1968; Fagg and Foster 1983; Storm-Mathisen and Ottersen 1987) as well as in primary afferent terminals, as demonstrated by immunolabeling of granular vesicles following rhizotomy (DeBiasi and Rustioni 1988). Upon noxious cutaneous stimulation or low- or high-intensity electrical stimulation to peripheral nerves, glutamate is released (Skilling et al. 1988), where it may act via several receptors (Schoepp et al. 1990a; Watkins et al. 1990). The ionotropic group of receptors, including α-amino-3-hydroxy-5-isoxazole-4-propionate (AMPA) and N-methyl-D-aspartate (NMDA) types, have been extensively studied and it is now well established that the NMDA receptor is involved in hypersensitized states such as long-term potentiation (LTP) in the hippocampus (Collingridge 1992) and wind-up in the spinal cord (Davies and Lodge 1987; Dickenson and Sullivan 1987, 1990; Thompson et al. 1990). A metabotropic group of glutamate receptors (mGlu), linked to G-proteins, also may be involved in such transmission. Studies have demonstrated a role for mGlu receptors, including a role in an NMDA receptor-independent model of LTP (Bortolotto and Collingridge 1993). Previous studies have demonstrated that 1-amino-cyclopentane-1,3-dicarboxylic acid (ACPD), a metabotropic glutamate receptor agonist (Irving et al. 1990), can augment the actions of ionotropic agonist-induced activity in spinal cord preparations (Cerne and Randic 1992; Bleakman et al. 1992), although the cellular mechanism responsible has yet to be elucidated.

In our study, we used a prolonged noxious chemical stimulus to investigate the involvement of NK_1, NK_2, mGlu receptors, and protein kinase C (PKC) in the sustained activation of dorsal horn neurons. The model used is topical cutaneous application of mustard oil (allyl isothiocyanate), a chemical irritant that selectively activates C (and occasionally some A-delta) afferent fibers (Heapy et al. 1987).

METHODS

ELECTROPHYSIOLOGY

We conducted experiments on male Wistar rats (250–340 g) anaesthetized with intravenous α-chloralose (60 mg/kg) and urethane (1200 mg/kg) after induction with halothane. Supplementary doses of α-chloralose were given as required. Rectal temperature was continuously monitored and maintained between 37–38°C. The rats respired spontaneously, but oxygen was supplied to the area of the tracheal cannula to enrich the inspired air.

The thoraco-lumbar spinal column was supported by clamps under the lateral processes and a laminectomy (segments L1–L4) was performed. To increase the recording stability, a 2% agar solution was injected under the spinal bone at the rostral end of the laminectomy and then poured over the exposed cord. A core of agar was removed from above the recording region, the dura carefully cut, and a pool of liquid paraffin applied to the region.

Extracellular recordings were made via the central barrel (4 M NaCl pH 4.0–4.5) of a seven-barreled glass microelectrode. One side barrel contained 1 M NaCl (pH 4.0–4.5) for automatic current balancing and current controls. Another side barrel contained Pontamine Sky Blue (2% in 0.5 M sodium acetate) for determination of neuronal location by ejection at the recording site followed by histological examination. The other barrels of the electrode contained NK_1, NK_2 or mGlu receptor antagonists or PKC inhibitors, which were applied locally by ionophoresis over a range of currents (10–80nA) for several minutes. NK_1 (L668,169) and NK_2 (L659,874) antagonists were prepared as 0.15 mM solutions in distilled water with 0.3% dimethylformamide, and the NK_1 antagonist GR82334 was a 1 mM aqueous solution; all were pH 4.5–5.0. Metabotropic glutamate (mGlu) antagonists (L- and D-2-amino-3-phosphoproprionate, L- and D-AP3) and (RS)-4-carboxy-3-hydroxyphenylglycine (CHPG) were 10 mM aqueous solutions pH 8.0–8.5. PKC inhibitors chelerythrine (1 mM aqueous solution) and GF109203X (0.2 mM aqueous solution with 0.2% dimethylformamide) were pH 4.0.

All neurons were located in dorsal horn laminae IV/V, had excitatory receptive fields on the ipsilateral hindlimb (excluding glabrous skin), and were multireceptive (i.e., displayed responses to both noxious and innocuous stimuli). Neurons were initially found by their responsiveness to widespread manual brushing of the ipsilateral hindlimb. Cutaneous receptive fields of the

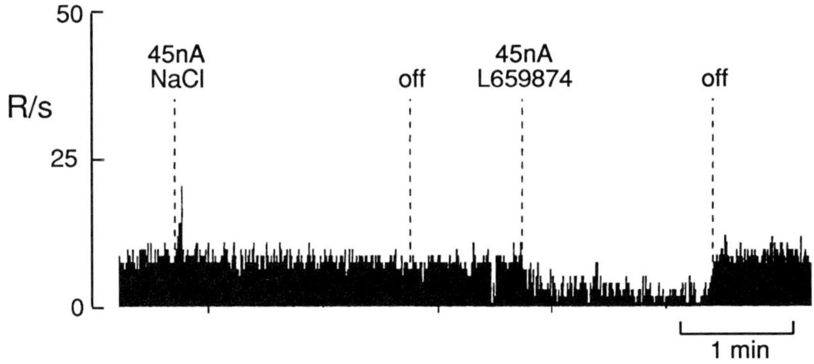

Fig. 1. Typical inhibitory effects of the NK_2 antagonist L659,874 on mustard oil–evoked activity of laminae IV/V dorsal horn neurons. Ionophoretic application of NaCl had no effect, whereas L659,874 consistently caused greater than 50% inhibition of evoked activity.

neurons were first localized by responses to manual brush, then the more restricted pinch and noxious heat fields were identified. The mustard oil (5–20% in paraffin oil) was applied topically with a paintbrush to the receptive fields.

BIOCHEMISTRY

To examine the subcellular translocation of protein kinase C (PKC, a facet of its activation in response to external stimuli), we performed the following [^{3}H]PDBu binding assay in spinal cord tissue ipsilateral/contralateral to mustard oil stimulation.

Male Wistar rats (273–330 g) were briefly anaesthetized with halothane, and mustard oil (7–20%) was applied three times to the left hindfoot and leg over a 15-minute period. This treated leg was bandaged to avoid cross-contamination and after one hour the rats were killed and the spinal cords removed and hemisected.

Each side of the spinal cord was separately homogenized in 0.4 ml of ice-cold buffer containing 20 mM Tris-HCl at pH 7.5, 50 mM 2-mercaptoethanol, 2 mM EDTA and 1 mM phenylmethylsulphonylfluoride with 0.01% leupeptin and 20 μM trans-epoxysuccinyl-L-leucylamido-(4-guanidino)butane (E-64). The samples were then centrifuged at 25,000 × g for 20 minutes at 4°C. The supernatant and pellet were carefully separated and the pellet was rehomogenized in 0.3 ml Tris-BSA (50 mM Tris HCl, pH 7.4), with 4 mg/ml essential fatty acid–free bovine serum albumin. While membrane binding was carried out in Tris-BSA, cytosolic binding assays additionally contained 1 mM $CaCl_2$ and 75 mM magnesium acetate and 1.35 mg/ml sonicated

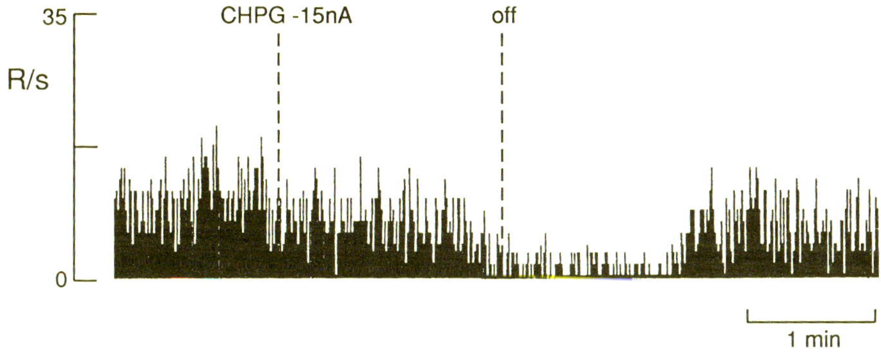

Fig. 2. An example of the inhibition of mustard oil–induced firing of a dorsal horn neuron by the metabotropic glutamate receptor antagonist CHPG. In this case recovery was observed within two minutes of termination of ionophoresis of the antagonist.

phosphatidylserine, sodium salt. Assays were conducted in a total volume of 275 µl (30 min, 37°C), with 5 nM [^{3}H]PDBu (approximately 0.03 µCi per tube) and dimethylformamide (0.5% final) or 10 µM PDBu in dimethylformamide for total and nonspecific binding measurements, respectively. Tissue samples gave a total binding of less than 10% of total radioactivity present. Protein was precipitated at 4°C by the addition of 100 µl of 12 mg/ml bovine gamma globulin and 300 µl of 24% polyethyleneglycol 8000 in 50 mM Tris-HCl (pH 7.4). After 20 minutes on ice, assay tubes were centrifuged (12,000 × g, 5 min, 4°C), the supernatant aspirated, and the [^{3}H] radioactivity in each pellet determined after solubilization.

All laboratory chemicals were from Sigma Chemical Co., Poole, Dorset, UK, except phosphatidyl serine from Lipid Products Ltd., Nutfield, Sussex, UK. Radioligand was from Du Pont NEN, Stevenage, Herts., UK. Drugs were from Cambridge Research Biochemicals Ltd., Northwich, Cheshire, UK; Calbiochem-Novabiochem, Nottingham, Notts., UK; Tocris Neuramin, Churchill Building, Langford House, Langford, Bristol, Avon, UK; or were gifts from Merck, Sharp and Dohme and Glaxo Group Research.

RESULTS

After application of the C-nociceptor-selective chemical algogen mustard oil, virtually all the multireceptive neurons showed a large and prolonged increase in activity (149 ± 36-fold of background, mean ± S.E.M.). In most cases, the steady elevated firing rate was achieved by repeated application of mustard oil 3–5 times to the same site over a period of 10–15 minutes.

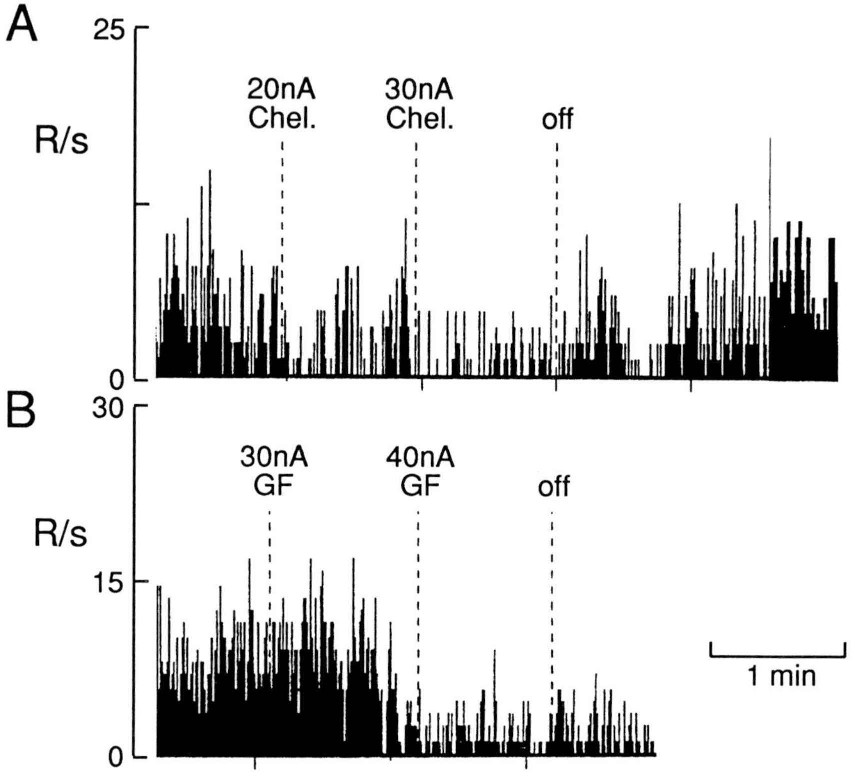

Fig. 3. The selective PKC inhibitors (**A**) chelerythrine and (**B**) GF109203X caused marked, yet recoverable inhibition of mustard oil–evoked activity.

The selective NK_2 antagonist L-659,874 (10–80 nA) caused a clear and maintained inhibition of the elevated activity, to 50 ± 7% mean ± S.E.M., of prior control level in 23 of 24 cells (Fig. 1). Recovery was observed in 13 of 17 cases examined after terminating ionophoresis of L659,874. In contrast, the two selective NK_1 antagonists L668,169 and GR82334 (20–80 nA) rarely inhibited mustard oil–evoked activity (in 1 of 11 and 3 of 11 cases, respectively). The mustard oil–evoked activity in many cells (n = 15) was unaffected by NK_1 antagonists but was inhibited by the NK_2 antagonist L659,874 (Munro et al. 1993).

Selective antagonists for mGlu (L-AP3 and CHPG) and NK_2 (L659,874) receptors also reliably inhibited the mustard oil–induced wind-up of neuronal activity. L-AP3 (–15 to –50 nA) and CHPG (–15 to –55 nA) inhibited the

Table I
Mustard oil–induced translocation of specific [^{3}H] PDBu binding sites
(% of total specific binding on control contralateral side)

	Cystolic Fraction	Membrane Fraction
Control (contralateral to mustard oil)	73.7 ± 2.5	26.2 ± 2.4
Test (ipsilateral to mustard oil)	37.6 ± 5.0	40.5 ± 4.8

Note: The proportion of [^{3}H] PDBu binding sites in the membrane fraction was significantly greater on the test side (mean 52%) than on the control side (mean 26%) $P < 0.05$, Wilcoxon test). Values are the means ± S.E.M. from nine separate experiments.

mustard oil–evoked activity (by 68 ± 7% and 56 ± 9% mean ± S.E.M.) in 11 of 16 and 7 of 8 cells, respectively (Fig. 2). Recovery was sometimes but not always observed. The stereoisomer of L-AP3, D-AP3 (which has a much lower affinity for mGlu receptors; Schoepp et al. 1990b) (–15 to –55 nA) had no effect in 5 of 5 cells.

The selective PKC inhibitors chelerythrine and GF109203X caused marked inhibition of mustard oil–induced activity in 8 of 9 and 8 of 8 cases respectively (Fig. 3). Rapid recovery was seen in the majority of cases after removal of the PKC inhibitor. In contrast, activity evoked by continuous innocuous brushing was completely unaffected by the PKC inhibitors (data not shown, n = 5).

In rats treated with mustard oil to one distal hindlimb, a significant translocation of specific [^{3}H]PDBu binding sites from the cytosolic to membrane fraction was observed in ipsilateral spinal segments L1–L5 in comparison with the contralateral (control) side (Table I).

DISCUSSION

These results indicate that both NK_2 and mGlu receptors play a crucial role in mediating the sustained excitation of lamina IV/V dorsal horn neurons elicited by cutaneous application of mustard oil. As mustard oil excites largely C-fibers (Heapy et al. 1987), this implies a role for NK_2 and mGlu receptors in the transmission of nociceptive information. For tachykinins, this finding agrees with our previous studies showing that ionophoretic administration of NK_2 but not NK_1 receptor antagonists inhibited the responses of both rat and cat dorsal horn neurons to brief noxious thermal stimuli applied to their cutaneous receptive fields (Fleetwood-Walker et al. 1990, 1991, 1992a,b).

This evidence for a role of mGlu receptors in sustained cutaneous nociceptive inputs that lead to hyperalgesia is novel and contrasts with data from Thompson et al. (1992) who found no evidence for inhibition by L-AP3 of ventral root potentials evoked by high-intensity stimulation of dorsal roots in an in vitro spinal cord preparation. Despite several reports of the attenuation of wind-up by NMDA receptor antagonists (Davies and Lodge 1987; Dickenson and Sullivan 1987, 1990; Thompson et al. 1990), we found no evidence for attenuation of mustard oil–evoked responses by the D-isomer of AP3 (which is a weak antagonist at the NMDA receptor [Schoepp et al. 1990b]). This may simply be a consequence of low potency of the antagonist or it may indicate a genuine mechanistic difference in the present case.

We also carried out a preliminary investigation of the intracellular mechanisms underlying the sensitization of spinal dorsal horn neurons brought about by the repeated application of mustard oil. The role of PKC in this model was clearly indicated by two separate approaches: (1) the inhibition of electrophysiological responses by ionophoretic administration of selective PKC inhibitors, and (2) translocation/activation of PKC in response to mustard oil. Although many other mechanisms may contribute to the processing of sustained nociceptive inputs and the integral sensitization of dorsal horn neurons which they bring about, this preliminary evidence clearly identifies a crucial role of PKC. Since both NK_2 and some mGlu receptors bring about hydrolysis of phosphoinositides, it seems likely that either or both of these receptors could well contribute to PKC activation by means of elevation of cellular diglyceride contact.

REFERENCES

Bleakman, D., Rusin K.I., Chard P.S., Glaum S.R. and Miller R.J., Metabotropic glutamate receptors potentiate ionotropic glutamate responses in rat dorsal horn, Molec. Pharmacol., 42 (1992) 192–196.

Bortollotto, Z.A. and Collingridge, G.L., Characterisation of long term potentiation induced by the activation of glutamate metabotropic receptors in area CA1 of the hippocampus, Neuropharmacology, 32 (1993) 1–9.

Cerne, R. and Randic, M., Modulation of AMPA and NMDA responses in rat spinal dorsal horn neurons by trans-ACPD, Neurosci. Letts., 144 (1992) 180–184.

Coderre, T,J., Katz, J., Vaccarino, A.L. and Melzack, R., Contribution of central neuroplasticity to pathological pain: review of clinical and experimental evidence, Pain, 52 (1993) 259–285.

Collingridge, G.L., The mechanism of induction of NMDA receptor-dependant long-term potentiation in the hippocampus, Exp. Physiol., 77 (1992) 771–797.

Cridland, R.A. and Henry, J.L., Comparison of the effects of substance P, neurokinin A, physalaemin and eledoisin in facilitating a nociceptive reflex in the rat, Brain Res., 381 (1986) 93–99.

Davies, S.N. and Lodge D., Evidence for involvement of NMDA receptors in "wind-up" of class 2 neurons in the dorsal horn of the rat, Brain Res., 424 (1987) 402–406.

DeBiasi, S. and Rustioni A., Glutamate and substance P coexist in primary afferent terminals in superficial laminae of the spinal cord, Proc Nat Acad Sci,USA, 85 (1988) 7820–7824.

Dickenson, A.H. and Sullivan A.F., Evidence for a role of the NMDA receptor in the frequency dependent potentiation of deep dorsal horn nociceptive neurons following C fibre stimulation, Neuropharmacology, 26 (1987) 1235–1238

Dickenson, A.H. and Sullivan A.F., Differential effects of excitatory amino acid antagonists on dorsal horn nococeptive neurons in the rat, Brain Res., 506 (1990) 331–39.

Duggan, A.W., Hope, P.J., Jarrott, B., Schaible, H.G. and Fleetwood-Walker, S.M., Release, spread and persistence of immunoreactive NKA in the dorsal horn of the cat following noxious cutaneous stimulation, Studies with antibody microprobes, Neuroscience, 35(1) (1990) 195–202.

Fagg G.E. and Foster A.C., Amino acid neurotransmitters and their pathways in mammalian CNS, Neuroscience, 9 (1983) 701–719.

Fleetwood-Walker, S.M., Mitchell, R., Hope, P.J., El-Yassir, N., Molony, V. and Bladon, C.M., The involvement of neurokinin receptor subtypes in somatosensory processing in the superficial dorsal horn of the cat, Brain Res., 519 (1990) 169–182.

Fleetwood-Walker, S.M., Hope, P.J., Parker, R.M.C. and Mitchell, R., Effects of antagonists selective for $neurokinin_1$ and $neurokinin_2$ receptors on somatosensory responses of rat dorsal horn neurons, Br. J. Pharmacol., 104 (1991) 472.

Fleetwood-Walker, S.M., Mitchell, R., Hope, P.J., El-Yassir, N., Molony, V. and Bladon, C.M., The involvement of neurokinin receptor subtypes in somatosensory processing in the superficial dorsal horn of the cat: corrigendum, Brain Res., 579 (1992a) 357.

Fleetwood-Walker, S.M., Parker, R.M.C., Munro, F.E., Hope, P.J. and Mitchell, R., Evidence for a role of NK_2 receptors in mediating brief nociceptive inputs to rat dorsal horn (laminae III–V) neurons, Eur. J. Pharmacol., 242 (1992b) 173–181.

Heapy, C.G., Jamieson, A. and Russell, N.J.W., Afferent C fibre and A-delta activity in models of inflammation, Br. J. Pharmacol., 90 (1987) 164P.

Henry, J.L., Effects of substance P on functionally-identified units in cat spinal cord, Brain Res., 114 (1976) 439–451.

Hope, P.J., Lang, C.W. and Duggan, A.W., Persistence of immunoreactive neurokinins in the dorsal horn of barbiturate anaesthetised and spinal cats, following release by tibial nerve stimulation, Neurosci. Letts., 118 (1990) 25–28.

Irving A.J., Schofield J.G., Watkins J.C., Sunter D.C. and Collingridge G.L., 1S,3R ACPD stimulates and L-AP3 blocks calcium mobilization in rat cerebellar neurons, Eur. J. Pharmacol., 186 (1990) 363–365.

Maggi, C.A., Patacchini, R., Rovero, P. and Giachetti, A., Tachykinin receptors and tachykinin receptor antagonists, J. Auton. Pharmacol., 13 (1993) 23–93.

Munro, F.E., Fleetwood-Walker, S.M., Parker, R.M.C. and Mitchell, R., The effects of neurokinin receptor antagonists on mustard oil-evoked activation of rat dorsal horn neurons, Neuropeptides, 25 (1993) 299–305.

Ogawa, T., Kanazawa, I. and Kimura, S., Regional distribution of substance P, neurokinin a and neurokinin b in rat spinal cord, nerve roots and dorsal root ganglia, and the effects of dorsal root section or spinal transection, Brain Res., 359 (1985) 152–157.

Petermann, J., Fischer, J.A., Theodorsson-Norheim, E. and Lundberg, J.M. Simultaneous release of several tachykinins and calcitonin gene-related peptide from rat-spinal cord slices, Neurosci. Letts., 63 (1986) 310–312.

Rizzoli, A.A., Distribution of glutamic acid, aspartic acid, GABA and glycine in six areas of cat spinal cord before and after transection, Brain Res., 11 (1968) 11–18.

Saria, A., Gamse, R., Petermann, J., Fischer, J.A., Theodorsson-Norheim, E. and Lundberg, J.M., Simultaneous release of several tachykinins and calcitonin gene-related peptide from rat-spinal cord slices. Neurosci. Letts., 63 (1986) 310–312.

Schoepp, D.D., Bockaert, J. and Sladeczek, F., Pharmacological and functional characteristics of metabotropic excitatory amino acid receptors, Trends in Pharmacological Sciences, 11 (1990a) 508–515.

Schoepp, D.D., Johnson, B.G., Smith E.C.R. and McQuaid, L.A., Stereoselectivity and mode of inhibition of phosphoinositide-coupled excitatory amino acid receptors by 2-amino-3-phosphopropionic acid, Molec. Pharmacol., 38 (1990b) 222–228.

Skilling, S.R., Smullin, D.H., Beitz, A.J. and Larson, A.A., Extracellular amino acid concentrations in the dorsal spinal cord of freely moving rats following veratridine and nociceptive stimula-

tion, J. Neurochem., 51 (1988) 127–132.
Storm-Mathisen, J. and Ottersen, O.P., Tracing of neurons with glutamate or GABA as putative transmitters, Biochem. Soc., 15 (1987) 210–213.
Takeda,Z. and Krause, J.E., Pharmacological and molecular biological studies on the diversity of rat tachykinin NK_2 receptor subtypes in rat CNS, duodenum, vas deferens and urinary bladder, Annals of the New York Academy of Sciences, 632 (1991) 479–482.
Thompson S.W.N., Gerber G., Sivilotti L.G. and Woolf C.J., Activity-dependent changes in rat ventral horn neurons in vitro: summation of prolonged evoked postsynaptic depolarizations produce D-APV sensitive wind-up, Eur. J. Neuroscience, 2 (1990) 638–649.
Thompson, S.W.N., Gerber, G., Sivilotti, G. and Woolf, C.J., Long duration ventral root potentials in the neonatal rat spinal cord in vitro: the effects of ionotropic and metabotropic excitatory amino acid receptor antagonists, Brain Res., 595 (1992) 87–97.
Urban, L. and Dray, A., Synaptic activation of dorsal horn neurons by selective C-fibre excitation with capsaicin in the mouse spinal cord *in vitro,* Neuroscience, 47 (1992) 693–702.
Watkins, J.C., Krogsgaard-Larsen, P. and Honore, T., Structure-activity relationships in the development of excitatory amino acid receptor agonists and antagonists, Trends in Pharmacological Sciences, 11 (1990) 25–27.
Yashpal, K., Dam, T.-V. and Quirion, R., Quantative autoradiographic distribution of multiple neurokinin binding sites in rat spinal cord, Brain Res., 506 (1990) 259–266.

Correspondence to: S.M. Fleetwood-Walker, PhD, Department of Preclinical Veterinary Sciences, Royal (Dick) School of Veterinary Studies, University of Edinburgh, Summerhall, Edinburgh EH9 1QH, UK. Tel: 44-31-650-6091; Fax: 44-31-650-6576.

Proceedings of the 7th World Congress on Pain,
Progress in Pain Research and Management, Vol. 2,
edited by G.F. Gebhart, D.L. Hammond, and T.S.
Jensen, IASP Press, Seattle, © 1994.

24

Differential Effects of Skin Inflammation, Extrasynaptic Substance P, and Noxious Skin Heating on Rhythmicity, Synchrony, and Nonlinear Dynamics in Rat Spinal Dorsal Horn

Jürgen Sandkühler, Antonio A. Eblen-Zajjur, and Xianguo Liu

II. Physiologisches Institut, Universität Heidelberg, Heidelberg, Germany

INTRODUCTION

Inflammation of the skin or other peripheral tissues and the concomitant excitation of fine primary afferents results in the release of various neuromediators, including neuropeptides, into the spinal cord. After excessive release, neuropeptides such as substance P and neurokinin A are distributed widely throughout the superficial and in some cases also throughout the deep dorsal horn (Duggan and Hendry 1986; Duggan et al. 1990). This extrasynaptic spread of chemical signals, which has been termed *volume transmission* (Agnati et al. 1986), clearly does not mediate the classical fast synaptic transmission of information, but may be relevant for long-term changes in the spinal dorsal horn induced by inflammation (Sandkühler 1993). Volume transmission not only will affect individual postsynaptic neurons (e.g., by increasing their excitability), but also may modify the properties of the neuronal network in the spinal cord (e.g., by facilitating or depressing specific synaptic pathways).

To assess parameters of functional plasticity in the spinal dorsal horn in addition to well-documented increases in excitability of individual neurons (e.g., Cook et al. 1987; Schaible et al. 1987; Dubner and Ruda 1992), we have simultaneously recorded from pairs of multireceptive neurons before and after inflammation of the skin or controlled superfusion of the cord dorsum with substance P. We searched for changes in the temporal correlation of discharges (e.g., the appearance or disappearance of synchronizations), which strongly facilitates the information transmission through converging neurons and which may be involved in use-dependent changes of synaptic gain (Cook 1991). It also may play a role for assembly coding of information (Singer 1993). We determined spectral discharge patterns and the dimensionality of discharges. Changes in discharge patterns may affect transmitter release and may modify the effect on postsynaptic neurons independent of changes in mean discharge rates. The determination of dimensionality of discharge patterns provides a quantitative measure for the number of independent variables that govern the process of spike generation and may thus be a sensitive indicator for functional changes of cellular or circuit properties.

METHODS

Principal experimental procedures have been described in detail elsewhere (Sandkühler et al. 1991b). We performed experiments on 37 male Sprague-Dawley rats (250–400 g body weight) under deep pentobarbital anesthesia. Tungsten microelectrodes placed in all laminae of the lumbar spinal dorsal horn recorded activity from single or pairs of multireceptive neurons. Action potentials of individual neurons were identified off-line in multineuron recordings by the principal component method based on the shape of the waveform. Spike occurrence times of background and evoked activity were determined with a resolution of 0.1 ms and analyzed further only after passing conventional tests for stationarity. We analyzed discharges consisting of at least 1000, but typically of more than 5000 action potentials.

Fourier analysis of the autocorrelation functions (bin width 1 ms, time window 0–5000 ms) revealed autospectra. Cross-correlograms of discharges of simultaneously recorded pairs of neurons were plotted with a bin width of 1 ms. We (Debus and Sandkühler, in preparation) have developed a phase-space portrait to graphically analyze discharge patterns that can be described by the differences (I') of neighboring interspike intervals (I; $I' = I_{n+1}-I_n$). To construct the phase-space portrait we plot I'_{n+1} on the ordinate versus I'_n on the abscissa. From a set of interspike interval differences $\{I' = |n = 1..N\}$, a time-delay vector $X_n=(I'_n, I'_{n+1}, I'_{n+m-1})$ is formed in an m-dimensional embedding space. These time-delay vectors are used to calculate the correlation function and to determine the D_2 correlation dimension (Grassberger and Procaccia 1983).

We used calibrated von Frey hairs (67 mN) to determine size and locations of cutaneous mechanoreceptive fields. Prolonged noxious radiant heating of the glabrous skin at the hindpaw consisted of 100-second pulses of 48°C. Inflammation of the glabrous skin was induced by repetitive, prolonged noxious radiant skin stimulations (3–5 × 48°C or 50°C for 100 seconds). A ring of specially prepared silicon rubber was placed onto the cord dorsum to control superfusion at the recording site (Sandkühler et al. 1991a). Substance P was dissolved in artificial cerebrospinal fluid at concentrations of 1, 10, or 100 μM and was applied to the cord dorsum for 30 minutes without exchanging of the pool content (≤ 200 ml). At the end of each experiment an electrolytic lesion was made at the recording site.

RESULTS

Results were obtained from 125 multireceptive neurons located in laminae I–VI of the lumbar spinal cord. No search stimuli were used, so we encountered only neurons with at least some background activity (range 0.3–60 impulses per second).

HARMONIC OSCILLATIONS

Inflammation of the skin induced harmonic oscillations in 11 of 19 (incidence: 57.9%) previously nonrhythmically discharging multireceptive neurons (Fig. 1A) and depressed rhythmicity in 3 of 11 (27.3%) previously oscillating neurons. Similar results were obtained by superfusions of the cord dorsum with substance P at 10 μM, which induced rhythmicity in 14 of 34 neurons (41.2%; Fig. 1B) and depressed rhythmicity in 3 of 9 (33.3%). In contrast, prolonged noxious skin heating predominantly depressed rhythmicity (9 of 15 neurons, 60%, Fig. 1C) and induced rhythmicity in only 2 of 35 neurons (5.7%).

NONLINEAR DYNAMICS

Inspection of the phase-space portraits and quantitative determination of the D_2 correlation dimension revealed that 7 of 11 neurons (63.6%) had clearly deterministic discharge patterns (D_2 correlation dimensions ranged

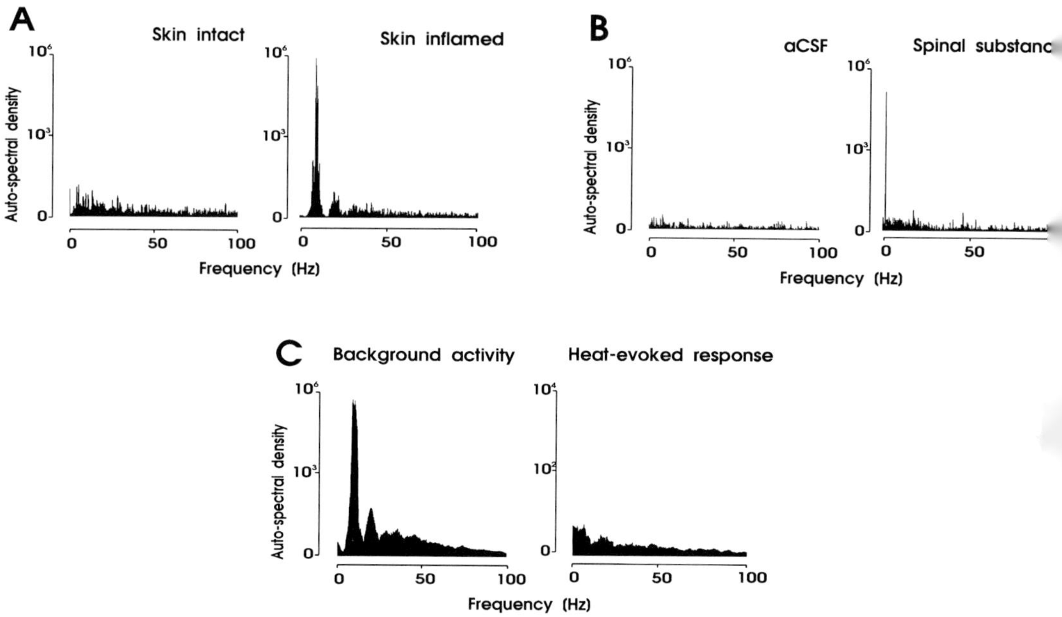

Fig. 1. Autospectra of three different multireceptive spinal dorsal horn neurons. **A:** the transition from nonrhythmic background activity with the skin intact to oscillating background activity throughout the recording period of four hours following inflammation of the skin. **B:** a neuron with nonrhythmic background activity became rhythmic after spinal substance P superfusion (10 µM), as revealed by a narrow but high peak in the autospectrum. **C:** rhythmic background activity of a neuron was replaced by nonrhythmic, noxious heat-evoked response (50°C, 100 seconds).

between 1.5 and 11; e.g., Fig. 2C). The complexity of the discharge patterns of 9 of 11 multireceptive neurons (81.8%) was reduced following inflammation of the skin (Fig. 2 A and B); dimensionality of 2 of 11 neurons (18.2%) remained unchanged, and increases in dimensionality were never seen after inflammation. In contrast, prolonged noxious skin heating produced increases (Fig. 2 C and D), decreases, or no changes in the D_2 correlation dimension with approximately the same incidence. We are presently investigating the effects of extrasynaptic substance P on nonlinear dynamics of discharge patterns.

TEMPORAL CORRELATION OF DISCHARGES

Skin inflammation induced *qualitative* changes in the temporal correlation of discharges of 5 of 13 (38.5%) simultaneously recorded pairs of multireceptive spinal dorsal horn neurons, e.g., a gain (Fig. 3A) or a loss of synchronization. In contrast, extrasynaptic substance P failed to induce quali-

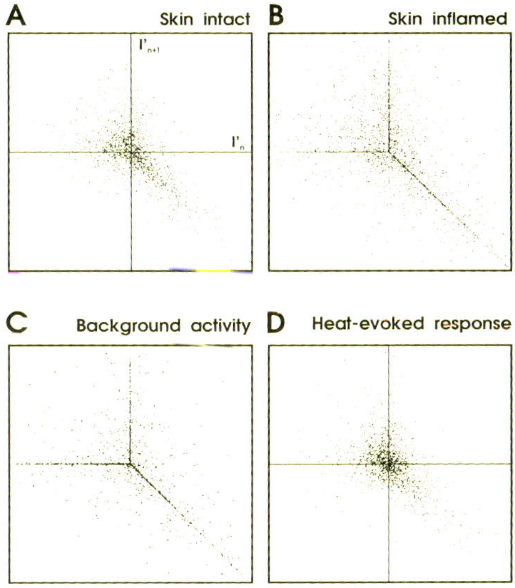

Fig. 2. Phase-space portraits of background activity of a multireceptive neuron before (**A**) and 3 hours after induction of skin inflammation (**B**) are shown (axes in A from –400 to +400 ms, in B from –700 to +700 ms). The axes in B and C are omitted to avoid eclipsing the points that are lined up along the axes. Skin inflammation evokes a transition from an apparently random discharge pattern (**A**; $D_2 > 20$) to a deterministic pattern (**B**; $D_2 = 7.5$), which was present throughout the remaining recording period of 5 hours. **C** shows the phase-space portrait (axes from –200 to +200 ms) of clearly deterministic background activity of another neuron ($D_2 = 1.53$). This pattern is lost during steady-state, noxious heat-evoked response, which displayed an apparently random pattern (**D**; $D_2 > 20$).

tative changes in the temporal correlation of 23 of 25 pairs of neurons (92.0%) and produced a loss of synchronization in 2 of 25 pairs (8.0%). During prolonged noxious skin heating 8 of 37 pairs of neurons (21.6%) qualitatively changed the temporal correlation of their discharges; four were *de*synchronized (Fig. 3C).

CUTANEOUS RECEPTIVE FIELDS

Following inflammation of the skin 23 of 34 neurons (67.6%) displayed enlarged cutaneous receptive fields. Five of six (83.3%) pairs of simultaneously recorded multireceptive neurons with previously completely (*n = 1*) or partially *(n = 4)* separate receptive fields developed completely overlapping receptive fields (Fig. 4). Seven other pairs of neurons had completely overlapping receptive fields before and after skin inflammation (Fig. 4). Following substance P superfusions, cutaneous receptive fields increased in 17 of 22 neurons (77.3%). New receptive fields were seen in 2 of 22 and discontinuous receptive fields were seen in two other neurons following superfusions with substance P. Four neurons initially showed an increase and then a decrease in receptive field size; only one neuron had a stable receptive field before, during, and after substance P superfusion. One pair with previously completely separate cutaneous receptive fields displayed completely overlapping receptive fields.

DISCUSSION

Our study has provided evidence that inflammation of the skin and extrasynaptic substance P may change properties of the functional neuronal network in the spinal dorsal horn. Spectral discharge pattern, phase-space portrait, dimensionality of discharges, and the temporal correlation of discharges of simultaneously recorded pairs of neurons were differentially affected by skin inflammation, extrasynaptic substance P, and noxious skin heating, suggesting that substance P may mediate some, but not all of the long-term effects that are induced by inflammation of the skin.

VOLUME TRANSMISSION IN THE SPINAL DORSAL HORN

Despite the widespread, extrasynaptic distribution of neuropeptides in the spinal cord following massive endogenous release, a high topographical order of action is achieved by binding to high-affinity receptors, which have a very distinct distribution in the spinal cord (Yashpal et al. 1990). While iontophoresis and pressure microinjections are suitable means to study neuropeptide effects on single neurons, the controlled superfusion of the cord dorsum best reproduces the widespread extrasynaptic distribution and dorso-ventral concentration gradient of the neuropeptides in the spinal cord following massive endogenous release induced by inflammation of various peripheral tissues (Beck et al. 1992). Thus, the controlled superfusion of the cord dorsum is a suitable means to study the effects of individual neuropeptides on functions of the neuronal network in the spinal dorsal horn.

HARMONIC OSCILLATIONS

Skin inflammation and extrasynaptic spinal substance P induce harmonic oscillations of background activity of some multireceptive spinal dorsal horn neurons. Oscillatory activity, which has been identified in neurons throughout

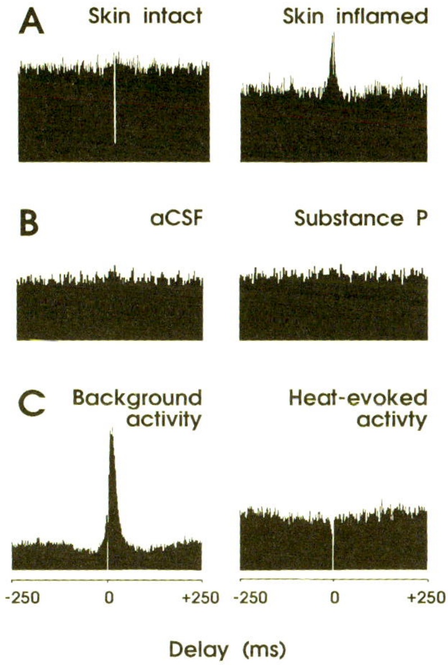

Fig. 3. Cross-correlograms of three different pairs of multireceptive spinal dorsal horn neurons. Flat correlograms indicate absence of any synchronization in the discharges; central peaks centered around zero delay represent the number of actions potentials that are discharged by one neuron shortly before (negative delays) or after an action potential occurred in the other neuron. Cross-correlograms of background activity before and 1–3 hours after induction of skin inflammation (**A**) or substance P superfusion (**B**) are shown. C: Synchronized background activity was followed by nonsynchronized, noxious heat-evoked activity. aCSF: superfusion with artificial cerebrospinal fluid.

the peripheral and central nervous system, usually results from reciprocal interactions between excitatory and inhibitory mechanisms. Such interactions may not only be realized by the neuronal circuitry with negative feedback connections, but also within single neurons by coupling between excitatory and inhibitory membrane conductances (Singer 1993). Thus, opening of reverberant pathways and changes in membrane potential that allow intrinsic pacemaker potentials to be expressed may be the underlying mechanisms for oscillations induced by substance P and by inflammation. For thalamo-cortical relay neurons it has been suggested that oscillations prevent the transmission of sensory information and indicate presence of a transfer block. Neurons may switch to the transfer mode by discharging nonrhythmically (McCormick and Feeser 1990). This hypothesis is consistent with our finding that noxious skin heating rarely induced rhythmicity but often depressed oscillations. Regular second messenger pulses are apparently more efficient than stochastic pulses

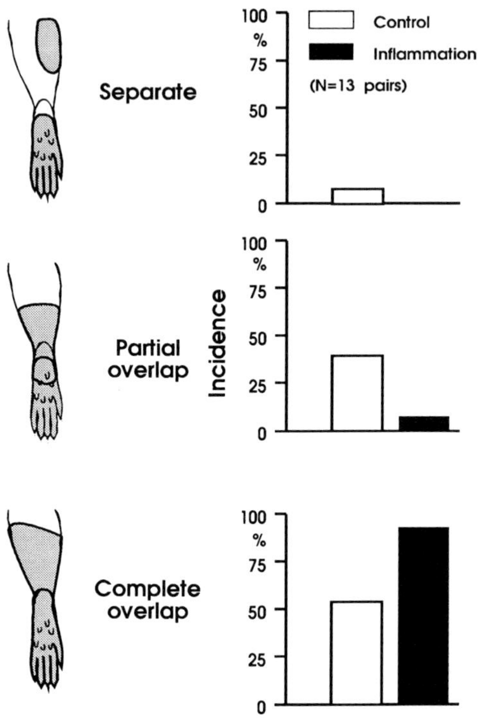

Fig. 4. Summary of the effect of skin inflammation on the cutaneous receptive fields of 13 simultaneously recorded pairs of multireceptive spinal dorsal horn neurons. One to four hours after inflammation the incidence of separate (**top**) or partially overlapping (**center**) receptive fields is strongly reduced, and almost all pairs of neurons had completely overlapping receptive fields (**bottom**).

to trigger cellular events (Li and Goldbeter 1992); thus, we might speculate that oscillations induced by inflammation of the skin or extrasynaptic substance P may enhance second messenger-mediated effects in higher-order neurons (e.g., the expression of immediate-early-genes such as c-*fos* or *jun* B; Table I).

NONLINEAR DYNAMICS OF DISCHARGE PATTERNS

Nonlinear dynamics of discharge patterns can not be detected by spectral analysis or counting statistics. We thus developed a phase-space portrait for neuronal discharges and determined the correlation dimension D_2 that provides a quantitative measure for the minimal number of degrees of freedom underlying the spike generation process (Debus and Sandkühler, unpublished data). This may be used as a sensitive indicator for changes in the functional state of individual neurons and/or the embedding neuronal network. It is generally assumed that action potentials are generated at random intervals, constituting a simple renewal process, because some of the mechanisms underlying spike generation are apparently stochastic processes, as revealed by the open

Table I
Summary of differential effects of skin inflammation, substance P superfusions, and prolonged noxious skin heating on multireceptive neurons in the spinal dorsal horn

Parameter	Skin Inflammation	Spinal Substance P	Skin Heating
Rhythmicity	↑↑	↑	↓↓
Correlation dimension	↓↓↓	n.d.	↑↓
Synchronization	↑↓	∅	↑↓
RF overlap	↑↑↑	↑	n.d.
Discharge rate*	↑↓	↑↓	↑↑↑
c-Fos-IR**	↑↑	↑↑	↑↑
jun-B-IR**	↑↑	↑↑	↑↑

Note: The predominant effects are indicated by arrows: ↑ for an increase, ↓ for a decrease. ∅ indicates no effect; n.d. indicates effect not determined. RF: cutaneous mechanoreceptive field; c-Fos-IR or jun-B-IR: numbers of cells with c-Fos or jun-B immunoreactivity; *data not shown; **data from Beck and Sandkühler 1993.

and closing times of ion channels (Colquhoun and Hawkes 1981) and peak amplitudes of unitary postsynaptic potentials (Stern et al. 1992). However, more than half of the multireceptive neurons in our sample displayed background activity with clearly deterministic patterns. Thus, background activity can no longer be considered to be purely stochastic noise. This conclusion is in line with recent data showing that transmitter release also may be a deterministic process and not, as previously believed, a purely random event (Kriebel et al. 1990). We might expect that skin inflammation would increase the number of degrees of freedom of discharge patterns (e.g., due to additional synaptic input from nociceptors, interneurons, or descending inhibitory or excitatory pathways). However, inflammation of the skin even further *reduced* the number of degrees of freedom in the discharges of most of the neurons. Decreases in dimensionality were independent of changes in mean discharge rates and are thus probably not simply epiphenomena of changes in excitability. Other pathophysiological conditions such as epileptic seizure or fibrillation of the heart (Pool 1989; Kaplan and Cohen 1990) also reduce the complexity of the corresponding electrophysiological process. In contrast, encoding of noxious skin heating had no consistent effect on dimensionality. At present we can only speculate on the underlying mechanisms that reduce the degrees of freedom in neuronal discharge patterns. Possibly, simple reverberant pathways are opened that dominate spike generation and prevent other afferents from contributing to the excitation of the cell. Perhaps kinetics of voltage- or ligand-gated ion channels, which are involved in spike generation, are modified via second messenger cascades triggered by extrasynaptic substance P and/or other neuromediators.

SYNCHRONIZATION OF DISCHARGES

Synchronization of discharges of convergent neurons is a highly effective way to enhance the degree of spatial summation at the postsynaptic membrane, especially when neurons are discharging with long interspike intervals. Thus, changes in the synchronization may be an efficient way to modulate information transfer without changes in mean discharge rates and for long periods of time. Brief but strong increases in mean discharge rates (e.g., during noxious skin heating) would benefit less from synchronization. Here, inflammation of skin, but not extrasynaptic substance P, produced long-lasting qualitative changes in the temporal correlation of pairs of simultaneously recorded multireceptive neurons, often without major changes in mean discharge rates. Synchronization of discharges can be achieved by direct or indirect excitatory connections between the neurons under study or by common excitatory or inhibitory inputs. Common input from (heat-sensitive) cutaneous nociceptors is probably not the cause for synchronized discharges observed here, as prolonged skin heating never produced synchronization but rather desynchronized discharges. We suggest that the qualitative changes in the pattern of the cross-correlograms may reflect changes in the functional connectivity within the spinal dorsal horn. Extrasynaptic substance P, which may relatively selectively enhance release of glutamate but not of other amino acids, failed to reproduce the effects of skin inflammation on cross-correlograms. Other neuromediators may be involved, possibly calcitonin gene-related peptide, which modulates release of glutamate, aspartate, and asparagine (Kangrga and Randic 1990).

Opening of suprathreshold synaptic pathways between neighboring dorsal horn neurons should have additive effects on their receptive fields, resulting in completely overlapping fields. And indeed, following inflammation of the skin, cutaneous receptive fields of almost all pairs of simultaneously recorded neurons completely overlapped, including receptive fields of neurons with previously completely separate fields. The large increase in receptive field size following skin inflammation or extrasynaptic substance P cannot be explained solely as a result of increased excitability with subthreshold input now becoming suprathreshold (Woolf and King 1989). Opening of excitatory synaptic pathways between dorsal horn neurons provides an additional plausible explanation for enlargements of receptive fields.

ACKNOWLEDGMENT

This work was supported by a grant from the Deutsche Forschungsgemeinschaft (SA 435).

REFERENCES

Agnati, L.F., Fuxe, K., Zoli, M., Ozini, I., Toffano, G. and Ferraguti, F., A correlation analysis of the regional distribution of central enkephalin and b-endorphin immunoreactive terminals and of opiate receptors in adult and old male rats. Evidence for the existence of two main types of communication in the central nervous system: the volume transmission and the writing transmission, Acta Physiol. Scand., 128 (1986) 201–207.

Beck, H. and Sandkühler, J., Role of volume transmission for spinal nociception: extrasynaptic mediators of immediate early gene expression. In: Abstracts: 7th World Congress on Pain, IASP Publications, Seattle, 1993, pp. 472.

Beck, H., Schröck, H. and Sandkühler, J., Distribution of neurokinin A during controlled superfusion of the rat spinal cord dorsum, Soc. Neurosci. Abstr., 18 (1992) 132.

Colquhoun, D. and Hawkes, A.G., On the stochastic properties of single ion channels, Proc. R. Soc. Lond. (Biol.), 211 (1981) 205–235.

Cook, A.J., Woolf, C.J., Wall, P.D. and McMahon, S.B., Dynamic receptive field plasticity in rat spinal cord dorsal horn following C-primary afferent input, Nature, 325 (1987) 151–153.

Cook, J.E., Correlated activity in the CNS: a role on every timescale? Trends Neurosci., 14 (1991) 397–401.

Dubner, R. and Ruda, M.A., Activity-dependent neuronal plasticity following tissue injury and inflammation, Trends Neurosci., 15 (1992) 96–103.

Duggan, A.W. and Hendry, I.A., Laminar localization of the sites of release of immunoreactive substance P in the dorsal horn with antibody-coated microelectrodes, Neurosci. Lett., 68 (1986) 134–140.

Duggan, A.W., Hope, P.J., Jarrott, B., Schaible, H.-G. and Fleetwood-Walker, S.M., Release, spread and persistence of immunoreactive neurokinin A in the dorsal horn of the cat following noxious cutaneous stimulation. Studies with antibody microprobes, Neuroscience, 35 (1990) 195–202.

Grassberger, P. and Procaccia, I., Characterization of strange attractors, Am. Phys. Soc., 50 (1983) 346.

Kangrga, I. and Randic, M., Tachykinins and calcitonin gene-related peptide enhance release of endogenous glutamate and aspartate from the rat spinal dorsal horn slice, J. Neurosci., 10 (1990) 2026–2038.

Kaplan, D.T. and Cohen, R.J., Is fibrillation chaos? Circ. Res., 67 (1990) 886–892.

Kriebel, M.E., Vautrin, J. and Holsapple, J., Transmitter release: prepackaging and random mechanism or dynamic and deterministic process, Brain Res. Rev., 15 (1990) 167–178.

Li, Y.-X. and Goldbeter, A., Pulsatile signaling in intracellular communication periodic stimuli are more efficient than random or chaotic signals in a model based on receptor desensitization, Biophys. J., 61 (1992) 161–171.

McCormick, D.A. and Feeser, H.R., Functional implications of burst firing and single spike activity in lateral geniculate relay neurons, Neuroscience, 39 (1990) 103–113.

Pool, R., Is it healthy to be chaotic? Science, 243 (1989) 604–607.

Sandkühler, J., Volume transmission in the spinal dorsal horn: role of neuropeptides in spinal nociception, Physiological Society Magazine, 7 (1993) 39–42.

Sandkühler, J., Fu, Q.-G. and Stelzer, B., Propriospinal neurons are involved in the descending inhibition of lumbar spinal dorsal horn neurons from the mid-brain. In: M.R. Bond, J.E. Charlton and C.J. Woolf, (Eds.), Proceedings of the VIth World Congress on Pain. Pain Research and Clinical Management, Vol. 4. Elsevier, Amsterdam, 1991a, pp. 313–318.

Sandkühler, J., Willmann, E. and Fu, Q.-G., Characteristics of midbrain control of spinal nociceptive neurons and nonsomatosensory parameters in the pentobarbital-anesthetized rat, J. Neurophysiol., 65 (1991b) 33–48.

Schaible, H.-G., Schmidt, R. and Willis, W., Enhancement of the responses of ascending tract cells in the cat spinal cord by acute inflammation of the knee joint, Exp. Brain Res., 66 (1987) 489–499.

Singer, W., Synchronization of cortical activity and its putative role in information processing and learning. In: J.F. Hoffman (Ed.), Annual Review of Physiology, Vol. 55. Annual Reviews Inc., Palo Alto, 1993, pp.349–374.
Stern, P., Edwards, F.A. and Sakmann, B., Fast and slow components of unitary EPSCs on stellate cells elicited by focal stimulation in slices of rat visual cortex, J. Physiol. (Lond.), 449 (1992) 247–278.
Woolf, C.J. and King, A.E., Subthreshold components of the cutaneous mechanoreceptive fields of dorsal horn neurons in the rat lumbar spinal cord, J. Neurophysiol., 62 (1989) 907–916.
Yashpal, K., Dam, T.-V. and Quirion, R., Quantitaive autoradiographik distribution of multiple neurokinin binding sites in rat spinal cord, Brain Res., 506 (1990) 259–266.

Correspondence to: Priv.-Doz. Dr. J. Sandkühler, II. Physiologisches Institut, Universität Heidelberg, Im Neuenheimer Feld 326, 69120 Heidelberg, Germany. Tel: 49-6221-564052; Fax: 49-6221-564049.

Proceedings of the 7th World Congress on Pain,
Progress in Pain Research and Management, Vol. 2,
edited by G.F. Gebhart, D.L. Hammond, and T.S.
Jensen, IASP Press, Seattle, © 1994.

25

Central Control of Peripheral Joint Inflammation and Heat Hyperalgesia

Kathleen A. Sluka, William D. Willis, and Karin N. Westlund

Marine Biomedical Institute and Department of Anatomy and Neurosciences, University of Texas Medical Branch, Galveston, Texas, USA

INTRODUCTION

Arthritis is a common and disabling problem in our population. Joint inflammation, arthritis, is associated with behavioral changes such as limping, guarding, decreased range of motion, and an increased response to peripheral noxious stimuli (hyperalgesia). For these reasons, experimental animal models have been designed to study various arthritic conditions. The injection of a mixture of kaolin and carrageenan into the knee joint is a model designed to study the acute inflammatory response. These irritants produce a localized joint inflammation and limping and guarding of the limb (Coggeshall et al. 1983; Sluka and Westlund 1992). This arthritis model has been studied in the anesthetized cat (Schaible et al. 1987; Neugebauer and Schaible 1990), anesthetized monkey (Dougherty et al. 1992b; Sluka et al. 1992; Sorkin et al. 1992; Westlund et al. 1992), and awake rat (Sluka and Westlund 1992, 1993a,b,c,d). Neural changes have been observed in both the peripheral and central nervous systems. Sensitization of articular primary afferent fibers (Coggeshall et al. 1983) and dorsal horn neurons (Dougherty et al. 1992b; Neugebauer and Schaible 1990; Schaible et al. 1987) to cutaneous and joint stimuli occurs after induction of arthritis.

From the symptomatic point of view, arthritis can be divided into two components: (1) the inflammation itself (redness, swelling, increased temperature) in and around the joint, and (2) the pain that accompanies this inflammation. Blood-borne or local factors have been considered the sole players in the development of inflammation (Hurley 1983) until relatively recently. There is clear evidence that both the peripheral somatic and sympathetic nervous systems are involved in a variety of inflammatory conditions (see Levine et al. 1988). For example, primary afferent fibers are known to release the inflammatory neuropeptides, substance P (SP) and calcitonin gene-related peptide (CGRP), into the knee joint (Yaksh et al. 1988; Larsson et al. 1991). These neuropeptides have been found in the exudate in both human arthritic conditions and in animal models of arthritis (Applegren et al. 1991; Larsson et al. 1991; Marshall et al. 1990). In adjuvant arthritis, a chronic inflammatory model, chemical sympathectomies decrease the severity of the arthritis (Levine et al. 1986).

We used the kaolin and carrageenan model of inflammation in our experiments to investigate the involvement of:

1. spinal excitatory amino acid (EAA) receptors of the non–N-methyl-D-aspartate (non-NMDA) (n = 8) and NMDA (n = 8) types,
2. spinal gamma-aminobutyric $acid_A$ ($GABA_A$) receptors (n = 8),
3. primary afferent fibers (unilateral dorsal rhizotomy) (n = 6), and
4. the sympathetic nervous system (surgical and/or chemical sympathectomy) (n = 6)

In rats, the knee joint is injected with a mixture of 0.1 cc of 3% kaolin and 3% carrageenan while animals are briefly anesthetized (Sluka and Westlund 1992). Following induction of arthritis, we assessed pain-related behaviors using paw withdrawal latency (PWL) to radiant heat and a subjective pain rating scale. The degree of inflammation was determined by measuring joint circumference and with thermography. Additionally, we assessed the effects of non-NMDA and NMDA receptors on excitatory amino acid (EAA) release in the dorsal horn. Antagonists were infused into the spinal cord through a microdialysis fiber implanted into the dorsal horn (lamina III–IV of the lumbar [L3–L6] spinal cord). As a control for the localization of the effects of receptor antagonists, a microdialysis fiber was placed into the sacral spinal cord. Untreated arthritic (n = 10) and saline-injected control animals (n = 4) were used for comparison. All experiments were approved by the Animal Care and Use Committee at our institution.

EXCITATORY AMINO ACID RELEASE

The release of the EAAs, aspartate (ASP) and glutamate (GLU), in the deep dorsal horn of the spinal cord was studied by measuring changes in their concentrations in extracellular fluid collected via a microdialysis fiber (Skilling et al. 1988; Sluka and Westlund. 1992; Sorkin et al. 1988) in awake rats during the development of the inflammation. An initial increase in ASP and GLU concentration was observed upon injection of the irritants (Fig. 1). Subsequently, a prolonged release of ASP and GLU in the deep dorsal horn began after three hours and persisted throughout the collection period (eight hours). If animals were pretreated either with the non-NMDA receptor antagonist, 6-cyano-7-nitroquinoxaline-2,3-dione (CNQX; 1.1 mM), or the NMDA receptor antagonist, DL-2-amino-7-phosphonoheptanoic acid (AP7; 2 mM), the increased release of ASP and GLU was blocked both at the time of injection and in the prolonged release phase. In fact, ASP concentrations fell significantly below baseline in the CNQX-treated arthritic animals. The antagonists—CNQX and AP7—had no effect on baseline levels of ASP or GLU (Fig. 1).

BEHAVIORAL CHANGES ASSOCIATED WITH JOINT INFLAMMATION

Arthritic animals treated with a non-NMDA, an NMDA, or a $GABA_A$ receptor antagonist did not display the increased sensitivity to radiant heat applied to the paw (heat hyperalgesia) that is characteristic of arthritic rats (cf. Hargreaves et al. 1988). In untreated arthritic rats, a faster withdrawal to radiant heat (1–2 seconds) occurs by four hours and is maintained through 24 hours (Sluka and Westlund 1993d) (Fig. 2). This hyperalgesia represents a central neuronal sensitization because the paw itself was not inflamed, but is now responsive to stimuli that were previously innocuous. The blockade of hyperalgesia by CNQX, AP7, or bicuculline implies that polysynaptic mechanisms are involved in the development of heat hyperalgesia. In contrast, arthritic animals sympathectomized by surgery and/or by phentolamine (1 mg/kg) were still hyperalgesic, similar to the untreated arthritic group.

In another model, the heat hyperalgesia associated with inflammation of the paw by carrageenan appears to be reversed by posttreatment with intrathecal injection of NMDA receptor antagonists and not of non-NMDA antagonists (Ren et al. 1992). This may reflect the time when the antagonists were delivered, i.e., pretreatment vs. posttreatment. We pretreated animals with the antagonists. If the animal is already hyperalgesic (as in the study by Ren and

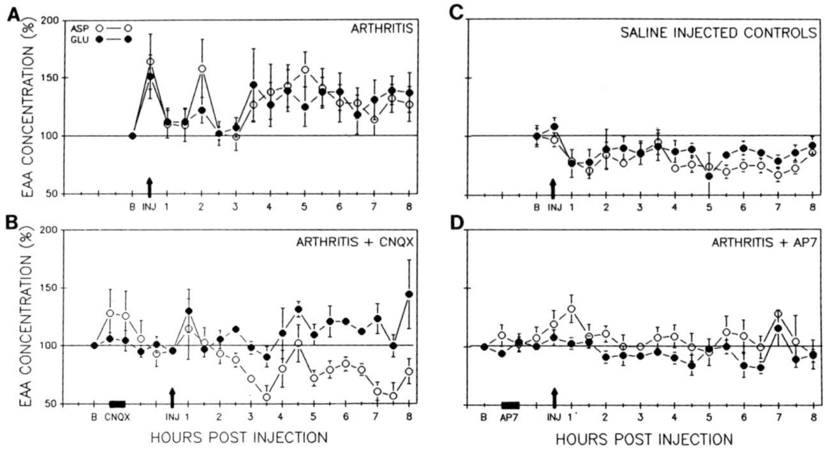

Fig. 1. The release of ASP and GLU in the dorsal horn of the spinal cord before and eight hours after induction of arthritis is represented in panel **A**. At the time of injection (arrow) there was a significant increase in the release of ASP (ANOVA; $P = 0.04$) and GLU ($P = 0.04$). A transient increase in ASP at two hours is followed by a prolonged increase in release of ASP and GLU beginning at 3.5 hours and continuing for at least eight hours. The increase in the prolonged release phase (3.5–8 hours) was significant for ASP ($P = 0.01$) and GLU ($P = 0.02$). In saline-injected control animals (**C**), no change occurred at the time of injection for either ASP or GLU. Interestingly, there was a significant decrease in release of ASP ($P = 0.0008$) in the prolonged-release phase. Animals were pretreated for one hour with either CNQX (2 mM; dissolved in artificial CSF and filtered; Research Biochemicals), a non-NMDA receptor antagonist, or AP7 (2 mM; dissolved in ACSF; Sigma), an NMDA receptor antagonist, followed by one hour of washout for CNQX or 30 minutes for AP7 before injection of the knee joint with 0.1 cc 3% kaolin and 3% carrageenan, (**B** and **D**, respectively). In the group of animals pretreated with CNQX (**B**; thick bar), no release at the time of injection (arrow) occurred. In the prolonged-release phase, delayed and attenuated release of GLU ($P = 0.02$) occurs with a significant decrease in the release of ASP ($P = 0.04$). If the animals were pretreated with AP7 (**D**; thick bar), no increase in ASP or GLU occurs at the time of injection (arrow), although there is a delayed peak in ASP between 30 minutes and one hour. No change in ASP or GLU concentration occurred in response to delivery of either CNQX or AP7.

colleagues), the further activation of the non-NMDA receptor may not be a requirement for continued sensitization of central neurons. NMDA receptor activation is necessary for wind-up (Davies and Lodge 1987) and also is involved in reducing the hyperexcitability of already sensitized dorsal horn neurons (Schaible et al. 1991). Therefore, the differences between the two studies suggest a critical time of non-NMDA receptor activation during the initial stages of the development of the inflammation, while the secondary hyperalgesia, once developed, is maintained by activation of the NMDA receptor. Another likely explanation concerns methodological differences between the delivery of the drugs to the superficial dorsal horn by intrathecal administration versus the deeper dorsal horn by microdialysis.

The injection of kaolin and carrageenan into the knee joint cavity results in guarding of and decreased weight bearing on the limb. To quantify these behavioral changes, the animals were graded by a subjective pain rating scale (0–5) modified from Guilbaud and colleagues (Attal et al. 1990) where: 0 is normal; 1 is curling of toes; 2 is eversion of foot; 3 is partial weight bearing; 4 is non–weight bearing and guarding; and 5 is avoidance of any contact with the limb. The untreated arthritic animals were graded 4.6 ± 0.15; they exhibited avoidance of contact with the limb by lying on the opposite flank in the cage and/or they would not walk on the limb at the end of eight hours. In contrast, scores of CNQX-treated arthritic animals averaged 1.5 ± 0.5 and those of bicuculline-treated arthritic animals averaged 1.2 ± 0.2. These animals all exhibited curling of the toes and some exhibited eversion of the foot. None of the animals in either group limped or guarded the limb. Similar to the untreated arthritic animals, subjective pain ratings for AP7-treated arthritic animals averaged 4.25 ± 0.4 and the sympathectomized animals averaged 4.3 ± 0.2. All of these animals demonstrated guarding of the limb and no weight bearing during ambulation of the limb. Therefore, the behavioral manifestations were greatly decreased only by treatment with the non-NMDA and the $GABA_A$ receptor antagonists and not by treatment with the NMDA receptor antagonist or by sympathectomy, which is consistent with a decrease in the degree of peripheral inflammation.

CENTRAL CONTROL OF JOINT INFLAMMATION

One of the most surprising findings was that spinal cord administration of either a non-NMDA (CNQX; 1.1 mM) or a $GABA_A$ (bicuculline; 0.01 mM) receptor antagonist prior to induction of arthritis significantly reduced the extent of joint inflammation compared to untreated arthritic animals (Fig. 3). Measurement of knee joint circumference revealed that the joint circumferences in animals pretreated with a non-NMDA or a $GABA_A$ receptor antagonist were significantly reduced compared to untreated arthritic animals. Similarly, following unilateral dorsal rhizotomy (L2–L6, 2–3 days) the joint circumferences of inflamed knees were significantly less than those in untreated arthritic animals (Fig. 3). In contrast, treatment of the spinal cord with an NMDA receptor antagonist did not reduce the degree of peripheral joint inflammation when compared to untreated arthritic animals. Nor did a combination of surgical and chemical (phentolamine, 1 mg/kg) sympathectomies reduce the degree of inflammation.

As a control for systemic effects, the microdialysis fiber was placed into the sacral spinal cord and the antagonist (CNQX or bicuculline) administered

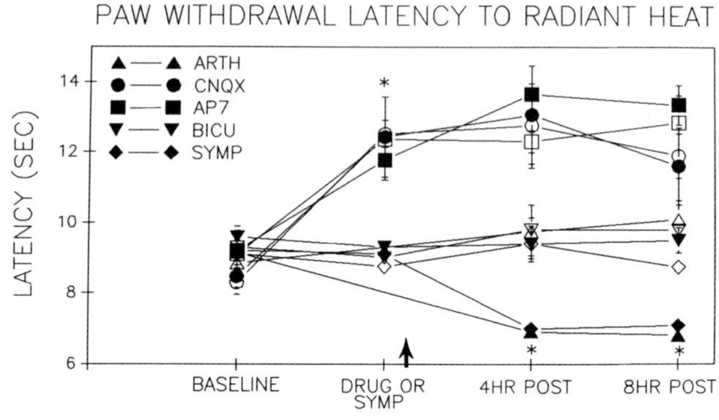

Fig. 2. This graph shows paw withdrawal latency (PWL) to radiant heat for animals that were untreated (triangles), CNQX-treated (circles), AP7-treated (squares), bicuculline-treated (inverse triangles), and sympathectomized (diamonds) arthritic animals. The response latency of the hindpaw ipsilateral to the inflamed knee joint is represented by filled symbols whereas the contralateral side is represented by unfilled symbols. Before the induction of arthritis or infusion of the antagonists, the withdrawal latencies averaged between 8 and 10 seconds. The receptor antagonists were infused for the duration of the experiment to account for differences in length of effectiveness of the drugs. After one hour infusion of either CNQX (non-NMDA) or AP7 (NMDA) through the dialysis fiber, the PWL increased significantly for both the ipsilateral and the contralateral sides when compared to baseline (paired *t* test; $P \leq 0.05$), suggesting the animals were hypoalgesic. Following the induction of arthritis, untreated and sympathectomized arthritic animals showed a 1–2 second decrease in PWL to radiant heat when compared to baseline at four and eight hours after injection of kaolin and carrageenan. In the animals treated with either CNQX or AP7, there was no further decrease in withdrawal times of either the ipsilateral or contralateral paws after induction of arthritis when compared to the withdrawal times induced by the application of the antagonists. Therefore, the heat hyperalgesia seen in untreated arthritic animals is blocked by the treatment of the spinal cord with either a non-NMDA (CNQX), an NMDA (AP7), or a $GABA_A$ (bicuculline) receptor antagonist.

in the same manner as in all other experiments. In these animals the degree of joint inflammation and the behavioral changes were similar to those of untreated arthritic animals. Therefore, the application of CNQX and bicuculline must be into the levels of the spinal cord receiving articular inputs to interfere with the progression of the inflammation and the resultant behavioral changes. Further, this finding demonstrated that application to the spinal cord through the microdialysis fiber remained confined regionally. Additionally, in animals (n = 3) in which methylene blue dye was passed through the fiber for the duration of infusion of the antagonist, the spread of the dye did not extend beyond one spinal segment or ventrally into the motor neuron pool.

Thermographic readings taken before and after induction of arthritis revealed that a major temperature increase occurs in the knee joint with inflammation. Similar changes were evident for arthritic animals after receiving treatment with the NMDA receptor antagonist or following sympathectomy. Treatment of the spinal cord with a non-NMDA or a $GABA_A$ receptor antagonist, however, reduced the thermal increases typical in knee joint inflammation. The thermal increases also were reduced following dorsal rhizotomy. The reduction in the severity of the inflammatory events by CNQX, bicuculline, or dorsal rhizotomy and not by AP7 or sympathectomy, as determined by thermographic and knee joint circumference measurements, suggest that differential control mechanisms are involved for the peripheral inflammatory and nociceptive events. This finding is consistent with the decrease in the degree of inflammatory exudate present in the knee joints of animals treated with CNQX, bicuculline, or dorsal rhizotomy.

DISCUSSION

These data support a contribution by central pathways to the development of peripheral joint inflammation. The central pathway(s) involves spinal non-NMDA (Sluka and Westlund 1993b) and $GABA_A$ (Sluka et al. 1993) receptors as well as the central terminals of primary afferent fibers. These data demonstrate that a central neuronal pathway exists that when blocked at the spinal cord level, not only reduces the transmission of nociceptive information but also influences the development of peripheral inflammation. Consequent behavioral manifestations of the arthritis also are decreased. Peripheral joint inflammation is reduced by dorsal rhizotomy, spinal application of CNQX or bicuculline, but not by AP7 or sympathectomy. Efferent activity was recorded in knee joint afferents in response to mechanical stimulation of the hindlimb following induction of acute arthritis (Rees et al. 1994). Thus, we hypothesize that the central pathway for increasing peripheral inflammation involves primary afferent depolarization of terminals in the dorsal horn and the consequent dorsal root reflexes (DRRs). The central terminals of primary afferent fibers must be intact for the joint inflammation to develop fully. The peripheral terminals of these afferents may directly release neuropeptides into the joint when invaded by antidromic nerve impulses (DRRs) triggered by primary afferent depolarization (PAD).

There is substantial evidence for the involvement of the peripheral nervous system in the inflammatory process. Peripherally, changes in content of fibers labeled for SP and CGRP occur in both human inflammatory conditions and animal models of inflammation (Mapp et al. 1990; Pereira da Silva and Foneseca 1990; Weihe et al. 1988). A peripheral release of SP and CGRP occurs in the inflammatory exudate of the joint (Appelgren et al. 1991; Larsson et al. 1991; Marshall et al. 1990) and these peptides increase the inflamma-

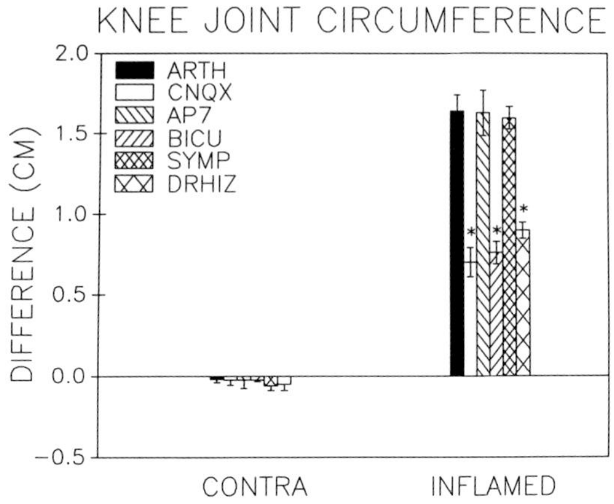

Fig. 3. The circumference of the knee joint was measured before and eight hours after induction of arthritis for the inflamed and the contralateral knee joints. The inflamed knee joint significantly (paired *t* test; $P < 0.05$) increased in girth when compared to its own size before induction of arthritis. The sympathectomized arthritic animals and those treated with AP7, an NMDA receptor antagonist, were significantly increased from baseline for the inflamed knee and were not significantly different from the untreated arthritic group. In animals treated with the non-NMDA (CNQX) or the $GABA_A$ (bicuculline) receptor antagonist, the increase in girth was approximately half of the untreated arthritic animals and was significantly less than that of untreated arthritic animals. Difference from untreated arthritic animals (Scheffé test) is represented by an asterisk (*).

tory events in the periphery (Levine et al. 1984; Brain and Williams 1985). This indicates that primary afferent neurons are involved in tissue extravasation during arthritis. Additionally, denervation of the knee joint or intra-articular injection of capsaicin, which depletes SP and CGRP, reduces peripheral joint inflammation (Lam and Ferrell 1989a,b).

Centrally, an early depletion of SP followed by a later increase of SP and CGRP are observed after induction of arthritis (Sluka et al. 1992; Sluka and Westlund 1993d). These dorsal horn changes occur across the entire superficial dorsal horn (Sluka et al. 1992; Sluka and Westlund 1993d). This includes not only the termination sites of the knee joint afferents (Craig et al. 1988), but also areas receiving input from cutaneous, muscle, and other joint primary afferent fibers. Dorsal horn CGRP is solely of primary afferent origin (Chung et al. 1988), so widespread release suggests long-term facilitatory events are occurring that affect a large number of primary afferent fibers. The increased degree of inflammation mediated through non-NMDA and $GABA_A$ mechanisms in the spinal cord and the widespread changes in GLU, SP, and CGRP (Sluka et al. 1992; Sluka and Westlund 1993d) that occur following induction of arthritis may be the result of PAD, which occurs through $GABA_A$ synapses on the central terminals of primary afferent fibers (Eccles et al. 1963; Jiminez et al. 1987). This is consistent with the reduction in the peripheral inflammation by spinal application of a $GABA_A$ receptor antagonist, bicuculline. Increased extracellular potassium concentration also results in PAD (Svobada et al. 1988), and a small increase $[K^+]$ has been shown in this arthritis model (Heinemann et al. 1990). Additionally, activation of descending pathways causes a depolarization of primary afferent fibers (Carpenter et al. 1963; Martin et al. 1979). This central pathway influencing joint inflammation is further supported by recent studies that demonstrated: (1) an increased release of neuropeptides into the knee joint on the side contralateral to the inflammation (Bileviciute et al. 1993), and (2) a blockade of the spread of inflammation to the contralateral limb following capsaicin pretreatment of either sciatic nerve (Donaldson et al. 1993).

Another alternative is increased activity in muscle efferents, which would result in behavioral signs similar to those observed in this model, i.e., limping, and guarding of the limb. Indeed, an increase in activity in muscle efferents has been observed in a variety of nociceptive conditions (Woolf 1983; Woolf and Wall 1986; Woolf and Thompson 1991). However, though many mechanisms may be responsible for the central control of peripheral joint inflammation, we believe that DRRs triggered by PAD are likely to play a major role.

The increased central EAA release and content of GLU, SP, and CGRP (Schaible et al. 1990; Sluka and Westlund 1992, 1993d; Sorkin et al. 1992) may contribute to the sensitization of dorsal horn neurons. In fact, the release and increased content of GLU is blocked by spinal application of either a non-NMDA or an NMDA receptor antagonist, while the increase in SP is blocked only by non-NMDA receptor antagonists (Sluka and Westlund 1993c). In addition, the changes in PWL have been correlated with the changes in GLU immunoreactivity in the superficial dorsal horn (Sluka and Westlund 1993d), further implicating GLU in the development of heat hyperalgesia. Lastly, central sensitization can be reduced by iontophoretic application of an NMDA receptor antagonist (Schaible et al. 1991). Increased responsiveness of nociceptive neurons due to sensitization would lead to an increased firing of the neurons and therefore an increased transmission of nociceptive information to higher centers.

The heat hyperalgesia of the paw that develops in these arthritic animals reflects a central neuronal sensitization because the inflammation itself is localized to the knee joint and does not include the sensitized paw. The sensitization of central neurons (Dougherty et al. 1992b) could be a result of the increased spinal release and content of EAAs (Sorkin et al. 1992; Sluka et al.

1992; Sluka and Westlund 1992, 1993a,c) and of neuropeptides (Schaible et al. 1990; Sluka et al. 1992; Sluka and Westlund 1993d). The heat hyperalgesia of the paw does not occur if EAA release and content are blocked by both non-NMDA and NMDA receptor antagonists (Sluka and Westlund 1993a,b,c). Previous studies have demonstrated involvement of NMDA (Aanonsen and Wilcox 1987; Ault and Hildebrand 1993; Ren et al. 1992; Schaible et al. 1991; Nasstrom and Karlsson 1992) and non-NMDA (Ault and Hildebrand 1993; Dougherty et al. 1992a,b; Nässtrröm et al. 1992; Sluka and Westlund 1993a) receptors in a variety of nociceptive events.

In summary, these studies indicate that there are central neuronal networks not only for processing nociceptive information but also for activating events resulting in peripheral inflammation. Transmission of the nociceptive information involves the release of the EAAs, ASP, and GLU, as well the activation of both non-NMDA and NMDA receptors. In contrast, the development of the peripheral inflammation and the behavioral manifestations (guarding and limping) are affected differentially by the two EAA receptor types. The joint inflammation is also reduced by spinal administration of a $GABA_A$ receptor antagonist and dorsal rhizotomy. The central pathway initially involves the activation of non-NMDA receptors in the spinal cord that in turn activate $GABA_A$ synapses on the central terminals of primary afferent fibers. Activation of these terminals would cause PAD and dorsal root reflexes that would produce a peripheral release of inflammatory neuropeptides into the joint. Clinically, these data seem to suggest that recovery time following surgical trauma and joint inflammation could be significantly reduced with preemptive treatment of the anticipated pain and inflammatory events.

ACKNOWLEDGMENTS

We thank Heidi Jordan for surgical assistance with the microdialysis experiments. This was supported by NIH grants NS11255 and NS01445, RO1 NS28064, and an unrestricted grant from the Bristol-Myers Squibb Company.

REFERENCES

Aanonsen, L.M. and Wilcox, G.L., Nociceptive action of excitatory amino acids in the mouse: effects of spinally administered opioids, phencyclidine and sigma agonists, J. Pharmacol. Exp. Ther., 243 (1987) 9–19.

Appelgren, A., Appelgren, B., Eriksson, S., Kopp, S., Lundeberg, T., Nylander, M. and Theodorsson, E., Neuropeptides in temporomandibular joints with rheumatoid arthritis: a clinical study, Scand. J. Dent. Res., 99 (1991) 519–521.

Attal, N., Jazat, F., Kayser, V. and Guilbaud, G., Further evidence for "pain-related" behaviours in a model of unilateral peripheral mononeuropathy, Pain, 41 (1990) 235–251.

Ault, B. and Hildebrand, L.M., Effects of excitatory amino acid receptor antagonists on a capsaicin-evoked nociceptive reflex: a comparison with morphine, clonidine, and baclofen, Pain, 52 (1993) 341–349.

Bileviciute, I., Lundeberg, T., Edblom, A. and Theodorssan, E., Bilateral changes of substance P-, neurokinin A-, calcitonin gene-related peptide- and neuropeptide Y-like immunoreactivity in rat knee joint synovial fluid during acute monoarthritis, Neurosci. Lett., 153 (1993) 37–40.

Brain, S.D. and Williams, T.J., Inflammatory oedema induced by synergism between calcitonin gene-related peptide (CGRP) and mediators of increased vascular permeability, Br. J. Pharm., 86 (1985) 855–860.

Carpenter, D., Lundberg, A. and Norrsell, U., Primary afferent depolarization evoked from the sensorimotor cortex, Acta Physiol. Scand., 59, (1963) 126–142.

Chung, K., Lee, W.T. and Carlton, S.M., The effects of dorsal rhizotomy and spinal cord isolation on calcitonin gene-related peptide-labeled terminals in the rat lumbar dorsal horn, Neurosci. Lett., 90 (1988) 27–32.

Coggeshall, R.E., Hong, K.A.P., Langford, L.A., Schaible, H.-G. and Schmidt, R.F., Discharge characteristics of fine medial articular afferents at rest and during passive movements of inflamed knee joints, Brain Res. 272 (1983) 185–188.

Craig, A.D., Heppelmann, B. and Schaible, H.-G., The projection of the medial and posterior articular nerves of the cat's knee to the spinal cord, J. Comp. Neurol., 276 (1988) 279–288.

Davies, S.N., and Lodge, D., Evidence for involvement of N-methylaspartate receptors in "wind-up" of class 2 neurons in the dorsal horn of the rat, Brain Res., 424 (1987) 402–406.

Donaldson, L.F., McQueen, D.S. and Seckl, J.R., Inhibition of spread of inflammation by perineural capsaicin: involvement of the nervous system in experimental arthritis. Abstract, XXXII Congress of the International Union of Physiological Sciences, 1993.

Dougherty, P.M., Palecek, J., Palecekova, V., Sorkin, L.S. and Willis, WD., The role of NMDA and non-NMDA excitatory amino acid receptors in the excitation of primate spinothalamic tract neurons by mechanical, chemical, thermal, and electrical stimuli, J. Neurosci., 12 (1992a) 3025–3041.

Dougherty, P.M., Sluka, K.A., Sorkin, L.S., Westlund, K.N. and Willis W.D., Neural changes in acute arthritis in monkeys. I. Parallel enhancement of responses of spinothalamic tract neurons to mechanical stimuli and excitatory amino acids, Brain Res. Rev., 17 (1992b) 1–13.

Eccles, J.C., Schmidt, R.F. and Willis, W.D., Pharmacological studies on presynaptic inhibition, J. Physiol., 168 (1963) 500–530.

Hargreaves, K., Dubner, R., Brown, F. and Flores, C., A new and sensitive method for measuring thermal nociception in cutaneous hyperalgesia, Pain, 32 (1988) 77–88.

Heinemann, U., Schaible, H.-G. and Schmidt, R.F., Changes in extracellular postassium concentration in cat spinal cord in response to innocuous and noxious stimulation of legs with healthy and inflamed knee joints, Exp. Brain Res., 79 (1990) 283–292.

Hurley, J.V., Acute Inflammation, Churchill Livingstone, New York, 1983.

Jimenez, I., Rudomin, P. and Solodkin, M., Mechanisms involved in the depolarization of cutaneous afferents produced by segmental and descending inputs in the cat spinal cord, Exp. Brain Res., 69 (1987) 195–207.

Lam, F.Y. and Ferrell, W.R., Inhibition of carrageenan induced inflammation in the rat knee by substance P antagonist, Ann. Rheum. Dis., 48 (1989a) 928–932.

Lam, F.Y. and Ferrell, W.R., Capsaicin suppresses substance P-induced joint inflammation in the rat, Neurosci. Lett., 105 (1989b) 155–158.

Larsson, J., Ekblom, A., Henriksson, K., Lundeberg, T. and Theodorsson, E., Concentration of substance P, neurokinin A, calcitonin gene-related peptide, neuropeptide Y and vasoactive intestinal polypeptide in synovial fluid from knee joints in patients suffering from rheumatoid arthritis, Scand. J. Rheumatol., 20 (1991) 326–335.

Levine, J.D., Clark, R., Devor, M., Helms, C., Moskowitz, M.A. and Basbaum, A.I., Intraneuronal substance P contributes to the severity of experimental arthritis, Science, 226 (1984) 547–549.

Levine, J.D., Dardick, S.J., Roizen, M.F., Helms, C. and Basbaum, A.I., Contribution of sensory afferents and sympathetic afferents to joint injury in experimental arthritis, J. Neurosci., 6 (1986) 3423–3429.
Levine, J.D., Coderre, T.J., and Basbaum, A.I. The peripheral nervous system and the inflammatory process. In: R. Dubner, G.F. Gebhart and M.R. Bond (Eds.), Proceedings of the Vth World Congress on Pain. Pain Research and Clinical Management, Vol. 3. Elsevier, Amsterdam, 1988, pp. 33–43.
Mapp, P.I., Kidd, B.L., Gibson, S.J., Terry, J.M., Revell, P.A., Ibrahim, N.B.N., Blake, D.R. and Polak, J.M., Substance P-, calcitonin gene-related peptide- and C-flanking peptide of neuropeptide Y-immunoreactive fibres are present in normal synovium but depleted in patients with rheumatoid arthritis, Neuroscience, 37 (1990) 143–153.
Marshall, K.W., Chiu, B. and Inman, R.D., Substance P and arthritis: analysis of plasma and synovial fluid levels, Arthritis Rheum., 33 (1990) 87–90.
Martin, R.F., Haber, L.H. and Willis, W.D., Primary afferent depolarization of identified cutaneous fibers following stimulation in medial brain stem, J. Neurophys., 42 (1979) 779–790.
Nässtrōm, J., Karlsson, U. and Post, C., Antinociceptive actions of different classes of excitatory amino-acid receptor antagonists in mice, Europ. J. Pharmacol., 212 (1992) 21–29.
Neugebauer, V. and Schaible, H.-G., Evidence for a central component in the sensitization of spinal neurons with joint input during development of acute arthritis in cat's knee, J. Neurophys., 64 (1990) 303–310.
Pereira da Silva, J.A. and Carmo-Fonseca, M., Peptide containing nerves in human synovium: immunohistochemical evidence for decreased innervation in rheumatoid arthritis, J. Rheumatol., 17 (1990) 1592–1599.
Rees, H., Sluka, K.A., Westlund, K.N. and Willis, W.D., Do dorsal root reflexes augment peripheral inflammation? Neuroreport, 5 (1994) 821–824.
Ren, K., Williams, G.M., Hylden, J.L.K., Ruda, M.A. and Dubner, R., The intrathecal administration of excitatory amino-acid receptor antagonists selectively attenuated carrageenan-induced behavioral hyperalgesia in rats, Europ. J. Pharmacol., 219 (1992) 235–243.
Schaible, H.-G., Schmidt, R.F. and Willis, W.D., Enhancement of the responses of ascending tract cells in the cat spinal cord by acute inflammation of the knee joint, Exp. Brain Res., 66 (1987) 466–489.
Schaible, H.-G., Jarrot, B., Hope, P.J. and Duggan, A.W., Release of immunoreactive substance P in the spinal cord during development of acute arthritis in the knee joint of the cat: a study with antibody microprobes, Brain Res., 529 (1990) 214–223.
Schaible, H.-G., Grubb, B.D., Neugebauer, V. and Oppman, M., The effects of NMDA antagonists on neuronal activity in cat spinal cord evoked by acute inflammation in the knee joint, Europ. J. Neurosci., 3 (1991) 981–991.
Skilling, S.R., Smullin, H.D., Beitz, A.J. and Larsson, A.A., Extracellular amino acid concentrations in the dorsal spinal cord of freely moving rats following veratridine and nociceptive stimulation, J. Neurochem., 51 (1988) 127–132.
Sluka, K.A. and Westlund, K.N., An experimental arthritis in rat: dorsal horn aspartate and glutamate increases, Neurosci. Lett., 145 (1992) 141–144.
Sluka, K.A. and Westlund, K.N., An experimental arthritis in rat: the effects on non-NMDA and NMDA receptor antagonists, Neurosci. Lett., 149 (1993a) 99–102.
Sluka, K.A. and Westlund, K.N., Centrally administered non-NMDA but not NMDA receptor antagonists block peripheral knee joint inflammation, Pain, 55 (1993b) 217–225.
Sluka, K.A. and Westlund, K.N., Spinal cord amino acid release and content in an arthritis model: the effects of pretreatment with non-NMDA, NMDA, and NK1 receptor antagonists, Brain Res., 627 (1993c) 89–103.
Sluka, K.A. and Westlund, K.N., Behavioral and immunohistochemical changes in an experimental arthritis model in rats, Pain, 55 (1993d) 367–377.

Sluka, K.A., Dougherty, P.M., Sorkin, L.S., Willis, W.D., and Westlund, K.N., Neural changes in acute arthritis in monkeys. III. Changes in substance P, calcitonin gene-related peptide and glutamate in the dorsal horn of the spinal cord, Brain Res. Rev., 17 (1992) 29–38.

Sluka, K.A., Willis, W.D. and Westlund, K.N., Joint inflammation and hyperalgesia are reduced by spinal bicuculline, Neuroreport, 5 (1993) 109–112.

Sorkin, L.S., Steinman, J.L., Hughes, M.G., Willis, W.D. and McAdoo, D.J., Microdialysis recovery of serotonin released in spinal cord dorsal horn, J. Neurosci. Methods, 23 (1988) 131–138.

Sorkin, L.S., Sluka, K.A., Dougherty, P.M., Westlund, K.N. and Willis, W.D., Neural changes in acute arthritis in monkeys. IV. Time-course of amino acid release into the lumbar dorsal horn, Brain Res. Rev., 17 (1992) 39–50.

Svoboda, J., Motin, V., Hajek, I. and Sykova, E., Increase in extracellular potassium level in rat spinal dorsal horn induced by noxious stimulation and peripheral injury, Brain Res., 458 (1988) 97–105.

Weihe, E., Nohr, D., Millan, M.J., Stein, C., Müller, S., Gramsch, C. and Herz, A., Peptide neuroanatomy of adjuvant-induced arthritic inflammation in rat, Agents Actions, 25 (1988) 255–259.

Westlund, K.N., Sun, Y.C., Sluka, K.A., Dougherty, P.M., Sorkin, L.S. and Willis, W.D., Neural changes in acute arthritis in monkeys. II. Increased glutamate immunoreactivity in the medial articular nerve, Brain Res. Rev., 17 (1992) 15–27.

Woolf, C.J., Evidence for a central component of post-injury pain hypersensitivity, Nature, 306 (1983) 686–688.

Woolf, C.J. and Thompson, S.W.N., The induction and maintenance of central sensitization is dependent on N-methyl-D-aspartic acid receptor activation; implications for the treatment of post-injury pain hypersensitivity states, Pain, 44 (1991) 293–299.

Woolf, C.J. and Wall, P.D., Relative effectiveness of C primary afferent fibers of diffferent origins in evoking a prolonged facilitation of the flexor reflex in the rat, J. Neurosci., 6 (1986) 1433–1442.

Yaksh, T.L., Bailey, J., Roddy, D.R. and Harty, G.J., Peripheral release of substance P from primary afferents. In: R. Dubner, G.F. Gebhart and M.R. Bond (Eds.), Proceedings of the Vth World Congress on Pain. Pain Research and Clinical Management, Vol. 3. Elsevier, Amsterdam, 1988, pp. 51–54.

Correspondence to: Karin N. Westlund, Marine Biomedical Institute, Department of Anatomy and Neurosciences, 200 University Blvd., University of Texas Medical Branch, Galveston, TX 77555-0843, USA. Tel: 409-772-2124; Fax: 409-762-9382.

Proceedings of the 7th World Congress on Pain,
Progress in Pain Research and Management, Vol. 2,
edited by G.F. Gebhart, D.L. Hammond, and T.S.
Jensen, IASP Press, Seattle, © 1994.

26

Anatomical and Pharmacological Evidence for a Contribution of Protein Kinase C to Persistent Nociception and Hyperalgesia after Noxious Chemical and Thermal Stimulation

Terence J. Coderre,[a,b,c] Kiran Yashpal,[a,d]
Graham M. Pitcher,[a] and Rémi Quirion[d,e]

[a]Pain Mechanisms Laboratory, Clinical Research Institute of Montreal; [b]Centre de Recherche en Sciences Neurologiques et Département de Médecine, Université de Montréal; [c]Department of Psychology and [d]Department of Psychiatry, McGill University, Montreal; and [e]Douglas Hospital Research Center, Verdun; Quebec, Canada

INTRODUCTION

Intense nociceptive inputs not only elicit direct synaptic responses in spinal and other central neurons, but also induce changes in excitability in these neurons that persist beyond the direct activation. Such changes, given terms such as wind-up, plasticity, or sensitization, cannot be fully explained as being mediated by long actions of peptides, such as substance P, or excitatory amino acids (EAA), because the persistent changes last much longer than do the direct synaptic events. Synaptic activation of N-methyl-D-aspartate (NMDA) and neurokinin-1 (NK-1) receptors produces brief effects lasting at most milliseconds to seconds for NMDA receptors (Gerber et al. 1991) and seconds to minutes for NK-1 receptors (Urban and Randic 1984; De Koninck and Henry 1991). Thus, it is unlikely that NMDA or NK-1 receptor activation by themselves can account for the prolonged changes in neuronal excitability that follow peripheral tissue injury. More likely, these prolonged changes in excitability depend on the ability of EAA and NK-1 receptor activation to stimulate the production of various intracellular messengers in neuronal cells (Watson and Downes 1983; Sugiyama et al. 1987).

Earlier studies from our laboratory have shown that protein kinase C (PKC), an intracellular product of EAA and NK-1 receptor activation, contributes to persistent pain in the formalin test (Coderre 1992). In the present study, we further assess the role of PKC in the development of central sensitization, persistent nociception, and secondary hyperalgesia following tissue injury. Thus, we compared the effects of pharmacological inhibition of PKC with PKC[19–36] or chelerythrine on persistent pain following formalin injury, with its effects on the mechanical hyperalgesia that develops in the hindpaw contralateral to a thermal injury. Furthermore, we conducted autoradiographic studies on rat spinal cords to assess the changes in the levels of membrane-associated PKC in response to both formalin and thermal injury. Binding sites for [^{3}H]-phorbol 12,13-dibutyrate ([^{3}H]-PDBu), which is a putative marker of membrane-bound PKC, were quantified at various times after the noxious stimulation was applied.

METHODS

These experiments were performed on male Long Evans hooded rats (Charles River) weighing 300–350 g. They were maintained under controlled lighting conditions with food and water available ad libitum. The guidelines described in the *Guide to the Care and Use of Experimental Animals* of the Canadian Council of Animal Care, Vols. I and II, were strictly followed in all experiments.

PHARMACOLOGICAL STUDIES

For chemical nociception, rats were given a subcutaneous injection of 50 μl of 2.5% formalin into the plantar surface of one hindpaw. For nociceptive testing, animals were placed in a 30 cm × 30 cm × 30 cm Plexiglas box with a mirror below the surface at a 45° angle to allow an unobstructed view of the paws. Scoring of nociceptive behaviors began immediately after formalin injection and continued for 50 minutes. A nociceptive score was determined for each five-minute time block by measuring the amount of time spent in each of the following behavioral categories: 0, the injected paw is not favored; 1, the injected paw has little or no weight placed on it; 2, the injected paw is elevated and is not in contact with any surface; 3, the injected paw is licked, bitten, or shaken. A weighted, average nociceptive score, ranging from 0 to 3, was calculated by multiplying the time spent in each category by the category weight, summing these products, and then dividing by the total time for each five-minute time block. All the rats were acclimatized to the test chamber before testing began.

The noxious thermal stimulus consisted of the immersion of one hindpaw into water maintained at 55°C for 15 seconds, while rats were briefly anesthetized with halothane inhalation anesthesia. Following the noxious thermal stimulation, mechanical hyperalgesia in the contralateral hindpaw was measured using the Randall Selitto apparatus, which exerts an accelerating force to a focused point on the rat's hindpaw. After baseline recordings for a flexion reflex response to the mechanical stimulus, the rat was anesthetized, and one of the rat's hindpaws was immersed in the 55°C water for 15 seconds. After recovery from the halothane anesthesia, mechanical flexion reflexes were measured again at 2, 5, 10, and 30 minutes, as well as 3, 12, and 36 hours, and 3 days following the noxious thermal stimulation. Mechanical flexion reflex thresholds for baseline and posttreatment trials were based on an average of four tests after eliminating the highest and lowest scores. Scores are given as change from baseline using the standard formula for percentage maximum possible effect {MPE = [(post drug score – baseline score)/(cutoff – baseline)] × 100} (Yaksh and Rudy 1977).

The two agents known to inhibit PKC included PKC[19–36] (4–40 μg) and chelerythrine (20–50 μg). PKC [19–36] was dissolved in 0.9% saline while chelerythrine was dissolved in 10% dimethyl sulfoxide (DMSO) in 0.9% saline, and both agents were given intrathecally in 30-μl volume by lumbar puncture between the L5 and L6 vertebrae, while the rats were under brief halothane anesthesia. For both formalin and secondary hyperalgesia trials, testing began 45–60 minutes after treatment with either a vehicle of 10% DMSO in 0.9% saline, PKC[19–36] or chelerythrine.

ANATOMICAL STUDIES

After the chemical injury (intraplantar injection of 50 μl of 5.0% formalin to one hindpaw), three animals were decapitated at each of three time points (5, 25, and 60 minutes). Rats were conscious following the injury and their behavior was observed up to the time of sacrifice. Similarly, in the case of thermal injury, three rats were decapitated at each of three time points (1, 10, and 30 minutes) after immersion of one hindpaw in 55°C water for 90 seconds. For thermal injury, rats were anesthetized with chloral hydrate (200 mg/kg ip.) during the noxious thermal stimulation and until sacrifice. Control rats received no injury.

After decapitation, spinal cords were rapidly removed, dissected into specific segments, and snap-frozen at –40°C in 2-methylbutane. Tissue blocks were fixed to microtome chucks and serial transverse sections (20 μm) were cut at –18°C using a cryostat microtome. Sections were then thaw mounted onto gelatin-coated microscope slides, dried overnight under a vacuum, and stored at –80°C until autoradiographic processing.

[^{3}H]-PDBu (17 Ci/mmol, New England Nuclear, Boston, Mass.) binding assay was performed by preincubating sections for one hour at 4°C in a buffer containing 50 mM Tris-HCl (pH 7.7), 100 mM NaCl, and 1 mM $CaCl_2$, as described by Worley et al. (1986). Incubations were then carried out in the same buffer containing bovine serum albumin (0.1%, Boehringer Mannheim) and 2.5 nM [^{3}H]-PDBu for one hour at 33°C. Nonspecific labeling was assessed by adding excess of unlabeled PDBu (1 μM, Sigma) to the incubation solution. At the end of the incubation period, sections were washed twice in ice-cold distilled water and immediately dried under a stream of cold air. Under these conditions, specifically bound [^{3}H]-PDBu represented the totality of bound ligand. Autoradiograms were generated by opposing 3H-Hyperfilm (Amersham) to slides for seven days. Binding of [^{3}H]-PDBu to sections was quantitated by microcomputer image analysis (MCID system) using tritium-labeled standards (Amersham) for film calibration. The regions sampled included superficial dorsal horn (laminae I–II), central canal (lamina X), and ventral horn for samples taken from the lumbar region of the spinal cord.

RESULTS

PHARMACOLOGICAL STUDIES

Nociceptive scores in the formalin test for the controls and two groups of rats treated with PKC[19–36] or with chelerythrine are shown in Fig. 1. The control group, treated with vehicle, exhibited the typical biphasic response after formalin injection to one hind paw. The first early phase, occurring maximally at five minutes, was followed by the intermediate phase (5–10 minutes) of relatively low nociceptive scores and then by the second nociceptive phase, which started at about 20 minutes after formalin injection and continued until the completion of testing at 50 minutes.

In the groups pretreated with PKC inhibitors, there was a significant reduction in the typical nociceptive responses. Thus, intrathecal administration of 4 μg of PKC[19–36] significantly reduced nociceptive scores during the

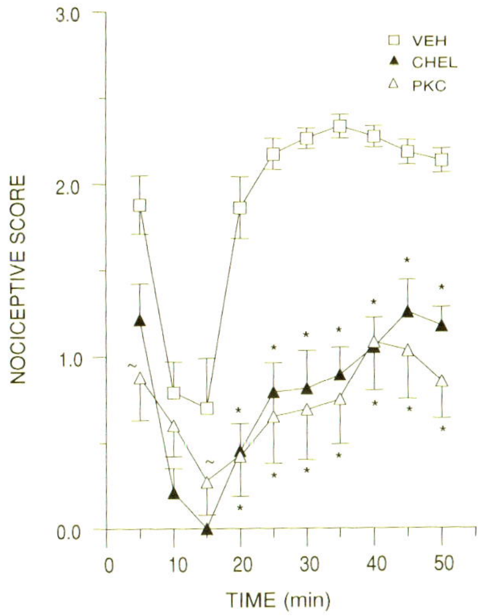

Fig. 1. Nociceptive responses (± S.E.M.) induced by injection of 50 µl of 2.5% formalin in rats pretreated with PKC [19–36] (4 µg, N = 5) or chelerythrine (20 µg, N = 5) or vehicle (N = 6). Repeated measures ANOVA reveals significant effects of drug treatment [$F(2,13) = 51.8$, $P < 0.001$] and time [$F(9, 117) = 16.9$, $P < 0.001$], as well as a significant treatment by time interaction [$F(18, 117) = 2.36$, $P < 0.01$]. Significant differences from the vehicle control group: ~ $P < 0.05$; * $P < 0.01$, Dunnett *t*.

early (0–5 minutes) and the late (10–50 minutes) phases of the formalin test. Intrathecal pretreatment with 20 µg of chelerythrine did not significantly reduce nociceptive scores during the early (0–5 minutes) phase, but did significantly reduce nociceptive scores during the late (15–50 minutes) phase of the formalin test.

Fig. 2 illustrates the mechanical flexion reflex measured by the Randall-Selitto test in one hind paw after the thermal injury to the contralateral hind paw. In the control group, there was an initial brief antinociception with thresholds significantly higher than baseline at the 0.5-minute time point after injury. This initial antinociception was followed by a persistent hyperalgesia, with thresholds significantly lower than baseline between 30 minutes and 12 hours after the injury. Mechanical flexion reflex thresholds returned to normal levels by the 36-hour measurement and remained so at the three-day recording. In the group pretreated with PKC[19–36], both the initial antinociceptive effect and the persistent hyperalgesia between 30 minutes and 12 hours was significantly attenuated. In the group given chelerythrine, the antinociception was significantly increased, and the persistent hyperalgesia was significantly attenuated at 30 minutes, 3, and 12 hours after the injury. Not only was the hyperalgesia blocked, but there may also have been a small degree of analgesia produced by chelerythrine.

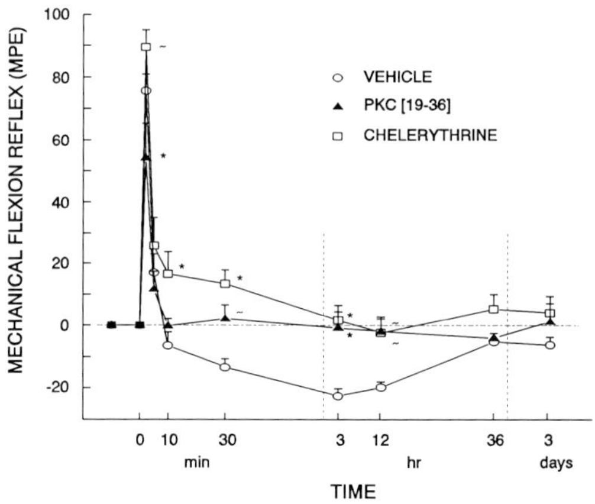

Fig. 2. Percentage maximum possible effect (MPE ± S.E.M.) for mechanical flexion reflex on Randall Selitto apparatus after thermal injury of the contralateral hind paw in rats pretreated with either PKC [19–36] (40 µg, N = 6), chelerythrine (50 µg, N = 6) or vehicle (N = 8). Repeated measures ANOVA reveals significant main effects for treatment group [$F(2,23) = 8.9$, $P < 0.01$] and time [$F(7, 161) = 136.4$. $P < 0.001$], as well as a significant group by time interaction [$F(14, 161) = 3.18$, $P < 0.001$]. Significant differences from the vehicle control group: ~ $P < 0.05$; * $P < 0.01$, Dunnett *t*.

ANATOMICAL STUDIES

Fig. 3 shows the distribution of binding sites for [^{3}H]-PDBu in the lumbar spinal cord of a control rat. Of the three regions (i.e., dorsal horn LI–II; central canal, LX; ventral horn) quantified densities in the superficial dorsal horn were the highest. Moderate amounts of [^{3}H]-PDBu binding were also detected in the central canal region, and the lowest amounts were found in the ventral horn.

The distribution of [^{3}H]-PDBu binding in the lumbar spinal cord of the rats sacrificed at 5, 25, and 60 minutes after the injection of formalin is also shown in Fig. 3. Quantification of the data reveals that [^{3}H]-PDBu binding increased in the superficial layers of the dorsal horn as early as five minutes after the formalin injection (at five minutes 1864.1 ± 32.1, n = 40 vs. controls 1413.0 ± 34.2 fmol/mg tissue, n = 12, $P < 0.01$). This increase remained significantly high, peaking at 25 minutes (1974.9 ± 41.1 fmol/mg tissue, n = 21, $P < 0.01$), but returned toward normal values, such that it was not significantly different than control, at 60 minutes (at 60 minutes 1565.5 ± 27.3, n = 8 vs. controls 1413.0 ± 34.2 fmol/mg tissue, n = 10, $P > 0.05$). The maximum level of membrane-bound PKC, as determined by the [^{3}H]-PDBu binding assay, appeared to occur at 25 minutes after the chemical injury,

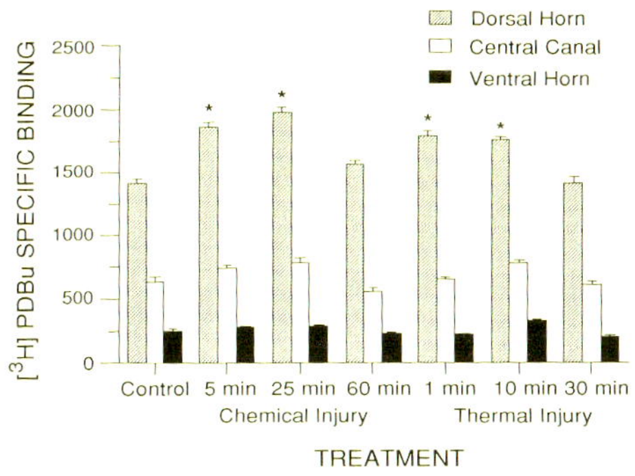

Fig. 3. Quantitative autoradiographic analysis of the distribution of [^{3}H]-PDBu binding in the lumbar spinal cord of control rats and experimental rats at specific times after noxious chemical (5, 25, and 60 min) or thermal (1, 10, and 30 min) stimulation. Each histogram represents specific [^{3}H]-PDBu binding as expressed as mean ± S.E.M. in fmol/mg tissue, obtained from 10–18 sections at each segmental level of spinal cords from three rats. ANOVA revealed a significant main effect of treatment group in the dorsal horn [$F(6,136) = 27.1$, $P < 0.001$], central canal [$F(5,32) = 4.6$, $P < 0.001$], and ventral horn [$F(6,132) = 14.2$, $P < 0.001$] regions. Significant differences from the control group are indicated by the asterisks (* $P < 0.01$, Scheffé).

which coincides with the peak behavioral responses to formalin injury.

The other regions besides the dorsal horn (laminae I and II) that were quantified included the central canal region (lamina X) and the ventral horn (Fig. 3). Quantification of these areas and their statistical analysis showed no significant differences at any time point when compared to control values (central canal: at 5 minutes 738.5 ± 23.6, n = 16; at 25 minutes 782.8 ± 35.8, n = 9; at 60 minutes 529.7 ± 33.6, n = 4; vs. controls 630.4 ± 43.6 fmol/mg tissue, n = 7). The binding densities were lowest for the ventral horn region, and as stated no significant difference was seen at any time period after formalin injection when compared to controls (ventral horn: at 5 minutes 281.0 ± 7.9, n = 40; at 25 minutes 286.4 ± 14.4, n = 13; at 60 minutes 231.4 ± 8.0, n = 8 vs. controls 253.9 ± 12.8 fmol/mg tissue, n = 12).

An immediate increase in [^{3}H]-PDBu binding was seen in laminae I and II of the dorsal horn of the lumbar segment when one of the hind paws of the rat was immersed in hot water at 55°C for 90 seconds (Fig. 3). These levels were significantly higher than the control values at one minute and remained significantly high until 10 minutes after the noxious thermal stimulus was applied (at 1 minute 1789.8 ± 42.2, n = 18; at 10 minutes 1762.6 ± 22.2, n = 14 vs. controls 1413.0 ± 34.2 fmol/mg tissue, n = 12). [^{3}H]-PDBu binding returned to the control levels by 30 minutes after the stimulus was given (at 30 minutes 1413.6 ± 50.1, n = 14 vs. controls 1413 ± 34.2 fmol/mg tissue, n = 12).

Along the lamina X (central canal) region, no significant change from control values was observed at 1, 10, or 30 minutes after the thermal stimulation (at 1 minute 649.9 ± 17.3, n = 11; at 10 minutes 775.0 ± 23.3, n = 16; at 30 minutes 606.0 ± 26.7, n = 8; vs. controls 630.4 ± 43.6 fmol/mg tissue, n = 7, $P > 0.05$) (Fig. 5A). In the ventral horn of the lumbar cord there was once again no significant change from control values in [^{3}H] PDBu binding either at 1 minute, 10 minutes, or 30 minutes after the thermal stimulation (at 1 minute 223.4 ± 6.8, n = 20; at 10 minutes 328.0 ± 13.1, n = 32; and at 30 minutes 206.9 ± 12.0 vs. controls 253.9 ± 12.8 fmol/mg tissue, n = 12, $P > 0.05$).

In summary, the density of [^{3}H]-PDBu binding in the dorsal horns of the lumbar region was increased at 1 and 10 minutes after thermal injury, and 5 and 25 minutes after formalin injury. Binding returned to control values by 30 minutes after thermal, and 60 minutes after formalin injury. No significant changes in [^{3}H]-PDBu binding were found in the central canal region and ventral horn at any time point after thermal or formalin injury.

DISCUSSION

The results from our present study provide evidence for a contribution of PKC to the persistent nociceptive responses induced by noxious chemical or thermal stimulation to one hind paw of the rat. The experiments provide not only pharmacological evidence with our two physiological models of nociception, but also anatomical evidence using a highly specific radioligand, [^{3}H]-phorbol-12,13 dibutyrate, as an autoradiographic probe for membrane-bound PKC. Both types of analysis suggest a participation of PKC in the mechanisms of persistent nociception. Thus, the pharmacological experiments indicate that intrathecal administration of each of the two inhibitors of PKC—PKC [19–36] and chelerythrine—attenuated the persistent nociception induced by formalin injection and blocked the contralateral hyperalgesia produced by immersion of a hind paw in hot water. Activation of PKC by noxious peripheral stimulation was also apparent in the autoradiographic data, which showed an increase in [^{3}H]-PDBu binding or translocation of membrane-bound PKC predominantly in the dorsal horn of the lumbar spinal cord.

Earlier studies from our laboratory have demonstrated an enhancement of nociceptive scores in the formalin test by intrathecal pretreatment with phorbol esters, activators of PKC, as well as a reduction of formalin-induced nociceptive behaviors with intrathecal pretreatment with a relatively nonspecific protein kinase inhibitor, H-7 (Coderre 1992). Experiments presented here indicate that administration of PKC [19–36] and chelerythrine, much more selective inhibitors of PKC, reduce the nociceptive scores in the late phase of formalin testing, and for PKC [19–36] also the early phase. In the case of thermal injury, these agents reduce the persistent hyperalgesia that develops in the hindpaw contralateral to a thermal injury. Importantly, the presence of the PKC inhibitor at the time of injury blocks the expression of secondary hyperalgesia between 30 minutes and 12 hours after the injury. Significantly, the intracellular events triggered here appear to be less involved in the initial responses to noxious stimulation, but rather, are critically involved in mediating the plastic changes and sensitization of neurons leading to prolonged nociception. A confirming point is that the inhibitors of PKC used in the present experiments are not analgesic themselves in noninjurious measures of mechanical and thermal reflexes (Coderre and Yashpal 1994). This finding provides further support to the notion that PKC is involved in persistent neural sensitization but is not involved in responses to brief noxious stimulation (Coderre 1992).

Our data on quantification of membrane-bound PKC in control rats support previous evidence demonstrating high densities of [^{3}H]-PDBu binding sites (Worley et al. 1986) as well as dense PKC-like immunoreactivity (Saito et al. 1988; Nagashima et al. 1991) in the dorsal horn of the lumbar spinal cord. In particular, we observed high densities in the superficial layers of the spinal cord dorsal horn (laminae I and II), very low densities in the ventral horn, and intermediate levels in lamina X (Fig. 3). We also showed that noxious chemical and thermal stimulation of a rat's hind paw produces increases in membrane-bound PKC in lumbar spinal cord. Noxious chemical stimulation produced a prolonged increase (at least 5–25 minutes) in [^{3}H]-PDBu binding in the lumbar spinal cord dorsal horn, while noxious thermal stimulation produced a brief increase (1–10 minutes) in [^{3}H]-PDBu binding in the dorsal horn of the lumbar spinal cord. Participation of PKC in persistent nociception is further supported by evidence that gangliosides, which inhibit the translocation and activation of PKC (Vaccarino et al. 1987), reduce nociceptive behaviors and thermal hyperalgesia that develop in the rats with constriction injury of the sciatic nerve (Hayes et al. 1992). In addition, spinal cord administration of GM1 ganglioside reverses both increased levels of membrane-bound PKC and pain-related behaviors following nerve-constriction injury (Mao et al. 1992).

A role of PKC in persistent nociception should not be unexpected given the growing evidence for the involvement of EAA and NK-1 receptors in persistent nociception, and for the contribution of EAAs and substance P to the generation of intracellular events that lead to the translocation and activation of PKC. In particular, persistent nociception in the formalin test is enhanced by intrathecal administration of L-glutamate, L-aspartate (Coderre and

Melzack 1992), and substance P (Yashpal et al. 1993); intrathecal administration of the selective NMDA receptor antagonist AP5 (Cahusac et al. 1984), or the nonpeptide NK-1 receptor antagonist CP-96,345 (Yashpal et al. 1993), attenuates nociceptive responses to tonic noxious stimuli. Furthermore, both persistent nociceptive responses in the formalin test, as well as remote secondary hyperalgesia following thermal injury, are dependent on NMDA (Murray et al. 1991; Coderre and Melzack 1991, 1992; Yamamoto and Yaksh 1992) and NK-1 receptor activity (Yashpal et al. 1991; Yamamoto and Yaksh 1992; Yashpal et al. 1993).

While evidence that EAAs and substance P are involved in persistent nociception is growing, it is also apparent that activation of EAA and NK-1 receptors produces an activation of various intracellular messengers. In particular, EAA (Sladeczek et al. 1985; Sugiyama et al. 1987) and NK-1 (Watson and Downes 1983) receptor activation increases the hydrolysis of phosphatidylinositol, which eventually leads to an increased translocation and activation of PKC (Vaccarino et al. 1987; Koizumi et al. 1992). The stimulation of PKC can in turn produce protein phosphorylation (Swope et al. 1992), which is an important post-translational system in regulation and maintenance of changes in synaptic efficacy and plasticity (Lynch et al. 1988; Linden and Routtenberg 1989). Recently, Gerber et al. (1989) have shown that activators of PKC enhance the basal and evoked release of glutamate and aspartate in the spinal cord slice, as well as depolarizing responses of dorsal horn neurons to exogenous glutamate and NMDA. Furthermore, Chen and Huang (1992) have demonstrated that PKC increases NMDA-activated currents in isolated trigeminal cells by increasing the probability of channel openings and by reducing the voltage-dependent Mg^{2+} block of NMDA receptor channels.

ACKNOWLEDGMENTS

The authors thank Dr. A. Parent for advice regarding the binding assay in this manuscript. A special thank you to Dr. J.G. Chabot for his time and help with the image analysis system. Thanks also to Dr. J.L. Henry for reviewing the manuscript. This work was supported by grants from the MRC and FRSQ to T.J.C. and from MRC to R.Q.

REFERENCES

Cahusac, P.M.B., Evans, R.H., Hill, R.G., Rodriquez, R.E. and Smith, D.A.S., The behavioural effects of an N-methylaspartate receptor antagonist following application to the lumbar spinal cord of conscious rats, Neuropharmacology, 23 (1984) 719–724.

Chen, L. and Huang, L.-Y.M., Protein kinase C reduces Mg^{2+} block of NMDA-receptor channels as a mechanism of modulation, Nature, 356 (1992) 521–523.

Coderre, T.J., Contribution of protein kinase C to persistent nociception following tissue injury in rats, Neurosci. Lett., 140 (1992) 181–184.

Coderre, T.J. and Melzack, R., Central neural mediators of secondary hyperalgesia following heat injury in rats: neuropeptides and excitatory amino acids, Neurosci. Lett., 131 (1991) 71–74.

Coderre, T.J. and Melzack, R., The contribution of excitatory amino acids to central sensitization and persistent nociception after formalin-induced tissue injury, J. Neurosci., 12 (1992) 3665–3670.

Coderre, T.J. and Yashpal, K., Intracellular messengers contributing to persistent nociception and hyperalgesia induced by L-glutamate and substance P in the rat formalin pain model, Eur. J. Neurosci. (1994) in press.

DeKoninck, Y. and Henry, J.L., Substance P-mediated slow EPSPs elicited in dorsal horn neurons in vivo by noxious stimulation, Proc. Natl. Acad. Sci. USA, 88 (1991) 11344–11348.

Gerber, G., Kangrga, I., Ryu, P.D., Larew, J.S.A. and Randic, M., Multiple effects of phorbol esters in the rat spinal dorsal horn, J. Neurosci., 9 (1989) 3606–3617.

Gerber, G., Cerne, R. and Randic, M., Participation of excitatory amino acid receptors in the slow excitatory synaptic transmission in rat spinal dorsal horn, Brain Res., 561 (1991) 236–251.

Hayes, R.L., Mao, J., Price, D.D., Germano, A., D'Avella, D., Fiori, M. and Mayer, D.L., Pretreatment with gangliosides reduces abnormal nociceptive responses associated with a rodent peripheral mononeuropathy, Pain, 48 (1992) 391–396.

Koizumi, H., Tanaka, H., Fukaya, T. and Ohkawara, T., Substance P induces intracellular calcium release and translocation of protein kinase C in epidermis, Br. J. Dermatol., 127 (1992) 595–599.

Linden, D.J. and Routtenberg, A., The role of protein kinase C in long-term potentiation: a testable model, Brain Res. Brain Res. Rev., 21 (1989) 279–296.

Lynch, G., Muller, D., Seubert, P. and Larson, J., Long-term potentiation: persisting problems and recent results, Brain Res. Bull., 21 (1988) 363–372.

Mao, J., Price, D.D., Mayer, D.J. and Hayes, R.L., Pain-related increases in spinal cord membrane-bound protein kinase C following peripheral nerve injury, Brain Res., 588 (1992) 144–149.

Murray, C.W., Cowan, A. and Larson, A.A. Neurokinin and NMDA antagonists (but not a kainic acid antagonist) are antinociceptive in the mouse formalin model, Pain, 44 (1991) 179–185.

Nagashima, T., Tanabe, H., Fujioka, Y., Nagashima, K. and Hidaka, H., Immunohistochemical localization of protein kinase C isozymes in human cerebellum, hippocampus and spinal cord, Acta Histochem. Cytochem., 24 (1991) 441–446.

Saito, N., Kikkawa, U., Nishizuka, Y. and Tanaka, C., Distribution of protein kinase C-like immunoreactive neurons in rat brain, J. Neurosci., 8 (1988) 369–382.

Sladeczek, F., Pin, J.-P., Recasens, M., Bockaert, J. and Weiss, S., Glutamate stimulates inositol phosphate formation in striatal neurons, Nature, 317 (1985) 717–719.

Sugiyama, H,. Ito, I. and Hirono, C., A new type of glutamate receptor linked to inositol phospholipid metabolism, Nature, 325 (1987) 531–533.

Swope, S.L., Moss, S.J., Blackstone, C.D. and Huganir, R.L., Phosphorylation of ligand-gated ion channels: a possible mode of synaptic plasticity, FASEB J., 6 (1992) 2514–2523.

Urban, L. and Randic, M., Slow excitatory transmission in rat dorsal horn: possible mediation by peptides, Brain Res., 290 (1984) 336–341.

Vaccarino, F., Guidotti, A. and Costa, E., Ganglioside inhibition of glutamate-mediated protein kinase C translocation in primary cultures of cerebellar neurons, Proc. Natl. Acad. Sci. USA, 84 (1987) 8707–8711.

Watson, S.P. and Downes, C.P., Substance P-induced hydrolysis of inositol phospholipids in guinea-pig ileum and rat hypothalamus, Eur. J. Pharmacol., 93 (1983) 245–253.

Worley, P.F., Baraban, J.M. and Snyder, S.H., Heterogeneous localization of protein kinase C in rat brain: autoradiographic analysis of phorbol ester receptor binding, J. Neurosci., 6 (1986) 199–207.

Yaksh, T.L. and Rudy, T.A., Studies on the direct spinal action of narcotics in the production of analgesia in the rat, J. Pharmacol. Exp. Ther., 202 (1977) 411–428.

Yamamoto, T. and Yaksh, T.L., Stereospecific effects of a nonpeptide NK-1 selective antagonist, CP-96,345: antinociception in the absence of motor dysfunction, Life Sci. 49 (1991) 1955–1963.

Yamamoto, T. and Yaksh, T.L., Comparison of the antinociceptive effects of pre- and post-treatment with intrathecal morphine and MK-801, an NMDA antagonist, on the formalin test in the rat, Anesthesiology, 77 (1992) 757–763.

Yashpal, K., Radhakrishnan, V. and Henry, J.L., NMDA receptor antagonist blocks the facilitation of the tail-flick reflex in the rat induced by intrathecal administration of substance P and by noxious cutaneous stimulation, Neurosci. Lett., 128 (1991) 269–272.

Yashpal, K., Radhakrishnan, V., Coderre, T.J. and Henry, J.L., CP-96,345, but not its stereoisomer, CP-96,344, blocks the nociceptive responses to intrathecally administered substance P and to noxious thermal and chemical stimuli in the rat, Neuroscience, 52 (1993) 1039–1047.

Correspondence to: Terence J. Coderre, PhD, Director, Pain Mechanisms Laboratory, Clinical Research Institute of Montreal, 110 Pine Ave. W., Quebec, Canada, H2W 1R7. Tel: 514-987-5750; Fax: 514-987-5624.

Proceedings of the 7th World Congress on Pain,
Progress in Pain Research and Management, Vol. 2,
edited by G.F. Gebhart, D.L. Hammond, and T.S.
Jensen, IASP Press, Seattle, © 1994.

27

Gene Delivery to Mouse Sensory Neurons Using Herpes Virus Vectors

Gudarz Davar,[a] Martha F. Kramer,[d] David Garber,[c] Alfred L. Roca,[b] Julie K. Andersen,[a,b] William Bebrin,[d] Donald M. Coen,[d] Magdalena Kosz-Vnenchak,[c] David M. Knipe,[c] Xandra O. Breakefield,[a,b] and Ole Isacson[a,b,e]

[a]*Neurology Service, Massachusetts General Hospital, Boston, Massachusetts, USA;* [b]*Neuroscience Program,* [c]*Department of Microbiology and Molecular Genetics, and* [d]*Department of Biological Chemistry and Molecular Pharmacology, Harvard Medical School, Boston, Massachusetts, USA; and* [e]*McLean Hospital, Belmont, Massachusetts, USA*

INTRODUCTION

The delivery of functional genes to the nervous system is recognized as a possible method of treatment for a variety of neurologic conditions (Breakefield and Geller 1987; Geller et al. 1991; Martuza et al. 1991; Breakefield et al. 1992). In animals and in humans, gene delivery could be used to alter function (Ho et al. 1993) or to correct underlying defects in gene expression in targeted neurons. In the somatosensory nervous system, for example, the delivery of toxic genes to sensory neurons might produce a cell-specific injury that mimics the pathology observed in some forms of painful neuropathy in humans (Watson 1989; Cornblath and McArthur 1988). Alternatively, the delivery of genes encoding analgesic neuropeptides to sensory neurons may eventually be useful for the treatment of some forms of persistent pain in humans (Davar et al. 1993).

Neurotropic viruses have potential method for delivering functional genes to sensory neurons (Loewy et al. 1991). Herpes simplex virus (HSV), a 150-kilobase, double-stranded, neurotropic DNA virus, is taken up by the terminals of primary sensory neurons and transported by fast axonal transport to the cell nucleus (Cook and Stevens 1973). Within the cell nucleus, it is capable of entering a lytic cycle, during which all kinetic classes of herpes virus genes are expressed (Roizman and Sears 1990) and viral progeny are produced. HSV can also enter a latent state in which the virus persists in the cell nucleus, most likely in an episomal form (Rock and Fraser 1983; Efstathiou et al. 1986; Mellerick and Fraser 1987), but no viral replication occurs, and transcription is largely limited to a specific region of the HSV genome (latency-associated transcripts [LATs]; Croen et al. 1987; Rock et al. 1987; Spivak and Fraser 1987; Stevens et al. 1987; Javier et al. 1988; Wagner et al. 1988). Despite this limited transcriptional activity from the HSV genome, foreign genes inserted into the HSV genome can be stably expressed during latency (Ho and Mocarski 1992; Dobson et al. 1989; Dobson et al. 1990). These foreign genes may be reporter genes such as *E. coli lacZ*, or other genes that have the potential to affect the physiology of either the neurons in which they are expressed or their synaptic targets.

Foreign genes can be inserted into the HSV genome using recombinant DNA methods (Tackney et al. 1984). Full-length recombinants are made by co-transfection of suitable cells with a plasmid containing the gene of interest, flanked by HSV genomic sequences, and infectious HSV genomic DNA. Recombinants are selected and are used in cell culture or in vivo to deliver the foreign gene to targeted cell populations. To further limit the toxicity associated with HSV infection, we used recombinants in which functional genes had been inserted into the HSV thymidine kinase (*tk*) coding region (Fig. 1). Such TK^- viruses are replication-defective in neurons but are capable of establishing latency during which long-term expression of foreign genes can been achieved (Efstathiou et al. 1989; Coen et al. 1989). These TK^- viruses were used to deliver the reporter gene, *lacZ*, to trigeminal ganglion neurons from their site of inoculation on the mouse cornea and snout.

METHODS

For a detailed description of the methods used and experimental results, please see Davar et al. 1994.

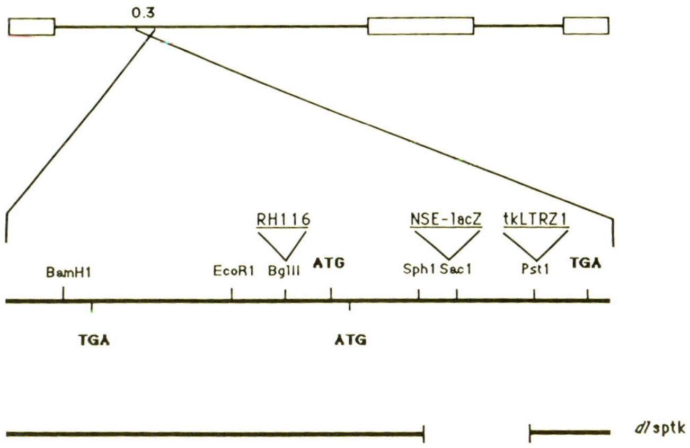

Fig. 1. Diagram of the herpes simplex virus (HSV) genome. **Upper:** the location of the thymidine kinase (*tk*) gene at map coordinate 0.3 is shown. Long diagonal lines connect to an expanded view of the 3.6 kb BamHI Q fragment encompassing the *tk* coding region and upstream regions with selected restriction endonuclease sites indicated. Short diagonal lines indicate the locations of the insertion mutations within (vectors NSE-*lacZ-tk*, *tk*LTRZ1, and *tk*LTRdyn) and outside (vector RH116) the *tk* protein coding region. The ATG and TGA marked above the line represent the initiation and termination codons of the *tk* coding region; the ATG and TGA marked below the line represent the initiation and termination codons of the adjacent UL24 coding region. **Lower:** the location of the deletion mutation in mutant *dls*ptk is shown. (Reprinted with permission from Davar et al. 1994)

VIRUS VECTORS

TK^- HSV vectors were constructed in a wild-type HSV type 1 (KOS strain) DNA background. They were TK^- due to the insertion of foreign elements into, and/or a deletional mutation of, the *tk* gene. These vectors all carried the reporter gene *lacZ*, inserted downstream of viral or mammalian promoter elements. They included RH116 (insertional mutant; *lacZ* downstream of the HSV β8 promoter; kindly provided by Drs. Ho and Mocarski, Stanford University; Ho and Mocarski, 1988), *tk*LTRZ1 (insertional mutant; *lacZ* downstream of the Moloney murine leukemia virus long terminal repeat promoter; Davar et al. 1992), and the neuron-specific enolase NSE-*lacZ-tk* (insertional mutant; *lacZ* downstream of the mammalian NSE promoter; Andersen et al. 1992) (Fig. 1). In addition to the *lacZ*+ vectors used in these experiments, a non–*lacZ*-containing deletion mutant, *dls*ptk was also tested (Coen et al. 1989).

Prior to inoculation, all viruses were maintained in 15% glycerol or tissue culture media (DMEM [Gibco] with 10% FCS, 100 μM/ml penicillin, and 100 μM/ml streptomycin). Titration of viruses was performed on Vero cell monolayer to obtain an estimate of the number of plaque-forming units (PFU) per ml.

INOCULATION PROCEDURES AND HISTOCHEMISTRY

Male Swiss Webster mice 10–16 weeks of age were anesthetized with a 1:1 solution of ketamine and xylazine. The corneal surface and snout were lightly scarified prior to inoculation of 10^6–10^8 PFU of one of the three *lacZ*+ vectors onto these surfaces. Control animals were inoculated with 10^7 PFU of *dl*sptk or received scarification alone (Fig. 2).

At 4, 14, 30, or 60 days after inoculation, animals were deeply anesthetized and perfused/fixed with 2% paraformaldehyde in 0.1 M phosphate buffer pH 7.2–7.4. The ipsilateral and contralateral trigeminal ganglia were removed, post-fixed for 1–2 hours in 2% paraformaldehyde, and incubated overnight at 37°C in 1% X-Gal solution. Histochemically reacted ganglia were transferred to sucrose and then cut in the coronal plane at 10–40 μM. Serial sagittal sections from the trigeminal ganglia of four additional animals were used to calculate a correction factor for estimation of neuronal cell counts (Abercrombie 1946; Burstein et al. 1990). Sections were mounted onto prepared glass slides,

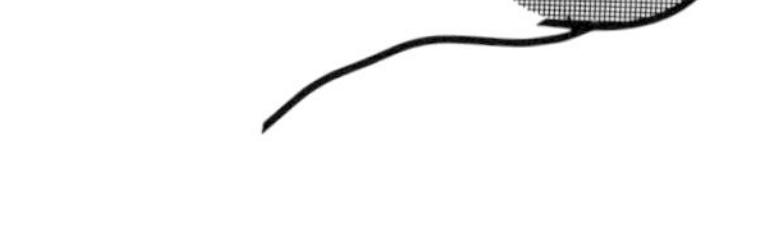

Fig. 2. Schematic of the mouse cornea and vibrissal pad, indicating the scarified (hatched lines) sites of inoculation of the different TK$^-$ HSV vectors used. A simplified sketch of the trigeminal ganglion, the three divisions of the trigeminal nerve, and the peripheral terminations of the first and second divisions of the trigeminal nerve is also shown.

counterstained with Neutral Red and examined under bright field in a light microscope.

In several other additional animals, sections were processed for immunocytochemistry with polyclonal antisera to *E. coli* β-galactosidase (5 Prime to 3 Prime, Inc.), or for in situ hybridization with an ^{35}S-labeled probe to the gene encoding LATs. As a control for the distribution of neurons labeled after corneal and snout inoculation of *lacZ*+ HSV vectors, two additional animals were inoculated with 20 μl of a 4% solution of Fluoro-Gold (Fluorochrome Inc.), and their ganglia removed 4 days after inoculation, sectioned, and examined for Fluoro-Gold labeling under fluorescence microscopy.

RESULTS

Light microscopic examination of histochemically reacted ganglia from animals inoculated with the three *lacZ*+ HSV vectors revealed labeled neurons ranging in size (longitudinal diameter) ranging from 8 to 48 μm. Several different intracellular labeling patterns were observed, including a dense blue stain filling the cytoplasm and, at times, extending into branching peripheral processes, and a speckled cytoplasmic staining pattern with or without nuclear labeling (Fig. 3).

The largest number of labeled neurons was observed 4 days following inoculation with vector *tk*LTRZ1. These neurons were in a rostromedial and central distribution within the trigeminal ganglion (data not shown) in regions of the trigeminal ganglion known to contain the cell bodies of sensory neurons innervating the cornea (Lavail et al. 1993) and snout (Bigotte and Olsson 1987). Labeling was observed for up to 60 days after inoculation with this vector, and the number of labeled neurons gradually declined with time (Fig. 4).

Significantly smaller numbers of trigeminal ganglion neurons were labeled 4 days after inoculation of the other two *lacZ*+ vectors (RH116 and NSE-*lacZ*-tk) tested. No labeling was observed with these vectors 14 days after inoculation (data not shown).

Immunocytochemistry, with polyclonal antisera to *E. coli* β-galactosidase, and in situ hybridization with a probe to LATs demonstrated labeled neurons in regions of the trigeminal ganglion similar to those observed by histochemistry with X-Gal (data not shown). This distribution of neuronal labeling was also observed after inoculation of the retrograde tracer Fluoro-Gold onto the mouse cornea and snout (data not shown).

Labeling was not observed in the trigeminal ganglion after inoculation of the TK^- HSV vector, *dls*ptk, or after scarification alone.

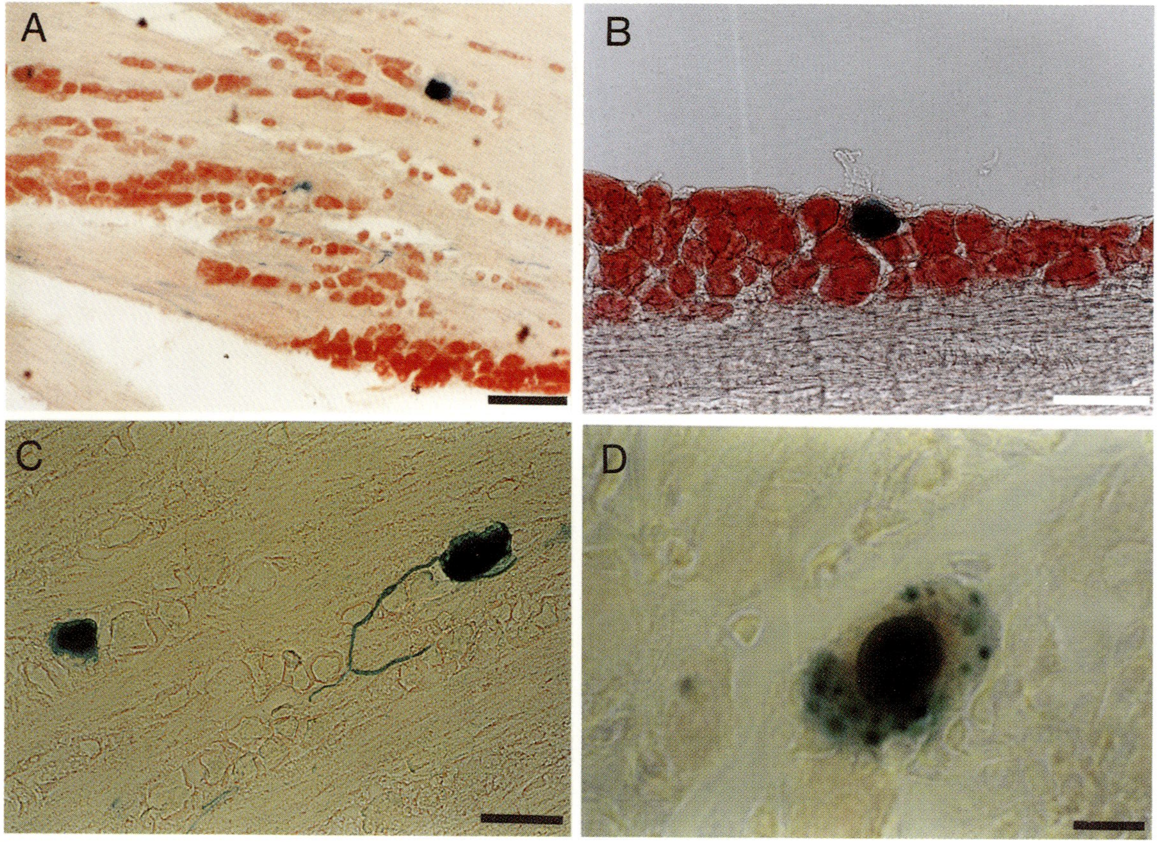

Fig. 3. Bright field photomicrographs of X-Gal–labeled neurons in coronal sections from trigeminal ganglion obtained 4 days after inoculation with vector *tk*TRZ1. **A–D** counterstained with Neutral Red; dense cytoplasmic labeling of neurons can be seen in **A–C**. Granular cytoplasmic labeling is also shown with nuclear labeling (**D**). A branching peripheral process, which originates from a densely labeled neuron, is seen in **C.** Scale bars: A, 100 μm; B, 50 μm; C, 50 μm; D, 10 μm.

DISCUSSION

These experiments demonstrated that retrogradely transported HSV vectors can be used to deliver the reporter gene *lacZ* to mouse trigeminal ganglion neurons in an anatomically predictable fashion. When vectors containing different viral and mammalian promoter elements upstream of *lacZ* were compared, vector *tk*LTRZ1 gave the greatest number and longest duration of labeling. This effect was most likely a result of the strong promoter element used in this vector (the Moloney murine leukemia virus long terminal repeat promoter; Price et al. 1987; Dobson et al. 1990). Smaller numbers of labeled neurons were observed after inoculation with vector RH116, at least partly because of the β8 promoter, which can drive the expression of *lacZ* at low levels and for short duration (Ho and Mocarski 1988). The low numbers of neurons labeled with vector NSE-*lacZ-tk* may also have resulted from low levels of activity of this promoter as well. The NSE promoter is known to have different levels of activity within different regions of the nervous system (Forss-Petter et al., personal communication). In addition, Marangos and Schmechel (1987) have demonstrated relatively low levels of NSE in the peripheral nervous system in contrast with levels in the central nervous system. Although weak promoter activity may explain the low numbers of neurons labeled with these two vectors, small amounts of *E. coli* β-galactosidase may have been present that could not be detected with our histochemical methods.

The slow decline in numbers of labeled neurons over time observed with vector *tk*LTRZ1 may be attributable to a gradual loss of promoter function. This promoter has been shown to turn off gradually in some in vivo situations (Palmer et al. 1991). The site of placement of this promoter within the *tk* gene may have also contributed to the decline in expression observed with time. Alternate placements of this promoter within the HSV genome may result in longer duration of expression of *lacZ* (Dobson et al. 1990; Bloom et al. 1993). The gradual loss of labeling observed with vector tkLTRZ1 could also have been the result of cell death. However, TK^- vectors are known to be replication-defective in neurons, and their use was not associated with evidence of degeneration or death of trigeminal ganglion neurons at any time point after inoculation.

The results obtained in these experiments with *lacZ* are currently being extended. We are in the process of constructing additional TK^- HSV vectors which will contain genes encoding analgesic neuropeptides such as enkephalin and prodynorphin (Davar et al. 1993). Similar to the results we have observed with our *lacZ*-containing TK^- HSV vectors, these new vectors may also be capable of delivering opioid peptide genes to sensory neurons in an anatomi-

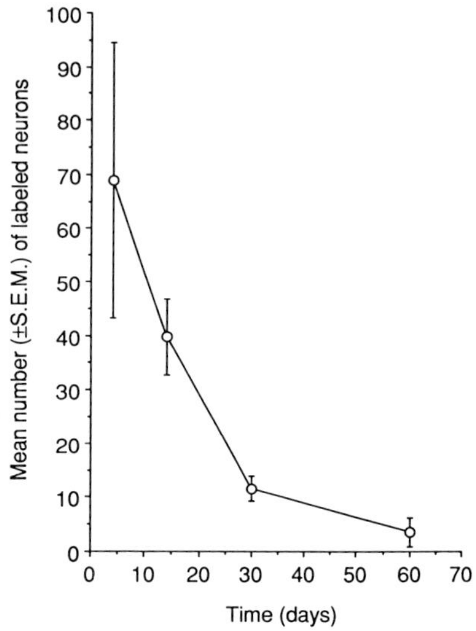

Fig. 4. Time course of X-Gal labeling of neurons with vector *tk*LTRZ1. The greatest mean number of labeled neurons was found at 4 days post-inoculation. (Reprinted with permission from Davar et al. 1994)

cally predictable fashion (Davar et al. 1993). The expression and subsequent release of their products may alter the physiology of postsynaptic neurons in spinal dorsal horn, potentially modulating nociceptive transmission at this level.

ACKNOWLEDGMENTS

The authors are grateful to D. Ho and E. Mocarski for the gift of vector RH116 and to C. Cepko for the gifts of pJ3β-gal and pJ4w. We also acknowledge the technical assistance of Steve R. Bossi, Olga Falkowski, and Wendy West, as well as Dr. B.P. Vos's assistance with the statistical analyses. This work was supported by NIH grants 1KO8NS01497 (G.D.), NS29178 (O.I.), AT24010 (D.K. and M. K.-V.), T32 CA09595 (M.K.), K15 DE00240 (W.B.), PO1AI24010 and RO1AI26126 (D.C.), and NS24279 (X.O.B.).

REFERENCES

Abercrombie, M., Estimation of nuclear population from microtome sections, Anat. Rec., 94 (1946) 239–247.

Andersen, J.K., Garber, D.A., Meaney, C.A. and Breakefield, X.O., Gene transfer into mammalian CNS using herpes virus vectors: long-term expression of bacterial *lac Z* in neurons using the neuron-specific enolase promoter, Hum. Gene Ther., 3 (1992) 487–499

Bigotte, L. and Olsson, Y., Degeneration of trigeminal ganglion neurons caused by retrograde axonal transport of doxorubicin, Neurology, 37 (1987) 985–992.

Bloom, D.C., Lokensgard, J.R., Maidment, N.T., Feldman, L.T. and Stevens, J.G., Long-term expression of genes in vivo using non-replicating HSV vectors, Gene Therapy, 1, Suppl. 1 (1994) 536–538.

Breakefield, X.O. and Geller, A.I., Gene transfer into the nervous system, Molec. Neurobiol. Rev., 1 (1987) 339–371.

Breakefield, X.O., Huang, Q., Andersen, J.K., Kramer, M.F., Bebrin, W., Davar, G., Vos, B., Garber, D.A., DiFiglia, M. and Coen, D.M., Gene transfer into neurons using recombinant herpes virus vectors. In: Gage R.H. and Y. Christen (Eds.), Gene Transfer and Therapy. Fondation IPSEN Proceedings. Springer-Verlag, Berlin, 1992, pp. 118–132.

Burstein, R., Dado, R.J. and Giesler, G.J., Jr., The cells of origin of the spinothalamic tract of the rat: a quantitative reexamination, Brain Res., 511 (1990) 329–337.

Coen, D.M., Kosz-Vnenchak, M., Jacobson, J.G., Leib, D.A., Bogard, C.L., Schaffer, P.A., Tyler, K.L. and Knipe, D.M., Thymidine kinase-negative herpes simplex virus mutants establish latency in mouse trigeminal ganglia but do not reactivate, Proc. Natl. Acad. Sci. USA, 86 (1989) 4736–4740.

Cook, M.L. and Stevens, J.G., Pathogenesis of herpetic neuritis and ganglionitis in mice: evidence for intra-axonal transport of infection, Infect. Immun., 7 (1973) 272–288.

Cornblath, D.R. and McArthur, J.C., Predominantly sensory neuropathy in patients with AIDS and AIDS-related complex, Neurology, 38 (1988) 794–796.

Croen, K.D., Ostrove, J.M., Dragovic, L.J., Smialek, J.E. and Strauss, S.E., Latent herpes simplex virus in human trigeminal ganglia: detection of an immediate early gene "anti-sense" transcript by in situ hybridization, N. Engl. J. Med., 317 (1987) 1427–1432.

Davar, G., Bebrin, W. Day, R., Dupuy, A., Coen, D.M. and Breakefield, X.O., Opioid peptide gene delivery to neurally derived cells using herpes virus vectors, Proc. Soc. Neurosci., 23 (1993) 577.2.

Davar, G., Kramer, M.F., Garber, D., Roca, A.L., Andersen, J.K., Bebrin, W., Coen, D.M., Kosz-Vnenchak, M., Knipe, D.M., Breakefield, X.O. and Isacson, O., Comparative efficacy of expression of genes delivered to mouse sensory neurons with herpes virus vectors, J. Comp. Neurol., 339 (1994) 3–11.

Dobson, A.T., Sederati, F., Devi-Rao, G., Flanagan, W.M., Farrell, M.J., Stevens, J.G., Wagner, E.K. and Feldman, L.T., Identification of the latency-associated transcript promoter by expression of rabbit beta-globin mRNA in mouse sensory nerve ganglia latently infected with a recombinant herpes simplex virus, J. Virol., 63 (1989) 3844–3851.

Dobson, A.T., Margolis, T.P., Sedarati, F., Stevens, J.G. and Feldman, L.T., A latent, nonpathogenic HSV-1-derived vector stably expresses β-galactosidase in mouse neurons, Neuron, 5 (1990) 353–360.

Efstathiou, S., Minson, A.C., Field, H.J., Anderson, J.R. and Wildy, P., Detection of herpes simplex virus-specific DNA sequences in latently infected mice and humans, J. Virol., 57 (1986) 446–455.

Efstathiou, S., Kemp, S., Darby, G. and Minson, A.C., The role of herpes simplex thymidine kinase in pathogenesis, J. Gen. Virol, 70 (1989) 869–879.

Geller, A.I., Bryan, J., Ashe, O., During, M.J. and Neve, R.L., Expression of an unregulated protein kinase C in cortical neurons from an HSV-1 vector, causes a long term, activity dependent increase in neurotransmitter release, Proc. Soc. Neurosci., 17 (1991) 240.12.

Ho, D.Y. and Mocarski, E.S., β-Galactosidase as a marker in the peripheral and neural tissues of the herpes simplex virus-infected mouse, Virology, 167 (1988) 279–283.

Ho, D.Y., Mocarski, E.S. and Sapolsky, R., Altering central nervous system physiology with a defective herpes simplex virus vector expressing the glucose transporter gene, Proc. Soc. Neurosci., 22 (1992) 304.2.

Javier, R.T., Stevens, J.G., Dissette, V.B. and Wagner, E.K., A herpes simplex virus transcript abundant in latently infected neurons is dispensable for establishment of the latent state, Virology, 166 (1988) 254–257.

LaVail, J.H., Johnson, W.E. and Spencer, L.E., Immunohistochemical identification of trigeminal ganglion neurons that innervate the mouse cornea: relevance to intercellular spread of herpes simplex virus, J. Comp. Neurol., 327 (1993) 133–140.

Loewy, A.D., Bridgman, P.C. and Mettenleiter, T.C., β-galactosidase expressing recombinant pseudorabies virus for light and electron microscopic study of retrograde transneuronally labeled CNS neurons, Proc. Soc. Neurosci., 17 (1991) 603.15.

Marangos, P.J. and Schmechel, D.E., Neuron-specific enolase, a clinically useful marker for neurons and neuroendocrine cells, Annu. Rev. Neurosci., 10 (1987) 269–297.

Martuza, R.L., Malick, A., Markert, A.M., Ruffner, K.L. and Coen, D.M., Experimental therapy of human glioma by means of a genetically engineered virus mutant, Science, 252 (1991) 854–856.

Mellerick, D.M. and Fraser, N.W., Physical state of the latent herpes simplex virus genome in a mouse model system: evidence suggesting an episomal state, Virology, 158 (1987) 265–275.

Palmer, T.D., Rosman, G.J., Osborne, W.R.A. and Miller, A.D., Genetically modified skin fibroblasts persist long after transplantation but gradually inactivate introduced genes. Proc. Natl. Acad. Sci. USA, 88 (1991) 1330–1334.

Price, J., Turner, D. and Cepko, C., Lineage analysis in the vertebrate nervous system by retrovirus-mediated gene transfer, Proc. Natl. Acad. Sci. USA, 84 (1987) 156–160.

Rock, D.L. and Fraser, N.W., Detection of HSV-1 genome in central nervous system of latently infected mice, Nature, 302 (1983) 523–525.

Rock, D.L., Nesburn, A.B., Ghiasi, H., Ong, J., Lewis, T.L., Lokensgard, J.R. and Wechsler, S.L., Detection of latency-related viral RNAs in trigeminal ganglia of rabbits, latently infected with herpes simplex virus type 1, J. Virol., 61 (1987) 3820–3826.

Roizman, B. and Sears., A.E., Herpes simplex viruses and their replication. In: B.N. Fields, M. Knipe, R.M. Chanock, M.S. Hirsch, J.L. Melnick, T.P. Monath and B. Roizman (Eds.), Fields Virology, 2nd ed., Vol. 2. Raven Press, New York, 1990, pp. 1795–1843.

Spivak, J.G. and Fraser, N.W., Detection of herpes simplex virus type 1 transcripts during latent infection in mice, J. Virol., 61 (1987) 3841–3847.

Stevens, J.G., Wagner, E.K., Devi-Rao, G.B., Cook, M.L. and Feldman, L.T., RNA complementary to a herpes virus alpha gene mRNA is prominent in latently infected neurons, Science, 235 (1987) 1056–1059.

Tackney, C., Cachianes, G. and Silverstein, S. Transduction of the Chinese hamster ovary *aprt* gene by herpes simplex virus, J. Virol., 52 (1984) 606–614

Wagner, E.K., Devi-Rao, G.B., Feldman, L.T., Dobson, A.T., Zhang, Y.-F., Flanagan, W.M. and Stevens, J.G., Physical characterization of the herpes simplex virus latency-associated transcript in neurons, J. Virol., 62 (1988) 1194–1202.

Watson, C.P.N., Postherpetic neuralgia. In: R.K. Portenoy (Ed.), Pain: Mechanisms and Syndromes. Neurologic Clinics of North America. W.B. Saunders, Philadelphia, 1989, pp 231–248.

Correspondence to: Gudarz Davar, Department BCMP, Harvard Medical School, 240 Longwood Ave., Boston, MA 02115, USA. Tel: 617-432-1789; FAX: 617-432-3833.

Proceedings of the 7th World Congress on Pain,
Progress in Pain Research and Management, Vol. 2,
edited by G.F. Gebhart, D.L. Hammond, and T.S.
Jensen, IASP Press, Seattle, © 1994.

28

Glutaminergic Neurotransmission, Proto-Oncogenes, and Pain

Masaya Tohyama, Hiroshi Kiyama, Kohji Satoh, Toshiyuki Araki, Hiroshi Maeno, Hiroko Oyamada, and Eiji Kondo

Department of Anatomy and Neuroscience, Osaka University Medical School, Osaka, Japan

PRIMARY SENSORY AFFERENTS RECEIVE GLUTAMINERGIC INNERVATION

Pharmacological studies have suggested the presence of glutamate receptors in primary sensory afferent neurons. For example, Davies et al. (1979) reported that kainic acid (KA) depolarizes sensory fibers of the dorsal root ganglion (DRG) of newborn rats. Subsequent studies suggested that this effect on primary sensory afferent C-fibers occurs via a specific receptor (Agrawal and Evans 1986; Evans et al. 1987; Lewis et al. 1987; Huetter 1990; Jeftinija et al. 1991). In addition, the existence of other types of glutamate receptors, such as α-amino-3-hydroxy-5-methyl-4-isoxazole proprionic acid (AMPA) receptors and N-methyl-D-aspartate (NMDA) receptors, on DRG neurons has also been suggested (Lovinger and Weight 1988; Huettner 1990). It is not clear , however, whether small or large cells, or both, in the DRG express AMPA, KA, and NMDA receptors. Although recent molecular biological techniques have revealed that these ionotropic receptors are composed of several subunits, the precise nature of the subunit types expressed in the DRG remains obscure. In this chapter, we describe the cellular expression of GluR1–4 (subunits of the AMPA receptor), GluR5 (a subunit of the KA receptor), and NR1 (a subunit of the NMDA receptor) (Sato et al. 1993a).

Fig. 1 shows the location of GluR1-like immunoreactivity (IR; Fig. 1A), GluR2/3-IR (Fig. 1B), and GluR4-IR (Fig. 1C) in the rat DRG in consecutive

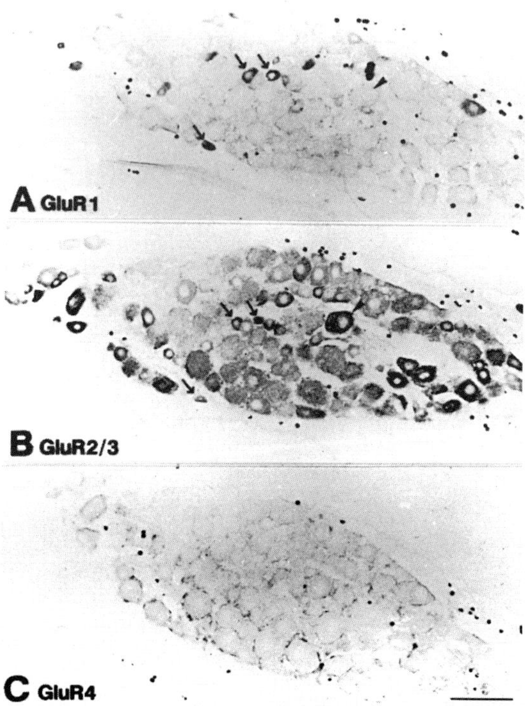

Fig. 1. Bright-field photomicrographs showing GluR-IR (A), GluR2/3-IR (B) and GluR4-IR (C) in dorsal root ganglion cells in three serial sections. Arrows and arrowheads in A and B are identical neurons. The GluR1 antibody labeled only small neurons, while the GluR2/3 antibody labeled both small and large neurons. No neurons labeled by the GluR4 antibody could be found. Dotted structures are erythrocytes. Bar = 100 μm. (From Sato et al. 1993)

thin sections. Antiserum used for detection of GluR2 or 3 recognizes both subunits (specificities of the antisera have been described elsewhere [Petralia and Wenthold 1992; Wenthold et al. 1992]). Some small ganglion neurons were labeled by the antiserum against GluR1 (Fig. 1A). Most of the ganglion neurons, however, both small and large, were positive for GluR2/3 with different intensities (Fig. 1B). We therefore concluded that neurons containing both GluR1-IR and GluR2/3-IR were always small (Fig. 1A and B, arrows). Large neurons with GluR2/3-IR were devoid of GluR1-IR (Fig. 1A and B, arrowhead). The antiserum against GluR4 did not label any DRG neurons (Fig. 1C).

DRG neurons expressing GluR5 mRNA are shown in Fig. 2A and B, a bright-field photomicrograph. Labeled cells were always small (thin arrows), whereas large neurons were always devoid of hybridization signals. However, all ganglion cells exhibited very strong expression of NR1 mRNA (Fig. 2C).

These results suggest that small neurons in the DRG express at least three different types of glutamate receptors: AMPA (GluR1, GluR2/3), KA (GluR5), and NMDA (NR1) (Fig. 3). However, many large cells express AMPA (GluR2/3) and NMDA receptors (NR1) but not GluR5 subunit (Fig. 3).

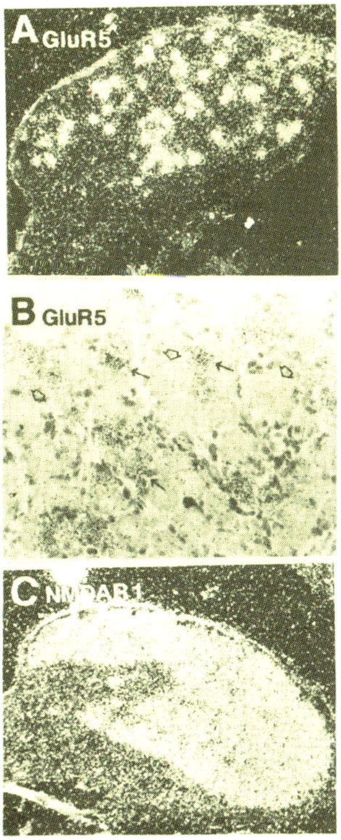

Fig. 2. **A** and **B:** Expression of GluR5 mRNA in the DRG. Small neurons were labeled strongly with the GluR5 probe (**B**, thin arrows), while large neurons lacked GluR5 mRNA (**B**, thick arrows). **C:** Expression of NR1 mRNA in the DRG. All DRG neurons were strongly labeled. Bar = 200 μm (A,C); 80 μm (B). (From Sato et al. 1993)

Since NR1 mRNA is expressed in all neurons in the DRG (both small and large), glutaminergic regulation via NMDA receptors in the DRG may be related to the activation of primary sensory afferents.

Pharmacological research has suggested that the KA receptor is expressed in primary afferent C-fibers (Davies et al. 1979; Schneider and Pearl 1985; Agrawal and Evans 1986; Evans et al. 1987; Lewis et al. 1987; Huettner 1990; Jeftinija et al. 1991). The present study provides direct morphological evidence supporting this, and further clarifies that GluR5, a subunit of the KA receptor, is predominantly expressed in small neurons. Thus, it may be that glutaminergic regulation of nociceptive primary sensory neurons occurs via KA receptors containing at least the GluR5 subunit (Fig. 3).

AMPA receptors are also expressed in both small and large neurons. The subunit composition of this receptor, however, is different between small and large neurons. Small neurons express both GluR1-IR and GluR2/3-IR, whereas large neurons express GluR2/3-IR but not GluR1-IR. Therefore, glutamate stimulation via AMPA receptors is probably different between nociceptive (small) and other (large) neurons.

In addition, Araki et al. (1993) reported that the metabotropic receptor-1 (mGluR1)-IR is expressed in the trigeminal ganglion, irrespective of cell size. It is therefore likely that primary sensory neurons express at least four types of glutamate receptors: AMPA, KA, NMDA, and metabotrophic receptors.

There are three different origins of glutamate that could bind to the glutamate receptors expressed in sensory ganglion neurons. First, glutamate could be released from spinal or supraspinal axons. In this case, primary sensory afferent neurons would receive glutaminergic input axo-axonically at the level of the dorsal horn (Fig. 4). The second possibility is release from sensory ganglion neurons themselves, as it has been established that glutamate is a neurotransmitter of both small and large neurons of the sensory ganglion (see Furuyama et al. 1993 for review). In this case, glutamate receptors expressed in the DRG could act as autoreceptors (Fig. 4). In both cases, glutamate should act as an inhibitory neurotransmitter. Glutamate is well known, however, as an excitatory neurotransmitter. This discrepancy should be solved. The third possibility is that circulating glutamate binds to the glutamate receptors expressed in sensory ganglion neurons (Fig. 4).

REGION-SPECIFIC EXPRESSION OF SUBUNITS OF IONOTROPIC GLUTAMATE RECEPTORS (GLUR1–5 AND NR1) IN THE SPINAL CORD, WITH SPECIAL REFERENCE TO NOCICEPTION

Because glutamate is contained in both small and large neurons of the sensory ganglion, it is probable that glutamate is not solely related to nociception but is involved in fundamental mechanisms of sensory transmission. However,

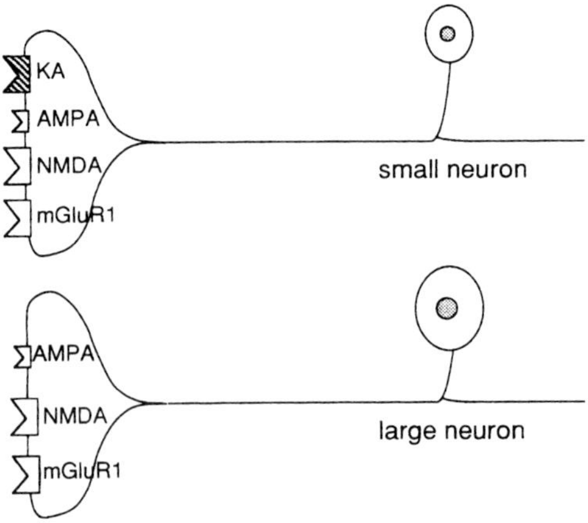

Fig. 3. Schematic drawing of the pattern of expression of AMPA, KA, and NMDA receptors on primary sensory afferents. The KA receptor is specifically expressed on small neurons related to nociception. NMDA receptors are widely expressed on both small and large neurons. Although the AMPA receptor is also expressed on both small and large neurons, the subunit composition of this receptor is different between small and large neurons (see text).

a study using in situ hybridization histochemistry (Sato et al. 1993b) revealed marked heterogeneity in the subunit composition of AMPA receptors. It is likely that the postsynaptic effect of glutaminergic transmission is characterized by the composition of different glutamate receptor subunits. In the present study, we aimed to elucidate the subunit composition of glutamate receptors in the superficial part of the dorsal horn, a region concerned with nociceptive processing (Furuyama et al. 1993).

Figs. 5 and 6 show the location of GluR1–4 mRNA in the cervical spinal cord. There were marked differences in GluR1-4 mRNA expression patterns according to each subunit and spinal region. In lamina II and the superficial part of lamina III, where afferents relating to nociception terminate, expression of GluR2 mRNA was strong (Fig. 5B). Many neurons here expressed GluR1 mRNA moderately (Fig. 5A). Scattered neurons moderately expressing GluR3 mRNA were also observed in these regions, while GluR4 mRNA expression was very low (Fig. 5C and D). In the remaining part of the dorsal horn, where non-nociceptive and nociceptive afferents terminate, expression of all the subunits was moderate (Fig. 5). The patterns of expression of GluR1-4 mRNA in motor neurons was considerably different from those in the dorsal horn (Fig. 6). Motor neurons in the ventral horn were labeled strongly by both GluR3 and GluR4 probes (Fig. 6C,D) and moderately by the GluR2 probe (Fig. 6B), while labeling of the motor neurons for GluR1 mRNA was weak (Fig. 6A).

In situ hybridization histochemistry (ISH) results were confirmed by immunohistochemistry. Fig. 7 shows the location of GluR1-, GluR2/3-, and

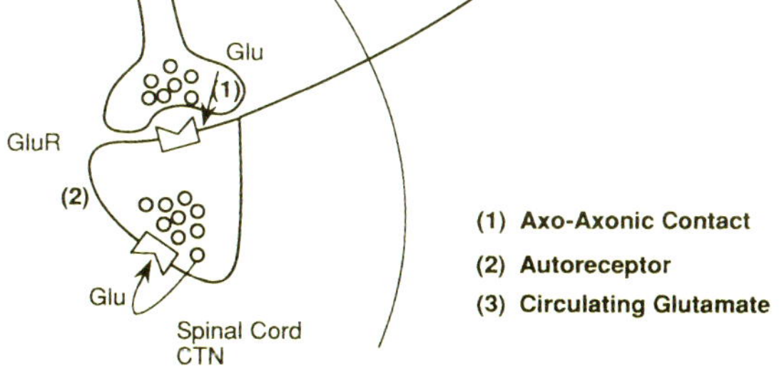

Fig. 4. Schematic drawing of the possible glutaminergic inputs to the primary sensory afferents.

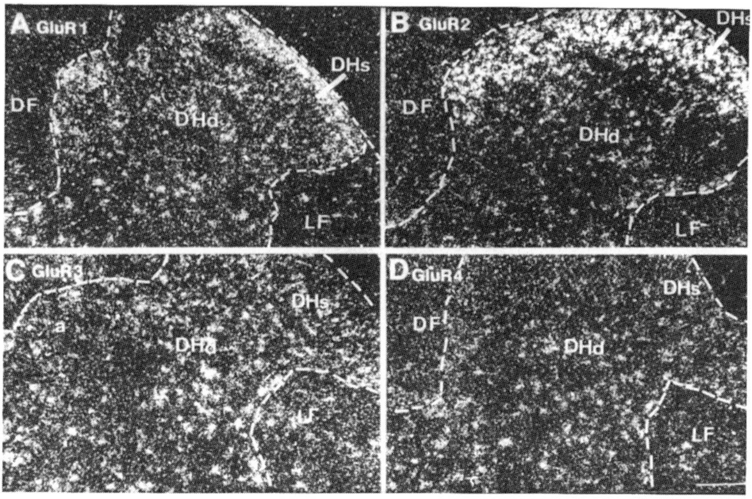

Fig. 5. Expression of GluR1–4 mRNAs in the dorsal horn (DH) of the cervical spinal cord. Expression of GluR2 is particularly high in lamina II and in the superficial part of lamina III. The dotted line outlines the border between the white and gray matter of the spinal cord. DF, dorsal funiculus; DHd, deep layers (laminae IV–VI) of the DH; DHs, superficial layers (laminae I–III) of the DH; LF, lateral funiculus. Bar = 200 μm. (From Furuyama et al. 1993)

GluR4-IR in the cervical cord. A large number of neurons with GluR1- and GluR2/3-IR were concentrated in lamina II and the superficial part of lamina III (Fig. 7A,C), with a predominance of GluR2/3 in both number and intensity. Dendrites from these neurons formed a dense plexus in lamina II (Figs. 7A,C). In addition, moderately labeled cells were scattered throughout lamina III–VI. We found few neurons and fibers containing GluR4-IR in the dorsal horn (Fig. 7E). Motor neurons were labeled strongly with the antibodies against GluR2/3 and GluR4 (Fig. 7D,F). Anti-GluR1 antibody, however, labeled motor neurons less intensely than did the other two (Fig. 7B).

Both dorsal and ventral horn expressed GluR5 mRNA at very low levels. NR1 mRNA was expressed strongly throughout the entire gray matter of the spinal cord. However, expression of NR1 in motor neurons was much more intense than in the dorsal horn. In the dorsal horn, expression of NR1 occurred rather evenly, and we observed no regional differences among lamina II, the superficial part of the lamina III, and remaining dorsal horn areas.

In the present study, we examined the expression of GluR1-4 subunits (AMPA receptor), GluR5 subunits (KA receptor), and NR1 subunits (NMDA receptor) in the spinal cord and showed that there was a region-specific expression. The patterns of expression are considerably different among regions

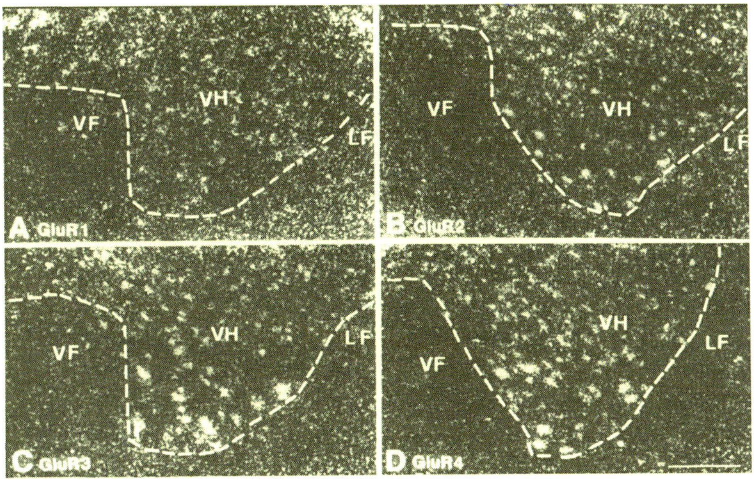

Fig. 6. Expression of GluR1–4 mRNAs in the ventral horn (VH) of the cervical spinal cord. The dotted line outlines the border between the white and gray matter. Expression of GluR3 and GluR4 was high. VF, ventral funiculus; LF, lateral funiculus. Bar = 200 μm. (From Furuyama et al. 1993)

of the spinal cord relating to nociception and those relating to other sensations, as well as in motor neurons; the region-specific type of expression was particularly marked for AMPA receptors. Although all four subunits of AMPA receptors were expressed in the spinal cord, their expression patterns differed considerably among lamina II and the superficial part of lamina III, the deep part of lamina III and lamina IV–VI, and the ventral horn. In lamina II and the superficial part of lamina III, expression of GluR2 was especially high, suggesting that such high expression is a characteristic of the AMPA receptor involved in nociception. In the remaining part of the dorsal horn, expression of the four subunits was fairly even. These data suggest that, although glutamate is contained in both small and large neurons of the DRG and is involved in various sensory conduction pathways, the subunit composition of the AMPA receptor in the spinal cord is different between neurons principally involved in conducting nociception and those neurons involved in other sensations. This is in contrast to the distribution of KA (GluR5) and NMDA (NR1) receptors; GluR5 and NR1 were evenly expressed throughout the dorsal horn.

The subunit composition of the AMPA receptor in lamina II, the superficial part of lamina III, and the remaining areas of the dorsal horn is also different from that in motor neurons. In the latter, the expression of GluR3 and GluR4 was especially high. This profile may be characteristic of AMPA receptors in motor neurons.

NEURONS EXPRESSING AMPA RECEPTORS IN THE SUBSTANTIA GELATINOSA MAY NOT PROJECT TO THE THALAMUS

As described above, substantia gelatinosa neurons express AMPA receptors in which GluR2 is highly expressed. Since primary sensory afferents contain glutamate, these neurons probably receive direct input from primary sensory afferents. Using combined immunocytochemistry for detection of GluR2/3-IR and the retrograde tracer method using fluoro-gold (FG), we investigated whether these neurons project to the thalamus or are local circuit neurons.

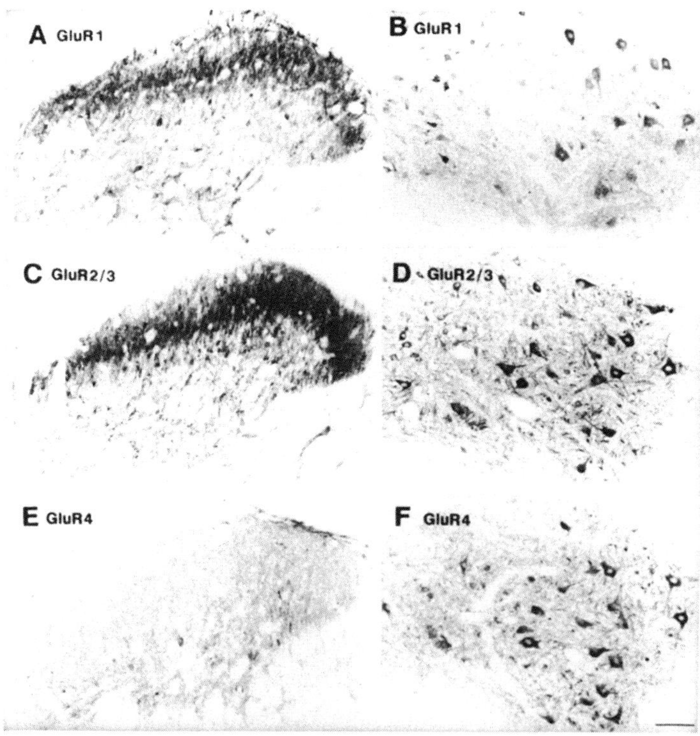

Fig. 7. Bright-field photomicrographs showing the location of GluR1-IR, GluR2/3-IR, and GluR4-IR in the cervical spinal cord. Lamina II and the superficial part of lamina III are strongly labeled by the antibody against GluR2/3 (**C**) and moderately by that against GluR1 (**A**). However, labeling of the dorsal horn by the GluR4 antibody is very weak (**E**). Motor neurons are strongly labeled by the antibody against GluR2/3 (**D**) and GluR4 (**F**), but moderately to weakly by that against GluR1 (**B**). Note the many cells labeled by GluR2/3 antiserum in lamina II and the superficial part of lamina III (**C**). Bar = 100 μm. (From Furuyama et al. 1993)

Injection of FG into the ventral posteromedial nucleus (VPM) of the rat resulted in labeling of scattered neurons in the contralateral marginal layer of the caudal trigeminal spinal nucleus (TNC). Neurons expressing GluR2/3 were located mainly in the substantia gelatinosa of this nucleus. We found no double-labeled neurons, indicating that neurons expressing AMPA receptors in the TNC substantia gelatinosa are likely local circuit neurons.

A PART OF NEURONS EXPRESSING AMPA RECEPTORS IN THE SUBSTANTIA GELATINOSA SHOW ENKEPHALIN-IR

Various neuropeptides synthesized in neurons in the substantia gelatinosa of the dorsal horn and TNC are considered to be localized in local circuit neurons that are involved in the modulation of pain transmission. Among these peptides, changes in opioid peptides and galanin have been extensively studied. The synthesis of galanin and opioid peptides such as enkephalin (Enk) and dynorphin (Dyn) has been shown to increase in response to noxious stimuli (Cesselin et al. 1980; Faccini et al. 1984; Millan et al. 1986; Hollt et al. 1987; Le Bars et al. 1987; Bourgoin et al. 1988; Iadarola et al. 1988; Ruda et al. 1988; Noguchi et al. 1989; Weihe et al. 1989; Tokunaga et al. 1992). It is generally agreed that these changes are due to trans-synaptic activation via primary sensory afferents, because morphological studies have shown that Enk neurons are postsynaptic to primary sensory afferents (Bennett et al. 1982; Glazer and Basbaum 1983). Neurons expressing AMPA receptors in the substantia gelatinosa, however, are local circuit neurons which receive glutaminergic projections from primary sensory neurons. It is therefore likely that neurons expressing AMPA receptors in the substantia gelatinosa contain at least some of these neuropeptides. By analyzing serial sections, we found that some neurons with GluR2/3-IR in the substantia gelatinosa also exhibit Enk-IR. This suggests that activation of Enk neurons in the substantia gelatinosa

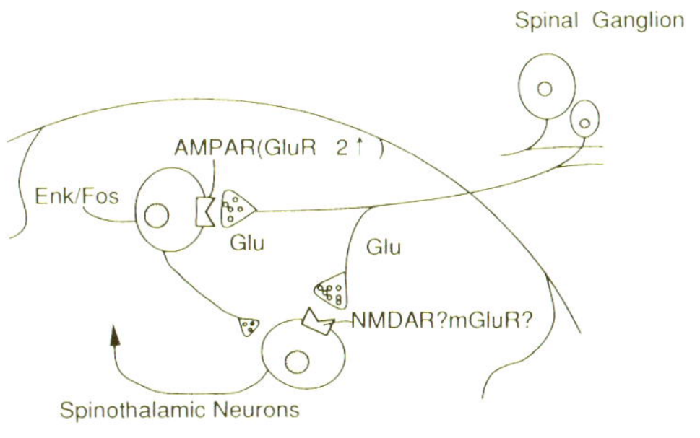

Fig. 8. Schematic illustration of the interaction of glutaminergic primary sensory afferents and Enk-containing local circuit neurons (which coexpress *fos*) in the substantia gelatinosa via the AMPA receptor. The possibility that spinothalamic neurons express NMDA- or metabotropic glutamate receptors is suggested.

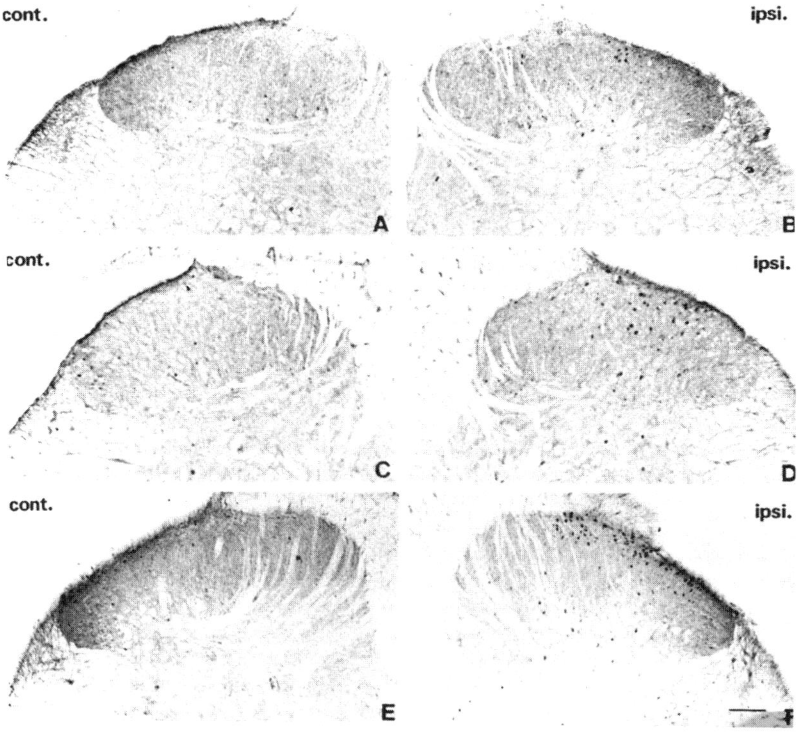

Fig. 9. Photomicrographs showing neurons with *fos*-IR nuclei in the dorsal horn of the spinal cord after the application of saline (**A,B**), histamine at 200 mg/ml (**C,D**), or histamine at 1 g/ml (**E,F**) to the leg skin and scratching with forceps. *Fos*-IR neurons are increased in the ipsilateral dorsal horn (**B,D,F**) compared to the contralateral side (**A,C,E**), and the change shows dose-dependency for histamine. Bar = 10 μm. (From Yao et al. 1992)

may occur by stimulation of glutaminergic primary sensory afferents via AMPA receptors in which GluR2 is highly expressed (Fig. 8).

EXPRESSION OF C-*FOS* IN THE SUBSTANTIA GELATINOSA AFTER NOXIOUS STIMULI: CORRELATION WITH ENK-IR

The proto-oncogene c-*fos* is a cellular immediate early gene linked to genomic events that control long-term changes in the nervous system (Goelet et al. 1986; Curran and Morgan 1987). In the rat spinal cord, *fos*-IR occurs rapidly and transiently in dorsal horn neurons following various kinds of noxious stimulation (Hunt et al. 1987; Menetrey et al. 1989; Fitzgerald 1990; Tolle et al. 1990; Williams et al. 1990; Yao et al. 1992).

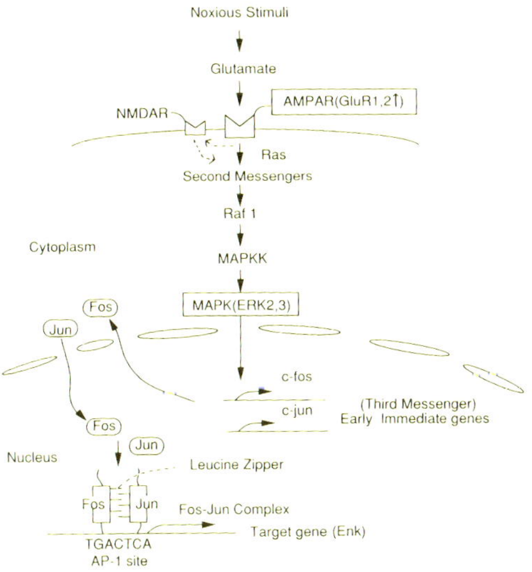

Fig. 10. Hypothesis for expression of Enk in substantia gelatinosa neurons through proto-oncogene activation after noxious stimulation (see text).

We investigated changes in *fos*-IR in the spinal cord after histamine application to the skin (Yao et al. 1992). Fig. 9 shows *fos*-IR neurons in the rat dorsal horn in saline- and histamine-treated rats. In the animals treated with saline and scratched, we observed a small number of nuclei with *fos*-IR bilaterally in the dorsal horns, but with ipsilateral predominance (Fig. 9A,B). Application of histamine to the lower limb caused a marked dose-dependent increase in *fos*-IR neurons in the dorsal horn, with marked ipsilateral predominance (Fig. 9C–F). In animals treated with histamine without scratching, we saw significantly fewer immunoreactive neurons in the dorsal horn compared with animals treated with the same dose of histamine and scratched. However, the number was still significantly greater than that in control rats treated with saline and not scratched. In the animals pretreated with morphine (16 mg/kg, ip.) before the application of histamine, the number of *fos*-IR neurons was reduced to one third of the number observed in rats pretreated intraperitoneally with saline. The number of *fos*-IR neurons in the deeper laminae was also markedly decreased in rats pretreated with morphine.

Researchers have shown that neurons which increase the production of Enk and Dyn in the dorsal horn after noxious stimuli exhibit *fos*-IR (Naranjo et al. 1991; Noguchi et al. 1991a,b). Increases in *fos*-IR precede those of Enk, Dyn, and galanin. A *fos-jun* complex has been shown to bind to the AP-1 site on the upstream enhancer regions of the proEnk (Sonnenberg et al. 1989) and proDyn (Naranjo et al. 1991) genes. Together with *jun*, *fos*, which is produced by activation of the c-*fos* gene, enhances the transcription of proEnk and proDyn genes by binding to the AP-1 sites.

MECHANISM OF ACTIVATION OF C-*FOS* AND PROENK GENES

Primary sensory afferents contain glutamate and make synaptic contacts with local circuit neurons in the substantia gelatinosa, increasing the production of *fos* and Enk after noxious stimuli (Fig. 10). In addition, local circuit neurons in the substantia gelatinosa express AMPA receptors in which expression of GluR2 is very high, and a proportion also probably contain Enk (Fig. 10). These findings suggest that stimulation of the AMPA receptor in local circuit neurons is the first important step in the enhancement of transcription of the proEnk gene (Fig. 10). Primary sensory afferents also contain substance P (SP) and calcitonin gene-related peptide (CGRP). SP increases intracellular Ca^{2+} levels in dorsal horn neurons (Womack et al. 1988). Since it has been shown that an increase in intracellular Ca^{2+} is crucial for c-*fos* expression (Morgan and Curran 1986), involvement of SP in the enhancement of *fos* and Enk expression cannot be excluded. It should be noted, however, that although the spinal trigeminal nucleus and dorsal horn contain a huge amount of SP-IR fibers, they contain only a few cells expressing NK-1 receptor mRNA (Maeno et al. 1993a). Furthermore, the possibility of the involvement of NMDA receptor cannot be excluded, because NR1 mRNA-containing cells also exist in the dorsal horn and interaction between SP or CGRP and NMDA receptors has been suggested (see Furuyama et al. 1993 for review).

Binding of glutamate and other neuromodulators to their receptors is associated with a variety of different intracellular mechanisms. Protein phosphorylation by kinases is one of the key mechanisms for the conveyance of intracellular signals. Microtubule-associated protein kinase (MAP-2 kinase) or mitogen-activated protein kinase (MAP kinase), which was later renamed extracellular signal-regulated kinase (ERK) 1, is a major intracellular kinase. It forms ERK families (ERK1–5), which are activated by hormone or growth factor stimulation, causing induction of the proto-oncogene (see Boulton et al. 1991 for review).

Researchers have examined expression of ERK family mRNAs in the brain and spinal cord (Maeno et al. 1993b). In the spinal cord, ERK1 mRNA is preferentially expressed in oligodendroglia, and expression of ERK1 in neurons is low. Conversely, expression of ERK3 mRNA is high in neurons but low in glial cells. ERK2 expression is intermediate between ERK1 and ERK3. Therefore, among the ERK family, it is possible that ERK2 and ERK3 are closely related to expression of c-*jun* and c-*fos* in the substantia gelatinosa.

REFERENCES

Agrawal, S.G. and Evans, R.H., The primary afferent depolarizing action of kainate in the rat, Br. J. Pharmacol., 87 (1986) 345– 355.

Araki, T., Kenimer, J.G., Hishimune, A., Sugiyama, H., Yoshimura, R. and Kiyama, H., Identification of the metabotropic glutamate receptor 1 protein in the rat trigeminal ganglion, Brain Res., 627 (1993) 341–346.

Bennett, G.J., Ruda, M.A., Gobel, S. and Dubner, R., Enkephalin immunoreactive stalked cells and lamina IIb islet cells in cat substantia gelatinosa, Brain Res., 240 (1982) 162–166.

Boulton, T.G., Nye, S.H., Robbins, D.J., Ip, N.Y., Radziejewska, E., Morgenbesser, S.D., DePinho, R.A., Panayotatos, N. Cobb, M.H. and Yancopoulos, D.Y., ERKs: a family of protein-serine/threonin kinases that are activated and tyrosine phosphorylated in responses to insulin and NGF, Cell, 65 (1991) 663–675.

Bourgoin, S., Le Bars, D., Clot, A.M., Hamon, M. and Cesselin, F., Spontaneous and evoked release of met-enkephalin–like material from the spinal cord of arthritic rat in vivo, Pain, 32 (1988) 107–114.

Cesselin, F., Montastruc, J.L., Gros, C., Bourgoin, S. and Hamon, M., Met-enkephalin levels andopiate receptors in the spinal cord of chronic suffering rats, Brain Res., 191 (1980) 289–293.

Curran, T. and Morgan, J.I., Memories of fos, Bioessays, 7 (1987) 255–258.

Davies, J., Evans, R.H., Francis, A.A. and Watkins, J.C., Excitatory amino acid receptors and synaptic excitation in mammalian central nervous system, J. Physiol. (Paris), 75 (1979) 641–654.

Evans, R.H., Evans, S.J., Pook, P.C. and Sunter, D.C., A comparison of excitatory amino acid antagonists acting at primary afferent C fibers and motoneurons of the isolated spinal cord of the rat, Br. J. Pharmacol., 91 (1987) 531–537.

Faccini, E., Uzumaki, H., Govoni, S., Missale, C., Spano, P.F., Covelli, V. and Trabucchi, M., Afferent fibers mediate the increase of met-enkephalin elicited in rat spinal cord by licalized pain, Pain, 18 (1984) 25–31.

Fitzgerald, M., C-Fos and the changing face of pain, Trends Neurosci., 13 (1990) 439–440.

Furuyama, T., Kiyama, H., Sato, K., Park, H.W., Maeno, H., Takagi, H. and Tohyama, M., Region-specific expression of subunits of ionotropic glutamate receptors (AMPA-type, KA-type and NMDA receptors) in the rat spinal cord with special refrence to nociception, Mol. Brain Res., 18 (1993) 141–151.

Glazer, E.J. and Basbaum, A.I., Opiate neurons and pain modulation: an ultrastructural analysis of enkephalin in cat superficial dorsal horn, Neuroscience, 10 (1983) 357–376.

Goelet, P., Castelluci, V.F., Schacher, S. and Kandel, E.R., The long and the short of long-term memory: a molecular framework, Nature, 332 (1986) 419–422.

Hollt, V., Haarmann, I., Millan, M.J. and Herz, A., Prodynorphin gene expression is enhanced in the spinal cord of chronic arthritic rats, Neurosci. Lett., 73 (1987) 90–94.

Huettner, J.E., Glutamate receptor channels in rat DRG neurons: activation by kainate and quisqualate and blockade of desensitization by Con A, Neuron, 5 (1990) 255–266.

Hunt, S.P., Pini, A. and Evan, G., Induction of c-fos–like protein in spinal cord neurons following sensory stimulation, Nature, 328 (1987) 632–634.

Iadarola, M.J., Douglass, J., Civelli, O. and Naranjo, R., Differential activation of spinal cord dynorphin and enkephalin neurons during hyperalgesia: evidence using cDNA hybridization, Brain Res., 455 (1988) 205–212.

Jeftinija, S., Jeftinija, K., Liu, F., Skilling S.R., Smullin D.H. and Larson, A.A., Excitatory amino acids are released from rat primary afferent neuronbs in vitro, Neurosci. Lett., 125 (1991) 191–194.

Le Bars, D., Bourgoin, S., Clot, A.M., Hamon, M. and Cesselin, F., Noxious mechanical stimuli increase the release of met-enkephalin–like material heterosegmentally in the rat spinal cord, Brain Res., 402 (1987) 188–192.

Lewis, S.J., Cincotta, M., Verberne, A.J.M., Jarrott, B., Lodge, D. and Beart, P.M., Receptor autoradiography with [^{3}H]L-glutamate reveals the presence and axonal transport of glutamate receptors in vagal afferent neurons of the rat, Eur. J. Pharmacol., 144 (1987) 413–415.

Lovinger, D.M. and Weight, F.F., Glutamate induces a depolarization of adult rat dorsal root ganglion neurons that is mediated predominantly by NMDA receptors, Neurosci. Lett., 94 (1988) 314–320.

Maeno, H., Kiyama, H. and Tohyama, M., Distribution of the substance P receptor (NK-1 receptor) in the central nervous system, Mol. Brain Res., 18 (1993a) 43–58.

Maeno, H., Kiyama, H. and Tohyama, M., Expression of mRNAs of ERK family in the rat brain and spinal cord, Neurosci Res., 17, Suppl. (1992) S122.

Menetrey, D., Gannon, A., Levine, J.D. and Basbaum, A.I., Expression of c-fos protein in interneu-

rons and projection neurons of the rat spinal cord in response to noxious somatic, articular, and visceral stimulation, J. Comp. Neurol., 285 (1989) 177–195.
Millan, M.J., Millan, M.H., Czlonkowski, A., Hollt, V., Pilcher, C.W.T., Herz, A. and Colpaert, F.C., A model of chronic pain in the rat: response of multiple opioid systems to adjuvant-induced arthritis, J. Neurosci., 6 (1986) 899–906.
Morgan, J.I. and Curran, T., Role of ion flux in the control of c-fos expression, Nature, 322 (1986) 552–555.
Naranjo, J.R., Mellstrom, B., Achaval, M. and Sassone-Corsi, P., Molecular pathways of pain: Fos/Jun-mediated activation of a noncannonical AP-1 site in the prodynorphin gene, Neuron, 6 (1991) 607–617.
Noguchi, K., Morita, Y., Kiyama, H., Sato, M., Ono, K. and Tohyama,M., Preproenkephalin gene expression in the rat spinal cord after noxious stimuli, Mol. Brain Res., 5 (1989) 227–234.
Noguchi, K., Dubner, R. and Ruda, M.A., Preproenkephalin mRNA in spinal dorsal horn neurons is induced by peripheral inflammation and is colocalized with Fos and Fos-related proteins, Neurosci., 46 (1991a) 561–570.
Noguchi, K., Kowalski, K., Traub, R., Solodkin, A., Iadarola, M.J. and Ruda, M.A., Dynorphin expression and Fos-like immunoreactivity following inflammation induced hyperalgesia and colocalized in spinal cord neurons, Mol. Brain Res., 10 (1991b) 227–233.
Petralia, R.S. and Wenthold, R.J., Light and electron immunocytochemical localization of AMPA-selective glutamate receptors in the rat brain, J. Comp. Neurol., 318 (1992) 329–354.
Ruda, M.A., Iadarola, M.J., Cohen, L.V., Young, W.S., III., In situ hybridization histochemistry and immunocytochemistry reveal an increase in spinal dynorphin biosynthesis in a rat model of peripheral inflammation and hyperalgesia, Proc. Natl. Acad. Sci. USA, 85 (1988) 622–626.
Sato, K., Kiyama, H., Park, H.P. and Tohyama, M., AMPA, KA and NMDA receptors are expressed in the rat DRG neurons, Neuroreport, 4 (1993a) 1263–1265.
Sato, K., Kiyama, H. and Tohyama, M., The differential expression patterns of messenger RNAs encoding non–N-methyl-D-aspartate glutamate receptor subunits (GluR1–4) in the rat brain, Neurosci., 52 (1993b) 515–539.
Schneider, S.P. and Pearl, E.R., Selective excitation of neurons in the mammalian spinal cord by aspartate and glutamate in vitro: correlation with location and excitatory input, Brain Res., 360 (1985) 339–343.
Sonnenberg, J.L., Rauscher, F.J., III., Morgan, J.I. and Curran, T., Regulation of proenkephalin by fos and jun, Science, 246 (1989) 1622–1625.
Tokunaga, A., Senba, E., Manabe, Y., Shida, T., Ueda, U. and Tohyama, M., Orofacial pain increases mRNA level for galanin in the trigeminal nucleus caudalis of the rat, Peptides, 13 (1992) 1067–1072.
Tölle, T.R., Castro-Lopes, J.M., Coimbra, A. and Zieglgansberger, W., Opiates modify induction of c-fos proto-oncogene in the spinal cord of the rat following noxious stimulation, Neurosci. Lett., 111 (1990) 73–81.
Weihe, E., Millan, M.J., Hollt, V., Nohr, D. and Herz, A., Induction of the gene encoding pro-dynorphin by experimentally induced arthritis enhances staining for dynorphin in the spinal cord of rats, Neuroscience, 31 (1989) 77–95.
Wenthold, R.J., Tokotani, N., Doi, K. and Wada, K., Immunochemical characterization of the non-NMDA glutamate receptor using subunit-specific antibodies, J. Biol. Chem., 267 (1992) 501–507.
Williams, S., Evan, G.I. and Hunt, S.P., Changing patterns of c-fos induction in spinal neurons following thermal cutaneous stimulation in the rat, Neuroscience, 36 (1990) 73–81.
Womack, M.D., MacDermott, A.B. and Jessell, T.M., Sensory transmitters regulate intracellular calcium in dorsal horn neurons, Nature, 334 (1988) 351–353.
Yao, G.L., Tohyama, M. and Senba, E., Histamine-caused itch induces Fos-like immunoreactivity in dorsal horn neurons: effect of morphin pretreatment, Brain Res., 599 (1992) 333–337.

Correspondence to: Masaya Tohyama, MD, PhD, Department of Anatomy and Neuroscience, Osaka University Medical School, 2-2 Yamadaoka, Suita-shi Osaka, 565, Japan. Tel: 81-6-879-3221; Fax: 81-6-879-3229.

Proceedings of the 7th World Congress on Pain,
Progress in Pain Research and Management, Vol. 2,
edited by G.F. Gebhart, D.L. Hammond, and T.S.
Jensen, IASP Press, Seattle, © 1994.

29

C-*fos* Protein, Prodynorphin mRNA, and Protein Kinase C Are Altered with Distinct Spatial and Temporal Patterns in the Spinal Cord of Monarthritic Rats

Thomas R. Tölle,[a] Annemarie Ableitner,[b]
José M. Castro-Lopes,[c] and Walter Zieglgänsberger[a]

[a]Clinical Neuropharmacology, Max-Planck-Institute of Psychiatry, Clinical Institute, Munich, Germany; [b]Department of Pharmacology, Faculty of Veterinary Medicine, University of Munich, Germany; and [c]Faculty of Medicine, Institute of Histology and Embryology, Porto, Portugal

INTRODUCTION

Synaptic excitation evoked by noxious stimulation triggers sets of neuronal events that last from milliseconds to weeks. While the earliest short-term responses are reflected in rapid changes in neuronal discharge activity as a consequence of transmembrane ion fluxes, the long-term changes most commonly require alterations in gene expression. Eucaryotic gene expression is regulated at the level of the initiation of transcription by transcription factors that are encoded by immediate-early genes (IEGs; Evan 1991; Morgan and Curran 1991). C-*fos* and c-*jun* are such nuclear phosphoproteins that can act as constituents in heterodimeric transcription factors interacting with the AP-1 consensus sequence of target genes. While members of the *fos* family require dimerization with *jun* proteins for function, *jun* proteins can form both homo- and heterodimers. The various *jun-fos* complexes possess different binding affinities for DNA consensus sequences and variable transcriptional activities (Evan 1991; Morgan and Curran 1991). IEGs are thought to participate as third messengers in the stimulus transcription cascade, altering gene expression and translation of the corresponding protein products such as enzymes, receptors, or neurotransmitters, thus contributing to the adaptive changes involved in neuronal plasticity and memory formation (Goelet et al. 1986).

In the spinal cord of the rat, IEGs of the *fos*-family, *jun*-family, and Krox-24/NGF1-a are rapidly induced in neurons following acute noxious peripheral stimulation (Hunt et al. 1987; Menetrey et al. 1989; Herdegen et al. 1991b; Tölle et al. 1990, 1994) or peripheral inflammation with complete Freund's adjuvant (Abbadie and Besson 1992; Lantéri-Minet et al. 1993; Tölle et al. 1994). The number, the anatomical distribution of neurons, as well as the time course in which neurons express IEGs depend on the specific stimulus parameters (Wisden et al. 1990; Williams et al. 1990; Herdegen et al. 1991a). Although a causal relationship between peripheral stimulation, IEG induction, and long-term changes in the expression of target genes is still lacking, circumstantial evidence indicates that at least some long-term effects triggered by noxious stimuli on central neurons may have their starting point in genetic events initiated by transactivation of IEGs. The list of possible targets for the action of the c-*fos* protein in the signaling cascade is growing. Among the best studied examples for activity-dependent neuronal plasticity in the central nervous system (CNS) is the increase of opioid synthesis in spinal neurons during experimental polyarthritis (Höllt et al. 1987) and localized hind limb inflammation (Iadarola et al. 1988; Ruda et al. 1988; Dubner and Ruda 1992). The enhanced opioid synthesis in spinal cord neurons parallels the behavioral hyperalgesia associated with the inflammation and is preceded by an ipsilateral increase in c-*fos* expression (Draisci and Iadarola 1989; Naranjo et al. 1991a). Furthermore, c-*fos*, prodynorphin, and proenkephalin mRNA are co-localized in some of these neurons (Weihe et al. 1990; Noguchi et al. 1991, 1992).

Recent behavioral studies indicate that protein kinase C (PKC) may act as a cellular link in neuronal plasticity evoked by noxious stimuli (Coderre 1992; for review see Coderre et al. 1992). This calcium-dependent protein kinase is activated in the presence of membrane lipids (diacylglycerol and phosphatidylserine) and phosphorylates a wide variety of substrates, including ion channel proteins (Nishizuka 1986). Molecular cloning studies have identified a least seven isoforms of PKC that are the products of three distinct (gamma, beta, and alpha) genes (Nishizuka 1986). Autoradiographic as well as immunohistochemical mapping with monoclonal antibodies showed a heterogeneous localization in the rat brain, with a particular enrichment in the substantia gelatinosa of the spinal cord (Worley et al. 1986; Mori et al. 1990).

In our study we induced monarthritis in rats and investigated the time courses of the expression of c-*fos* protein and prodynorphin mRNA as well as changes in the binding intensity and the laminar distribution of PKC in the spinal cord dorsal horn.

MATERIALS AND METHODS

We used female rats, 150 g in weight at the start of the induction of inflammation, and followed ethical guidelines for investigation of experimental pain in conscious animals (Zimmermann 1983). Monarthritis was induced by intraarticular injection of 50 μl of complete Freund's adjuvant (CFA) according to the method described by Butler et al. (1992). The same volume of saline was injected in control animals. The severity of the inflammation was assessed daily by subjective ratings (score 0–4) that considered redness, paw swelling, hyperalgesia to mechanical pressure, and the reduction of locomotor activity. Score 0 indicated no inflammatory signs, while score 4 indicated severe inflammation and persistent flexion of the knee joint (Castro-Lopes et al. 1992).

Following survival times of two hours to 28 days after injection of CFA or saline, animals were randomly chosen from a pool of inflamed and noninflamed control animals and processed for the detection of (1) the IEG c-*fos* with immunohistochemical methods, (2) expression of prodynorphin mRNA by in situ hybridization, and (3) receptor-autoradiography with [^{3}H]phorbol 12,13 dibutyrate (PDBu), which binds and activates the diacylglycerol (DAG) binding site on PKC.

In brief, for c-*fos* detection, following deep halothane anesthesia, animals were perfused intracardially with sodium phosphate-buffered saline followed by 4% paraformaldehyde. From every animal, cryostat coronal serial sections (40 μm) were obtained from lumbar segments L2 to S1 and every consecutive fifth section was incubated for 12 hours with a polyclonal c-*fos* antibody (Cambridge Research Biochemicals). The avidin-biotin-HRP method using diaminobenzidine (DAB) as a chromogene was employed to visualize the immunostained neuronal nuclei. Counterstaining with cresyl violet and viewing against a standard plan with the boundaries of the spinal laminae (Paxinos and Watson 1982) was used to assign the immunostained neurons to Rexed's laminae. Regardless of staining intensity, ranging from lightly brown to dark brown/black, neurons were termed c-*fos* positive if the nuclei showed the characteristic staining of oxidized DAB and a clear distinction from the background at low and high magnifications. The average number of c-*fos* positive neurons from five randomly derived sections from lumbar regions L4–L5 were quantified for the number of nuclei in the various laminae of the spinal dorsal horn.

For in situ hybridization and [^{3}H]PDBu binding, animals were deeply anesthetized with halothane, followed by decapitation, and the lumbar spinal cords were quickly removed and stored at –70°C. Sections (12 µm) cut on a cryostat were processed with minor modifications as described previously for in situ hybridization (Wisden et al. 1991) and for [^{3}H]PDBu-binding (Worley et al. 1986). The in situ hybridization was performed with an ^{35}S-labeled prodynorphin probe. The oligonucleotide probe consisted of 45 bases complementary to bases 864–909 of the prodynorphin mRNA sequence (Civelli et al. 1985). Oligonucleotides were labeled with α35 SdATP (1200 Ci/mmol, NEN) using terminal transferase (Boehringer Mannheim) and a 30:1 molar ratio of dATP:oligonucleotide. Sections were hybridized in 50% formamid, 4× saline sodium citrate (SSC), 10% dextran sulfate at 42°C for 12 hours, and were washed in 1× SSC at 55°C. Sections were dipped in Ilford K5 emulsion for eight weeks. Controls for specificity included incubating sections with a 100-fold excess of unlabeled probe with the corresponding ^{35}S-labeled probe.

After development, sections were counterstained with thionine. Prodynorphin positive neurons were counted and quantified with an image analyzer (OPTIMAS-BIOscann). Neurons showing less than two silver grains per μ^2 were termed lightly labeled. Neurons showing a grain density above two silver grains per μ^2 were termed heavily labeled. Background silver grain density was below 0.24 grains per μ^2. For quantification and anatomical localization, the number of lightly and heavily labeled neurons in three L4–L5 sections were counted and camera lucida plotted. For ^{3}H-PDBu binding, the thaw-mounted sections were gradually brought up to room temperature and incubated for 60 minutes in a solution consisting of 50 mM Tris-HCl (pH 7.4)/100 mM NaCl, 1 mM $CaCl_2$ and 2.5 nM ^{3}H-PDBu (NEN, specific activity 13.2 Ci/mmol). Nonspecific binding was determined by adding 1 µM PDBu to the incubation buffer. Following incubation, the sections were rinsed twice for two minutes in ice-cold buffer, finally in ice-cold distilled water (five seconds) and dried under a stream of cold air. Autoradiograms were prepared by apposing the sections to LKB Ultrofilm for seven days at 4°C together with a set of spinal cord paste sections (12 µm) containing serial dilutions of the radiolabel. Optical density (OD) measurements of the autoradiograms were made within a frame set on laminae I–III of the dorsal horn of each side of the spinal cord and on the area around the central canal using an image analyzer (Quantimet 520). The ODs obtained were related to picomoles per gram of tissue by reference to the OD of spinal cord paste sections with known content of the radiolabel.

For statistical analysis the differences between the experimental groups for the various variables investigated (paw volume, inflammation score, c-*fos* and prodynorphin expression, [^{3}H]PDBu binding) were tested with analysis of variance (ANOVA) followed by Duncan posthoc tests or Newmann-Keul's multiple-range test.

RESULTS

EXPERIMENTAL MONARTHRITIS

Intraarticular CFA caused an inflammatory reaction leading to an increase in paw volume that was apparent 4–8 hours after the injection, reached maximum values two weeks later, and remained elevated throughout the period investigated (Fig. 1A). The inflammation score, as a subjective rating procedure reflecting the inflammatory state induced in the animal, followed a similar time course (Fig. 1B). One-way ANOVA revealed no significant differences between the groups of animals processed for c-*fos* or prodynorphin and PKC.

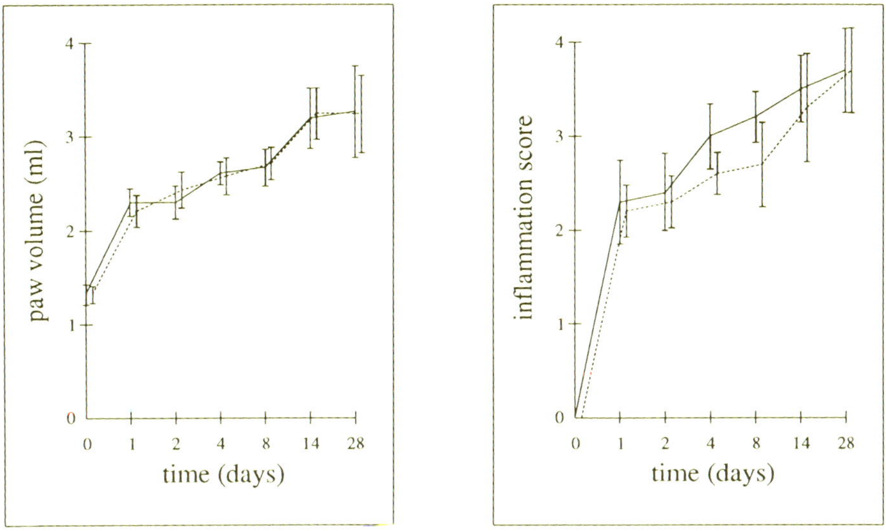

Fig. 1. Development of paw volume **(left)** and inflammation score **(right)** in rats after injection of complete Freund's adjuvant into the tibio-tarsal joint of one hind limb. Solid lines show averaged values ± SD obtained from animals processed for the IEG c-*fos*; dashed lines resemble data from animals processed for prodynorphin mRNA and protein kinase C. No significant difference between the two groups (N = 5 each time point) for both variables were detected (ANOVA).

C-*FOS* AND PRODYNORPHIN EXPRESSION

In animals sacrificed two hours two hours after CFA injection only a few neurons immunoreactive for c-*fos* protein (11 ± 7 per 5 × 40 μm sections) could be observed in the dorsal horn ipsilateral to the treated paw. Immunoreactive neurons were found from L2 to L6, showing a maximum in L4–L5. Although at this early point most labeled neurons occurred in laminae I–II, some neurons in deeper laminae also showed immunostained nuclei. At 24 hours postinjection the number of c–*fos* immunoreactive neurons substantially increased, and the pattern of the dorsoventral distribution also changed (Fig. 2). C–*fos* positive neurons were now scattered ipsilateral to the injection site at higher density in deep laminae (III–VI; 80 ± 5 neurons per 5 × 40 μm sections) than in the superficial laminae (I–II; 20 ± 3 neurons per 5 × 40 μm sections). This pattern persisted for more than 48 hours after CFA injection. Thereafter, the number of immunoreactive neurons started to decay. Two weeks after CFA injection, no significant difference from control expression could be detected. Four weeks after CFA, only 1–2 neurons per 5 × 40 μm section could be observed (Fig. 2); at every time point investigated only a few neurons (1–3 per 5 × 40 μm sections) were found in the superficial and deep laminae of the dorsal horn contralateral to the injection site.

In control animals prodynorphin mRNA was detected in 50–80 lightly labeled neurons per 3 × 12 μm sections located preferentially in superficial laminae of the dorsal horn. Prodynorphin neurons occurred also in deeper laminae (IV–VI), but were far less abundant (Fig. 3). Following induction of monarthritis, an enhanced expression of prodynorphin mRNA emerged, as evidenced by increased silver grain density overlying the neuronal cell bodies. At day 2 of CFA-inflammation, 30–40 heavily labeled neurons per 3 × 12 μm sections could be detected strictly ipsilateral to the side of peripheral inflammation. These heavily prodynorphin-expressing neurons (1–2 neurons per 3 × 12 μm sections in control animals) were primarily located in the medial two-thirds of laminae I–II and in the middle of laminae IV–VI. The maximal number of heavily labeled neurons was found at lumbar segments L4–L5. This distribution agrees with the known projection of primary endings from the inflamed joint. The number of heavily labeled neurons peaked four days after CFA injection. To the end of the 28-day observation period, the number of heavily labeled neurons slightly decreased to values of 20–30 neurons per 3 × 12 μm sections (Fig. 3).

[^{3}H]PDBU BINDING

In control animals the highest binding for [^{3}H]PDBu was found in laminae I–II of the dorsal horn (Fig. 4; 1050 ± 40 pmol/g tissue). Compared to

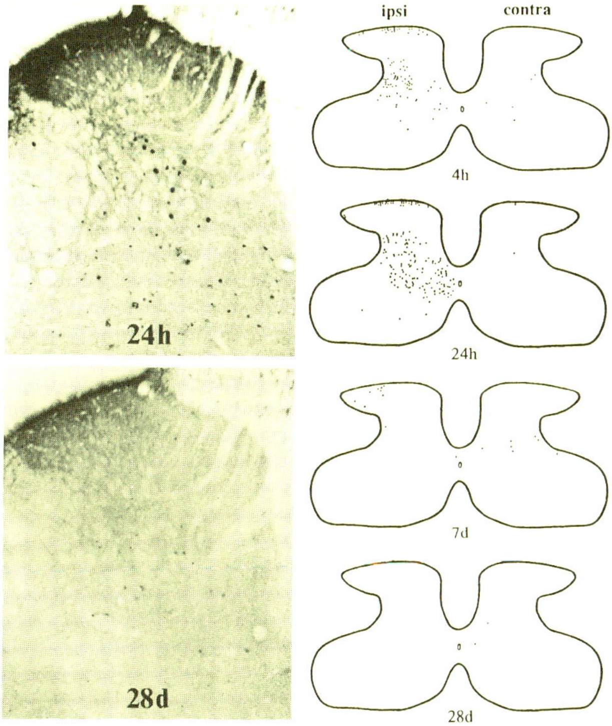

Fig. 2. Bright-field photomicrographs (24 hours and 28 days) and camera lucida reconstructions (4 hours, 24 hours, 7 days, and 28 days) of c-*fos* immunostained lumbar spinal cord sections illustrating the distribution of neurons ipsilateral and contralateral to an inflammation induced by injection of complete Freund's adjuvant into the tibio-tarsal joint of one hind limb. Each drawing represents the nuclei observed in five randomly depicted 40-μm sections obtained from the lumbar segments L4–L5 (each dot represents one labeled nucleus).

these values, binding in the area adjacent to the central canal (lamina X of Rexed) was moderate (400 ± 30 pmol/g tissue). With the sensitivity of the applied biochemical detection system, other spinal structures showed no quantifiable binding (Fig. 4A). After CFA, the ipsilateral and the contralateral dorsal horn showed enhanced binding of [^{3}H]PDBu (Fig. 4). The observed increase in specific binding was significant on the ipsilateral side on day 4 and on the contralateral side on day 14. The maximal increase of binding was observed at day 14, reaching values of about 1340 ± .50 pmol per g tissue on both sides of the spinal cord. The changes of specific binding around the central canal did not reach significance. Beside the increase in binding in superficial laminae I–II of the dorsal horn, binding sites were now observed in deeper laminae III and IV of the dorsal horn (Fig. 4).

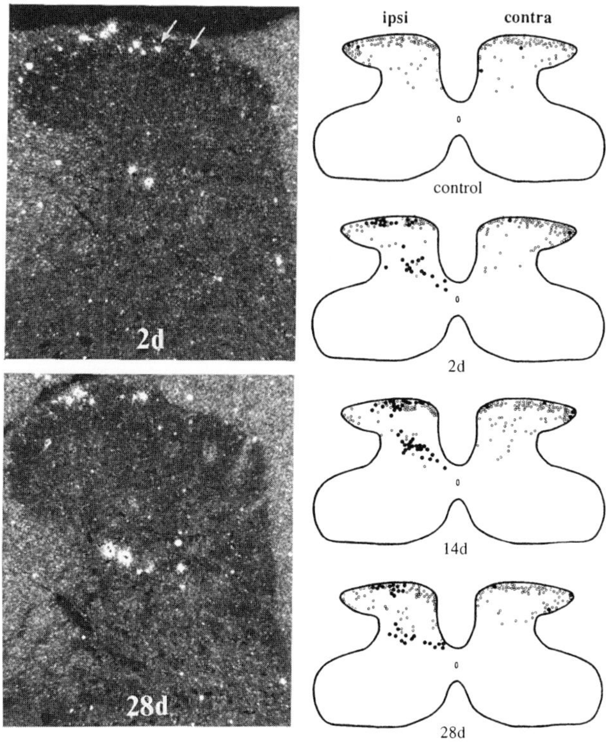

Fig. 3. Dark-field photomicrographs (2 and 28 days) and camera lucida reconstructions (control, 2, 14, and 28 days) of spinal cord sections following in situ hybridization with an ^{35}S-labeled prodynorphin probe. They illustrate the distribution of prodynorphin mRNA-containing neurons ipsilateral and contralateral to an inflammation induced by injection of complete Freund's adjuvant into the tibio-tarsal joint of one hind limb. Arrowheads in the upper photomicrograph indicate neurons that were termed lightly and heavily expressing neurons (for details see Methods). Each drawing represents all neurons observed in three randomly depicted 12 μm sections obtained from the lumbar segments L4–L5 (filled symbol = one heavily labeled neuron; open symbol = three lightly labeled neurons). During the whole 28 days of monarthritis a considerable amount of heavily prodynorphin mRNA-expressing neurons, showing an increased density of silver grains overlying the neurons, could be detected ipsilaterally in superficial and deep laminae.

DISCUSSION

Our study illustrates that in CFA-induced monarthritic animals the dynamic alterations in the signaling cascade follow distinct temporal and spatial patterns and do not remain strictly ipsilateral to the side of inflammation.

In the few studies that have investigated the effect of prolonged noxious stimulation on c-*fos* expression in the spinal cord (Menetrey et al. 1989; Noguchi et al. 1991, 1992) the observations were limited to the first 72 hours after injection of the inflammatory agent. Only recently has c-*fos* expression been studied in CFA polyarthritic rats for up to 22 weeks (Abbadie and Besson 1992). In that study c-*fos* followed the time course of the clinical signs of arthritis and peaked simultaneously with hyperalgesia three weeks after inoculation (Abbadie and Besson 1992). In our, the number of c-*fos* neurons had already decreased to low levels (3–7 neurons per 5 × 40 μm sections) seven days after CFA injection, and c-*fos* positive neurons were completely absent after two weeks, a time when hyperalgesia was still demonstrable in this model of monarthritis (Butler et al. 1992). These observations suggest that in monarthritic rats the degree of hyperalgesia and the expression of c-*fos* follow different time courses, underlining the limited value of IEGs as mere activity markers in this model. However, another study that employed chronic somatic inflammation and showed an evoked c-*fos* expression only during the first two days postinjection, reported *jun* B expression for two weeks and *fos* B, c-*jun*, and *jun* D expression until 6, 9, and 15 weeks, respectively. Furthermore, all IEG proteins were expressed in deep dorsal horn neurons during the whole disease period (Lantéri-Minet et al. 1993).

Induction of the IEG c-*fos* and the gene encoding for prodynorphin or preproenkephalin has been observed in the same neurons following inflammation (Noguchi et al. 1991, 1992). The consecutive appearance of both genes in the same neurons and the demonstration of AP-1 sequences in the prodynorphin gene promotor region are further evidence in favor of a functional link (Naranjo et al. 1991b). To define which DNA regions could mediate trans-synaptic regulation of gene induction, a recent study in transgenic mice demonstrated that increased expression of preproenkephalin mRNA in the spinal cord in response to pain acts through a 193 base-pair promotor region (Takemura et al. 1992). Further evidence for a high degree of functional connectivity between c-*fos* and prodynorphin induction can be derived from an in vitro study in cultured spinal cord neurons where the transactivation of prodynorphin was completely blocked with a c-*fos* antisense oligonucleotide (Lucas et al. 1993). In our monarthritic model, enhanced expression of prodynorphin mRNA was still detectable in the same subset of spinal cord neurons for weeks after c-*fos* protein was no longer detectable. These findings suggest, considering a half-life of prodynorphin mRNA in the range of hours, that transactivation of the prodynorphin gene is achieved at these later times by other IEG products. Whether other IEGs, partly co-induced in some neurons (Naranjo et al. 1991b), subserve the ongoing prodynorphin transactivation or another not yet defined nuclear machinery is at work, can not be answered. Whether c-*fos* could serve

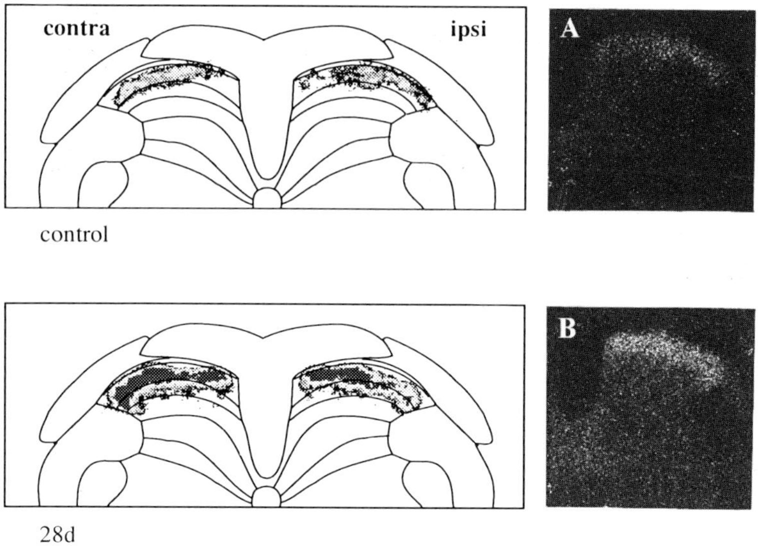

Fig. 4. X-ray film autoradiographs of lumbar rat dorsal horn sections (12 µm) illustrating the distribution of [^{3}H]PDBu binding in control animals (**A**) and following 28 days (**B**) of inflammation induced with injection of complete Freund's adjuvant into the tibio-tarsal joint of one hind limb. Photomicrographs show the dorsal horn quadrant of a spinal cord section ipsilateral to the side of inflammation. The computerized black/white autoradiographs of the [^{3}H]PDBu binding fit to a schematic slice showing the boundaries of Rexed's laminae and reveal the preferential location of the [^{3}H]PDBu binding to superficial laminae of the dorsal horn. Following 28 days of inflammation, the [^{3}H]PDBu binding shows bilaterally (1) a considerable increase in binding, as evidenced by the dark gray areas, and (2) binding in deeper laminae III–IV of the dorsal horn.

only to initialize transcription, while other IEG-derived (*fos* B, c-*jun* and *jun* D) transcription complexes with a low level of expression (Herdegen et al. 1991b; Lantéry-Minet et al. 1993; Tölle et al. 1994) maintain transactivation of target genes remains to be shown.

The present study revealed a bilateral increase of [^{3}H]PDBu binding and an expansion of [^{3}H]PDBu binding to deeper laminae of the dorsal horn following unilateral inflammation. Electrophysiological studies suggest that in the rat spinal dorsal horn activators of PKC such as the phorbol ester PDBu, which binds to and activates the DAG binding site on protein kinase C (Worley et al. 1986), enhance the basal and evoked release of amino acid neurotransmitters (Gerber et al. 1989) and also may be involved in the regulation of postsynaptic NMDA- and NK_1 receptors (Chen et al. 1992; Swartz et al. 1993; Munro et al. 1993) and calcium currents (Rane et al. 1989). A recent study reported that a splice variant of the rat NMDA-receptor, which shows a distinct distribution of subunit genes in the spinal cord (Tölle et al. 1993; and unpublished observations), possesses a different sensitivity to activators of PKC, resulting in a 20-fold increase of the NMDA response (Durand et al. 1992). A synopsis of these findings suggests PKC as a crucial mediator of intracellular changes that can induce enhanced excitability of neurons. Recent behavioral studies indicate that nociceptive responses to formalin injury are suppressed following intrathecal application of an inhibitor of PKC, and are enhanced after treatment with phorbol esters (Coderre 1992; Coderre et al. 1993; Yashpal et al. 1993). The pathophysiological significance of a bilateral increase in [^{3}H]PDBu binding is further suggested by the observation that persistent pain produced by formalin injury and mechanical hyperalgesia in the hindpaw contralateral to a thermal injury are influenced by PKC inhibitors (Coderre et al. 1993). Whether the increased binding of [^{3}H]PDBu resembles de novo target-gene derived synthesis of PKC or functional activation of nonactive forms of PKC can not be resolved from the present data. It remains to be elucidated whether the increased binding of [^{3}H]PDBu and/or the detection of [^{3}H]PDBu in deeper laminae of the dorsal horn is based on an increase of all PKC subspecies (Mori et al. 1990), or whether this increase is restricted to certain PKC subspecies with distinct biochemical properties.

REFERENCES

Abbadie, C. and Besson, J.-M., *C-fos* expression in rat lumbar spinal cord during the development of adjuvant-induced arthritis, Neurosci., 48, 4 (1992) 985–993.

Butler, St. H., Godefroy, F., Besson, J.-M. and Weil-Fugazza, J., A limited arthritic model for chronic pain studies in the rat, Pain, 48 (1992) 73–81.

Castro-Lopes, J.M., Tavares, I., Tölle, T.R., Coito, A. and Coimbra, A., Increase in GABAergic cells and GABA levels in the spinal cord in unilateral inflammation of the hindlimb in the rat, Eur. J. Neurosci., 4 (1992) 296–301.

Chen, L. and Mae Huang, L-Y., Protein kinase C reduces Mg^{2+} block of NMDA-receptor channels as a mechanism of modulation, Nature, (1992) 521–523.

Civelli, O., Douglass, J., Goldstein, A. and Herbert, E., Sequence and expression of the rat prodynorphin gene, Proc. Natl. Acad. Sci., 82, Neurobiology (1985) 4291–4295.

Coderre, T.J., Contribution of protein kinase C to central sensitization and persistent pain following tissue injury, Neurosci. Lett., 140 (1992) 181–184.

Coderre, T.J., Katz, J., Vaccarino, A.L. and Melzack, R., Contribution of central neuroplasticity to pathological pain: review of clinical and experimental evidence, Pain, 52 (1993) 259–285.

Coderre, T.J., Pitcher, G.M. and Yashpal, K., Pharmacological and anatomical evidence for a contribution of protein kinase C to persistent pain and hyperalgesia following tissue injury in rats, Abstracts: 7th World Congress on Pain, IASP Publications, Seattle, 1993, p. 223.

Draisci, G. and Iadarola, M.J., Temporal analysis of increases in c-fos, preprodynorphin and preproenkephalin mRNAs in rat spinal cord, Mol. Brain Res., 6 (1989) 31–37.

Dubner, R. and Ruda, M.A., Activity-dependent neuronal plasticity following tissue injury and inflammation, TINS, 15 (1992) 96–103.

Durand, G.M., Gregor, P., Zheng, Y., Bennett, M.V.L., Uhl, G.R. and Zukin R.S., Cloning of an apparent splice variant of the rat N-methyl-D-aspartate receptor NMDAR1 with altered sensitivity to polyamines and activators of protein kinase C, Proc. Natl. Acad. Sci. USA, 89 (Neurobiology) (1992) 9359–9363.

Evan, G., Regulation of gene expression, Br. Med. Bull., 47 1 (1991) 116–135.

Gerber, G., Kangrga, I., Ryu, P.D., Larew, J.S.A. and Randic, M., Multiple effects of phorbol esters in the rat spinal dorsal horn, J. Neurosci., 9 (1989) 3606–3617.

Goelet, P., Castellucci, V.F., Schacher, S. and Kandel, E.R., The long and the short of long-term memory: a molecular framework, Nature, 322 (1986) 419–422.

Herdegen, T., Tölle, T.R., Bravo, R., Zieglgänsberger, W. and Zimmermann, M., Sequential expression of JUN B, JUN D and FOS B proteins in rat spinal neurons: cascade of transcriptional operations during nociception, Neurosci. Lett., 129 (1991a) 221–224.

Herdegen, T., Kovary, K., Leah, J. and Bravo, R., Specific temporal and spatial distribution of JUN, FOS, and KROX-24 proteins in spinal neurons following noxious transsynaptic stimulation, J. Comp. Neurol., 313 (1991b) 178–191.

Höllt, V., Haarmann, I., Millan, M.J. and Herz, A., Prodynorphin gene expression is enhanced in the spinal cord of chronic arthritic rats, Neurosci. Lett., 73 (1978) 90–94.

Hunt, S.P., Pini, A., Evan, G., Induction of *c-fos*–like proteins in spinal cord neurons following sensory stimulation, Nature, 328 (1987) 632–634.

Iadarola, M., Douglass, J., Civelli, O. and Naranjo, J., Differential activation of spinal cord dynorphin and enkephalin neurons during hyperalgesia: evidence using cDNA hybridization, Brain. Res., 455 (1988) 205–212.

Lantéri-Minet, J., de Pommery, J., Herdegen, T., Weil-Fugazza, J., Bravo, R. and Menétrey, D., Differential time course and spatial expression of Fos, Jun, and Krox-24 proteins in spinal cord of rats undergoing subacute or chronic somatic inflammation, J. Comp. Neurol., 333 (1993) 223–235.

Lucas, J.J., Mellström, B., Colado, M.I. and Naranjo, J.R., Molecular mechanisms of pain: serotonin-1A receptor agonists trigger transactivation by c-*fos* of the prodynorphin gene in spinal cord neurons, Neuron, 10 (1993) 599–611.

Menetrey, D., Gannon, A., Levine, J.D., and Basbaum, A.J., The expression of *c-fos* protein in presumed nociceptive interneurons and projection neurons of the rat spinal cord: anatomical mapping of the central effect of noxious somatic, articular and visceral stimulation, J. Comp. Neurol., 285 (1989) 177–195.

Morgan, J.I. and Curran, T., Stimulus-transcription coupling in the nervous system: involvement of the inducible proto-oncogenes *fos* and *jun*, Ann. Rev. Neurosci., 14 (1991) 421–451.

Mori, M., Kose, A., Tsujino, T. and Tanaka, C., Immunocytochemical localization of protein kinase C subspecies in the rat spinal cord: light and electron microscopic study, J. Comp. Neurol., 299 (1990) 167–177.

Munro, F., Young, M., Fleetwood-Walker, S., Parker, R. and Mitchell R., Receptor and cellular mechanisms involved in mustard oil–induced activation of dorsal horn neurons. In: Abstracts: 7th World Congress on Pain, IASP Publications, Seattle, 1993, p. 467.

Naranjo, J.R., Mellström, B., Achaval, M. and Sassone-Corsi, P., Molecular pathways of pain: Fos/Jun-mediated of a noncanonical AP-1 site in the prodynorphin gene, Neuron, 6 (1991a) 607–617.

Naranjo, J.R., Mellström, B., Achaval, M., Lucas, J.J., Del Rio, J. and Sassone-Corsi, P., Co-induction of jun B and c-*fos* in a subset of neurons in the spinal cord, Oncogene, 6 (1991b) 223–227.

Nishizuka, Y., Studies and perspectives of protein kinase C, Science, 233 (1986) 305–312.

Noguchi, K., Kowalski, K., Traub, R., Solodkin, A., Iadorola, M.M., and Ruda, M.A., Dynorphin expression and fos-like immunoreactivity following inflammation induced hyperalgesia are colocalized in spinal cord neurons, Mol. Brain Res., 10 (1991) 227–233.

Noguchi, K., Dubner, R. and Ruda, M.A., Preproenkephalin mRNA in spinal dorsal horn neurons is induced by peripheral inflammation and is co-localized with fos and fos-related proteins, Neuroscience, 46, 3 (1992) 561–570.

Paxinos, G. and Watson, C., The Rat Brain in Stereotaxic Coordinates, Academic Press, Sydney, 1982.

Rane, St.G., Walsh, M.P., McDonald, J.R. and Dunlap, K., Specific inhibitors of protein kinase C block transmitter-induced modulation of sensory neuron calcium current, Neuron, 3 (1989) 239–245.

Ruda, M.A., Iadarola, M.J., Cohen, L.V. and Young, W.S., III, In situ hybridization histochemistry and immunocytochemistry reveal increase in spinal dynorphin biosynthesis in a rat model of peripheral inflammation and hyperalgesia, Proc. Natl. Acad. Sci. USA, 85 (1988) 622–626.

Swartz, K.J., Merritt, A., Bean, B.P. and Lovinger, D.M., Protein kinase C modulates glutamate receptor inhibition of Ca^{2+} channels and synaptic transmission, Nature, 361 (1993) 165–168.

Takemura, M., Donovan, D.M. and Uhl, G.R., Primary afferent stimulation acts through a 193 base pair promoter region to upregulate preproenkephalin expression in dorsal horn of transgenic mice, Brain. Res. Mol. Brain. Res., 13 (1992) 207–212.

Tölle, T.R., Castro-Lopes, J.M., Coimbra, A. and Zieglgänsberger, W., Opiates modify induction of c-fos proto-oncogene in the spinal cord of the rat following noxious stimulation, Neurosci. Lett., 111 (1990) 46–51.

Tölle, T.R., Berthele, A., Zieglgänsberger, W., Seeburg, P.H. and Wisden, W., The differential expression of 16 NMDA and non-NMDA receptor subunits in the rat spinal cord and in periaqueductal grey, J. Neurosci., 13, 12 (1993) 5009–5028.

Tölle, T.R., Herdegen, T., Schadrack, J., Bravo, R., Zimmermann, M. and Zieglgänsberger, W., Application of morphine prior to noxious stimulation differentially modulates expression of Fos, Jun and Krox-24 proteins in rat spinal cord neurons, Neuroscience, 58, 2 (1994) 305–327.

Tölle, T.R., Castro-Lopes, J.M. and Zieglgänsberger, W., Nociceptive stimulation induces immediate early gene expression and increases GABA immunoreactivity in spinal neurons. In: T. Hökfelt, H.-G. Schaible and R.F. Schmidt (Eds.), Neuropeptides, Nociception and Pain, VCH-Verlag, Weinheim, 1994 (in press).

Wang, Lu-Yang, Salter, M.W. and MacDonald, J.F., Regulation of kainate receptors by cAMP-dependent protein kinase and phosphatases, Science, 253 (1991) 1132–1135.

Weihe, E., Iadarola, J.J., Nohr, D., Müller, S., Millan, M.J., Yanaihara, N., Stein, C. and Herz, A., Sustained expression and colocalization of proenkephalin and prodynorphin opioids and *c-fos* protein in dorsal horn neurons revealed in arthritic rats. In: J.M. van Ree, A.H. Mulder, V.M. Wiegant and T.B. van Wimersma Greidanus (Eds.), New Leads in Opioid Research, Elsevier, Amsterdam, 1990, pp. 92–94.

Williams, S., Evans, G.I. and Hunt, S.P., Changing patterns of c-fos induction in spinal neurons following thermal cutaneous stimulation in the rat, Neuroscience, 36 (1990) 73–81.

Wisden, W., Errington, M.L., Williams, W., Dunnett, S.B., Waters, C., Hitchcock, D., Evan, G., Bliss, T.V.P. and Hunt, S.P., Differential expression of immediate early genes in the hippocampus and spinal cord, Neuron, 4 (1990) 603–614.

Wisden, W., Morris, B.J. and Hunt, S.P., In situ hybridization with synthetic DNA probes. In: J. Chad and H. Wheal (Eds.), Molecular Neurobiology: A Practical Approach, Oxford University Press/IRL Press, New York, 1991.

Worley, P.F., Baraban, J.M. and Snyder, S.H., Heterogeneous localization of protein kinase C in rat brain: autoradiographic analysis of phorbol ester receptor binding, J. Neurosci., 6, 1 (1986) 199–207.

Yashpal, K. and Codere, T.J., Contribution of nitric oxide, arachidonic acid and protein kinase C to persistent pain following tissue injury in rats. In: Abstracts: 7th World Congress on Pain, IASP Publications, Seattle, 1993, p. 224.

Zimmermann, M., (Chair, IASP Committee on Research and Ethical Issues) , Ethical guidelines for investigations of experimental pain in conscious animals, Pain, 16 (1983) 109–110.

Correspondence to: T.R. Tölle, Clinical Neuropharmacology, Max-Planck-Institute of Psychiatry, Clinical Institute, Kraepelinstrasse 10, D-80804 München, Germany. Tel: 49-89-30622-350; Fax: 49-89-30622-402.

Proceedings of the 7th World Congress on Pain,
Progress in Pain Research and Management, Vol. 2,
edited by G.F. Gebhart, D.L. Hammond, and T.S.
Jensen, IASP Press, Seattle, © 1994.

30

C-*fos* Activation by Noxious Input of Spinal Neurons Projecting to the Nucleus of the Tractus Solitarius in the Rat

Deolinda Lima, Filomena Esteves,
and Antonio Coimbra

Institute of Histology and Embryology, Faculty of Medicine and Center of Experimental Morphology of the University of Oporto, Porto, Portugal

INTRODUCTION

The nucleus of the tractus solitarius (NTS) was recently shown to be part of the supraspinal antinociceptive system. Electrical stimulation (Lewis et al. 1987; Morgan et al. 1989; Aicher and Randich 1990; Du and Zhou 1990; Ren et al. 1990) or glutamate injection (Morgan et al. 1989; Du and Zhou 1990; Ren et al. 1990) into the NTS depresses nociceptive reflexes (Lewis et al. 1987; Morgan et al. 1989; Aicher and Randich 1990) and inhibits the responses of dorsal horn neurons to noxious input (Du and Zhou 1990; Ren et al. 1990). Considering the well-known involvement of the NTS in viscerosensory processing (Kalia and Mesulam 1980; Altschuler et al. 1989) and cardiovascular control (Lipski et al. 1975; Loewy and Burton 1978; Ciriello et al. 1981; Donoghue et al. 1982, 1984; Ross et al. 1985; Hancock 1988), it is possible that modulation of nociceptive transmission by the NTS is elicited by changes in autonomic parameters. In fact, raising the blood pressure results in an increased pain threshold (Zamir and Sogal 1979; Zamir and Shuber 1980) mediated by baroreceptors (Dworkin et al. 1979), while stimulation of the vagus nerve produces NTS-mediated inhibition of spinal nociceptive cells and decreases the tail-flick response to radiant heat (Randich and Aicher 1988; Ren et al. 1990).

The possibility that noxious messages ascending from the spinal cord trigger analgesic mechanisms in the NTS, as has been suggested for other antinociceptive areas (Basbaum and Fields 1984), can not be excluded. The NTS receives massive projections from spinal neurons (Menétrey and Basbaum 1987; Esteves et al. 1993) which, according to their location in lamina I and the dorsal horn neck, are likely to process nociceptive input (Christensen and Perl 1970; Cervero et al. 1976; Menétrey et al. 1977; Kumazawa and Perl 1978). On the other hand, electrical stimulation of the sciatic nerve inhibits NTS cells activated by baroreceptors (McMahon et al. 1992). The NTS thus may also participate in the genesis of autonomic responses to pain recently demonstrated in research studies. Increases in heart rate and blood pressure were recorded following muscular ischemia (Maixner et al. 1990) or during noxious cooling or heating of the skin (Abram et al. 1983).

We evaluated the participation of several spinal neuronal groups in the transmission of nociceptive input to the NTS by combining immunodetection of the *fos* protein following cutaneous noxious stimulation with retrograde neuronal tracing.

MATERIALS AND METHODS

For all experiments we used Male Wistar rats, weighing from 280–310 g, from the colony of the Gulbenkian Institute of Science. We followed ethical guidelines for the investigation of experimental pain in conscious animals. Animals were injected stereotaxically under halothane anesthesia with 4% fluorogold in the caudal third of the left NTS, following the coordinates of Paxinos and Watson (1982). Two injections of equal volume (0.2µl each) were made in rostrocaudal sequence. Four days later, the rats were given chloral hydrate anesthesia (1 ml/kg body weight, intraperitoneally), and noxious stimulation by chemical, mechanical, or thermal agents was applied to a well-delimited area of hairy skin in the proximal internal aspect of the right thigh. Chemical stimulation consisted of a subcutaneous injection of 0.4 ml of 5% neutral formalin (four rats). Mechanical stimulation consisted of pinching for two hours, at two minute intervals, successive points of the skin with a rat tooth forceps (four rats). Thermal stimulation consisted of 20-second pulses of radiant heat at 65°C (which corresponded to 58°C intradermally at the depth of 0.1 mm) at two-minute intervals, for two hours (four rats). Control animals were subjected to fluorogold injections into the NTS followed four days later by two hours of chloral hydrate anesthesia without noxious stimulation (two rats), subcutaneous injection of 0.4 ml of saline (two rats), rubbing the skin during two hours, at two-minute intervals, with a piece of cotton (two rats) or pressing the skin at 10 mg/mm^2 using a 4-mm^2 probe (Lima et al. 1993) every two minutes for two hours (two rats). Two hours after the beginning of stimulation, rats were perfused through the ascending aorta with 100 ml of phosphate buffered-saline (PBS) followed by 1000 ml of 4% paraformaldehyde in 0.1M phosphate buffer, pH 7.4. The medulla oblongata and spinal segments T13, L1, L2, and L3 were removed and immersed in fixative overnight and in 30% sucrose in phosphate buffer for 24 hours. Coronal 40-μm thick frozen sections were cut from the injection site and each spinal cord segment. All spinal sections were immunoreacted with an anti-*fos* antibody raised in sheep (Cambridge Research Biochemicals) at 1/1500 revealed by a fluorescein-conjugated rabbit anti-sheep. The sections were mounted in 75% glycerin in phosphate buffer and observed with an epifluorescent microscope under an excitation light of 330–380 nm wavelength to visualize fluorogold and 450–490 nm to visualize fluorescein. Control rats did not exhibit *fos*-immunostaining except for a few lamina I cells following subcutaneous injection of saline (89 cells in segments T13–L3), or rubbing the skin (46). Spinal cells retrograde-labeled with fluorogold, immunoreactive for the *fos*-protein, or presenting both fluorogold and *fos* staining (double-labeled cells) were counted in all Rexed's laminae of the right half of all sections of segments T13, L1, L2, and L3. Spinal laminae were delimited in the epifluorescent microscope by measuring their width with an eyepiece with reticular holder. The widths of laminae I, IV–V, VII, and X in immunostained sections were calculated from the widths measured in formol-thionin stained sections of an additional rat (Donovick 1974) by applying a factor of 1.3. This was the ratio between the maximal dorsoventral extension of gray matter (from a point midway between the medial and lateral ends of the dorsal gray contour and the ventral tip of the dorsal horn) in immunoreacted and formol-thionin stained sections. Laminar widths did not vary significantly between the segments examined. The laminar location of stained cells in five sections randomly taken from each segment was plotted on laminar diagrams of the same segment obtained from the formol-thionin stained sections. Lamina I cells labeled with fluorogold or double-labeled were characterized morphologically according to Lima and Coimbra (1983, 1986). Percentages of double-labeled cells in the population of fluorogold-labeled or *fos*-positive cells were compared by the test of the exact probability of Fisher.

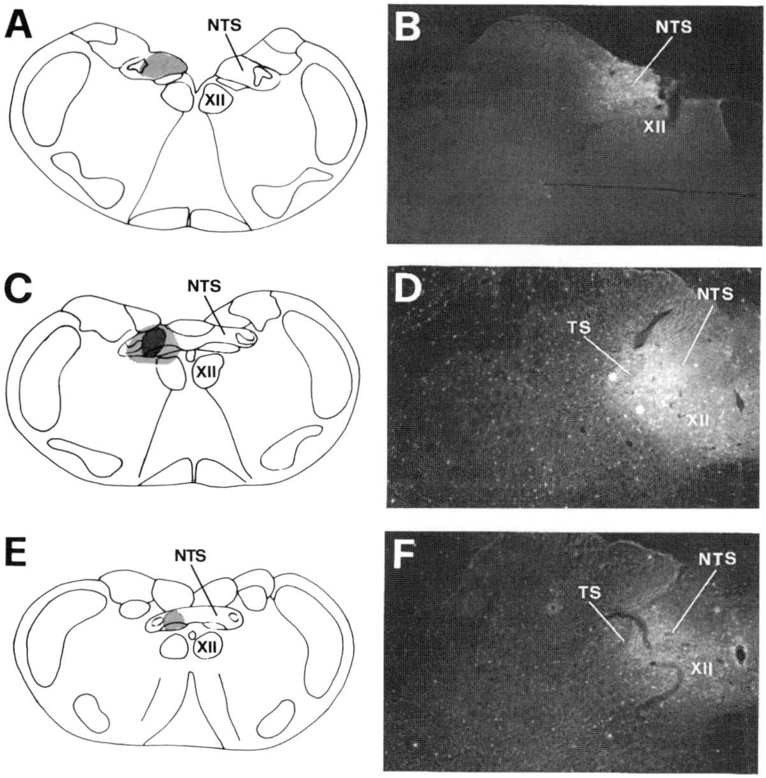

Fig. 1. Diagrammatic representation (**A, C, E**) and respective photomicrographs (**B, D, F**) of the injection site from one experiment at –4.3 (**A, B**), –4.8 (**C, D**), and –5.3 mm (**E, F**) from the interaural line. The peripheral halo of the injection site is marked with an asterisk (**D**).

RESULTS

INJECTION SITES

Fluorogold injection sites were centered in the caudal two-thirds of the left NTS (Fig. 1). They consisted of a central core that filled the lateral portion of the commissural subnucleus; a slightly dense halo without neuronal staining (asterisks in Fig. 1D) encroached on the motor nucleus of the vagus nerve (X), the dorsal portion of the nucleus of the hypoglossal nerve (XII), and the most medial part of the dorsal reticular nucleus (DRt). Spinal labeling

Table I
Numbers of retrograde-labeled cells (± SD) per Rexed's lamina

Lamina	Stimulation		
	Chemical	Mechanical	Thermal
I	891 ± 160 (5)	695 ± 145 (5)	863 ± 144 (5)
IV–V	9003 ± 460 (51)	8045 ± 2045 (54)	9185 ± 466 (54)
VII	6381 ± 696 (36)	5521 ± 1460 (37)	6326 ± 106 (37)
X	1326 ± 326 (8)	545 ± 145 (4)	628 ± 316 (4)

Note: Percentage per lamina is given in parentheses; n = 4.

in our study can not be attributed to the injection of the motor nucleus of the Xth cranial nerve or of the nucleus of the XIIth nerve, because none has been known to receive spinal projections in the rat (Esteves et al. 1993). Moreover, the spinal-DRt pathway was not labeled because no lamina I cells of the multipolar type, which project massively to the DRt (Lima and Coimbra 1990), were stained.

RETROGRADE LABELING

Total numbers of spinal cells retrograde-labeled by fluorogold in segments T13 to L3 averaged 16,510 ± 2,276 per animal. Cells were distributed through laminae I, IV–V, VII, and X, bilaterally (Table I; Fig. 2), which agrees with previous data obtained with wheat-germ agglutinin-HRP (Menétrey and Basbaum 1987) or cholera toxin subunit b (CTb) (Esteves et al. 1993). The distribution of labeled cells per lamina (Table I) did not vary in animals subject to the three stimuli. It was, however, slightly different from that observed previously with CTb (15%, 33%, 23%, and 8%; Esteves et al. 1993). Cells labeled in lamina I were either pyramidal (45%), with the characteristic triangular perikarya and primary dendrites oriented dorsally and lateromedially (Fig. 3A,B); flattened (37%); presenting oval perikarya and dendrites oriented lateromedially (Fig. 3D,E); or fusiform (18%), with round perikarya often

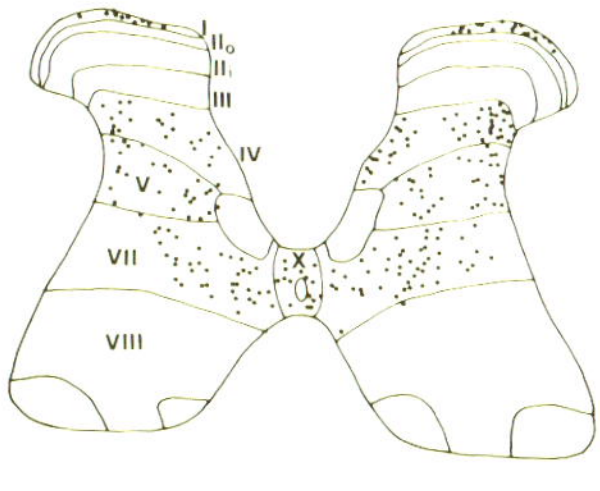

Fig. 2. Distribution per Rexed's laminae of neurons retrograde-labeled with fluorogold in five sections of spinal segment L1 of one rat.

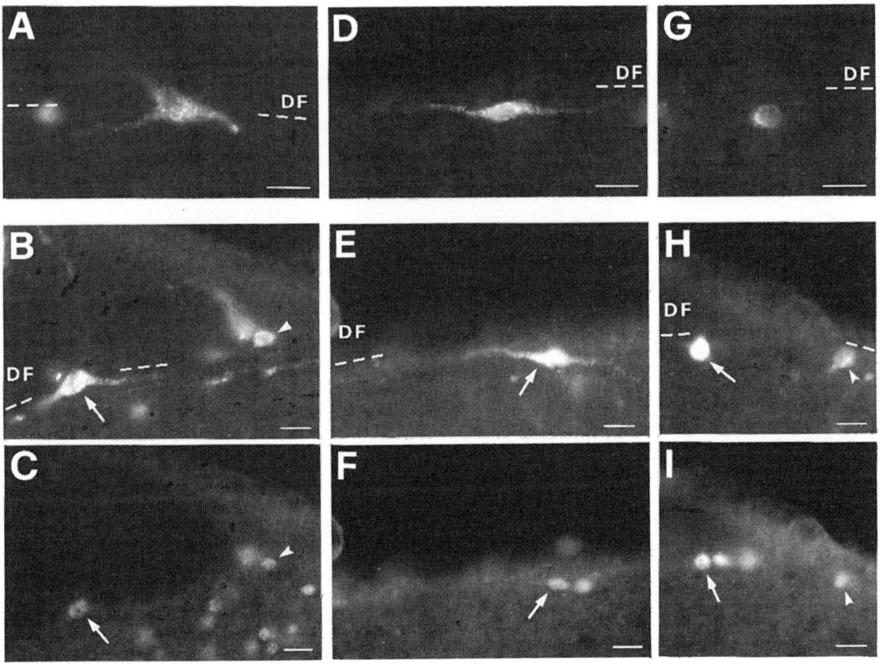

Fig. 3. Lamina I cells retrograde-labeled with fluorogold (**A, D, G**) or double-labeled (**B, C, E, F, H, I**) following mechanical (**B, C**) or chemical (**E, F, H, I**) stimulation. Photomicrographs **B, E, H** were made with an excitation light of 330–380 nm to visualize fluorogold staining, and **C, F, I** with 450–490 nm to visualize *fos*-stained nuclei. Cells in **A** and **B-C** (arrows) are pyramidal, in **D** and **E-F** are flattened, and in **G** and **H-I** are fusiform. Arrow heads in **B-C** and **H–I** point to double-labeled fusiform cells that are slightly out of focus. Magnification bar = 15 μm.

missing primary dendritic trunks due to the orientation of the latter perpendicular to the plane of section (Fig. 3G,H). The same cell groups were previously labeled in similar proportions (38%, 37%, and 25%, respectively) with CTb in the cervical and lumbar enlargements (Esteves et al. 1993).

CELLS IMMUNOREACTIVE TO THE *FOS*-PROTEIN

Following all stimuli, *fos*-positive cells occurred on the side of the spinal cord ipsilateral to the area of skin that had been stimulated, except for formalin injections after which a few cells also occurred on the contralateral dorsal horn (Fig. 4). In consonance with previous data (Lima et al. 1993), the distribution of *fos*-immunoreactive cells per Rexed's laminae varied according to the noxious stimulus used. Numbers of *fos*-positive cells were similar in lamina I

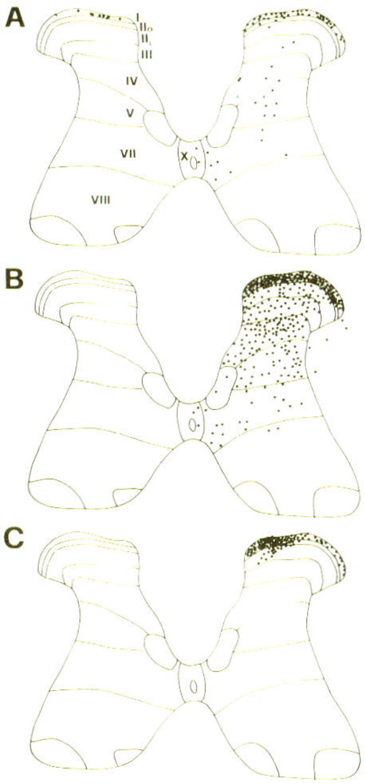

Fig. 4. Distribution per Rexed's laminae of *fos*-immunoreactive cells occurring in five sections of spinal segment L1 following chemical (**A**), mechanical (**B**), or thermal (**C**) stimulation.

following all stimuli but varied considerably in the remaining laminae. Following chemical stimulation (Fig. 4A), *fos*-cells occurring in laminae IV–V, VII, and X were few (Table II). Mechanical stimulation activated large numbers of cells in the deep laminae, with marked prevalence in IV–V (Table II; Fig. 4B). Following thermal stimulation no *fos*-positive cells occurred in the ventralmost laminae.

DOUBLE-LABELED CELLS

Most cells expressing both fluorogold staining and *fos*-immunoreaction (double-labeled cells) following all stimuli were located in lamina I (Table III). In laminae IV–V and VII, double-stained cells occurred only after mechanical or chemical stimulation. Percentages of double-labeled cells in the population of retrograde-labeled cells were relatively high in lamina I after all stimuli, but negligible in the other laminae (Table III). Percentages of double-labeled cells in the population of *fos*-positive cells following chemical or mechanical stimulation (Table III) were not statistically different between laminae but varied significantly between stimuli in lamina I ($P < 0.001$).

Double-labeled cells in lamina I (Fig. 3B,C,E,F,H,I) following all stimuli belonged to the three morphological groups that project to the nucleus of the

Table II
Numbers of fos-positive cells (± SD) per Rexed's lamina

	Stimulation		
Lamina	Chemical	Mechanical	Thermal
I	1146 ± 343	1019 ± 111	893 ± 191
IV–V	38 ± 9	556 ± 180	0
VII	65 ± 12	108 ± 37	0
X	4 ± 3	14 ± 4	0

Note: n = 4.

tractus solitarius (Esteves et al. 1993). Chemical stimulation activated fewer cells of each group than did mechanical or thermal stimulation (Fig. 5). Flattened cells were activated in lesser amounts than were pyramidal or fusiform cells following all stimuli (Fig. 5).

DISCUSSION

Under our experimental conditions, spinal cells immunoreactive for the *fos*-protein following subcutaneous injection of saline or innocuous mechanical stimulation were few or nil, which agrees with previous data showing that induction of the proto-oncogene c-*fos* monitors the activation of spinal neurons by noxious input (Hunt et al. 1987; Bullitt 1990; Williams et al. 1989;

Table III
Distribution of double-labeled cells per Rexed's lamina

	Stimulation		
Lamina	Chemical	Mechanical	Thermal
I	139 ± 34 (16) (12)	157 ± 21 (23) (15)	188 ± 60 (22) (21)
IV–V	2 ± 2 (0.02) (5)	77 ± 19 (1) (14)	0
VII	8 ± 3 (0.1) (12)	18 ± 5 (0.3) (17)	0
X	0.3 ± 0.5 (0.02) (8)	0.6 ± 1 (0.1) (4)	0

Note: Percentages of double-labeled cells in retrograde-labeled cells are given in parentheses on the left; percentages of double-labeled cells in fos-cells are given in parentheses on the right; n = 4.

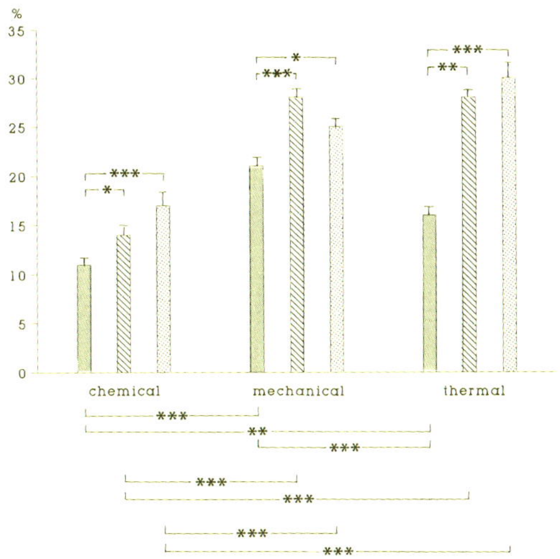

Fig. 5. Percentages of double-labeled lamina I cells that are flattened (gray bars), pyramidal (hatched bars), or fusiform (dotted bars) within retrograde-labeled cells of the same groups, following chemical, mechanical, or thermal stimulation (* $P < 0.05$; ** $P < 0.01$; *** $P < 0.001$).

Lima et al. 1993). Our findings indicate that spinal cells projecting to the NTS are driven by noxious input from the skin. The NTS thus appears to play a role in the processing of somatic nociceptive information in addition to its well-known function as a relay for visceral input conveyed by the vagus and glossopharyngeal nerves (Lipski et al. 1975, 1977; Kalia and Mesulam 1980; Ciriello et al. 1981; Donoghue et al. 1982, 1984; Altschuler et al. 1989), and as a center for cardiovascular control (Loewy and Burton 1978; Ross et al. 1985; Hancock 1988). Considering the antinociceptive role that has been recently attributed to the NTS (Lewis et al. 1987; Morgan et al. 1989; Aicher and Randich 1990; Du and Zhou 1990; Ren et al. 1990), the somatic noxious input reaching the NTS may trigger integrated modulatory actions on pain transmission and visceral functions.

The number of retrograde-labeled cells, though considerable in lamina I, was much greater in laminae IV–VII. In contrast, cells expressing the *fos*-protein prevailed markedly in lamina I regardless of the stimulus. As the proportion of double-labeled cells within the population of *fos*-positive cells was similar from lamina to lamina, net numbers of spinal-NTS cells sensitive to noxious stimulation were higher in lamina I. This finding indicates that spinal-NTS cells processing noxious input from the skin are concentrated in lamina I. This conclusion was amply confirmed by the high proportion of fluorogold-labeled neurons that were double-labeled in lamina I, averaging 20% against less than 1% in deeper laminae. Most NTS-projecting cells in laminae IV–VII may thus be either innocuous or activated from deep tissues. In fact, in the cat, $A_{\alpha\beta}$ low-threshold mechanoreceptors are known to terminate in the dorsal horn neck, whereas primary afferents originating in deep tissues arborize mainly in the ventral horn (Brown 1981).

The proportion of fluorogold-labeled or *fos*-stained lamina I cells that were double labeled varied according to the nature of the stimulus. This was probably not due to differences in stimulus intensity, because the numbers of *fos*-positive cells occurring in lamina I after each kind of stimulus were similar. Although there are no electrophysiological data pointing out that spinofugal systems are differentially activated by different kinds of noxious input, our findings suggest that it may occur in the spinal-NTS system. However, although particularly numerous (Esteves et al. 1993), NTS-projecting flattened cells were activated to a lesser extent than were pyramidal or fusiform cells, irrespective of the noxious stimulus applied. Curiously, spinothalamic flattened cells also were activated in lesser amounts (16–23%) than were spinomesencephalic pyramidal or fusiform cells (22–35%) by the same stimuli (Lima et al. 1992). Future studies are needed to explain why flattened cells may be less effective in transmitting noxious input supraspinally.

ACKNOWLEDGMENTS

We are grateful to Prof. Joaquim Maia for the important advice on statistical analysis. This work was supported by JNICT grant no. PMCT/C/SAU/31/90.

REFERENCES

Abram, S.E., Kostreva, D.R., Hopp, F.A. and Kampine, J.P., Cardiovascular responses to noxious radiant heat in anesthetized cats, Am. J. Physiol., 245 (1983) R576–R580.

Aicher, S.A. and Randich, A., Antinociception and cardiovascular responses produced by electrical stimulation in the nucleus tractus solitarius, nucleus reticularis ventralis, and the caudal medulla, Pain, 42 (1990) 103–119.

Altschuler, S.M., Bao, X, Bieger, D., Hopkins, D.A. and Miselis, R.R., Viscerotopic representation of the upper alimentary tract in the rat: sensory ganglia and nuclei of the solitary and spinal trigeminal tracts, J. Comp. Neurol., 283 (1989) 248–268.

Basbaum, A.I. and Fields, H.L., Endogenous pain control systems: brainstem spinal pathways and endorphin circuitry, Ann. Rev. Neurosci., 7 (1984) 309–338.

Brown, A.G., The organization of the dorsal horn. In: A.G. Brown (Ed.), Organization in the Spinal Cord, Springer-Verlag, Berlin, 1981, pp. 136–153.

Bullit, E., Expression of *C-fos*-like protein as a marker for neuronal activity following noxious stimulation in the rat, J. Comp. Neurol., 296 (1990) 517–530.

Cervero, F., Iggo, A. and Ogawa, H., Nociceptor-driven dorsal horn neurones in the lumbar spinal cord of the cat, Pain, 2 (1976) 5–24.

Christensen, B.N. and Perl, E.R., Spinal neurons specifically excited by noxious or thermal stimuli: marginal zone of the dorsal horn, J. Neurophysiol., 33 (1970) 293–307.

Ciriello, J., Hrycyshyn and Calaresu, F.R., Horseradish peroxidase study of brainstem projections of carotid sinus and aortic depresor nerves in the cat, J. Autonom. Nerv. Syst., 4 (1981) 43–61.

Donoghue, S., Garcia, M., Jordan, D. and Spyer, K.M. Identification and brain-stem projections of aortic baroreceptor afferent neurones in nodose ganglia of cats and rabbits, J. Physiol., 322 (1982) 337–352.

Donoghue, S., Felder, B., Jordan, D. and Spyer, K.M., The central projections of carotid baroreceptors and chemoreceptors in the cat: a neurophysiological study, J. Physiol., 347 (1984) 397–409.

Donovick, P.J., A metachromatic stain for neural tissue, Stain Technol., 49 (1974) 49–51.

Du, H. J. and Zhou, S.Y., Involvement of solitary tract nucleus in control of nociceptive transmission in cat spinal cord neurons, Pain, 40 (1990) 323–331.

Dworkin, B.R., Filewich, R.J., Miller, N.E., Craigmyle, N. and Pickering, T.G., Baroreceptor activation reduces reactivity to noxious stimulation: implications for hypertension, Science, 205 (1979) 1299–1301.

Esteves, F., Lima, D. and Coimbra, A., Structural types of spinal cord marginal (lamina I) neurons projecting to the nucleus of the tractus solitarius in the rat, Somatosens. Mot. Res., 10 (1993) 203–216.

Hancock, M.B., Evidence for direct projections from the nucleus of the solitary tract onto medullary adrenaline cells, J. Comp. Neurol. 276 (1988) 460–467.

Hunt, S.P., Pini, A. and Evan, G., Induction of *c-fos*-like protein in spinal cord neurons following sensory stimulation, Nature, 328 (1987) 632–634.

Kalia, M. and Mesulam, M.-M., Brain stem projections of sensory and motor components of the vagus complex in the cat: II. Laryngeal, tracheobronchial, pulmonary, cardiac, and gastrointestinal branches, J. Comp. Neurol., 193 (1980) 467–508.

Kumazawa, T. and Perl, E.R., Excitation of marginal and substantia gelatinosa neurons in the primate spinal cord: indications of their place in dorsal horn functional organization, J. Comp. Neurol., 177 (1978) 417–434.

Lewis, J.W., Baldrighi, G. and Akil, H., A possible interface between autonomic function and pain control: opiod analgesia and the nucleus tractus solitarius, Brain Res., 424 (1987) 65–70.

Lima, D. and Coimbra, A., The neuronal population of the marginal zone (lamina I) of the rat spinal cord. A study based on reconstructions of serially sectioned cells, Anat. Embryol., 167 (1983) 273–288.

Lima, D. and Coimbra, A., A Golgi study of the neuronal population of the marginal zone (lamina I) of the rat spinal cord, J. Comp. Neurol., 244 (1986) 53–71.

Lima, D. and Coimbra, A., Structural types of marginal (lamina I) neurons projecting to the dorsal reticular nucleus of the medulla oblongata, Neuroscience, 34 (1990) 591–606.

Lima, D., Avelino, A. and Coimbra, A., Differential participation of marginal cells in the transmission of nociceptive input to the thalamus and mesencephalon, Eur. J. Neurosci., Suppl. 5 (1992) 2057.

Lima, D., Avelino, A. and Coimbra, A., Differential activation of c-fos in spinal neurones by distinct classes of noxious stimuli, Neuroreport, 4 (1993) 747–750.

Lipski, J., McAllen, R.M. and Spyer, K.M., The sinus nerve and baroreceptor input to the medulla of the cat, J. Physiol., 251 (1975) 61–78.

Lipski, J., McAllen, R.M. and Spyer, K.M., The carotid chemoreceptor input to the respiratory neurones of the nucleus of tractus solitarius, J. Physiol., 269 (1977) 797–810.

Loewy, A.D. and Burton, H., Nuclei of the solitary tract: efferent projections to the lower brain stem and spinal cord of the cat, J. Comp. Neurol., 181 (1978) 421–450.

Maixner, C., Gracely, R.H., Zuniga, J.R., Humphrey, C.B. and Bloodworth, G.R., Cardiovascular and sensory responses to forearm ischemia and dynamic hand exercise, Am. J. Physiol., 259

(1990) R1156–R1163.
McMahon, S.E., McWilliam, P.N., Robertson, J.C. and Kaye, J.C., Inhibition of carotid sinus baroreceptor neurones in the nucleus tractus solitarius of the anaesthetized cat by electrical stimulation of hindlimb afferent fibers, J. Physiol., 452 (1992) 224P.
Menétrey, D. and Basbaum, A.I., Spinal and trigeminal projections to the nucleus of the solitary tract: a possible substrate for somatovisceral and viscerovisceral reflex activation, J. Comp. Neurol. 255 (1987) 439–450.
Menétrey, D., Giesler, G.J., Jr. and Besson, J.-M., An analysis of response properties of spinal cord dorsal horn neurones to nonnoxious and noxious stimuli in the spinal rat, Exp. Brain Res., 27 (1977) 15–33.
Morgan, M.M., Sohn, J.-H., Lohof, A.M., Ben-Eliyahu, S. and Liebeskind, J.C., Characterization of stimulation-produced analgesia from the nucleus tractus solitarius in the rat, Brain Res., 486 (1989) 175–180.
Paxinos, G. and Watson, C., The Rat Brain in Stereotaxic Coordinates, Academic Press, Sydney, 1982.
Randich, A. and Aicher, S.A., Medullary substrates mediating antinociception produced by electrical stimulation of the vagus, Brain Res., 445 (1988) 68–76.
Ren, K., Randich, A. and Gebhart, G.F., Modulation of spinal nociceptive transmission from nuclei tractus solitari: a relay for effects of vagal afferent stimulation, J. Neurophysiol., 63 (1990) 971–986.
Ross, C.A., Ruggiero, D.A. and Reis, D.J., Projections from the nucleus tractus solitari to the rostral ventrolateral medulla, J. Comp. Neurol., 242 (1985) 511–534.
Williams, S., Pini, A., Evan, G. and Hunt, S.P., Molecular events in the spinal cord following sensory stimulation. In: F. Cervero, G.J. Bennett and P.M. Headley (Eds.), Processing of Sensory Information in the Superficial Dorsal Horn of the Spinal Cord. Series A: Life Sciences, 176, Plenum Press, New York, 1989, pp. 273–283.
Zamir, N. and Shuber, E., Altered pain perception in hypertensive humans, Brain Res., 201 (1980) 471–474.
Zamir, N. and Sogal, M., Hypertension induced analgesia: changes in pain sensitivity in experimental hypertensive rats, Brain Res., 160 (1979) 170–173.

Correspondence to: Deolinda Lima, Institute of Histology and Embryology, Faculty of Medicine, 4200 Porto, Portugal. Tel: 351-2-591468; Fax: 351-2-598119.

Part VI

Neuropathic Pain

Proceedings of the 7th World Congress on Pain,
Progress in Pain Research and Management, Vol. 2,
edited by G.F. Gebhart, D.L. Hammond, and T.S.
Jensen, IASP Press, Seattle, © 1994.

31

Multiple Mechanisms of Neuropathic Pain: A Clinical Perspective

Howard L. Fields and Michael C. Rowbotham

Department of Neurology, University of California, San Francisco, California, USA

The management of neuropathic pain is in a transitional phase. Advances in our knowledge of the basic mechanisms of pain transmission (Wall and Melzack 1994), the development of new animal models (Bennett, this volume), and the systematic examination of patients have all contributed to better understanding of the mechanisms that underlie neuropathic pain. In addition, controlled clinical trials in well-defined patient populations have proven the efficacy of some treatments.

Despite this progress, the gap between the relatively well understood animal models of neuropathic pain and the clinical conditions they are meant to mimic remains significant. Our knowledge of the mechanisms of neuropathic pain in patients, although growing, is still fragmentary, and many patients continue to suffer severe pain despite optimal use of currently available treatments. However, for some conditions there is meaningful and therapeutically relevant information about contributory mechanisms. A prominent example is the syndrome of sympathetically maintained pain for which sympatholysis represents a straightforward and effective therapy (Campbell et al. 1992; Blumberg, this volume). For many other patients, however, the pain-generating mechanism is a complete mystery and therapeutic options are limited. An example of this is the steady pain that occasionally results from lesions of the central nervous system (Leijon and Boivie 1989a,b; Cassinari and Pagni 1969).

The focus of this chapter is upon treatments that are effective for patients with specific types of neuropathic pain. We will discuss these treatments in the context of neural mechanisms that are thought to contribute to pain following peripheral nervous system injury or dysfunction. Some of these mechanisms are operative under physiological conditions and contribute to pain even when there is no neural damage or dysfunction. Other mechanisms come into play only when the nervous system is damaged. Regardless of whether pathological or physiological, each contributory mechanism offers a potential point for therapeutic intervention. To the extent possible, we will relate therapeutic interventions to particular pain mechanisms and review the available clinical evidence for the efficacy of such treatments. Finally, we will discuss current therapeutic options in the context of a treatment trials algorithm for peripheral neuropathic pain.

MECHANISMS OF NEUROPATHIC PAIN

This subject is reviewed elsewhere (chapters by Bennett, Blumberg, and Willis in this volume; Fields 1987, 1990) and will not be reviewed in detail in this chapter. Some of the neural mechanisms thought to contribute to neuropathic pain are as follows:

- Nervi nervorum activation
- Spontaneous ectopic activity in damaged primary afferent nociceptors (PANs)
- Increased mechanical or thermal sensitivity of PANs
- Adrenergic receptor mediated sensitization of PANs
- Neurogenic inflammation
- Loss of central inhibitory effect of myelinated primary afferents
- Reorganization of spinal cord connectivity
- Spontaneous activity in deafferented spinal pain transmission neurons (SPTNs)
- Prolonged excitation of SPTNs

This chapter will focus on the clinical evidence that relates particular treatment approaches to different pain mechanisms.

Before discussing each mechanism and the relevant treatments, it is worth emphasizing that more than one pain generating mechanism is likely to be operative in an individual patient. It is also likely that even in patients with the same diagnosis, different pain-generating mechanisms contribute to different degrees. For example, some patients with postherpetic neuralgia (PHN) have lancinating pain, minimal sensory deficit, cutaneous hyperalgesia, and allodynia. Other PHN patients have constant pain, virtually complete cutaneous anesthesia, and no cutaneous hypersensitivity. While many PHN patients may have a mixture of these two types of sensory abnormalities, it seems likely that the pain associated with each type of abnormality has a distinct mechanism. In support of this concept, PHN associated with profound sensory loss appears to be less responsive to currently available treatments (Rowbotham and Fields 1989).

If multiple mechanisms are involved in generating neuropathic pain, it is likely that a variety of pharmacologically distinct drugs, targeted upon these different mechanisms, will be effective. Furthermore, if the mechanism or combination of mechanisms that contribute to the pain differs among patients, it is likely that they will respond to different drugs or combinations of drugs.

The challenge that confronts both the clinician and the clinical scientist is to match specific treatments to different pain-generating mechanisms. At present this is not possible because our knowledge of such mechanisms is fragmentary at best and there are few controlled clinical trials of mechanism-based treatments. However, careful clinical investigations of mechanisms in individual patients and controlled clinical trials to establish efficacy for different classes of pharmacological agents are beginning to appear. These two approaches to the study of neuropathic pain are complementary because establishing the efficacy of a mechanism-specific pharmacological agent can provide critical support for a particular hypothesis of pain generation. For example, the fact that sympathetic blockade can relieve pain in some patients is the strongest evidence that sympathetic activity can generate a pain signal.

PRIMARY AFFERENT NOCICEPTOR ACTIVITY IN NEUROPATHIC PAIN

Any pathological process that leads to increased discharge in primary afferent nociceptors (PANs) should produce pain, provided their central connections are intact. Although loss of function is the more frequent correlate of nervous system injury or disease, there are two distinct classes of nerve pathology that could cause increased PAN activity (Asbury and Fields 1984): physiological activation of nociceptive nervi nervorum and abnormal activity in damaged primary afferent nociceptors.

Nervi Nervorum

Peripheral nerves have an extrinsically derived innervation via the neurovascular bundle and there is immunocytochemical evidence that at least some of the innervation is by unmyelinated nociceptors (Appenzeller et al. 1984; Bahns et al. 1986; Zochodne 1993). An inflammatory process involving the nerve could, for example, activate chemosensitive PANs that normally innervate the connective tissue sheath. Although there is no direct evidence to support this mechanism, acute inflammatory demyelinating neuropathy (Guillain-Barré syndrome) is an example of a condition that could elicit pain through activity in the nervi nervorum. Because the pathology is demyelination, unmyelinated axons are relatively spared and pain sensation in these patients is typically normal in clinical testing. This indicates that the axons of PANs that run with the nerve are intact. Guillain-Barré syndrome is commonly painful. The pain these patients report is usually deep and has an aching quality more typical of pains of musculoskeletal origin (Asbury and Gilliatt 1984). Although anti-inflammatory agents would be expected to relieve the pain in Guillain-Barré syndrome, this approach has not been systematically studied.

Damaged PANs: Spontaneous and/or Ectopic Impulse Generation

A second set of mechanisms for nociceptor activation are brought into play when PAN axons in the nerve trunk are directly damaged. In patients, damage to unmyelinated and small diameter myelinated fibers is usually revealed by a sensory deficit to thermal and noxious stimuli. This may be confusing to evaluate clinically because hyperalgesia and hypoesthesia may coexist in many patients (Lindblom and Verrillo 1979).

Although evidence of clinical damage to PANs is one of the most ubiquitous features of patients with neuropathic pain, this correlation does not prove that activity in the dysfunctional PANs generates the pain signal. The evidence that favors this idea is derived primarily from studies in a variety of animal models. These studies show that some damaged PAN axons exhibit spontaneous activity, sensitization and increased mechanical sensitivity (Devor and Rappaport 1990; Scadding 1981; Tanelian and MacIver 1991; Kajander and Bennett 1992; Cline et al. 1989).

Extensive but anecdotal clinical experience indicates that similar phenomena occur in patients. Thus, spontaneous pain is present in a variety of axonal polyneuropathies that affect unmyelinated axons (Thomas 1974). Although persistent pain is not the rule following nerve trauma, unpleasant mechanical hypersensitivity is common, particularly near neuromata or sites of entrapment (Dawson et al. 1983). In two patients with postamputation phantom limb pain, Nystrom and Hagbarth (1981) demonstrated by microneurography that there was spontaneous ectopic activity in primary afferents innervating the painfully sensitive neuroma. That a pain signal can be generated in or near a neuroma is supported by Chabal's demonstration in patients that local perfusion of a neuroma with lidocaine can provide significant relief (Chabal et al. 1989).

Ochoa and his colleagues (Cline et al. 1989) have provided direct clinical evidence that dysfunctional PANs can generate a pain signal in the absence of a noxious stimulus. They have described a small number of patients who complain of burning cutaneous pain and have a reduced threshold to heat pain. This pain appears to be C-fiber mediated because it persists during compression block of myelinated axons and, importantly, spontaneous C-fiber discharge has been recorded in primary afferents innervating the painful region. Interestingly, the skin of these patients is painful and hyperalgesic primarily in regions that are objectively warmer than surrounding normal skin. The authors propose that the pain and warmth in these patients are due to spontaneous activity in sensitized PANs with peripheral release of vasodilating peptides such as substance P. Moderate cooling of the skin relieves the burning pain which is consistent with the notion that spontaneous activity in nociceptors sensitized to thermal stimuli is crucial to pain generation in these patients. We also have observed that some patients with postherpetic neuralgia have coextensive regions of spontaneous pain, mechanical hyperalgesia, and objective warmth (Rowbotham and Fields 1989b).

Several other clinical observations support the idea that spontaneously active C-mechanothermal nociceptors are generating a pain signal in some PHN patients. First, PHN patients often volunteer that icing their skin provides relief. Second, we have recently completed a controlled clinical trial demonstrating that cutaneous application of lidocaine produces relief in PHN patients with cutaneous hyperalgesia (Rowbotham et al. 1992). Finally, some PHN patients are relieved by topical application of capsaicin, a neurotoxin that selectively inactivates unmyelinated primary afferents, primarily nociceptors (Lynn 1990; Holzer 1991). These clinical observations support the idea that, in some patients with neuropathic pain, spontaneous activity arising in the peripheral terminals of dysfunctional PANs is critical for generating a pain signal.

The clinical and experimental evidence reviewed above indicates that when a peripheral nerve is damaged the PANs develop spontaneous activity and can become sensitized to both thermal and mechanical stimulation. Clinically relevant sites along the dysfunctional PAN where abnormal impulses can be generated include its axon just proximal to an interruption (usually in a neuroma) and at its terminals in the tissue that it normally innervates. Experimental evidence also shows that ectopic impulses can be generated near the cell body of a damaged primary afferent (Devor and Rappaport 1990; Burchiel

1984; Wall and Devor 1983), though there is no clinical evidence for the relevance of this observation.

It is of interest and potential clinical importance that spontaneous ectopic impulses in damaged primary afferents are sensitive to blockade by use-dependent blockers of voltage-sensitive sodium channels (Burchiel 1984; Chabal et al. 1989; Devor et al. 1992; Dougherty et al. 1992). Prominent drugs of this class are the local anesthetics and their congeners. Oral and parenteral administration of these drugs are most commonly used to treat cardiac arrhythmias. The proven efficacy of such drugs for pain in defined patient groups such as diabetic neuropathy (mexiletine; Dejgard et al. 1988; Stracke et al. 1992), traumatic neuropathy (mexiletine; Chabal et al. 1992a), and postherpetic neuralgia (lidocaine; Rowbotham et al. 1991) in which there may be spontaneous ectopic activity in damaged PANs is consistent with an etiological role of such activity in these diseases. However, parenteral use of local anesthetics appears to have broad analgesic efficacy including painful conditions unassociated with obvious PAN damage (Glazer and Portenoy 1991). Furthermore, there is some evidence that parenteral lidocaine can inhibit spinal cord nociceptive neurons (Woolf and Wiesenfeld-Hallin 1985).

Sympathetically Maintained Pain

Among the mechanisms that have been proposed to contribute to neuropathic pain, the best established clinically is sympathetic efferent activation of PANs (Blumberg this volume). Since Leriche reported the efficacy of surgical sympathectomy in the treatment of causalgia (1939), an immense clinical and experimental literature has accumulated (Loh and Nathan 1978; Bonica 1979) that largely supports the view that in certain patients sympathetic postganglionic neurons, through the release of noradrenaline, can activate or sensitize PANs either in peripheral tissues or at a site of damage in a peripheral nerve.

The key clinical observations are those demonstrating pain relief by a variety of sympatholytic procedures or adrenergic blocking agents. These include perivascular or paraspinal surgical sympathectomy or local anesthetic block, regional intravascular perfusion with guanethidine (Hannington-Kiff 1974), bretylium (Hord et al. 1992) or reserpine (Rocco et al. 1989), intravenous phentolamine (Arner et al. 1991; Raja et al. 1991), and oral phenoxybenzamine (Ghostine et al. 1984) or prazosin (Abram 1981).

In addition to the vast literature on sympathetic block, there are important and intriguing observations in patients that support the idea that sympathetically maintained pain (SMP) involves a change in the stimulus response function of PANs. Thus, Walker and Nulsen (1948) observed that following sympathectomy, stimulating the decentralized sympathetic chain reproduced the pain in patients who had had causalgia prior to surgery. Such stimulation did not produce pain in patients undergoing sympathectomy for vascular insufficiency. In patients who had obtained relief of pain by sympathetic block, Wallin et al. (1976) were able to reproduce the pain by injecting norepinephrine into formerly affected areas of skin. Davis et al. (1991) reported a similar result with the alpha-1 agonist phenylephrine. Norepinephrine does not produce pain when injected into normal skin. In a related study, Chabal and coworkers (1992b) demonstrated that infiltration of epinephrine, but not saline, into the area around a postamputation neuroma produces pain with a burning and shooting quality.

These clinical studies provide critical support for the concept that in patients with sympathetically maintained pain, PANs in damaged peripheral nerve acquire increased sensitivity to α-adrenergic agents. This phenomenon has been documented in animal models of SMP (e.g., Devor and Jänig 1981; Scadding 1981; Wall and Devor 1983; Sato and Perl 1991). If this concept is correct, then normal or even *decreased* sympathetic activity could be sufficient to produce pain in these patients. It is even possible that pain could arise in sympathetically denervated tissues if circulating catecholamines were in sufficient concentration to sensitize nociceptors. The clinical syndrome of postsympathectomy neuralgia might be an example of such a phenomenon (Raskin et al. 1974).

In summary, there is a wealth of clinical and experimental evidence to support the hypothesis that some neuropathic pains are maintained by increased activity in dysfunctional PANs. Factors such as sensitization, spontaneous ectopic impulse generation, and increased alpha adrenergic sensitivity may contribute to this increased activity. Positive results in controlled clinical trials with treatment approaches such as topical application of the PAN neurotoxin capsaicin, and lidocaine, have provided important evidence supporting a contribution to pain by these mechanisms.

To the extent that PAN activity contributes to neuropathic pain, it follows that neuropathic and nonneuropathic pain share an essential neural mechanism. It also leads to the prediction that some centrally acting analgesic drugs, such as opioids, also should relieve PAN-mediated neuropathic pain, though perhaps to a different degree than nonneuropathic pain. This issue is controversial (Arner and Meyerson 1988; Max et al. 1988), but we and others have demonstrated significant opioid efficacy for relief of neuropathic pain (Portenoy and Foley 1986; Rowbotham et al. 1991; Jadad et al. 1992).

LOSS OF THE CENTRAL INHIBITORY ACTION OF MYELINATED PRIMARY AFFERENTS

Most natural stimuli to the skin activate a broad range of primary afferents. Selective blockade of myelinated afferent axons in a peripheral nerve leads to a loss of fine spatiotemporal discrimination of skin stimuli. In addition to this loss of function under conditions of myelinated afferent axon block, activation of intact unmyelinated primary afferents even by normally innocuous cold and pressure stimuli produces a severe, usually burning pain that outlasts the stimulus (Landau and Bishop 1953). Clearly, activation of myelinated afferents has a significant inhibitory effect on the intensity of pain produced by concurrently active PANs. Importantly, some innocuous stimuli are capable of eliciting pain mediated by unmyelinated afferent axons when myelinated afferents innervating the same cutaneous region are blocked. Observations such as these contributed to the gate control hypothesis of Melzack and Wall (1965), which postulated that myelinated afferents activate an inhibitory interneuron in the substantia gelatinosa (the "gate"), which modulated the pain transmission neuron receiving input from unmyelinated PANs. The similarity between the sensations reported by some neuropathic pain patients to those elicited in normal subjects by selective myelinated afferent fiber block led Melzack and Wall to propose that predominant myelinated fiber block was the cause of pain in some of these patients.

Although the gate control hypothesis gave rise to a number of clinical studies of selective myelinated fiber activation, the question of whether such a mechanism contributes to any clinical syndrome remains open. Furthermore, despite promising anecdotal reports, analgesic efficacy has not been proven for any treatment method based on this concept. The most extensively studied methods using this approach are transcutaneous electrical nerve stimulation (TENS; Woolf 1989) and dorsal column or spinal stimulation (Marchand et al. 1991; North et al. 1993). Although occasional patients report dramatic relief, the efficacy appears to wear off over time in many patients. Furthermore, because stimulation produces a characteristic sensation, it has been difficult to study this type of method in a truly double-blind manner (Marchand et al. 1993). Patient selection also may be a significant problem. On the other hand, TENS is safe and virtually without side effects so there is little harm in using it.

In summary, loss of the inhibitory effect on pain of myelinated afferent input remains an intriguing but unproven contributing mechanism in neuropathic pain. Convincing clinical trials of large-fiber stimulation in well-selected patient populations have yet to be carried out.

INCREASED EXCITABILITY OF CENTRAL PAIN TRANSMISSION NEURONS

A variety of changes are known to occur in central somatosensory neurons as a result of damage to primary afferent neurons. Some of these are listed above (see Mechanisms of Neuropathic Pain). Because of the obvious difficulty in determining the relevance of such mechanisms to painful human disease, this subject will not be reviewed in detail in this chapter. We will, however, review two mechanisms, deafferentation hyperactivity and central sensitization, that offer relevant therapeutic options.

Deafferentation Hyperactivity

Experimental studies have shown that some deafferented dorsal horn neurons, including putative somatosensory projection neurons, develop high levels of spontaneous activity following dorsal rhizotomy (Lombard and Larabi 1983). Whether this actually occurs in patients is unclear; however, one of the best examples of a human deafferentation syndrome is brachial plexus avulsion. The majority of patients with this condition have significant pain (Wynn-Parry 1980). Consistent with the idea that hyperactive dorsal horn neurons are generating a pain signal is the observation that dorsal root entry zone lesions that destroy most of the dorsal horn (Nashold 1979) appear to be one of the few consistently effective treatments for this condition.

Nociceptor Induced Prolonged Central Excitation

It is well established that prolonged or repetitive input from unmyelinated PANs produce progressive increases in dorsal horn neuronal and subjective responses to subsequent cutaneous stimuli. Wind-up is a well-established example of this phenomenon. Wind-up refers to the observation in dorsal horn nociceptive neurons that repeated identical inputs from unmyelinated PANs is associated with a progressive increase in the discharge produced by each stimulus. Wind-up can be suppressed by opioids, substance P receptor antagonists, and NMDA receptor ion channel blockers (Chapman and Dickenson 1992; Mao et al. 1993; Tal and Bennett 1993; Sakurada et al. 1993). A phenomenon similar to wind-up has been observed in the responses of human subjects to repeated near-threshold noxious thermal stimuli (Price et al. 1978).

The increased excitability of dorsal horn neurons by volleys in unmyelinated PANs may represent a prolonged depolarization due to entry by both peptides and calcium via the NMDA receptor ion channel. There is some evidence that nitric oxide also contributes to this prolonged increase in excitability (Meller and Gebhart 1993).

Although this phenomenon is probably a normal consequence of any prolonged noxious input, it could play a major role in the maintenance of neuropathic pain, particularly if there is a persistent peripheral source of input via unmyelinated PANs. As discussed earlier in this chapter, there is reason to believe that this is indeed the case for many patients with neuropathic pain. If substance P and excitatory amino acids acting at the NMDA receptor contribute significantly to neuropathic pain, antagonists for these actions could represent a significant advance for the management of neuropathic pains.

One area of active clinical investigation is the study of drugs acting at the NMDA receptor ion channel (see above). Ketamine is of particular interest because it has an NMDA receptor ion channel blocking effect, is in clinical use, and has analgesic actions (Dich-Nielsen et al. 1992). The issue of the analgesic efficacy of NMDA blockers for neuropathic pain is now under active investigation (Mao et al. 1993; Tal and Bennett 1993).

CURRENT TREATMENT OF NEUROPATHIC PAIN

The evidence reviewed above clearly demonstrates that neuropathic pain is not a unitary phenomenon. Just as there are multiple causes for neural injury, there are multiple pain-generating mechanisms. Each different mechanism provides a potential opportunity for a pain relieving intervention by the clinician. The current armamentarium for the treatment of neuropathic pain includes a variety of procedures and drugs, some with established efficacy and others whose efficacy is unsupported by empirical proof. Each of these therapies targets a particular pain-generating or pain-modulating mechanism. Unfortunately, it usually is not possible to determine with certainty the pain-generating mechanism in a particular patient. Clearly, the current challenge for the clinician is to provide help for patients in the face of diagnostic uncertainty and a limited range of proven therapies.

Our current approach is the algorithm outlined in Fig. 1. This flow diagram is meant as a general guide for a treatment-oriented clinical evaluation of neuropathic pain. It is not necessary to use this approach in patients who have a clear-cut diagnosis for which well-accepted and effective treatments are available. For example, an elderly, otherwise healthy and neurologically intact patient with shooting pains in the lower trigeminal divisions may be presumed to have trigeminal neuralgia and should be treated immediately with carbamazepine. A patient with hypothenar pain, progressive loss of sensory and motor function in the ulnar distribution, and conduction slowing of the ulnar nerve at the elbow should be considered for early decompressive surgery. If the clinical features do not suggest a diagnosis that has an established

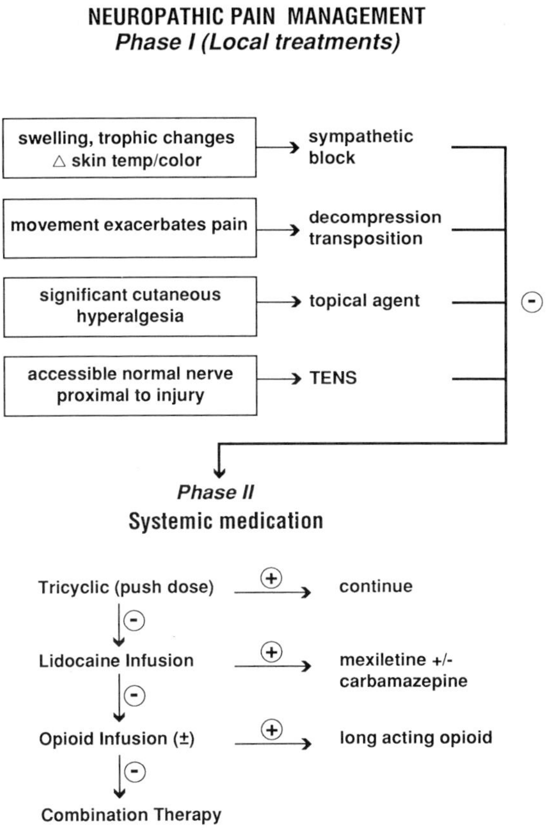

Fig. 1. Neuropathic pain management.

effective treatment, this algorithm can provide a useful framework for reducing the time and degree of suffering. The goal is to achieve optimal therapy in the minimum time.

PHASE I: LOCAL TREATMENTS

In the initial phase of evaluation the emphasis should be on uncovering pain-generating factors that are potentially reversible or can be effectively managed with local therapies. The goal of this approach is to avoid, where possible, committing the patient to a long-term course of systemic drugs, all of which have significant and/or occasionally dangerous side effects.

In patients with extremity pain associated with swelling, temperature change, and cutaneous hypersensitivity, the diagnosis of sympathetically maintained pain should be considered and rapidly assessed with a diagnostic sympathetic block. We use intravenous phentolamine initially because it is a relatively noninvasive sympatholytic method and is reversible. However, if this test is negative, we do not hesitate to carry out local anesthetic blockade of the sympathetic chain. This type of block is more sensitive than iv. phentolamine, but less specific because of the possibility of either somatic blockade or systemic redistribution of the absorbed local anesthetic and action at a distance. A positive response calls for a program of physical therapy, repeated blocks, and possibly oral sympatholytic drugs (Ghostine et al. 1984).

Surgical approaches to peripheral nerve pain such as neurolysis, decompression, transposition, or neurotomy should be considered in patients with traumatic or entrapment neuropathies that are exacerbated by movement (Dawson et al. 1983). TENS is most effective for traumatic and compressive mononeuropathies when the stimulating electrodes can be placed on a relatively normal stretch of nerve that is proximal to the site of injury (Meyer and Fields 1972). However, because it is harmless, a short trial of TENS is warranted in any patient.

Patients with significant cutaneous hypersensitivity, especially with thermal hyperalgesia and warm skin, are the most likely to benefit from topical therapy. Topical capsaicin preparations are occasionally of benefit if the patients can put up with the burning sensations that are common early in treatment. Clinical trials suggest that some patients with postherpetic neuralgia (Watson et al. 1988; Bernstein et al. 1989), diabetic neuropathy (Scheffler et al. 1991; Tandan et al. 1992), and postmastectomy pain (Watson and Evans 1992) achieve benefit with capsaicin, especially the 0.075% preparation. Topical preparations of aspirin and NSAIDs (King 1988; De Benedittis et al. 1992) and others containing lidocaine (Rowbotham and Fields 1989a; Stow et al. 1989; Kissin et al. 1989) may be helpful for patients with neuropathic pain and cutaneous hypersensitivity; however, only the eutectic mixture of local anesthetics (EMLA, prilocaine/lidocaine) is commercially available.

PHASE II: ORAL MEDICATIONS

Although some patients achieve satisfactory relief with local therapies, most are left with significant residual pain. Our next step is to initiate therapy with a tricyclic antidepressant. Tricyclics antidepressants are clearly effective for the two most common forms of neuropathic pain, diabetic neuropathy (Max et al. 1992) and postherpetic neuralgia (Kishore-Kumar et al. 1990). A variety of other pain syndromes also respond. Our own experience is that, in addition to those conditions, many patients with chronic pain due to traumatic mononeuropthies have a good response to tricyclic antidepressants.

Amitriptyline, desipramine, and imipramine are the most extensively studied of the antidepressant drugs (Onghena and Van Houdenhove 1992). Unfortunately, these drugs have a variety of pharmacologic actions (blockade of 5-HT and norepinephrine uptake, antagonism of histamine, alpha adrenergic, and muscarinic cholinergic receptors; Richelson 1990). Their mechanism of analgesic action is uncertain. There is some evidence that antidepressants that are relatively selective for the blockade of 5-HT reuptake are ineffective for the treatment of chronic neuropathic pain (Max et al. 1992).

Because of the broad range of side effects, tricyclic antidepressants are often unpleasant for patients and are associated with sedation, orthostatic hypotension, cardiac conduction block, urinary retention, and memory disturbance. Patient compliance is a significant problem. Warning the patients about the side effects and initiating therapy with a very low dose is essential.

If patients continue to experience significant pain following dose optimization with tricyclic antidepressants, we proceed to a lidocaine infusion (Rowbotham et al. 1991). Intravenous lidocaine provides significant relief for postherpetic neuralgia and other neuropathic pains. With a positive response to the lidocaine infusion we proceed to a therapeutic trial of Mexiletine. We will increase the dose of oral mexiletine up to 1200 mg per day, provided plasma levels are within the therapeutic range. Gastrointestinal side effects are common, but can be handled with symptomatic treatment in most patients. It is often the case that the relief obtained with mexiletine is disappointing despite a dramatic response to lidocaine. In these patients we may add an anticonvulsant such as carbamazepine or switch to an alternative antiarrhythmic such as tocainide.

A significant number of patients continue to have pain despite full exploitation of the approach outlined above. We offer these patients the option of long-term opioid therapy. There is no question that some patients with neuropathic pain obtain significant relief with opioids (Rowbotham et al. 1991). This response is not surprising considering the likelihood that in many patients neuropathic pains have shared neural mechanisms with nonneuropathic pains (see above). It must be admitted that the long-term efficacy of opioids in neuropathic pain has not been tested rigorously in a prospective clinical trial.

SUMMARY AND CONCLUSION

This is an exciting time for those of us who manage patients with neuropathic pain. There has been steady progress in our understanding of mechanism of pain generation and in the availability of good quality clinical trials that establish efficacy for certain drugs. It is clear that a large number of patients with neuropathic pain have hyperactive, dysfunctional PANs, and there is clinical evidence that therapies expected to reduce such activity (PAN neurotoxins and both systemic and topical local anesthetics) effectively reduce neuropathic pain. The role of more traditional analgesic therapies such as opioids, tricyclic antidepressants, anticonvulsants, and sympatholysis are becoming more clearly defined. Finally, new therapies, rationally targeted upon recently discovered mechanisms (e.g., NMDA channel activation, spinal neurokinin release) are on the horizon.

ACKNOWLEDGMENTS

The authors thank Janet Supár. This work supported by a grant from the USPHS, NS21445.

REFERENCES

Abram, S.E. and Lightfoot, R.W., Treatment of long-standing causalgia with prazosin, Reg. Anesth., 6 (1981) 79–81.

Appenzeller, O., Dhital, K.K., Cowen, T. and Burnstock, G., The nerves to blood vessels supplying blood to nerves: the innervation of vasa nervorum, Brain Res., 304 (1984) 383–386.

Arner, S., Intravenous phentolamine test: diagnostic and prognostic use in reflex sympathetic dystrophy, Pain, 46 (1991) 17–22.

Arner, S. and Meyerson, B., Lack of analgesic effect of opioids on neuropathic and idiopathic forms of pain, Pain, 33 (1988) 11–23.

Asbury, A.K. and Fields, H.L., Pain due to peripheral nerve damage: a hypothesis, Neurology, 34 (1984) 1587–1590.

Asbury, A.K. and Gilliatt, R.W., Peripheral Nerve Disorders, Butterworths, London, 1984, pp. 21–44.

Bahns, E., Ernsberger, U., Jänig, W. and Nelke, A., Discharge properties of mechanosensitive afferents supplying the retroperitoneal space, Pfluger's Arch., 407 (1986) 519–525.

Bernstein, J.E., Korman, N.J., Bickers, D.R., Dahl, M.V. and Milliken, L.E., Topical capsaicin treatment of chronic postherpetic neuralgia, J. Am. Acad. Dermatol., 21 (1989) 265–270.

Bonica, J.J., Causalgia and other reflex sympathetic dystrophies, Adv. Pain Res. Ther., 3 (1979) 141–161.

Burchiel, K.J., Effects of electrical and mechanical stimulation on two foci of spontaneous activity which develop in primary afferent neurons after peripheral axotomy, Pain, 18 (1984) 249–265.

Campbell, J.N., Meyer, R.A. and Raja, S.N., Is nociceptor activation by alpha-1 adrenoreceptors the culprit in sympathetically maintained pain? APS Journal, 1 (1992) 3–11.

Cassinari, V. and Pagni, C.A., Central Pain, A Neurosurgical Survey, Harvard University Press, Cambridge, 1969, 192 pp.

Chabal, C., Russell, L.C. and Burchiel, K.J., The effect of intravenous lidocaine, tocainide, and mexiletine on spontaneously active fibers originating in rat sciatic neuromas, Pain, 38 (1989) 333–338.

Chabal, C., Jacobson, L., Mariano, A., Chaney, E. and Britell, C.W., The use of oral mexiletine for the treatment of pain after peripheral nerve injury, Anesthesiology, 76 (1992a) 513–717.

Chabal, C., Jacobson, L., Russel, L.C. and Burchiel, K.J., Pain responses to perineuromal injection

of normal saline, epinephrine, and lidocaine in humans, Pain, 49 (1992b) 9–12.
Chapman, V. and Dickenson, A.H., The combination of NMDA antagonism and morphine produces profound antinociception in the rat dorsal horn, Brain Res., 573 (1992) 321–323.
Cline, M.A., Ochoa, J. and Torebjörk, H.E., Chronic hyperalgesia and skin warming caused by sensitized C nociceptors, Brain, 112 (1989) 621–647.
Davis, K.D., Treede, R.D., Raja, S.N., Meyer, R.A. and Campbell, J.N., Topical application of clonidine relieves hyperalgesia in patients with sympathetically maintained pain, Pain, 47 (1991) 309–317.
Dawson, D.M., Hallett, M. and Millender, L.H., Entrapment Neuropathies, Little Brown, Boston, 1983, 302 pp.
De Benedittis, G., Besana, F. and Lorenzetti, A., A new topical treatment for acute herpetic neuralgia and post-herpetic neuralgia: the aspirin/diethyl ether mixture. An open-label study plus a double-blind controlled clinical trial, Pain, 48 (1992) 383–390.
Dejgard, A., Petersen, P. and Kastrup, J., Mexiletine for the treatment of chronic painful diabetic neuropathy, Lancet, 29 (1988) 9–11.
Devor, M. and Jänig, W., Activation of myelinated afferents ending in neuroma by stimulation of the sympathetic supply in the rat, Neurosci. Lett., 24 (1981) 43–47.
Devor, M. and Rappaport, Z.H., Pain and the pathophysiology of damaged nerve. In: H.L. Fields (Ed.), Pain Syndromes in Neurology, Butterworths, London, 1990, pp. 47–84.
Devor, M., Wall, P.D. and Catalan, N., Systemic lidocaine silences ectopic neuroma and DRG discharge without blocking nerve condition, Pain, 48 (1992) 261–268.
Dich-Nielsen, J.O., Svendsen, L.B. and Berthelsen, P., Intramuscular low-dose ketamine versus pethidine for post operative pain treatment after thoracic surgery, Acta. Anaesthesiol. Scand., 36 (1992) 583–587.
Dougherty, P.M., Garrison, C.J. and Carlton, S.M., Differential influence of local anesthetic upon two models of experimentally induced peripheral mononeuropathy in the rat, Brain Res., 570 (1992) 109–115.
Fields, H.L., Pain, McGraw-Hill, New York, 1987, pp. 133–170.
Fields, H.L., Pain Syndromes in Neurology, Butterworths, London, 1990, 286 pp.
Ghostine, S.Y., Comair, Y.G., Turner, D.M., Kassell, N.F. and Azar, C.G., Phenoxybenzamine in the treatment of causalgia: report of 40 cases, J. Neurosurg., 60 (1984) 1263–1268.
Glazer, S. and Portenoy, R.K., Systemic local anesthetics in pain control, J. Pain Sympt. Manage., 6 (1991) 30–39.
Hannington-Kiff, J.G., Intravenous regional sympathetic block with guanethidine, Lancet, (1974) 1019–1020.
Holzer, P., Capsaicin: cellular targets, mechanisms of action, and selectivity for thin sensory neurons, Pharmacol. Rev., 43 (1991) 143–201.
Hord, A.H., Rooks, M.D., Stephens, B.O., Rogers, H.G. and Fleming, L.L., Intravenous regional bretylium and lidocaine for treatment of reflex sympathetic sydtrophy: a randomized, double-blind study, Anesth. Analg., 74 (1992) 818–821.
Jadad, A.R., Carroll, D., Glynn, C.J., Moore, R.A. and McQuay, H.J., Morphine responsiveness of chronic pain: double-blind randomised crossover study with patient-controlled analgesia, Lancet, 339 (1992) 1367–1371.
Kajander, K.C. and Bennett, G.J., Onset of a painful peripheral neuropathy in rat: a partial and differential deafferentation and spontaneous discharge in Aβ and Aδ primary afferent neurons, J. Neurophysiol., 68 (1992) 734.
King, R.B., Concerning the management of pain associated with herpes zoster and of postherpetic neuralgia, Pain, 33 (1988) 73–78.
Kishore-Kumar, R., Max, M.B., Schafer, S.C., Gaughan, A.M., Smoller, B., Gracely, R.H. and Dubner, R., Desipramine relieves post-herpetic neuralgia, Clin. Pharmacol. Ther., 47 (1990) 305–312.
Kissin, I., McDanal, J. and Xavier, A.V., Topical lidocaine for relief of superficial pain in postherpetic neuralgia, Neurology, 39 (1989), 1132–1133.

Landau, W. and Bishop, G.G., Pain from dermal, periosteal and fascial endings and from inflammation, Arch. Neurol. Psychiatry, 69 (1953) 490–504.
Leijon, G. and Boivie, J., Central post-stoke pain: a controlled trial of amitriptyline and carbamazepine, Pain, 36 (1989) 27–36.
Leijon, G., Boivie, J. and Johansson, I., Central post-stroke pain: neurological symptoms and pain characteristics, Pain, 36 (1989) 13–25.
Leriche, R. (Ed.), The Surgery of Pain, Bailliere, Tindall and Cox, London, 1939.
Levine, J.D., Fields, H.L. and Basbaum, A.I., Peptides and primary afferent nociceptors, J. Neurosci., 13 (1993) 2273–2286.
Lindblom, U. and Verrillo, R.T., Sensory functions in chronic neuralgia, J. Neurol. Neurosurg. Psychiatry., 42 (1979) 422–435.
Loh, L. and Nathan, P.W., Painful peripheral states and sympathetic blocks, J. Neurol. Neurosurg. Psychiatry., 41 (1978) 664–671.
Lombard, M.C. and Larabi, Y., Electrophysiological study of cervical dorsal horn cells in partially deafferented rats. In: J.J. Bonica, U. Lindblom and A. Iggo (Eds.),Proceedings of the Third World Congress on Pain. Advances in Pain Research and Therapy, Vol. 5. Raven Press, New York, 1983, pp. 147–154.
Lynn, B., Capsaicin: actions on nociceptive C-fibres and therapeutic potential, Pain, 41 (1990) 61–69.
Mao, J., Price, D.D., Hayes, R.L., Lu, J., Mayer, D.J. and Frenk, H., Intrathecal treatment with dextrorphan or ketamine potently reduces pain-related behaviors in a rat model of peripheral mononeuropathy, Brain Res., 605 (1993) 164–168.
Marchand, S., Bushnell, M.C., Molina-Negro, P., Martinez, S.N. and Duncan, G.H., The effects of dorsal column stimulation on measures of clinical and experimental pain in man, Pain, 45 (1991) 249–257.
Marchand, S., Charest, J., Li, J., Chenard, J.-R., Lavignole, B. and Laurencelle, L., Is TENS purely a placebo effect? A controlled study on chronic low back pain, Pain, 54 (1993) 99–106.
Max, M.B., Schafer, S.C., Culnane, M., Dubner, R. and Gracely, R.H., Association of pain relief with drug side effects in postherpetic neuralgia: a single dose study of clonidine, codeine, ibuprofen and placebo, Clin. Pharmacol. Ther., 43 (1988) 363–371.
Max, M.B., Lynch, S.A., Muir, J., Shoaf, S.E., Smoller, B. and Dubner, R., Effects of desipramine, amitriptyline, and fluoxetine on pain in diabetic neuropathy, N. Engl. J. Med, 326 (1992) 1250–1256.
Meller, S.T. and Gebhart, G.F., Nitric oxide (NO) and nociceptive processing in the spinal cord, Pain, 52 (1993) 127–136.
Melzack, R. and Wall, P.D., Pain mechanisms: a new theory, Science, 150 (1965) 971–978.
Meyer, G.A. and Fields, H.L., Causalgia treated by selective large fibre stimulation of peripheral nerve, Brain, 95 (1972) 163–168.
Mitchell, S.W., Injuries of Nerves and Their Consequences, Dover Publications, New York, 1965.
Nashold, B.S. Jr. and Ostdahl, R.H., Dorsal root entry zone lesions for pain relief, J. Neurosurg., 51 (1979) 59–69.
North, R.B., Kidd, D.H., Zahurak, M., James, C.S. and Long, D.M., Spinal cord stimulation for chronic, intractable pain: experience over two decades, Neurosurgery, 32 (1993) 384–394.
Nystrom, B., Hagbarth, K.E., Microelectrode recordings from transected nerves in amputees with phantom limb pain, Neurosci. Lett., 27 (1981) 211–216.
Ochoa, J.L., Yarnitsky, D., Mechanical hyperalgesias in neuropathic pain patients: dynamic and static subtypes. Ann. Neurol., 33 (1993) 465–472.
Onghena, P. and Van Houdenhove, B., Antidepressant-induced analgesia in chronic non-malignant pain: a meta-analysis of 39 placebo-controlled studies, Pain, 49 (1992) 205–220.
Portenoy, R. and Foley, K., Chronic use of opioid analgesics in non-malignant pain: report of 38 cases, Pain, 25 (1986) 171–186.
Price, D.D., Hayes, R.L., Ruda, M.A. and Dubner, R:, Spatial and temporal transformations of input to spinothalamic tract neurons and their relation to somatic sensations, J. Neurophysiol.,

41 (1978) 933–947.

Raja, S.N., Treede R.-D., Davis, K.D., Campbell, J.N., Systemic alpha-adrenergic blockade with phentolamine: A diagnostic test for sympathetically maintained pain. Anesthesiology, 74 (1991) 691–698.

Raskin, N.H., Levinson, S.A., Hoffman, P.M., Pickett, J.B.E. and Fields, H.L., Postsympathectomy neuralgia, Am. J. Surg., 128 (1974) 75–78.

Richelson, E., Antidepressants and brain neurochemistry, Mayo Clin. Proc., 65 (1990) 1227–1236.

Rocco, A.G., Kaul, A.F., Reisman, R.M., Gallo, J.P. and Lief, P.A., A comparison of regional intravenous guanethidine and reserpine in reflex sympathetic dystrophy. a controlled, randomized, double-blind crossover study, Clin. J. Pain, 5 (1989) 205–209.

Rowbotham, M.C. and Fields, H.L., Topical lidocaine reduces pain in post-herpetic neuralgia, Pain, 38 (1989a) 297–302.

Rowbotham, M.C. and Fields, H.L., Postherpetic neuralgia: the relation of pain complaint, sensory disturbance, and skin temperature, Pain, 39 (1989b) 129–144.

Rowbotham, M.C., Reisner, L.M. and Fields, H.L., Both intravenous lidocaine and morphine reduce the pain of post–herpetic neuralgia, Neurology, 41 (1991) 1024–1028.

Rowbotham, M.C., Miller, K.V., Davies, P., Reisner-Keller, L. and Fields, H.L., Topical lidocaine for post-herpetic neuralgia pain: results of a double blind, vehicle controlled trial, Neurology, 42 (1992) 390.

Sakurada, T., Katsumata, K., Yogo, H., Tan-No, K., Sakurada, S. and Kisara, K., Antinociception induced by CP 96, 345, a non-peptide NK-1 receptor antagonist, in the mouse formalin and capsaicin tests, Neurosci. Lett., 151 (1993) 142–145.

Sanjue, H. and Jun, Z., Sympathetic facilitation of sustained discharges of polymodal nociceptors, Pain, 38 (1989) 85–90.

Sato, J. and Perl, E.R., Adrenergic excitation of cutaneous pain receptors induced by peripheral nerve injury, Science, 251 (1991) 1608–1610.

Scadding, J.W., Development of ongoing activity, mechanosensitivity, and adrenaline sensitivity in severed peripheral nerve axons, Exp. Neurol., 73 (1981) 345–364.

Scheffler, N.M., Sheitel, P.L. and Lipton, M.N., Treatment of painful diabetic neuropathy with capsaicin 0.075%, J. Am. Podiatr. Med. Assoc., 81 (1991) 288–293.

Stow, P.J., Glynn, C.J. and Minor, B., EMLA cream in the treatment of post-herpetic neuralgia. Efficacy and pharmacokinetic profile, Pain, 39 (1989) 301–305.

Stracke, H., Meyer, U.E., Schumacher, H.E. and Federlin, K., Mexiletine in the treatment of diabetic neuropathy, Diabetes Care, 15 (1992) 1550–1555.

Tal, M. and Bennett, G.J., Dextrorphan relieves neuropathic heat-evoked hyperalgesia in the rat, Neurosci. Lett., 151 (1993) 107–110.

Tandan, R., Lewis, G.A., Krusinski, P.B., Badger, G.B. and Freis, T.J., Topical capsaicin in painful diabetic neuropathy. Controlled study with long-term follow-up, Diabetes Care, 15 (1992) 8–14.

Tanelian, D.L. and MacIver, M.B., Analgesic concentrations of lidocaine suppress tonic A-delta and C fiber discharges produced by acute injury, Anesthesiology, 74 (1991) 934–936.

Thomas, P.K., The anatomical substratum of pain, Can. J. Neurol. Sci., May (1974) 92–97.

Walker, E.A. and Nulson, F., Electrical stimulation of the upper thoracic portion of the sympathetic chain in man, Arch. Neurol. Psychiat., 59 (1948) 559–560.

Wall, P.D. and Devor, M., Sensory afferent impulses originate from dorsal root ganglia as well as from the periphery in normal and nerve injured rats, Pain, 17 (1983) 321–339.

Wall, P.D. and Gutnick, M., Ongoing activity in peripheral nerves: the physiology and pharmacology of impulses originating from a neuroma, Exp. Neurol., 43 (1974) 580–593.

Wall, P.D. and Melzack, R., (Eds.), Textbook of Pain, 3rd ed., Churchill Livingstone, Edinburgh, 1994.

Wallin, G., Torebjörk, E. and Hallin, R., Preliminary observations on the pathophysiology of hyperalgesia in the causalgic pain syndrome. In: Y. Zotterman (Ed.), Sensory Functions of the Skin in Primates, Pergamon, New York, 1976, pp. 489–502.

Watson, C.P. and Evans, R.J., The postmastectomy pain syndrome and topical capsaicin: a randomized trial, Pain, 51 (1992) 375–379.
Watson, C.P.N., Evans, R.J. and Watt, V.R., Post-herpetic neuralgia and topical capsaicin, Pain, 33 (1988) 333–340.
Willis, W.D., Jr., Hyperalgesia and allodynia, Raven Press, New York, 1992.
Woolf, C.J., Segmental afferent fibre-induced analgesia: transcutaneous electrical nerve stimulation and vibration. In: P.D. Wall and R. Melzack (Eds.), Textbook of Pain, 2nd ed., Churchill Livingstone, Edinburgh, 1989, pp. 884–896.
Woolf, C.J. and Wiesenfeld-Hallin, Z., The systemic administration of local anaesthetics produces a selective depression of C-afferent fibre evoked activity in the spinal cord, Pain, 23 (1985) 361–374.
Wynn-Parry, C.B., Pain in avulsion lesions of the brachial plexus, Pain, 9 (1980) 41–53.
Zochodne, D.W., Epineurial peptides: a role in neuropathic pain? Can. J. Neurol. Sci., 20 (1993) 69–72.

Correspondence to: Howard L. Fields, MD, PhD, Box 0114–Neurology, University of California, San Francisco, CA 94143 USA. Tel: 415-476-4201; Fax: 415-476-9386.

Proceedings of the 7th World Congress on Pain,
Progress in Pain Research and Management, Vol. 2,
edited by G.F. Gebhart, D.L. Hammond, and T.S.
Jensen, IASP Press, Seattle, © 1994.

32

Clinical Phenomenology and Mechanisms of Reflex Sympathetic Dystrophy: Emphasis on Edema

Helmut Blumberg,[a] Ulrike Hoffmann,[b] Mohsen Mohadjer,[a] and Rudolf Scheremet[a]

Departments of [a]Neurosurgery and [b]Anesthesiology, University of Freiburg, Germany

INTRODUCTION

Reflex sympathetic dystrophy (RSD) is a generic and descriptive term that includes causalgia, Sudeck's atrophy, algodystrophy, and other conditions (Lankford 1980; Schwartzmann and McLellan 1987; Stanton-Hicks et al. 1989; Jänig et al. 1991). Leading symptoms of RSD are pain and swelling, which are often associated with various motor disturbances (Kozin et al. 1976; Davidoff et al. 1986; Blumberg 1991; Deuschl et al. 1991). These disturbances, like the other symptoms of RSD, develop predominantly at the distal part of the affected extremities.

The cause and treatment of RSD and the involvement of the sympathetic nervous system have become a focus of interest in basic and clinical research during the past decade (Jänig 1985; Devor et al. 1991; Jänig and Schmidt 1992). In spite of this interest, the mechanisms of edema in RSD have not been clarified. In the few long-term clinical studies to address this symptom both sympatholytic and corticoid treatment were followed by reduction of the edema (Christensen 1982; Davidoff et al. 1988; Kozin et al. 1976). The question therefore remained as to whether the sympathetic nervous system plays a major role in the development of this symptom of RSD.

As part of a more general model on the generation of RSD in which a vicious circle with a sympathetic contribution is assumed (Jänig 1985, 1990;

Devor et al. 1991), a specific hypothesis has been formulated regarding edema in RSD (Blumberg 1988). The crux of this hypothesis is the assumption that sympathetic neurons increase vasoconstriction on the postcapillary side as compared with the precapillary side. The reduced venous return that accompanies this phenomenon leads to the edema in RSD.

According to this hypothesis, a sympathetic block would necessarily be immediately followed by a decrease of the edema. This could be clinically studied by observing the size of an affected extremity before, during, and directly after sympatholytic interventions. So far, such an acute effect of sympathetic blocks has not been shown in cases with typical RSD. This effect is demonstrated below using four representative case reports from an ongoing study of the mechanisms of the edema in RSD.

CLINICAL PHENOMENOLOGY OF RSD

According to a recent consensus statement for the diagnosis of RSD (Jänig et al. 1991), the symptoms of RSD can be described by a triad of autonomic (sympathetic), motor, and sensory disturbances. In almost all cases they develop after a noxious event. Typically, the triad develops irrespective of the type and site of the preceding lesion at the extremities or even in the viscera or centrally (for ref. see Schwartzmann and McLellan 1987). The RSD symptoms are not confined to a nerve zone or dermatome, but in most cases appear distally generalized in one extremity. In rare cases, a so-called localized form of RSD may occur, which affects, for instance, only a lesioned thumb (see case report in Blumberg et al. 1993). RSD may occasionally affect more than one extremity (Bentley and Hameroff 1980).

TYPES OF SYMPTOMS

Based on a clinical approach described elsewhere (Blumberg 1991), the triad of RSD symptoms, which can be rated on a scale from 1 to 3 (see below), ensues from the following findings (Table I).

1. Autonomic Symptoms

The distal part of the affected extremity shows generalized swelling, which is nearly always prominent on the dorsal side. The affected extremity is warmer or colder than the contralateral one, with the skin temperature difference being most prominent at the palmar or plantar tips of the fingers or toes. The skin is often reddish or marbled, or cyanotic. Sweating may be increased or decreased,

Table I
Type, incidence, and mean score of RSD symptoms with respect to duration of RSD

	RSD Duration	
	≤ 10 days (n = 24)	0.35 to 168 months (n = 157)
I. Autonomic Symptoms (%)		
Distally generalized swelling	96	96
Warm or cold affected extremity	75	78
Hypohydrosis or hyperhydrosis	42	52
II. Motor Symptoms (%)		
Active movement reduced	88	8
Muscular strength diminshed	92	89
Tremor (postural or action)	33	47
III. Sensory Symptoms (%)		
Deep spontaneous pain	75	75
Hypoalgesia or hyperalgesia	87	76
Hypoesthesia or hyperesthesia	83	71
Mechanical allodynia	0	8
Mean RSD Score	14 ± 3	14 ± 3
Mean RSD Duration (months)	0.1 ± 0.1	6 ± 16

Source: Modified from Blumberg and Jänig 1994.

usually on the palmar or plantar side. Most patients report a strange reaction of the skin temperature to changes of environmental temperature (for example, the affected hand in comparison with the healthy hand cools too slowly—or too quickly—when exposed to cold). Consistent with such reports, experimental investigations showed an abnormal (side-different) response of skin blood flow upon thermal stimulation in RSD patients (Blumberg 1988).

The skin temperature was measured on the palmar or plantar tips of fingers or toes of the affected and the contralateral extremity, using a fast-reading infrared thermometer (Blumberg 1991). A warm or cold affected extremity was noted (Table I) when a so-called systematic side difference of skin temperature was found, i.e., all fingers or toes of the affected extremity showed higher or lower values than the corresponding contralateral ones.

2. Motor Symptoms

Typically, the active range of motion of the affected extremity is reduced (e.g., the inability to close the fist and/or to oppose the tips of thumb and fifth finger). Muscular strength is usually reduced (paresis) or even lost (plegia), commonly involving all muscles of the affected distal extremity. Furthermore, tremor (postural or action) in the hand is seen in roughly half of all cases. The postural tremor associated with RSD has been characterized experimentally as increased physiological tremor (Deuschl et al. 1991). Motor symptoms, especially tremor, are more pronounced in an affected hand than in an affected foot.

3. Sensory Symptoms

A prominent symptom in most RSD patients is spontaneous pain. It is usually felt diffusely deep inside the hand or foot. Most characteristically, this pain shows an orthostatic component, with the pain increasing when the extremity is lowered and decreasing when it is elevated. Interestingly, according to the history, a number of patients noted this phenomenon at the onset of RSD, if combined with a warm extremity. Later, however, with the occurrence of a cold extremity, the phenomenon had disappeared. The pain in RSD is usually more severe at night. In addition to the spontaneous pain, movement-related pain can occur in one or several joints, even when these were not involved in the preceding lesion.

Other sensory disturbances include changes in skin algesia (hyper- and hypoalgesia) and skin esthesia (hyper- and hypoesthesia). Such changes are usually more pronounced on the palmar and plantar side than on the dorsal side of the hand and foot. Mechanical allodynia (pain elicited by light, brief touch of the skin; Merskey et al. 1986) was not observed in the first days after the onset of RSD and in general is a rare symptom of RSD (Table I; Blumberg 1991; Blumberg and Jänig 1994).

Trophic Disturbances

Trophic disturbances—such as disturbed nail and hair growth, thin glossy skin, and osteoporosis—are not present at the onset of RSD. Therefore, in our opinion they should be judged as late consequences of RSD and cannot serve as criteria for early diagnosis of RSD (Blumberg 1991). Passive movement disturbances (stiff joints) develop later in patients with RSD and are considered to be primarily due to trophic changes in joints and tendons. However, they may also be the expression of some kind of functional motor disturbance.

RSD SCORE

To allow an interindividual comparison, an index has been proposed to assess the clinical picture of RSD (Blumberg 1991). This index includes only the nine most common symptoms and signs of RSD. They are weighted according to their clinical relevance and are assigned the following values: swelling/decreased active range of motion/spontaneous pain = 3 each; systematic side difference of skin temperature/paresis or plegia/disturbed algesia = 2 each; side difference in sweating/tremor/disturbed esthesia = 1 each. Thus, a full RSD-syndrome will have a maximum score of 18 points.

ONSET AND MAJOR SYMPTOMS OF RSD

Among the triad, the major symptoms of RSD at its onset are pain, swelling, and difference of skin temperature between the distal extremities. Early diagnosis of RSD (≤ 10 days after the initiating event) can be facilitated by considering the way this pain develops, its characteristics, and the distribution of the swelling.

Initially, the pain is localized at the site of the preceding lesion. After a variable period of time (hours to weeks), the typical diffuse deep spontaneous pain of RSD with its orthostatic component develops distally (Blumberg 1988, 1991). In many patients the initial pain has almost disappeared at this stage.

The spontaneous pain of RSD characteristically can be suppressed by bandaging the distal part of the affected extremity and applying suprasystolic compression just proximal to the bandage—a procedure called the *ischemia test* (Blumberg and Hoffmann 1992). Similar observations have been made by other investigators (Loh et al. 1981; Gracely et al. 1990). According to recent findings, pain suppression will occur under test conditions only if the pain shows an orthostatic component (Hoffmann and Blumberg, unpublished observations). However, the ischemia test, which can be used as a bedside test, requires independent confirmation before it can be generally recommended for early diagnosis of RSD. In some cases, spontaneous pain can be absent at the onset of RSD, despite otherwise typical onset and symptoms (Blumberg 1991; Table I; case I below).

The swelling is identified to be a symptom of RSD if it is distally generalized without direct spatial connection to the site of a preceding lesion. This is most evident in patients in whom no or only a strictly localized or minor lesion had occurred distally. Such a distribution of swelling also indicates the onset of RSD if it occurs in an acute manner days or even weeks after the occurrence of a lesion (e.g., following a radial fracture treated with plaster cast, which may have put local pressure on the extremity for a few days, or following a persisting local painful skin lesion[case III below]). In cases with severe and extensive distal lesions (for example, when the entire hand has been squeezed), however, the accompanying acute distal edema may be a direct posttraumatic event.

In general, with respect to type, incidence, and mean score of RSD symptoms, there are no relevant differences between cases seen early (during the first 10 days) or later after the onset of RSD with regard to the difference in clinical phenomenology (Table I; case reports below).

EFFECT OF SYMPATHOLYTIC STRATEGIES ON THE EDEMA IN RSD

In an ongoing study at our institution on the mechanisms of edema in RSD, various sympatholytic interventions—distal blockade of postganglionic noradrenaline release by means of regionally applied guanethidine (see below), proximal blockade of sympathetic activity by means of conventional block of stellate ganglion, and spinal anesthesia—are applied in RSD patients. The following four cases are typical of how the edema in RSD responds to sympatholytic treatment, especially in patients with early RSD.

They are also representative for several other important features of RSD. Usually, the disorder develops acutely (cases I–IV). It nearly always affects primarily unlesioned regions. This can best be demonstrated in cases with a minor preceding lesion (cases I, III, IV). RSD characteristically presents with a distally generalized distribution of symptoms, irrespective of the site of the preceding lesion, which may occur distally (cases III, IV), more proximally (case I), or even at visceral regions (case II). There are no relevant differences in the clinical picture between early (cases I–III) and late (case IV) RSD. These four cases illustrate the effect of various sympatholytic strategies on the edema in upper (cases I and III) and lower extremities (cases II and IV) with minor (case III) up to most severe (case II) expression of the edema.

For the regional guanethidine blockade, the technique as described by Hannington-Kiff (1989, 1994) was somewhat modified. The cuff was applied distally (just proximal to the hand or foot joint) to allow dose reduction of guanethidine. Following intravenous injection of the drug, physiological saline was injected repeatedly to improve the distribution of guanethidine inside the symptomatic area (Hoffmann and Blumberg 1994).

CASE I: DISTAL BLOCKADE OF POSTGANGLIONIC NORADRENALINE RELEASE IN RSD WITH DISTAL EDEMA FOLLOWING MINOR PROXIMAL LESION

A 37-year-old healthy male accidentally banged his left elbow while doing work around the house. Noticing no lesion, he continued to work. About one hour later, he lay down for a nap. Upon waking about two hours later, he noticed severe swelling of the left hand, accompanied by diffuse numbness of the entire hand. On the same day, he reported to the Department of Surgery, where no evidence of a fracture or nerve or vascular lesion was found. Under the suspicion of RSD following a minor lesion he was referred to us.

On neurological investigation 2 days later, the typical triad of RSD was found with distally generalized autonomic, motor, and sensory symptoms (RSD score: 10). Edema of the entire left hand and reduced active range of motion, mainly affecting extension of fingers, were the leading signs (Photo 1a). Neither spontaneous pain nor hyperalgesia nor allodynia was present. There was no evidence of a nerve lesion. There was no edema and no obstruction of elbow movement at the site of the initial injury.

Before treatment, a 2-day observation period was initiated with the hand kept elevated, which had no significant effect on the edema. Afterward, a 2.5-mg guanethidine block was applied to the left hand. Directly following this intervention, the edema started to decrease, as evidenced by the onset of skin shrinkage. Because the edema did not completely regress, two additional blockades were applied at 4-day intervals. Finally, 8 days after the onset of treatment, the edema was entirely gone and motor function had been restored (Photo 1b). There were no other symptoms of RSD (RSD score: zero). The patient returned to work. At follow-up 3 weeks later, the same normal findings were obtained.

CASE II: DISTAL BLOCKADE OF POSTGANGLIONIC NORADRENALINE RELEASE IN RSD WITH EDEMA OF THE ENTIRE AFFECTED EXTREMITY FOLLOWING A HIGH PROXIMAL INJURY

A 50-year-old male patient on chronic dialysis for disturbed renal function underwent surgery for a retroperitoneal hematoma. After coming out of the general anesthesia, he complained of pain radiating down to the left leg. On the next day, a slight root (S 1) compression syndrome was assumed. Because of this, no special treatment was considered.

The next day, 2 days after surgery, the pain sensation changed. The patient mainly complained about diffuse pain in the left foot, accompanied by warm skin. An increase in size of the left thigh was documented for the first time. The pain in the left foot increased during the following days, accompanied

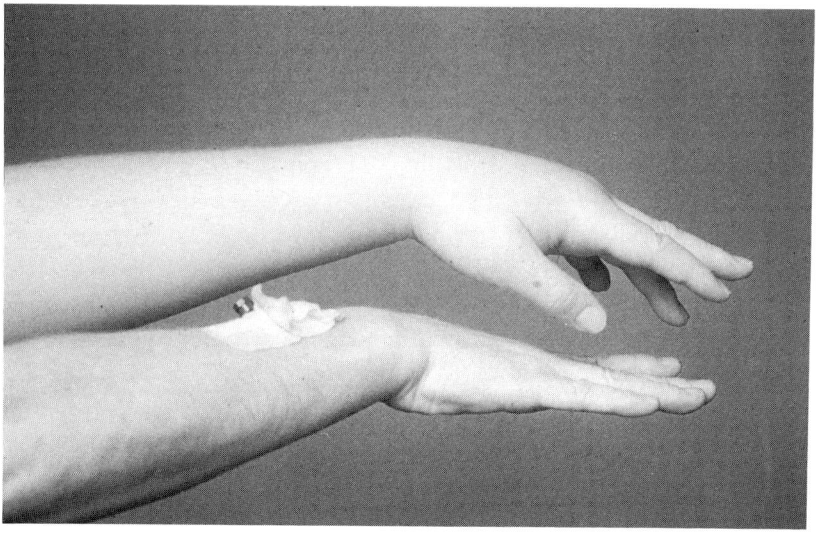

Photo 1a. RSD in the left hand (top) in case I. Note the severe edema and the decreased active range of motion (extension) of the affected fingers. The right lower arm was cannulated to take a blood sample.

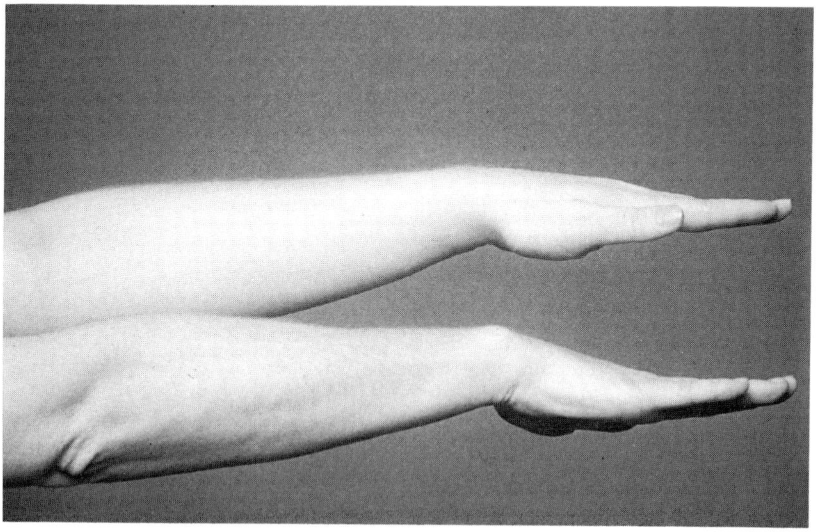

Photo 1b. The hands in case I after guanethidine treatment, 8 days after Photo 1a. Note the disappearance of the edema and the restored motor function in the left hand.

by a drastic increase in the size of the entire left leg, with proximal emphasis. The previously normal skin of the left lower leg and of the dorsal side of the foot acutely developed blisters. This was considered to be due to the strong tension of the skin related to the sudden increase of the edema. The blisters were treated locally. Thorough investigations, including phlebography (not illustrated [the authors hold supporting documents for all items noted as "not illustrated"]), gave no explanation for the nature of the edema. Nine days after the intervention, RSD was assumed and the patient was referred to us.

On neurological investigation, the typical triad of RSD was found (RSD score: 12). The leading sign was edema of the entire left lower leg (Photo 2a). The pain was felt deeply and diffusely inside the left foot, showing an orthostatic component. There was no allodynia or hyperalgesia. Pain was completely suppressed by the ischemia test. Bone scanning showed a diffuse increase in uptake at the left leg compared with the right leg (not illustrated).

The course of the disorder with the behavior of the edema before, during, and after treatment is shown in Fig. 1. Following the diagnosis of RSD, a 3-day control period was introduced with the left leg kept elevated. During these days, the size of the upper leg remained stable. Directly after the first

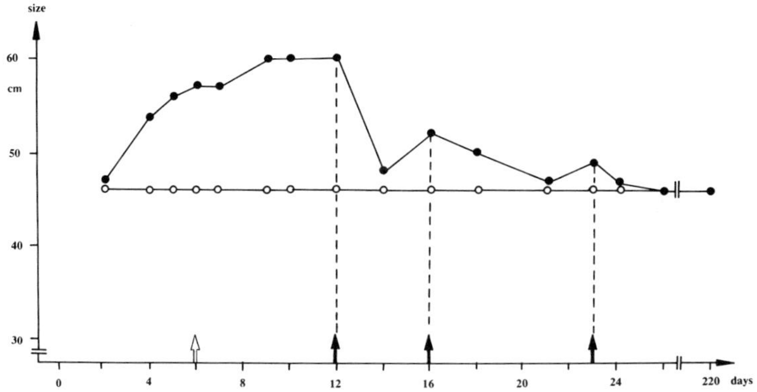

Fig. 1. Effect of distal guanethidine blockade on the edema in RSD (case II). Following a visceral surgical intervention, a severe swelling of the entire left leg developed over a period of days according to repeated measurements of the size of the affected upper leg. RSD was diagnosed after thorough investigations, including phlebography (unfilled arrow), gave no explanation for the edema. Following the diagnosis of RSD, a 3-day control period (left leg elevated) was initiated. During that period, the edema in the left leg did not increase. A distal guanethidine block was applied on day 12 (filled arrow) and the edema began to decrease over the next 2 days. After two similar blockades (days 16 and 23, filled arrows), each applied after the edema began to return, the edema disappeared permanently (observation period: 7 months). Filled circles = size of left upper leg. Unfilled circles = size of healthy right upper leg.

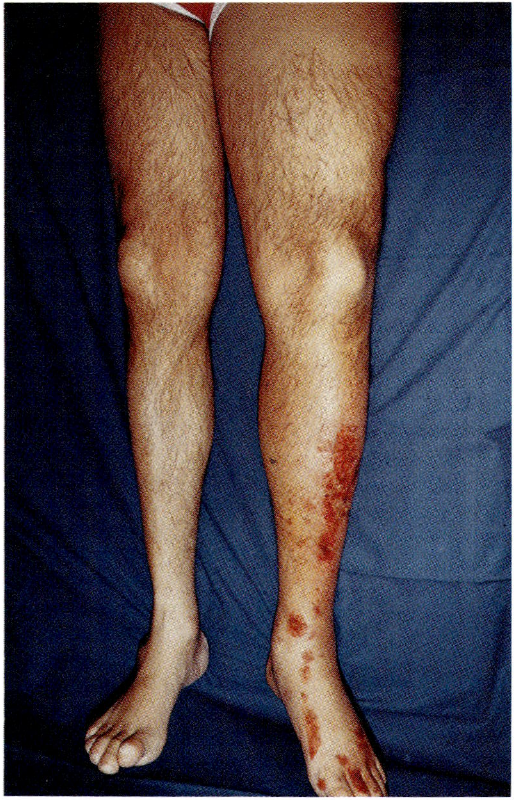

Photo 2a (left). RSD in the left lower leg in case II. Note the severe edema of the left leg, most pronounced in the upper part of the leg. The red color of the skin of left lower leg and dorsal side of left foot is due to local treatment of underlying blisters, which had developed during the drastic increase in edema (see Fig. 1).

Photo 2b (right). The legs in case II, 7 months after treatment. Note the disappearance of all signs in the left lower leg.

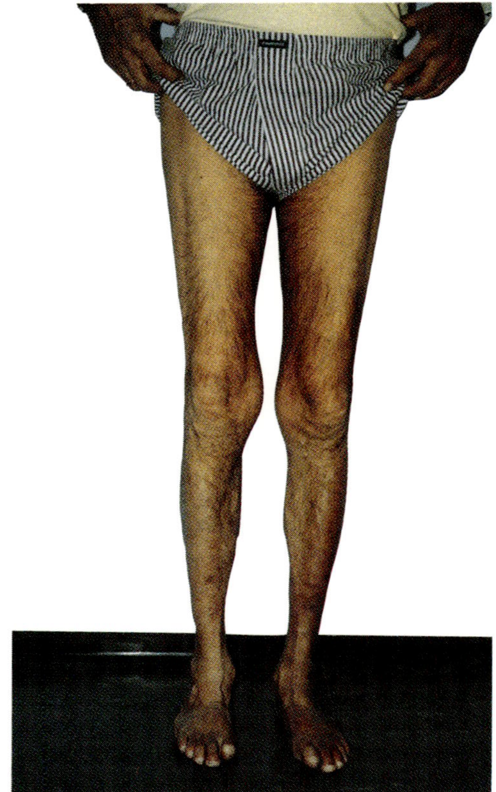

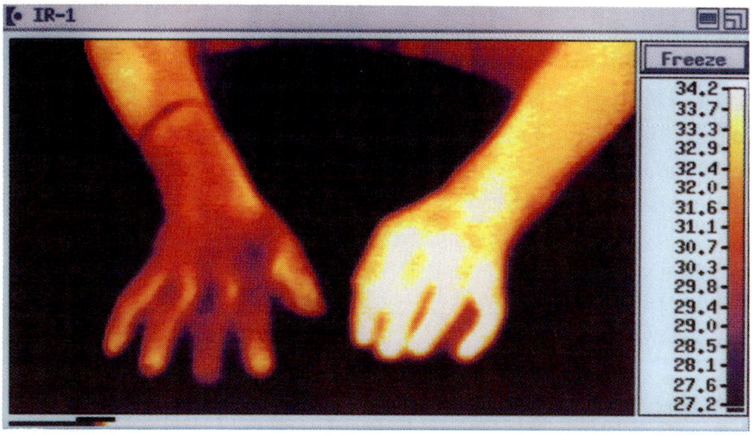
IR-1
Freeze
34.2
33.7
33.3
32.9
32.4
32.0
31.6
31.1
30.7
30.3
29.8
29.4
29.0
28.5
28.1
27.6
27.2

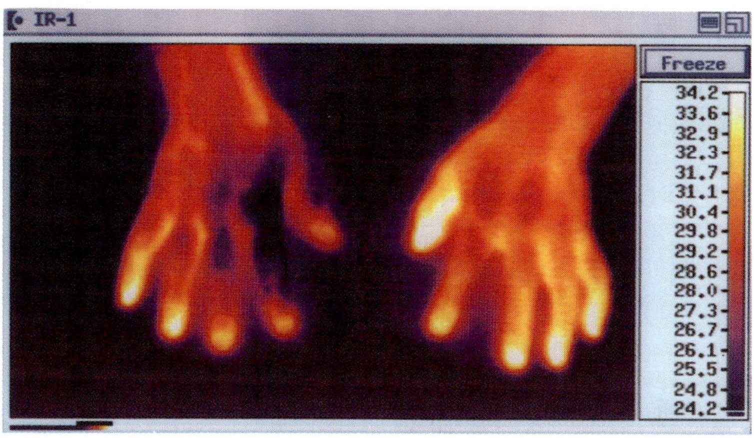
IR-1
Freeze
34.2
33.6
32.9
32.3
31.7
31.1
30.4
29.8
29.2
28.6
28.0
27.3
26.7
26.1
25.5
24.8
24.2

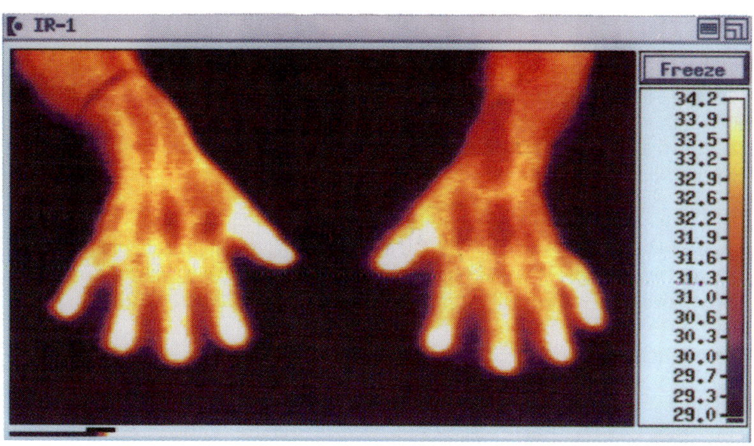
IR-1
Freeze
34.2
33.9
33.5
33.2
32.9
32.6
32.2
31.9
31.6
31.3
31.0
30.6
30.3
30.0
29.7
29.3
29.0

distal 5-mg guanethidine block, a decrease in edema could be observed, which continued during the next 2 days. During that time, there was no spontaneous pain. The pain and swelling returned, however, so a second blockade was applied, and then a third after the symptoms had returned again.

After the third and final blockade, the edema and pain disappeared permanently, and the other RSD symptoms improved (RSD score: 6). In the meantime, the skin lesions (blisters) started to heal with no special treatment. At follow-up 3 months later, three-phase bone scanning showed normal findings (not illustrated). At this time, as well as 7 months later (Photo 2b), no symptoms of RSD were present, and the skin at the previously lesioned areas was normal (RSD score: zero).

CASE III: PROXIMAL BLOCKADE OF SYMPATHETIC ACTIVITY IN RSD WITH DISTAL EDEMA FOLLOWING LOCAL SKIN LESIONS ON THE LEFT HAND

For about one month, this 51-year-old female secretary suffered from inflammatory skin lesions between the left second and third and the third and fourth fingers and at the middle joint of the fourth finger. She had been seeing a dermatologist for this condition. She had throbbing pain at the site of the lesions between the third and fourth fingers and in the adjacent area. There

Overleaf:

Thermogram 1 (top). Skin blood flow side differences in RSD (case III). The investigation is done under room temperature conditions. In this and subsequent thermograms, values on the scale at the right indicate °C. White/yellow color indicates relatively high temperatures compared with blue/black color on the scale and in the figure. Temperatures above 34.2 and below 27.2°C (see scale) cannot be determined because of the externally applied range of skin temperature illustrated. Basically, the same procedure (with somewhat different values) was applied for the subsequent thermograms. Note that the entire left hand and the distal lower left arm showed considerably higher skin temperatures compared with the healthy right side. Note also the impaired motor function of the left hand (impaired spreading and extension of fingers) compared with the healthy right hand. (Thermography system: Agema, Thermovision 900).

Thermogram 2 (center). Same case as Thermogram 1 (case III) 12 days after sympathetic block. Note the decrease in side differences of skin temperature compared with Thermogram 1. Note also the improved motor function of the left hand (better extension and spreading of fingers) compared with Thermogram 1. Compare also with Photo 3b, same patient. For methods and technical details see legend of Thermogram 1.

Thermogram 3 (bottom). Same case as Thermograms 1 and 2 (Case III) 7 months after sympathetic block. At this time, no relevant side differences in skin blood flow could be seen. Note also the restored motor function of the left hand. For methods and technical details see legend of Thermogram 1.

were no motor disturbances, edema, or skin temperature changes outside the area of the skin lesions, and the patient continued to go to work.

With no obvious reason, fingers two to five and nearly the entire dorsal side of the hand suddenly began to swell. This was accompanied by diffuse burning pain, which in addition to the localized throbbing pain was felt diffusely deep inside the swollen area. At the same time, the left hand became very warm in comparison with the right hand. The active range of motion of the fingers became reduced so that the patient was unable to work. The next day, dermatological examination determined considerable increased redness at the sites of the local lesions, which was related to the generalized reaction of the hand. RSD was therefore assumed, and the patient was referred to us.

On neurological investigation 4 days following the onset of the diffuse swelling and pain, the typical triad of RSD was found (RSD score: 12). Leading symptoms were pain and swelling (Photo 3a). Extension and spreading of the fingers (Thermogram 1) and the fist grip were impaired (Photo 4a). The entire left hand and left distal lower arm were warmer than the healthy right side (Thermogram 1; thermography, used to document the state of skin blood flow in RSD before and after therapy and to prove the technical success of applied sympathetic blocks, was available only for this case in the study). Bone scanning showed a diffuse increase in uptake in the left hand compared with right hand (not illustrated). The diffuse burning pain was completely suppressed by the ischemia test, which also caused an acute improvement in the ability to move the fingers. The local throbbing pain, however, was not influenced by the test (Fig. 2, A and B).

To determine whether one or both types of the spontaneous pain might be related to the sympathetic nervous system, a blockade of the ipsilateral stellate ganglion, using 5 ml bupivacaine 0.5%, was applied. Based on a neurological investigation, this did not induce any blockade of afferent (plexus or root) fibers supplying the affected arm. Directly after the onset of sympatholysis (increase of skin temperature up to around 36°C), which was documented thermographically (not illustrated), the diffuse burning pain was completely relieved. In sharp contrast, and like the situation during the previous ischemia test performed by an independent investigator, the local pain was not influenced by the blockade (Fig. 2, C and D). At the same time and still under the action of the block, the edema started to decrease, as was seen clinically by the onset of shrinkage of the skin inside the area of the diffuse edema.

About 24 hours later, the diffuse deep pain was still absent, and the edema had disappeared entirely. However, the local pain remained unchanged. At follow-up 12 days later, swelling was still absent (Photo 3b), and the diffuse pain had not returned. On that occasion, fist grip was regular (Photo 4b)

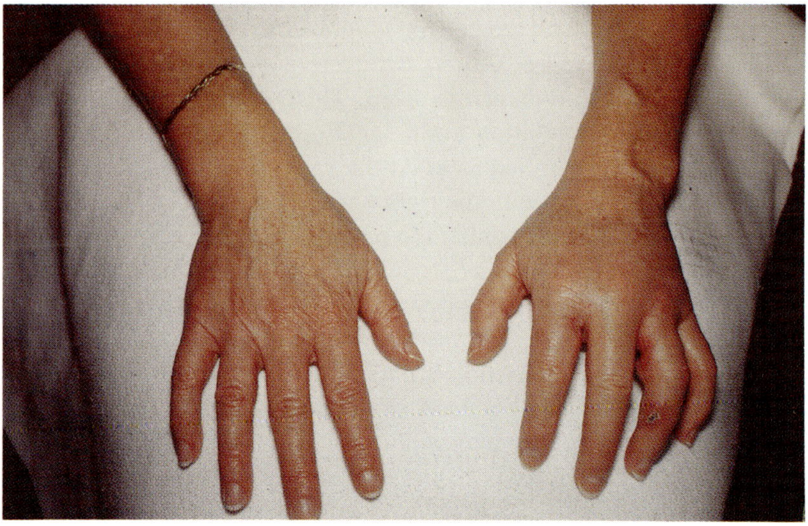

Photo 3a. RSD in the left hand in case III. Note the diffuse edema of the left hand and the local skin lesions.

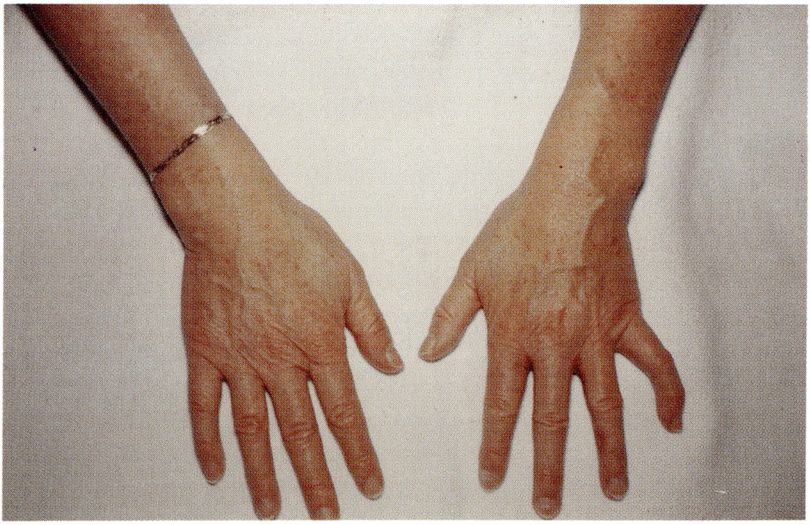

Photo 3b. The hands in case III, 12 days after stellate ganglion block. Note the disappearance of the edema of left hand, compared with Photo 3a.

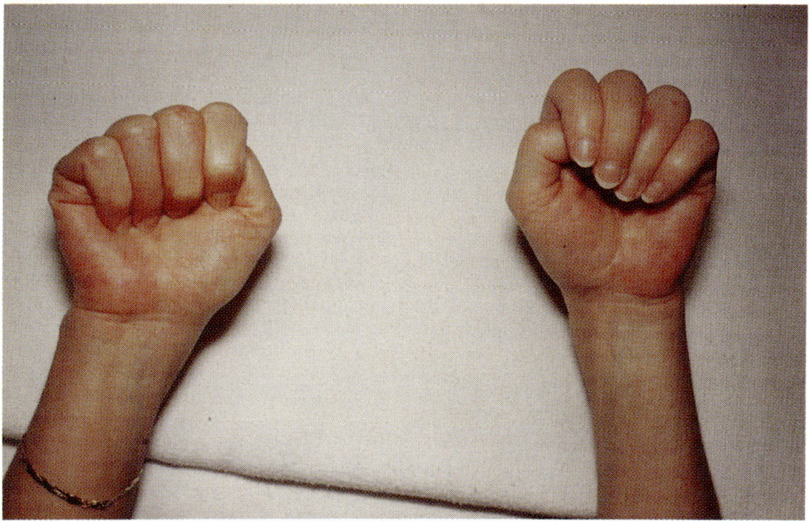

Photo 4a. The hands in case III, on the same day as Photo 3a. Note the inability to completely close the fist of the left hand.

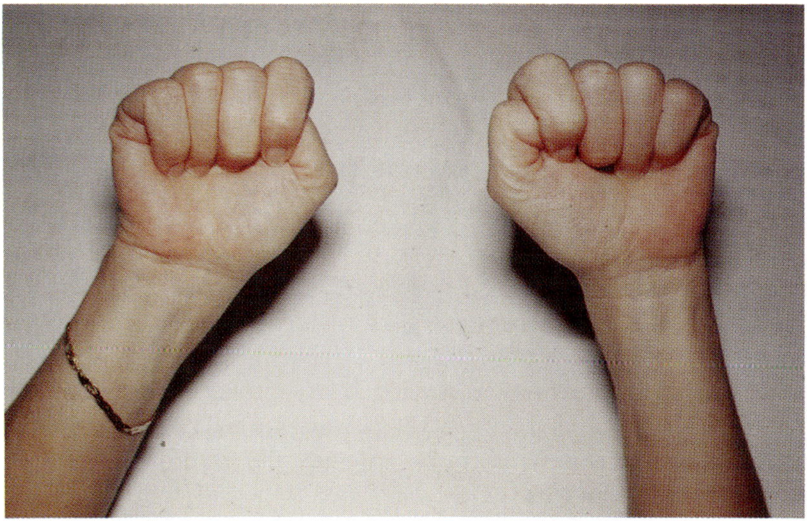

Photo 4b. The hands in case III, 12 days after stellate ganglion block. Note the normal fist grip, compared with Photo 4a.

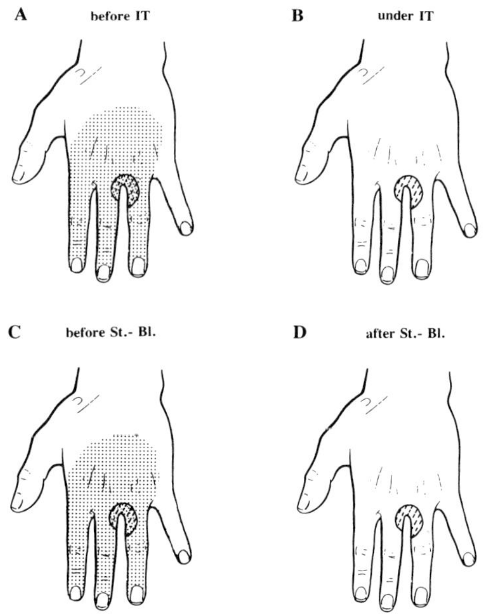

Fig. 2. Illustration of the different kinds of spontaneous pain in RSD during the ischemia test (under IT) and following ipsilateral stellate ganglion block (St.-Bl.) in case III (see text). The deep burning pain, which was closely related to the area of the edema of RSD (see Photo 3a), was totally suppressed during the ischemia test (A/B) and was relieved by the sympathetic block (C/D). In contrast, the throbbing pain localized to an interdigital skin lesion (see Photo 3a) was affected neither by the ischemia test (A/B) nor by the sympathetic block (C/D). Shaded region = area of diffuse burning pain. Circled hatched region = area of the local pain.

and, except for a—reduced—side difference in skin temperature (Thermogram 2), there were no other symptoms of RSD (RSD score: 2). In the following course, the skin lesions finally improved with dermatological treatment, and the local pain subsided. At a last investigation 7 months later, normal conditions were seen in the left hand (RSD score: zero), including a loss of relevant skin temperature side differences as seen thermographically (Thermogram 3).

CASE IV. CONTINUOUS SUPPRESSION OF PREGANGLIONIC SYMPATHETIC ACTIVITY IN RSD OF THE LEFT LOWER LEG FOLLOWING MINOR FOOT LESION

While at school this healthy 15-year-old girl banged the dorsal part of her right foot. No visible skin lesion developed. During the night, diffuse pain developed in the left foot, accompanied by warm skin and diffuse swelling, which steadily increased during the next 24 hours. The foot became paretic. Examinations on the next day, including X-ray, produced no evidence of a bony or other lesion. Laboratory findings were normal. Because the edema continued to increase until it finally affected the entire lower right leg, phlebography was performed. This also failed to provide an explanation for the swelling.

During the next 2 months, the symptoms could not be influenced by physical or oral drug therapy, including non-steroidal anti-inflammatory drugs. During that time, the patient went to school but kept the right leg elevated, since this alleviated the spontaneous pain somewhat. No diagnosis could be established until finally a severe diffuse osteoporosis was found in the right foot by means of X-ray (not illustrated). In addition, bone scanning showed a diffuse increase in uptake at the left foot compared with the right (not illustrated). At that stage, she was unable to move the right foot at all (plegia) and felt deep pain when standing on the right foot. Because of these findings, RSD was diagnosed and peridural anesthesia was applied for treatment. Following that procedure, the spontaneous pain disappeared and the edema regressed slightly; however, the pain when standing remained unchanged. Because treatment was only partially successful, the patient was referred to us.

On neurological investigation 3 months following the initial injury, RSD was confirmed (RSD score: 10). In addition to plegia of the right foot, swelling of the right leg with distal dominance was the leading sign (Photo 5). Standing on the right foot caused deep pain, for the most part felt at the heel bone. She did not complain of spontaneous pain, and there was no skin allodynia or skin hyperalgesia. Continuous sympatholysis via spinal anesthesia was considered to be the treatment of choice, and 4 days later the patient was admitted to the Department of Pediatrics. The course of the edema before, during, and after treatment of this case is shown in Fig. 3.

On the first day of admission, a spinal catheter system was implanted; the tip of the catheter was positioned at TH 10 (not illustrated). This intervention was followed by a 3-day control period with the right leg kept elevated. During that period, no obvious changes in the size of the right leg were seen. Afterward, spinal anesthesia with 1.4 ml 0.5% bupivacaine per hour for 43 hours was applied in the intensive care unit of the Department of Anesthesiology. During that time, paraplegia accompanied by sensory loss below TH 8 developed, including loss of bladder and bowel control.

The onset of sympatholysis brought about by spinal anesthesia was indicated by an increase in toe-tip temperatures from about 26°C and 23°C in the affected and the healthy foot, respectively, to around 36°C (maximum: 36.4°C) on both sides. This is illustrated for the affected side in Photo 6. Some 15 minutes after the onset of sympatholysis, edema reduction could be observed for the first time by the occurrence of skin shrinkage. This was followed by a more or less continuous edema regression. One day after the beginning of treatment, most of the edema had disappeared (Photo 7). Twenty hours later treatment was stopped after nearly complete regression of the edema. The next day edema returned to a lesser degree, with spontaneous remission during the next couple of days. The edema had not returned at the end of an observation

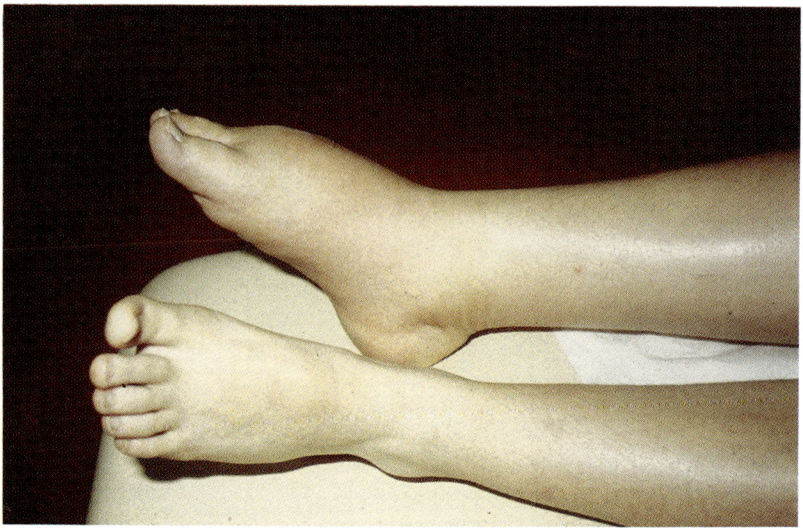

Photo 5. RSD in the right lower leg in case IV. Note the severe edema of the right foot and distal part of right leg. Compare also Fig. 3.

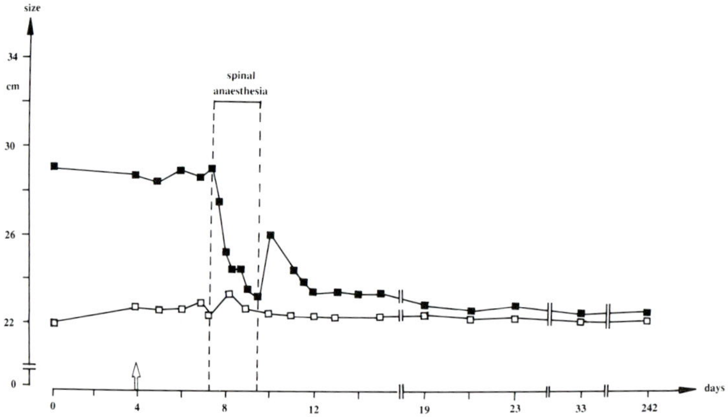

Fig. 3. Effect of continuous spinal anesthesia on the edema in RSD; case IV. To treat the edema, a spinal catheter system was implanted neurosurgically (unfilled arrow), followed by a 3-day control period (right leg elevated). Then spinal anesthesia was applied (for details see text). As measured by the size of the right foot shortly after the onset of sympatholysis (increase in skin temperature at toetips to around 36 °C; see also Photos 6 and 7), swelling of the right foot decreased continuously. Treatment was stopped when the feet reached about equal size. On the next day, the edema returned slightly and regressed spontaneously over the following days. The edema did not return during the entire observation period (8 months). Filled squares = size of affected right foot. Unfilled squares = size of healthy left foot.

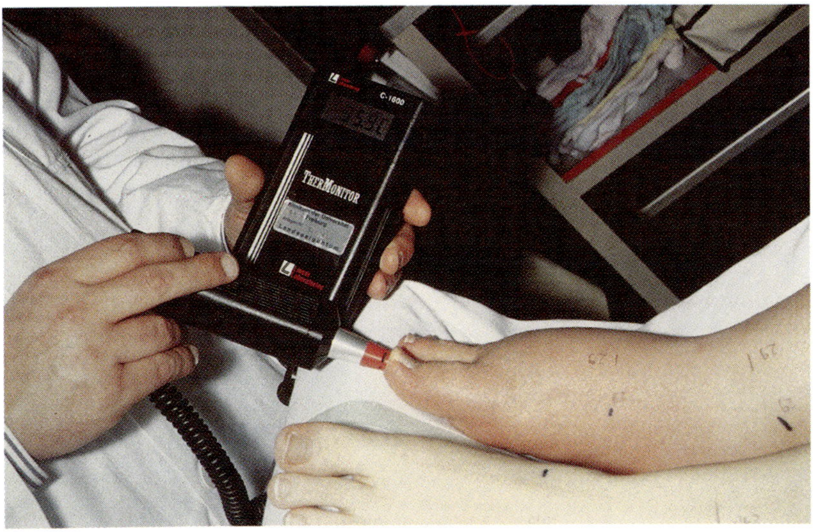

Photo 6. The right foot in case IV at the onset of spinal anesthesia. Sympatholysis is indicated by increase in skin temperature of both legs to about 36°C, here documented for the right big toe (see value on the infrared thermometer shown).

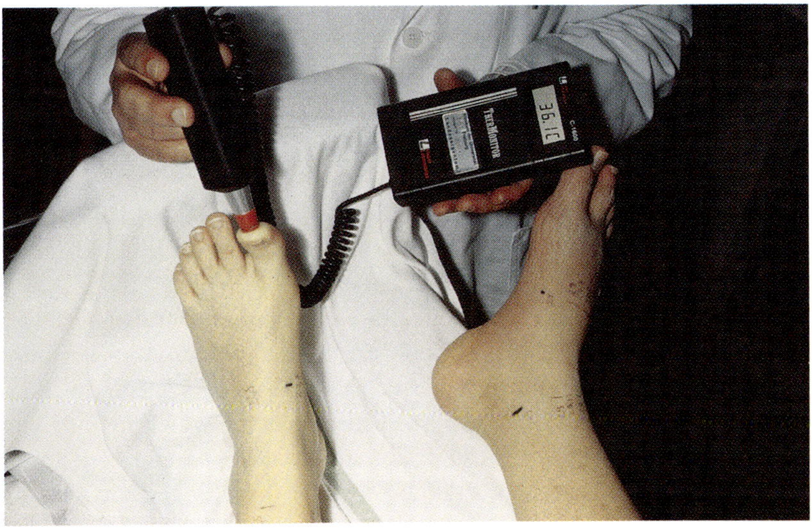

Photo 7. The right foot in case IV, 23 hours after the onset of sympatholysis with maintained high skin temperature of both legs, here documented for the left big toe (see value on the infrared thermometer shown). At that time, most of the edema of the right foot had disappeared (compare with Photos 5 and 6; see also Fig. 3).

period of 8 months (Fig. 3). Motor disturbances and pain on standing gradually resolved during that time. Except for slightly discolored skin of the right foot, no symptoms of RSD were left at final examination (RSD score: zero), at which time the catheter system was removed.

DISCUSSION

In four representative cases of RSD with edema as its major symptom, various sympatholytic strategies were applied for its treatment. In all cases this treatment was immediately followed by regression of the edema. Such an effect of sympatholytic therapy in RSD has not been shown before. These results must be discussed with respect to the mechanisms underlying the cause and regression of the edema. Before possible specific (sympathetic) mechanisms for these phenomena are discussed, other more general mechanisms are considered.

GENERAL CONSIDERATIONS REGARDING THE MECHANISMS OF THE EDEMA IN RSD

For generation of the edema in RSD, known mechanisms (e.g., myocardial or renal dysfunction) can be excluded because the edema occurs unilaterally. Deep-vein thrombosis as a possible source for a unilateral edema, especially in the legs, could be ruled out in two of our cases. Phlebography in these cases produced normal findings for the affected lower leg.

Classical mechanisms of inflammation are also unlikely to be responsible. The edema in RSD develops acutely and is distally generalized when distally there is only a minor, non-inflammatory preceding lesion (case IV). It may also occur distally following proximal lesions (cases I, II), which in a similar case may even be associated with an extremity affected by cold (see case report in Blumberg 1991).

In addition, mechanisms of neurogenic inflammation (release of vasoactive peptides from excited nociceptors and subsequently from surrounding cells) must be considered for the edema in RSD (for ref. see Handwerker and Reeh 1991; Szolcsány et al. 1992). Such mechanisms, which include vasodilation combined with enhanced plasma extravasation, should act first at the lesioned area. For this reason, they can not be initially responsible for the edema in RSD, which characteristically develops in unlesioned areas (distally generalized) from the onset of the disorder (cases I–IV). However, if the edema were caused by another mechanism, which at the same time activated nociceptors in unlesioned areas (see below), the mechanisms of neurogenic inflammation could contribute to the edema in RSD.

Spontaneous remission must be considered responsible for the reduction of edema in RSD, since this may happen in early RSD (Blumberg, unpublished observations). This, however, is unlikely to be the case in at least two of our patients with early RSD (cases I, II). The repeated effect of guanethidine blocks tend to suggest a treatment-related effect. In the patient with a longer duration of RSD (3 months, case IV), however, spontaneous remission can be ruled out.

The observations made during the treatment of our four patients give reason to consider the role of the sympathetic nervous system in the development of edema in RSD. The notion of such a role is supported by animal experiments that have shown that edema in an unlesioned extremity which was elicited by a contralateral lesion (Denko and Petricevic 1978) could be diminished by sympathectomy (Levine et al. 1985). However, since direct evidence for a sympathetically generated edema in humans is lacking, the discussion must include hypothetical mechanisms.

HYPOTHESIS OF A SYMPATHETIC CONTRIBUTION TO THE EDEMA IN RSD

A hypothesis is presented to explain the cause and relief of the edema in our cases (Blumberg 1988; Fig. 4). This hypothesis is merely a specification of a general model concerning the pathophysiology of RSD, which also includes a key role of the sympathetic nervous system in RSD (Devor et al. 1991; Jänig 1985, 1990).

According to this hypothesis, nociceptive afferent input, which is generated by the preceding lesion, sensitizes spinal circuits. This sensitization also affects the spinal circuits of the sympathetic nervous system and leads to an abnormal discharge pattern in vasoconstrictor neurons. This generates the edema by an increased vasoconstriction on the postcapillary side with respect to the precapillary side, leading to an increased filtration pressure. The related increased interstitial pressure is presumed to activate afferent fibers (e.g., deep nociceptors) in nonlesioned tissues. Thus, an indirect coupling between the sympathetic and the afferent nervous systems takes place via the vascular system, by which the central sensitization process is maintained. A vicious circle has been produced, which has become independent of the type and site of the initial lesion. This lesion simultaneously may—or may not—persist.

Regarding the key element of this hypothesis, there are two main possible mechanisms by which the sympathetic nervous system may mediate the proposed enhanced vasoconstriction on the postcapillary side compared with the precapillary side. First, each section of the vascular bed is separately innervated by postganglionic vasoconstrictor neurons. This in principle would enable the sympathetic nervous system to regulate differentially the caliber of pre- and postcapillary vessels. Experimental evidence of this phenomenon is lacking, however. Second, pre- and postcapillary vessels react differently to the same activity in postganglionic vasoconstrictor neurons. Animal experiments support this concept—it has been shown that upon sympathetic activity the stimulus-response relationship of capacitance vessels is much steeper than that of resistance vessels (Mellander 1960; Hainsworth 1986; Hottenstein and Kreulen 1987). Thus, any abnormal discharge pattern of sympathetic vasoconstrictor neurons may predominantly act on the venous side (for further discussion see Jänig 1990).

Based on this hypothesis, and as regards the edema and the spontaneous pain in RSD, sympathetic blocks should lead to enhanced venous return, mainly by interrupting vasoconstrictor activity and thereby opening the venules. As a direct and acute effect of sympatholysis, this should be followed by a decrease in the edema. Because of the accompanying decrease in interstitial pressure, the activity of the afferent fibers, especially of the nociceptors, becomes reduced. As a result, central sensitization becomes diminished or abolished. This interrupts the vicious circle, as an indirect and possibly also lasting effect of sympatholysis, and sympathetic outflow is no longer disturbed.

THE HYPOTHESIS AS APPLIED TO THE CASE REPORTS

In all four cases, sympatholytic treatment was immediately followed by a decrease in the edema. This is consistent with the hypothesis in that the opening of the venules by the sympatholytic action would result in enhanced venous return, which would in turn diminish the edema.

Following sympatholytic interventions, the edema disappeared permanently in all four cases. Therefore, the interventions must have induced long-lasting changes of some kind, for instance, through an interruption of the proposed vicious circle.

Interestingly, in two of our patients with proximal preceding lesions (cases I and II), the region of this lesion was not treated by sympatholysis (and did not show symptoms of RSD). This means that any possible afferent input from the lesioned site is of no importance for maintaining the vicious circle in RSD. This idea is supported by an additional important observation. In one of our patients (case III, see also below), the vicious circle including the RSD-type pain was stopped, despite persisting nociceptive input from the site of the preceding lesion. The hypothesis takes this into account, stating that the vicious circle in RSD, once initiated, becomes independent of the site (and type)

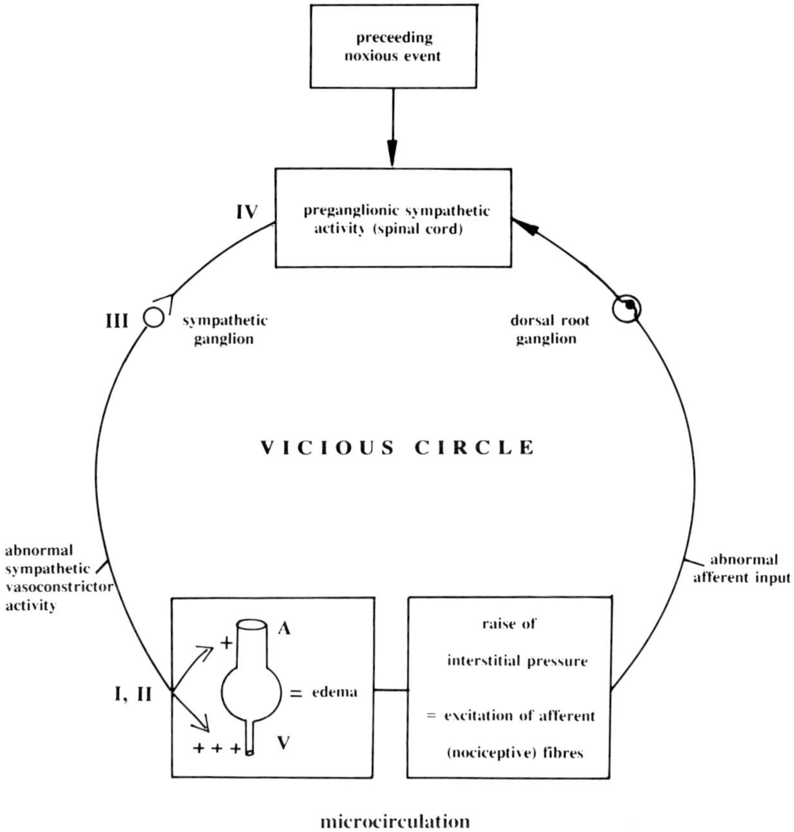

Fig. 4. Hypothesis on the sympathetic contribution to the edema in RSD. Following a noxious event, an abnormal sympathetic discharge pattern develops centrally. Peripherally, this generates edema via an increased level of veno-vasoconstriction compared with the level of arterio-vasoconstriction, leading to reduced venous return. The associated increase in interstitial pressure activates afferent (nociceptive) fibers. The resulting abnormal afferent input by reflex maintains the abnormal sympathetic outflow. A vicious circle has been initiated (for details see text). This vicious circle can be interrupted by sympathetic blocks applied at various sites (I–IV; the numbers also refer to case reports above). A = arteriole; V = venule.

of preceding lesion which may—or may not—produce any afferent (nociceptive) input.

The suggested abnormal discharge pattern of sympathetic vasoconstrictor neurons may have disappeared after the vicious circle was interrupted. In other words, the peripheral therapeutic action has caused central neuronal changes (so called central desensitization). It is uncertain, however, which afferent neuronal event caused by this action (e.g., conduction block, increase or decrease of afferent activity) mediated such central changes in RSD.

Conduction block of afferent fibers can be ruled out in three of our cases. Neither guanethidine (as used in two of these cases) nor anesthetizing the stellate ganglion resulted in any signs of such a block of nerves or roots supplying the affected extremity. This was, however, a major side effect of treatment in the patient with spinal anesthesia (case IV). Thus, considering both types of sympatholytic strategies (with or without accompanying afferent fiber block), such a block as well as changes in afferent activity could be the relevant neuronal event to mediate the central changes in RSD.

Experimental evidence is lacking for both theories. Therefore, it also remains open as to which type of afferent fibers—nociceptive or non-nociceptive—may be involved in the possible changes in afferent activity as a consequence of sympatholysis in RSD.

Two of the cases presented also support the notion that spontaneous pain in RSD may be sympathetically mediated, since the typical pain (deep, diffuse, showing an orthostatic component) in these cases disappeared acutely after sympatholytic treatment. This is consistent with common experiences (for ref. see Bonica 1990). The hypothesis also offers an explanation for these findings, stating that the reduction of interstitial pressure accompanying the decrease in edema also reduces the excitation of nociceptors. However, because the two other patients who also suffered from severe edema did not complain (case I) or no longer complained (case IV) of spontaneous pain, this part of the hypothesis is questioned (Devor et al. 1991).

On the other hand, pain sensation in RSD does not necessarily have to be sympathetically mediated. Instead, it may be of other origins (e.g., associated nerve [root] compression or inflammation), or different kinds of pain might be present in a given case with RSD (Price et al. 1989). The latter possibility must be considered for one of our patients (case III), who suffered from pain with different characteristics: deep diffuse pain with an orthostatic component—the RSD type of pain—and localized pain, without such a component and showing a spatial connection to the skin lesions.

In this patient, the ischemia test and the sympathetic block influenced only the typical RSD-type pain. This indicates specific (sympathetic) mechanisms for this pain compared with the other (inflammatory) pain. This observation also indicates that the ischemia test, as well as the sympathetic block, may provide information about a sympathetic pain mechanism. Indeed, in a systematic diagnostic study on the behavior of the pain in RSD, the pain was only relieved by a guanethidine block if it was also suppressed by the ischemia test. Accordingly, both kinds of interventions resulted in about the same degree of pain relief (Blumberg and Hoffmann 1994).

SUMMARY

This chapter introduces the clinical phenomenology of RSD, with edema as one of its leading symptoms. To demonstrate the effect of various sympatholytic strategies on this edema, which has never been done before, four representative cases of RSD were illustrated. In all four cases, immediate and lasting relief of the edema was achieved by this kind of treatment. Possible mechanisms underlying the generation of this edema and its relief are discussed. A hypothesis of a major role of the sympathetic nervous system is presented. As part of a vicious circle in RSD, which is initiated by its preceding lesion, abnormal sympathetic activity induces increased vasoconstriction on the postcapillary side compared with the precapillary side. This leads to the edema in RSD, which causes an abnormal afferent (nociceptive) input. Centrally, this maintains the sympathetic changes. Sympatholytic interventions interrupt the vicious circle, which brings about immediate and lasting relief of the edema.

ACKNOWLEDGMENTS

This work was financed by the Bundesministerium für Forschung und Technologie, supporting an interdisciplinary study on the pathophysiology of the edema in RSD at our institution. We thank Annette Böger-Koch for her technical assistance and Gabriele Kinzer for typing the manuscript. A special thanks is given to Prof. Dr. W. Seeger, Head of the Department of Neurosurgery, University of Freiburg, for his support. We also thank Prof. W. Jänig, who made very valuable suggestions for improving the chapter.

REFERENCES

Bentley, J.B. and Hameroff, S.R., Diffuse reflex sympathetic dystrophy, Anaesthsiology, 53 (1980) 256–257.

Blumberg, H., Zur Entstehung und Therapie des Schmerzsyndroms bei der sympathischen Reflexdystrophie, Der Schmerz, 2 (1988) 125–143.

Blumberg, H., A new clinical approach for diagnosing reflex sympathetic dystrophy. In:. M.R. Bond, J.E. Charlton and C.J. Woolf (Eds.), Proceedings of the VIth World Congress on Pain. Pain Research and Clincial Management, Vol. 4. Elsevier, Amsterdam, 1991, pp. 395–403.

Blumberg, H. and Hoffmann, U., Der "Ischämie-Test": ein neues Verfahren in der klinischen Diagnostik der sympathischen Reflexdystrophie (Kausalgie, M.Sudeck), Der Schmerz, 6 (1992) 196-198.

Blumberg, H. and Hoffmann, U., Zur Diagnostik der sympathischen Reflexdystrophie: Vergleich von Ischämie-test und modifizierter Guanethidin-Blockade. Nervenarzt 6 (1994), in press.

Blumberg, H. and Jänig, W., Clinical manifestations of reflex sympathetic dystrophy and sympathetically maintained pain. In: P.D. Wall and R. Melzack (Eds.), Textbook of Pain, 3rd ed., Churchill Livingstone, Edinburgh, 1994, pp. 685–698..

Blumberg, H. Wakhloo, A.K., Hoffmann, U. and Wokalek, H., Die lokalisierte Form einer sympathischen Reflexdystrophie: ein Fallbericht, Der Schmerz, 6 (1993) 178–181.

Bonica, J.J., Causalgia and other reflex sympathetic dystrophies. In: J.J. Bonica (Ed.), The Management of Pain, 2nd ed., Lea and Febiger, Philadelphia, 1990, pp. 220-243.

Christensen, K., Jensen, E.M. and Noer, I., The reflex dystrophy syndrome: response to treatment with systemic corticosteroids, Acta Chir. Scand., 148 (1982) 653–655.

Davidoff, G., Morey, K., Amann, M. and Stamps, J., Pain measurement in reflex sympathetic dystrophy syndrome, Pain, 32 (1988) 27–34.

Denko, C.W. and Petricevic, M., Sympathetic or reflex footpad swelling due to crystal-induced inflammation in the opposite foot, Inflammation, 3 (1978) 81–86.

Deuschl, G., Blumberg, H. and Lücking, C.H., Tremor in reflex sympathetic dystrophy, Arch. Neurol., 48 (1991) 1247–1252.

Devor, M., Basbaum, A.J., Bennett, G.J., Blumberg, H., Campbell, C.N., Dembowsky, K.P., Guilbaud, G., Jänig, W., Koltzenburg, M., Levine, J.D., Otten, U.H. and Portenoy, R.K., Mechanisms of neurophatic pain following peripheral injury. In: A.J. Basbaum and J.-M. Besson (Eds.), Towards a new pharmacotherapy of pain. Dahlem workshop reports, J. Wiley and Sons, Chichester, 1991, pp. 417–440.

Gracely, R.H., Lynch, S. and Bennett, G.J., Ischemic block of large fiber function in reflex sympathetic dystrophy: a paradox, Soc. Neuro. Sci. Abstr., 16 (1990) 1280.

Hainsworth, R., Vascular capacitance: its control and importance, Rev. Physiol. Biochem. Pharmacol., 105 (1986) 101–173.

Handwerker, H.O. and Reeh, P.W., Pain and inflammation. In: M.R. Bond, J.E. Charlton and C.J. Woolf (Eds.), Proceedings of the VIth World Congress on Pain. Pain Research and Clinical Management, Vol. 4. Elsevier, Amsterdam, 1991, pp. 59–70.

Hannington-Kiff, J.G., Intravenous regional sympathetic blocks. In: J.G. Stanton-Hicks, W. Jänig and R.A. Boas (Eds.), Reflex sympathetic dystrophy, Kluwer Academic, Boston, 1989, pp.113–124

Hannington-Kiff, J.G., Sympathetic nerve blocks in painful limb disorders. In: P.D. Wall and R. Melzack (Eds.), Textbook of Pain, 3rd ed., Churchill Livingstone, Edinburgh, 1994, pp. 1035–1051.

Hoffmann, U. and Blumberg, H., Modifikationen der Guanethidin-Blockade zur Diagnostik der sympathischen Reflexdystrophie, Der Schmerz, 8 (1994), in press.

Hottenstein, O.D. and Kreulen, D.L., Comparison of the frequency dependence of venous and arterial responses to sympathetic nerve stimulation in guinea-pig, J. Physiol., 384 (1987) 153–167.

Jänig, W., Causalgia and reflex sympathetic dystrophy: in which way is the sympathetic nervous system involved? TINS, 8 (1985) 471–477.

Jänig, W., The sympathetic nervous system in pain: physiology and pathophysiology. In: M. Stanton-Hicks (Ed.), Pain and the Sympathetic Nervous System, Kluwer Academic, Boston, 1990, pp. 17–89.

Jänig, W. and Schmidt, F.R., Reflex Sympathetic Dystrophy: Pathophysiological Mechanisms and Clinical Implications, VCH, Weinheim, 1992.

Jänig, W., Blumberg, H., Boas, R.A. and Campbell, J.A., The reflex sympathetic dystrophy syndrome: consensus statement and general recommendations for diagnosis and clinical reseach. In: M.R. Bond, J.E. Charlton and C.J. Woolf (Eds.), Proceedings of the VIth World Congress on Pain. Pain Research and Clinical Management, Vol. 4. Elsevier, Amsterdam, 1991, pp. 372–375

Kozin, F., McCarty, D.J., Sims, J. and Genant, H., The reflex sympathetic dystrophy syndrome. I. Clinical and histologic studies: evidence of bilateral response to corticosteroids and articular involvement, Am. J. Med., 60 (1976) 321–331.

Lankford, L.L., Reflex sympathetic dystrophy. In: G.E. Ohmer and M. Spinner (Eds.), Manage-

ment of Peripheral Nerve Problems, Saunders, Philadelphia, 1980, pp. 216–244.
Levine, J.D., Dardick, S.J., Basbaum, A.I. and Scipio, E., Reflex neurogenic inflammation. I. Contribution of the peripheral nervous system to spatially remote inflammatory responses that follow injury, J. Neurosci., 5 no. 5 (1985) 1380–1386.
Loh, L., Nathan, P.W. and Schott, G.D., Pain due to lesions of central nervous system removed by sympathetic block, BMJ, 282 (1981) 1026–1028.
Mellander, S., Comparative studies on the adrenergic neuro-hormonal control of restistance and capacitance blood vessels in the cat, Acta Physiol. Scand., 50 Suppl. 176 (1960) 1–86.
Merskey, H. (Ed.), Classification of chronic pain, Pain, Suppl. 3 (1986) S216–S222.
Price, D.D., Bennett, G.J. and Raffii, A., Psychophysical observations on patients with neuropathic pain relieved by a sympathetic block, Pain, 36 (1989) 273–288.
Schwartzmann, R.J. and McLellan, T.L., Reflex sympathetic dystrophy, Arch. Neurol., 44 (1987) 555–561.
Stanton-Hicks, R.J., Jänig, W. and Boas, R.A., Reflex sympathetic dystrophy, Kluwer Academic, Boston, 1989.
Szolcsány, E., Pintér, E. and Pethö, G., Role of unmyelinated afferents in regulation of microcirculation and its chronic distortion after trauma and damage. In: W. Jänig and R.F. Schmidt (Eds.), Reflex sympathetic dystrophy: pathophysiolgical mechanisms and clinical implications, VCH, Weinheim, 1992.

Correspondence to: PD Dr. med. Helmut Blumberg, Neurochirurgische Klinik der Universität Freiburg, Hugstetter Str. 55, 79106 Freiburg, Germany. Tel: 49-761-270-5027; Fax: 49-761-553-521.

Proceedings of the 7th World Congress on Pain,
Progress in Pain Research and Management, Vol. 2,
edited by G.F. Gebhart, D.L. Hammond, and T.S.
Jensen, IASP Press, Seattle, © 1994.

33

Pathophysiological Spectrum of Organic and Psychogenic Disorders in Neuropathic Pain Patients Fitting the Description of Causalgia or Reflex Sympathetic Dystrophy

José L. Ochoa,[a] Renato J. Verdugo,[b]
and Mario Campero[a]

[a]*Departments of Neurology and Neurosurgery, Good Samaritan Hospital and Oregon Health Sciences University, Portland, Oregon, USA, and*
[b]*Department of Neurological Sciences, Faculty of Medicine, Universidad de Chile, Santiago, Chile*

INTRODUCTION

Patients with chronic painful syndromes featuring variable combinations of spontaneous pains, mechanical or thermal hyperalgesias, cutaneous hypoesthesia, muscle weakness, spasms, and vasomotor changes are usually qualified as neuropathic and are categorized under the purely descriptive diagnostic terms of causalgia and reflex sympathetic dystrophy (RSD). We prefer to define these patients with a term that simply reiterates the clinical components without presuming pathophysiological significance: *Chronic pains* (plural) associated with various (and variable) combinations of negative and positive *sensory, motor, and, vasomotor* phenomena (much less so sudomotor). This lengthy description calls for an acronym: CPSMV (Ochoa 1993).

We analyzed a series of 270 rigorously evaluated CPSMV patients referred to the Neuromuscular Unit, Good Samaritan Hospital (GSH) & Medical Center and Oregon Health Sciences University, Portland, Oregon. Our study population included 168 females (62.2%) and 102 males (37.7%); 12–82 years of age (mean 43 years). Behind the relatively monotonous clinical profile expressed by these patients, there may exist any of multiple possible primary pathophysiological derangements at the peripheral or central nervous system level, certainly inclusive of the brain-mind. It is unfortunate that the spectrum of pathophysiological mechanisms that may operate in these patients often is not recognized. Encouraged by current diagnostic classifications, they undergo scores of (sometimes mutilating) ineffective therapies. Such classifications, which are based on simplistic overinterpretation of clinical phenomena and are equivocally assumed to be supported by ad-hoc animal models of organic neuropathy, typically carry a gratuitous pathophysiological connotation.

SOCIOECONOMIC AND HEALTH IMPACT

Our study population illustrates the socioeconomic impact of CPSMV: a work-related injury triggered the painful syndrome in 172 patients (63.7%) and 119 (44.1%) were receiving worker's compensation benefits at the time of evaluation. Furthermore, 49 patients (18.1%) were involved in court litigation related to the painful syndrome. At the time of first consultation to our department the mean duration of illness as measured from the onset of symptoms was 41.4 months for the 270 patients. Before evaluation at GSH these patients had consulted an average of 17 doctors each and had been given multiple diagnoses. Significant previous therapies included TENS unit, which gave transient partial relief in only 3 of 74 patients. Different modalities of physical therapy were given to 183 patients (67.7%), but only 8 obtained useful partial relief, and just transiently. One hundred and forty patients (51.9%) had undergone some ineffective surgery, including 12 patients (4.4%) who had sympathectomies. Sympathetic blocks were given to 69 patients (26.%), with partial and typically transient relief in two thirds.

CLINICAL APPROACH

Clinical evaluation of these patients at Good Samaritan Hospital included a detailed medical and social history followed by a thorough general and neurological examination. Fig. 1 summarizes key manifestations of the painful syndrome. Patients frequently reported subjective manifestations that could not be corroborated through examination. This observation was particularly striking for swelling of the affected segment and for changes in skin tempera-

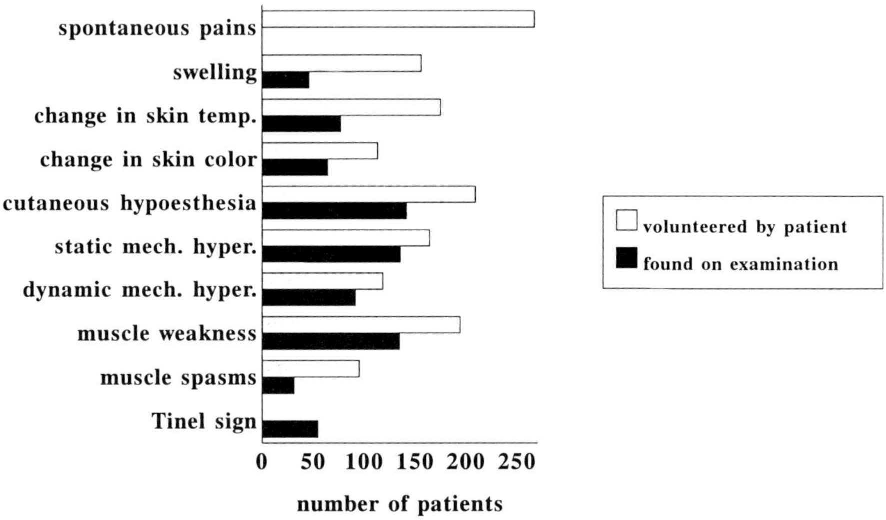

Fig. 1. Frequency distribution of the main clinical symptoms and signs in 270 patients with chronic pains associated with combinations of positive and negative sensory, motor, and vasomotor phenomena (CPSMV), fitting the descriptive terms of causalgia and RSD. Mech = mechanical; hyper = hyperalgesia.

ture, anomalies that were found on examination in less than half the patients who reported them. This discrepancy suggests either that these symptoms are paresthetic or, alternatively, that they emanate from a distorted body image perceived at brain-mind level. Cutaneous hypoesthesia was found on examination in 141 patients (52.2%), but it followed a normal anatomical distribution, as classically described for peripheral nerves and roots, in only 72 of them (51%). Mechanical hyperalgesia was also a frequent finding; it followed normal anatomical distribution in only 70 patients (46%). In all patients who reported nonanatomical areas of hypoesthesia or mechanical hyperalgesia, we also tested the whole spectrum of sensory and motor pathways through a multidisciplinary approach to find evidence of absence of nerve injury behind the complaints.

LABORATORY

After clinical evaluation, patients went through the following laboratory protocol. Conventional sensory and motor nerve conduction, needle EMG, and somatosensory evoked potentials were measured for evaluation of function of large-caliber afferent pathways and motor fibers (Kimura 1989). A quantitative somatosensory thermotest (QST) was administered to evaluate noninvasively the function of small-caliber afferent pathways (Fruhstorfer et al. 1976; Verdugo and Ochoa 1992a). Thermography and laser Doppler capillary flowmetry allowed evaluation of function of vasomotor sympathetic fibers and possible antidromic vasodilation (Pulst and Haller 1981; Ochoa 1986; Jones 1987; Cline et al. 1989; Triplett and Ochoa 1990; Thomas and Ochoa 1993). Placebo-controlled diagnostic somatic nerve block was a critically useful test to investigate the origin and mechanisms of pains (Boas and Cousins 1988; Verdugo and Ochoa 1993; submitted). Blocks were always combined with thermography for objective specification of the patient's private vasoconstrictor nerve territories (Campero et al. 1993; Verdugo and Ochoa 1993). Placebo-controlled diagnostic IV phentolamine sympathetic block (Raja et al. 1991; Verdugo and Ochoa 1994a) was another critical test applied to assess the hypothetical presence of sympathetically maintained pain. Microneurography and intraneural microstimulation were administered to qualified patients to explore abnormal neurological mechanisms of positive sensory phenomena (Torebjörk and Ochoa 1980; Ochoa and Torebjörk 1980; Ochoa et al. 1982; Cline et al. 1989; Burke 1992). We also performed compression-ischemia differential nerve block in some patients to determine the type of fibers mediating certain clinical manifestations (Campbell et al. 1988; Ochoa et al. 1989; Yarnitsky and Ochoa 1990; Ochoa and Yarnitsky 1993).

PATHOPHYSIOLOGICAL CATEGORIES

At the end of such a comprehensive evaluation we identified an organic neuropathic lesion as the cause of the complaints in 92 patients (34.1%), whereas we documented evidence of absence of nerve injury that might have caused the symptoms in 149 (55.2%) of these neuropathic patients. In the remaining 29 (10.7%) we detected organic neuropathy, but these lesions could not possibly account for a disproportionate assortment of major complaints.

Among the patients with nerve injury, we identified several distinct pathophysiological categories.

SENSITIZATION OF PERIPHERAL C-NOCICEPTORS

The syndrome of sensitization of peripheral polymodal nociceptors (ABC syndrome; Ochoa 1986; Cline and Ochoa 1986; Cline et al. 1989) was identified in four patients (1.5%) (three women, one man; 43 to 69 years, average 55.5). Only two had been previously evaluated by a neurologist even when their painful syndrome had lasted an average of 6.9 years at the time of the evaluation at the Neuromuscular Unit. The painful syndrome involved both feet in three patients who harbored a predominantly sensory neuropathy, and the radial dorsum of the hand in another patient. All four patients complained of the characteristic spontaneous burning pain and mechanical hyperalgesia; in three patients both symptoms were worsened by exposure to heat.

At the time of examination three patients had static mechanical hyperalgesia and one also expressed dynamic mechanical hyperalgesia. In all, mechanical hyperalgesia followed classic anatomical distribution consistent with a peripheral polyneuropathy (three patients) or with superficial radial nerve dysfunction (one patient). In all four patients the skin temperature of the symptomatic segment was abnormally increased, and three exhibited characteristic reddish discoloration. All four showed evidence of available vasomotor sympathetic activity as measured by changes in thermal emission profile or laser Doppler capillary flowmetry in response to reflex maneuvers, or as shown by further warming of the skin after anesthetic block of a nerve supplying the symptomatic segment. The QST showed hypoesthesia to warm stimuli in all four patients, associated with heat hyperalgesia in three, in keeping with sensitization of C-polymodal nociceptors (Cline and Ochoa 1986; Cline et al. 1989; Verdugo and Ochoa 1992a). Routine electrophysiological study was normal in two patients and revealed axonal impairment of large caliber afferent fibers in two. The sural nerve biopsy of these last two patients confirmed an axonal polyneuropathy affecting myelinated and unmyelinated fibers. Microneurographic recording was performed in two patients, it showed sensitization of polymodal C-nociceptors in one, and was inconclusive in the other. Another case of sensitization of C-nociceptors was documented microneurographically soon after the closure of this series (Ochoa, Serra, and Campero, unpublished data).

TRIPLE COLD SYNDROME

Eight patients had probable central release of primary afferent input in response to low temperature (Triple Cold Syndrome, Ochoa and Yarnitsky 1990, 1994). This group included five women and three men, 48 to 80 years of age (mean 60.6 years). All eight patients complained of spontaneous pain, described as burning in four, as dull ache in four and as shooting pains superimposed on a constant pain in three. All patients also reported mechanical hyperalgesia. In four patients in this group, exposure to cold clearly worsened the symptoms, and skin temperature was abnormally hypothermic in four patients. Cutaneous hypoesthesia was shown in seven patients, always following anatomical distribution. Mechanical hyperalgesia was shown in four patients, two of the static and two of the dynamic subtype (Ochoa and Yarnitsky

1993). The QST showed clear-cut cold hyperalgesia in four patients and paradoxical hot burning sensation in response to low temperature stimulation in all eight patients. The cause of the neurological disease behind the syndrome was a sensory polyneuropathy in seven patients and a thalamic stroke in one.

ECTOPIC GENERATION OF IMPULSES

The group of patients with nerve injury in whom abnormal ectopic generation (or ephaptic transmission) of nerve impulses was assessed to be the cause of the painful syndrome is likely heterogeneous: more than one primary abnormal biophysical mechanism probably will be identified for them in the future. These 80 patients (39 women, 41 men; 20 to 82 years of age, mean 48.2 years) expressed varied combinations of spontaneous pains, mechanical and thermal hyperalgesias, cutaneous hypoesthesia, muscle weakness, and changes in color and temperature of the skin. They all had clear evidence of an organic peripheral nerve injury documented through nerve conduction study (53 patients), needle EMG (17 patients), QST patterns that were consistent upon repetition and in keeping with peripheral nerve dysfunction (56 patients, Verdugo and Ochoa 1992a), and thermograms in keeping with antidromic discharges of C-nociceptors, recent sympathetic vasomotor denervation, or sympathetic denervation supersensitivity (28 patients).

ABSENCE OF NERVE INJURY BEHIND THE COMPLAINTS

The remaining patients, the majority, had absolute evidence of absence of neuropathic organic disorder (149 patients, 55.2%) or had a minor neuropathic lesion that could not possibly account for many complaints (29 patients, 10.7%) that were not anatomically or physiologically commensurate. In 117 neuropathic patients (78.5%) with evidence of absence of nerve injury, the painful syndrome was triggered by a work-related injury; 104 (70%) were on worker's compensation benefits at the time of evaluation and 40 (26.8%) were in court litigation. Like the patients with documented nerve injury, these pseudoneuropathic patients also complained of various combinations of spontaneous pains (of burning causalgic quality in 33.6% of patients), dynamic and static mechanical hyperalgesias, changes in color and temperature of the skin, swelling, cutaneous hypoesthesia, muscle weakness, and spasms.

The clinical presentation of these patients closely resembled the clinical picture of patients with nerve injury, even in certain objective findings such as mild swelling of the symptomatic parts (18 patients, 12%), mild abnormalities of the color of the skin (30 patients, 20.1%), or local hypothermia as shown by thermography (33 patients, 33.1%). Nevertheless, laboratory evaluation invariably showed complete normality of function of a wide spectrum of peripheral nerve fibers. Conventional sensory and motor conduction studies obtained in 146 patients were always normal for the nerves serving the symptomatic areas, and the same applied for needle EMG. QST, done in all patients, showed normal patterns, or inconsistent abnormalities not in keeping with neuropathic injuries (Verdugo and Ochoa 1992a). Thermography (141 patients) and laser Doppler capillary flowmetry (132 patients) always showed normality of vasomotor sympathetic reactivity even in those 33 patients who had a hypothermic symptomatic part at baseline. Additionally, these patients showed some bizarre phenomena that were observed only in this group, most of which amounted to positive evidence of nonorganic origin of the apparent neuromuscular complaints:

1. Although on examination cutaneous hypoesthesia was found in 102 patients (68.5%), the areas of light touch and pinprick deficit expanded beyond anatomical textbook territories for peripheral nerves and roots in 86 patients (84.3%). This phenomenon was never observed in patients with documented nerve injury. Furthermore, while blindfolded, some patients punctually signaled with a "no" every tactile stimulus applied to the hypoesthetic or anesthetic part.

2. Dynamic or static mechanical hyperalgesia was found in 74 patients. In 58 (78.4%) the areas of mechanical hyperalgesia expanded beyond normal anatomical peripheral nerve territories, a phenomenon that is not observed in patients with documented nerve injury (Campero et al. 1992; Campero and Ochoa, submitted).

3. Needle EMG showed interrupted voluntary effort, in the absence of pain, in 49 patients (62% of patients who had EMG)—again a phenomenon not observed in patients with documented nerve injury.

4. Injection of saline close to the area of maximal pain, or lidocaine block of a nerve serving the area of pain, resulted in spectacular and organically unexplainable reversal of profound cutaneous hypoesthesia in 20 patients. In many patients relief of muscle weakness also was recorded. These behaviors were not observed in patients with documented nerve injury.

All these phenomena indicate that the clinical picture of most patients with neuropathic pain with sensory, motor, and autonomic manifestations, but without nerve injury, is specific and defines the disorder as a pseudoneuropathy of psychogenic origin (Ochoa 1993). Although recently it has been argued that perhaps subtle nerve injuries not detectable by the available diagnostic methods may be causing the complaints of these patients (Drummond et al. 1993; Gracely et al. 1992), such hypothetical microneuromas cannot account for any of the above listed manifestations. Besides, according to Drummond et al. (1993) microneuromas also are found in asymptomatic areas; thus, they probably have no pathophysiological role.

PLACEBO

To properly interpret responses to diagnostic/therapeutic interventions, such as local somatic and sympathetic nerve blocks, it is essential to keep in mind the high incidence of inert placebo response observable in chronic pain patients (Verdugo and Ochoa 1991, 1994b). In our study, 231 patients had subcutaneous injection of a few milliliters of saline close to the site of maximal pain for inert placebo control. A significant reduction of spontaneous pain (diminution of pain magnitude by 50% or more) was volunteered by 135 (57.7%) patients, which is in keeping with previous series (Verdugo and Ochoa 1991, 1994b). This high incidence of inert placebo response makes placebo control mandatory to validate interpretation of results of diagnostic-therapeutic procedures whose results rely heavily on the subjective reports of patients. In our study population we found no difference in the incidence of inert placebo response between patients with and without nerve injury; this finding affirms the concept that placebo response does not necessarily imply psychogenic origin for the complaints, although of course it does not rule it out either (see Ochoa 1993).

We administered local anesthetic nerve block of a nerve serving the area of maximal pain to 229 patients; 204 (89.1%) reported significant relief of pains during the block. Over and above the placebo response to an *inert* substance, it is essential to assess the possibility of an *active* placebo effect, a neglected phenomenon more difficult to evaluate. An active, or impure, placebo effect is the beneficial outcome of any active drug or procedure not obtained through specific mechanisms (Fellner 1958; Fingl and Woodbury 1965). In our study group we found evidence of an active placebo effect induced by a local anesthetic block in 121 patients (59.3% of those responding to a local nerve block). Criteria for operation of active placebo effect included: (1) relief of spontaneous pain and mechanical hyperalgesia beyond the area of lidocaine-induced hypoesthesia, even when no satisfactory nerve block was achieved, or when blocking a nerve not related to the area of pain; (2) normalization of areas of profound cutaneous *hypo*esthesia (Verdugo and Ochoa 1992b; Verdugo and Ochoa, submitted); (3) relief of muscle weakness, or relief of dystonia. In contrast to the inert placebo effect, active placebo effect was significantly greater among patients without nerve injury (95.6% of the lidocaine responders in this group) than among patients with nerve injury (27.2% of the responders).

The issue of placebo response is particularly relevant to sympathetic blocks. Diagnostic sympathetic blocks are routinely used in the clinic for diagnostic endorsement of sympathetically maintained pain, a concept circularly defined as "all pain syndromes that can be relieved by sympathetic blockade" (Treede et al. 1991). Unfortunately, sympathetic blocks are traditionally performed without placebo control. Furthermore, diagnostic-therapeutic procedures are usually carried out in such a way as "to maximize the placebo response" (Evans 1974), and there are no double-blind placebo-controlled observations to prove therapeutic usefulness of sympathetic blocks in nonvascular painful syndromes. Neither are there outcome studies on sympathectomy for treatment of patients with chronic neuropathic painful syndromes. Leriche (1928) himself denied its usefulness as early as 1928. Dotson et al. (1990) evaluated the clinical status of 30 neuropathic-RSD patients, concluding that "none of the thirty patients were permanently improved by diagnostic-therapeutic sympathetic blocks."

A recently published attempt to perform placebo control for phentolamine sympathetic diagnostic blocks (Raja et al. 1991) suffered flaws in the placebo phase. Specifically, the authors set a waiting period varying between 8 and 35 minutes (average 20 minutes), which, when tested, is not long enough (Verdugo et al. 1991; Verdugo and Ochoa 1994a; Blumberg, personal communication, 1993). When the placebo phase is extended to a minimum of 30 minutes, phentolamine by itself is no better than placebo for pain relief (Verdugo et al. 1991; Verdugo and Ochoa 1994a). Echoing our group discussion in Portland, Roberts himself, the author of the sympathetically maintained pain (SMP) hypothesis, also worries that the effect attributed by Raja et al. (1991) to phentolamine might simply be a placebo effect due to "too little time allowed for expression of placebo-induced pain relief prior to injection of phentolamine" (Roberts and Kramis 1992). Furthermore, double-blind administration of phenylephrine, before or after phentolamine infusion, not only failed to worsen the painful symptoms but led to an increase in the proportion of patients improved by the procedure, thus suggesting a cooperative active placebo effect (Verdugo and Ochoa 1994a).

Only a few studies have included placebo control for regional Bier's sympathetic blocks given to RSD patients (Glynn et al. 1981; Glynn and Jones 1990; McGlone et al. 1993). None showed convincing differences between control and active procedures. In our study population, placebo controlled phentolamine sympathetic block was administered to 96 patients, following a strict protocol that allowed at least 30 minutes of placebo phase (Verdugo and Ochoa 1994a). We found that 40 patients (41.7%) expressed significant inert placebo response and 26 patients (27.1%) appeared to be specific phentolamine responders. However, all the apparent responders simply sustained linearly a relief initiated during the inert placebo phase. There was no instance of legitimate phentolamine response and, therefore, not a single case of documented SMP occurred, although prior to their evaluation at Good Samaritan Hospital, two-thirds of 69 patients had experienced transient relief of pain after nonplacebo-controlled sympathetic block, and thus had been diagnosed in the illusory category of sympathetically maintained pain.

CONCLUSIONS

The analysis of these data allows the following conclusions:

1. Multiple organically based and psychogenically based neuropathic painful entities are diagnosable through objective multidisciplinary methods.
2. The differential diagnosis of these patients requires rigorous assessment through qualified clinical neurological evaluation and properly interpreted comprehensive laboratory testing.
3. Psychogenic pseudoneuropathy masquerades for organic disease. It is often misdiagnosed and labeled with the misleading term RSD.
4. The concept of sympathetically maintained pain becomes void when the criterion (response to sympathetic block) is corrected for inert and active placebo effect (Verdugo and Ochoa 1991, 1994a).
5. Conceptual chaos in this area deviates clinicians into misconstrued testing and aborted therapies (Ochoa 1994a).

ACKNOWLEDGMENTS

This study was supported by NIH grants numbers: RO1 NS 24766 and 28747

REFERENCES

Boas, R.A. and Cousins, M.J., Diagnostic Neural Blockade. In: M.J. Cousins and P.O. Bridenbaugh, (Eds.), Neural Blockade in Clinical Anesthesia and Management of Pain, 2nd ed., Lippincott, Philadelphia, 1988.

Burke, D., Microneurography, impulse conduction and paresthesias. Seventeenth Annual Edward

H. Lambert Lecture. American Association of Electrodiagnostic Medicine, Plenary Session II: Microneurography, 1992, pp 79–85.
Campbell, J.N., Raja, S.N., Meyer, R.A. and Mackinnon, S E., Myelinated afferents signal the hyperalgesia associated with nerve injury, Pain, 32 (1988) 89–94.
Campero, M., Ochoa, J.L. and Pubols, L., Receptive fields of hyperalgesia confine to districts of injured nerves; fields "expand" in "RSD" without nerve injury, Soc. Neurosci. Abstr., 18 (1992) 287.
Campero, M. and Ochoa, J.L., Areas of mechanical hyperalgesia in chronic neuropathic painful syndromes: clinical-pathophysiological dichotomy determined by presence and absence of nerve injury, (Submitted).
Campero, M., Verdugo, R.J. and Ochoa, J.L., Vasomotor innervation of the skin of the hand: a contribution to the study of human anatomy, J. Anat., 182 (1993) 361–368.
Cline, M. and Ochoa, J.L., Chronically sensitized C Nociceptors in skin. Patient with hyperalgesia, hyperpathia, and spontaneous pain, Soc. Neurosci. Abstr., 12 (1986) 331.
Cline, M.A., Ochoa, J.L. and Torebjörk, H.E., Chronic hyperalgesia and skin warming caused by sensitized C nociceptors, Brain, 112 (1989) 621–647.
Dotson, R., Ochoa, J.L., Cline, M.A. and Yarnitsky D., A reassessment of sympathetic blocks as long term therapeutic modality for "RSD," Pain, Suppl. 5 (1990) S490.
Drummond, P.D., Finch, P.M. and Gibbons, I.L., Microneuromas in reflex sympathetic dystrophy. In: Abstracts: 7th World Congress on Pain, IASP Publications, Seattle, 1993, pp 563–564.
Evans, F.J., The placebo response in pain reduction. In: J.J. Bonica, (Ed.), Advances in Neurology, Vol. 4, Pain, Raven Press, New York, 1974, pp 289–296.
Fellner, C.H., Tranquilizing drugs in general practice or the triumph of impure placebo, American Practitioner and Digest of Treatment, 9 (1958) 1265–1268.
Fingl, E. and Woodbury, D.M., General principles. In: L.S. Goodman and A. Gilman (Eds.), The Pharmacological Basis of Therapeutics, 3rd ed., MacMillan, New York, 1965, pp 1–36.
Fruhstorfer, H., Lindblom, U. and Schmidt, W.G., Method for quantitative estimation of thermal thresholds in patients, J. Neurol. Neurosurg. Psychiatry, 39 (1976) 1071–1075.
Glynn, C.J. and Jones, P., An investigation of the role of clonidine in the treatment of reflex sympathetic dystrophy, In: M. Stanton-Hicks, W. Jänig and R.A. Boas, (Eds.), Reflex Sympathetic Dystrophy, Kluwer Academic Publishers, Norwell, Mass., 1990, pp 187–196.
Glynn, C.J., Basedow, R.W. and Walsh, J.A., Pain relief following post-ganglionic sympathetic blockade with i.v. guanethidine, Br. J. Anesth., 53 (1981) 1297–1301.
Gracely, R.H., Lynch, S.A. and Bennett, C.J., painful neuropathy: altered central processing maintained dynamically by peripheral input, Pain, 51 (1992) 175–194.
Jones, D., Medical electro-optics: measurements in the human microcirculation, Phys. Technol., 18 (1987) 79–85.
Kimura, J., Electrodiagnosis in disease of nerve and muscle: principles and practice, F.A. Davis Company, Philadelphia, 1989.
Leriche, R., Surgery of the sympathetic system: indications and results, Ann. Surg., 88 (1928) 449–469.
McGlone, F., Dean, J. and Dhar, S., A sympathetic response to sympathetic block in RSD? In: Abstracts: 7th World Congress on Pain, IASP Publications, Seattle, 1993, p 350.
Ochoa, J.L., The newly recognized painful ABC syndrome: thermographic aspects, Thermology, 2 (1986) 65–107.
Ochoa, J.L., Essence, investigation and management of "neuropathic" pains: hopes from acknowledgement of chaos (Guest Editorial), Muscle and Nerve, 16 (1993) 997–1062.
Ochoa, J.L. and Torebjörk, H.E., Paresthesiae from ectopic impulse generation in human sensory nerves, Brain, 103 (1980) 835–853.
Ochoa, J.L. and Yarnitsky, D., Triple cold (CCC) painful syndrome, Pain, Suppl. 5 (1990) S278.
Ochoa, J.L. and Yarnitsky, D., Mechanical hyperalgesias in neuropathic pain patients: dynamic and static subtypes, Ann. Neurol., 33 (1993) 465–472.
Ochoa, J.L. and Yarnitsky, D., The Triple Cold (CCC) syndrome: cold hyperalgesia, cold

hypoesthesia and cold skin in peripheral nerve disease, Brain, 117 (1994) 185–197.
Ochoa, J.L., Torebjörk, H.E., Culp, W.J. and Schady, W., Abnormal spontaneous activity in single sensory nerve fibers in humans, Muscle and Nerve, 5 (1982) S74–S77.
Ochoa, J.L., Roberts, W.J., Cline, M.A., Dotson, R. and Yarnitsky, D., Two mechanical hyperalgesias in human neuropathy, Soc. Neurosci. Abstr., 15 (1989) 472.
Pulst, St.-M. and Haller, P., Thermographic assessment of impaired sympathetic function in peripheral nerve injuries, J. Neurol., 226 (1981) 35–42.
Raja, S.N., Treede, R.D., Davis, K. and Campbell, J.N., Systemic alpha-adrenergic blockade with phentolamine: a diagnostic test for sympathetically maintained pain, Anesthesiology, 74 (1991) 691–698.
Roberts, W.J. and Kramis, R.C., Adrenergic mediation of SMP: via nociceptive or non-nociceptive afferents or both? APS Journal, 1 (1992) 12–15.
Thomas, P.K. and Ochoa, J.L., Clinical features and differential diagnosis. In: P.J. Dyck, P.K. Thomas, J.W. Griffin, P.A. Low and J.F. Poduslo (Eds.), Peripheral Neuropathy, 3rd ed., WB Saunders, Philadelphia, 1993, pp 749–774.
Torebjörk, H.E. and Ochoa, J.L., Specific sensations evoked by activity in single identified sensory units in man, Acta Physiol. Scand., 110 (1980) 445–447.
Treede, R.D., Raja, S.N., Davis, K.D., Meyer, R.A. and Campbell, J.N., Evidence that peripheral alpha-adrenergic receptors mediate sympathetically maintained pain. In: M.R. Bond, J.E. Charlton and C.J. Woolf (Eds.), Proceedings of the VIth World Congress on Pain. Pain Research and Clinical Management, Vol. 4. Elsevier, Amsterdam, 1991, pp 377–382.
Triplett, B. and Ochoa, J.L., Contemporary techniques in assessing peripheral nervous system function, Am. J. EEG Technol., 30 (1990) 29–44.
Verdugo, R.J. and Ochoa, J.L., High incidence of placebo responders among chronic neuropathic pain patients, Ann. Neurol., 30 (1991) 229.
Verdugo, R.J. and Ochoa, J.L., Quantitative somatosensory thermotest: a key method for functional evaluation of small calibre afferent channels, Brain, 115 (1992a) 893–913.
Verdugo, R.J. and Ochoa, J.L., Hypoesthesia erased by somatic nerve block, or placebo: a pseudoneuropathic, psychogenic, sign in causalgia/RSD, Soc. Neurosci. Abstr., 18 (1992b) 287.
Verdugo, R.J. and Ochoa, J.L., Use and misuse of conventional electrodiagnosis, quantitative sensory testing, thermography and nerve blocks in the evaluation of painful neuropathic syndromes, Muscle and Nerve, 16 (1993) 1056–1062.
Verdugo, R.J. and Ochoa, J.L., Phentolamine sympathetic block questions the concept of "sympathetically maintained pain," I., Neurology, 44 (1994a), in press.
Verdugo, R.J. and Ochoa, J.L., Placebo response in chronic, causalgiform, "neuropathic" pain patients: study and review, Pain Reviews, 1 (1994b) 31–44.
Verdugo, R.J. and Ochoa, J.L., Reversal of hypoesthesia in response to nerve block, or placebo injection: a pseudoneuropathic sign, (submitted).
Verdugo, R.J., Rosenblum, S. and Ochoa, J.L., Phentolamine sympathetic blocks mislead diagnosis, Soc. Neurosci. Abstr., 17 (1991) 107.
Yarnitsky, D. and Ochoa, J.L., Release of cold-induced burning pain by block of cold specific afferent input, Brain, 113 (1990) 893–902.

Correspondence to: José L. Ochoa, DSc, MD, PhD, Neuromuscular Unit, Good Samaritan Hospital, 1040 NW 22nd, Suite 460, Portland, OR 97210, USA. Tel: 503-229-7294; Fax: 503-790-1201.

Proceedings of the 7th World Congress on Pain,
Progress in Pain Research and Management, Vol. 2,
edited by G.F. Gebhart, D.L. Hammond, and T.S.
Jensen, IASP Press, Seattle, © 1994.

34

Animal Models of Neuropathic Pain

Gary J. Bennett

Neurobiology and Anesthesiology Branch, National Institute of Dental Research, National Institutes of Health, Bethesda, Maryland, USA

INTRODUCTION

Human neuropathic pain syndromes are caused by trauma or disease-evoked damage to peripheral nerves, posterior roots, spinal cord, or to certain regions in the brain. These syndromes are characterized by several different kinds of abnormal pain sensations. Spontaneous pain is commonly present; it may be a continuous superficial burning pain, and/or a deep aching pain, or it may appear as episodic attacks of pain, which are often described as being like electric shocks. Abnormal evoked pains such as heat-, cold-, and mechano-hyperalgesia and heat-, cold-, and mechano-allodynia are also common and are frequently debilitating. In some cases the abnormal pains appear to be dependent on activity in the sympathetic nervous system, while in others they do not. The mechanisms responsible for neuropathic pains are poorly understood, and our ability to treat them is often unsatisfactory.

Clinical research on this problem is difficult. These are not common disorders, and statistically valid samples of patients homogenous for important variables (e.g., pain quality and severity, and responses to prior therapies) are difficult to obtain. Our progress in understanding these conditions and in discovering effective treatments would obviously be accelerated if the conditions could be produced in laboratory animals. The evidence reviewed below shows that we do have useful animal models for several neuropathic pain conditions. Work with these models has already made important contributions to our understanding and has given us new leads in our search for effective therapy. The tempo of this work is increasing rapidly, as shown clearly by the increase in the number of groundbreaking studies reported at the 7th World Congress on Pain compared to its predecessor three years ago. One can hope that at the next World Congress we will begin to see whether these laboratory studies will lead to the clinical advances that are our ultimate goal.

NEUROPATHIC PAIN FOLLOWING DAMAGE TO THE CENTRAL NERVOUS SYSTEM

The central pain syndromes in humans follow injury to certain parts of the brain and spinal cord. It is now clear that the so-called thalamic syndrome occurs with damage (usually from a cerebral vascular accident) in the thalamus, brainstem, or cortex. The common factor in these cases appears to be damage to some component of the spinothalamic system (Boivie et al. 1989; Leijon et al. 1989). There are relatively few studies of abnormal pain sensations in animals with comparable injuries. A notable exception is the dysesthesia syndrome that can be produced in monkeys (Levitt 1991).

Injuries confined to the spinal cord may give rise to particularly severe neuropathic pain. There are now two procedures for producing this in rats. The most extensively studied model is an experimental infarction of a short segment of the cord's superficial vasculature produced by laser excitation of a photosensitive dye, erythrosin B, which produces temporary vessel occlusion via a massive recruitment of platelets (Hao et al. 1991; Xu et al. 1992). Following such an episode of spinal ischemia, rats become extremely hypersensitive to touch in and around the affected dermatome, such that very gentle mechanical stimulation evokes vocalizations and avoidance behaviors. This mechano-allodynia is accompanied by increased sensitivity to cold. People with spinal cord damage complain of spontaneous pain or dysesthesia. It is not clear whether the rat model produces such sensations. An important series of pharmacological studies has shown that the mechano-allodynia is relatively resistant to opiates but is strongly suppressed by an antagonist of the cholecystokinin-B receptor (Xu et al. 1993).

Spinal cord injury resulting from intramedullary lesion has recently been modeled in the rat by intraspinal microinjection of the excitotoxin quisqualic acid (Yezierski and Park 1993). Such an injection produces intraspinal cavitation surrounded by degeneration, and the animals develop an extreme hypersensitivity to mechanical stimulation in and around the affected dermatome. Single unit analysis of spinal neurons adjacent to the lesion have shown markedly abnormal discharges following mechanical stimuli. There is a lowering of the cell's response threshold, and the stimuli evoke very prolonged afterdischarges. Increased levels of background spontaneous discharge are also found and may correspond to abnormal spontaneous sensations (pain and/or dysesthesia) in the awake animal. Work in mice (Defrin and Urca 1993) and rats (Wiesenfeld-Hallin et al. 1993) indicates a significant genetic contribution to the animal's susceptibility to abnormal pain following spinal cord injury.

Avulsion of the posterior roots, which commonly occurs with traumatic stretch injury to the upper limb, is often followed by intractable neuropathic pain. A similar condition can be produced in the rat by surgical transection of multiple dorsal roots. Rats with such an injury self-mutilate the deafferented limb (autotomy) and display several other behaviors indicative of abnormal pain sensations (Basbaum and Wall 1976; Albe-Fessard and Rampin 1991; Lombard and Besson 1991). In rhizotomized animals, somatosensory neurons in the spinal cord and thalamus develop obviously abnormal spontaneous discharges, including epileptiform bursting discharges. Identical abnormal discharges have been recorded in the spinal cord of a man whose roots were sectioned by an accident to the cauda equina (Loeser et al. 1967).

PAINFUL PERIPHERAL NEUROPATHIES DUE TO DISEASE

The most common neuropathic pain disorders due to peripheral nerve damage are caused by two diseases, shingles and diabetes.

Shingles is caused by reactivation of the varicella-zoster virus, which lies dormant within the nucleus of the primary afferent neuron's cell body (and/or the nuclei of its ensheathing satellite cells) following an attack of chicken pox. An attack of shingles is very painful, but in most cases the pain disappears as the cutaneous rash heals and the viral infection returns to its dormant state. In some people however, especially the elderly, abnormal spontaneous and evoked-pain sensations persist for months, years, and even decades after healing is complete. This is postherpetic neuralgia which is becoming increasingly common as medical advances prolong life into the later decades and as immunocompromised patients (e.g., those with organ transplantations and HIV infections) become more common. It is possible to infect animals with chicken pox and to establish a latent infection in the spinal ganglia, but it has not been possible to produce a reactivated infection like shingles. The absence of an animal model of postherpetic neuralgia is a serious deficiency.

Diabetic rodents are easily obtained. The inbred BB/Wistar strain of albino rat develops diabetes spontaneously. The so-called sand rat, actually a species of gerbil, develops diabetes when fed ordinary rat lab chow, which is highly caloric compared to the animal's natural desert-adapted diet. Diabetes can be produced easily by an injection of alloxan or streptozotocin, poisons that kill the insulin-secreting cells. Russell and Burchiel (1993) have demonstrated that the nerves of diabetic rats exhibit electrodiagnostic signs of sensory and autonomic neuropathy like those seen in humans, and that these signs develop despite attempts at good control over glucose levels. The hindpaws of diabetic rats have been shown to be allodynic to warmth and mechanical stimuli and to be hyperalgesic to noxious heat and pinch (Fig. 1; Courtiex et al. 1993; Wuarin-Bierman et al. 1987; Forman et al. 1986). There is evidence that the severity of the diabetic rat's pain syndrome is increased with uncontrolled hyperglycemia (Lee et al. 1990).

Ahlgren and her colleagues (Ahlgren et al. 1992, Ahlgren and Levine 1993a,b) have presented evidence showing that C-fiber nociceptors in diabetic rats have an abnormal hyper-responsiveness to prolonged high-intensity mechanical stimuli: they discharge more during the stimulus and have abnormally long afterdischarges. These abnormalities bear some resemblance to the ordinary nociceptor sensitization that occurs with tissue injury, but the differences are noteworthy. In the diabetic case there is no lowering of the response

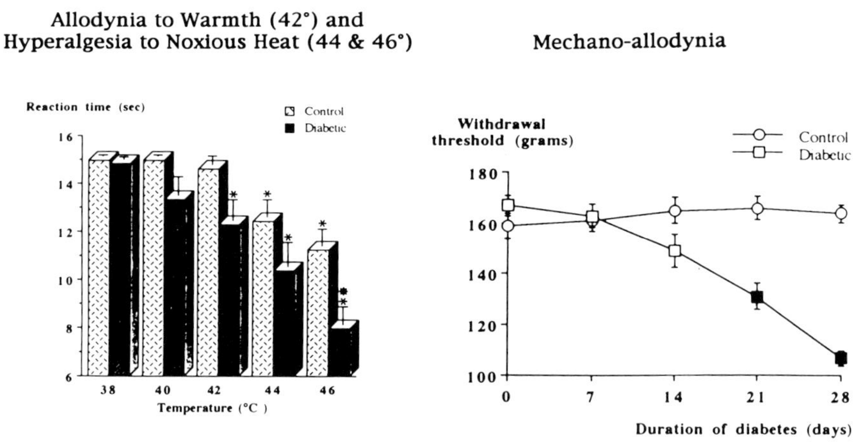

Fig. 1. Neuropathic pain sensations in rats made diabetic by an injection of streptozotocin. **Left:** Latencies of the nocifensive withdrawal reflex evoked by dipping the hindpaw in water of various temperatures. The control animals generally did not respond (relative to a 15 sec cutoff) to 38°, 40°, or 42° C water; these temperatures are thereby classified as non-noxious, and the withdrawal responses seen in the diabetic rats to the 42°C stimulus thus indicate the presence of warm-allodynia. The 44° and 46°C stimuli were noxious to the control animals, and the diabetic rats' significantly shorter latencies thus indicate heat-hyperalgesia. **Right:** There was a statistically significant (filled symbols) reduction in the amount of force needed to evoke a withdrawal reflex at 21 and 28 days after the initiation of diabetes. These forces never evoked nocifensive responses in the control rats, and the diabetics' responses thus indicate the presence of mechano-allodynia. (Reprinted with permission from Courteix et al. 1993)

threshold and no spontaneous discharge. Moreover, ordinary receptor sensitization is mediated by stimulatory G-proteins, which regulate a cAMP-dependent protein kinase. The hyper-responsiveness of C-fiber nociceptors in the diabetic rat also involves a cAMP-dependent protein kinase (probably protein kinase C), but in this case it does not appear to be dependent on stimulatory G-proteins.

Hyper-responsiveness in C-fiber nociceptors is clearly pertinent to the stimulus-evoked pains of the diabetic patient, but it does not appear to explain the patient's ongoing spontaneous pain. It is well known that diabetic nerve damage involves a dying-back neuropathy, that is, a degeneration of the distal end of the peripheral axon. Nerve cells with long axons are especially susceptible (hence the typical burning feet of the diabetic patient). A neuron with a partial functional impairment may not be able to sustain a long axon, but as axonal die-back progresses, a point may be reached where the cell's remaining capacity is sufficient to sustain its axon at a less than normal length. Fluctuations in the underlying disease process will result in waves of die-back followed by attempted regeneration. We would therefore expect to find a diabetic neuropathy patient's affected nerves to contain the sprouts of axons attempting to regenerate. Dying-back afferents cannot be directly involved in stimulus-evoked pain abnormalities (they are no longer connected to their receptors), but they may be involved in the production of spontaneous pain. Axonal sprouts that end in neuromas are known to have spontaneous discharge (Devor 1989), and there is evidence for spontaneous discharge in the nerves of diabetic rats (Burchiel et al. 1985).

Recent pharmacological experiments show that diabetic rats, like human patients, obtain partial pain relief with tricyclic antidepressants that block norepinephrine reuptake (Bardin et al. 1993). Exciting new animal studies suggest that prolonged relief from diabetic neuropathy pain may be achieved safely with vapreotide, a long-lasting analog of the endogenous neuropeptide somatostatin (Fialip et al. 1993).

PAINFUL PERIPHERAL NEUROPATHIES DUE TO TRAUMA

The "neuroma model" (Wall et al. 1979) has yielded critically important information about pathogenic mechanisms in damaged primary afferent neurons (for review see Devor 1989). For example, animal studies with this model suggested, and clinical studies in humans with transected nerves confirmed, that spontaneous and evoked activity in primary afferent sprouts was a significant source of abnormal pain sensations. Animal studies have also shown that not only the sprout of the damaged afferent neuron, but also its cell body in the dorsal root ganglion (DRG) was a source of ectopic discharge. Moreover, it has been shown that the DRG source is particularly sensitive to the effects of local anesthetics at doses well below those that block ectopic discharge in sprouts, and that both the DRG and sprout sources are blocked by doses far below those that block impulse propagation (Devor et al. 1992). The recognition of this low-dose effect of local anesthetics suggests a likely mechanism of action for the therapeutic effects of other sodium channel blockers, like mexiletine.

More recent work with the neuroma model points to significant pathogenic mechanisms in the CNS. For example, Seltzer and his colleagues (1991) have shown that a few seconds of C-fiber–strength electrical stimulation of the nerve before it is cut, accelerates the onset of autotomy and increases its severity (Fig. 2). Importantly, these effects are not evident until days after-

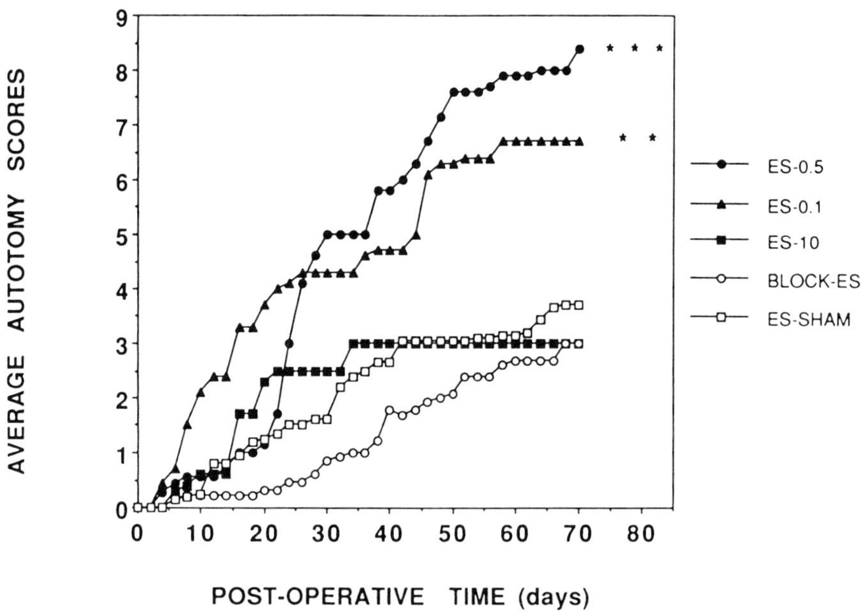

Fig. 2. The effects of primary afferent volleys just before sciatic nerve transection on the subsequent development of autotomy in the neuroma model. All groups marked "ES" received 150 nerve shocks just before transection. ES-0.5: shocks at 0.5 Hz, which produces the C-fiber–evoked wind-up effect. ES-0.1: shocks at 0.1 Hz, which produces a C-fiber volley after each shock. ES-10: shocks at 10 Hz; this frequency is too fast for C-fibers (but not A-fibers) to follow every shock and it thus yields less C-fiber input than the slower frequencies. Block-ES: shocks at 0.5 Hz, but with conduction blocked by bupivacaine pretreatment. ES-Sham: electrodes placed on the nerve, but no shocks delivered. Conditioning stimulation that produced large and consistent C-fiber volleys (ES-0.5 and ES-0.1) significantly decreased the time to onset and increased the severity of autotomy. **, *** significantly different compared to ES-Sham. (Reprinted with permission from Seltzer et al. 1991)

ward, indicating that the conditioning stimulation creates a persistent CNS effect that is not manifest until some other event occurs (in this case, probably the onset of primary afferent ectopic spontaneous discharge). Conversely, Feria and his colleagues (1993) have shown that a subcutaneous injection of magnesium at the time of the nerve transection retards the onset of autotomy and decreases its severity. Again, this is an effect that is not manifest until days afterwards. These and other studies in different nerve injury models show that the old question about painful neuropathy, Is it peripheral or is it central?, misses the point: peripheral *and* central mechanisms are of fundamental importance.

The perceptual consequences of the nerve injury in the neuroma model are inferred from the animal's self-inflicted damage to the denervated body part. It is reasonable to hypothesize that this behavior is the animal's response to the ongoing pain that humans describe in a phantom limb. This is, however, an inference, and definitive proof is lacking and perhaps unattainable. More importantly, the human conditions that interest us include those where there is at least some sparing of the innervation and where allodynic and hyperalgesic pains evoked from the periphery are major components of the patient's complaint. There are now several rat models of abnormal pain conditions after experimental nerve injuries that do not produce complete denervations (Table I).

It is important to note that these models are not redundant; the symptoms that they produce appear to differ in important ways (Table I), and this is probably due to different injuries producing different pathogenic mechanisms. For example, the partial nerve ligation model (PNL) of Seltzer and his colleagues (1990) and the spinal nerve transection (SNT) model introduced by Kim and Chung (1992) produce heat-hyperalgesia on both sides (greatest ipsilaterally), whereas contralateral heat-hyperalgesia is minor or absent in the chronic constriction injury (CCI; Bennett and Xie 1988; Attal et al. 1990). There are also several examples of particular symptoms being absent in a given model. Heat-hyperalgesia (ipsilateral) is prominent in the CCI, PNL, SNT, and peripheral neuritis models, but it is absent in the cryoneurolysis model. In contrast, the freeze injury yields a pronounced mechano-allodynia that is absent in the peripheral neuritis model. Additional evidence shows that sympathetically maintained pain is prominent in some models but not in others. The CCI model's abnormal pain sensations are only partly dependent on the sympathetic nervous system, and even this partial dependency is seen only in the first few days after the injury (Bennett and Xie 1988; Perrot et al. 1993). In the PNL and SNT models however, the abnormal pain symptoms are completely reversed by sympathectomy, even when the intervention is

Table I
Nerve injury models producing abnormal pain sensations

Model	Symptom						
	Spont	Auto	M-hyper	M-allo	H-hyper	C-allo	Lat
Collateral hyperalgesia (Markus et al. 1984)	?	+	+	+	?	?	uni
Chronic constriction injury (CCI) (Bennett and Xie 1988)	+	+*	+	+	+	+	uni†
Partial nerve ligation (PNL) (Seltzer et al. 1990)	+	–	+	+	+	–	bi
Spinal nerve transection (SNT) (Kim and Chung 1992)	+	–	?	+	+	+	bi
Peripheral neuritis (Maves et al. 1993a,b)	?	–	–	–	+	?	uni
Cryoneurolysis (DeLeo et al. 1994)	?	+	?	+	–	?	bi

Note: +, evidence that symptom is present; –, tested and not found; ?, no evidence; Spont, evidence, other than the presence of autotomy, for spontaneous pain or dysesthesia; Auto, autotomy; M-hyper, (mechano-hyperalgesia; M-allo, mechano-allodynia; H-hyper, heat-hyperalgesia; C-allo, cold-allodynia; Lat, laterality; uni, unilateral/ipsilateral; bi, definite symptoms on contralateral side.
* Autotomy is minor (confined mostly to the roots and claws) and present in a small minority
† One laboratory finds a relatively mild degree of contralateral heat-hyperalgesia and mechano-allodynia in a small percentage of cases.

done many weeks or months after the nerve injury (Shir and Seltzer 1991; Kim et al. 1993).

All of the models listed in Table I involve the sciatic nerve and produce abnormal pain in the hindpaw. The CCI injury has also been applied to the infraorbital nerve which produces abnormal pain sensations on the face, including the whisker pad (Vos and Maciewicz 1991; Kawamoto et al. 1993). Maves and his colleagues (1993a,b) have shown that an inflammation of the nerve sheath that causes little or no damage to the axons within the nerve can produce heat-hyperalgesia (but not mechano-hyperalgesia) that lasts for a week or two. It may be more appropriate to consider this as a model of a neuritis, rather than a model of nerve damage; although inflammation of the nerve sheath is likely to be a component of nerve damage due to trauma or disease (especially shingles). Cryoneurolysis is sometimes used to treat painful peripheral neuropathy, and rarely does it appear to create or worsen pain. It is thus interesting that nearly all rats receiving a freeze injury to the sciatic nerve exhibit autotomy and mechano-allodynia (DeLeo et al. 1994; Willenbring et al. 1993).

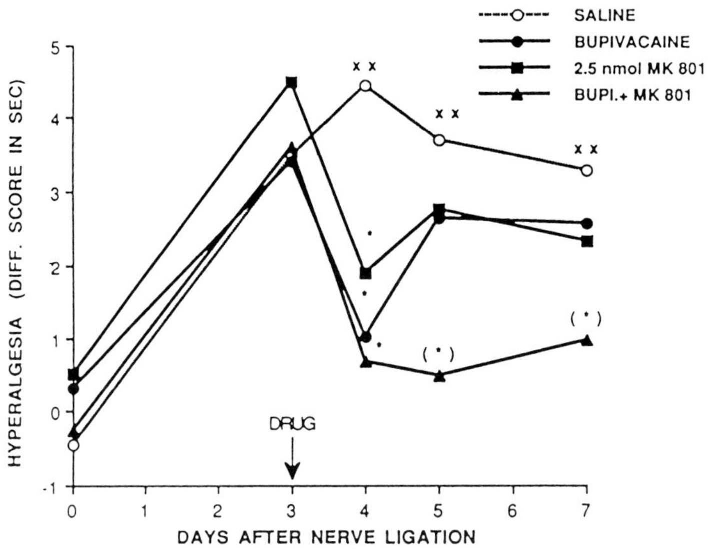

Fig. 3. The effects of a local anesthetic block (bupivacaine on the injured nerve proximal to the lesion), an intrathecal injection of an NMDA receptor antagonist (MK801), and the block and intrathecal injection combined, on heat-hyperalgesia in CCI rats. Prior to nerve injury (day 0), the difference between the latencies of the nocifensive withdrawal reflexes on both sides were not significantly different from zero, i.e., the pain thresholds were equal on the two hindpaws. Three days after creating the CCI, the latency (pain threshold) on the nerve-injured side is significantly shorter than on the control side, indicating the presence of heat-hyperalgesia. Drug treatments were given immediately after the test on day 3, and the animals were examined at 24-hour intervals thereafter. Saline injection had no effect. Local anesthetic block reduced heat-hyperalgesia 24 hours later (long after impulse conduction block had gone); an intrathecal injection of MK801 did the same (again, long after the expected duration of the pharmacological effect). Giving the NMDA antagonist and the nerve block simultaneously yielded at least 4 days of pain relief. * $P < 0.05$ compared to saline group; (*) $P < 0.05$ compared to each of the other three groups; ** $P < 0.01$ significant main effect in ANOVA. (Reprinted with permission from Mao et al. 1992b.)

It has been known for many years that afferents in intact neighboring nerves will emit collateral sprouts and invade the territory of a nerve that has been completely transected. Markus and his colleagues (1984) were the first to show that the collaterally innervated territory is the source of abnormal pain sensations. Attempts to explain this pain on the basis of the response properties of the collateral sprouts (and their de novo receptor innervation) have been unsuccessful; it is possible that the phenomenon is largely of central origin (Kingery et al. 1989). It would be of great interest to know whether collateral sprouts also invade a partially denervated territory.

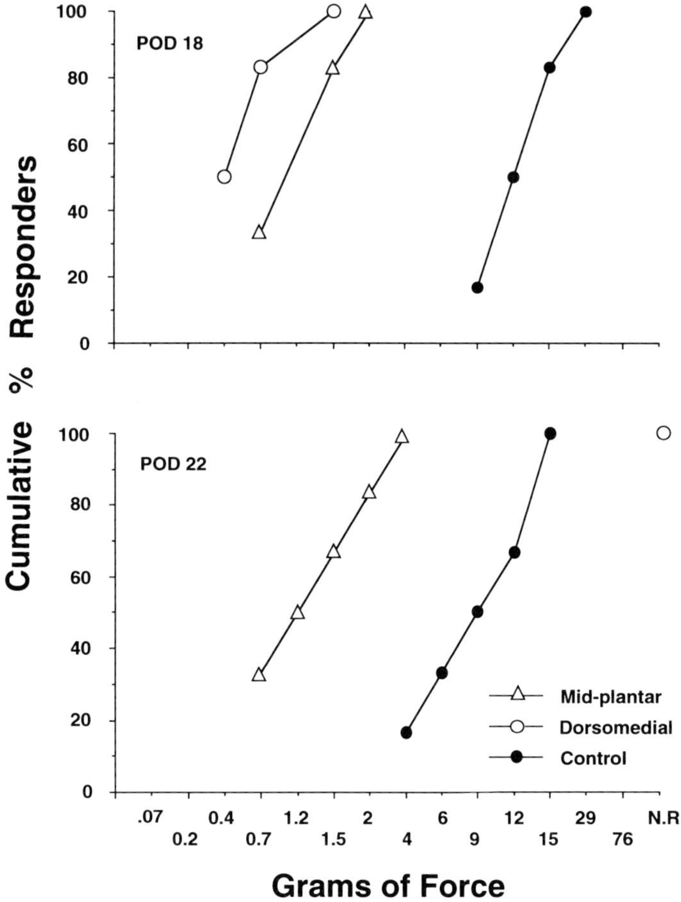

Fig. 4. Mechano-allodynia with a stocking-like distribution in CCI rats. The graphs show the cumulative percentage of rats (n = 6) with threshold responses to a series of von Frey hair stimuli (zero percent responses omitted for clarity). Grams of force exerted by each hair when depressed to the bending point is shown on the abscissa (N.R.: no response to any hair tested). Responses on the control, sham-operated side (filled circles) were not different from those obtained from both sides prior to nerve injury. **Top:** On postoperative day 18, (POD 18), there is statistically significant mechano-allodynia on the nerve-injured side (open symbols) when testing the midplantar hindpaw (the sciatic nerve's territory) and the dorsomedial hindpaw (the uninjured saphenous nerve's territory). **Bottom:** After cutting the saphenous nerve, there is no significant change in the allodynia seen in the sciatic nerve's territory, but no responses can be evoked from the saphenous territory. Therefore, the mechano-allodynia in the saphenous territory was mediated via input from the saphenous nerve (rather than an overlapping innervation from the injured sciatic nerve) and the extraterritorial mechano-allodynia is almost certainly due to a CNS mechanism. (Adapted from Tal and Bennett 1994.)

Table II
Therapeutic effects of NMDA receptor antagonists on
painful peripheral neuropathies in the rat

Drug	Model	Route	Symptom	Reference
MK-801	CCI	ip.*	H-hyper	Davar et al. 1991
	CCI	it.	H-hyper	Yamamoto and Yaksh 1992
	CCI	it.	H-hyper, Spont	Mao et al. 1992a
	SNT	it.	M-allo	Chaplan et al. 1993
AP-5	CCI	it.	H-hyper	Yamamoto and Yaksh 1992
	SNT	it.	M-allo	Chaplan et al. 1993
Ketamine	CCI	it.	H-hyper	Yamamoto and Yaksh 1992
	CCI	it.	H-hyper, Spont	Mao et al. 1993
Dextrorphan	CCI	ip., it.	H-hyper	Tal and Bennett 1993
	CCI	it.	H-hyper	Mao et al. 1993
	SNT	it.	M-allo	Chaplan et al. 1993
Memantine	SNT	it.	M-allo	Chaplan et al. 1993
	CCI	ip.	H-hyper	Eisenberg et al. 1993

Note: CCI, chronic constriction injury model of Bennett and Xie (1988); SNT, spinal nerve transection model of Kim and Chung (1992); ip.*, 10 daily injections (all other studies tested after a single bolus); it., intrathecal administration ; H-hyper, heat-hyperalgesia; Spont, spontaneous pain, other than autotomy; M-allo, mechano-allodynia.

WHAT CAN ANIMAL MODELS CONTRIBUTE TO MEDICAL PRACTICE?

A great deal of work has been performed on the models described above, even though many of them are of quite recent origin. It is impossible to review all of this work here; instead, I note a few observations that seem to me to be particularly good examples of the importance of research in animals for clinical practice.

Clinicians have long noted that a local anesthetic nerve block can give a patient days or weeks of relief. This result is very difficult to understand in terms of the known duration of the pharmacological effect, and it is sometimes suspected to be a supernormal placebo effect, or presumptive evidence that the patient is neurotic or malingering. It is therefore of interest that rats with the CCI obtain prolonged relief after a single nerve block (Fig. 3). They also get prolonged relief from a single intrathecal bolus injection of an N-methyl-D-aspartate (NMDA) receptor antagonist, and giving the intrathecal injection and the nerve block simultaneously gives an even longer period of relief (Mao et al. 1992b). Prolonged relief in these cases makes no more sense in terms of pharmacokinetics than the effects seen in patients, but we can be confident that the rats' responses are not placebo, neurosis, or malingering. The explanation for the prolonged relief in the rat is not known, although a hypothesis developed for the human case may be applicable (Gracely et al. 1992). Whatever the explanation, the significance of the animal work is that it validates the possibility of a physiologic explanation for the puzzling clinical finding.

Clinicians have often noted another puzzling finding in patients with painful post-traumatic neuropathy: the area of spontaneous pain and abnormal evoked-pain sometimes does not correspond to the individual or aggregate territories of nerves or roots. When the extremities are involved (and they usually are), the presentation is often of pain in a glove- or stocking-like distribution. There are few events in the history of medicine more dramatic than Charcot's revelation of the psychogenic cause of hysterical paralysis, and every medical student is taught to look for the telltale paralysis with a glove- or stocking-like distribution. It is not surprising that a neurosis is often considered as a diagnosis for the patient with pain in an extraterritorial distribution, especially when the physician is unable to discover any other plausible cause, and when the patient is refractory to all treatment and displays obvious emotional distress. (And, I am sad to suspect, often when the patient is a woman or has a socioeconomic and educational status quite different from the physician's.) It is therefore of importance that rats with a painful peripheral neuropathy (the CCI model) have been shown to have pain in a stocking-like distribution (Tal and Bennett 1994; Kingery et al. 1994). The CCI damages the sciatic nerve but not the saphenous nerve, which innervates a strip of skin along the dorsomedial edge of the paw. Heat-hyperalgesia, mechano-hyperalgesia and mechano-allodynia occur in both the sciatic and saphenous territories of CCI rats. The abnormal pain responses to mechanical stimulation have similar latencies to onset and severity in both nerve territories (Fig. 4). No sensations are evoked from the saphenous nerve's territory if the saphenous nerve is subsequently cut, which shows that the abnormal pain sensations were due to input from the undamaged nerve, rather than an overlapping innervation from the injured sciatic nerve (Tal and Bennett 1994). The explanation for the stocking-like distribution of pain in the rats will not be found on the psychiatrist's couch. A great deal of evidence has been found for significant CNS pathophysiology in the CCI model (Bennett 1993). Extraterritorial pain is easily explained if there is pathophysiology in the somatosensory processing regions of the spinal cord, thalamus or cortex. For example, in the spinal cord dorsal horn, the body surface is represented by a somatotopic map which is an emergent property of the spatial distribution of the receptive fields of individual spinal neurons. Adjacent neurons have adjacent, and often partially overlapping, receptive fields. Importantly, it is common for spinal neurons to be excited by input from more than one nerve or root. A dysfunction in spinal neuron function will therefore manifest itself as pain in an area corresponding to the aggregate of the receptive fields of the affected neurons; this will be a portion of the map, and it need not correspond to a nerve territory or dermatome. The animal work is important because it shows that a neurosis is not the only reasonable explanation for pain with a non-anatomic distribution.

The greatest contribution of animal models of neuropathic pain may lie in their use in tests of the efficacy of new and old drugs. For example, tricyclic antidepressants reduce the pain seen in the CCI and diabetic rat models (Ardid and Guilbaud 1992; Bardin et al. 1993). Opioids are also effective in the CCI model, although there are important differences in their ability to block different kinds of abnormal pain sensations: they are very effective against mechano-allodynia but markedly less effective against cold- and warm-allodynia (Desmeules et al. 1993). This differential sensitivity may explain at least some of the controversy about the efficacy of opiates in neuropathic pain patients.

Another example of potentially great importance is the use of NMDA receptor antagonists. Data from six laboratories and tests using five different NMDA receptor antagonists (Table II) show that these drugs suppress the abnormal pain sensations seen in the CCI and SNT models. Studies have shown repeatedly that the site of action lies in the spinal cord and that profound pain relief can be obtained without obvious side effects if the intrathecal route is used. Research has also demonstrated the prophylactic efficacy of NMDA receptor antagonists (Davar et al. 1991; Mao et al. 1992a; Eisenberg et al. 1993). It is firmly established that NMDA receptor antagonists have little or no effect on the pain sensitivity of the paw contralateral to the nerve injury. Thus, these drugs are not analgesics in the usual sense; instead, their action is specifically anti-hyperalgesic, and traditional animal pain models like the tail-flick assay would never have detected their potential usefulness. Preliminary investigations in patients and in normal human subjects support the hypothesis that NMDA blockers may be clinically useful in the treatment of neuropathic pain (Kristenson et al. 1992; Byas-Smith et al. 1993; Park et al. 1993; Backonja et al. 1994).

REFERENCES

Ahlgren, S.C. and Levine, J.D., Mechanical hyperalgesia in streptozotocin-diabetic rat, Neuroscience, 52 (1993a) 1049–1055.

Ahlgren, S.C. and Levine, J.D., Reduction of C-fiber mechanical hyperexcitability in the streptozotocin-diabetic rat by protein kinase C inhibition. In: Abstracts: 7th World Congress on Pain, IASP Publications, Seattle, 1993b, pp. 453–454.

Ahlgren, S.C., White, D.M. and Levine, J.D., Increased responsiveness of sensory neurons in the

saphenous nerve of the streptozotocin-diabetic rat, J. Neurophysiol., 68 (1992) 2077–2085.
Albe-Fessard, D. and Rampin, O., Neurophysiological studies in rats deafferented by dorsal root sections. In: B.S. Nashold and J. Ovelmen-Levitt (Eds.), Deafferentation Pain Syndromes: Pathophysiology and Treatment, Raven Press, New York, 1991, pp. 125–139.
Ardid, D. and Guilbaud, G., Antinociceptive effects of acute and chronic injections of tricyclic antidepressant drugs in a new model of mononeuropathy in rats, Pain, 49 (1992) 279–287.
Attal, N., Jazat, F., Kayser, V. and Guilbaud, G., Further evidence for "pain-related" behaviours in a model of unilateral peripheral mononeuropathy, Pain, 41 (1990) 235–251.
Backonja, M., Arndt, G., Gombar, K.A., Check, B. and Zimmermann, M., Response of chronic neuropathic pain syndromes to ketamine: a preliminary study, Pain, 56 (1994) 51–57.
Bardin, M., Courteix, C., Chantelauze, C., Lavarenne, J. and Eschalier, A., Pharmacological sensitivity of the animal model of painful diabetes. In: Abstracts: 7th World Congress on Pain, IASP Publications, Seattle, 1993, p. 528.
Basbaum, A.I. and Wall, P.D., Chronic changes in the responses of cells in adult dorsal horn following partial deafferentation: the appearance of responding cells in a previously non-responding region, Brain Res., 116 (1976) 181–204.
Bennett, G.J., An animal model of neuropathic pain: a review, Muscle Nerve, 16 (1993) 1040–1048.
Bennett, G.J. and Xie, Y.-K., A peripheral mononeuropathy in rat that produces disorders of pain sensation like those seen in man, Pain, 33 (1988) 87–107.
Boivie, J., Leijon, G. and Johansson, I., Central post-stroke pain: a study of the mechanisms through analyses of the sensory abnormalities, Pain, 37 (1989) 173–185.
Burchiel, K.J., Russell, L.C., Lee, R.P. and Sima, A.A.F., Spontaneous activity of primary afferent neurons in diabetic BB/Wistar rats, Diabetes, 34 (1985) 1210–1213.
Byas-Smith, M.G., Max, M.B., Gracely, R.H. and Bennett, G.J., Intravenous ketamine and alfentanil in patients with chronic causalgic pain and allodynia. In: Abstracts: 7th World Congress on Pain, IASP Publications, Seattle, 1993, p. 454.
Chaplan, S.R., Pogrel, J. and Yaksh, T.L., Pharmacologic modulation of tactile allodynia in a rat neuropathy model. In: Abstracts: 7th World Congress on Pain, IASP Publications, Seattle, 1993, p. 37.
Courteix, C., Eschalier, A. and Lavarenne, J., Streptozotocin-induced diabetic rats: behavioral evidence for a model of chronic pain, Pain, 53 (1993) 81–88.
Davar, G., Hama, A., Deykin, A., Vos, B. and Maciewicz, R., MK-801 blocks the development of thermal hyperalgesia in a rat model of experimental painful neuropathy, Brain Res., 553 (1991) 327–330.
Defrin, R. and Urca, G., Kainate induced spinal cord lesions: an animal model of central neuropathic pain of spinal origin. In: Abstracts: 7th World Congress on Pain, IASP Press, Seattle, 1993, pp. 28–29.
DeLeo, J.A., Coombs, D.W., Willenbring, S., Colburn, R.W., Fromm, C., Wagner, R. and Twitchell, B.B., Characterization of a neuropathic pain model: sciatic cryoneurolysis in the rat, Pain, 56 (1994) 9–16.
Desmeules, J.A., Kayser, V. and Guilbaud, G., Selective opioid receptor agonists modulate mechanical allodynia in an animal model of neuropathic pain, Pain, 53 (1993) 277–285.
Devor, M., The pathophysiology of damaged peripheral nerves. In: P.D. Wall and R. Melzack (Eds.), Textbook of Pain, 2nd ed., Churchill Livingstone, Edinburgh, 1989, pp. 63–81.
Devor, M., Wall, P.D. and Catalan, N., Systemic lidocaine silences ectopic neuroma and DRG discharge without blocking nerve conduction, Pain, 48 (1992) 261–268.
Eisenberg, E., LaCross, S. and Strassman, A.M., The prophylactic and therapeutic effects of the clinically tested NMDA receptor antagonist memantine on hyperalgesia induced by chronic constriction injury to the sciatic nerve in the rat. In: Program Book of American Pain Society 12th Annual Scientific Meeting, Nov. 4–7, 1993, Orlando, Fla., USA, p. 64.
Feria, M., Abad, F., Sánchez, A. and Abreu, P., Magnesium sulphate injected subcutaneously suppresses autotomy in peripherally deafferented rats, Pain, 53 (1993) 287–293.
Fialip, J., Betoin, F., Lavarenne, J., Duchene-Marullaz, P. and Eschalier, A., Behavioral evidence for a very long-lasting antinociceptive effect of systemic vapreotide, involving an opioidergic

mechanism. In: Abstracts: 7th World Congress on Pain, IASP Publications, Seattle, 1993, p. 527.
Forman, L.J., Estilow, S., Lewis, M. and Vasilenko, P., Streptozotocin diabetes alters immunoreactive ß-endorphin levels and pain perception after 8 weeks in female rats, Diabetes, 35 (1986) 1309–1313.
Gracely, R.H., Lynch, S. and Bennett, G.J., Painful neuropathy: altered central processing, maintained dynamically by peripheral input, Pain, 51 (1992) 175–194.
Hao, J.-X., Xu, X.-J., Aldskogius, H., Seiger, A. and Wiesenfeld-Hallin, Z., Allodynia-like effects in rats after ischaemic spinal cord injury photochemically induced by laser irradiation, Pain, 45 (1991) 175–186.
Hao, J.-X., Xu, X.-J., Seiger, A. and Wiesenfeld-Hallin, Z., Antagonists of the AMPA and NMDA excitatory amino acid receptors relieve mechanical allodynia after transient spinal cord ischemia. In: Abstracts: 7th World Congress on Pain, IASP Publications, Seattle, 1993, p. 222.
Kawamoto, H., Imamura, Y., Nakanishi, O. and Nishi, M., Hyperalgesia in rats with trigeminal mononeuropathy. In: Abstracts: 7th World Congress on Pain, IASP Publications, Seattle, 1993, p. 39.
Kim, S.H. and Chung, J.M., An experimental model for peripheral neuropathy produced by segmental spinal nerve ligation in the rat, Pain, 50 (1992) 355–363.
Kim, S.H., Na, H.S., Sheen, K. and Chung, J.M., Effects of sympathectomy on a rat model of peripheral neuropathy, Pain, 55 (1993) 85–92.
Kingery, W.S. and Vallin, J.A., The development of chronic mechanical hyperalgesia, autotomy and collateral sprouting following sciatic nerve section in rat, Pain, 38 (1989) 321–332.
Kingery, W.S., Lu, J.D., Roffers, J.A. and Kell, D.R., The resolution of neuropathic hyperalgesia following motor and sensory functional recovery in sciatic axonotometic mononeuropathies, Pain, (1994) in press.
Kristenson, J.D., Svensson, B. and Gordh, T., The NMDA receptor antagonist CPP abolishes neurogenic 'windup pain' after intrathecal administration in humans, Pain, 51 (1992) 249–253.
Lee, J.H., Cox, D.J., Mook, D.J. and McCarty, R.C., Effect of hyperglycemia on pain threshold in alloxan-diabetic rats, Pain, 40 (1990) 105–107.
Leijon, G., Boivie, J. and Johansson, I., Central post-stroke pain: neurological symptoms and pain characteristics, Pain, 36 (1989) 13–25.
Levitt, M., Chronic dysesthesias of central neural origin in subhuman primates. In: B.S. Nashold and J. Ovelmen-Levitt (Eds.), Deafferentation Pain Syndromes: Pathophysiology and Treatment, Raven Press, New York, 1991, pp. 229–238.
Loeser, J.D., Ward, A.A. and White, L.E., Chronic deafferentation of human spinal cord neurons, J. Neurosurg., 29 (1968) 48–50.
Lombard, M.-C. and Besson, J.-M., Behavioral and physiopharmacological aspects of the deafferentation syndrome due to dorsal rhizotomy in the rat. In: J.-M. Besson and G. Guilbaud, (Eds.), Lesions of Primary Afferent Fibers as a Tool for the Study of Clinical Pain, Excerpta Medica, Amsterdam, 1991, pp. 83–99.
Mao, J., Price, D.D., Hayes, R.L., Lu, J. and Mayer, D.J., Differential roles of NMDA and non-NMDA receptor activation in induction and maintenance of thermal hyperalgesia in rats with painful peripheral mononeuropathy, Brain Res., 598 (1992a) 271–278.
Mao, J., Price, D.D., Mayer, D.J., Lu, J. and Hayes, R.L., Intrathecal MK 801 and local nerve anesthesia synergistically reduce nociceptive behaviors in rats with experimental peripheral mononeuropathy, Brain Res., 576 (1992b) 254–262.
Mao, J., Price, D.D., Hayes, R.L., Lu, J., Mayer, D.J. and Frenk, H., Intrathecal treatment with dextrorphan or ketamine potently reduces pain-related behaviours in a rat model of peripheral mononeuropathy, Brain Res., 605 (1993) 164–168.
Markus, H., Pomeranz, B. and Krushelnycky, D., Spread of saphenous somatotopic projection map in spinal cord and hypersensitivity of the foot after chronic sciatic denervation in adult rat, Brain Res., 296 (1984) 27–39.
Maves, T.J., Pechman, P.S., Gebhart, G.F. and Meller, S.T., Continuous infusion of acidified saline around the rat sciatic nerve produces a reversible thermal hyperalgesia. In: Abstracts: 7th World Congress on Pain, IASP Publications, Seattle, 1993a, p. 31.

Maves, T.J., Pechman, P.S., Gebhart, G.F. and Meller, S.T., Possible chemical contribution from chronic gut sutures produces disorders of pain sensation like those seen in man, Pain, 54 (1993b) 57–69.

Park, K.M., Max, M.B., Robinovitz, E., Gracely, R.H. and Bennett, G.J., Effects of intravenous ketamine and alfentanil on hyperalgesia induced by intradermal capsaicin. In: Abstracts: 7th World Congress on Pain, IASP Publications, Seattle, 1993, p. 454.

Perrot, S., Attal, N., Ardid, D. and Guilbaud, G., Are mechanical and cold allodynia in mononeuropathic and arthritic rats relieved by systemic treatment with calcitonin or guanethidine? Pain, 52 (1993) 41–47.

Russell, L.C. and Burchiel, K.J., Abnormal activity in diabetic rat saphenous nerve, Diabetes, 42 (1993) 814–819.

Seltzer, Z., Dubner, R. and Shir, Y., A novel behavioral model of neuropathic pain disorders produced in rats by partial sciatic nerve injury, Pain, 43 (1990) 205–218.

Seltzer, Z., Beilin, B., Ginzburg, R., Paran, Y. and Shimko, T., The role of injury discharge in the induction of neuropathic pain behavior in rats, Pain, 46 (1991) 327–336.

Shir, Y. and Seltzer, Z., Effects of sympathectomy in a model of causalgiaform pain produced by partial sciatic nerve injury in rats, Pain, 45 (1991) 309–320.

Tal, M. and Bennett, G.J., Dextrorphan relieves neuropathic heat-evoked hyperalgesia, Neurosci. Lett., 151 (1993) 107–110.

Tal, M. and Bennett, G.J., Extra-territorial pain in rats with a peripheral mononeuropathy: mechano-hyperalgesia and mechano-allodynia in the territory of an uninjured nerve, Pain, (1994), in press.

Vos, B. and Maciewicz, R., Behavioral changes following ligation of the infraorbital nerve in rat: an animal model of trigeminal neuropathic pain. In: J.-M. Besson and G. Guilbaud (Eds.), Lesions of Primary Afferent Fibers as a Tool for the Study of Clinical Pain, Excerpta Medica, Amsterdam, 1991, pp. 147–158.

Wall, P.D., Devor, M., Inbal, R., Scadding, J.W., Schonfeld, D., Seltzer, Z. and Tomkiewicz, M.M., Autotomy following peripheral nerve lesions: experimental anesthesia dolorosa, Pain, 7 (1979) 103–113.

Wiesenfeld-Hallin, Z., Hao, J.-X., Xu, X.-J., Aldskogius, H. and Seiger, A., Genetic factors influence the development of mechanical hypersensitivity, motor deficits and morphological damage after transient spinal cord ischemia in the rat, Pain, 55 (1993) 235–241.

Willenbring, S., DeLeo, J.A. and Coombs, D.W., Further behavioral characterization of the sciatic cryoneurolysis neuropathic pain model in the rat. In: Program Book of American Pain Society 12th Annual Scientific Meeting, Nov. 4–7, 1993, Orlando, Fla., USA, p. 68.

Wuarin-Bierman, L., Zahnd, G.R., Kaufmann, F., Burcklen, L. and Adler, J., Hyperalgesia in spontaneous and experimental models of diabetic neuropathy, Diabetologia, 30 (1987) 653–658.

Xu, X.-J., Hao, J.-X., Aldskogius, H., Seiger, A. and Wiesenfeld-Hallin, Z., Chronic pain-related syndrome in rats after ischemic spinal cord lesion: a possible animal model for pain in patients with spinal cord injury, Pain, 48 (1992) 279–290.

Xu, X.-J., Hao, J.-X., Seiger, A., Hughes, J., Hokfelt, T. and Wiesenfeld-Hallin, Z., Chronic pain-related behaviors in spinally injured rats: evidence for altered function of the endogenous cholecystokinin and opioid systems. In: Abstracts: 7th World Congress on Pain, IASP Publications, Seattle, 1993, p. 265.

Yamamoto, T. and Yaksh, T.L., Spinal pharmacology of thermal hyperesthesia induced by constriction injury of sciatic nerve: excitatory amino acid antagonists, Pain, 49 (1992) 121–128.

Yezerski, R. and Park, S.H., Altered mechanosensitivity of spinal sensory neurons following the injection of quisqualic acid. In: Abstracts: 7th World Congress on Pain, IASP Publications, Seattle, 1993, pp. 470–471.

Correspondence to: G.J. Bennett, PhD; NAB, NIDR, NIH; Bldg. 49, Room 1A11; 9000 Rockville Pike; Bethesda, MD 20892, USA. Tel: 301-496-6804; Fax: 301-402-0667.

Proceedings of the 7th World Congress on Pain,
Progress in Pain Research and Management, Vol. 2,
edited by G.F. Gebhart, D.L. Hammond, and T.S.
Jensen, IASP Press, Seattle, © 1994.

35

The Properties of Unmyelinated Nociceptive Afferents Change in a Painful Chronic Constriction Neuropathy

Martin Koltzenburg, Stefan Kees, Stephan Budweiser, Günter Ochs, and Klaus V. Toyka

Department of Neurology, University of Würzburg, Germany

INTRODUCTION

Several lines of evidence indicate that abnormal receptive functions of unmyelinated primary afferents are an important cause of neuropathic pain in patients. First, pain often can be abolished or significantly reduced by local anesthetic block of the damaged peripheral nerve (Arnér et al. 1990) or affected skin (Rowbotham and Fields 1989). This indicates that neural activity arising distally in the nerve or even in the receptive endings contributes significantly to the symptoms. Second, the continuous background pain and many forms of stimulus-induced pain sensations persist during a differential nerve fiber block that selectively eliminates conduction in myelinated fibers (Koltzenburg et al. 1992; Campbell et al. 1992; Ochoa and Yarnitzky 1993). Finally, psychophysical experiments suggest that unmyelinated nociceptive afferents probably develop ongoing activity that correlates with the level of continuous background pain and some forms of hyperalgesia (Gracely et al. 1992; Koltzenburg et al. 1992). We investigated the receptive properties of unmyelinated nociceptors in a rat model of neuropathic pain that produces disorders of sensations similar to those seen in humans (Bennett and Xie 1988; Attal et al. 1990).

There is also evidence that the pain and hyperalgesia in some neuropathic pain states are generated and maintained by the sympathetic nervous system (Bonica 1990; Koltzenburg and McMahon 1991; Campbell et al. 1992). Pain relief can be afforded by local or regional sympatholytic treatment, suggesting that the abnormal receptive functions of primary afferents are the key element in sympathetically maintained pain states (Bonica 1990; Davis et al. 1991; Wahren et al. 1991). Moreover, in some patients who have obtained significant relief by sympatholytic therapy, pain and hyperalgesia can be rekindled by intracutaneous injections of noradrenaline into previously symptomatic skin (Wallin et al. 1976; Davis et al. 1991). Importantly, such noradrenaline-evoked pain can be elicited during a differential nerve block when only unmyelinated fibers are conducting (Torebjörk et al. 1993), further emphasizing the important role of abnormal C-fiber function in the generation and maintenance of neuropathic pains. Thus, we also studied the responses of unmyelinated fibers to application of noradrenaline to their receptive terminals.

METHODS

As a model for a painful neuropathy we produced a modified chronic constriction injury (CCI) as described by Bennett and Xie (1988). Instead of the sciatic nerve, the constriction was induced in the saphenous nerve of Sprague-Dawley rats by application of four loose chromic gut ligatures (4-0) 3–107 days prior to the recordings. The ligatures retarded but did not arrest epineural blood flow, and the constriction of the nerve was verified histologically. Both the constriction and the chromic suture material are thought to be responsible for initiating the pain behavior (Maves et al. 1992), which is maximal at the end of the first postoperative week and which decreases gradually during the following weeks. Although we have not studied the behavioral consequences of this lesion in detail, we have noticed exaggerated reflex responses in awake or lightly anaesthetized animals following pinprick stimuli applied to the paw supplied by the lesioned nerve. We also studied C-fibers in normal control rats.

Unmyelinated primary afferents were recorded in vitro as described previously (Reeh 1986; Kress et al. 1992). Briefly, the saphenous nerve and the attached skin were dissected and mounted corium-side up in an organ bath that was constantly superfused with oxygenated HEPES-buffered electrolyte solution. Using a dissecting microscope and sharpened watchmaker forceps, we repeatedly split the saphenous nerve proximal to the ligatures until single-unit activity could be recorded from fine strands using standard electrophysiological techniques. Only unmyelinated afferents (conduction velocity < 2.0 m per second) that could be excited by electrical and mechanical stimulation applied distal to the ligatures were studied in detail. Following electrical identification, the receptive fields of identified units were isolated from the organ bath with self-sealing metal rings and the units were fully characterized using standard natural stimuli consisting of graded mechanical forces exerted with calibrated von Frey's hairs (1–362 mN), feedback-coupled heat ramps (32–47° C in 15 seconds), and cold stimuli (application of ice-cold electrolyte solution). After establishing the functional properties, we tested the units with superfusion of either noradrenaline or lidocaine. Noradrenaline (NA) was applied in an ascending series of concentrations (1, 10, 100 µM each for one minute) and in a concentration of 100 µM for five minutes. Lidocaine was superfused onto the receptive field in an ascending series of concentrations (0.1, 1, 10 mM each for 10 minutes) until electrically evoked conduction of the units was abolished.

RESULTS

We studied 1018 single unmyelinated units. In 861 units we recorded only the presence or absence of ongoing activity, while in the remaining 157 units we studied the receptive properties in detail. We studied 31 C-fibers from normal control animals and 126 units 3–107 days after creation of the constriction neuropathy. The afferents sampled from normal animals did not differ significantly in conduction velocity, distribution of receptor classes, and mechanical or thermal responses from results in an extensive investigation published previously (Kress et al. 1992).

ALL TYPES OF NOCICEPTIVE C-FIBERS PRESENT IN THE NORMAL SAPHENOUS NERVE WERE RECORDED FOLLOWING CONSTRICTION INJURY

In normal cutaneous nerves of the rat, mechano-heat-sensitive C-fibers (CMH unit) are the most frequent class of nociceptor. The features of these units recorded from normal and neuropathic rats are illustrated in Fig. 1. In normal animals CMH units have no spontaneous activity; they are activated by noxious heat stimuli but not by noxious cold. Essentially the same pattern was observed in CMH units recorded from neuropathic rats, except that the units exhibited a variable degree of ongoing activity prior to application of any stimuli; spontaneous activity was often inhibited by application of cold stimuli.

All types of nociceptors that are present in normal nerve also were recorded in the constriction neuropathy. Of all the mechano-sensitive units, 47% responded to heat and were consequently classified as mechano-heat-responsive

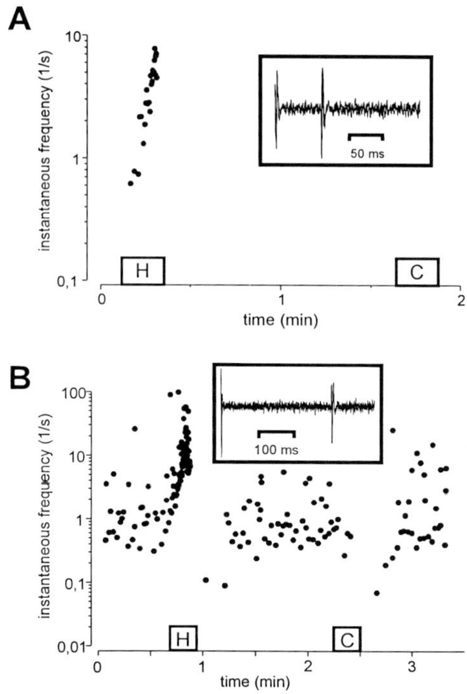

Fig. 1. Representative examples of CMH units in (**A**) normal control animals (c.v. 0.58 m/s) and (**B**) a neuropathic animal (28 days po.; c.v. 0.22 m/s). Insets show the identification using electrical stimulation of the receptive terminal. H, heat ramp; C, cold stimulation.

(CMH) C-fibers. Of the remaining units, around 15% responded to cold (CMC units) but not to heat while about 11% were excited by both thermal stimuli (CMHC units). The rest of the mechano-sensitive units failed to respond to either thermal stimulus (CM units). The relative distribution of nociceptor subtypes remained relatively stable during the postoperative period and there was no significant difference in the distribution of nociceptor subtypes in the normal or neuropathic condition (Fig. 2).

C-FIBERS HAVE A SLOWER CONDUCTION VELOCITY AND HIGHER INCIDENCE OF ONGOING ACTIVITY FOLLOWING CONSTRICTION INJURY

Following constriction injury, unmyelinated fibers had a conduction velocity of 0.41 ± 0.02 m/s (mean ± S.E.M., n = 116), which was significantly slower ($P < 0.001$, *t* test) than the average 0.60 ± 0.05 m/s (mean ± S.E.M., n = 31) found in normal controls (Fig. 3). This finding is consistent with the notion that the units sampled in our study were indeed affected by the constriction and not simply normal units that survived the constriction.

Moreover, the proportion of fibers exhibiting resting activity and the rate

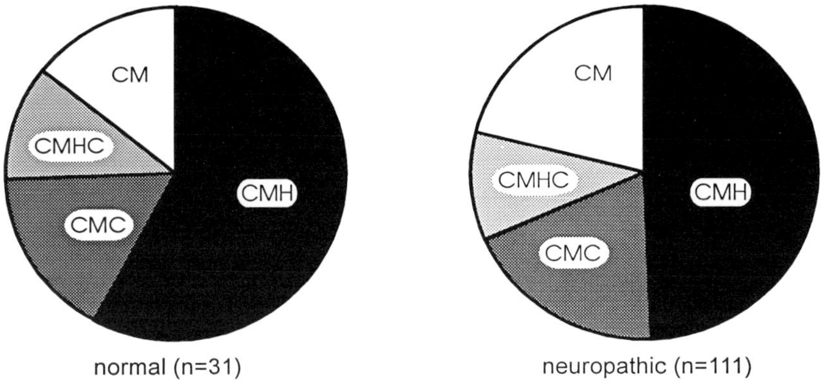

Fig. 2. Relative distribution of different nociceptor subtypes in normal and neuropathic animals. CMH, mechano-heat responsive; CMC, mechano-cold responsive; CMHC, mechano-heat-cold responsive; CM, mechano-sensitive.

of this activity were conspicuously higher following constriction injury compared to normal animals. In this preparation spontaneous activity was seen in 2% of normal C-fibers, some of which where cold-sensitive non-nociceptive fibers that showed the typical bursting discharge at the 32° C of the organ bath (Kress et al. 1992). Yet, following constriction we observed a higher incidence of spontaneously active fibers exceeding 10% during the first post-operative week. This was followed by a gradual decline of the rate of spontaneously active fibers to normal levels during the next three weeks. However, we also noticed a second peak with a high incidence of spontaneously active units two to four months after the ligation.

Units with ongoing activity also had a significantly lower average conduction velocity than did those fibers without ongoing activity (Fig. 3). Conversely, the level of ongoing activity was significantly higher in fibers with conduction velocity below 0.4 m/s compared to faster conducting C-fibers.

THE RECEPTIVE PROPERTIES OF C-FIBERS FOLLOWING CONSTRICTION INJURY

Except for their ongoing activity, nociceptive C-fibers recorded from the CCI model also differed in their receptive properties from those of normal animals. There was a significant ($P < 0.05$, Wilcoxon test) increase of the median mechanical threshold force from 13.6 mN (quartile range 58) to 64 mN (quartile range 204). This finding indicates that reductions of the mechanical threshold of unmyelinated nociceptors are an unlikely explanation for the behavioral manifestations of mechanical hyperalgesia observed in this model.

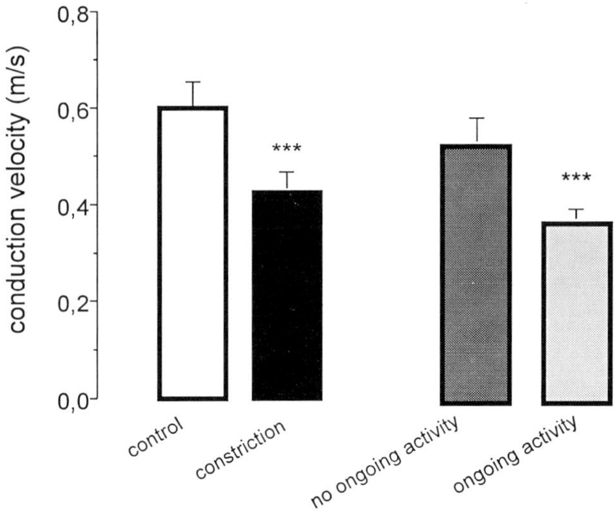

Fig. 3. Conduction velocity of unmyelinated fibers recorded in control and neuropathic conditions. Fibers from neuropathic animals have a significantly lower conduction velocity than do units in normal animals ($P < 0.001$; t test). In neuropathic animals, units with ongoing activity have a significantly lower conduction velocity than do those without such activity. ($P < 0.001$, t test)

In contrast, the mean heat response tended to be increased after constriction injury. In normal animals a standard heat stimulus evoked 23.0 ± 5.4 (mean ± S.E.M.) spikes, and this response increased to 30 ± 3.5 (mean ± S.E.M.) in the second postoperative week when the behavioral correlates of heat hyperalgesia are most prominent. Furthermore, in some 5% of the units unusual heat afterdischarges were observed. It is unclear whether the afterdischarges in the few units could contribute to the prolonged flexion reflexes found behaviorally (Bennett and Xie 1988) or to the heat afterdischarges recorded in some spinothalamic tract neurons (Palecek et al. 1992).

Although behavioral studies have documented an increased pain response to noxious cold stimuli (Attal et al. 1990), there was no change of the C-fiber responsiveness to noxious cold stimuli.

NORADRENALINE CAN EXCITE C-FIBERS WITH LOW ONGOING ACTIVITY FOLLOWING CONSTRICTION INJURY

We tested 74 fibers with noradrenaline in the CCI model. The units had a resting activity ranging from 0 to 1.5 impulses per second, with 36 units having a low rate (< 0.1 impulses per second) while 21 exhibited a high rate of spontaneous activity (> 0.5 impulses per second). Noradrenaline appeared to have a differential effect on these two populations. Units with no or low ongoing activity often could be excited during superfusion of the receptive field with noradrenaline (Fig. 4A). In contrast, units that had high initial ongoing activity were either unchanged or inhibited. This finding indicates that an increased excitability of a nociceptor as judged by the level of ongoing activity does not necessarily correlate with an increased responsiveness to catecholamines. Among the fibers that responded to noradrenaline, the response magnitude was maximal during the second postoperative week (Fig. 4B).

Superfusion with noradrenaline did not significantly change the response of units to noxious heat or cold stimuli. We also noted a further increase in the mechanical threshold from 64 mN to 318 mN following noradrenaline application. Thus, while catecholamines can increase the ongoing activity in a subpopulation of nociceptive afferents, they do not mediate a generalized increase in the excitability of the receptive endings following a constriction injury.

LIDOCAINE SUPERFUSION OF THE RECEPTIVE TERMINALS INDICATES THAT NOCICEPTORS CONTAIN MULTIPLE GENERATORS OF THE SPONTANEOUS ACTIVITY

Superfusion of the receptive field with lidocaine was used as a tool to localize the generator of ectopic activity in spontaneously active C-fibers. The excitation of C-fibers elicited by electrical stimulation of the receptive terminal could be blocked by virtually identical concentrations of lidocaine in both normal or neuropathic conditions.

In 17 units with ongoing activity recorded from neuropathic rats, the resting activity could be completely abolished in nine fibers, suggesting that the generator for these fibers is the receptive terminal proper or the axon in its immediate vicinity. In contrast, there was no quantitative change of the level of ongoing activity in three fibers when electrical conduction from the receptive field was completely blocked. This means that the generator for the ongoing activity was located proximally in the nerve, possibly at the constriction site. In the remaining five fibers ectopic spontaneous activity was significantly reduced, but not completely eliminated, when conduction from the receptive terminals was blocked. This finding suggests that there are multiple generators of ectopic activity in single nociceptive afferents under neuropathic conditions (Fig. 5).

Lidocaine also had a differential effect on the generation of spontaneous activity and the ability of C-fibers to conduct action potentials. In 17 of 28 fibers, superfusion of the receptive field with lidocaine abolished or reduced

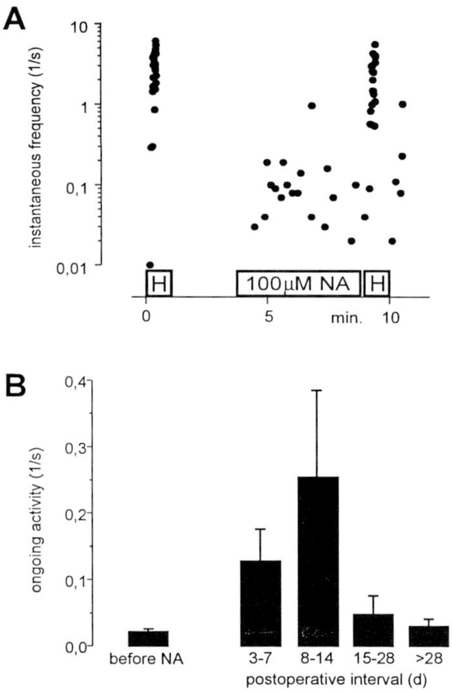

Fig. 4. A: response of a CMH fiber to superfusion of the receptive field with noradrenaline (100 µM for five minutes). H, heat stimulus. **B:** time course of the mean activity evoked by superfusion of the receptive field in units without or with low (< 0.1 impulses per second) ongoing activity.

ongoing activity prior to production of a conduction block. This could mean that the mechanisms that are responsible for the generation of ectopic activity differ from those of action potential propagation.

DISCUSSION

The principal finding of our investigation is that several important changes occur in the functional properties of unmyelinated nociceptors in a chronic constriction neuropathy that produces pain behavior. The percentage of spontaneously active fibers and the rate of ongoing activity significantly increased. The development of ongoing activity confirms the prediction made from patient studies that the level of ongoing activity correlates with the magnitude of stimulus-independent background pain in neuralgia (Koltzenburg et al. 1992). Furthermore, because activity of C-fibers induces secondary changes of somatosensory processing (Dubner and Ruda 1992; Wall 1992), it is likely that the increased C-fiber input initiates and maintains several central nervous system changes that have been observed in this model.

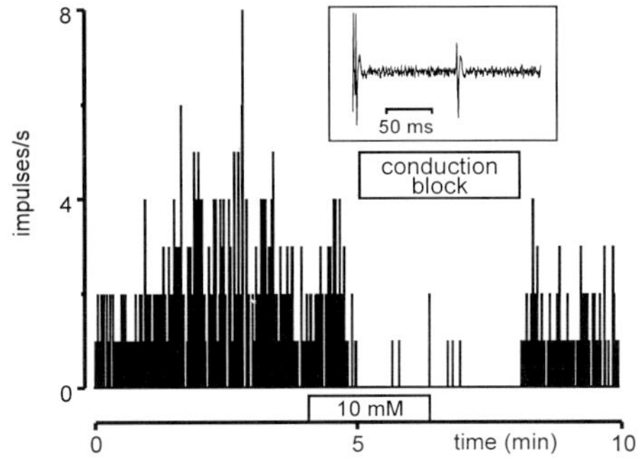

Fig. 5. Ongoing activity of a CMH fiber (17 days po., c.v. 0.28 m/s) during superfusion of the receptive terminal with lidocaine. When conduction from the receptive terminal, as tested with electrical stimuli, was blocked, the spontaneous activity of the unit was significantly reduced, but not completely abolished. Inset shows the identification of the unit using electrical stimulation of the receptive field.

Spontaneous activity has been found in both myelinated and unmyelinated fibers following axotomy. This ongoing activity can either arise from the tips of axotomized nerve fibers or is generated in the soma of the injured nerve cells. Our study revealed a third possibility, namely that ongoing activity also can arise from the receptive terminals of unmyelinated nerve fibers that run in a damaged nerve. Ectopic activity arising distally in the terminals of nociceptors has not been noted previously, and the lidocaine superfusion experiments determined that ectopic activity can be generated at different segments even in a single unmyelinated nerve fiber. The generation of ectopic activity in this animal model correlates well with clinical observations that local anesthetic nerve blocks distal to a partial nerve lesion (Kibler and Nathan 1960) or even local cutaneous anesthesia (Rowbotham and Fields 1989) can often provide pain relief.

The reasons for the appearance of ongoing activity are not fully understood and it is possible that several factors contribute. One possibility is that afferents in the damaged nerve start to produce increased amounts of sodium channels or decreased numbers of potassium channels, which eventually will result in ectopic activity (Devor et al. 1993; Matzner and Devor 1992). However, at least in the early stages of the nerve injury, there is a genuine inflammatory reaction with a massive invasion of macrophages (Griffin et al. 1992), and the local production of excitatory agents might contribute to the ongoing excitation of nociceptive units.

It has been previously hypothesized that peripheral nerve lesions might produce changes in the receptive properties of primary afferents supplying the innervation territory of a damaged nerve (Jänig and Koltzenburg 1991). While we have shown that ongoing activity is one such possibility, we also have determined that the receptive properties of nociceptive afferents can change to some extent although the relative distribution of nociceptor subtypes is not altered. The number of action potentials evoked by a standard heat stimulus increased with a peak during the second postoperative week. This time course appears to be similar to the behavioral changes of heat hyperalgesia that also are fully developed during the second postoperative week (Bennett and Xie 1988). However, the increased heat sensitivity is not indicative of a generalized excitability increase of nociceptive afferents. The response of nociceptors to noxious cold changed little in the neuropathy model. Moreover, there was a significant increase in the mechanical threshold of fibers in neuropathic nerves, indicating that the mechanical or cold hyperalgesia observed in this model is probably not the consequence of a reduction in threshold of nociceptive afferents. Thus, the changes in the receptive properties observed in our study are probably not sufficient to explain all behavioral manifestations of neuropathic pain in these animals. Alternatively, central nervous system changes that are induced and probably maintained by a barrage of nociceptive afferents could account for some forms of hyperalgesia in neuropathic conditions.

Many clinical observations have shown repeatedly that the pain and hyperalgesia in some neuropathic pain states are generated and maintained by the sympathetic nervous system, while they are independent in other conditions with identical clinical presentation (Bonica 1990; Koltzenburg and McMahon 1991; Campbell et al. 1992). Previous studies have determined that axotomized nociceptive afferents acquire a sensitivity to catecholamines (Devor and Jänig 1981; Häbler et al. 1987). Our study also directly showed that a subpopulation of nociceptive afferents can be excited by application of noradrenaline to the receptive endings. As the studies were conducted in vitro, we can exclude the possibility that the effects were secondary to vascular changes. The catecholamine sensitivity was most prominent in fibers without or with low initial ongoing activity, while units exhibiting high levels of ongoing activity where inhibited. Such differential effect also has been reported for the resting activity that develops in axotomized primary afferents. This could mean that the balance of excitatory and inhibitory effects is important whether a pain condition is sympathetically dependent or not.

The excitatory effects of noradrenaline were maximal during the second postoperative week, a finding also noted in other models of partial nerve injury (Sato and Perl 1991; Selig et al. 1993). Importantly, this sensitivity was not found in axotomized fibers, but probably reflects a genuine alteration of undamaged afferents. Little is known about the mechanisms that regulate catecholamine sensitivity of primary sensory neurons, but such knowledge would be of some importance if we are to understand the factors that precipitate sympathetically maintained pain syndromes.

CONCLUSION

Our study showed changes in nociceptive afferents following a chronic constriction neuropathy in the rat that produces pain behavior similar to symptoms found in human neuralgia. (1) Nociceptive afferents develop ongoing ectopic activity that is mainly generated in the receptive terminals, but also proximally along the damaged nerve. (2) While the heat response of nociceptive units increases, there are no corresponding changes in the excitability to noxious cold or mechanical stimuli. (3) A subpopulation of unmyelinated afferents with low ongoing activity can be excited by application of noradrenaline to the receptive terminals.

ACKNOWLEDGMENTS

We thank Sabine Müller for technical assistance. This work was supported by the Wilhelm Sander-Stiftung.

REFERENCES

Arnér, S., Lindblom, U., Meyerson, B.A. and Molander, C., Prolonged relief of neuralgia after regional anesthetic blocks. A call for further experimental and systematic studies, Pain, 43 (1990) 287–297.

Attal, N., Jazat, F., Kayser, V. and Guilbaud, G., Further evidence for pain-related behaviours in a model of unilateral peripheral mononeuropathy, Pain, 41 (1990) 235–251.

Bennett, G.J. and Xie, Y.K., A peripheral mononeuropathy in rat that produces disorders of pain sensation like those seen in man, Pain, 33 (1988) 87–107.

Bonica, J.J., Causalgia and other sympathetic reflex dystrophies. In: J.J. Bonica (Ed.), The Management of Pain, Lea and Febiger, Philadelphia, 1990, pp. 220–243.

Campbell, J.N., Meyer, R.A. and Raja, S.N., Is nociceptor activation by alpha-1 adrenoreceptors the culprit in sympathetically maintained pain, APS Journal, 13 (1992) 344–350.

Davis, K.D., Treede, R.D., Raja, S.N., Meyer, R.A. and Campbell, J.N., Topical application of clonidine relieves hyperalgesia in patients with sympathetically maintained pain, Pain, 47 (1991) 309–317.

Devor, M. and Jänig, W., Activation of myelinated afferents ending in a neuroma by stimulation of the sympathetic supply in the rat, Neurosci. Lett., 24 (1981) 43–47.

Devor, M., Govrin Lippmann, R. and Angelides, K., Na^+ channel immunolocalization in peripheral mammalian axons and changes following nerve injury and neuroma formation, J. Neurosci., 13 (1993) 1976–1992.

Dubner, R. and Ruda, M. Activity-dependent neuronal plasticity following tissue injury and

inflammation, Trends Neurosci., 15 (1992) 96–103.
Gracely, R.H., Lynch, S.A. and Bennett, G.J., Painful neuropathy: altered central processing, maintained dynamically by peripheral input, Pain, 51 (1992) 175–194.
Griffin, J.W., George, R., Lobato, C., Tylor, W.R., Yan, L.C. and Glass, J.D., Macrophage response and myelin clearance during Wallerian degeneration: relevance to immune-mediated demyelination, J. Neuroimmunol., 40 (1992) 153–165.
Häbler, H.-J., Jänig, W. and Koltzenburg, M., Activation of unmyelinated afferents in chronically lesioned nerves by adrenaline and excitation of sympathetic efferents in the cat, Neurosci. Lett., 82 (1987) 35–40.
Jänig, W. and Koltzenburg, M., What is the interaction between the sympathetic terminal and the primary afferent fiber. In: A.I. Basbaum and J.-M. Besson (Eds.), Towards a New Pharmacotherapy of Pain, John Wiley, Chichester, 1991, pp. 331–352.
Kibler, R.F. and Nathan, P.W., Relief of pain and paraesthesiae by nerve block distal to a lesion, J. Neurol. Neurosurg. Psychiatry, 23 (1960) 91–98.
Koltzenburg, M. and McMahon, S.B. The enigmatic role of the sympathetic nervous system in chronic pain, Trends Pharmacol. Sci., 12 (1991) 399–402.
Koltzenburg, M., Wahren, L.K. and Torebjörk, H.E., Plasticity of mechanical hyperalgesia in chronic neuralgia and acute chemogenic pain, Soc. Neurosci. Abstr., 18 (1992) 384.
Kress, M., Koltzenburg, M., Reeh, P.W. and Handwerker, H.O., Responsiveness and functional attributes of electrically localized terminals of cutaneous C-fibers in vivo and in vitro, J. Neurophysiol., 68 (1992) 581–595.
Matzner, O. and Devor, M., Na+ conductance and the threshold for repetitive neuronal firing, Brain Res., 597 (1992) 92–98.
Maves, T.J., Pechman, P.S., Gebhart, G.F. and Meller, S.T., Possible chemical contribution from chromic gut sutures produces disorders of pain sensation like those seen in man, Pain, 54 (1992) 57–69.
Ochoa, J.L. and Yarnitzky, D., Mechanical hyperalgesias in neuropathic pain patients: dynamic and static subtypes, Ann. Neurol., 33 (1993) 465–472.
Palecek, J., Paleckova, V., Dougherty, P.M., Carlton, S.M. and Willis, W.D., Responses of spinothalamic tract cells to mechanical and thermal stimulation of skin in rats with experimental peripheral neuropathy, J. Neurophysiol., 67 (1992) 1562–1573.
Reeh, P.W., Sensory receptors in mammalian skin in an in vitro preparation, Neurosci. Lett., 66 (1986) 141–147.
Rowbotham, M.C. and Fields, H.L., Topical lidocaine reduces pain in post-herpetic neuralgia, Pain, 38 (1989) 297–301.
Sato, J. and Perl, E.R., Adrenergic excitation of cutaneous pain receptors induced by peripheral nerve injury, Science, 251 (1991) 1608–1610.
Selig, D.K., Meyer, R.A. and Campbell, J.N., Noradrenaline excitation of cutaneous nociceptors two weeks after ligation of spinal nerve L7 in monkey, Soc. Neurosci. Abstr., 19 (1993) 326.
Torebjörk, H.E., Wahren, L.K. and Koltzenburg, M., Noradrenaline applications can provoke pain and hyperalgesia in some patients with sympathetically maintained pain. In: Abstracts: 7th World Congress on Pain, IASP Publications, 1993, 346.
Wahren, L.K., Torebjörk, E. and Nyström, B., Quantitative sensory testing before and after regional guanethedine block in patients with neuralgia in the hand, Pain, 46 (1991) 23–30.
Wall, P.D., Neuropathic pain and injured nerve: central mechanisms, Br. Med. Bull., 47 (1992) 631–643.
Wallin, B.G., Torebjörk, H.E. and Hallin, R.G., Preliminary observations on the pathophysiology of hyperalgesia in the causaligic pain syndrome. In: Y. Zotterman (Ed.), Sensory Functions of the Skin in Primates, Pergamon Press, Oxford, 1976, pp. 489–499.

Correspondence to: Dr. Martin Koltzenburg, Department of Neurology, University of Würzburg, Josef-Schneider-Str. 11, D-97080 Würzburg, Germany. Tel: 49-931-201-2621; Fax: 49-931-201-2697.

Part VII

Opioids and Analgesia

Proceedings of the 7th World Congress on Pain,
Progress in Pain Research and Management, Vol. 2,
edited by G.F. Gebhart, D.L. Hammond, and T.S.
Jensen, IASP Press, Seattle, © 1994.

36

Where and How Do Opioids Act?

Anthony H. Dickenson

Department of Pharmacology, University College London, UK

The aim of this chapter is to examine current knowledge on the mechanisms of action of opioids relevant to the relief of pain, to report new developments on how and why opioid controls can be altered in different pain states, and how this basic research could lead to improved therapy.

By using selective probes for the mu, delta, and kappa opioid receptors, we are gaining understanding of their relative roles in physiological functions and the involvement of the endogenous opioids in different pain states. The very recent isolation and cloning of the delta receptor followed by the mu and kappa receptors will in time provide important information on the location and mode of activation of effects mediated by the receptors and eventually the production of useful new pharmacological tools for the probing of function.

The recent findings that the morphine metabolites are not inactive has lead to a reappraisal of the effects of long-term morphine dosing. In particular, morphine-6-glucuronide is a remarkably active metabolite, whereas the other metabolite, the 3-glucuronide, may interfere with the actions of opioids.

One of the most intriguing areas of research on opioids has been the accumulating evidence for plasticity in opioid controls—opioid actions are not immutable but are subject to modulation by other transmitter systems in the spinal cord. We are now in a position to begin to understand, based on animal models, why and how opioid analgesia can vary in different pain states.

The factors that alter opioid actions can be divided into pathological changes in the circuitry and pharmacological factors. The best example of the former is the loss of opioid receptors on the primary afferent C-fiber terminals as a result of their degeneration following section of the peripheral nerve by rhizotomy. The main candidate systems that are potentially able to reduce opioid analgesia are the nonopioid peptides cholecystokinin (CCK) and F8a and the N-methyl-D-aspartate (NMDA) receptor for the excitatory amino acids. The latter has been implicated in nociceptive transmission in several models of prolonged pain including inflammation, neuropathy, and ischemia. A rationale for preemptive analgesic strategies may be the prevention of the induction of these systems, a topic discussed in the chapter by McQuay. These three transmitter systems, which can interfere with opioid analgesia in the short term, also may influence the longer term development of opioid tolerance. There is good evidence that opioid analgesia in nociceptive states where these transmitters are active is improved by coadministration of the opiate with local anesthetics or either CCK and NMDA receptor antagonists.

By contrast, opiates show an increased effectiveness in some inflammatory states, partly due to novel peripheral sites in inflamed tissue. In addition, enhanced spinal opioid actions may result from reduced CCK release and/or altered descending controls. In this latter case activation of spinal alpha-2 adrenoceptors produces synergistic antinociception with mu opiates.

The studies cited above provide a rationale for the use of opioids with other drugs so that the combined actions of the opioid and adjunct will provide clinical benefits. The pharmacological agents used with opioids could thus be NMDA antagonists, local anesthetics, CCK antagonists, or alpha-2 adrenoceptor agonists. Many basic science studies have shown beneficial effects of these combinations by either enhancing or restoring opioid actions.

Many years have elapsed since the discovery of the existence of an opioid receptor, which was closely followed by the isolation and identification of the endogenous opioid peptides, the natural transmitters (Kosterlitz 1985). These events were undoubtedly major breakthroughs in the understanding of the actions of opioids, but since then no novel opioids have been introduced into clinical medicine and the desirable effects of the opioids have not been separated from the unwanted actions. It is to be hoped that this situation will alter in the not too distant future because there is now ample evidence for different opioid receptors and detailed information on the effects of opioids in many animal models of different pain states (Yaksh and Nouiehed 1985; Dickenson 1991a,b). The use of electrophysiological and behavioral techniques to study the roles of opioids in different models of pain have produced insights into their roles in central nervous system (CNS) function. The increasing dialogue and interactions between basic scientists and clinicians will surely translate to a better treatment of pain by using opioids in different ways and in concert with adjuncts designed to target some of the pharmacological systems now known to be the basis for altered opioid actions (McQuay and Dickenson 1990).

What then is the current state of opioid research? The breadth of this field restricts this chapter to covering only some of the more important areas relating to the actions and effects of opioids. The focus will be on the mechanisms of action in producing analgesia at numerous sites, the factors that can alter the efficacy of opioid controls on pain, and finally the way in which opioid interactions with other transmitter systems can be used as a basis for improving analgesia by combination therapy.

HOW AND WHERE DO OPIOIDS ACT?

Opioids act by interacting with the three opioid receptors: the mu, the delta, and the kappa (Table I). The endogenous opioid peptides—the enkephalins, dynorphins, and endorphin family—are not specific for any one receptor. Thus, the enkephalins at higher concentrations will activate the mu receptor as well as the delta receptor for which they have highest affinity (Kosterlitz 1985). These three main families of opioids are derived from different precursors so that the propeptides for the endorphins, enkephalins, and dynorphins are quite separate. Immunohistochemical stains for the messenger RNA for the propeptides have allowed unequivocal identification of the neurons containing the different opioids; the levels of mRNA serve as a measure of opioid peptide synthesis under various conditions. One area of interest has been the finding that opioid peptide synthesis can be altered in animal models of different pain states so that dynorphin levels in the spinal cord during inflammation are increased enormously due to the turning on of the gene for the synthesis of the parent propeptide (Ruda et al. 1988; Dubner and Ruda 1992). The physiological consequence remains unclear (Stanfa and Dickenson 1994), but the availability of selective antagonists for the three opioid receptors provides good tools to answer questions of this nature (Table I).

The high susceptibility of the opioids, particularly the enkephalins, to

Table I
Properties of the three opioid receptors

	Mu	Delta	Kappa
Endogenous ligand	endorphins	enkephalins	dynorphins
Selective agonists	DAMGO morphine	DPDPE dstbulet	U69593 C1977
Antagonists	CTAP	naltrindole	nor-BNI
Effector	cAMP G protein opens potassium channel	cAMP G protein opens potassium channel	G protein closes calcium channel
Subtypes	1 and 2	1 and 2	1, 2, and 3

peptidase degradation means that their biological lifetimes are short, which can cause problems in the measurement of tissue levels of the peptides and the study of their function. It is now possible to protect the enkephalins from breakdown by the use of peptidase inhibitors that are active systemically (Roques et al. 1993). This advance together with the synthesis of stable analogues of the endogenous opioids, which have far greater selectivity than do the endogenous opioids themselves, has provided the means to study of the roles and function of opioids and their receptors (Table I). The development of selective antagonists has been of great importance in assigning roles to the different opioid receptors in various models of pain. It is to be hoped that these derivatives will lead to clinically useful agents, based on the premise that drugs that act on receptors other than the morphine site could lack the morphine-like side effects that can cause problems in humans.

As is the case with any transmitter system, the greater the number of receptors the greater the chance that the desirable effects can be separated from the unwanted effects. In the case of the opioid receptors, a further division from the main three has been proposed. Thus, the mu receptor may consist of a mu 1 and a mu 2 subtype, the delta has been similarly subdivided, and the kappa receptor has been divided into three subtypes (Pasternak and Wood 1986; Traynor 1989; Jiang et al. 1991). Whether these subtypes have functional consequences remains to be seen; the physiological consquences are still hazy except for the delta subtypes, where there is evidence for differential effects of the two receptors (Jiang et al. 1991). It has been suggested that one of the delta receptors is in a complex with the mu receptor, an interesting proposition that needs further study (Porrecca et al. 1991). The delta opioid receptor has recently been isolated and cloned and seems to have the same seven-membrane spanning conformation as other second-messenger linked receptors. The advent of selective ligands has allowed the location and relative distribution of opioid receptor subtypes to be gauged. The recent cloning of the opioid receptors will further facilitate this task because probes based on the receptor sequence will provide unequivocal proof of location of the particular receptor and important insights into the mechanisms of opioid actions and the existence of subtypes (Evans et al. 1992; Keiffer et al. 1992; Chen et al. 1993).

Table I lists the current state of knowledge about selective drugs that act at the opioid receptors. Morphine has been listed as a selective agonist for the mu receptor. This drug has high affinity for the mu receptor, a relative affinity of 50 times less for the delta receptor, and minimal affinity for the kappa receptor. Thus, relatively nonselective effects could occur with very high doses such as those achieved in vitro and in binding studies where non-mu effects of morphine have been reported. However, in vivo, doses of spinal morphine that are sufficient to abolish the C-fiber evoked responses of dorsal horn nociceptive neurons are entirely mu-receptor mediated. Naltrindole, the delta receptor antagonist, at doses that block delta-receptor mediated antinociceptive, has no effect at all on the inhibitory effects of morphine (Sullivan and Dickenson; in preparation). Likewise, physiological studies provide no evidence for mu-delta cross-tolerance (Kalso et al. 1993). Thus, it appears that morphine produces its physiological effects by actions at the mu receptor.

There is intriguing evidence that morphine itself may be endogenous because the plant synthetic pathway is present in the mammal and there are regional differences in the levels of traces of morphine in the CNS (Kosterlitz 1987). In addition, in patients receiving L-DOPA therapy for Parkinson's disease, the levels of plasma morphine (presumed to be endogenous because the patients were not taking opiate drugs) are higher than in normal subjects. The synthetic pathway for morphine is present in the kidney, and L-DOPA can act as a precursor. This evidence suggests that the pathway for the production of morphine can be induced in humans (Matsubara et al. 1992).

There has been hope that agonists acting at the delta and kappa receptors will be useful analgesics while lacking some of the undesirable effects of drugs such as morphine and other mu agonists. The pharmaceutical industry is pursuing these non-mu agonists, but it is too early to determine if they will have clinical utility.

Opioids act by three common mechanisms. These underlying events by which opioids interfere with the transmission of pain are the same as the mechanisms by which opioids cause their other actions, including side effects. The three main mechanisms are:

1. A presynaptic action on the terminals of neurons whereby activition of opioid receptors reduces the release of transmitters from the terminals.

2. A postsynaptic hyperpolarization that can affect cell bodies of output neurons, interneurons, or dendrites, and reduces evoked activity in the neuronal pathways.

3. A disinhibition in a circuit of two inhibitory neurons where the second cell is held in check by the other inhibitory neuron; inhibition of the first neuron by the opioid allows the second cell to become active, with a resultant inhibition of activity.

The presynaptic action results from an opening of potassium channels (mu and delta receptors) or a closing of calcium channels (kappa), both of which lead to a reduction in calcium influx into C-fiber terminals, thus diminishing transmitter release (Duggan and North 1984; McFadzean 1988; North 1989). C-fibers release several transmitters including the tachykinins, excitatory amino acids, and excitatory peptides that act on multiple receptors. Consequently, this presynaptic action reducing the release of many transmitters will be a highly effective route to analgesia because it will be equivalent to the block of multiple postsynaptic receptors.

Evidence for functional opioid actions at postsynaptic receptors is based on electrophysiological and behavioral approaches (Hylden and Wilcox 1983; Duggan and North 1984; Lombard and Besson 1989). Postsynaptic hyperpolarizations again result via the opening of potassium ion channels or the closing of calcium channels (Duggan and North 1984). These receptors could hyperpolarize the dendrites of projection neurons, interneurons, or the cell body of projection cells. In the former two cases the action of the opioids would be selective for noxious transmission as is observed in electrophysiological studies. However, in the latter case actions on the cell body may not be selective for nociceptive inputs.

An important indirect postsynaptic action is the opioid disinhibitory effect mediated via GABA and enkephalin neurons in the substantia gelatinosa, which in turn leads to an inhibition of output neurons. Both morphological and electrophysiological evidence supports this action (see Magnuson and Dickenson 1991).

These three effects of opioids underlie both analgesia and the unwanted effects produced by opioids acting at numerous sites in the central nervous system; the spinal cord is possibly the best understood simply because it can be accessed independently of the rest of the CNS.

SPINAL ANALGESIA

Opioid receptors in the spinal cord are a critical site in the production of analgesia, as has been clearly shown by the demonstration of opioid inhibition of nociceptive neurons in the spinal cords of animals and direct analgesia following epidural and intrathecal opioids in animals and then subsequently in humans (Besson and Chaouch 1987; Yaksh and Nouiehed 1985). This is an excellent example of how basic research in animals can have a rapid and important application to the clinical relief of pain. Researchers have devoted considerable efforts to the study of opioid receptor subtypes in the spinal cord, using both electrophysiological and behavioral approaches. The recent studies on the spinal opioid systems have begun to address the extent of plasticity in opioid spinal function, with indications that opioid activity and function are not immutable even to the extent of activation of opioid peptide genes by particular stimuli (Dickenson 1991b; Dubner and Ruda 1992).

Present studies using labeled selective ligands show that the highest levels of opioid receptors in the spinal cord are around the C-fiber terminal zones in lamina 1 and the substantia gelatinosa, with lower levels found in deeper layers. The best current estimates suggest that the mu receptor forms 70%, the delta 24%, and the kappa 6% of the total opioid sites in the rat spinal cord (Besse et al. 1990). The idea that kappa levels are higher in the mouse and guinea pig spinal cord has been put forward. However, studies in species other than the rat have not been carried out with the most selective ligands for the receptors and so may not represent the true relative distribution of the receptors. It is surprising that the availability of selective ligands for the three receptors has not led to systematic quantitative studies in several species on the relative distribution of the receptors in a variety of CNS sites.

Cutting the dorsal roots and waiting for degeneration of the primary afferents will result in loss of the presynaptic opioid receptors. Consequently, we can calculate the relative numbers of pre- and postsynaptic receptors. The presynaptic sites predominate. The proportions of presynaptic sites in the spinal cord vary from 70–50% for the subtypes based on drops in levels after rhizotomy; more than 70% of the total mu receptor sites are on the afferent terminals (Besse et al. 1990). The presynaptic action of opioids has been demonstrated for mu and delta agonists but not kappa on the basis of a reduced release of the primary afferent transmitters present in C-fibers. Evidence for a presynaptic action of opioids comes from studies of opioid inhibition of C-fiber evoked release of transmitters (substance P and glutamate) and from in vitro and in vivo electrophysiological studies (Hirota et al. 1985; Aimone and Yaksh 1989; Kangra et al. 1991; Hori et al. 1992), although some studies have failed to demonstrate this action (Lang et al. 1991). Capsaicin can elicit the release of these transmitters, so at least a proportion of the release must be from C-fiber afferents. The expected axo-axonic morphological basis for this interaction, enkephalin neurons making synaptic contact onto the afferent terminals, has not been seen. Consequently, there may be nonsynaptic actions of opioids released from distant neurons and diffusing to the receptors on the afferent terminals. The association of opioid receptors with C-fiber but not large A-fiber terminals allows for the observed selective effects of spinal opioids on noxious evoked activity (Duggan and North 1984; Dickenson and Sullivan 1986; Besson and Chaouch 1987).

However, opioids can have facilitatory effects on C-fiber transmission at low doses, probably due to release of excitatory transmitters from the afferent terminals. A characteristic of mu receptor agonists is that the lowest doses of all intrathecal mu opioids enhance C-fiber activity. However, inhibitions occur and then predominate as the dose is increased (Dickenson and Sullivan 1986; Dickenson et al. 1987b; Crain and Shen 1990; Wiesenfeld-Hallin et al. 1990). This mild increase in C-fiber activity elicited by low doses could explain the itching around the extremities of the spinal morphine injection that occurs in humans. These effects may be the one exception to the primary inhibitory actions of opioids (Crain and Shen 1990).

The postsynaptic actions of opioids are harder to interpret because any direct hyperpolarization of a cell soma would inhibit all responses of the cell including the innocuous inputs onto convergent or multireceptive cells. However, many of the opioid receptors in the substantia gelatinosa could be on the dendrites of the deep cells penetrating into the C-fiber terminal zone; inhibitory effects here also would be selective. Another possibility is based on the observation that the responses of substantia gelatinosa cells are enhanced by opioids following various routes of administration. This enhancement appears to be via $GABA_A$-mediated disinhibition of enkephalin interneurons, or vice versa; the net result is the same (Magnuson and Dickenson 1991). If these disinhibited cells fed onto the output cells, excitatory interneurons, or dendrites, they would be an additional source of inhibition of nociceptive transmission. Whatever the case, these different mechanisms will have overall similar final effects, but pathological damage to the afferents will remove the presynaptic receptors on the terminals, which has relevance to the treatment by opioids of neuropathic pain.

Comparative studies in animals with and without the presynaptic sites provide electrophysiological evidence that the postsynaptic actions of opioids require higher doses of morphine than do the presynaptic effects (Lombard and Besson 1989). Consequently, if the loss of the presynaptic receptors contributes to any reduced opioid sensitivity of postamputation pain, dose escalation should overcome this spinal problem. In addition, the supraspinal sites of action of opioids will not be perturbed by primary afferent damage or dysfunction. Fig. 1 shows these spinal actions of opioids.

Most mu and delta opioids have similar dose ranges after intrathecal application but the most potent opioids are the mu ligands, presumably reflecting the many mu opioid sites in the spinal cord. Efficacy also is a factor. The relative lack of tolerance seen with the mu opioid DAGOL compared to less potent mu opioids has been attributed to a large pool of spare receptors; fewer receptors will need to be activated to produce maximal analgesia with this highly potent peptide (Stevens and Yaksh 1989). The clinical selection of opioids and the dose for spinal analgesia must consider the clear inverse relationship between lipophilicity and potency for a range of synthetic opioids (McQuay et al. 1989; Dickenson et al. 1990). In these studies the most potent spinal opioid was morphine, which is the least lipophilic; drugs such as fentanyl were relatively ineffective. This relationship is probably due to nonspecific binding of the lipophilic opioids in the lipid-rich fiber tracts capping the cord, or to efficient vascular redistribution that reduces the dose of opioid reaching the receptors in the gelatinosa. This relationship has been confirmed in humans.

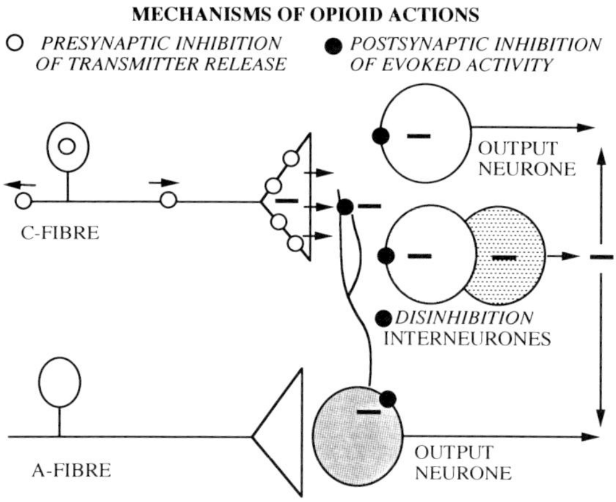

Fig. 1. The analgesic actions of opioids. The three modes of action, namely presynaptic inhibition of transmitter release, postsynaptic inhibition of evoked activity, and postsynaptic disinhibition are shown in relation to the circuitry of the spinal cord. Note that opioid receptors are synthesized in dorsal root ganglia of C-fibers but not large A-fibers. The text provides further details.

Antagonists for the opioid receptors have demonstrated the independence of mu, delta, and kappa receptors at the spinal level in terms of antinociception (Porreca et al. 1984; Schmauss and Yaksh 1984; Sullivan et al. 1989a), although some studies have failed to demonstrate reversal of kappa receptor agonist effects by kappa antagonists. The independent analgesic effects following activation of non-mu receptors indicated that there is potential for opioid analgesics that are delta or kappa agonists. In general, there is little evidence to suggest modality-selective effects of opioids (Parsons and Headley 1989); they are effective in most circumstances against cutaneous, chemical inflammatory, visceral, and other stimuli (Yaksh and Nouiehed 1985; Dickenson 1991b; Maves and Gebhart 1992). In contrast, in models of neuropathic pain states—whether the nerve damage is central or peripheral—reduced effects of opioids are observed in animals and in man (Arner and Meyerson 1988; Portenoy et al. 1990; Jadad et al. 1992; Dickenson 1994).

The studies quoted so far have used synthetic drugs, some of which are analogues of the endogenous opioids because the latter have only limited selectivity for the three opioid receptors. However, it is possible to use antagonists to study the roles of the opioid peptides mediated by actions at particular receptors. The enkephalins are rapidly degraded by membrane-bound peptidases, which curtail their actions. The synthesis of peptidase inhibitors has been a successful strategy. Kelatorphan, a mixed peptidase, inhibits at least two of the important breakdown enzymes, affording almost complete protection to the enkephalins (Roques et al. 1993). The spinal application of the inhibitor reduces nociceptive responses of cells (Dickenson et al. 1987a); the pool of enkephalins protected by the inhibitor is likely to derive from both a segmental release and from descending pathways activated by the stimulus. The inhibitions are reversed by a selective delta antagonist. Behavioral studies have shown similar effects with another peptidase inhibitor. The recent reports of a systemically active mixed peptidase inhibitor, RB101, is the next stage toward the clinical application of this novel approach to pain relief. Interestingly, the side effect profile of RB101 appears to be unlike that of morphine in physical and psychological dependence (Roques et al. 1993).

Dynorphin, the endogenous kappa opioid receptor agonist, has some effects that differ from the typical opioid actions. It promoted action of some neurons and inhibits other nociceptive neurons when applied spinally (Knox and Dickenson 1987). The up-regulation in spinal dynorphin seen in inflammation due to gene induction (Ruda et al. 1988; Dubner and Ruda 1992) probably has physiological relevance. Spinal application of a kappa receptor antagonist increases and decreases individual neuronal activity in normal animals but is considerably more effective in animals with inflammation (Stanfa and Dickenson 1994). The consequences for pain transmission are not understood.

NOVEL PERIPHERAL ANALGESIA

Opioids have no peripheral actions at cutaneous sites in undamaged tissue, but there is now good evidence that the consequences of inflammation can induce a novel site of opioid action that appears rapidly after the induction of the inflammation. The synthesis of opioid receptors occurs in dorsal root ganglion cells as well as other locations in the body. These receptors are transported in the fine afferent fibers in both directions; the centrally directed receptors become the presynaptic receptors and the peripherally transported receptors somehow become active only following inflammation. The relative effectiveness of mu, delta, and kappa receptor activation to elicit peripheral analgesia varies between models, but all three are active in arthritic states (Stein et al. 1989). Alongside the appearance of the peripheral opioid receptors on afferent nerves, the arrival of endogenous opioid peptides at the injury site seems to be related to immune-cell proliferation. Thus, opioids unable to penetrate the CNS and consequently devoid of central side effects may be good analgesics in inflammatory states via these peripheral sites. The chapter by Stein discusses this topic in detail. Interestingly, the same models of inflammation show clear parallel increases in the spinal effects of opioids (Hylden et al. 1991; Stanfa et al. 1992).

SUPRASPINAL ANALGESIA

The first demonstration of opioid actions within the central nervous system was the analgesia seen following intraventricular morphine. Supraspinal sites of opioid analgesia are now well established and have been localized to areas in the medial brain stem around the nucleus raphe magnus and extending rostrally to periaqueductal and periventricular gray areas (Yaksh et al. 1988). The roles of these areas in morphine analgesia have been based on microinjection studies and the ability of locally applied naloxone to reduce the effects of systemic morphine (Yaksh et al. 1988; Fields et al. 1988). Mu and delta receptors are effective in eliciting analgesia at brain stem sites (kappa have not been widely tested), and intraventricular administration of kappa opioids in the rat produces analgesia (Millan 1990).

The mechanisms of opioid action at these supraspinal levels, and in particular how they interact with descending inhibitory controls are still unclear. Many studies have reported both opioid-induced increases and decreases in descending inhibitory controls. Examination of the anatomy and pharmacology of the descending systems may provide a basis for these disparate results. First, descending controls originate from many different areas of the brain stem and the midbrain and a complex pharmacology exists in these pathways. Noradrenaline, 5-HT, enkephalin, and substance P are involved, with the last three coexisting in some neurons. The monoamines have numerous receptors at the spinal terminal sites that, when activated, could inhibit or excite depending on the receptor. Whether or not the postsynaptic receptors are on excitatory or inhibitory elements also will be important. Consequently, the problem is not the direction of effect of opioids on these systems but to understand the physiological roles and consequences of the mixed opioid actions on these multiple pathways.

Many of the sites of opioid actions at supraspinal sites overlap with areas where descending inhibitory controls originate; the simplest situation is that supraspinal opioids increase descending inhibitions and these in turn block spinal pain transmission. The clearest demonstration that morphine increases supraspinal descending inhibitory controls is the finding that the spinal induction of c-*fos*, used as a marker of noxious evoked activity, is clearly reduced by intraventricular morphine (Gogas et al. 1991).

Other findings, however, do not show this direction of effect. Diffuse noxious inhibitory controls (DNIC) are descending controls induced by heterosegmental noxious stimulation and partly involve both opioid and serotonergic mechanisms. Morphine reduces these descending controls. DNIC are thought to establish a contrast between a discrete pool of activated nociceptive neurons that trigger the system and a surrounding pool of inhibition of ongoing innocuous activity in other segments of the cord. It has been proposed that this differential activity forms the message perceived by the brain as noxious; as supraspinal PAG and intraventricular morphine reduce DNIC, the perception of pain decreases (Le Bars and Villeneuva 1988). The direct spinal actions of opioids in blocking the spinal transmission of pain would prevent the initial activation of DNIC and so reduce both the segmental excitations and these descending controls.

Fields and colleagues have provided evidence for a theory that is not exclusive of the first, in that certain cells in the brain stem are turned off by noxious stimuli; this inhibition is presumed to remove inhibitory influences on the cord, allowing a reflex to occur. Morphine turns on these cells, probably via disinhibiting GABA interneurons, so no reflex results. At the same time, morphine inhibits a second group of cells that are activated by a noxious stimulus, so the overall effect would be a reduction in descending controls (Fields et al. 1988). Both concepts thus rely on two distinct effects of morphine on two pools of cells.

We face considerable difficulties in arriving at a simple consensus as to the direction of effect of opioids on descending control systems. However, as discussed above, the multiplicity of these descending controls in their anatomical locations, pharmacology, and spinal projections forms a framework within which to incorporate the various directions of effect of opioids. There is no doubt that whatever the mechanism, supraspinal opioids produce behavioral analgesia.

Opioid receptors occur at many other sites in the brain stem, midbrain, and at higher centers. Whereas some of these receptors will underlie analgesia, the others will influence the centrally mediated side effects of opioids such as respiratory depression, cough suppression, nausea, and dependence.

CHANGES IN OPIOID SYSTEMS

Substantial clinical and animal data support the idea that the effects of opioids, particularly with regard to analgesia, are not invariable but will differ in different pain states. The major problem is the treatment of pain where there is a reduced opioid sensitivity. Neuropathic pains are frequently in this category, but substantial animal evidence shows that inflammatory pains are accompanied by opposite opioid effect—an increased sensitivity to opioids. There are several possible explanations for changes in opioid actions. Knowledge of these systems will greatly benefit the treatment of difficult pain. The following list of possibilities reflects the current knowledge; these are not exclusive systems and it is possible that there will be multiple causes even in a single pain state.

1. A loss of opioid receptors would be expected to contribute to a reduction in opioid sensitivity. One well-established example is the reduction in spinal opioid receptor number seen after nerve section, which may explain the poor opioid sensitivity of postamputation pain.
2. The ability of exogenous application of the nonopioid peptides, FLFQPQRFamide (F8Fa) or cholecystokinin (CCK), either spinally or supraspinally, to act as negative influences on opioid actions. There is now evidence that this has physiological relevance and that the levels of CCK in the cord can determine the potency of morphine.
3. Overexcitability of spinal neurons, thus inducing a hypersensitive state against which opioid controls are insufficiently efficacious. The N-methyl-D-aspartate (NMDA) receptor is a strong candidate for generation of hyperalgesic states in inflammatory, neuropathic, and ischemic pain models. An associated reduction in opioid effects has frequently been observed.
4. The transmission of painful messages via the normally innocuous A-fiber population as a result of pathological changes in peripheral and/or central processes. There are no opioid receptors on the central terminals of these fibers.
5. An accumulation of morphine-3-glucuronide, the major metabolite and a purported antagonist of morphine.

These five possibilities are not mutually exclusive and there may well be common sites of interactions between these different pharmacological systems that can alter the excitability of the dorsal horn and reduce opioid sensitivity. Changes in afferent activity above and below the normal level are important in their genesis because it is clear in many animal models and in humans that the spinal manifestation of these changes occurs as a result of, and not independently of, peripheral afferent activity (Dickenson 1991b; Gracely et al. 1993).

LOSS OF OPIOID RECEPTORS

Sectioning of a peripheral nerve will lead to degeneration of the nerve and loss of receptors found on the nerve itself. In the case of a C-fiber, the mu receptor for morphine on the presynaptic terminals in the spinal cord (Fig. 1) will be reduced by 70% (Besse et al. 1990). In animal models where the presynaptic opioid receptors have been removed by prior rhizotomy, in electrophysiological studies with systemic morphine (Lombard and Besson 1989), and behavioral studies with spinal application (Xu and Wiesenfeld-Hallin

1991), higher doses (twofold) than in normal animals are required to produce antinociception. The reduced antinociceptive effects of morphine are not surprising because although nerve section will reduce opioid sites, the spinal postsynaptic receptors are still available as are the supraspinal sites. Thus, when opioid receptors are lost due to either peripheral or central lesions, there will be at most a reduction in opioid action, which should predictably be overcome by dose escalation.

ANTI-OPIOID PEPTIDES

The exogenous spinal application of both FLFQPQRFamide and CCK, nonopioid peptides found within intrinsic neurons in the spinal cord and elsewhere in the brain, will prevent mu- but not delta-mediated neuronal inhibitions at doses that have little effect on the neuronal responses (Baber et al. 1989; Dickenson 1991a,b). Both reduce intrathecal morphine analgesia in behavioral studies (Xu et al. 1993; Zhou et al. 1993). In addition to their ability to reduce the actions of morphine at the spinal level, there is considerable evidence that they are effective in reducing the analgesia elicited by mu opioids acting at supraspinal sites, thus making them potential causes of global reductions in morphine analgesia. In situations where there is a release of these peptides we would expect a reduction in morphine effects without requiring any change in opioid receptor number. In fact, the ability of these peptides to interfere with analgesia is not restricted to the effects of opioids but also includes alpha-adrenoceptor agonist actions (Dickenson 1991a).

The mechanism whereby these peptides interfere with the effects of drugs such as morphine is unclear, as are the circumstances behind their release. However, there is some evidence that morphine itself can cause a release of CCK and as such there is good reason to believe that this mechanism may underlie tolerance (Zhou et al. 1993). Nociceptive inputs into the spinal cord in physiopathological states may release the peptide and produce concomitant reduced opioid effectiveness. In the case of the other peptide, F8amide, there is similar evidence for both morphine and afferent activity-induced release, at least at the spinal level. Preventing the actions of the peptides with antagonists or antibodies both potentiates the analgesic effects of morphine and reduces tolerance (Baber et al. 1989; Stanfa and Dickenson 1993; Xu et al. 1993; Zhou et al. 1993). More is known about CCK and it is likely that the receptors, the CCK-B subtype, are located on presynaptic terminals in the spinal cord and also on postsynaptic elements, both probably close to the opioid receptor sites. At supraspinal sites the widespread distribution of CCK receptors includes some sites rich in opioid receptors. CCK does not bind to opioid receptors so the mechanisms of interference with opioid analgesia are thought to be indirect; either the binding of CCK to the CCK-B receptor induces an allosteric change in the mu receptor that reduces the actions of morphine, or the peptide produces intracellular changes that oppose those following activation of the mu receptor. Opioids decrease calcium levels in terminals to reduce transmitter release; the recent demonstration that CCK will mobilize intracellular calcium is one possible basis for the interference with opioid actions (Wang et al. 1992).

Two different studies have recently provided evidence for a physiological role for CCK as a factor in altered opioid actions. The effects of spinal morphine are reduced after peripheral nerve section and this is associated with a marked up-regulation of CCK in primary afferent terminals (Xu et al. 1993). This finding points to a presynaptic action of CCK in reducing opioid actions; the administration of CCK-B antagonists restores opioid sensitivity. Exactly the opposite occurs following the induction of peripheral inflammation where the spinal actions of morphine (Stanfa et al. 1992) are increased, apparently due to reduced levels of the peptide (Stanfa and Dickenson 1993). It is fascinating evidence that the CCK control of opioid analgesia is dependent on the behavioral state of the animal (Wiertelak et al. 1992). If this finding applies to patients, some of the variability in opioid analgesia may be explained by environmental factors.

Opioid analgesia could be enhanced if the potential role of CCK as an "antagonist" of morphine applies to the clinical situation in pain states with reduced opioid sensitivity. CCK antagonists are being developed (Baber et al. 1989) and should be useful adjuncts to opioids (Table II).

These peptides are not the only factors in the spinal cord that can alter opioid actions; galanin (Wiesenfeld-Hallin et al. 1990) and adenosine (Sawynok and Yaksh 1993) may well play important roles.

NMDA RECEPTORS

Nociceptive stimulation can cause a persistent enhancement of the excitability of the spinal cord (Woolf 1983). The NMDA receptor, one of the receptors for the excitatory amino acid glutamate, which is widely used in the central nervous system as a transmitter, has been strongly implicated in the responses of dorsal horn neurons to prolonged stimulation (Dickenson 1990; Woolf and Thompson 1991; Dubner and Ruda 1993) as well as in other aspects of neurotransmission in the CNS (Daw et al. 1993). In addition to this role in the transmission of painful messages over long periods of time, the activation of this receptor is associated with alterations in opioid responsiveness seen in different pain states (Dickenson 1990; 1991b; 1994;

Table II
Summary of the effects of changing cholecystokinin levels on opioid analgesia and tolerance

Increased Levels	Decreased Levels
Reduced opioid actions after nerve section	Increased opioid actions after inflammation
Morphine tolerance	CCK-B antagonists potentiate analgesia
	CCK-B antagonists reduce tolerance

McQuay and Dickenson 1990).

Wind-up is an important spinal mechanism mediated by the activation of the NMDA receptor, which exaggerates the C-fiber induced activity of dorsal horn nociceptive neurons (Dickenson and Sullivan 1987). The expected constant neuronal response to a constant C-fiber stimulation is transformed to an enhanced and prolonged response following activation of the NMDA receptor following a short series of stimuli (Fig. 2). Consequently, this may be one of the events underlying prolonged and/or chronic pain and the production of so-called central hypersensitive states (Dickenson 1990,1991b; Dubner and Ruda 1992; Woolf and Thompson 1991). There is now evidence from animal studies that this is the case for the induction and maintenance of hyperalgesia in models of inflammatory pain, ischemic pain, and neuropathic pains (Haley et al. 1990; Sher and Mitchell 1990; Schaible et al. 1991; Seltzer et al. 1991; Yamamoto and Yaksh 1992; Mao et al. 1993; Ren et al. 1992; Stanfa et al. 1992).

In many of these studies, involvement of the NMDA receptor in the transmission of nociception is associated with reduction in sensitivity of the response to opioids. Exceptions to this are the carrageenan model of inflammation (Hylden et al. 1991; Stanfa et al. 1992) and mechanical nociception in a model of neuropathy (Attal et al. 1991) with enhanced opioid actions (Table III). In the former model, as discussed in the previous section, the changes in CCK may predominate and overcome the influence of the NMDA activity.

In all other models NMDA receptor activation reduces opioid sensitivity. Opioids, presumably by their ability to reduce the release of primary afferent transmitters or to inhibit interneurons early in nociceptive pathways, initially reduce or block the C-fiber inputs onto the deeper dorsal horn nociceptive neurons (Dickenson and Sullivan 1986; Chapman and Dickenson 1992). However, as the peripheral stimulation continues, wind-up then breaks through the inhibitions of input and the cells start to respond. Thus, at moderate doses, opioids delay the onset of wind-up without inhibiting the process itself (Fig. 2). With wind-up, the rightward shift in the opioid dose-response curve is particularly marked at the lower end of the curve and so dose escalation can

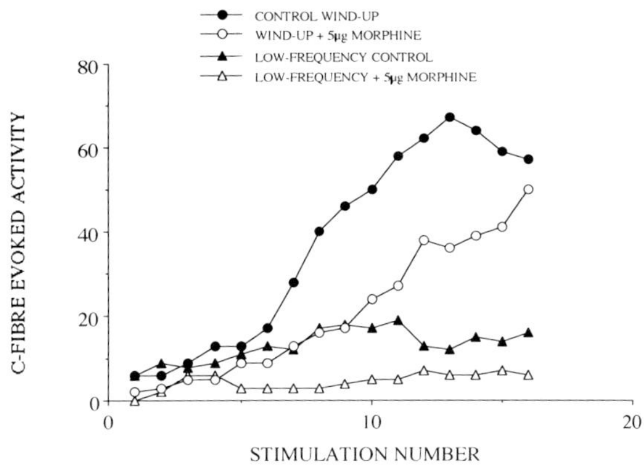

Fig. 2. NMDA receptor activation reduces opioid effectiveness. A neuronal recording from the dorsal horn of the anesthetized rat showing wind-up elicited by constant C-fiber stimulation at 0.5 Hz (control wind-up). Low-frequency stimulation, although at the same intensity, does not activate the NMDA receptor, so no wind-up occurs (low-frequency control). Spinal morphine almost abolishes this response (low frequency + morphine), but in the same neuron when the stimulation is changed to 0.5 Hz, inducing wind-up, the neuronal activity now breaks through the opioid inhibitions (wind-up + morphine).

overcome the reduced opioid effectiveness (Dickenson and Sullivan 1986; Chapman and Dickenson 1992). This is also the case for pain-related behavior after nerve section where the threshold for opioid inhibitions is raised (Xu and Wiesenfeld-Hallin 1991).

Neuropathic pain can be difficult to treat with opioids (Arner and Meyerson 1988; Portenoy et al. 1990; Jadad et al. 1992) and the same holds for at least some of the measures in the animal models of neuropathic pain. Complicated changes occur in the sensitivity of the inflammatory models; after carrageenan inflammation there is a clear involvement of the NMDA receptor in the hyperalgesia and the neuronal response changes observed (Hylden et al. 1991; Stanfa et al. 1992; Ren et al. 1992), yet a clear increase in spinal opioid sensitivity (Stanfa et al. 1992). However, in the formalin model of inflammation there is a reduced sensitivity of the second prolonged and NMDA-mediated phase of the response to opioids when they are administered once the activity is established compared to the same dose given prior to the induction of the response (Dickenson and Sullivan 1989). Again, increases in the dose of the opioid will restore the ability to block the response. C-fiber evoked NMDA-mediated hypersensitivity of the flexion reflex is (Woolf and Thompson 1991), like the formalin response, less sensitive to morphine once the enhanced state is established (Woolf and Wall 1986).

All of these studies on pain that is poorly responsive to opioids have

Table III
Opioid sensitivity and NMDA receptor involvement in animal models

Type of Model	Sensitivity and Receptor Involvement
Wind-up	reduced
C-fiber induced reflex hypersensitivity	reduced
Second inflammatory phase of the formalin response	reduced
Thermal hyperalgesia after peripheral neuropathy	reduced
Allodynia after spinal disinhibition	reduced
Carrageenan inflammation	enhanced

emphasized mu opioids, especially morphine, but mu and delta opioids and alpha-2 antagonists all have similar effects on wind-up (Dickenson 1991; Dickenson and Sullivan 1986). It is unlikely that these three systems would have different effects on MNDA receptor-mediated events. Drugs such as clonidine are thus unlikely to be alternatives to morphine, at least for spinal events that implicate the NMDA receptor.

In contrast to the effects of opioids on the mechanisms of wind-up, NMDA antagonists have no effect on the initial inputs onto the cells, but abolish wind-up. The potentiated response then reverts to a constant response to the constant stimulus (Davies and Lodge 1987; Dickenson and Sullivan 1987a, 1990). NMDA antagonists thus could be antinociceptive agents alone, but possibly more usefully in combination with opioids. Profound inhibitions of nociceptive responses can be elicited with threshold doses of morphine combined with low doses of NMDA antagonists (Chapman and Dickenson 1992). Low doses of both drugs can produce the powerful synergistic effects and could have low side effect liability. The potentiation probably results from the combination of presynaptic opioid inhibitions that reduce afferent inputs onto the cells and the postsynaptic NMDA block that reduces wind-up. In addition, in a model of neuropathic pain in which morphine is inoperative, the coapplication of an NMDA antagonist restores the ability of morphine to inhibit the response (Yamamoto and Yaksh 1992). Two drugs with current clinical usages, ketamine and dextromethorphan, are NMDA channel blockers and are effective at reducing NMDA-mediated responses in these dorsal horn nociceptive systems (Davies and Lodge 1987; Haley et al. 1990; Dickenson et al. 1991). Recent behavioral evidence from studies in neuropathic pain in animals has convincingly shown that dextrorphan and ketamine are effective against the hyperalgesia and spontaneous pain (Mao et al. 1993; Tal and

Bennett 1993). These drugs are important because they both block the channel associated with the receptor and appear to lack some of the adverse effects of the most potent experimental channel blocker, MK801. They also are in current clinical use.

Aside from directly influencing the NMDA-mediated responses by agents directed at the receptor or channel, another tactic to improve morphine analgesia would be to reduce the resultant excitability via the pharmacologically nonspecific actions of spinal local anesthetics. These synergize with spinal morphine as shown in many investigations ranging from electrophysiology stidoes in which the potentiation is partly due to the ability of the former to reduce NMDA-mediated activity (Fraser et al. 1992), to behavioral approaches (Akerman et al. 1988; Maves and Gebhart 1992), and to clinical studies.

PAIN VIA A-FIBERS

Doses of morphine that abolish C-fiber activity in normal animals have only minor effects on A-fiber activity (Dickenson and Sullivan 1986). Consequently, in circumstances where A-fiber stimulation can induce sensations of pain as a result of either pathological changes in the periphery and/or the central processing of the nociceptive messages, opioid sensitivity would be low. Allodynia may be one manifestation. Bearing this out, the allodynia produced by the spinal application of GABA and glycine antagonists in behavioral studies is reduced by NMDA antagonism but is morphine insensitive (Yaksh 1989). Wind-up is only induced by C-fiber stimulation, but the resultant hyperactivity is postsynaptic. Many neurons receive both A and C-fiber inputs, and A-fiber inputs will impinge upon the hyperexcitable neuron, which may underlie some forms of allodynia. If the allodynia and some of the hyperalgesias are transmitted through A-fiber afferents, a poor sensitivity to opioids would not be surprising because presynaptic opioid receptors are only associated with C-fibers (Besson and Chaouch 1987). A few opioid receptors located on the output neurons (Fig. 1) are the only opioid control on these pathways.

MORPHINE METABOLITES

The glucuronidation of morphine produces two major metabolites, morphine-3-glucuronide (M3G) and morphine-6-glucuronide (M6G) (see Sullivan et al. 1989b; Smith et al. 1990; Gong et al. 1992). They have remarkably different actions. The 6-glucuronide is more potent than morphine itself, and although the degree of this enhanced action varies from study to study, it is at least 10-fold more effective in tests of analgesia (Sullivan et al. 1989b). The reasons for this are not obvious at present because the affinity of M6G for the mu receptor is not appreciably greater than that of morphine itself. However, the morphine-3-glucuronide metabolite has no affinity for the mu receptor, and being unable to bind to the receptor, has no opioid actions. Nevertheless, results of behavioral studies suggest that morphine-3-glucuronide is a factor that contributes to reduced opioid sensitivity (Smith et al. 1990; Gong et al. 1992). In both studies M3G reduced the effects of morphine to some extent, but an appreciable analgesia still occurred. One of the studies stated that the metabolite given by the intraventricular route caused marked behavioral agitation that interfered with the behavioral tests. In contrast to these studies, electrophysiological evidence (where nonspecific effects are less likely to interfere with the results) shows that even with dose ratios of 100:1 of the metabolite to morphine, morphine-3-glucuronide has absolutely no effect on the inhibitory effects of morphine on spinal nociceptive neurons (Hewett et al. 1993; Table IV). The spinal site of action of morphine is a major contributor to systemic analgesia, and in renal insufficiency where the metabolite will accumulate, opiate effects tend to be enhanced rather than reduced. The contribution of morphine-3-glucuronide to pain poorly responsive to opioid remains to be determined.

OPIOID INTERACTIONS WITH OTHER TRANSMITTER SYSTEMS

The preceding section indicates how the concomitant activation of other transmitter systems such as the NMDA and CCK can reduce opioid actions and how this mechanism can be manipulated by blocking this interference. The activation of nonopioid inhibitory controls also can be harnessed to increase opioid analgesia (Table V).

Table IV
Properties of morphine metabolites

Morphine-6-glucuronide	Morphine-3-glucuronide
More potent than morphine	Not analgesic
Unexpected penetration into CNS	Unexpected penetration into CNS
	No affinity for opioid receptors
	Can cause hyperexcitability
	No antagonism of spinal opioid analgesia
	Antagonism at supraspinal sites?

The section on supraspinal analgesia presented considerable evidence for an interaction between morphine and other opioids and descending control systems. However, in addition to the interactions between opioids at supraspinal sites and descending controls involving noradrenaline and 5-hydroxytryptamine (5-HT), the level of activity in descending controls has a bearing on the spinal actions of opioids. The number and complexity of 5-HT receptors has made it difficult to interpret the spinal interactions between morphine and serotonergic systems. For noradrenaline, the spinal target site has been clearly established as the alpha-2 receptor, located in similar areas to the opioid receptors. Alpha-2 receptor activation results in a selective inhibition of the spinal transmission of nociceptive information and behavioral analgesia. In addition to the effects of alpha-2 and opiate agonists alone, there is considerable evidence that the coadministration of drugs acting at these separate receptors can produce supra-additive or synergistic effects (Dickenson and Sullivan 1993).

The analgesic effects of a threshold dose of morphine are markedly increased in the presence of clonidine, and the combination of inactive doses of dexmedetomidine with threshold doses of morphine cause almost complete, naloxone-reversible inhibitions of the neurons. Thus, when morphine and an alpha-2 agonist at low doses, which would be expected to produce minor side effects, are applied spinally the resultant analgesia will be profound. Interestingly, there was no potentiation of the weaker inhibitory effects of the two on the tactile A-beta fiber evoked responses of the same cells (Dickenson and Sullivan 1993). Thus, with an increase in descending noradrenergic activity we would expect an increase in opiate effectiveness due to the synergistic interactions between the opiate and the alpha-2 agonist. This goal can be achieved with exogenous alpha-2 agonists (Fig. 3).

The enhancement of noradrenaline function in the brain is associated with

Table V
Transmitter system interactions with opioid actions

Transmitter System	Effect
Local anesthetics	positive
Alpha-2-adrenoceptor agonists	positive
Morphine-6-glucuronide	positive
NMDA receptor activation	negative
Cholecystokinin and F8Fa	negative
Morphine-3-glucuronide	negative

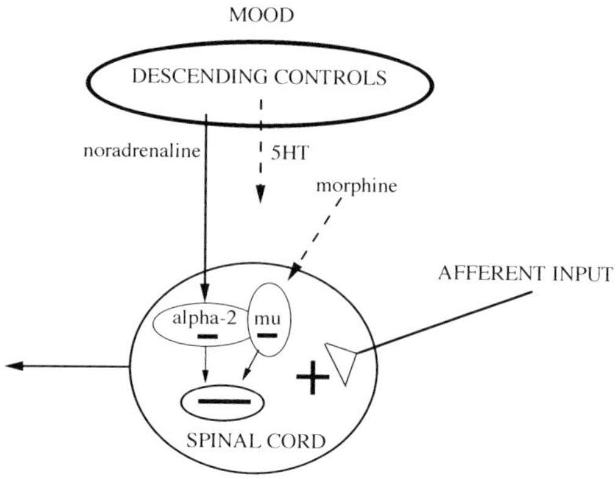

Fig. 3. Descending monoamine systems can alter pain transmission and opioid actions. The synergy between alpha-2 adrenoceptor activation and morphine at the spinal level is particularly well understood. Further details are given in the text.

elevations in mood; many antidepressants act by increasing the synaptic levels of the catecholamine. The levels of noradrenaline in the central nervous system will reflect the person's mood and level of stress. Noradrenaline may thus form a link between emotion, pain, and opioid analgesia. Increases in noradrenaline in the spinal cord will not only have the potential to reduce the transmission of pain, but also could increase opioid effectiveness by merit of the synergy between the opioid and alpha-2 agonist.

Table VI
Examples of ways in which analgesic outcomes can be improved by combination of morphine with other agents

Morphine with
Agents that reduce excitability
Local anesthetics
Ketamine and NMDA antagonists
NSAIDs
Agents that increase inhibitions
Alpha-2 adrenoceptor agonists

To conclude, the recent advances in our understanding of how and where opioids act and the factors that can influence the efficacy of opioids form a basis for improving the clinical outcomes of opioid use. Opioid receptors are but part of the vast pharmacological repertoire of neurons in the nervous system, and the ways in which the concurrent activation of other transmitter systems can alter opioid actions reflect the integrated function of the CNS.This recent knowledge of the biology of opioids can be harnessed through combination therapy (Table VI) and by recognizing the potential of timing and routes of administration to influence opioid actions. There is little doubt that opioids are, and will remain, a subject area of great activity, and it is to be hoped that this emerging basic knowledge of their actions will benefit the patient.

ACKNOWLEDGMENTS

The author's work is supported by the Medical Research Council, The Wellcome Trust, and The Pain Society. The help, advice, and experimental contributions of Ann Sullivan, Louise Stanfa, Vicky Chapman, Henry McQuay, Eija Kalso, and Jane Haley are gratefully acknowledged.

REFERENCES

Aimone, L.D. and Yaksh, T.L., Opioid modulation of capsaicin evoked release of substance P from rat spinal cord in vivo, Peptides, 10 (1989) 1–5.

Akerman, B., Arwestrom, E. and Post, C., Local anesthetics potentiate spinal morphine analgesia, Anesth. Analg., 67 (1988) 943–948.

Arner, S. and Meyerson, B.A., Lack of analgesic effect of opioids on neuropathic and idiopathic forms of pain, Pain, 33, (1988) 11–23.

Attal, N., Chen, Y.L., Kayser, V. and Guilbaud, G.L., Behavioural evidence that systemic morphine may modulate a phasic pain-related behaviour in a rat model of peripheral mononeuropathy, Pain, 47 (1991) 65–70.

Baber, N.S., Dourish, C.T. and Hill, D.R., The role of CCK, caerulein, and CCK antagonists in nociception, Pain, 39 (1989) 307–328.

Besse, D., Lombard, M.C., Zakac, J.M., Roques, B.P. and Besson, J.-M., Pre- and postsynaptic distribution of mu, delta and kappa opioid receptors in the superficial layers of the cervical dorsal horn of the rat spinal cord, Brain Res., 521 (1990) 15–22.

Besson, J.-M. and Chaouch, A., Peripheral and spinal mechanisms of nociception, Physiol. Rev., 67 (1987) 67–186.

Chapman, V. and Dickenson, A.H., The combination of NMDA antagonism and morphine produces profound antinociception in the rat dorsal horn, Brain Res., 573 (1992) 321–323.

Chen, Y., Mestek, A., Liu, J., Hurley, J.A. and Yu, L., Molecular cloning and functional expression of a mu-opiopid receptor from rat brain, Mol. Pharm., 44 (1993) 8–12.

Crain, S.M. and Shen, K.F., Opioids can evoke direct receptor mediated excitatory effects on sensory neurones, Trends Pharmacol. Sci., 11 (1990) 77–81.

Davies, S.N. and Lodge, D., Evidence for involvement of N-methyl-D-aspartate receptors in "wind-up" of class 2 neurones in the dorsal horn of the rat, Brain Res., 424 (1987) 402–406.
Daw, N.W., Stein, P.S.G. and Fox, K., The role of NMDA receptors in information processing, Ann. Rev. Neurosci., 16 (1993) 207–222.
Dickenson, A.H., A cure for wind-up: NMDA receptor antagonists as potential analgesics, Trends Pharmacol. Sci., 11 (1990) 307–309.
Dickenson, A.H., Recent advances in the physiology and pharmacology of pain: plasticity and its implications for clinical analgesia, J. Psychopharm., 5 (1991a) 342–351.
Dickenson, A.H., Mechanisms of the analgesic actions of opiates and opioids, Br. Med. Bull., 47 (1991b) 690–702.
Dickenson, A.H., The pharmacology of opioid poorly responsive pain, Cancer Reviews, in press.
Dickenson, A. H. and Sullivan, A.F., Electrophysiological studies on the effects of intrathecal morphine on nociceptive neurones in the rat dorsal horn, Pain, 24 (1986) 211–222.
Dickenson, A.H. and Sullivan, A.F., Evidence for a role of the NMDA receptor in the frequency dependent potentiation of deep dorsal horn neurones following C-fibre stimulation, Neuropharmacology, 26 (1987) 1235–1238.
Dickenson, A.H. and Sullivan, A.F., Subcutaneous formalin induced activity of dorsal horn neurones in the rat:differential response to an intrathecal opiate administered pre or post formalin, Pain, 30 (1989) 349–360.
Dickenson, A.H. and Sullivan, A.F., Combination therapy in analgesia; seeking synergy, Current Opinion in Anaesthesiology, 6 (1993) 861-865.
Dickenson, A.H., Sullivan, A.F., Fournie-Zaluski, M.-C. and Roques, B., Prevention of degradation of endogenous enkephalins produces inhibition of nociceptive neurones in rat spinal cord, Brain Res., 408 (1987a) 185–191.
Dickenson, A.H., Sullivan, A.F., Knox, R.J., Zajac, Z. and Roques, B.P., Opioid receptor types in the rat spinal cord: electrophysiological studies with μ and δ opioid receptor agonists in the control of nociception, Brain Res., 413 (1987b) 649–652.
Dickenson, A.H., Sullivan, A.F. and McQuay, H.J., Intrathecal etorphine, fentanyl and buprenorphine on spinal nociceptive neurones in the rat, Pain, 42 (1990) 227–234.
Dickenson, A.H., Sullivan, A.F. Stanfa, L.C. and McQuay, H., Dextromethorphan and levorphanol on dorsal horn nociceptive neurones in the rat, Neuropharmacology, 30 (1991) 1303–1308.
Dubner, R and Ruda, M.A., Activity dependent neuronal plasticity following tissue injury and inflammation, Trends Neurosci., 15 (1992) 96–103.
Duggan, A.W. and North, R.A. Electrophysiology of opioids, Pharmacol. Rev., 35 (1984) 219–281.
Evans, C.J., Keith, D.E., Morrisson, H., Magendzo, K. and Edwards, R.H., Cloning of a delta receptor by functional expression, Science, 258 (1992) 1952–1955.
Fields, H.L., Barbaro, N.M. and Heinricher, M. M., Brain stem neuronal circuitry underlying the antinociceptive action of opiates. In: H.L. Fields and J.-M. Besson, (Eds.), Pain Modulation, Progress in Brain Research, Vol. 77. Elsevier, Amsterdam, 1988, pp 245–258.
Fitzgerald, M., C-Fos and the changing face of pain, Trends Neurosci., 13 (1990) 439–440.
Fraser, H., Chapman, V. and Dickenson, A.H., Spinal local anaesthetic actions on afferent evoked responses and wind-up of nociceptive neurones in the rat spinal cord: combination with morphine produces marked potentiation of antinociception, Pain, 49 (1992) 33–41.
Gogas, K.R., Presley, R.N., Levine, J.D. and Basbaum, A.I., Antinociceptive action of suppressed spinal opioids results from an increase in descending inhibitory control: correlation of nociceptive behavior in c-*fos* expression, Neuroscience, 42 (1991) 617-628.
Gong, Q.L., Hedner, J., Bjorkman, R. and Hedner, T., Morphine-3-glucuronide may functionally antagonize morphine-6-glucuronide induced antinociception and ventilatory depression in the rat, Pain, 48 (1992) 249–255.
Gracely, R., Lynch, S.A. and Bennett, G.J., Painful neuropathy: altered central processing maimtained dynamically by peripheral input, Pain, 52 (1993) 251–253.
Haley, J. E., Sullivan, A.F. and Dickenson, A. H., Evidence for spinal N-methyl-D-aspartate receptor involvement in prolonged chemical nociception in the rat, Brain Res., 518 (1990)

218–226.

Hewett, K., Dickenson A.H. and McQuay H.J., Lack of effect of morphine-3-glucuronide on the spinal antinociceptive actions of morphine in the rat: an electrophysiological study, Pain, 53 (1993) 59–63.

Hirota, N., Kuraishi, Y., Hino, Y., Satoh, M. and Takagi, H., Met-enkephalin and morphine but not dynorhin inhibit noxious stimuli induced release of substance P from rabbit dorsal horn in situ, Neuropharmacology, 24 (1985) 567–570

Hori, Y., Endo, K. and Takahashi, T., Presynaptic inhibitory action of enkephalin on excitatory transmission in superficial dorsal horn of rat spinal cord, J. Physiol., 450 (1992) 673–685

Hylden, J.L.K. and Wilcox, G.L., Pharmacological characterization of Substance P induced nociception in mice: modulation by opioid and noradrenergic agonists at the spinal level, J. Pharmacol. Exp. Ther., 226 (1983) 398–404.

Hylden, J.L.K., Thomas, D.A., Iadorola, M.J., Nahin, R.L. and Dubner, R., Spinal opioid analgesic effects are enhanced in a model of unilateral inflammation/hyperalgesia: possible involvement of noradrenergic mechanisms, Eur. J. Pharmacol., 194 (1991) 135–143.

Jadad, A.R., Carroll, D., Glynn, C.J., Moore, R.A., McQuay, H.J., Morphine responsiveness of chronic pain: double-blind randomized crossover study with patient-controlled analgesia, Lancet, 339 (1992) 1367–1371.

Jiang, Q.A.E., Takemori, A.E., Sultana, M., Portoghese, P.S., Bowen, W.D., Mosberg, H.I. and Porreca, F., Differential antagonism of opioid delta antinociception by [D-Ala2, Leu5, Cys6] enkephalin and naltrindole 5′-isothiocynanate: evidence for delta receptor subtypes, J. Pharmacol. Exp. Ther., 257 (1991) 1069–1077.

Kalso E.A., Sullivan, A.F., McQuay, H.J., Dickenson, A.H. and Roques, B.P., Cross-tolerance between mu opioid and alpha-2 adrenergic receptors, but not between mu and delta opioid receptors in the spinal cord of the rat, J. Pharmacol. Exp. Ther., 265 (1993) 551–558.

Kangra, I. and Randic, M., Outflow of endogenous aspartate and glutamate from the rat spinal dorsal horn in vitro by activation of low- and high-threshold primary afferent fibres. Modulation by m opioids, Brain Res. 553 (1991) 347–352.

Kieffer, B.L., Befort, C., Gavieraux, C. and Hirth, C.G., The δ-opioid receptor: isolation of a cDNA by expression cloning and pharmacological characterization, Proc. Natl. Acad. Sci. USA., 89 (1992) 12048–12052.

Knox, R.J. and Dickenson, A.H., Effects of selective and non-selective κ opioid agonists on cutaneous C-fibre evoked responses of rat dorsal horn neurones, Brain Res., 415 (1987) 21–29.

Kosterlitz, H.W., Opioid peptides and their receptors, Proc. R. Soc. Lond. (Biol.), 225 (1985) 27–40.

Kosterlitz, H.W., Biosynthesis of morphine in the animal kingdom, Nature, 330 (1987) 606–607.

Lang, C.W., Duggan, A.W. and Hope, P., Analgesic doses of morphine do not reduce noxious stimulus evoked release of immunoreactive neurokinins in the dorsal horn of the spinal cat, Br. J. Pharmacol., 103 (1991) 1871–1876

Le Bars, D. and Villaneuva, L., Electrophysiological evidence for the activation of descending inhibitory controls by nociceptive afferent pathways, In: H.L. Fields and J.-M. Besson, (Eds.), Pain Modulation, Progress in Brain Research, Vol. 77, Elsevier, Amsterdam, 1988, pp 275–300.

Lodge, D. and Johnson, K. M., Noncompetitive excitatory amino acid receptor antagonists, Trends Pharmacol. Sci., 11 (1990) 81–86.

Lombard, M.C. and Besson, J.-M., Attempts to gauge the relative importance of pre-and postsynaptic effects of morphine on the transmission of noxious messages in the dorsal horn of the rat spinal cord, Pain, 37 (1989) 335–346.

Magnuson, D.S.K. and Dickenson, A.H., Lamina-specific effects of morphine and naloxone in dorsal horn of rat spinal cord in vitro, J. Neurophysiol., 66 (1991) 1941–1950.

Magnuson, D.S.K., Sullivan, A.F., Simmonet,G., Roques, B.P. and Dickenson, A.H., Differential interactions of cholecystokinin and FLQPQRFamide with μ and δ opioid antinociception in rat spinal cord, Neuropeptides, 16 (1990) 213–218.

Mao, J., Price, D.D., Hayes, R.L., Lu, J., Mayer, D.J. and Frank, H., Intrathecal treatment with dextrophan or ketamine potently reduces pain-related behaviours in a rat model of peripheral mononeuropathy, Brain Res., 605 (1993) 164–168.

Matsubara, K., Fukushima, S., Akane, A., Kobayashi, S. and Shiono, H., Increased urinary morphine, codeine and tetrahydropapaveroline in Parkinsonian patient undergoing L-3,4-dihydroxyphenyalanine therapy: a possible biosynthetic pathway of morphine from L-3,4-dihydroxyphenyalanine in humans, J. Pharmacol. Exp. Ther., 260 (1992) 974–978.

Maves, T.J. and Gebhart, G.F., Antinociceptive synergy between intrathecal morphine and lidocaine during visceral and somatic nociception in the rat, Anesthesiology, 76 (1992) 91–99.

McFadzean,I., The ionic mechanisms underlying opioid actions, Neuropeptides, 11 (1988) 173–180.

McQuay, H. and Dickenson, A.H., Implications of central nervous system plasticity for pain management, Anaesthesia, 45 (1990) 101–102.

McQuay, H.J., Sullivan, A.F., Smallman, K. and Dickenson, A.H., Intrathecal opioids, potency and lipophilicity, Pain, 36 (1989) 111–115.

Millan, M.J., k opioid receptors and analgesia, Trends Pharmacol. Sci., 11 (1990) 70–76.

North, R.A., Drug receptors and the inhibition of nerve cells, Br. J. Pharmacol., 98 (1989) 13–28.

Parsons C.G. and Headley P.M., Spinal antinociceptive actions of μ- and κ-opioids; the importance of stimulus intensity in determining 'selectivity' between reflexes to different modalities of noxious stimulus, Br. J. Pharmacol., 98 (1989) 523–532.

Pasternak, G.W. and Wood, P.J., Multiple opioid receptors, Life Sci., 28 (1986) 1889–1893.

Porreca, F., Mosberg H.I., Hurst R., Hruby V.J. and Burks T.F., Roles of mu, delta and kappa opioid receptors in spinal and supraspinal mediation of gastrointestinal transit effects and hot-plate analgesia in the mouse, J. Pharmacol. Exp. Ther., 230 (1984) 341–348.

Porreca, F., Jiang, Q. and Mosberg, H.I., Modulation of μ opioid potency and efficacy by opioid δ agonists: dissociation of antinociception from development of antinociceptive tolerance. In: M.R. Bond, J.E. Charlton and C.J. Woolf (Eds.), Proceedings of the VIth World Congress on Pain. Pain Research and Clinical Management, Vol 4. Elsevier, Amsterdam, 1991, 145–150.

Portenoy, R.K., Foley,. K.M. and Inturrisi, C.E., The nature of opioid responsiveness and its implications for neuropathic pain: new hypotheses derived from studies of opioid infusions, Pain, 43 (1990) 273–286.

Ren, K., Hylden, J.L.K., Williams, G.M., Ruda, M.A. and Dubner, R., The effects of a non-competitive NMDA receptor antagonist, MK-801, on behavioural hyperalgesia and dorsal horn neuronal activity in rats with unilateral inflammation, Pain, 50 (1992) 331–344.

Roques, B.P., Noble, F., Dauge V., Fournie-Zaluski, M.C. and Beaumont, A., Neutral endopeptidase 24.11: structure, inhibition and experimental and clinical pharmacology, Pharmacol. Rev., 45 (1993) 88–146.

Ruda, M.A., Iadorala, M.J., Cohen, L.V. and Young, W.S., III, In situ hybridisation histochemistry and immunocytochemistry reveal an increase in spinal cord dynorphin biosynthesis in a rat model of peripheral inflammation and hyperalgesia, Proc. Natl. Acad. Sci. USA, 85 (1988) 622–626.

Sawynok, J. and Yaksh, T.L., Caffeine as an analgesic adjuvant: a review of pharmacology and mechanisms of action, Pharmacol. Rev., 45 (1993) 43–82.

Schaible, H.G., Grubb, B.D., Neugebauer, V. and Oppmann, M., The effects of NMDA antagonists on neuronal activity in cat spinal cord evoked by acute inflammation in the knee joint, Eur. J. Neurosci., 3 (1991) 981–991.

Schmauss, C. and Yaksh, T.L., In vivo studies on spinal opiate receptor systems mediating antinociception. II. Pharmacological profiles suggesting a differential association of μ, δ, κ receptors with visceral chemical and cutaneous thermal stimuli in the rat, J. Pharmacol. Exp. Ther., 228 (1984) 1–12

Seltzer, Z., Cohn, S., Ginzburg, R. and Beilin, B.Z., Modulation of neuropathic pain in rats by spinal disinhibition and NMDA receptor blockade of injury discharge, Pain, 45 (1991) 69–76.

Sher, G. and Mitchell, D., N-methyl-D-aspartate receptors mediate responses of rat dorsal horn neurones to hindlimb ischaemia, Brain Res., 522 (1990) 55–62.

Smith, M.T., Watt, J.A. and Cramond, T., Morphine-3-glucuronide: a potent antagonist of morphine analgesia, Life Sci., 47 (1990) 579–585.

Stanfa, L.C. and Dickenson, A.H., Cholecystokinin as a factor in the enhanced potency of spinal morphine following carrageenan inflammation, Br. J. Pharmacol., 108 (1993) 967–973.

Stanfa, L.C. and Dickenson, A.H., Electrophysiological studies on the spinal roles of endogenous opioids in carrageenan inflammation, Pain, 56 (1994) 185-191.

Stanfa, L.C., Sullivan, A.F.and Dickenson, A.H., Alterations in neuronal excitability and the potency of spinal mu, delta and kappa opioids after carrageenan-induced inflammation, Pain, 50 (1992) 345–354.

Stein, C., Millan, M.J., Shippenberg, T. S., Peter, K. and Herz, A., Peripheral opioid receptors mediating antinociception in inflammation. Evidence for involvement of mu, delta and kappa receptors, J. Pharmacol. Exp. Ther., 248 (1989) 1269–1275.

Stevens, C.W. and Yaksh,T.L., Time course characteristics of tolerance development to continously infused antinociceptive agents in rat spinal cord, J. Pharmacol. Exp. Ther., 251 (1989) 216–223.

Sullivan, A.F., Dickenson, A.H. and Roques,B.P., δ-opioid mediated inhibitions of acute and prolonged noxious-evoked responses in rat dorsal horn neurones, Br. J. Pharmacol., 98 (1989a) 1039–1049.

Sullivan, A.F., McQuay, H.J., Bailey, D. and Dickenson, A.H., The spinal antinociceptive actions of morphine metabolites morphine-6-glucuronide and normorphine in the rat, Brain Res., 482 (1989b) 219–224.

Tal, M. and Bennett, G.J., Dextrophan relieves neuropathic heat-evoked hyperalgesia in the rat, Neurosci. Lett., 151 (1993) 107–110.

Traynor, J., Subtypes of the κ opioid receptor: fact or fiction? Trends Pharmacol. Sci., 10 (1989) 52–53.

Wang, J., Ren, M. and Han, J., Mobilization of calcium from intracellular stores as one of the mechanisms underlying the antiopioid effects of cholecystokinin octapeptide, Peptides,13 (1992) 947–951.

Wiertelak, E.P., Maier, S.F. and Watkins, L.R., Cholecystokinin antianalgesia: safety cues abolish morphine analgesia, Science, 256 (1992) 830–833.

Wiesenfeld-Hallin, Z., Xu, X.-J., Villar, M.J. and Hokflet, T., Intrathecal galanin potentiates the spinal analgesic effect of morphine; electrophysiological and behavioural studies, Neurosci. Lett., 109 (1990) 217–221.

Woolf, C. J., Evidence for a central component of post-injury pain hypersensitivity, Nature, 221 (1983) 313–328.

Woolf, C, J. and Thompson, S.W.N., The induction and maintenance of central sensitization is dependent on N-methyl-D-aspartic acid receptor activation; implications for the treatment of post-injury hypersensitivity states, Pain 44 (1991) 293–299.

Woolf, C, J. and Wall, P.D., Morphine sensitive and morphine insensitive actions of C-fibre input on the rat spinal cord, Neurosci. Lett., 64 (1986) 221–225.

Xu, X.-J. and Wiesenfeld-Hallin, Z., The threshold for the depressive effect of intrathecal morphine on the spinal noccieptive flexor reflex is increased during autotomy after sciatic nerve section in rats, Pain, 46 (1991) 223–229.

Xu, X.-J., Puke, M.J.C., Verge, V.M.K., Wiesenfeld-Hallin, Z., Hughes, J. and Hokfelt, T., Up-regulation of cholecystokinin in primary sensory neurons is associated with morphine insensitivity in experimental neuropathic pain in the rat, Neurosci. Lett., 152 (1993) 129–132.

Yaksh, T. L., Behavioural and autonomic correlates of the tactile evoked allodynia produced by spinal glycine inhibition: effects of modulatory receptor systems and excitatory amino acid antagonists, Pain, 37 (1989) 111–123.

Yaksh, T.L. and Nouiehed, R., Physiology and pharmacology of spinal opiates, Ann. Rev. Pharmacol. Toxicol., 25 (1985) 433–462.

Yaksh, T.L., Al-Rodhan, N.R.F. and Jenson, T.S., Sites of action of opiates in production of analgesia. In: H.L. Fields and J.-M. Besson, (Eds.), Progress in Brain Research, Elsevier,

Amsterdam, 1988, pp 371–394.
Yamamoto, T. and Yaksh, T.L., Studies on the spinal interaction of morphine and the NMDA antagonist MK-801 on the hyperesthesia observed in a rat model of sciatic mononeuropathy, Neurosci. Lett., 135 (1992) 67–70.
Zhou, Y., Sun, Y.-H., Zhang, Z.-W. and Han, J.-S., Increased release of immunoreactive cholecystokinin octapeptide by morphine and potentiation of mu opioid analgesia by CCK-B receptor antagonist L-365,260 in rat spinal cord, Eur. J. Pharmacol., (1993) 234, 147–154.

Correspondence to: Anthony H. Dickenson, Department of Pharmacology, University College London, London WC1E 6BT, UK. Tel: 44-71-387-7050; Fax: 44-71-380-7298.

Proceedings of the 7th World Congress on Pain,
Progress in Pain Research and Management, Vol. 2,
edited by G.F. Gebhart, D.L. Hammond, and T.S.
Jensen, IASP Press, Seattle, © 1994.

37

Endogenous Opioid Systems in the Modulation of Pain: Behavioral Studies in Rat Models of Persistent Hyperalgesia

Valérie Kayser

Unité de Recherches de Physiopharmacologie du Système Nerveux
INSERM U 161, Paris, France

The question of the functional role of endogenous opioid peptides in pain modulation was first addressed in the mid-1970s after the discovery of opioid receptors and endogenous substances with morphine-like properties (Kosterlitz and Hughes 1975; Goldstein et al. 1976). Several researchers attempted to identify the putative controls exerted by endogenous opioid peptides on nociceptive messages using naloxone, the best opioid receptor antagonist at that time. Results obtained in numerous studies were highly controversial; they varied in dose, species, general methodology, and nociceptive behavioral test. In fact, there was no clear evidence for the existence of these controls, at least in normal animals (references in Kayser et al. 1988b). However, looking back to the clinical literature, two studies from Lasagna (1965) and Levine et al. (1979) reported ambivalent effects of naloxone on postoperative pain: according to the dose, naloxone induced hypo- or hyperalgesic effects.

This finding led us to determine the effect of the drug in rat models of clinical pain. We used three models of inflammatory and neuropathic pain that have been extensively investigated over the past decade: (1) a model of diffuse, persistent inflammatory pain in rats rendered polyarthritic by a Freund's adjuvant injection into the tail (Pearson et al. 1961; Gouret et al. 1976); (2) a model of more localized and acute inflammatory pain in rats with an intraplantar injection of carrageenan (Winter et al. 1962; Vinegar et al. 1969; Di Rosa et al. 1971); and more recently, (3) a model of unilateral, persistent neuropathic pain produced by moderate constriction of one sciatic nerve (Bennett and Xie 1988). Interestingly, the antinociceptive effect of morphine and other opioid agonists administered systemically is greater in these animals than in normal rats, as gauged with the vocalization threshold to paw pressure test (Kayser and Guilbaud 1983; Neil et al. 1986; Kayser et al. 1990; Attal et al. 1991; Desmeules et al. 1993). In addition, changes in endogenous opioid peptides occur in these models, so that both their levels and biosynthesis increase in the dorsal horn of the spinal cord (Cesselin et al. 1980; Faccini et al. 1984; Millan 1986; Höllt et al. 1987; Kajander et al. 1990; Draisci et al. 1991; Dubner and Ruda 1992).

As a nociceptive test, we used the measure of the vocalization threshold to paw pressure, a centrally integrated test (Kayser et al. 1985; Kayser and Guilbaud 1990). The threshold for vocalization was measured using the Basile analgesimeter (Apelex). Increasing pressure was applied to the hindpaw until a squeak was elicited. Prior to the test phase, rats had no experience with the testing apparatus. In neuropathic rats, we also measured the score of spontaneous pain (Attal et al. 1990a). In some experiments, we recorded thalamic neuronal activities in halothane/N_2O-anesthetized rats (Guilbaud et al. 1982; Kayser et al. 1988a).

The guidelines proposed by the Committee for Research and Ethical Issues of the IASP (1980) have been followed. In particular, the duration of the experiment was as short as possible and the number of rats used was kept to a minimum.

EFFECTS OF HIGH DOSES OF NALOXONE

POLYARTHRITIC RATS

We first determined the effects of relatively high doses of naloxone (1 and 3 mg/kg iv.) in polyarthritic rats. These animals exhibit a clear decrease in their vocalization threshold to paw pressure, maximal between three and four weeks after the beginning of the disease. At this time, naloxone produced a further increase in the initial hyperalgesia with behavioral modifications; the rats became more sensitive to handling and vocalized to touch (Kayser and Guilbaud 1981, 1987; Kayser et al. 1986a, 1988b). For 1 mg per kg naloxone, the threshold was further decreased by about 40% at the moment of maximum effect. A greater dose (3 mg/kg iv.) produced no greater effect and this action was highly reproducible; we observed the same decrease and the same time course in different experimental series (Fig. 1). These doses of naloxone also enhanced the activity of spinal dorsal horn neurons in arthritic rats (Lombard and Besson 1989).

This finding suggests a tonic activity of endogenous opioid systems in this model of pain. These effects were not observed in normal rats, but appear to

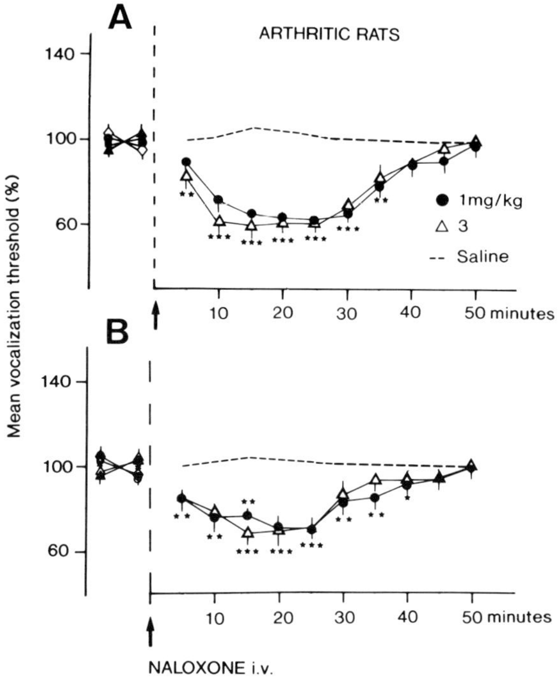

Fig. 1. Mean curves of naloxone effects on the threshold for vocalization (± S.E.M.) expressed as percentage of the control in arthritic rats (n = 9 in each group of rats) in two different experimental series. The mean curves obtained with Fixanal (pH equivalent to that of the naloxone solution), not illustrated, were similar to those of saline. * $P < 0.05$; ** $P < 0.01$; *** $P < 0.001$; Student's *t* test. (Panel **A** adapted from Kayser et al. 1986a; panel **B** adapted from Kayser and Guilbaud 1987b)

be related to persistent pain. However, we thought that these effects could be due to the diffuse inflammation. For these reasons, we investigated the effects of naloxone in a model of more localized inflammatory pain, carrageenan-injected rats.

CARRAGEENAN-INJECTED RATS

In this model, the intraplantar injection of carrageenan produced a clear decrease of the vocalization threshold to paw pressure. This decreased about 30% four hours after the beginning of the inflammation (Kayser and Guilbaud 1987a). Naloxone (1 mg/kg iv.) significantly enhanced the carrageenan-induced hyperalgesia (the mean threshold was further decreased by 40% at 20 minutes after the injection) with a total recovery 40 minutes later (Kayser and Guilbaud 1991). Thus, this effect of naloxone also exists in a model of localized inflammatory pain, but in this case it could be related to the inflammatory process. This possibility led us to determine the effects of naloxone in a model of noninflammatory pain. We chose a model of mononeuropathy recently proposed by Bennett et al. (1988) and extensively developed by our group (Attal et al. 1990a).

MONONEUROPATHIC RATS

The neuropathy is produced by four loose ligatures around one sciatic nerve. One week after the ligature, the rats exhibit a clear decrease of around 30% in the vocalization threshold to paw pressure (Attal et al. 1989). We observed that naloxone produced a further decrease in this threshold lasting 40 minutes; during this period, the rats would vocalize to touch (Attal et al. 1989, 1990b). In this model, it also was possible to measure a score of spontaneous pain, calculated using the abnormal position of the affected paw. It was possible to rate the position of this paw from 0, the normal position, to 5, an absolutely abnormal position in which the rat licked its paw. Using the formula proposed by Dennis and Melzack (1979) for the formalin test, we calculated a score taking into account the time spent in each position in a five-minute period. The mean score was between two and three at week two after the nerve ligature. At this time, naloxone (1 mg/kg iv.) produced a further increase in this score, a clear hyperalgesic effect; the rats were often licking their paw, a position that is unusual in the absence of naloxone (Jazat and Guilbaud 1991).

Thus, even in a model of noninflammatory pain, the hyperalgesic effect of naloxone could be observed. This suggests that in these models of clinical pain, naloxone suppressed tonically active inhibitory systems involving opioid peptides.

CHARACTERISTICS OF THE EFFECT

The use of models of localized hyperalgesia (carrageenan- and mononeuropathic rats) with a time course that can be followed allowed us to determine some characteristics of this effect. At 24 hours after the beginning of the inflammation, some carrageenan-injected rats were not hyperalgesic, in spite of a steady inflammation and a noticeable level of sensitizing substances in the exudate (Di Rosa et al. 1971). Although it appears that a clear relationship between edema (roughly unmodified over 96 hours) and hyperalgesia does not necessarily exist (Winter and Flataker 1965; Kayser and Guilbaud 1987), we suggested that, in these rats, inhibitory controls modulating the noxious peripheral inputs were triggered by the initial excitatory influences, leading to a reduction in the initial hyperalgesia. We hypothesized that tonic endogenous opioid control systems were responsible for this inhibition. We then tested rats 24 hours after injection of carrageenan. When naloxone (1 mg/kg iv.) was injected, we observed a significant negative relation between the effect of the high dose of naloxone and the degree of the initial hyperalgesia (Fig. 2). Naloxone induced a consistent hyperalgesic effect only in the rats that had recovered from their initial carrageenan-induced hyperalgesia.

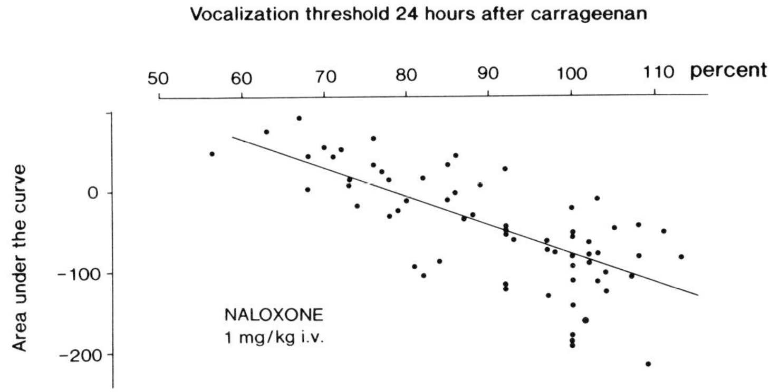

Fig. 2. Relation between the hyperalgesic effect of naloxone 24 hours after carrageenan (areas under the curves obtained for each rat) and the vocalization thresholds to paw pressure obtained just before injection (expressed as percentages of pre-carrageenan control values). Each point represents an individual animal. ($Y = -3.59x + 278.85$, $r = 0.69$, $P < 0.01$, $n = 60$). (Adapted from Kayser and Guilbaud 1991)

Inversely, the more hyperalgesic the animals were 24 hours after carrageenan, the less effective naloxone was, suggesting that the tonically active endogenous opioidergic systems were weaker in this group of rats.

Comparable data were obtained using the same nociceptive test in rats with a peripheral mononeuropathy. Naloxone two weeks after the sciatic injury induced no mean significant effect in these animals. However, there was an effect in a few rats that had recovered from the neuropathic hyperalgesia measured with the vocalization threshold to paw pressure (Attal et al. 1990b).

These results strongly suggest that the potency of the endogenous opioid inhibitory controls can vary between animals. This finding is important in the light of previous studies performed in animals and in humans, reporting that in conditions of both experimentally induced and clinical pain, high doses of naloxone induced a state of hyperalgesia, and this seemed to set off a tonically active system involving opioid peptides, which ensures a certain level of pain insensitivity. For example, Buchsbaum et al. (1983) found that subjects who were relatively pain-insensitive experienced electrical shock as being more painful after naloxone, while subjects relatively pain-sensitive felt less pain. Satoh et al. (1979) showed that naloxone reversed, in a dose-dependent manner, an adaptation of the flexor reflexes to repeated nociceptive stimuli in the rat (injection of bradykinin into common iliac artery of the rat), while the drug, even at a greater dose, produced little or no hyperalgesic effects in rats which did not show such an adaptation.

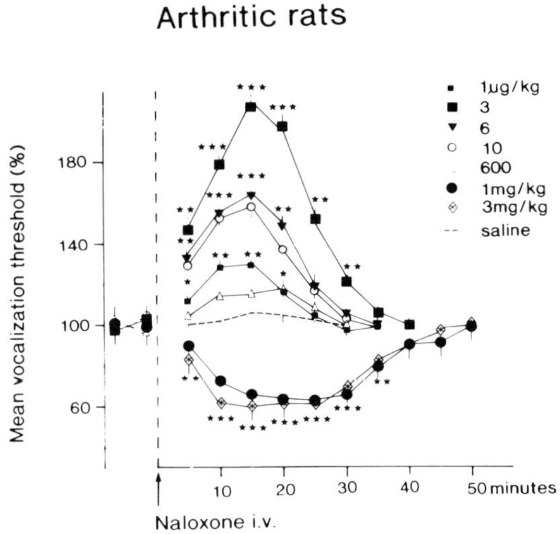

Fig. 3. Mean curves of naloxone effects (3 µg/kg to 1 mg/kg) on the threshold for vocalization (± S.E.M.) expressed as percentage of the control in arthritic rats (n = 9 in each group of rats). * $P < 0.05$, ** $P < 0.01$, *** $P < 0.001$, Student's *t*-test. (Adapted from Kayser et al. 1986a)

WHICH RECEPTOR COULD MEDIATE THE EFFECT?

To determine which opioid receptor could mediate this effect, we used morphine-tolerant arthritic rats (Kayser and Guilbaud 1985; Kayser et al. 1986a,b). In these animals, the hyperalgesia induced by naloxone (1 and 3 mg/kg iv.) remained unmodified in comparison with saline-pretreated arthritic rats, whether the rats were rendered tolerant using high or low doses of morphine (Kayser et al. 1986a; Kayser and Guilbaud 1987b). This suggests that mu-opioid receptors are not important in this effect.

We then determined the effect of naloxone (1 mg/kg iv.) co-injected with specific kappa- or delta-opioid receptor antagonists. These experiments were performed in arthritic and neuropathic rats, using various antagonists (Cattaneo et al. 1993; Attal et al. 1993). In the two models, with a kappa-antagonist (MR-2266, 0.2 mg/kg iv. or nor-binaltorphimine, 1 mg/kg iv.), the hyperalgesic effect of naloxone remained unchanged. In sharp contrast, with a delta-antagonist (ICI-174,864, 10 mg/kg iv. or naltrindole, 1 mg/kg iv.), this effect was considerably reduced (by about three- to fourfold when gauged by the mean areas under the curves). This suggests that the effects exerted by endogenous opioid peptides are, to some extent, mediated via opioid receptors with delta characteristics.

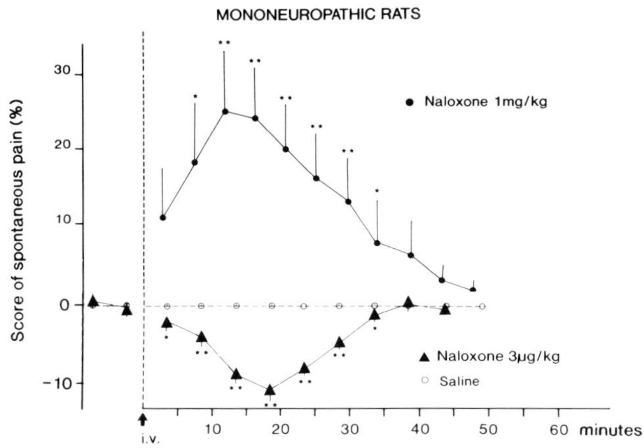

Fig. 4. Effects of the two doses of naloxone (3 μg/kg and 1 mg/kg iv.) on the spontaneous pain-related behavior, expressed as percentage of the mean values obtained just before the injection, one week after the nerve ligation (n= 9 rats in each group). The open circles represent the behavior after saline injection (n = 4); * $P < 0.05$, ** $P < 0.01$, Student's *t* test. (Jazat and Guilbaud 1991)

EFFECTS OF LOW DOSES OF NALOXONE

Decreasing the doses of naloxone produced unexpected results. In fact, extremely low doses of naloxone produced paradoxical potent antinociceptive effects and a significant decrease in thalamic neuronal activities.

POLYARTHRITIC RATS

Fig. 3 illustrates the effects of naloxone on the vocalization threshold to paw pressure in arthritic rats given a large range of doses from 3 mg/kg to 1 μg/kg iv. In contrast to the effect of high doses, lower doses (from 600 to 1 μg/kg) induced a progressive increase in the threshold, consequently a clear antinociceptive effect that peaked at the extremely low dose of 3 μg/kg iv. For this dose, the paradoxical antinociceptive effect is potent; the threshold is increased by 90%, an effect comparable in intensity to that produced by 1 mg/kg iv. morphine in these animals (Kayser and Guilbaud 1983). The rats appeared quiet and free of evident pain-related behavior. We found the electrophysiological counterpart of this antinociceptive action. In halothane/N_2O-anesthetized rats, low doses of naloxone induced a powerful and dose-dependent depressive effect on ventrobasal (VB) thalamic neuronal responses elicited by stimulation applied to the joints (Guilbaud et al. 1982).

CARRAGEENAN- AND MONONEUROPATHIC RATS

We also found this antinociceptive effect of naloxone in models of localized pain produced in carrageenan-injected and neuropathic rats (Kayser et al. 1989; Attal et al. 1989, 1990a,b); Jazat and Guilbaud 1991). As an example, Fig. 4 illustrates the effect obtained on the score of spontaneous pain in neuropathic rats. In sharp contrast with the effect of 1 mg/kg iv naloxone, the low dose of 3 µg/kg iv. produced a clear decrease in this score, corresponding to a hypoalgesic effect. At the moment of the maximum effect, some animals were able to put their paw normally on the floor and the rats appeared very quiet and even drowsy (Jazat and Guilbaud 1991). Fig. 5 represents an example of one ventrobasal (VB) neuronal response in rats 24 hours after injection of carrageenan, induced by moderate pressure of the inflamed paw in halothane/N_2O-anesthetized rats. The low dose of 3 µg/kg iv. naloxone rapidly depressed the VB neuronal responses, with spontaneous recovery 35 minutes later (Kayser et al. 1988a).

Thus, from various experiments performed in rat models of clinical pain, it is clear that extremely low doses of naloxone can have a paradoxical analgesic effect, while high doses induce the expected hyperalgesia. This effect, not seen in normal rats, is reminiscent of the biphasic effect of naloxone in postoperative pain in humans, as mentioned previously (Lasagna 1965; Levine et al. 1979).

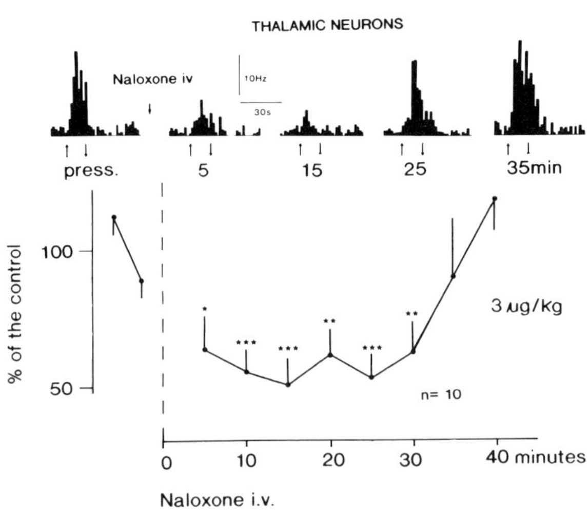

Fig. 5. Top: Depressive effect of naloxone (3 µg/kg iv.) on responses of a VB neuron, elicited by moderate pressure of the inflamed joints in a 24-hour post-carrageenan-injected rat. **Bottom:** mean curve of the depressive effect obtained with all the neurons used in this study * $P < 0.05$, $P < 0.01$, $P < 0.001$; Student's *t*-test. (Adapted from Kayser et al. 1987)

CHARACTERISTICS OF THE EFFECT

The use of these models of localized pain, with a time course that can be followed, allowed us to determine some characteristics of this antinociceptive effect.

We demonstrated that the paradoxical antinociceptive effect of naloxone increased with the duration and degree of the initial hyperalgesia. Indeed, in carrageenan-injected rats, we noted that the effect of 3 µg/kg iv. naloxone, only slight and transient one hour after carrageenan, increased over the following 4 to 24 hours (Kayser et al. 1987). In addition, when we compared the individual effect of naloxone in rats 24 hours after injection of carrageenan, we determined that the effect of the drug was clearly related to the degree of the initial hyperalgesia (Fig. 6). In neuropathic rats, we made comparable observations. In the rats with a high degree of hyperalgesia, with a potent reduction in their threshold one week after surgery, the low dose of naloxone had a more potent action (Attal et al. 1989). The same rats had a more pronounced effect at week two than at week one (Attal et al. 1990b).

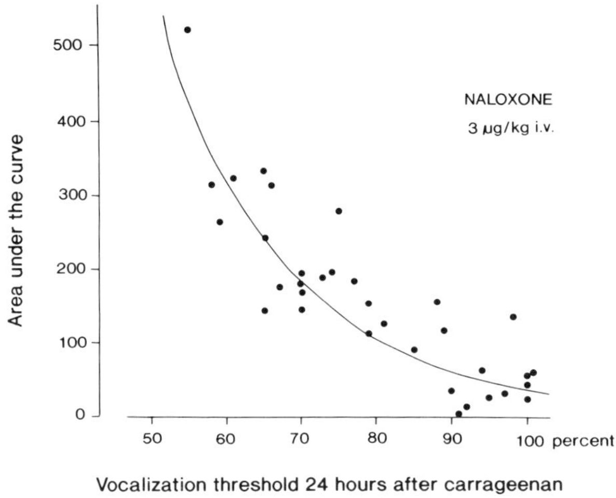

Fig. 6. Relation between the analgesic effect of naloxone 24 hours after carrageenan (areas under the curves obtained for each rat) and the vocalization thresholds to paw pressure obtained just before injection (expressed as percentage of pre-carrageenan control value). Each point illustrates an individual animal ($Y = 8377.19e^{-0.05x}$, $r = 0.77$, $P < 0.01$, n = 34). (Kayser et al. 1988)

PUTATIVE INHIBITORY CONTROL OF ENDOGENOUS OPIOID RELEASE

To explain the paradoxical antinociceptive effect of low doses of naloxone, we suggested (Kayser et al. 1986a, 1988b) that the endogenous opioid peptide release could be controlled by negative feedback mechanisms, comparable to those observed for others neuromediators (Langer 1981; Starke 1981; Arrang et al. 1983). According to this hypothesis, which supported by biochemical studies (Giros et al. 1983; Ueda et al. 1986, 1987; Bourgoin et al. 1991; Collin et al. 1992), extremely low doses of naloxone, interacting with putative highly sensitive receptors, could increase the spontaneous release of endogenous opioids modulated by these receptors and thus generate an antinociceptive effect in conditions of persistent pain (Fig. 7).

WHICH RECEPTOR(S) COULD MEDIATE THE EFFECT?

Studies in Morphine-Tolerant Arthritic Rats

We showed that in the rats rendered tolerant to morphine's antinociceptive effects with repeated administration of high or low doses of morphine (Kayser et al. 1986a,b; Kayser and Guilbaud 1987b), the paradoxical antinociceptive effect of low doses of naloxone (1,3,6,10 µg/kg iv.) was dramatically and dose-dependently decreased, while the high doses of naloxone still induced hyperalgesia, as seen previously.

These results emphasize that the receptors involved in the two opposite effects of naloxone not only are differentially sensitive to naloxone, but also that they are of different types, and that mu-opioid receptors could mediate the paradoxical antinociceptive effect of naloxone.

Effects of Extremely Low Doses of Morphine in Arthritic Rats

According to this hypothesis, we suggested (Kayser et al. 1987) that extremely low doses of morphine could mimic the effects of endogenous opioids and decrease the spontaneous release of endogenous opioids modulated by these putative receptors, thus inducing a paradoxical hyperalgesic effect. For this purpose, we tested the effects of extremely low doses of morphine from 50 to 3 µg/kg iv. on the vocalization threshold to paw pressure in arthritic rats (Fig. 8). Still present at 50 µg/kg, the antinociceptive effect of morphine completely disappeared at 30 µg/kg; lower doses from 10 to 3 (but mainly 6) µg/kg iv. produced a significant decrease in the threshold. Thus, a clear hyperalgesic effect occurred at very low doses. Simultaneously, we observed a

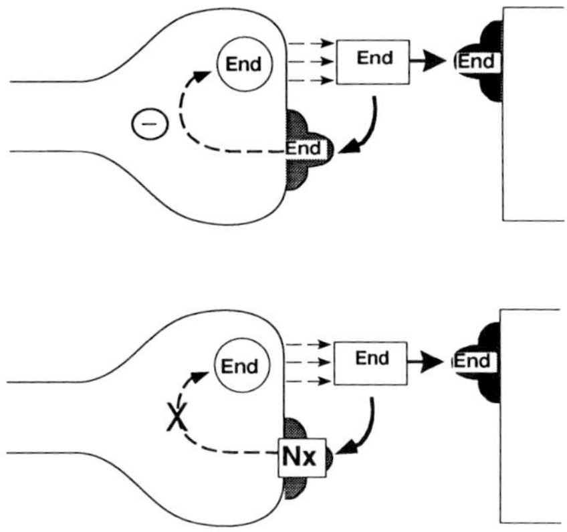

Fig. 7. Schematic representation of a putative inhibitory control of endogenous opioid release. End = endogenous opioids; Nx = naloxone.

modification of behavior; the animals became more reactive to manipulation and vocalized readily in response to touch. These results again suggest the involvement of mu-opioid receptors in the putative inhibitory control of endogenous opioid peptide release.

Studies with Specific Delta- and Kappa-Opioid Receptor Antagonists

In further experiments with specific antagonists for delta- and kappa-opioid receptors in arthritic and neuropathic rats, we showed that delta-antagonists, ICI 174,864 (10 mg/kg iv.) or naltrindole (1 mg/kg iv.), did not modify the antinociceptive action of the low dose of 3 µg/kg iv. naloxone (Cattaneo et al. 1993; Attal et al. 1993). This finding suggests that delta-opioid receptors are not important in the putative negative feedback control of the endogenous opioid release. These data appear to contradict other studies using ICI-174,864 in normal rats Taiwo et al. 1989) or naltrindole in diabetic mice (Kamei et al. 1992), suggesting that the paradoxical analgesia produced by naloxone could be mediated by interaction at a site with characteristics of the delta-opioid receptor. In normal rats, only very weak antinociceptive effects of naloxone were seen following intrathecal injection of naloxone (Taiwo et al. 1989). In the particular case of diabetic mice (Kamei et al. 1992), very high doses of naloxone (5 mg/kg sc.) were used to produce analgesia.

In direct contrast to these results, use of kappa-antagonists, MR-2266 (0.2 mg/kg iv.) or nor-binaltorphimine (1 mg/kg iv.), produced almost a complete suppression of the naloxone antinociceptive effect (Cattaneo et al. 1993; Attal et al. 1993). These data support the involvement of kappa-opioid recep-

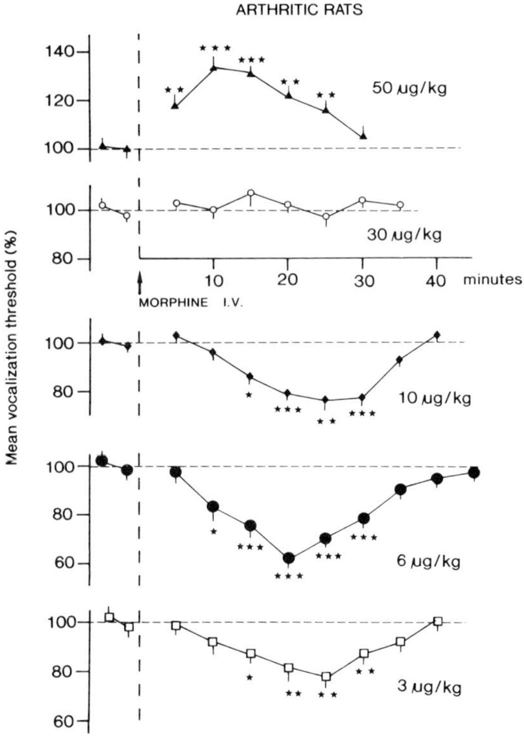

Fig. 8. Effects of extremely low doses (3 µg/kg to 50 µg/kg) of morphine (mean ± S.E.M.) in arthritic rats (n = 9 in each group of rats). * $P < 0.05$, ** $P < 0.01$, $P < 0.001$; student's *t* test. (From Kayser et al. 1987)

tors in the paradoxical effect of naloxone in these models of persistent pain, and thus in the putative inhibitory control of endogenous opioid peptide release.

The apparent high sensitivity of opioid sites with kappa characteristics to extremely low doses of naloxone is somewhat puzzling. In fact, it appears that kappa-receptor sites could participate in a complex modulation of nociceptive messages, in particular in models of inflammatory pain (references in Cattaneo et al. 1993). The possible involvement of mu-opioid receptors suggests that the two types of opioid receptors may participate (Fig. 9), and it is possible that there is some coupling between mu and kappa sites at least in these pathological conditions.

CONCLUSION

Using various doses of naloxone and different opioid receptor antagonists in models of clinical pain, we revealed the existence of tonic inhibitory con-

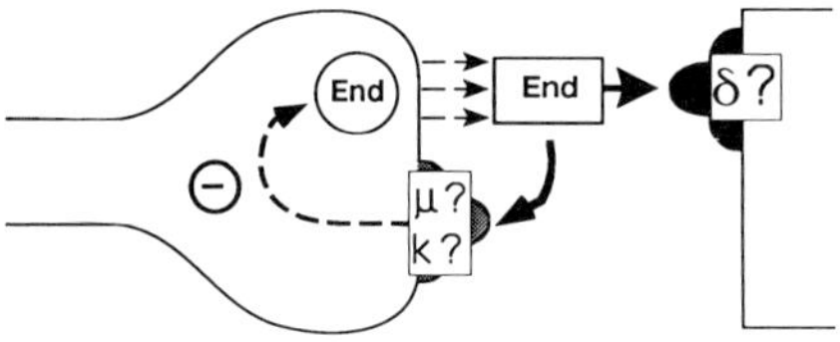

Fig. 9. Receptors involved in the tonic inhibitory control exerted by endogenous opioid peptides on nociceptive messages and in the putative negative feedback control of their release; μ= mu-, δ = delta-, k = kappa-opioid receptors.

trols exerted by endogenous opioids, which appeared to be mediated by delta-opioid receptors. Recent experiments showed effectively that high doses of delta-antagonists can produce hyperalgesic effects. In all cases, extremely low doses of naloxone revealed the existence of a putative inhibitory control of endogenous opioid release, which appeared to be mediated by mu- and/or kappa- opioid receptors.

Our finding that the paradoxical antinociceptive effect of naloxone is enhanced in the presence of pain, which relates to the degree and duration of pain, could suggest that the putative inhibitory control of endogenous opioid release itself increases with the severity and duration of hyperalgesia and thus could be a possible component of a vicious circle leading to the establishment of persistent pain.

This hypothesis does not exclude other hypotheses proposed by authors who found biphasic effects of naloxone in normal rats and with intrathecal or iontophoresis application (Woolf 1980; Dickenson et al. 1981; Crain and Shen 1991). Whatever the exact mechanism, our results suggest that a future therapeutical strategy might not only increase the levels of endogenous opioids by using inhibitors of their degrading enzymes (Refs in Roques et al. 1993), but also to try to abolish or reduce the putative inhibitory control of their release.

ACKNOWLEDGMENTS

We are indebted to Drs. G. Guilbaud and J.M. Besson for their interest in and support of these studies. Dr. A.H. Dickenson is gratefully thanked for English language revision.

REFERENCES

Arrang, J.M., Garbarg, M. and Schwarz, J.C., Autoinhibition of brain histamine release mediated by a novel class (H3) of histamine receptors, Nature (Lond.), 302 (1983) 832–837.

Attal, N., Kayser, V., Jazat, F. and Guilbaud, G., Behavioral evidence for a bidirectional effect of systemic naloxone in a model of experimental neuropathy in the rat, Brain Res., 494 (1989) 276–284.

Attal, N., Jazat, F., Kayser, V. and Guilbaud, G., Further evidence for a "pain-related" behaviours in a model of unilateral peripheral mononeuropathy, Pain, 41 (1990a) 235–251.

Attal, N., Kayser, V. and Guilbaud, G., The bidirectional dose-dependent effect of systemic naloxone is also related to the intensity and duration of pain-related disorders: a study in a rat model of peripheral mononeuropathy, Brain Res., 525 (1990b) 170–174.

Attal, N., Chen, Y.L., Kayser, V. and Guilbaud, G., Behavioural evidence that systemic morphine may modulate a phasic pain-related behaviour in a rat model of peripheral mononeuropathy, Pain, 47 (1991) 65–70.

Attal, N., Kayser, V. and Guilbaud, G., Use of opioid antagonists to characterize the modifications in opioid endogenous systems in a model of persistent "pain" due to nerve constriction injury. In: Abstracts: 7th World Congress on Pain, IASP Publications, Seattle, 1993. p. 34.

Bennett, G.J. and Xie, Y.K., A mononeuropathy in rat that produces abnormal pain sensation like those seen in man, Pain, 33 (1988) 87–107.

Bourgoin, S., Collin, E., Benoliel, J.J., Chantrel, D., Mauborgne, A., Pohl, M., Hamon, M. and Cesselin, F., Opioid control of the release of Met-enkephalin-like material from the rat spinal cord, Brain Res., 551 (1991) 178–184.

Buchsbaum, M.S., Davies, G.C., Naber, D. and Pickar, D., Pain enhances naloxone-induced hyperalgesia in human as assessed by somatosensory evoked potentials, Psychopharmacology, 79 (1983) 99–103.

Cattaneo, I., Kayser, V. and Guilbaud, G., Differential effects of specific delta and kappa opioid receptor antagonists on the bidirectional dose-dependent effect of systemic naloxone in arthritic rats, an experimental model of persistent pain, Brain Res., 623 (1993) 201–207.

Cesselin, F., Montastruc, J.L., Gros, C., Bourgoin, S. and Hamon, M., Met-enkephelin levels and opioid receptors in the spinal cord of chronic suffering rats, Brain Res. 191 (1980) 25–31.

Collin, E., Bourgoin, S., Ferhat, L., Hamon, M. and Cesselin, F., κ-opioid receptor stimulation abolishes μ- but not δ-mediated inhibitory control of spinal Met-enkephalin release, Neuroscience Lett., 134 (1992) 238–242.

Crain, S.M. and Shen, K.F., Opioids can evoke direct receptor-mediated excitatory effects on sensory neurons, TIPS, 11 (1991) 77–81.

Dennis, S.G. and Melzack, R., Comparison of phasic and tonic pain in animals. In: J.J. Bonica Bonica, J.C. Liebeskind and D. Albe-Fessard (Eds.). Proceedings of the Second World Congress on Pain. Advances in Pain Research and Therapy, Vol. 3. Raven Press, New York, 1979, pp. 747–760.

Desmeules, J., Kayser, V. and Guilbaud, G., Selective opioid receptor agonists modulate mechanical allodynia in an animal model of neuropathic pain, Pain, 53 (1993) 277–285.

Dickenson, A.H., Le Bars, D. and Besson, J.M., Endogenous opiates and nociception: a possible functional role in both pain inhibition and detection as revealed by intrathecal naloxone, Neurosci. Lett., 24 (1981) 161–164.

Di Rosa, M., Giroud, J.P. and Willoughby, D.A., Studies of the mediators of the acute inflammatory response induced in rats in different sites by carrageenan and turpentine, J. Pathol., 104 (1971) 15–29.

Draisci, G., Kajander, K.C., Dubner, R., Bennett, G. and Iadarola, M.J., Up-regulation of opioid gene expression in spinal cord evoked by experimental nerve injuries and inflammation, Brain Res., 560 (1991) 186–192.

Dubner, R. and Ruda, M.A., Activity-dependent plasticity following tissue injury and inflamma-

tion, TINS, 15 (1992) 96–103.
Faccini, E., Uzumaki, H., Govoni, S., Missale, C., Spano, P.F., Covelli, V. and Trabucchi, M., Afferent fibers mediate the increase of Met-enkephalin elicited in rat spinal cord by localized pain, Pain, 18 (1984) 25–31.
Giros, B., De La Baume, S., Gros, C. and Schwartz, J.C., Inhibition de la liberation évoquée de (Met5) enképhaline de coupes de globus pallidus en présence de thiorphan et de bestatine, C.R.Acad. Sci. III, 297 (1983) 609–612.
Goldstein, A., Pryor, G.T., Otis, L.S. and Larsen, F., On the role of endogenous opioid peptides: failure of naloxone to influence shock escape threshold in the rat, Life Sci., 18 (1976) 599–604.
Gouret, C., Mocquet, G. and Raynaud, G., Use of Freund's adjuvant arthritis test in anti-inflammatory drug screening in the rat: value of animal selection and preparation at the breeding center, Lab. Anim. Sci., 26 (1976) 281–287.
Guilbaud, G., Benoist, J.M., Gautron, M. and Kayser, V., Effects of systemic naloxone upon ventrobasal thalamus neuronal responses in arthritic rats, Brain Res., 243 (1982) 59–66.
Höllt, V., Haarman, I., Millan, M.J. and Herz, A., Prodynorphin gene expression is enhanced in the spinal cord of chronic arthritic rats, Neurosci. Lett., 73 (1987) 90–94.
Jazat, F. and Guilbaud, G., The "tonic" pain-related behaviour seen in mononeuropathic rats is modulated by morphine and naloxone, Pain, 44 (1991) 97–102.
Kajander, K.C., Sahara, Y., Iadarola, M.J. and Bennett, G., Dynorphin increases in the dorsal spinal cord in rats with a painful peripheral neuropathy, Peptides, 11 (1990) 719–728.
Kamei, J., Kawashima, N. and Kasuya, Y., Paradoxical analgesia produced by naloxone in diabetic mice is attributable to supersensitivity of d-opioid receptors, Brain Res., 592 (1992) 101–105.
Kayser, V. and Guilbaud, G., Dose-dependent analgesic and hyperalgesic effects of systemic naloxone in arthritic rats, Brain Res., 226 (1981) 344–348.
Kayser, V. and Guilbaud, G., The analgesic effect of morphine, but not those of the enkephalinase inhibitor thiorphan, are enhanced in arthritic rats, Brain Res., 267 (1983) 131–138.
Kayser, V. and Guilbaud, G., Can tolerance to morphine be induced in arthritic rats? Brain Res., 334 (1985) 335–338.
Kayser, V. and Guilbaud, G., Local and remote modifications of nociceptive sensitivity during carrageenan-induced inflammation in the rat, Pain, 28 (1987a) 99–108.
Kayser, V. and Guilbaud, G., Cross-tolerance between analgesic low doses of morphine and naloxone in arthritic rats, Brain Res., 405 (1987b) 123–129.
Kayser, V. and Guilbaud, G., Differential effects of various doses of morphine and naloxone on two nociceptive test threshold in arthritic and normal rats, Pain, 41 (1990) 353–363.
Kayser, V. and Guilbaud, G., Physiological relevance and time-course of a tonic endogenous opioid modulation of nociceptive messages, based on the effects of naloxone in a rat model of localized hyperalgesic inflammation, Brain Res., 567 (1991) 197–203.
Kayser, V., Peschanski, M. and Guilbaud, G., Neuronal loss in the ventrobasal complex of the rat thalamus alters behavioral responses to noxious stimulation. In: H.L. Fields, R. Dubner and F. Cervero (Eds.), Proceedings of the Fourth World Congress on Pain. Advances in Pain Research and Therapy, Vol. 9. Raven Press, New York, 1985.
Kayser, V., Besson, J.M. and Guilbaud, G., Analgesia produced by low doses of the opiate antagonist naloxone in arthritic rats is reduced in morphine-tolerant animals, Brain Res., 371 (1986a) 37–41.
Kayser, V., Neil, A. and Guilbaud, G., Repeated low doses of morphine induce a rapid tolerance in arthritic rats but a potentiation of opiate analgesia in normal animals, Brain Res., 383 (1986b) 392–396.
Kayser, V., Besson, J.M. and Guilbaud, G., Paradoxical hyperalgesic effect of exceedingly low doses of systemic morphine in an animal model of persistent pain (Freund's adjuvant-induced arthritic rats), Brain Res., 414 (1987) 155–157.
Kayser, V., Benoist, J.M., Neil, A., Gautron, M. and Guilbaud, G., Behavioral and electrophysiological studies on the paradoxical analgesic effects of an extremely low dose of naloxone in an

experimental model of acute and localized inflammation, Exp. Brain Res., 73 (1988a) 402–410.
Kayser V., Besson, J.M. and Guilbaud, G, Paradoxical effects of low doses of naloxone in experimental models of inflammatory pain. In: H.L. Fields and J.M. Besson (Eds), Pain modulation. Progress in Brain Research, Vol. 77. Elsevier, Amsterdam, 1988b, pp. 301–312.
Kayser, V., Chen, Y.L. and Guilbaud, G., Behavioural evidence for a peripheral component in the enhanced antinociceptive effect of a low dose of systemic morphine in carrageenan-induced hyperalgesic rats, Brain Res., 560 (1991) 237–244.
Kosterlitz, H.W. and Hughes, J., Some thoughts on the significance of enkephalin, the endogenous ligands, Life Sci., 17 (1975) 91–96.
Langer, S.Z., Presynaptic regulation of the release of catecholamine, Pharmacol. Rev., 32 (1981) 337–362.
Lasagna, L., Drug interaction in the field of analgesic drugs, Proc. R. Soc. Med., 58 (1965) 978–983.
Levine, J.D., Gordon, N.C. and Fields, H.L., Naloxone dose-dependently produces analgesia and hyperalgesia in post-operative pain, Nature (Lond.), 278 (1979) 740–741.
Lombard, M.C. and Besson, J.M., Electrophysiological evidence for a tonic activity of the spinal cord intrinsic opioid systems in a chronic pain model, Brain Res., 477 (1989) 48–56.
Millan, M.J., Multiple opioid systems and pain, Pain, 27 (1986) 303–347.
Neil, A., Kayser, V., Gacel, G., Besson, J.M. and Guilbaud, G., Opioid receptor types and antinociceptive activity in chronic inflammation: both kappa and mu opiate agonistic effects are enhanced in arthritic rats, Eur. J. Pharmacol., 130 (1986) 203–208.
Pearson, C.M., Waksman, B.H. and Sharp, J.J., Studies of arthritis and other lesions induced in rats by injection of mycobacterial adjuvant. Changes affecting the skin and mucous membranes. Comparison of the experimental process with human disease, J. Exp. Med., 113 (1961) 485–509.
Roques, B.P., Noble, F., Daugé, V., Fournié-Zaluski, M.C. and Beaumont, A., Neutral endopeptidase 24.11: structure, inhibition, and experimental and clinical pharmacology, Pharmacol. Rev., 45 (1993) 87–133.
Satoh, M., Kawajiri, S.I., Yamamoto, M., Makino, H. and Takagi, H., Reversal by naloxone of adaptation of rats to noxious stimuli, Life Sci., 24 (1979) 685–690.
Starke, K., Presynaptic receptors, Annu. Rev. Pharmacol. Toxicol., 21 (1981) 7–30.
Taiwo, Y.O., Basbaum, A.I., Perry, F. and Levine, J.D., Paradoxical analgesia produced by low doses of the opiate-antagonist naloxone is mediated by interaction at a site with characteristics of the delta-opioid receptor, JPET, 249 (1989) 97–100.
Ueda, H., Fukushima, N., Kitao, T.G.M. and Takagi, H., Low doses of naloxone produce analgesia in the mouse by blocking presynaptic autoinhibition of enkephalin release, Neurosci. Lett., 65 (1986) 247–252.
Ueda, H., Fukushima, N., Ge, M., Takagi, H. and Satoh, M., Presynaptic opioid κ-receptor and regulation of the release of Met-enkephalin in the rat brainstem, Neurosci. Lett., 81 (1987) 309–313.
Vinegar, R., Schreiber, W. and Hugo, R., Biphasic development of carrageenan edema in rats, J. Pharmacol. Exp. Ther., 166 (1969) 96–103.
Winter, C.A., Risley, E.A. and Nuss, G.W., Carrageenan-induced edema in hind paw of the rat as an assay for anti-inflammatory drugs, Proc. Soc. Exp. Biol. Med., 111 (1962) 544–547.
Winter, C.A. and Flataker, L., Reaction thresholds to pressure in oedematous hind paw of rats: responses to analgesic drugs, J. Pharmacol. Exp. Ther., 148 (1965) 373–379.
Woolf, C.J., Analgesia and hyperalgesia produced in the rat by intrathecal naloxone, Brain Res., 189 (1980) 593–597.

Correspondence to: Valérie Kayser, Unité de Recherches de Physiopharmacologie du Système Nerveux, INSERM U 161, 2, Rue d'Alésia, 75014 Paris, France. Tel: 33-1-45-89-3662; Fax: 33-1-45-88-1304.

Proceedings of the 7th World Congress on Pain,
Progress in Pain Research and Management, Vol. 2,
edited by G.F. Gebhart, D.L. Hammond, and T.S.
Jensen, IASP Press, Seattle, © 1994.

38

Combining Opioids with Other Drugs: Challenges in Clinical Trial Design

Mitchell B. Max

*Chief, Clinical Trials Unit, Neurobiology and Anesthesiology Branch,
National Institute of Dental Research, National Institutes of Health,
Bethesda, Maryland, USA*

INTRODUCTION

The two centuries of clinical analgesic research have often been likened to the search for the Holy Grail—a quest for a molecule with potent analgesic effects, yet without the troublesome side effects or dependence liability of the mu receptor opioid agonists (Mather 1990). The recent explosive development of the basic neuropharmacology of pain and analgesia has intensified this focus on single agents. Unfortunately, results of clinical trials have not fulfilled all the hopes engendered by basic science discoveries. For chronic pain in particular, pain relief is usually incomplete at nontoxic dose levels of opioids (Arner and Meyerson 1988; Cherny et al. 1994), antidepressants (Max 1994), adrenergic agonists (Zeigler et al. 1992), or oral congeners of local anesthetics (Dejgard et al. 1988; Chabal et al. 1992). Optimists might say that the availability of cloned receptor structures will allow synthesis of more selective drugs that will increase the therapeutic ratio of these therapies. I would consider it equally likely, however, that given the multiple pathways for pain generation, no single agent will ever prove to be a panacea.

Elsewhere in this volume, Professor Besson refers to the despair provoked by such slow progress. The despondent researcher might profit from the counsel of a seasoned clinical pharmacologist. "Look at the history of therapy in hypertension, congestive heart failure, cancer, and infectious diseases," the pharmacologist might say. "In each of these fields clinicians encountered the same problem of modest but insufficient efficacy for single agents pushed as high as toxicity would allow. Dramatic advances have come from systematic clinical research into combinations of agents working through different mechanisms."

In this chapter, I will argue that the time is ripe for rigorous clinical research into drug combinations, which until now have received only cursory attention. I will provide some illustrations of the challenges posed by these clinical trials, and highlight some recent studies that illustrate solutions.

CLINICALLY USEFUL COMBINATIONS

For basic researchers, research into drug combinations has become an active topic indeed. An example of this interest is the current controversy about how to determine that a drug combination is synergistic for analgesia (Tallarida 1992; Miaskowski and Levine 1992; Plummer 1993; Laska et al. 1994). While the appropriate experimental designs and statistical methods needed to establish synergism are in dispute, all agree that synergism refers to supra-additive analgesic effects of a combination—greater than the total analgesic effect predicted by the doses of the components.

For the clinical researcher, however, the crucial issue is *clinical usefulness* rather than analgesic synergism. To be clinically useful, the combination must have a more favorable therapeutic ratio than do the components. A specific criterion is that the combination have fewer unwanted side effects than either component when one compares dose levels of each that produce equivalent pain relief (equianalgesic doses). The components need not be synergistic for analgesia; they may be merely additive or even subadditive, as long as side effects show even *less* additivity in the combination.

Combining opioids with other drugs is not a new idea in pain research (Table I). Several classes of drugs are widely accepted to improve on opioids alone in some clinical situations, including nonsteroidal anti-inflammatory drugs (NSAIDs) or acetaminophen (American Pain Society 1992), amphetamine-like drugs in selected cancer patients (Bruera et al. 1987), and low concentrations of epidural local anesthetics (Hogan et al. 1991). Several other combinations have lingered in the gray area, "clinical usefulness uncertain," despite a solid grounding in animal experiments and at least one clinical trial for each showing that the combination produces more pain relief than does the opioid alone. Such adjuvants to opioids include hydroxyzine and other antihistamines (Beaver and Feise 1976; Kantor and Steinberg 1976; Hupert et al. 1980; Stambaugh and Lane 1983), tricyclic antidepressants (Levine et al. 1986; Max et al. 1992, Gordon et al. 1993, Kerrick et al. 1993), cholecystokinin (CCK) antagonists (Price et al. 1985; Lavigne et al. 1989; Lehmann et

Table I
Drugs reported to enhance opioid analgesia in at least one clinical trial

Clinically Useful	Usefulness Uncertain
NSAIDs, acetaminophen	Hydroxyzine
Amphetamines	Tricyclic antidepressants
Spinal local anesthetics	CCK antagonists
	Clonidine
	μ + k opioid combinations

al. 1989), clonidine (Mogensen et al. 1992; Gordon et al. 1992), and non–μ receptor opioids (Levine and Gordon 1988). For these classes of adjuvants, the missing experiment has been the test of clinical usefulness described above, a comparison of the toxicity of the combination with a dose of the opioid alone that gives equal analgesia.

Clinical research into combinations of opioids and tricyclic antidepressants provides an example of the preliminary nature of work in analgesic drug combinations. For two decades, a leading hypothesis of pain research has been that opioid analgesia is mediated in large part by descending pathways from the brainstem that release norepinephrine and serotonin (Basbaum and Fields 1978; Dubner and Bennett 1983). Many laboratories have shown that in animals, drugs that increase activity of these monoamine systems increase opioid analgesia. Among them are the tricyclic antidepressants, which block synaptic reuptake of norepinephrine and serotonin, prolonging their inhibitory actions (Taiwo et al 1985; Kellstein et al. 1988).

Levine et al. (1986) and Gordon et al. (1993) have presented the most convincing data that tricyclic antidepressants increase opioid analgesia in humans. Levine et al. pretreated groups of 10 oral surgery patients for one week with the norepinephrine reuptake blocker desipramine, 75 mg/day; the mixed reuptake blocker, amitriptyline, 75 mg/day; or placebo. After surgery, patients reporting pain received morphine, 6 mg intravenously. Fig. 1 shows that morphine alone, with placebo pretreatment, just held the pain steady for the 2½-hour study period, and amitriptyline had a similar result. In the group pretreated with desipramine, however, morphine caused a marked drop in pain levels. Gordon et al. (1993) replicated the desipramine-morphine effect in a second study.

These investigators hoped to validate the basic science concept that a

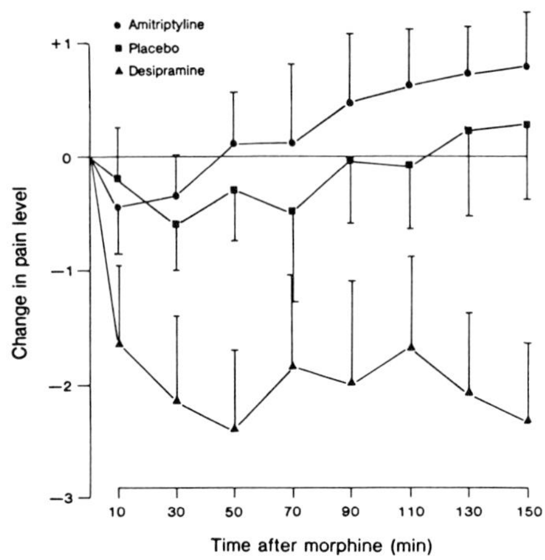

Fig. 1. Effect of desipramine and amitriptyline pretreatment on morphine analgesia following oral surgery (Levine et al., 1986). Groups of 10 patients each received desipramine or amitriptyline, 75 mg/day, or placebo for one week before surgery. Changes in postoperative pain intensity on a 10-cm visual analog scale are plotted against time after the morphine dose. The augmentation of morphine analgesia by desipramine was statistically significant. Although this was the first demonstration that a tricyclic antidepressant augments opioid analgesia, the study was not designed to examine whether the combination is clinically useful, i.e., less toxic than the higher dose of morphine alone that would produce the same level of analgesia.

norepinephrine reuptake blocker enhances opioid analgesia in humans. They achieved this well-circumscribed aim quite well, and no criticism is intended in pointing out that these studies leave unanswered the question of whether the combination is clinically useful. For example, side effects were not reported. Perhaps desipramine increases morphine side effects as much as, or more than, it enhances analgesia, either through a central nervous system mechanism, or merely by altering the distribution of metabolism of morphine. In that case, the combination would be no better than a higher dose of morphine alone.

Despite several other clinical studies addressing the opioid-tricyclic antidepressant combination, the question of clinical usefulness remains unanswered. Max et al. (1992) studied the effects of a single dose of desipramine on morphine analgesia, sedation, and nausea after inpatient orthopedic or gynecological surgery, but found no effect of that dose of desipramine on analgesia or side effects. This result does not contradict the positive findings of Levine and Gordon, who observed that a full week of desipramine pretreatment is necessary for the analgesic enhancement (Gordon et al. 1993). Similar to

Levine et al. (1986), Kerrick et al. (1993) reported that amitriptyline did not enhance postoperative morphine analgesia, but Kerrick et al. did not evaluate desipramine. Taken overall, the results leave open the possibility that patients taking opioids may benefit from the addition of desipramine, but the studies to confirm the clinical usefulness of the acute effects and extend the observations to chronic treatment remain to be done.

A classic design that is well suited to testing clinical usefulness of a combination is the relative potency assay (Laska and Meisner 1987). These designs were extensively used in the 1950s and 1960s to compare the efficacy of various opioids in relieving pain and depressing respiration, although they can be used to compare any effects (Bellville et al. 1968). As applied to drug combinations, a dose-response curve is determined for the opioid alone and for the opioid plus an adjuvant drug. A large dose range will ensure some overlap of the two curves (Fig. 2) and will allow the comparison of any type of side effect at equianalgesic dose levels (Max and Laska 1991).

An elegant example of the use of the relative potency design is a recent study in normal volunteers by Coda et al. (1993a) examining the effects of oral pretreatment with a serotonin-releasing drug, fenfluramine, on analgesia to experimental pain stimuli. Each of 10 subjects took part in four treatment sessions: placebo followed by saline infusion, fenfluramine followed by saline infusion, placebo followed by morphine infusion, and fenfluramine followed by morphine infusion. The investigators satisfied the requirements discussed above for supporting overall clinical usefulness of a drug. They prospectively measured side effects (visual analogue scales [VAS] for sedation, nausea, itching, and mood) and compared the combination to morphine alone at equianalgesic dose levels. An equianalgesic range of doses was ensured by providing a range of different morphine levels, using the laboratory's method of pharmacokinetic tailoring. As previously reported (Hill et al. 1990), they determined each subject's pharmacokinetic parameters for morphine after a single bolus dose given several weeks before the morphine-fenfluramine study sessions. For the four sessions of the drug combination study, they entered the morphine pharmacokinetic parameters into the computer program that controls the morphine pump. On each testing day, subjects were taken through three different targeted plasma levels of morphine (or saline control) spanning the usual therapeutic range, 16, 32, and 64 ng/ml. Plasma morphine determinations at each infusion rate showed that the targeted levels were precisely achieved, and that fenfluramine had no effect on morphine metabolism or distribution. The incorporation of individualized pharmacokinetic tailoring greatly reduces the variability that would otherwise be produced by the two- to fourfold variation in opioid disposition between subjects (Mather 1992).

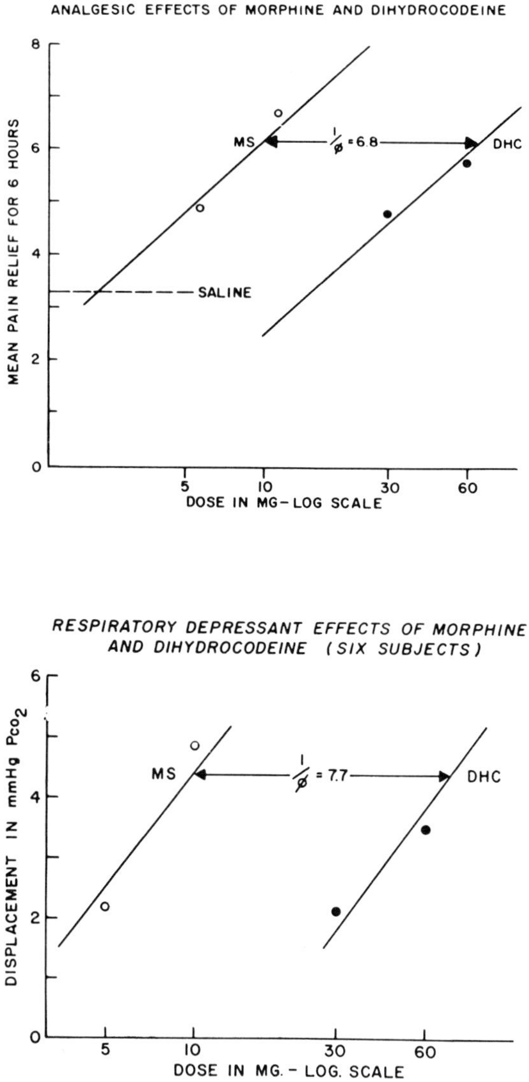

Fig. 2. The relative potency assay, a classic design well suited to comparing side effects and analgesic potencies of various treatments. In this study by Seed et al. (1958), intramuscular doses of morphine, 5 and 10 mg, were compared to dihydrocodeine, 30 and 60 mg, for pain relief (**top**; 5-point category scale summed over 6 hours) and respiratory depression (**bottom**). Relative potencies compared to morphine, denoted by 1/ø, were similar for analgesia and respiratory depression. In the analgesic study, a saline placebo (horizontal dotted line) was also one of the treatments, but was not an essential part of the design. If doses are chosen to ensure overlap of the analgesic effect ranges, this design can be used to compare side effects of a drug combination and its components at equianalgesic doses.

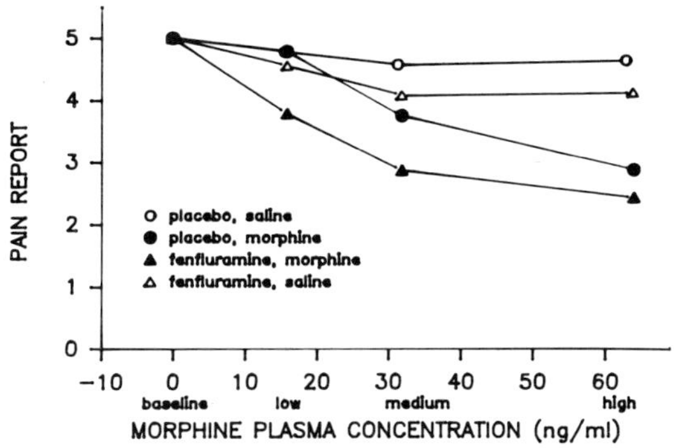

Fig. 3. Analgesic effects of placebo, fenfluramine, morphine, and morphine plus fenfluramine on ratings of electrical tooth pulp stimuli in normal subjects (from Coda et al. 1993a). Subjects participated in four testing sessions and received each of the treatments. During each session, subjects rated the experimental pain stimuli before morphine (or saline) infusion, and again at morphine (or saline) infusion rates targeted to produce morphine plasma concentrations of 16, 32, or 64 ng/ml. The addition of fenfluramine to morphine approximately doubled analgesic potency, relative to morphine alone. This is an example of a relative potency study; if the data had been plotted in terms of pain relief rather than pain intensity, the graph would have resembled Fig. 2.

Fig. 3 compares the amount of pain evoked by a series of electrical tooth pulp stimuli during the four experimental sessions. The open circles in the uppermost curve represent the placebo-saline session and show negligible lowering of pain ratings as the session proceeded. The open triangles represent fenfluramine-saline, which produced a small but statistically significant reduction in pain. The filled circles represent placebo-morphine, which caused a dose-related reduction in pain for the medium and high plasma morphine concentrations, but no effect for the low concentrations. The filled triangles, representing the fenfluramine-morphine combination, produced highly statistically significant reductions in pain scores. Note that at the low morphine concentration, where morphine alone had been ineffective, the combination was analgesic. Morphine analgesia at the two higher concentrations also was augmented by fenfluramine pretreatment. The graph shows roughly equal analgesia for the combination at the low morphine concentration and morphine alone at the medium concentration, as well as for the combination at the medium concentration and morphine alone at the highest level, corresponding to about a doubling of the analgesic potency of morphine by fenfluramine.

Fig. 4 shows that morphine side effects, in contrast to analgesia, were not substantially affected by fenfluramine pretreatment. Although subjects pre-

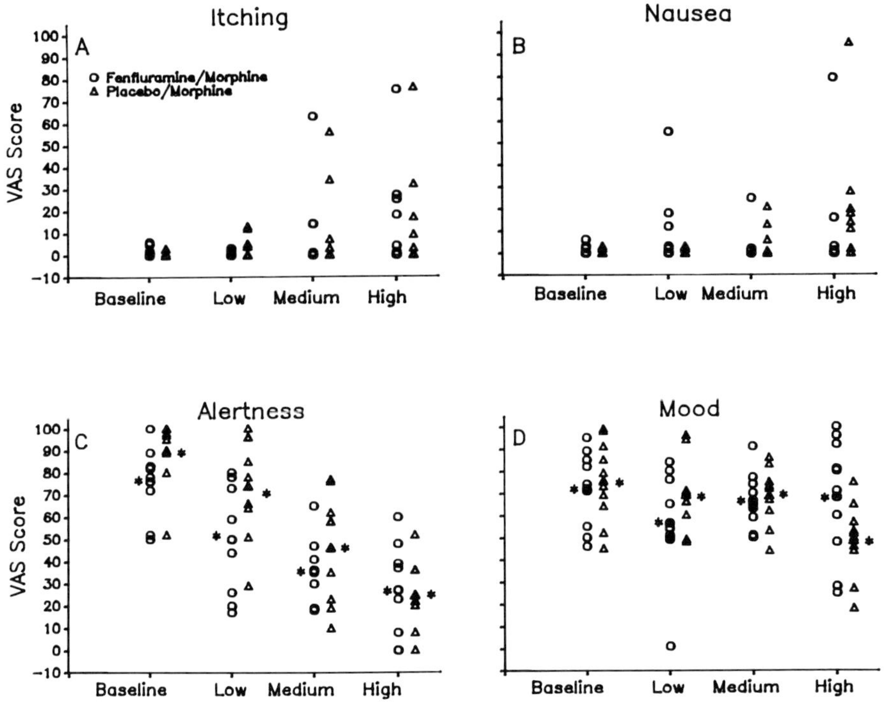

Fig. 4. Side effects of fenfluramine/morphine (circles) compared to morphine alone (triangles), from Coda et al. 1993a. Individual subjects' visual analog scale ratings are shown before morphine infusion and at the low, medium, and high morphine plasma concentrations. On the plots of alertness and mood, the asterisks indicate mean values for the group; itching and nausea did not show a normal distribution, so means were not calculated. The zero and 100-point extremes of the VAS scales were marked, respectively, "no itch" and "itch as bad as it could possibly be"; "no nausea" and "constant nausea"; "can't keep my eyes open" and "wide awake"; and "worst I've ever felt" and "best I've ever felt." Apart from a slight reduction in alertness in at the low morphine concentration, the addition of fenfluramine did not affect side effect scores, suggesting that the augmentation of morphine analgesia shown in Fig. 3 might be clinically useful.

treated with fenfluramine were slightly less alert than were placebo-pretreated patients at the low morphine concentration, this effect was not consistent across the three morphine concentrations, and fenfluramine did not increase morphine-associated itching, nausea, or mood change. Coda et al. (1993a) concluded that drugs that release or mimic serotonin are likely to be useful adjuvants to opioids. Fenfluramine itself may be limited for chronic pain treatment because after 24 hours of use it depletes neuronal serotonin stores (Shoulson and Chase 1975); nevertheless, this result encourages studies of other drugs with serotonergic mechanisms.

The clarity of the results of the fenfluramine-morphine study derives from the investigators' attention to methodological detail. This study suggests the value of expanding research in several areas, including the measurement of side effects and the use of experimental pain models in the early development of drug combinations.

MEASUREMENT OF SIDE EFFECTS

The clinical researcher who heeds the preceding admonitions to measure side effects will soon notice that the literature on analgesic side effect assessment is scant, and the commonly cited papers date from 20–30 years ago. Therefore, anyone doing sustained work on analgesic combinations will need to break some new methodological ground. Three research groups have made fresh contributions to the assessment of opioid side effects over the past several years, and illustrate the variety of approaches that might be taken. Working with patients with chronic cancer pain, Bruera et al. (1989, 1992) have been using a simple battery of tests including finger tapping speed, mental arithmetic, digit reversal, visual memory, and VAS for sedation. They reported that these measures were not affected by the patient's usual oral dose of opioids if the dose had been stable for two weeks. Impairment was demonstrable, however, after a recent and substantial dose increase (Bruera et al. 1989). A later study (Bruera et al. 1992) showed that many of these measures were sensitive to the cognitive improvement produced by a single dose of the stimulant methylphenidate.

In contrast to this bedside clinical approach, Banning, Sjogren, and coworkers have focused on a single automated measure—reaction time to an auditory pulse (Sjogren and Banning 1989; Banning and Sjorgen 1990; Banning et al. 1992). This measure appears more sensitive than Bruera's battery in that it is abnormal even in cancer patients on stable opioid doses. A possible drawback is that the clinical meaning of abnormalities is uncertain—e.g., it is not obvious that a prolongation of reaction time by several hundredths of a second is functionally significant for the patient. The broadest and most sophisticated approach in the recent literature is that of Coda et al. (1993b) and Kerr et al. (1991), who have used normal volunteers to study several opioid sensitive measures that closely parallel everyday activities. For example, they employed computer-assisted tools to measure reading speed and to assess performance of sensitive hand movements such as maintaining a constant level of force needed to hold a drinking glass.

EXPERIMENTAL PAIN MODELS

Experimental pain models offer promise for meeting the challenges posed by combination studies. Several type of experimental pain stimuli are sensitive to opioids (Gracely 1991). Experimental pain models have several advantages in the early stages of investigating opioid combinations, many of which were illustrated by the fenfluramine-morphine study described above. Investigators can readily do crossover studies, which control for the interindividual variation in opioid kinetics, as well as for the variations in pharmacodynamics, i.e., the physiological response to a given level of drug (Mather 1992). For normal subjects, more extensive data can be collected than is feasible in acutely ill patients. This would promote, for example, the development of new assessment measures for side effects. Finally, it is possible to do preliminary dose-finding studies without exposing patients to ineffective or toxic levels of drug. Unless an investigator has enough prior experience with the drugs to make some assumptions about doses, the need for dose-finding studies is even more extensive than discussed above. A complete assessment of a drug combination not only requires dose-response curves for the opioid alone and the combination, but the adjuvant alone, and possibly several other dose ratios for the combination (Levine and Gordon 1988; Goldstein and Brunelle 1991; Carter et al. 1988).

Several old and new experimental pain models chiefly used in studies of pain perception and neural mechanisms could be brought to bear on early drug development. Brief electrical, thermal, or pressure stimuli, and continuous pain evoked by cold pressor and tourniquet ischemia are sensitive to opioids (Gracely et al. 1991). Although these methods are subject to various types of bias, many of these potential confounds can be eliminated (Gracely et al. 1988). The most frequent error is to rely upon measurements of pain thresholds, which are far less sensitive to drugs are than the magnitudes of suprathreshold pain stimuli. Brennum et al. (1993) have shown that brief electrical, thermal, and mechanical stimuli are sensitive to epidural morphine, which could provide the basis for combination studies of drugs given by this route.

Pain models that focus on central nervous system (CNS) excitation with repeated stimuli could be useful for developing treatments for neuropathic and inflammatory pain. One interesting model of this type measures the allodynia and hyperalgesia produced by intradermal injection of capsaicin (Simone et al. 1989; LaMotte et al. 1991). Preliminary experiments by Park et al. (this volume) have shown that this model is sensitive enough to detect modest analgesic effects of an opioid and an N-methyl-D aspartate (NMDA) antago-

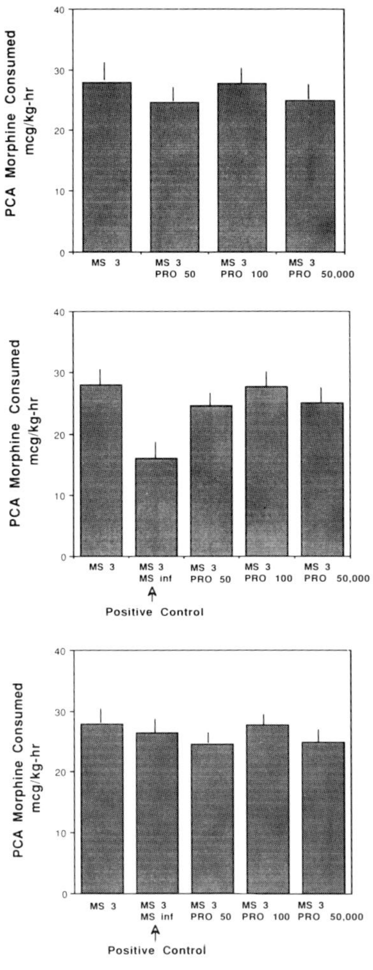

Fig. 5. Value of a positive control group in interpreting negative results. The top panel illustrates data from Lehmann et al. (1989), who studied the effects of adding various doses of the CCK antagonist proglumide to 3 mg boluses of intravenous morphine, administered by patient-controlled analgesia (PCA) devices following major abdominal or gynecological surgery. The mean ± S.E.M. hourly delivery of morphine over the 18-hour observation period is plotted for the four treatment groups, showing that the addition of various proglumide doses to the morphine boluses did not reduce consumption. Without a positive control group, however, we cannot reject the possibility that proglumide enhanced morphine analgesia and that the study methods were not sensitive to that level of treatment difference. The center and bottom panels add a hypothetical positive control treatment, in which patients were given no proglumide but received a continuous infusion of morphine in addition to the PCA boluses on demand. The finding that this intervention reduced the amount of morphine given by PCA, relative to the morphine bolus alone condition (center panel), would demonstrate that the assay is sensitive to an effective intervention and would confirm that proglumide was ineffective. If the supplementary morphine infusion did not reduce PCA morphine (bottom panel), these data would say little about proglumide as an opioid enhancer. We would conclude that the study methods were flawed in some manner that rendered the analgesic assay insensitive.

nist in a group of 12 normal subjects. Price et al. (1977) developed another attractive model showing that repeated painful thermal and electrical stimuli, if given as closely as three seconds apart, cause steady buildup of pain despite fatiguing of peripheral afferents, proving that there is a central wind-up mechanism. Because this wind-up phenomenon also can be demonstrated in patients with neuropathic pain (Price et al. 1992), studies of repeated stimuli in normal volunteers could be useful in developing treatments for these clinical conditions.

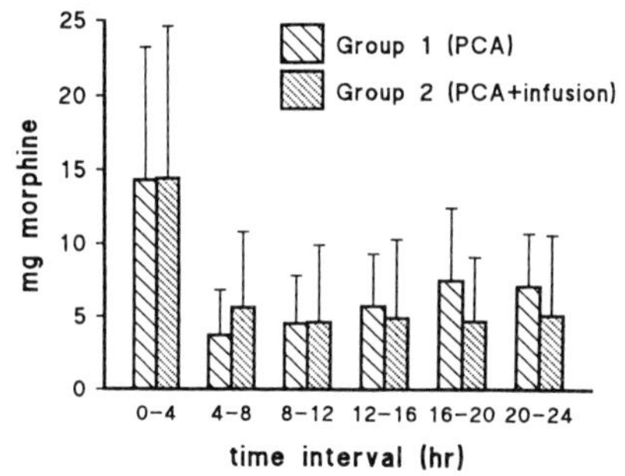

Fig. 6. Postoperative analgesic studies using the patient-controlled analgesia (PCA) model may have limited assay sensitivity. Russell et al. (1993) compared PCA alone (morphine, 1 mg boluses) to PCA plus a continuous morphine infusion at 1 mg/hr. The addition of the infusion amounted to an augmentation of the PCA alone regimen by about 60%. The mean PCA morphine consumption (excluding the infused amount) is plotted for the two treatment groups over time, showing that the addition of the infusion did not reduce the number of morphine boluses taken. Presumably, these study methods may also have failed to detect the effects of an analgesic potentiator that increased morphine potency by 60%.

GETTING DEFINITIVE ANSWERS: THE IMPORTANCE OF POSITIVE CONTROLS

Given the wealth of ideas for potential treatments emerging from basic neuropharmacology laboratories, it is crucial that our clinical studies lead to crisp positive or negative answers so that we can either move ahead with a drug or close the door and try other drug classes. Thus far, this chapter has focused on the question, "How do we know that a positive result for opioid enhancement is really positive—that is, clinically useful?" Before concluding, I would like to briefly discuss the complementary question: "How do we know that a negative result is really negative?"—often denoted by the term assay sensitivity.

To illustrate this problem, let us turn to another class of putative opioid enhancers, the CCK antagonists. After animal studies suggested that these drugs enhance opioid analgesia (Watkins et al. 1985), two clinical groups (Price et al. 1985; Lavigne et al. 1989) reported that 50 μg of the CCK inhibitor proglumide appeared to increase opioid analgesia. However, a group that has done exemplary studies using the postoperative patient-controlled analgesia (PCA) model (Lehmann 1991), reported a discouraging result. Lehmann et al. (1989) conducted a study of 80 abdominal surgery patients who received postoperative morphine via PCA. When patients pushed the control button for a dose, the control group received intravenous morphine, 3 mg alone, while the boluses for the three proglumide adjuvant groups consisted of morphine, 3 mg, plus either 50, 100, or 50,000 μg of proglumide (Fig. 5, top). None of the proglumide doses reduced the number of supplementary morphine boluses relative to the treatment group receiving morphine alone. Pain levels also were similar in the four groups (data not shown).

Is it possible that proglumide did enhance morphine analgesia *in this particular study,* but that the study methods were insufficiently sensitive to pick that up? I submit that we cannot rule out such a failure in assay sensitivity because published PCA studies, and multiple-dose chronic pain studies in general, fail to include a positive control in their design. For decades, analgesic studies experts have agreed that even in the best of hands, single-dose studies often fail to show effectiveness for established analgesics. A variety of factors might be responsible, including the nurse-observer, disruptive effects of ward routines, a confusing pain scale, or changes in the surgical procedure or patient population.

To protect against a false negative result that could threaten a promising drug development program, single-dose studies routinely incorporate a positive control to test whether the methods are sufficient to detect a treatment difference (Food and Drug Administration 1992; Max and Laska 1991). In the center panel of Fig. 5, I have taken the liberty of adding a hypothetical positive control group to the Lehmann et al. data—a group that, like the placebo group, received morphine, 3 mg, with every PCA demand, but also received a background morphine infusion of 30 μg/kg-hr, a dose approximately equal to PCA morphine consumption in the other four groups. If, as shown, this intervention caused a statistically significant decrease in PCA morphine demands, it would suggest that the study methods were sensitive enough to detect a doubling of morphine dose; therefore, the various proglumide doses did not appreciably augment morphine analgesia. If the positive control were not distinguishable from placebo (Fig. 5, bottom panel), we could conclude that the study methods were insensitive and disregard the negative result for proglumide.

Although studies by Lehmann et al. and other groups have often demonstrated the ability to distinguish various active treatments from each other (Einnolf et al. 1989; McCoy et al. 1993), several recently published PCA studies raise the question of the sensitivity of this method. All were clinical studies to test whether the addition of a continuous opioid infusion to an on-demand bolus regimen should be used after surgery. Russell et al. (1993) studied 62 patients following gynecological surgery, comparing intravenous PCA morphine alone (1 mg boluses) to PCA plus a continuous morphine infusion at 1 mg/hr. The addition of the infusion amounted to an augmentation of the PCA alone regimen by about 60%. Fig. 6 plots the mean PCA morphine consumption per patient for the two treatment groups over time, showing that the addition of the infusion did not reduce the number of morphine boluses taken. Pain levels at rest and with movement also were virtually identical in the two treatment groups (data not shown). This study shows that a sophisticated group of PCA investigators may fail to detect the effects of a manipulation that increases the effective morphine dose by 60%. Parker et al. (1991, 1992) have reported several large PCA studies that also showed insensitivity to the addition of a supplementary opioid infusion.

I conclude from these results that the assay sensitivity of the postoperative PCA model urgently needs attention, as PCA is the standard treatment method in many clinical settings for studies of treatments that might augment opioid analgesia. The same concern extends to other types of multiple-dose studies, particularly those dealing with chronic pain. If we are to efficiently screen and study analgesic combinations, we must develop ways to improve assay sensitivity and, optimally, test for it in every clinical trial.

CONCLUSIONS

In conclusion, I would like to reiterate the claim that the investigation of analgesic combinations will be one of the most important areas of clinical pain research over the next several decades. Coming to a crisp positive or negative conclusion about leads from basic science labs is essential if we are to continue to justify the funding going into pain research. We already have a wealth of hypotheses, a stream of ever more specific receptor agonists and antagonists that are entering human studies, human pain models, and well-established experimental designs for combination studies. In developing this research, it would be useful to reach out to other disciplines. For example, collaborations with clinical pharmacology groups will help us to tailor more efficient dosing regimens and to examine metabolic interactions of drugs. Statisticians, some of whom already are grappling with issues regarding the definition of drug synergy, might be enlisted in the effort to define statistical tests for the clinical usefulness of a combination as discussed above.

Another problem may be that research funding incentives do not favor the systematic development of drug combinations—e.g., regulatory systems make it cumbersome for drug companies to collaborate to develop combinations of new drugs, while grant review committees may view combinations of old drugs as less exciting than the newest basic science hypotheses. Our colleagues in cardiovascular diseases and oncology have shown that these barriers can be overcome. With a rigorous and determined approach to investigating drug combinations, we may yet achieve the long-sought goal of a selective increase in opioid analgesia.

REFERENCES

American Pain Society, Principles of Analgesic Use in the Treatment of Acute Pain and Cancer Pain, 3rd ed., American Pain Society, Skokie, Ill., 1992, 41 pp.

Arner, S. and Meyerson, B.A., Lack of analgesic effect of opioids on neuropathic and idiopathic forms of pain, Pain 33 (1988) 11–24.

Banning, A. and Sjogren, P., Cerebral effects of long-term oral opioids in cancer patients measured by continuous reaction time, Clin. J. Pain, 6 (1990) 91–95.

Banning, A., Sjogren, P. and Kaiser, F., Reaction time in cancer patients receiving peripherally acting analgesics alone or in combination with opioids, Acta Anaesthesiol. Scand., 36 (1992) 480–482.

Basbaum, A.L. and Fields, H.L., Endogenous pain control mechanisms: review and hypothesis, Ann. Neurol., 4 (1978) 451–462.

Beaver, W.T. and Feise, G., Comparison of the analgesic effects of morphine, hydroxyzine, and their combination in patients with postoperative pain. In: J.J. Bonica and D. Albe-Fessard (Eds.), Proceedings of the First World Congress on Pain. Advances in Pain Research and Therapy, Vol. 1. Raven Press, New York, 1976, pp. 553–557.

Bellville, J.W., Forrest, W.H., Elashoff, J. and Laska, E., Evaluating side effects of analgesics in a cooperative clinical study, Clin. Pharmacol. Ther., 9 (1968) 303–313.

Brennum, J., Arendt-Nielsen, L., Horn, A., Secher, N.H. and Jensen, T.S., Quantitative sensory examination during epidural anaesthesia and analgesia in man: effects of morphine, Pain, 52 (1993) 75–83.

Bruera, E., Chadwick, S., Brenneis, C., Hanson, J. and MacDonald, R.N., Methylphenidate associated with narcotics for the treatment of cancer pain, Cancer Treatment Reports, 71 (1987) 67–70.

Bruera, E., Macmillan, K., Hanson, J, and MacDonald, R.N., The cognitive effects of the administration of narcotic analgesics in patients with cancer pain, Pain, 39 (1989) 13–16.

Bruera, E., Miller, M.J., Macmillan, K. and Kuehn, N., Neuropsychological effects of methylphenidate in patients receiving a continuous infusion of narcotics for cancer pain, Pain, 48 (1992) 163–166.

Carter, W.H., Jr. and Carchman, R.A., Mathematical and biostatistical methods for designing and analyzing complex chemical interactions, Fundam. Appl. Toxicol., 10 (1988) 590–595.

Chabal, C., Jacobson, L., Mariano, A., Chaney, E. and Britell, C.W., The use of oral mexiletine for the treatment of pain after peripheral nerve injury, Anesthesiology, 76 (1992) 513–517.

Cherny, N.I., Thaler, H.T., Friedlander–Klar, H., Lapin, J., Foley, K.M., Houde, R. and Portenoy, R.K., Opioid responsiveness of cancer pain syndromes caused by neuropathic or nociceptive mechanisms: a combined analysis of controlled single dose studies, Neurology, 44 (1994) 857–861.

Coda, B.A., Hill, H.F., Schaffer, R.L., Luger, T.J., Jacobson, R.C. and Chapman, R.C., Enhancement of morphine analgesia by fenfluramine in subjects receiving tailored opioid infusions, Pain, 52 (1993a) 85–91.

Coda, B.A., Hill, H.F., Hunt, E.B., Kerr, E.B., Jacobson, R.C. and Chapman, R.C., Cognitive and motor function impairments during continuous opioid analgesic infusions, Human Psychopharmacology , 8 (1993b) 383–400.

Dejgard, A., Petersen, P. and Kastrup, J., Mexiletine for treatment of chronic painful diabetic neuropathy, Lancet, 1 (1988) 9–11.

Dubner, R. and Bennett, G.J., Spinal and trigeminal mechanisms of nociception, Ann. Rev. Neurosci., 6 (1983) 381–418.

Einnolf, C., Eberlein, H.J., Nabel, R. and Lehmann, K.A., Trandermal appliziertes fentanyl in der posoperativen schmerztherapie. Untersuchungen mit hilfe der on-demand analgesie, Anaethesist, 38, Suppl. 1 (1989) 556.

Food and Drug Administration, Guideline for the Clinical Evaluation of Analgesic Drugs, U.S.

Department of Health and Human Services, Rockville, Md., 1992, 26 pp.
Goldstein, D.J. and Brunelle, R.L., Dose-response model for combination analgesic drugs. In: M.B. Max, R.K. Portenoy and E.M. Laska (Eds.), The Design of Analgesic Clinical Trials. Advances in Pain Research and Therapy, Vol. 18. Raven Press, New York, 1991, pp. 125–132.
Gordon, N.C., Heller, P.H. and Levine, J.D., Enhancement of pentazocine analgesia by clonidine, Pain, 48 (1992) 167–170.
Gordon, N.C., Heller, P.H., Gear, R.W. and Levine, J.D., Temporal factors in the enhancement of morphine analgesia by desipramine, Pain 53 (1993) 273–276.
Gracely, R.H., Experimental pain models. In: M.B. Max, R.K. Portenoy and E.M. Laska (Eds.), The Design of Analgesic Clinical Trials. Advances in Pain Research and Therapy, Vol. 18. Raven Press, New York, 1991, pp. 33–47.
Gracely, R.H., Lota, L., Walther, D.J. and Dubner, R., A multiple random staircase method of psychophysical pain assessment, Pain, 32 (1988) 55–63.
Hill, H.F., Saeger, L., Bjurstrom, R., Donaldson, G., Chapman, C.R. and Jacobson, R., Steady-state infusions of opioids in human volunteers. I. Pharmacokinetic tailoring, Pain, 43 (1990) 57–67.
Hogan, Q., Haddox, J.D., Abram, S., Weissman, D., Taylor, M.L. and Janjan, N., Epidural opiates and local anesthetics for the management of cancer pain, Pain, 46 (1991) 326–344.
Hupert, C., Yacoub, M. and Turgeon, L.R., Effect of hydroxyzine on morphine analgesia for the treatment of postoperative pain, Anesth. Analg., 59 (1980) 690–696.
Kantor, T.G. and Steinberg, F.P., Studies of tranquilizing agents and meperidine in clinical pain: hydroxyzine and meprobamate. In: J.J. Bonica and D. Albe-Fessard (Eds.), Proceedings of the First World Congress on Pain. Advances in Pain Research and Therapy, Vol. 1. Raven Press, New York, 1976, pp. 567–572.
Kellstein, D.E., Malseed, R.T., Ossipov, M.H. and Goldstein, F.J., Effect of chronic treatment with tricyclic antidepressants upon antinociception induced by intrathecal injection of morphine and monoamines, Neuropharmacology, 27 (1988) 1–14.
Kerr, B., Hill, H., Coda, B., Calogero, M., Chapman, C.R., Hunt, E., Buffington, V. and Mackie, A., Concentration-related effects of morphine on cognition and motor control in human subjects, Neuropsychopharmacology, 5 (1991) 157–166.
Kerrick, J.M., Fine, P.G., Lipman, A.G. and Love, G., Low dose amitriptyline as an adjunct to opioids for postoperative orthopedic pain: a placebo-controlled trial, Pain, 52 (1993) 325–330.
LaMotte, R.H., Shain, C.N., Simone, D.A. and Tsai, E.-F.P., Neurogenic hyperalgesia: psychophysical studies of underlying mechanisms, J. Neurophysiol., 66 (1991) 190–211.
Laska, E.M. and Meisner, M.J., Statistical methods and applications of bioassay, Ann. Rev. Pharmacol. Toxicol., 27 (1987) 385–397.
Laska, E.M., Meisner, M., and Siegel, C., Simple designs and model-free tests for synergy, Biometrics (1994), in press.
Lavigne, G.J., Hargreaves, K.M., Schmidt, E.A. and Dionne, R.A., Proglumide potentiates morphine analgesia for acute postsurgical pain, Clin. Pharmacol. Ther., 45 (1989) 666–673.
Lehmann, K.A., Patient-controlled intravenous analgesia for postoperative pain relief. In: M.B. Max, R.K. Portenoy and E.M. Laska (Eds.), The Design of Analgesic Clinical Trials. Advances in Pain Research and Therapy, Vol. 18. Raven Press, New York, 1991, pp. 481–506.
Lehmann, K.A., Schlusener, M. and Arabatsis, P., Failure of proglumide, a cholecystokinin antagonist, to potentiate clinical morphine analgesia: a randomized double-blind postoperative study using patient-controlled analgesia (PCA). Anesth. Analg. 68 (1989) 51–56.
Levine, J.D. and Gordon, N.C., Synergism between the analgesic actions of morphine and pentazocine, Pain 33 (1988) 369–372.
Levine, J.D., Gordon, N.C., Smith, R. and McBryde, R., Desipramine enhances opiate postoperative analgesia, Pain, 27 (1986) 45–49.
Mather, L.E., Pharmacokinetics and pharmacodynamic profiles of opioid analgesics: a sameness amongst equals, Pain, 43 (1990) 3–6.
Mather, L.E., Pharmacokinetics and patient-controlled analgesia, Acta Anaesth. Belg., 43

(1992) 5–20.
Max, M.B., Antidepressants as analgesics. In: H.L. Fields and J.C. Liebeskind (Eds.), Pharmacological Approaches to the Treatment of Chronic Pain: New Concepts and Critical Issues, IASP Press, Seattle, 1994, pp. 229–246.
Max, M.B. and Laska, E.M., Single-dose analgesic comparisons. In: M.B. Max, R.K. Portenoy and E.M. Laska (Eds.), The Design of Analgesic Clinical Trials. Advances in Pain Research and Therapy, Vol. 18. Raven Press, New York, 1991, pp. 55–95.
Max, M.B., Zeigler, D., Shoaf, S.E., Craig, B.E., Benjamin, J., Li, S.-H., Buzzanell, C., Perez, M. and Ghosh, B.C., Effects of a single oral dose of desipramine on postoperative morphine analgesia, J. Pain Symptom Management, 7 (1992) 454–462.
McCoy, E.P., Furness, G. and Wright, P.M.C., Patient-controlled analgesia with and without background infusion: analgesia assessed using the demand : delivery ratio, Anaesthesia, 48 (1993) 256–265.
Miaskowski, C. and Levine, J.D., Comments on the evaluation of drug interactions using isobolographic analysis and analysis of variance, Pain, 51 (1992) 383–387.
Mogensen, T., Eliasen, K., Ejlersen, E., Vegger, P., Nielsen, I.K. and Kehlet, H., Epidural clonidine enhances postoperative analgesia from a combined low-dose epidural bupivacaine and morphine regimen, Anesth. Analg., 75 (1992) 607–610.
Parker, R.K., Holtmann, B. and White, P.F., Patient-controlled analgesia: does a concurrent opioid infusion improve pain management after surgery? JAMA, 266 (1991) 1947–1952.
Parker, R.K., Holtmann, B. and White, P.F., Effects of a nighttime opioid infusion with PCA therapy on patient comfort and analgesic requirements after abdominal hysterectomy, Anesthesiology, 76 (1992) 362–367.
Plummer, J.L., Analysis of variance in the study of drug interactions, Pain, 53 (1993) 357–361.
Price, D.D., Hu, J.W., Dubner, R. and Gracely, R.H., Peripheral suppression of first pain and central summation of second pain evoked by noxious heat pulses, Pain, 3 (1977) 57–68.
Price, D.D., Von der Gruen, A., Miller, J., Rafii, A. and Price, C., Potentiation of systemic morphine analgesia in humans by proglumide, a cholecystokinin antagonist, Anesth. Analg., 64 (1985) 801–806.
Price, D.D., Long, S. and Huitt, C., Sensory testing of pathophysiological mechanisms of pain in patients with reflex sympathetic dystrophy, Pain, 49 (1992) 163–173.
Russell, A.W., Owen, H., Ilsley, A.H., Kluger, M.T. and Plummer, J.L., Background infusion with patient-controlled analgesia: effect on postoperative oxyhaemoglobin saturation and pain control, Anaesth. Intens. Care, 21 (1993) 174–179.
Seed, J.C., Wallenstein, S.L., Houde, R.W. and Bellville, J.W., A comparison of the analgesic and respiratory effects of dihydrocodeine and morphine in man, Arch. Int. Pharmacodyn., 116 (1958) 293–339.
Shoulson, I. and Chase, T.N., Fenfluramine in man: hypophagia associated with diminished serotonin turnover, Clin. Pharmacol. Ther., 17 (1975) 616–621.
Simone, D.A., Baumann, T.K. and LaMotte, R.H., Dose-dependent pain and mechanical hyperalgesia in humans after intradermal injection of capsaicin, Pain, 38 (1989) 99–107.
Sjogren, P. and Banning, A., Pain, sedation and reaction time during long-term treatment of cancer patients with oral and epidural opioids, Pain, 39 (1989) 5–11.
Stambaugh, J.E. and Lane, C., Analgesic efficacy and pharmacokinetic evaluation of meperidine and hydroxyzine, alone and in combination, Cancer Invest., 1 (1983) 111–117.
Taiwo, Y.O., Fabian, A., Pazoles, C.J. and Fields, H.L., Potentiation of morphine antinociception by monoamine reuptake inhibitors in the rat spinal cord, Pain, 21 (1985) 329–337.
Tallarida, R.J., Statistical analysis of drug combinations for synergism, Pain, 49 (1992) 93–98.
Watkins, L.R., Kinscheck, I.B. and Mayer, D.J., Potentiation of morphine analgesia by the cholecystokinin antagonist proglumide, Brain Res., 327 (1985) 169–180.
Zeigler, D., Lynch, S.A., Muir, J., Benjamin, J. and Max, M.B., Transdermal clonidine versus placebo in painful diabetic neuropathy, Pain, 48 (1992) 403–408.

Correspondence to: Mitchell Max, MD, National Institutes of Health, Building 10, Room 3C-405, Bethesda, MD 20892, USA. Tel: 301-496-6695; Fax: 301-402-4347.

Proceedings of the 7th World Congress on Pain,
Progress in Pain Research and Management, Vol. 2,
edited by G.F. Gebhart, D.L. Hammond, and T.S.
Jensen, IASP Press, Seattle, © 1994.

39

Nimodipine, a Calcium Channel Blocker, Enhances Opiate Analgesia in Patients with Cancer Pain Tolerant to Morphine

Rosa Santillán,[a] José M. Maestre,[a] María A. Hurlé,[b] and Jesús Flórez[b]

Department of [a]Anesthesiology (Pain Unit), University Hospital, "M. de Valdecilla," and Departments of [b]Physiology and Pharmacology, University of Cantabria, Santander, Spain

INTRODUCTION

A major drawback in treating cancer pain with oral and spinal opiates is the need to increase the dose steadily, due to either an advanced progression of the disease or the development of tolerance. Tolerance to different side effects of opiates can be developed at different rates and with different intensity, so dosing should be maintained at the lowest level compatible with pain relief to reduce unacceptable toxicity. Previous studies with rats showed that nimodipine, a calcium channel antagonist of the dihydropyridine series, was able to potentiate the analgesic effect of mu-opioid agonists in both naive and tolerant conditions (Hoffmeister and Tettenborn 1986; Dierssen et al. 1990). In addition, when nimodipine was concurrently infused with sufentanil for seven days during the development of tolerance, the calcium channel antagonist not only prevented the progressive loss of the analgesic effect of the opiate, but it potentiated the analgesic activity much more markedly than in acute conditions (Dierssen et al. 1990). This effect of nimodipine was stereospecific. A parallel potentiation of the opiate-induced respiratory depression by calcium channel antagonists in rats has not been observed (Szikszay et al. 1986; Ruiz et al. 1993).

Based on these results, we conducted an open, preliminary clinical study to assess whether nimodipine would modify in a similar way the development of tolerance to morphine in cancer pain management, and to determine the effectiveness and safety of this drug combination.

METHODS

The study protocol was approved by the National Agency of Clinical Trials as an open-ended study. Twenty-three patients with a mean age of 68 years (range 35–79 years) receiving outpatient treatment for advanced cancer were included. All patients were diagnosed as having a stable tumor pain syndrome and gave their written informed consent prior to inclusion in the study. The following criteria had to be met: (1) patients with cancer untreatable by surgery or radiotherapy; (2) good pain control with regular administration of oral or spinal morphine; (3) a gradual escalation of the dose, suggesting tolerance. Tolerance was considered to be present when a patient, free of pain at rest, required at least two successive increments of the morphine dose to achieve pain relief without apparent clinical aggravation of the disease. The following exclusion criteria were adopted: (1) history of allergic reactions to or abuse of opiates; (2) history of drug or alcohol abuse; (3) chronic obstructive pulmonary disease (COPD), severe cardiac, hepatic, or renal insufficiency; (4) unable to give informed consent; (5) pregnancy; (6) increased intracranial pressure; (7) consumption of other calcium channel blockers; (8) hypersensitivity or intolerance to nimodipine.

Initially, the patients were visited weekly. Pain was assessed using a patient-completed visual analog scale (scores 0–10). The daily dose of morphine was prescribed to reach full relief of pain in resting conditions (pain scores 0–2). When a patient met the criteria for tolerance development and the last dose of morphine had remained stable for at least seven days, oral nimodipine was introduced in the treatment protocol, starting with a dose of 60 mg on the first day, and then increased up to 120 mg/day divided in four doses. Subsequently, the patients were visited daily and regular attempts were made to reduce the dose of morphine by a third of the previous dose, the criteria being maintained to get full relief of pain in resting conditions. The lowest dose of morphine achieved was the dose below which pain score would increase above 3; any increase in a patient's pain score was matched with daily morphine increments. Consequently, the assessment of daily morphine consumption was the primary effect parameter of the study.

Data are expressed as mean ± S.E.M. Statistical significance was evaluated by the Student's paired t test, with $P < 0.05$ at the level of significance.

RESULTS

Eight women and 15 men were included in the study. Nineteen patients had received increasing doses of oral morphine for periods ranging from 37 to 780 days, three patients received intrathecal morphine from an implanted infusion pump for periods of 21 to 97 days, and one patient received oral and intrathecal morphine for 127 days (Table I).

In 16 patients (69.5%), nimodipine was successful in controlling the progressive increment in the daily dose of morphine, so that a reduction of the dose was possible (Table I; Fig. 1). Thirteen of these patients were treated with oral morphine, two with intrathecal morphine, and one with both oral and intrathecal morphine. Nimodipine failed to modify the daily dose of morphine needed to relief pain in two patients, and it was withdrawn during the first week of treatment in an additional five patients due to intolerance in three cases (headache, gastrointestinal complaints, and hypotension) and natural aggravation of the disease in the remaining two.

In the 20 patients treated with oral morphine, the initial dose of the opiate was 88.4 ± 14.0 mg/day (range: 60–240 mg/day) and was steadily increased up to 254.7 ± 39.2 mg/day (range 120–720 mg/day). Excluding the five dropouts who did not tolerate nimodipine, the daily dose of morphine after we introduced the calcium channel antagonist was reduced from 282.6 ± 47.7 mg to a minimum of 158.7 ± 26.2 mg (range 60–420 mg); the difference with the pre-nimodipine dose of morphine was significant ($P < 0.001$; Fig. 2). This minimum dose was attained in 17.5 ± 4.9 days of treatment, and could be maintained for 73.4 ± 21.8 days in 9 of the 13 patients in whom nimodipine was effective. In the other four patients, nimodipine was withdrawn after two weeks of treatment due to intolerance in two patients (headache and gastric upset) and to aggravation of the disease in another two.

Two patients were treated with intrathecal morphine at a daily dose of 4 and 6 mg/day. After adding nimodipine, the dose of morphine was reduced to 3 and 4.5 mg/day, respectively, in one week, remaining at that level for at least 30 days. A third patient received oral and intrathecal morphine simultaneously. The doses had been progressively raised up to 240 mg/day p.o. and 24 mg/day intrathecally. After adding nimodipine, oral morphine could be withdrawn in 14 days and intrathecal morphine was reduced to 18 mg/day and remained stable for 21 days.

Nine patients showed a significant improvement in the quality of life after the addition of nimodipine, with a better general state of health, mood, mobility, and activity. Coadjuvant drugs could be either reduced or suppressed in eight patients. Nimodipine did not increase the side-effects of morphine.

Table I
Effects of nimodipine in cancer pain patients treated chronically with morphine

			Morphine Therapy Pre-nimodipine				Morphine Therapy Post-nimodipine			
			Daily Dose		Days of Therapy					
Patient	Age (yr)	Sex (M/F)	Initial (mg)	Final (mg)	Total Duration	At Final Dose	Minimal Daily Dose Attained (mg)	Elapsed Time to Minimal (days)	Treatment Time at Minimal (days)	Subjective Improvement
RESPONDERS										
Oral morphine										
A.C.	67	F	60	360	240	60	120	21	14	yes
M.T.	76	M	60	120	750	450	60	21	164	yes
A.J.	64	M	60	120	21	7	60	7	44	
F.S.	79	F	60	120	495	75	60	7	180	
I.G.	70	M	240	360	247	7	240	7	7*	
E.O.	69	F	60	240	540	120	120	7	7*	yes
M.H.	35	F	60	180	780	120	60	37	37	yes
J.F.	72	M	240	600	75	45	240	67	127	
A.P.	67	F	120	360	247	60	240	7	7†	yes
A.M.	63	M	60	120	247	7	60	14	51	yes
M.C.	70	M	180	720	67	15	420	4	14	yes

B.G.	72	M	60	180	37	7	120	7	7†	yes
A.D.	61	F	60	360	141	21	180	21	30	yes
P.S.	61	M	60	200	21	7	No response			
F.S.	75	M	60	200	80	14	No response			
Intrathecal Morphine										
M.D.	70	M	2	4	37	7	3	7	30	
J.A.	53	M	1	6	97	7	4.5	7	30	
C.A.	66	M	480/4‡	240/24‡	127	7	0/18‡	14	21	
NONRESPONDERS										
P.S.	61	M	60	200	21	7	No response			
F.S.	75	M	60	200	80	14	No response			
DROPOUTS DURING THE FIRST WEEK OF POST-NIMODIPINE										
J.R.	79	F	60	120	77	60	Aggravation of the disease			
J.A.	60	M	60	120	90	15	Intolerance			
M.B.	63	F	60	120	60	16	Intolerance			
A.G.	44	M	60	240	150	7	Aggravation of the disease			
J.H.	60	M	9§	15	21	7	Intolerance			

* Intolerance.; † aggravation of the disease.; ‡ oral/intrathecal; § intrathecal.

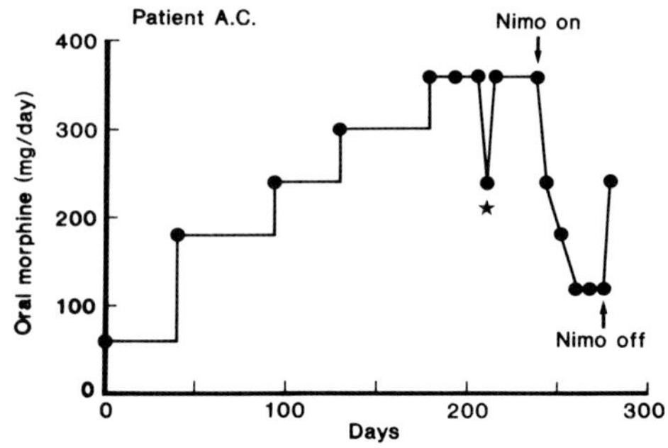

Fig. 1. Variations in the daily dose of oral morphine required to relieve pain in a cancer patient, before and after adding nimodipine (120 mg/day). At * an unsuccessful attempt was made to reduce the dose of morphine.

DISCUSSION

Our data show that nimodipine, a calcium channel blocker with relatively high affinity for the central nervous system, can enhance the analgesic activity of long-term treatment with morphine in cancer patients who required regular increments of the opiate to relieve pain. Whether the dose increments were the result of tolerance development or of the progression of the disease can not be ascertained, although the clinical assessment in some patients suggested that the disease remained stable. Introduction of nimodipine not only interrupted the escalation of the regular administration of morphine, but allowed substantial reduction of the daily dose for several weeks. Other clinical studies also have demonstrated that calcium channel antagonists induce a moderate potentiation of the analgesic and anesthetic activities of acutely administered opiates (Boldt et al. 1987; Carta et al. 1990; Pereira et al. 1993). In our patients, however, morphine had been administered chronically before nimodipine was added, thus providing the condition for the implementation of molecular mechanisms leading to the development of tolerance.

Several experimental reports have shown that calcium channel blockers can potentiate acute central effects of opiates (Dierssen et al. 1990, 1991). In addition, Dierssen et al. (1990) demonstrated in tolerant rats that nimodipine, when concurrently infused with chronic sufentanil, disturbed the expression of tolerance and potentiated the analgesic effect much more markedly than in acute conditions. Other investigators (Contreras et al. 1988) also have reported an antagonism of the opiate-induced tolerance to analgesia in rats. These results indicated that calcium channel antagonists can interfere with the development of calcium-related events that are known to be involved in the development of tolerance to opiates (Littleton and Little 1989). For example,

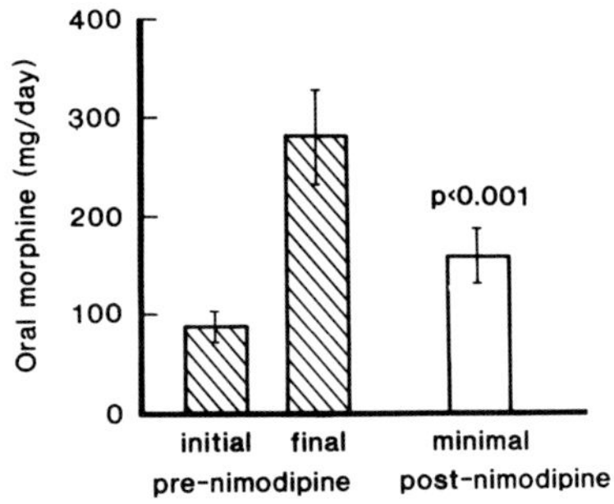

Fig. 2. Changes in the requirements of the daily dose of oral morphine (means and S.E.M.) in 13 patients with cancer pain, before and after adding nimodipine (120 mg/day).

chronic treatment with opiates up-regulates the dihydropyridine binding sites in brain membranes (Ramkumar and El-Fakahany 1984, 1988; Saito et al. 1985; Antkiewitz-Michaluk et al. 1990; Ohnishi et al. 1990; Díaz et al. 1992) and down-regulates the mu-opioid receptors (Tao et al. 1987; see Morris 1991). However, when the calcium channel blocker nimodipine is infused chronically and simultaneously with sufentanil in rats, the up-regulation of the dihydropyridine binding sites was further enhanced while the down-regulation of the opioid receptors was mitigated at both cortical and spinal levels (Díaz et al. 1992). These results suggest that some of the mechanisms involved in the development of tolerance to morphine can be disrupted by the sustained calcium channel blockade. Thus, it is possible that the calcium-related events elicited by the chronic administration of morphine and responsible for the development of tolerance in our patients, were counteracted by the action of nimodipine, thus leading to a partial reversal of tolerance development.

A pharmacokinetic interaction between morphine and nimodipine should not be disregarded. Although serum morphine levels were not monitored, the possibility that the enhanced analgesic activity were accounted for by a nimodipine-induced increment in morphine levels seems unlikely because: (1) no increment in the sufentanil plasma levels was observed in rats treated with chronic nimodipine and sufentanil, in which marked potentiation of analgesia had been attained (Dierssen et al. 1990); and (2) nine of our patients showed higher alertness and daily activity after adding nimodipine. Experiments are now in progress under double-blind conditions to examine this contingency.

REFERENCES

Antkiewicz-Michaluk, L., Michaluk, J., Romanska, L. and Vetulani, J., Cortical dihydropyridine binding sites and behavioral syndrome in morphine-abstinent rats, Eur. J. Pharmacol., 180

(1990) 129–139.
Boldt, J., Von Borman, B., Kling, D., Russ, W., Ratthey, K. and Hempelmann, G., Low-dose fentanyl analgesia modified by calcium channel blockers in cardiac surgery, Eur. J. Anaesthesiol., 4 (1987) 387–394.
Carta, F., Bianchi, M., Argenton, S., Cervi, D., Marolla, G., Tamburini, M., Breda, M., Fantoni, A. and Panerai, A.E., Effect of nifedipine on morphine-induced analgesia, Anesth. Analg., 70 (1990) 493–498.
Contreras, E., Tamayo, L. and Amigo, M., Calcium channel antagonists increase morphine-induced analgesia and antagonize morphine tolerance, Eur. J. Pharmacol., 148 (1988) 463–466.
Diaz, A., Hervás, R., Ruiz, F., Hurlé, M.A. and Pazos, A., Functional and biochemical interactions between the calcium channel blocker nimodipine and the μ-opiate agonist sufentanil. In: Proceedings of the 15th Annual Meeting of the European Neuroscience Association, Munich 1992, p. 193.
Dierssen, M., Flórez, J. and Hurlé, M., Calcium channel modulation by dihydropyridines modifies sufentanil-induced antinociception in acute and tolerant conditions, Naunyn Schmiedebergs Arch. Pharmacol., 342 (1990) 559–565.
Dierssen, M.M., Ruiz, F., Flórez, J. and Hurlé, M.A., Ca^{2+} channel modulation by dihydropyridines modifies sufentanil-induced respiratory depression in cats, Eur. J. Pharmacol., 198 (1991) 149–155.
Hoffmeister, F. and Tettenborn, D., Calcium agonists and antagonists of dihydropyridine type: Antinociceptive effects, interference with opiate-μ-receptor agonists and neuropharmacological actions in rodents, Psychopharmacology, 90 (1986) 299–307.
Littleton, J.M. and Little, H.J., Adaptation in neuronal calcium channels as a common basis for physical dependence on central depressant drugs. In: A.J. Goudie and M.W. Emmett-Oglesby (Eds.), Psychoactive Drugs: Tolerance and Sensitization, Humana Press, Clifton, N.J., 1989, pp. 461–518.
Morris, B.J., Modulation of central opioid receptors. In: O.F.X. Almeida and T.S. Shippenberg (Eds.), Neurobiology of Opioids, Springer-Verlag, Berlin 1991, pp. 185–197.
Ohnishi, T., Saito, K., Maeda, S., Matsumoto, K., Sajuda, M. and Inoki, R., Intracere-broventricular treatment of mice with pertussis toxin induces hyperalgesia and enhaces ^{3}H-nitrendipine binding to synaptic membranes: Similarity with morphine tolerance, Naunyn Schmiedebergs Arch. Pharmacol., 341 (1990) 123–127.
Pereira, I.T., Prado, W.A. and Dos Reis, M.P., Enhancement of the epidural morphine-induced analgesia by systemic nifedipine, Pain, 53 (1993) 341–345.
Ramkumar, V. and El-Fakahany, E.E., Increase in ^{3}H-nitrendipine binding sites on the brain in morphine tolerant mice, Eur. J. Pharmacol., 102 (1984) 371–372.
Ramkumar, V. and El-Fakahany, E.E., Prolonged morphine treatment increases rat brain dihydropyridine binding sites: possible involvement in development of morphine dependence, Eur. J. Pharmacol., 146 (1988) 73–83.
Ruiz, F., Dierssen, M., Flórez, J. and Hurlé, M.A., Potentiation of acute opiate respiratory depression and reversion of tolerance by the calcium antagonist nimodipine in awake rats, Naunyn Schmiedebergs Arch. Pharmacol., 348 (1993) 633–637.
Saito, K., Ishii, K., Fujita, N. and Inoki, R., Selective enhancement in striatal ^{3}H-nitrendipine following chronic treatment with morphine, Neurochem. Int., 7 (1985) 1033–1036.
Szikszay, M., Snyder, F.R. and London, E.D., Effects of diltiazem on morphine-induced respiratory decline, J. Pharm. Pharmacol., 38 (1986) 625–627.
Tao, P.-L., Law, P.-Y. and Loh, H.H., Decrease in delta and mu opioid receptor binding capacity in rat brain after chronic etorphine treatment, J. Pharmacol. Exp. Ther., 240 (1987) 809–817.

Correspondence to: Jesús Flórez, MD, PhD, Department of Physiology and Pharmacology, Faculty of Medicine, University of Cantabria, Avda. Herrera Oria, s/n, 39011 Santander, Spain. Tel: 34-42-201981; Fax: 34-42-201903.

Proceedings of the 7th World Congress on Pain,
Progress in Pain Research and Management, Vol. 2,
edited by G.F. Gebhart, D.L. Hammond, and T.S.
Jensen, IASP Press, Seattle, © 1994.

40

Opioid Tolerance and Responsiveness: Research Findings and Clinical Observations

Russell K. Portenoy

Pain Service, Department of Neurology, Memorial Sloan-Kettering Cancer Center, and Department of Neurology, Cornell University Medical College, New York, New York, USA

INTRODUCTION

Like many scientific pursuits directly applicable to medical treatment, the field of opioid pharmacology is characterized by gaps between the commonplace observations of clinical practice and the rapid advances in clinical and basic research. These gaps are exemplified by phenomena described by the terms *tolerance* and *efficacy*. Although there has been remarkable progress in the scientific understanding of the basic processes involved in these phenomena, the data sometimes appear tangential to the practice of clinicians who administer long-term opioid therapy, and conversely, some clinical events that may be highly relevant to an understanding of basic drug mechanisms appear to be poorly appreciated by researchers. The movement of new information from the laboratory to the clinic requires ongoing efforts to maintain communication between those who treat patients and those who study opioid drugs, beginning with an effort to document the disparities in their observations.

THE NOMENCLATURE OF OPIOID RESPONSE

Improved communication begins with clarity of the nomenclature used to describe opioid response. There is considerable imprecision in the use of terms, and accepted nomenclature may imply distinct processes to observers with varying frames of reference. It is, therefore, useful to define terminology as a first step.

TOLERANCE

The term *tolerance* refers to a phenomenon in which exposure to a drug results in the diminution of an effect or the need for a higher dose to maintain an effect (Jaffe 1985). The term *tachyphylaxis* is applied to a similar phenomenon that occurs with a shorter time course, typically within minutes.

Tolerance may be described from several perspectives. *Associative* tolerance refers to changes in the response to a drug that are presumably related to learning; a decline in drug effect due to operant conditioning, for example, would be labeled in this way. *Non-associative* or *pharmacological* tolerance denotes changes that are independent of learning. Pharmacological tolerance may, in turn, be described as *dispositional* or *pharmacodynamic*. The former term refers to a reduction in drug effect caused by pharmacokinetic changes, such as may occur if exposure to the drug induces activity in a metabolic pathway that eliminates it from the body. In contrast, pharmacodynamic tolerance refers to a decline in drug effect that is independent of disposition and is attributed to changes in neural systems.

Given the broad range of responses it encompasses, tolerance should be viewed as a descriptive label that indicates a change in the relation between dose (or concentration) and response but does not illuminate the underlying mechanisms. The label does imply, however, that exposure to the drug itself somehow "drives" the diminution in effect. If reduced effect, or more precisely, the need for higher doses to maintain an effect, occurs as a result of increasing pathology rather than drug exposure per se, the phenomenon should not be termed tolerance.

In animal models and in vitro preparations, progressive reduction in the magnitude of antinociceptive and other effects can be induced simply and reliably by repeated opioid exposure (Way 1993). Tolerance to antinociceptive effects, for example, has been studied in many experimental paradigms that incorporate brief noxious stimuli, such as the tail-flick or hot-plate tests (Cochin and Kornetsky 1964; Yaksh 1991; Stevens and Yaksh 1989). As discussed below, it is now generally accepted that this type of tolerance is predominantly pharmacodynamic. For the pharmacologist, therefore, opioid tolerance is often assumed to refer to a diminution of analgesic effects related to some process of neural adaptation, a process that is perceived to be directly relevant to human responses. The need for dose escalation that occurs in many street addicts is a well-recognized model for these responses.

In the clinical arena, clinicians often us the word tolerance less precisely, and this may confuse the salient issues. Many refer to the phenomenon only in terms of analgesic effects. They may describe as tolerant any patient who develops a need for dose escalation to retain analgesia, even if this is occurring with clear-cut evidence of worsening pathology. Conversely, the patient who has stable analgesia may be considered to be without evidence of tolerance, even if other opioid effects, such as sedation, never occurred or disappeared as doses were escalated.

Clinicians often fail to recognize that declining analgesic effects have a differential diagnosis. In contrast to animal models that apply controlled noxious stimuli, the clinical response to an opioid may reflect uncontrollable changes in the stimulus or any of numerous other processes independent of drug-receptor-effector interactions (Table I). Increasing activity in nociceptive pathways may occur with progression of a lesion or associated factors like inflammatory change or evolution of peripheral or central neuropathic processes. Worsening pain may also occur as a consequence of psychological processes, such as a changes in affect (e.g., anxiety or depression), cognitive state (which alters pain reporting or shifts the meaning attached to the pain), or the responses of significant others in the environment. Tolerance cannot be imputed to be the "driving force" for loss of analgesia in patients who have one or more alternative physical or psychological reasons for increasing pain. Although it is possible that pharmacodynamic tolerance to analgesic effects contributes to the need for dose escalation when these other processes exist,

Table I
A differential diagnosis for declining analgesic effects in the clinical setting

Increased activity in nociceptive pathways
Increased activation of peripheral nociceptors
due to mechanical factors (e.g., tumor growth)
due to biochemical changes (i.e., inflammation)
due to peripheral neuropathic processes (e.g., neuroma formation)
Increased activity in central nociceptive pathways
due to central neuropathic processes (e.g., sensitization, shift in receptive fields, change in modulatory processes)
Psychological processes other than conditioned responses to the drug
Increasing psychological distress (e.g., anxiety or depression)
Change in cognitive state leading to altered pain perception or reporting (e.g., delirium)
Conditioned pain behavior independent of the drug
Tolerance
due to pharmacodynamic processes
due to pharmacokinetic processes
due to psychological processes

and equally true that associative tolerance may be an appropriate label for some of the psychological processes that result in declining analgesia, it is not appropriate to assume that the clinical situation mirrors experimental models of tolerance when such complex events are occurring.

In the clinical setting, pharmacodynamic tolerance to opioid analgesia (of a type that may be fundamentally similar to the phenomena demonstrated in animal models) can be credibly inferred only if an alternative cause for increasing pain cannot be found and there is no evidence of pharmacokinetic or behavioral tolerance. Such an inference may be appropriate, for example, in the patient who has no apparent change in baseline physical or psychological condition and complains of a decline in the duration of analgesia after each opioid dose. There can be no definitive proof of this, of course, but the inference can be strong enough to warrant correlation with experimental models of tolerance.

The phenomenon of tolerance has a negative connotation in the clinic, which presumably derives from the tendency to equate the term with the loss of analgesia. Indeed, tolerance is often invoked as a reason to avoid early use of an opioid, because it is believed that exposure to the drug could reduce the potential for beneficial effects at a later time. It is seldom emphasized that phenomena other than tolerance may account for opioid dose escalation and that tolerance to the adverse effects produced by opioid drugs is a favorable clinical outcome, which may open the so-called therapeutic window and facilitate successful individualization of therapy through upward dose titration. If tolerance failed to develop to the respiratory depressant effects of the opioids, for example, the potential for clinical benefits from dose escalation would not exist to the extent it does.

DEPENDENCE

Dependence can describe widely varying phenomena and should not be used without clarification. Physical dependence refers to the potential for an abstinence syndrome following abrupt dose reduction, discontinuation of the drug, or administration of an antagonist drug (Jaffe 1985). This phenomenon has been extensively studied in both animals (Domino et al. 1987; Martin 1974; Redmond and Krystal, 1984) and humans (Creighton and Ghodse 1989; Heishman et al. 1989a; Heishman et al. 1989b; Jasinski 1977; Judson et al. 1980; Martin 1977; Martin and Jasinski 1989; Redmond and Krystal 1984).

In contrast to the well-described phenomenology of physical dependence in human experimental subjects without pain (Martin 1977; Jasinski 1977), the prevalence and patterns of abstinence responses in patients treated with opioids have not been clearly defined (Table II). Although clinicians usually

Table II
Signs and symptoms of opioid abstinence,
as described in addict populations

Signs	Symptoms
Hypertension	Pain (abdominal cramps, myalgia, allodynia)
Tachycardia	Dysphoria (fear, anger)
Tachypnea	Insomnia
Hyperthermia	Drug craving
Diarrhea	
Mydriasis	
Rhinorrhea	
Chills	

act on the assumption that opioid withdrawal similar to that observed in addicts is possible after a few days of repeated drug administration, there are no data that confirm this, and most clinicians actually have little experience with the abstinence syndrome because they make considerable efforts to prevent it in their patients. The diverse physiological and psychological components of withdrawal are occasionally encountered (usually after an error is made, such as the inadvertent administration of an antagonist), but the relation between such clinical events and the acute and protracted abstinence syndromes characterized in populations who undergo opioid exposure in the absence of pain is obscure (Martin 1977).

Lack of information about the phenomenology of physical dependence in pain patients complicates efforts to unravel the relation between tolerance and dependence. A strong link between these processes has been posited for many years. In the early addiction literature, tolerance and physical dependence were inextricably connected and were together viewed as the substrate for the development of addiction: tolerance led to the use of higher doses to maintain euphoric effects, and a conditioned avoidance response to the aversive experience of withdrawal helped to maintain drug seeking (Wikler 1980). More recently, data from animal models and in vitro preparations have been adduced to support the interrelation of these phenomena (Trujillo and Akil 1991a; Way 1993), and in the clinical setting, patients are still labeled "tolerant" or "dependent" in an almost interchangeable way.

Accumulating clinical experience suggests that this perceived link between tolerance and physical dependence does not reflect the complexity of the systems involved. The phenomenologies of tolerance and physical dependence are highly variable, and the defining characteristics of each may or may not coexist in individual patients. Although it is true that patients who are receiving relatively high doses of an opioid, and are presumably tolerant to at least some opioid effects, are also more likely to develop abstinence if an antagonist is administered, this observation suggests only that tolerance and physical dependence both relate to dose. The degree to which their clinical features and underlying mechanisms occur together remains speculative, particularly in patients who receive opioids for pain. The most appropriate nomenclature, therefore, should attempt to describe tolerance and physical dependence separately.

Another critical element of the dependence nomenclature is the persistent tendency of clinicians to mislabel physical dependence as psychological dependence or addiction. Psychological dependence implies the craving of a drug for its psychic effects and is most aptly considered to be an element of the addiction syndrome. Addiction is characterized by the association of psychological dependence and aberrant drug-related behaviors (Jaffe 1985; Portenoy and Payne 1992; Rinaldi et al. 1988). From a clinical perspective, the labeling of a pharmacological property of a drug (namely, physical dependence) with a term that connotes a highly aberrant psychological and behavioral syndrome (addiction) is a serious error. It encourages the stigma that continues to be associated with opioid use (Portenoy 1991) and could potentially contribute to patient distress or undertreatment.

The definitions of addiction developed from observation of addicts (Jaffe 1985; Rinaldi et al. 1988) have been problematic when applied to the types of responses observed in patients. The aberrant behaviors that have been associated with the addiction syndrome exist on a continuum and have not been adequately studied in patients who receive opioids for the treatment of painful diseases (Portenoy, in press). Some behavior that would be highly predictive of addiction in a person without a target symptom for a drug becomes less predictive if the drug is the source of relief of that symptom (Table III). For example, unsanctioned dose escalation by a patient who has not been specifically warned against this behavior and is experiencing unrelieved pain cannot, by itself, be interpreted as addiction. Efforts have been made to distinguish the responses of pain patients from those of addicts through the use of terms such as *pseudoaddiction* (Weissman and Haddox 1989) and *therapeutic dependence* (Cherny and Portenoy 1994). Clinicians and researchers alike must be strongly discouraged from applying the descriptors *addiction* or *psychological dependence* unless there is compelling evidence that the patient's drug use reflects a loss of control, compulsive use, and continued use despite harm (Portenoy and Payne 1992).

EFFICACY AND OPIOID RESPONSIVENESS

The uncertainties surrounding use of the terms *tolerance* and *dependence* are mirrored in other nomenclature applied specifically to analgesic response.

Table III
Aberrant drug-related behaviors that raise the suspicion of addiction in patients who are receiving opioids for the treatment of pain

Probably More Predictive	Probably Less Predictive
Selling prescription drugs	Complaining aggressively about the need for more drug
Forging prescriptions	Hoarding drug during periods of reduced symptoms
Stealing or "borrowing" drugs from others	Requesting specific drugs
Injecting oral formulations	Acquiring similar drugs from other medical sources
Obtaining prescriptions drugs from nonmedical sources	Unsactioned dose escalation once or twice
Concurrent abuse of illict drugs	Unapproved use of drug to treat another symptom
Multiple does escalations despite warnings	Reporting psychic effect not intended by the clinician
Multiple episodes of prescription "loss"	

Source: Adapted from Portenoy, in press.
Note: On the basis of clinical experience, these behaviors are divided into those that are probably less predictive of addiction and those that are probably more predictive.

Most important, confusion in the use of the terms *efficacy, responsiveness,* and *resistance* has impeded efforts to define the most important issues for investigation.

Efficacy has meanings that vary greatly with context, and consequently should not be used without explanation. At the most basic level, pharmacologists use the term to denote intrinsic efficacy, a construct that refers to the proportion of receptors in a given system that must be occupied by the drug to yield a given effect. Specifically, efficacy is a dimensionless factor that relates receptor occupancy to the receptor stimulus produced by an agonist drug; the receptor occupancy required for an agonist to yield a response is inversely proportional to its intrinsic efficacy.

In clinical pharmacology, the term efficacy also has been used to describe the effect produced by a given dose of a drug or the maximal effect that can be produced by the drug. These meanings of efficacy are often contrasted with *potency*, which indicates the dose required to produce a specified effect.

The maximal efficacy of an opioid could potentially be determined by the appearance of a ceiling effect for analgesia—a dose above which additional dosage increments fail to yield any additional analgesia. This phenomenon is observed during dose escalation with agonist-antagonist opioids, such as pentazocine. Most of the opioids used for long-term therapy are pure agonists, however, and do not demonstrate a clinical ceiling effect for analgesia. In most clinical situations, therefore, the maximal analgesic efficacy of an opioid drug can only be defined by the analgesic effects obtained at a dose associated with limiting toxicity. Thus, clinicians often use *efficacy* to describe an outcome in which a favorable balance between analgesia and side effects has been achieved during gradual dose titration.

Although therapeutically meaningful, this conventional usage of the term may complicate efforts to discern the connection between clinical observations and the findings of animal studies. Unlike observations in humans, experimental models can apply criteria that allow the evaluation of efficacy in terms of analgesia alone. Moreover, common clinical use of the term may or may not imply that a maximal effect has been identified.

To clarify this nomenclature, the term *responsiveness* has been used to characterize the balance between analgesia and side effects in the clinical setting (Portenoy et al. 1990). Opioid responsiveness indicates the probability that adequate analgesia (that is, satisfactory relief without intolerable and unmanageable side effects) can be attained during dose titration. Alternatively, the term could be used to define the degree of analgesia achieved at a dose associated with intolerable and unmanageable side effects (that is, maximal efficacy from a clinically relevant perspective). If a side effect criterion must be applied, as it must in any clinical discussion of analgesic outcome, it is less confusing to use the term responsiveness than efficacy.

Some authors have applied the term *resistance* to describe the clinical situation in which opioid administration produces intolerable side effects at a dose associated with little or no analgesia (Arner and Meyerson 1993). Although this, again, represents the laudable attempt to avoid the confusion surrounding the nomenclature of efficacy, it is also more problematic than the use of the term responsiveness. There clearly are risk factors that reduce the likelihood of a favorable analgesic response during long-term therapy with opioids (Bruera et al. 1989), and all clinicians encounter patients who develop dose-limiting toxicity without analgesia during repeated trials of opioid drugs; this potential is not in question. However, current data are inadequate to conclude that any type of pain or pain patient is inherently resistant to opioids (see below), and the unfortunate tendency to apply this label to entire groups of patients, such as those with neuropathic pain, has been counterproductive. It fails to highlight the observation that many such patients do respond well in the clinical setting, or that resistance to one opioid does not imply resistance to all (Galer et al. 1992), and in this way can diminish enthusiasm for aggressive dosing.

Two fundamental elements are implicit in the concept of opioid responsiveness (and indeed, in the clinical concept of efficacy): the need for dose titration and the recognition that the endpoints used to define the balance between analgesia and side effects are inherently subjective. Thus, investigations of opioid responsiveness require clearly defined criteria for dose escalation and monitoring of subjective responses for both analgesia and adverse effects. This type of methodology, which has been applied infrequently (Inturrisi et al. 1990; Jadad et al. 1992; McQuay et al. 1992; Kalso et al. 1991), may be useful to discern systematic differences in opioid responsiveness among various drugs or patient subgroups.

BASIC RESEARCH IN OPIOID TOLERANCE AND RELATED PHENOMENA

Recent reviews have detailed the rapidly advancing basic knowledge related to tolerance and other aspects of opioid response (Cox 1991; Foley 1993; Johnson and Fleming 1989; Martin 1977; Redmond and Krystal 1984; Smith et al. 1988; Trujillo and Akil 1991a; Vaught 1991; Way 1993; Yaksh 1991). Some of the most relevant findings can be summarized as follows:

1. Both associative and non-associative tolerance to opioid drugs can be readily demonstrated in the laboratory. These phenomena can be clearly distinguished in experimental models (Tiffany and Maude-Griffen 1988).

2. Non-associative tolerance has been studied extensively in a large number of in vivo or in vitro assays. These investigations have established that tolerance can be demonstrated after acute dosing or accrue more gradually with repeated dosing, and that different opioid effects manifest tolerance at varying rates (Ling et al. 1989). Pharmacokinetic processes do not contribute significantly to these phenomena; rather, pharmacodynamic processes predominate.

3. The degree and time course of experimental tolerance can be influenced by many factors. Recent studies have demonstrated that varying effects can be produced by different drugs, dosing schedules, routes of administration, and study paradigms (Dafters and Odber 1989; Vaught 1991; Yaksh 1991).

Studies of drug-selective differences in the capacity to induce experimental tolerance have yielded findings that could become relevant to the clinical setting if confirmed in humans. These investigations have established that drug-selective differences are determined, at least in part, by differences in intrinsic efficacy. In studies performed in several animal models, intrinsic efficacy could predict both the pattern of tolerance to antinociceptive effects and the degree of cross-tolerance conferred by alternative opioid drugs (Ivarsson and Neil 1989; Paronis and Holtzman 1992; Picker and Yarbrough 1991; Sosnowski and Yaksh 1990; Stevens and Yaksh 1989).

Although it could be postulated that ongoing nociception, such as can be experienced by patients with chronic pain, may be an important influence on the development of tolerance, this potential has not been systematically investigated in animal models. In a recent study that may be relevant to this issue (Lyness et al. 1989), rats with adjuvant-induced arthritis (a model of relatively prolonged nociception) demonstrated significantly less self-administration of morphine during a 29 day period (less drug overall and less escalation of the dose over time) than rats without a nociceptive lesion. This finding combined with the results of very limited additional nociceptive testing in these animals may suggest that nociception modulates or prevents the development of analgesic tolerance. However, the paradigm does not provide definitive evidence for this effect, and the potential interactions between tolerance and ongoing nociception remain conjectural (see below).

4. Pharmacodynamic tolerance is known to be receptor-selective. A mu-selective drug, for example, will induce only minimal cross-tolerance at kappa or delta receptors (Stevens and Yaksh 1992). One study demonstrated that rats chronically infused with levorphanol, a mu and kappa receptor agonist, developed substantial cross-tolerance to the antinociceptive effects of the mu-selective drug morphine, whereas rats made tolerant to morphine developed little cross-tolerance to levorphanol (Moulin et al. 1988). Recent studies further suggest that there may be important interactions among receptor subtypes. For example, delta receptor agonists can modulate the efficacy of morphine, a mu agonist, even after tolerance has been induced by prior morphine exposure (Jiang et al. 1990). The development of abstinence phenomena also appears to be receptor-selective (Adams and Holtzman 1990; Cowan et al. 1988; Fukagawa et al 1989).

5. On a theoretical basis, the mechanisms responsible for this receptor-selective pharmacodynamic tolerance to opioid drugs could relate to: (1) a reduction in the number of receptors, (2) uncoupling of the receptor from its second messengers, and/or (3) changes in parallel antagonistic or facilitatory systems. Presumably, the influence of intrinsic efficacy on tolerance development could be due to interaction with any or all of these processes, or to other distinct actions that are as yet unidentified. These mechanisms have been extensively investigated, and there is good evidence that the last two are prominently involved in the development of analgesic tolerance in experimental models. Although down-regulation of receptors can be demonstrated following chronic exposure to an opioid (Werling et al. 1989), changes in receptor number are not necessary for tolerance to occur (Cox 1991), and this phenomenon probably plays a minor role, if any, in tolerance or dependence. Similarly, although recent work has indicated that opioid exposure also reduces the production of some endogenous opioid peptides (Mocchetti and Costa 1986),

it is unlikely that such an action determines the development of tolerance. A role for the latter process has been postulated in the development of abstinence following withdrawal of exogenous opioid drugs (Trujillo and Akil 1991a).

A substantial body of work concludes that functional decoupling of opioid receptors from second messenger systems is a major factor in the development of pharmacodynamic tolerance. The three best characterized opioid receptor subtypes, mu, kappa, and delta, are coupled to second messenger systems by G proteins (guanine nucleotide-binding proteins). Decoupling of receptors from G proteins can inhibit G protein–mediated actions such as regulation of ion channels, and thereby inhibit cell function (Christie et al. 1987; Cox 1991; Puttfarcken et al. 1988). This process, which is reversible, can occur without change in receptor number.

There is also recent evidence that parallel systems are involved in tolerance and dependence. Studies have demonstrated that the development of tolerance can be attenuated by the administration of cholecystokinin antagonists (Dourish et al. 1988; Watkins et al. 1984) or dynorphin (Lee 1984). Others have established a role for excitatory amino acids with the demonstration that N-methyl-D-aspartate antagonists and a nitric oxide synthase inhibitor can block the development of tolerance or dependence (Kolesnikov 1992; Marek et al. 1991; Rasmussen et al. 1991; Tiseo and Inturrisi 1993; Trujillo and Akil 1991b).

6. The finding that phenomena related to tolerance and dependence are receptor-selective is particularly important in view of data that establish the existence of large genetic differences in sensitivity to receptor-selective drugs (Baran et al. 1975; Pick et al. 1991). Sensitivity to morphine, for example, varies remarkably among species, and among various strains within a single species. These differences presumably relate to variations in the densities or affinities of receptor subtypes. It can be postulated that similar variability exists in humans (Galer et al. 1992).

7. Given the likelihood that humans develop tolerance and dependence that are receptor-selective and that there are probably substantial individual differences in receptor number and affinity, the observed association between different pain mechanisms and effects produced by specific receptor subtypes is clearly relevant. One study (Schumass and Yaksh 1983) demonstrated that the analgesic efficacy of a delta receptor agonist and a kappa receptor agonist varied with the type of nociceptive stimulus (cutaneous thermal vs. visceral chemical); these interactions are complex, however, and may vary with changes in stimulus intensity or other factors (Millan 1989). Another study documented different patterns of change over time in the binding of mu-, delta-,

and kappa-selective drugs following the development of a unilateral experimental mononeuropathy (Stevens et al. 1991). Finally, studies suggest that the central changes that result from nerve injury may diminish the ability of morphine to inhibit activity in central neurons (Xu and Wiesenfeld-Hallin 1991). Although it may be postulated that these interactions between receptor subtypes and pain mechanisms may render some types of pain relatively more or less responsive to specific types of opioids, or that individuals who vary in the density or affinity of specific receptor subtypes may be more or less responsive to opioids for pains of different mechanisms, such implications have yet to be explored in either experimental models or the clinical setting.

RELEVANT CLINICAL INVESTIGATIONS OF TOLERANCE AND RESPONSIVENESS

Few studies in humans specifically address issues related to tolerance or responsiveness. Those extant raise numerous questions for future research. The major findings can be summarized as follows:

1. McQuay and coworkers (1981) have described in humans a phenomenon that may be akin to the acute tolerance observed in animal models. Varying intraoperative doses of fentanyl citrate that produced large differences in plasma opioid concentration were associated with similar pain and respiratory responses in the immediate postoperative period. This finding could be explained by the occurrence of a greater degree of tolerance to the higher doses than the lower doses. Heishman and coworkers (1989a,b) induced acute physical dependence after brief exposure to morphine in postaddicts, a finding that may not be directly relevant to mechanisms of tolerance but which similarly suggests the potential for rapid changes in the human neural substrate following exposure to an opioid.

In a pharmacokinetic-pharmacodynamic study of methadone, Inturrisi et al. (1990) addressed the issue of acute tolerance. They measured plasma concentration and effects from 16 patients with chronic cancer pain during and after a brief (approximately 3-hour) methadone infusion. All patients had been receiving opioids chronically before the study. The lack of a clockwise hysteresis suggested that acute tolerance, or any other process that would lessen analgesic efficacy during this brief period, did not occur. This finding contrasts with the study performed by McQuay et al. (1981), which evaluated a different drug in opioid-naive patients during the treatment of postoperative pain, and suggests the need for caution in generalizing the findings of clinical studies from one group of patients to another. Clearly, similar caution is needed in generalizing the results of short-term animal studies to any clinical setting.

2. Two small studies of cancer patients evaluated the development of tolerance and cross-tolerance in humans during a somewhat longer period of opioid administration. The patients in these studies had chronic pain and were receiving relatively low doses of opioid drugs when evaluated. In the first study, 10 patients received graded single doses of morphine in controlled fashion before and after two weeks of regular morphine therapy (Houde et al. 1966). A rightward shift in the dose response curve indicated the development of analgesic tolerance during this period. The second study evaluated 13 patients who underwent a controlled relative potency assay comparing morphine and metapon (an opioid compound not presently available) before and after approximately one week of regular dosing with either drug (Houde 1985). The dose response curves from the second assay showed a shift to the right for both drugs, with a larger change for the drug that was administered repeatedly during the interval since the first assay. This finding suggests that analgesic tolerance and cross-tolerance occur, and that cross-tolerance occurs less rapidly or less completely than direct tolerance.

3. In contrast to these few clinical studies, most of the extant data pertaining to tolerance and physical dependence in humans have been collected from subjects who had no pain. A large number of studies have been performed in postaddicts who received morphine or other opioids while monitored in an inpatient setting for weeks or months (Jasinski 1977; Martin 1977). In one group of studies, subjects were monitored for changes in vital signs, pupillary diameter, and other physiological and psychological functions while receiving gradually increasing doses of morphine for five weeks; the final daily dose of 240 mg was then maintained for up to 7 months, at which time the dose was tapered and abstinence monitored for another period of months. These studies confirmed that tolerance can develop to various nonanalgesic effects, that tolerance to different effects occurs at varying rates, and that all such processes are characterized by large intraindividual and interindividual variability. This variability has also been observed in longitudinal surveys of methadone maintenance patients; adverse opioid effects and hormonal changes wane in most, but not all, and the pattern of residual effects is variable (Kreek 1973, 1986).

4. Studies of opioid responsiveness are similarly sparse. Clinical observation and studies in both acute and chronic dosing paradigms suggest that the following factors may influence responsiveness:

- *Patient-related factors*: age, gender, psychological distress, prior opioid exposure (duration and recent consumption), existence of cognitive impairment and other factors predisposing to opioid side effects, history of psychological dependence or addiction.

- *Pain-related factors*: usual intensity, existence of breakthrough pain, rapid tempo of pain escalation, predominant mechanism.
- *Drug-selective effects.*

For example, a recent report described the influence of patient characteristics and opioid dosing regimen on analgesic response through a combined analysis of over 2600 administrations of standard morphine doses during a series of controlled single-dose opioid trials (Thaler et al. 1991). The population comprised cancer patients who had limited or no prior opioid use and were undergoing evaluation during the immediate postoperative period. Analysis of covariance revealed that a relatively strong analgesic response was associated with older age, female gender, lower pain, longer interval since surgery, time since last analgesic dose, length of prior opioid exposure, and opioid intake during the previous 48 hours. The influence of prior opioid consumption on this clinical response suggested the impact of tolerance, a finding replicated in a recent controlled single-dose relative potency study of hydromorphone and heroin (Wallenstein et al. 1990).

5. The influence of various factors in determining opioid responsiveness during chronic dosing has been similarly addressed in several studies. A validation survey for the Edmonton Staging System, an assessment method designed to identify cancer patients who are relatively less likely to attain satisfactory analgesia during opioid therapy (Bruera et al. 1989), demonstrated that the following characteristics predicted poor outcome after three weeks of intensive clinical management: inferred neuropathic mechanism for the pain, the presence of incident pain (pain induced by specific maneuvers), impaired cognitive function, a high level of psychological distress, the current use of relatively high opioid doses (more than that equivalent to 300 mg oral morphine), and the need for a rapid increase in opioid dose (more than 5% of the initial dose per day). Another recent survey of 130 patients with advanced cancer observed that poor analgesic responsiveness during the two months prior to death was associated with the occurrence of incident pain and relatively poor response during an initial four-day opioid test period (Mercadante et al. 1992). Although the influence of past and current opioid use suggests that tolerance is a factor in the responsiveness of some patients, the tenuous nature of this conclusion must be recognized. As discussed previously, the need for dose escalation can only be attributed to tolerance if other reasons for increasing pain, such as progression of a lesion or psychological distress, cannot be demonstrated. Furthermore, the association between opioid exposure and poor responsiveness may not indicate causality; both phenomena could be due to a third factor, such as a specific pain characteristic or mechanism.

6. Genetic factors can also be postulated to have a role in opioid respon-

siveness. Studies in animals have established the importance of genetic differences in determining the sensitivity to receptor-selective drugs (Baran et al. 1975; Pick et al. 1991). In humans, genetic differences have been demonstrated, for example, in the O-demethylation of codeine to morphine (Chen et al. 1988; Yue et al. 1989). Genetically determined differences in receptor densities, receptor affinities, or efficiency of coupling to second messenger systems must be considered as potential sources of the large variability observed in all clinical studies.

7. Several studies have attempted specifically to address the relation between inferred pain mechanism and opioid responsiveness (Arner and Meyerson 1993). Some data suggest that a neuropathic mechanism confers a relatively reduced responsiveness to opioid drugs (Arner and Meyerson 1988; Kupers et al. 1991), and reported clinical experience generally (Bruera et al. 1989; Moulin and Foley 1990), but not uniformly (Mercadante et al. 1992), supports the conclusion that patients with neuropathic pain are less likely to achieve a satisfactory balance between analgesia and toxicity than patients with other inferred pain mechanisms. Nonetheless, clinical surveys strongly suggest that some patients with neuropathic pain respond well to opioid therapy (Galer et al. 1992; Mercadante et al 1992; Portenoy and Foley 1986; Urban et al. 1986), and recent investigations have provided confirmatory evidence. A controlled clinical trial demonstrated that patients with postherpetic neuralgia obtain analgesia from morphine (Rowbotham et al. 1991), and a combined analysis of several controlled single-dose studies observed that pains inferred to have a neuropathic mechanism do respond to a standard opioid dose, but with relatively less analgesia than pains inferred to have nociceptive mechanisms (Cherny et al. 1994). Similarly, pharmacokinetic-pharmacodynamic analysis of brief opioid infusions has demonstrated the potential for a concentration-dependent analgesic response in patients with neuropathic pain (Portenoy et al. 1990).

The relative responsiveness of neuropathic and nociceptive pains also has been evaluated in a paradigm that incorporates patient-controlled analgesia to explore the balance between analgesia and side effects (Jadad et al. 1992; McQuay et al. 1992). These studies have confirmed that the spectrum of response is broad for both groups. Some patients with neuropathic pain achieve a favorable response to morphine, while others with nociceptive pain cannot attain a satisfactory balance between analgesia and side effects. Overall, the likelihood of favorable response is lower among those with neuropathic pain (McQuay et al. 1992). Together, these data suggest that a neuropathic mechanism may impart a relatively reduced opioid responsiveness but does not result in opioid resistance.

CLINICAL OBSERVATIONS RELEVANT TO TOLERANCE AND RESPONSIVENESS

Although the limited data from clinical investigations suggest that the phenomena produced in experimental models can occur in humans, it is evident that the complexity of human pain necessitates caution in extrapolating any of the findmgs from animal or human studies. Furthermore, many clinical observations that may be relevant to opioid tolerance and responsiveness in humans remain to be systematically studied. Researchers must be aware of these observations, since they may provide a context for the interpretation of data and the development of new investigations. Some of the most important are as follows:

1. Unlike animal models, which demonstrate the development of tolerance to antinociceptive effects within hours to days following the initiation of opioid administration (Cochin and Kornetsky 1964; Stevens and Yaksh 1989; Yaksh 1991), the typical clinical response to long-term opioid treatment is characterized by continued analgesia without dose escalation. Most patients who receive opioid drugs achieve a plateau of stable dosing that extends for a prolonged period (Brescia et al. 1992; Foley 1993; France et al. 1984; Kanner and Foley 1981; Onofrio and Yaksh 1990; Plummer et al. 1991; Portenoy and Foley 1986; Schug et al. 1992; Taub 1982; Twycross 1974; Urban et al. 1986). For example, opioid-naive patients who were allowed to self-administer morphine for acute oral pain due to mucositis increased doses for three days, then stabilized for the remaining weeks of treatment (Hill et al. 1990).

2. Most patients who receive opioid drugs for the treatment of chronic pain require dose escalation periodically, and some need continuously increasing doses to maintain analgesia. In most of these instances, however, the need for dose escalation can be attributed to a readily identifiable process sufficient to explain the progression of the pain, typically a worsening physical lesion capable of producing nociception (Gonzales et al. 1991; Schug et al. 1992). Thus, the clinical pattern that would be most clearly identified as a manifestation of analgesic tolerance and most closely parallel that observed in animal models—opioid dose escalation in the absence of a progressing physical or psychological disorder—is a distinctly uncommon event during the long-term treatment of patients with pain. From this perspective, the experimental finding that rats with adjuvant arthritis self-administer morphine less than control animals is particularly interesting (Lyness et al. 1989), suggesting the potential importance of the mechanisms responsible for pain as modulators of changing opioid requirement.

3. Whatever the driving force for dose escalation, it is commonly observed that doses can be increased gradually with limited occurrence, or even

complete lack, of many potential adverse effects, including respiratory depression and somnolence. Indeed, in the setting of persistent pain, opioid doses can be safely escalated to extraordinary levels, many tens of thousands of morphine equivalent milligrams per day (Coyle et al 1990). Moreover, after doses have been increased in this way, a bolus injection that would have been lethal in the nontolerant patient can be given without any adverse effects. In the absence of pharmacokinetic processes, which have never been demonstrated, these observations suggest either that pharmacodynamic tolerance to these nonanalgesic opioid effects (of a type that parallels analgesic tolerance in animal models) has occurred or that other factors are operating that allow the patient to tolerate the dose (see below).

4. The relevance of pain-related factors to changes in opioid response is further suggested by the observation that doses can be dramatically reduced if a nonopioid analgesic intervention is effective. For example, treatments that reduce central transmission of nociceptive afferent input, such as nerve blocks or cordotomy, can result in a prompt decline in the dose required to provide analgesia for residual pain (Macaluso and Foley 1988; Schug et al. 1992). Similarly, it has been observed that the opioid doses used to manage "crescendo" pain in some delirious cancer patients may be markedly reduced as the delirium improves with the administration of a neuroleptic (Coyle et al. 1994). This phenomenon may suggest that analgesic tolerance, as it is usually understood, was not actually occurring as doses were driven higher by progressive pathology. Alternatively, it is possible that whatever degree of analgesic tolerance was contributing to dose escalation in these cases reversed rapidly when other factors were removed. Rapid reduction of analgesic dose requirements in patients is also commonly observed following a brief cessation of drug use. Rather than the prolonged duration of tolerance that can be observed in animal models (Cochin and Kornetsky 1964), humans exposed to opioids appear to have a more rapid return of opioid sensitivity.

5. The complexity of the interaction between pain and changes in opioid response is further highlighted by the striking observation that some opioid-treated patients who undergo a procedure to eliminate pain, such as cordotomy, may immediately develop adverse opioid effects that were not present prior to the procedure. For example, a patient with poorly controlled pain who is receiving a stable opioid regimen and is alert and breathing normally may rapidly develop obtundation and respiratory depression after a cordotomy or nerve block. Clinicians have learned to address this risk by dose reduction and close monitoring after such procedures. The potential for this phenomenon, which occurs in some patients and not others, suggests that the ability of some patients to tolerate opioid dose escalation (that is, their lack of adverse effects as the dose increases) may not be due to neural changes driven by exposure to

the drug (that is, to tolerance as it is usually defined) but rather to mechanisms subserving the experience of pain itself, perhaps including both specific nociceptive processes and a nonspecific alerting response. Alternatively, a component of the tolerance produced by drug exposure could interact in some way with nociceptive processes, such that the elimination of the latter leads to rapid reversal of tolerance.

Most of the foregoing observations have not been systematically investigated. This further underscores the need for caution in generalizing experimental results to humans with pain. It is also evident that these clinical observations should not be overinterpreted. Analgesic tolerance may be a contributing factor to dose escalation even if an alternative explanation can be discerned, and it should not be inferred from clinical experience that pharmacodynamic tolerance to analgesic effects is rare or unimportant in patients. The extremely large variability that characterizes patient response to opioids suggests the possibility that tolerance may be prominent in some patients and minimal in others. It is also possible that analgesic tolerance may be clinically relevant (as the driving force for dose escalation) for a brief period after dosing begins, but thereafter becomes less important than other determinants of analgesic response.

6. Another clinical observation is relevant to the issues surrounding both tolerance and efficacy. A switch from one opioid to another is usually accompanied by some change in the balance between analgesia and side effects (Galer et al. 1992). As a result, the opioid responsiveness of a patient can vary remarkably from drug to drug. One drug may produce intolerable sedation at an effective dose, whereas another yields no adverse effects at a dose that provides equivalent analgesia. This observation, which suggests that there are differences in the degree of cross-tolerance to various opioid effects, may be consistent with the finding in animal studies that tolerance is receptor-selective. Presumably, a patient will experience a change from one drug to another as favorable if there is less cross-tolerance at the receptors mediating analgesia than at those mediating adverse effects. Indeed, in the absence of toxicity, the dose of the new drug may be able to be escalated to provide even higher levels of analgesia. Conversely, should the degree of cross-tolerance at receptors mediating side effects be less than that produced at receptors mediating analgesia, the overall balance between analgesia and side effects may shift in an unfavorable direction and the patient will not benefit from the change.

Variability in the outcome of sequential opioid trials also illustrates the confusion that can develop if the nomenclature applied to opioid response is not clarified. If analgesia is the only effect of interest, then a switch from one opioid to another may demonstrate that the second drug has a higher potency than would be expected on the basis of published relative potency estimates (Houde et al. 1966). That is, following a prolonged period of regular dosing with one opioid, equivalent analgesia may be attained with a dose of a second opioid that is smaller than that calculated from an equianalgesic dose table. This phenomenon, which justifies the usual recommendation that a switch from one opioid to another should be accompanied by a reduction in the equianalgesic dose (Cherny and Portenoy 1994), may indicate that there is a shift in the relative potency between drugs if one of the drugs is administered long enough for tolerance to develop. If this change over time in relative potency actually occurs, it may also indicate that analgesic tolerance does indeed commonly influence drug response, at least during the initial period of dosing with an opioid drug.

As noted previously, studies have demonstrated that the degree of analgesic cross-tolerance between opioids is related to differences in their intrinsic efficacies (Ivarsson and Neil 1989; Paronis and Holtzman 1992; Picker and Yarbrough 1991; Sosnowski and Yaksh 1990; Stevens and Yaksh 1989). This type of efficacy is, however, like potency itself, unrelated to the change in clinical efficacy that results from a switch from one opioid to another. Although the second drug may be more potent than expected, its clinical efficacy is not defined solely by analgesic effects but rather by the balance between analgesia and side effects. Furthermore, if fewer side effects occur following the switch, persistent pain may become manageable by increases in the dose of the second drug, thereby yielding a greater maximal efficacy for this drug. The varying uses of the term *efficacy* in this situation may be confusing, particularly since the overall change in the balance between analgesia and side effects might be entirely different if any of the numerous variables was changed, including the identity of the first or second opioid, their doses, the duration of treatment before the switch, or many other clinical factors specific to the patient. For these reasons, the term *responsiveness* is preferred.

CONCLUSIONS

The gaps between research findings and clinical observations pose a challenge to both investigators and clinicians. The data pertaining to opioid tolerance and efficacy acquired in laboratory studies and investigations of pain-free subjects may or may not be generalizable to patients who receive opioid drugs for pain. The limited data from studies of pain patients provide an interesting glimpse of the type of information that may be accessible in clinical trials, but have only begun to illuminate the underlying processes. Clinical observations are essential for the development of guidelines for patient care, but the degree to which they clarify the mechanisms of tolerance and efficacy is unknown. The disparities in the information available highlight the need for both researchers and clinicians to carefully define terms and to strive to remain informed about the observations that may provide insight into the complexities encountered either in the laboratory or in the clinic.

From the clinical perspective, several additional implications deserve emphasis. First, analgesic tolerance appears to be a rare limiting factor during opioid pharmacotherapy. Concern about tolerance should not impede the early administration of an opioid drug in a patient who is otherwise a candidate for this therapy. Second, tolerance to most adverse effects is both anticipated and welcomed, since a decline in dose-limiting toxicity opens the therapeutic window and increases the likelihood of a favorable balance between analgesia and side effects. Third, escalating pain in a patient receiving a previously stable opioid dose should never be attributed, a priori, to the development of analgesic tolerance. In cancer patients particularly, increasing pain should always be evaluated as presumptive evidence of recurrent or progressive disease. Fourth, any patient who is administered an opioid must be provided ongoing dose titration designed to identify the optimal balance between analgesia and side effects. Although factors that may predict opioid responsiveness have been identified, none presently alter the basic approach to clinical practice.

From the perspective of the investigator interested in issues related to opioid tolerance or efficacy, these imperatives of clinical practice suggest that new studies of these phenomena should include animal models capable of evaluating multiple opioid effects and chronic nociception or nerve injury. Controlled clinical investigations are needed that specifically address the phenomenology of opioid tolerance and responsiveness, particularly as it relates to effects that may be specific to different opioid drugs or characteristics of patients or pains. Studies that address variations in responsiveness must incorporate dosing paradigms that explore the dose-response relationship and evaluate both analgesia and side effects. In this manner, the insights gained into tolerance and responsiveness will be most relevant to the use of opioids in patients with pain.

REFERENCES

Adams, J.U. and Holtzman, S.G., Pharmacologic characterization of the sensitization to the rate-decreasing effects of naltrexone induced by acute opioid pretreatment in rats, J. Pharmacol. Exp. Ther., 253 (1990) 483–489.

Arner, S. and Meyerson, B.A., Lack of analgesic effect of opioids on neuropathic and idiopathic forms of pain, Pain, 33 (1988) 11–23.

Arner, S. and Meyerson, B., Opioids in neuropathic pain, Pain Digest, 3 (1993) 15–22.

Baran, A., Shuster, L., Elefterhiou, B.E. and Bailey, D.W., Opiate receptors in mice: genetic differences, Life Sci., 17 (1975) 633–640.

Brescia, F.J., Portenoy, R.K., Ryan, M., Drasnoff, L. and Gray, G., Pain, opioid use and survival in hospitalized patients with advanced cancer, J. Clin. Oncol., 10 (1992) 149–155.

Bruera, E., MacMillan, D., Hanson, J. and MacDonald, R.N., The Edmonton staging system for cancer pain: preliminary report, Pain, 37 (1989) 203–210.

Chen, Z.R., Somogyi, A.A. and Bochner, F., Polymorphic O-demethylation of codeine, Lancet, 2 (1988) 914–915.

Cherny, N.I. and Portenoy, R.K., Practical issues in the management of cancer pain. In: P.D. Wall and R. Melzack (Eds.), Textbook of Pain, 3rd ed., Churchill Livingstone, Edinburgh, 1994, pp. 1437–1468.

Cherny, N.I., Thaler, H.T., Friedlander-Klar., H, Lapin, J., Foley, K.M., Houde. R.W. and Portenoy, R.K., Opioid responsiveness of cancer pain syndromes caused by neuropathic or nociceptive mechanisms: a combined analysis of controlled single-dose studies, Neurology, 44 (1994) 857–861.

Christie, M.J., Williams, J.T. and North, R.A., Cellular mechanisms of opioid tolerance: studies in single brain neurons, Mol. Pharmacol., 32 (1987) 633–638.

Cochin, J. and Kornetsky, C., Development and loss of tolerance to morphine in the rat after single and multiple injections, J. Pharmacol. Exp. Ther., 145 (1964) 1–20.

Cowan, A., Zhu, X.Z., Mosberg, H.I., Omnaas, J.R. and Porreca, F., Direct dependence studies in rats with agents selective for different types of opioid receptor, J. Pharmacol. Exp. Ther., 246 (1988) 950–955.

Cox, B.M., Molecular and cellular mechanisms in opioid tolerance. In: A.I. Basbaum and J.-M. Besson (Eds.), Towards a New Pharmacotherapy of Pain, John Wiley and Sons, New York, 1991, pp. 137–156.

Coyle, N., Adelhardt, J., Foley, K.M. and Portenoy, R.K., Character of terminal illness in the advanced cancer patient: pain and other symptoms in the last 4 weeks of life, J. Pain Sympt. Manage., 5 (1990) 83–93.

Coyle, N., Weaver, S., Breitbart, W. and Portenoy, R.K., Delirium as a contributing factor to "crescendo" pain: three case reports, J. Pain Sympt. Manage., 9 (1994) 44–47.

Creighton, F.J. and Ghodse, A.H., Naloxone applied to conjuctiva as a test for physical opiate dependence, Lancet, 1 (1989) 748–750.

Dafters, R. and Odber, J., Effects of dose, interdose interval, and drug-signal parameters on morphine analgesic tolerance: implications for current theories of tolerance, Behav. Neurosci., 103 (1989) 1082–1090.

Domino, E.F., Dahlstrom, B.E., Domino, L.E. and Domino, S.E., Relation of plasma morphine concentration to severity of abrupt withdrawal in morphine-dependent monkeys, J. Pharmacol. Exp. Ther., 243 (1987) 138–143.

Dourish, C.T., Hawley, D. and Iversen, S.D., Enhancement of morphine analgesia and prevention of morphine tolerance in the rat by the cholecystokinin antagonist L-364,718, Eur. J. Pharmacol., 147 (1988) 469–472.

Foley, K.M., Clinical tolerance to opioids. In: A.I. Basbaum and J.-M. Besson (Eds.), Towards a New Pharmacotherapy of Pain, John Wiley and Sons, New York, 1991, pp. 181–204.

Foley, K.M., Changing concepts of tolerance to opioids: what the cancer patient has taught us. In: C.R. Chapman and K.M. Foley (Eds.), Current and Emerging Issues in Cancer Pain: Research and Practice, Raven Press, New York, 1993, pp. 331–350.

France, R.D., Urban, B.J. and Keefe, F.J., Long-term use of narcotic analgesics in chronic pain, Soc. Sci. Med., 19 (1984) 1379–1382.

Fukagawa, Y., Katz, J.L. and Suzuki, T., Effects of a selective k-opioid agonist, U-50,488H, on morphine dependence in rats, Eur. J. Pharmacol., 170 (1989) 47–51.

Galer, B.S., Coyle, N., Pasternak, G.W. and Portenoy, R.K., Individual variability in the response to different opioids: report of five cases, Pain, 49 (1992) 87–91.

Gonzales, G.R., Elliot, K.J., Portenoy, R.K. and Foley, K.M., The impact of a comprehensive evaluation in the management of cancer pain, Pain, 47 (1991) 141–144.
Heishman, S.J., Stitzer, M.L., Bigelow, G.E. and Liebson, I.A., Acute opioid physical dependence in humans: effect of varying the morphine-naloxone interval, J. Pharmacol. Exp. Ther., 250 (1989a) 485–491.
Heishman, S.J., Stitzer, M.L., Bigelow, G.E. and Liebson, I.A., Acute opioid physical dependence in postaddict humans: naloxone dose effects after brief morphine exposure, J. Pharmacol. Exp. Ther., 248 (1989b) 127–134.
Hill, H.F., Chapman, C.R., Kornell, J.A., Sullivan, K.M., Saeger, L.C. and Benedetti, C., Self-administration of morphine in bone marrow transplant patients reduces drug requirement, Pain, 40 (1990) 121–129.
Houde, R.W. and Nathan B., Eddy Memorial Lecture: The analgesic connection, In: L.S. Harris (Ed.), Problems of Drug Dependence. NIDA Research Monograph, 55. National Institute of Drug Abuse, Rockville, Md., 1985, pp. 4–13.
Houde, R.W., Wallenstein, S.L. and Beaver, W.T., Evaluation of analgesics in patients with cancer pain, In: L. Lasagna (Ed.), International Encyclopedia of Pharmacology and Therapeutics, sec. 6, vol. 1, Clinical Pharmacology, Pergamon Press, Oxford, 1966, pp. 59–98.
Inturrisi, C.E., Portenoy, R.K., Max, M.B., Colburn, W.A. and Foley, K.M., Pharmacokinetic-pharmacodynamic (PK-PD) relationships of methadone infusions in patients with cancer pain, Clin. Pharmacol. Ther., 47 (1990) 565–577.
Ivarsson, M. and Neil, A., Differences in efficacies between morphine and methadone demonstrated in the guinea pig ileum: a possible explanation for previous observations of incomplete opioid cross-tolerance, Pharm. Toxicol., 65 (1989) 368–371.
Jadad, A.R., Carroll, D., Glynn, C.J., Moore, R.A. and McQuay, H.J., Morphine responsiveness of chronic pain: double-blind randomised crossover study with patient-controlled analgesia, Lancet, 339 (1992) 1367–1371.
Jaffe, J.H., Drug addiction and drug abuse, In: A.G. Gilman, L.S. Goodman, T.W. Rall and F. Murad (Eds.), The Pharmacological Basis of Therapeutics, 7th ed., Macmillan, New York, 1985, pp. 532–581.
Jasinski, D.S., Assessment of the abuse potentiality of the morphinelike drugs (methods used in man). In: W.R. Martin (Ed.), Drug Addiction I. Handbook of Experimental Pharmacology, Vol 45. Springer-Verlag, New York, 1977, pp. 197–258.
Jiang, Q., Mosberg, H.I. and Porreca, F., Modulation of the potency and efficacy of mu-mediated antinociception by delta agonists in the mouse, J. Pharmcol. Exp. Ther., 254 (1990) 683–689.
Johnson, S.M. and Fleming, W.W.,Mechanisms of cellular adaptive sensitivity changes: applications to opioid tolerance and dependence, Pharmacol. Rev., 41 (1989) 435–488.
Judson, B.A., Himmelberger, D.U. and Goldstein, A., The naloxone test for opiate dependence, Clin. Pharmacol. Ther., 27 (1980) 492–501.
Kalso, E., Poyhia, R., Onnela, P., Linko, K., Tigerstedt, I. and Tammisto, T., Intravenous morphine and oxycodone for pain after abdominal surgery, Acta Anaesthesiol. Scand., 35 (1991) 642–646.
Kanner, R.M. and Foley, K.M., Patterns of narcotic drug use in a cancer pain clinic, Ann. N.Y. Acad. Sci., 362 (1981) 161–172.
Kolesnikov, Y.A., Pick, C.G. and Pasternak, G.W., Ng-nitro-l- arginine prevents morphine tolerance, Eur. J. Pharmacol., 221 (1992) 399–400.
Kreek, M.J., Medical safety and side effects of methadone in tolerant individuals, JAMA, 223 (1973) 665–668.
Kreek, M.J., Tolerance and dependence: implications for the pharmacological treatment of addiction. In: L.S. Harris (Ed.) Problems of Drug Dependence 1986. NIDA Research Monograph 76. National Institute of Drug Abuse, Rockville, Md., 1986, pp. 53–62.
Kupers, R.C., Konings, H., Adriaensen, H. and Gybels J.M., Morphine differentially affects the sensory and affective pain rating in neurogenic and idiopathic forms of pain, Pain, 47 (1991) 5–12.

Lee, N.M., The role of dynorphin in narcotic tolerance mechanisms. In: C.W. Sharp (Ed.), Mechanisms of Tolernce and Dependence. Natl. Inst. Drug Abuse, Rockville, Md., 1984, pp. 162–167.
Ling, G.S.F. Paul, D., Simantov, R. and Pasternak, G.W., Differential development of acute tolerance to analgesia, respiratory depression, gastrointestinal transit and hormone release in a morphine infusion model, Life Sci., 45 (1989) 1627–1636.
Lyness, W.H., Smith, F.L., Heavner, J.E., Iacono, C.U. and Garvin, R.D., Morphine self-administration in the rat during adjuvant-induced arthritis, Life Sci., 45 (1989) 2217–2224.
Macaluso, C. and Foley, K.M., Cordotomy for lumbosacral, pelvic and lower extremity pain of malignant origin: safety and efficacy, Neurology, 38 (1988) 110.
Marek, P., Ben–Eliyahu, S., Vaccarino, A.L. and Liebeskind, J.C., Delayed application of MK-801 attenuates development of morphine tolerance in rats, Brain Res., 558 (1991) 163–165.
Martin, W.R., Neuropharmacology and neurochemistry of subjective effects, analgesia, tolerance and dependence produced by narcotic analgesics. In: W.R. Martin (Ed.), Drug Addiction I. Handbook of Experimental Pharmacology, Vol 45. Springer-Verlag, New York, 1977, pp. 43–158.
Martin, W.R. and Jasinski, D.R., Physiological parameters of morphine dependence in man: tolerance, early abstinence, protracted abstinence, J. Psychiatr. Res., 7 (1989) 9–17.
Martin, W.R., Eades, C.G., Thompson, W.O., Thompson, J.A. and Flanary, H.G., Morphine physical dependence in the dog, J. Pharmacol. Exp. Ther., 189 (1974) 759–71.
McQuay, H.J., Bullingham, R.E.S. and Moore, R.A., Acute opiate tolerance in man, Life Sci., 28 (1981) 2513–2517.
McQuay, H.J., Jadad, A.R., Carroll, D., Faura, C., Glynn, C. J., Moore, R.A. and Liu, Y., Opioid sensitivity of chronic pain: a patient-controlled analgesia method, Anaesthesia, 47 (1992) 757–767.
Mercadante, S., Maddaloni, S., Roccella, S. and Salvaggio, L., Predictive factors in advanced cancer pain treated only by analgesics, Pain, 50 (1992) 151–155.
Millan, M.J., Kappa-opioid receptor-mediated antinocicepter in the rat. I. Comparative actions of mu-, and kappa-opioids against noxious thermal pressure and electrical stimuli, J. Pharmacol. Exp. Ther., 251 (1989) 334–341.
Mocchetti, I. and Costa, E., Down regulation of hypothalamic pro-opioimelanocortin system during morphine tolerance, Clin. Neuropharmacol., 9, Suppl 1. (1986) 125–127.
Moulin, D.E. and Foley, K.M., A review of a hospital-based pain service. In: K.M. Foley, J.J. Bonica and V. Ventafridda (Eds.), Second International Congress on Cancer Pain. Advances in Pain Research and Therapy, Vol 16. Raven Press, New York, 1990, pp. 413–428.
Moulin, D.E., Ling, G.S.F. and Pasternak, G.W., Unidirectional analgesia cross-tolerance between morphine and levorphanol in the rat, Pain, 33 (1988) 233–239.
Onofrio, B.M. and Yaksh, T.L., Long-term pain relief produced by intrathecal morphine infusion in 53 patients, J. Neurosurg., 72 (1990) 200–209.
Paronis, C.A. and Holtzman, S.G., Development of tolerance to the analgesic activity of mu agonists after continuous infusion of morphine, meperidine or fentanyl in rats, J. Pharmacol. Exp. Ther., 262 (1992) 1–9.
Pick, C.G., Cheng, J., Paul, D. and Pasternak, G.W., Genetic influences in opioid analgesic sensitivity in mice, Brain Res., 566 (1991) 295–298.
Picker, M.J. and Yarbrough, J., Cross-tolerance and enhanced sensitivity to the response rate-decreasing effects of opioids with varying degress of efficacy at the mu receptor, Psychopharmacology, 105 (1991) 459–466.
Plummer, J.L., Cherry, D.A., Cousins, M.J., et al, Long-term spinal administration of morphine in cancer and non-cancer pain: a retrospective study, Pain, 44 (1991) 215–220.
Portenoy, R.K., Chronic opioid therapy for persistent noncancer pain: can we get past the bias? American Pain Society Bulletin, 1 (1991) 1–5.
Portenoy, R.K., Iatrogenic addiction. In: J.H. Jaffe (Ed.), The Encyclopedia of Drugs and Alcohol, Macmillan, New York.

Portenoy, R.K. and Foley, K.M., Chronic use of opioid analgesics in non-malignant pain: report of 38 cases, Pain 25 (1986) 171–186.

Portenoy, R.K. and Payne, R., Acute and chronic pain, In: J.H. Lowinson, P. Ruiz, R.B. Millman (Eds.), Comprehensive Textbook of Substance Abuse, Williams and Wilkins, Baltimore, 1992, pp. 691–721.

Portenoy, R.K., Moulin, D., Rogers, A., Inturrisi, C.E. and Foley, K.M., Continuous intravenous infusion of opioids in cancer pain: review of 46 cases and guidelines for use, Cancer Treatment Reports, 7 (1986) 575–581.

Portenoy, R.K., Foley, K.M. and Inturrisi, C.E., The nature of opioid responsiveness and its implications for neuropathic pain: new hypotheses derived from studies of opioid infusions, Pain, 43 (1990) 273–286.

Puttfarcken, P.S., Werling, L.L. and Cox, B.M., Effects of chronic morphine exposure on opioid inhibition of adenyl cyclase in 731c cell membranes: a useful model for the study of tolerance at mu opioid receptors, Mol. Pharmacol., 33 (1988) 520–527.

Rasmussen, K., Fuller, R.W., Stockton, M.E., Perry, K.W., Swinford, R.M. and Ornstein, P.L., NMDA receptor antagonists suppress behaviors but not norepinephrine turnover or locus coeruleus unit activity induced by opiate withdrawal, Eur. J. Pharmacol., 197 (1991) 9–16.

Redmond, D.E and Krystal, J.H., Multiple mechanisms of withdrawal from opioid drugs, Ann. Rev. Neurosci., 7 (1984) 443–478.

Rinaldi, R.C., Steindler, E.M., Wilford, B.B. and Goodwin, D., Clarification and standardization of substance abuse terminology, JAMA, 259 (1988) 555–557.

Rowbotham, M.C., Reisner-Keller, L.A. and Fields, H.L., Both intravenous lidocaine and morphine reduce the pain of postherpetic neuralgia, Neurology, 41 (1991) 1024–1028.

Schmauss, C. and Yaksh, T.L., In vivo studies on spinal opiate receptor systems mediating antinociception. II. Pharmacological profiles suggesting a differential association of mu, delta and kappa receptors with visceral, chemical and cutaneous stimuli in the rat, J. Pharmacol. Exp. Ther., 228 (1983) 1–2.

Schug, S.A., Zech, D., Grond, S., Jung, H., Meurser, T.H. and Stobbe, B., A long-term survey of morphine in cancer pain patients, J. Pain Sympt. Manage., 7 (1992) 259–266.

Smith, A.P., Law, P.Y. and Loh, H.H., Role of opioid receptors in narcotic tolerance/dependence. In: G. Pasternak (Ed.), The Opiate Receptors, Humana, Clifton, N.J., 1988, pp. 441–485.

Sosnowski, M. and Yaksh, T.L., Differential cross-tolerance between intrathecal morphine and sufentanil in the rat, Anesthesiology, 73 (1990) 1141–1147.

Stevens, C.W. and Yaksh, T.L., Potency of infused spinal antinociceptive agents is inversely related to magnitude of tolerance under continuous infusion, J. Pharmacol. Exp. Ther., 250 (1989) 1–8.

Stevens, C.W. and Yaksh, T.L., Studies of morphine and D-ala2-D-leu5-enkephalin (DADLE) cross-tolerance after continuous intrathecal infusion in the rat, Anesthesiology, 76 (1992) 596–603.

Stevens, C.W., Kajander, K.C., Bennett, G.J. and Seybold, V.S., Bilateral and differential changes in spinal mu, delta and kappa opioid binding in rats with a painful, unilateral neuropathy, Pain, 46 (1991) 315–326.

Taub, A., Opioid analgesics in the treatment of chronic intractable pain of non-neoplastic origin. In: L.M. Kitahata and D. Collins (Eds.), Narcotic Analgesics in Anesthesiology, Williams and Wilkins, Baltimore, 1982, pp. 199–208.

Thaler, H.T., Friedlander-Klar, H., Cirrincione, C., Portenoy, R.K., Wallenstein, S.L., Foley, K.M and Houde, R.W., A statistical approach to measuring analgesic response. In: M.R. Bond, J.E. Charlton and C.J. Woolf (Eds.), Proceedings of the VIth World Congress on Pain. Pain Research and Clinical Management, Vol. 4. Elsevier, Amsterdam, 1991, pp. 539–542.

Tiffany, S.T. and Maude-Griffen, P.M., Tolerance to morphine in the rat: associative and nonassociative effect, Behav. Neurosci., 102 (1988) 534–543.

Tiseo, P.J. and Inturrisi, C.E., Attenuation and reversal of morphine tolerance by the competitive N-methyl-D-aspartate receptor antagonist, LY274614, J. Pharmacol. Exp. Ther., 264 (1993)

1090–1096.
Trujillo, K.A. and Akil, H., Opiate tolerance and dependence: recent findings and synthesis, New Biologist, 3 (1991a) 915–923.
Trujillo, K.A. and Akil, H., Inhibition of morphine tolerance and dependence by the NMDA receptor antagonist MK-801, Science, 251 (1991b) 85–87.
Twycross, R.G., Clinical experience with diamorphine in advanced malignant disease, Int. J. Clin. Pharmacol. Ther. Toxicol., 9 (1974) 184–198.
Urban, B.J., France, R.D., Steinberger, D.L., Scott, D.L. and Maltbie, A.A., Long-term use of narcotic/antidepressant medication in the management of phantom limb pain, Pain, 24 (1986) 191–197.
Vaught, J.L., What is the relative contribution of mu, delta, and kappa opioid receptors to antinociception and is there cross-tolerance. In: A.I. Basbaum and J.-M. Besson (Eds.), Towards a New Pharmacotherapy of Pain, John Wiley and Sons, New York, 1991, pp. 121–136.
Wallenstein, S.L., Houde, R.W., Portenoy, R.K., Lapin, J., Rogers, A. and Foley, K.M., Clinical analgesic assay of repeated and single doses of heroin and hydromorphone, Pain, 41 (1990) 5–13.
Watkins, L.R., Kinscheck, I.B. and Mayer, D.J., Potentiation of opiate analgesia and apparent reversal of morphine tolerance by proglumide, a cholecystokinin antagonist, Science, 224 (1984) 395–396.
Way, E.L., Opioid tolerance and physical dependence and their relationship. In: A. Herz (Ed.), Opioids II. Handbook of Experimental Pharmacology, Vol 104. Springer-Verlag, New York, 1993, pp. 573–595.
Weissman, D.E. and Haddox, J.D., Opioid pseudoaddiction: an iatrogenic syndrome, Pain, 36 (1989) 363–366.
Werling, L.L., McMahon, P.N. and Cox, B.M., Selective changes in mu receptor properties induced by chronic morphine exposure, Proc. Natl. Acad. Sci. USA, 86 (1989) 6393–6397.
Wikler, A., Opioid Dependence: Mechanisms and Treatment, Plenum Press, New York, 1980.
Xu, X.-J. and Wiesenfeld-Hallin, Z., The threshold for the depressive effect of intrathecal morphine on the spinal nociceptive flexor reflex is increased during autotomy after sciatic nerve section in rats, Pain, 46 (1991) 223–229.
Yaksh, T.L., Tolerance: factors involved in changes in the dose-effect relationship with chronic drug exposure. In: A.I. Basbaum and J.-M. Besson (Eds.), Towards a New Pharmacotherapy of Pain, John Wiley and Sons, New York, 1991, pp. 157–180.
Yue, O.Y., Svensson, J.O., Alm, C., Sjoqvist, F. and Sawe, J., Codeine O-demethylation co-segregates with polymorphic debrisoquine hydroxylation, Br. J. Clin. Pharmcol., 28 (1989) 639–645.

Correspondence to: Russell K. Portenoy, MD, Dept. of Neurology, Memorial Hospital, 1275 York Ave., New York, NY 10021, USA. Tel: 212-639-8702; Fax: 212-717-3081.

Proceedings of the 7th World Congress on Pain,
Progress in Pain Research and Management, Vol. 2,
edited by G.F. Gebhart, D.L. Hammond, and T.S.
Jensen, IASP Press, Seattle, © 1994.

41

Paradoxical and Other Pain Uncontrolled by Morphine

John S. Morley, Jon Watt, J. Chris Wells, Pauline. E. McKibbin, Lawrence Seabra, and John B. Miles

Pain Research Institute, Pain Relief Foundation, Liverpool, UK

INTRODUCTION

Morphine remains one of the most powerful analgesics and is the drug of choice in most hospices for the relief of severe pain in cancer sufferers. Occasionally, however, continuous use of morphine/diamorphine induces a state in which pain ceases to be relieved or is worsened by further administration of the drug. Detailed investigation of a recent case (Case History 1) led us to attribute the cause to increased differential metabolism of morphine (M) to morphine-3-glucuronide (M3G) (Morley et al. 1992).

> *Case History 1:* Male (47) disabled by pelvic and low back pain from disseminated metastases secondary to colonic carcinoma. During 30 days of increasingly larger doses of intrathecal (it.) morphine and oral diamorphine, the pain worsened and he became agitated. Analysis of his cerebrospinal (CSF) fluid showed high concentrations of M3G, but no morphine-6-glucuronide (M6G). The morphine and diamorphine administration was then stopped and he was given M6G (1 mg) it. on alternate days for five days. On each occasion full pain relief lasted for seven hours, and relief of the pelvic pain lasted two days.

We described this patient's pain as paradoxical because it worsened during the morphine/diamorphine treatment. After careful consideration of the definitive problems that arise (Bowsher 1993; Davis and Turner 1993; Hanks et al. 1993; Hardy 1993; Jessop 1993; Twycross 1993), the IASP Task Force on Taxonomy decided that it is premature to include this term in its list of definitions (personal communication from H. Merskey). Meanwhile, we use the term *morphine paradoxical pain* to describe pain that would normally be expected to respond to morphine, including pain that has previously been well-relieved by morphine; and that, at some time during the course of treatment with increasing doses of morphine/diamorphine actually seems to intensify; and that is associated with agitation and distress over and above that which might be expected from the pain alone (hyperalgesia/hyperesthesia or allodynia may be noted on examination).

In our follow-up study, we distinguished morphine paradoxical pain (as defined above) and other nociceptive pain which, during continuous use of morphine, *ceases to be adequately relieved* by oral morphine/diamorphine. Hereafter, the two types are collectively referred to as uncontrolled pain. Our purpose was to establish the incidence of the metabolic abnormality of the type found in case 1, and to test the validity of our speculation and a corollary—that a switch to the use of methadone should relieve pain in such cases.

METHODS

Cancer sufferers with uncontrolled pain were identified in collaboration with 140 U.K. Hospices. In each case the patient's case history and drug usage were recorded, and checks were made to ascertain if existing symptoms included the development of agitation or allodynia. When the latter symptoms existed, or if the pain itself had worsened as a result of the morphine treatment, the uncontrolled pain was judged to be paradoxical.

Plasma, and where possible, cerebrospinal fluid (CSF) samples were withdrawn, placed in lithium heparinized tubes, stored at – 40°C, and analyzed at the Pain Research Institute, Liverpool, within one week by the method we have described (Venn and Michalkiewicz 1990). Control plasma samples (and, in one case, CSF retrieved postmortem one hour after death) from cancer sufferers whose pain was being adequately controlled by morphine (subsequently referred to as patients with controlled pain) were similarly collected and analyzed. The sensitivities in our assay were M3G 2 nmol/l, M6G 4 nmol/l, and M 6 nmol/l.

We identified 36 patients with uncontrolled pain. The mean age was 55.4 (range 31–81); 26 were men and 10 were women. The mean daily dose of morphine (mainly MST Continus) in the 24 hours prior to sampling was 725 mg (median 600 mg; range 150–4200 mg). Except where otherwise stated, sampling was carried out 1–3 hours after the last morphine administration. The diagnoses were carcinomas of the gastrointestinal tract (6), pancreas (1), lung (7), kidney (2), pelvis (3), prostate (2), uterus (1), cervix (1), spine (6), and others (7). Of these, eight patients were judged to be suffering from paradoxical pain.

In addition, plasma (six cases) and CSF (one case) were withdrawn from seven patients whose nociceptive pain was controlled by morphine. CSF analyses obtained in an earlier study (Venn et al. 1990) on six patients with controlled pain (providing CSF data on seven patients in all) were included in determining mean CSF concentrations in controlled pain that are quoted in this paper.

RELEVANT METABOLIC SPECIES

There is general agreement that M6G contributes to the analgesia produced during morphine administration (Venn et al. 1990; Osborne et al. 1988; Portenoy et al. 1992). The proposition that *most* of the analgesic activity is due to M6G (Osborne et al. 1988; Venn et al. 1990) is, however, debatable. Animal tests of antinociceptive activity show that M6G is up to 620 times more potent than morphine (Paul et al. 1989), but when given intrathecally to humans it is reported to have only about twice the analgesic potency of morphine (Hanna et al. 1990). Thus, the summation of M6G and morphine concentrations may more accurately reflect analgesic species during peripheral administration of morphine. Accordingly, in this study we used the ratio M3G/M6G+M to try to assess the functional significance of M3G.

We explored two distinct features of our speculation by measuring this ratio in uncontrolled (both paradoxical and nonparadoxical) and controlled pain. First, we studied whether a sufficiently increased ratio (i.e., sufficiently high proportions of M3G) might cause complete antagonism of the analgesic activity of both morphine and M6G and thereby account for uncontrolled pain. This speculation is based on the reported potent antagonistic activity of M3G on the effect of morphine in the rat tail-flick test (Smith et al. 1990) and on the effect of M6G in the hot-plate, tail-flick, and writhing tests (Gong et al. 1992). However, these results are disputed by Suzuki et al. (1993), who report no significant effect of low-dose intrathecal M3G on morphine-induced antinociception in either the rat tail-flick or hot-plate tests. Hewett et al. (1993) also report that intrathecal M3G does not significantly antagonize the A-beta fiber and noxious C-fiber responses of convergent dorsal horn neurons to morphine. Second, we studied whether the ratio may be so excessively raised in some cases as to permit central stimulatory effects of M3G, accounting for the aggravation seen in paradoxical pain. This speculation is based on reports that intracerebroventricular (but not intravenous) administration of

M3G to rats elicits a variety of CNS excitatory effects (Jacquet et al. 1980; Yaksh et al. 1986) and hyperalgesia and allodynia (Smith et al. 1990).

Our speculation has been criticized on the grounds that "M3G does not bind to opiate receptors" (Hanks et al. 1993). But Chen et al. (1991) report that M3G has a Ki of 37.1 nM against opioid mu receptors, an affinity about the same as that of methadone, seven times greater than that of codeine, and only 1/30th that of morphine. Pasternak et al. (1987) found weaker affinity and attributed this to "the presence of trace amounts of morphine" in the M3G. Structure-activity relationships do indeed suggest that morphine derivatives with bulky groups at the 3 position should lack affinity for the opiate receptor, but there is now evidence that this generalization may not apply to M3G because, unlike most 3-substituted derivatives, it exists in folded conformers (Carrupt et al. 1991). The matter must be regarded as unresolved until new measurements are made using M3G of established purity.

RESULTS

PLASMA CONTENTS

The M3G/M6G+M ratios in the 36 patients with uncontrolled pain were divided into three groups. In 4 patients the ratio was greater than 10, in 16 it was 5–10, and in 16 it was less than 5. As expected, the plasma concentrations varied widely, but the mean plasma concentrations showed that the decrease in the ratio between the groups can be attributed to increased M6G and M concentrations rather than decreased M3G concentrations (Table I).

The mean ratio in all 36 patients with uncontrolled pain was 9.7 (range 1.2–133), while the mean ratio in the six patients with controlled pain was 4.1 (range 1.2–5.9). Within the uncontrolled pain group, the mean ratio for the eight patients with paradoxical pain was 7.8 (range 2.2–20.4), and the mean ratio for the 28 patients with nonparadoxical pain was 10.2 (range 1.2–133) (Table II).

CSF CONTENTS

The mean M3G/M6G+M ratios in the 12 patients with uncontrolled pain was 19.8 (range 3.7–140), while the mean ratio in the seven patients with controlled pain was 1.1 (range 0.3–2.4). Within the uncontrolled pain group, the mean ratio for the two patients with paradoxical pain was 77.0 (range 14.1–140) and the mean ratio for the 10 patients with nonparadoxical pain was 8.4 (range 3.7–17.4) (Table III).

Table I
Mean plasma levels of morphine (M) and its 3- and 6-glucuronides (M3G and M6G) in 36 patients whose pain was uncontrolled by morphine

	Mean Plasma Level (range) (nmol/l)		
Ratio M3G/M6G+M	M3G	M6G	M
> 10 (n = 4)	2601 (288–7483)	59 (<4–7023)	65 (<6–170)
5–10 (n = 16)	8880 (507–50,010)	1049 (46–7023)	175 (<6–1636)
< 5 (n = 16)	9166 (141–24,392)	2212 (30–5628)	1076 (<6–3514)

Note: The ratio M3G/M6G+M was calculated, and the results are divided into three groups according to the magnitude of the ratio.

DISCUSSION

Although the mean plasma M3G/M6G+M ratio in patients with controlled pain was lower than the mean ratio in patients with uncontrolled pain, the difference did not reach statistical significance. The range around the means (respectively, 1.2–133 and 1.2–5.9) precludes any diagnostic value of plasma ratios; a patient with paradoxical pain had a ratio of 2.2 and a patient with uncontrolled nonparadoxical pain had a ratio of 1.2, both falling within the lower range for controlled pain. Neither was the plasma ratio of value in distinguishing paradoxical pain from uncontrolled nonparadoxical pain; there was no significant difference in the mean plasma ratio of these two groups, and the overlap in range around the means (2.2–20.4 and 1.2–133, respectively) was considerable. In fact, the highest ratio (133) occurred in a patient with uncontrolled nonparadoxical pain.

Our data on CSF M3G/M6G+M ratios are necessarily restricted, particularly for patients whose pain is controlled by morphine. However, the mean ratio (19.8) in the 12 patients we studied with uncontrolled pain was very significantly higher than the mean ratio (1.1) in six patients with controlled pain. Moreover, there was no overlap in the range around these means (3.7–140 and 0.3–2.4, respectively). We tentatively conclude that uncontrolled pain is associated with CSF M3G/M6G+M ratios greater than 4, approximately, whereas in controlled pain, ratios are below 3. Within the uncontrolled pain group, the mean ratio for two paradoxical pain patients was much higher (77.0) than for ten nonparadoxical pain patients (8.4), but no conclusions can be drawn because of the small numbers of patients involved.

Our results confirm the wide variation in morphine metabolism in individual patients. Although only a small number of patients with controlled pain were included in this study, our results also confirm previous findings that the mean ratio of relevant metabolic species (M3G/M6G+M) is about 5 in plasma and 1 in CSF when pain is being adequately controlled by oral morphine (Table IV).

They also show that, when pain is uncontrolled by morphine, much higher plasma ratios sometimes arise, and that more consistent changes occur in CSF. The mean CSF ratio then increased twenty-fold, and the lowest CSF ratio was higher than any we found in controlled pain patients.

CONCLUSIONS

On the basis of these results, we conclude that nociceptive pain may be uncontrolled by oral morphine if: (a) a metabolic abnormality exists such that high amounts of M3G are formed relative to the amounts of analgesic species (M6G+M), and/or (b) access of M3G into the CSF is somehow promoted, or access of M6G or morphine is inhibited. This conclusion supports our speculation that high M3G concentrations effectively antagonized the action of analgesic species (M6G+M) at CNS opiate receptors and stresses that it is circulating CSF concentrations of the three species that are relevant. The possibility that increased access of M3G to the CSF may arise in cancer, rheumatoid arthritis, and other conditions as a result of changing pathology (e.g., developing vasculitis) is now being explored. Our further speculation that extremely high proportions of circulating M3G may induce paradoxical pain also is consistent with the results of this study, but no firm conclusions

Table II
Controlled vs. uncontrolled pain: comparison of morphine metabolite ratios in plasma

	Plasma Ratio MG/M6G+M	
	Mean	Range
Pain uncontrolled (n = 36)	9.7	1.2–133
Paradoxical (n = 8)	7.8	2.2–20.4
Nonparadoxical (n = 28)	10.2	1.2–133
Pain controlled (n = 6)	4.1	1.2–5.9

Note: Controlled vs. uncontrolled and paradoxical vs. nonparadoxical not significant (analysis of variance and nonparametric paired test).

can be drawn because CSF analyses were possible in only two of the paradoxical pain patients.

MORPHINE/METHADONE CONVERSION

A corollary of our speculation is that opioids that are incapable of metabolism to a 3-glucuronide derivative (those lacking a 3-hydroxy group) should relieve uncontrolled pain of the type we have investigated. Methadone, lacking hydroxyl groups, is such an opioid. We first examined the effect of a switch from morphine to methadone in a hospital patient suffering from paradoxical pain (Case History 2).

Case History 2: Male (57) with disseminated pelvic carcinoma, whose pain had been uncontrolled (VAS 61–100) for several weeks despite eventual use of epidural diamorphine (60 mg/day) and oral morphine (400 mg MST, b.i.d.). He was also severely agitated. Plasma concentrations were 7483 nmol/l M3G, 197 nmol/l M6G and 170 nmol/l morphine (M3G/M6G+M ratio 20.4). Replacement of the diamorphine and morphine with methadone (40 mg/day epidurally; 10 mg q.i.d. orally) resulted in immediate and sustained pain relief (VAS consistently below 12) and cessation of the agitation.

This satisfactory outcome, and the conclusions from our study of metabolic ratios, prompted us to encourage hospices to consider the switch to methadone in all situations where morphine/diamorphine ceases to be effective and dominant neuropathic pain is excluded. Recommended guidelines

Table III
Controlled vs.uncontrolled pain: comparison of morphine metabolite ratios in cerebrospinal fluid (CSF)

	CSF Ratio M3G/M6G+M	
	Mean	Range
Pain uncontrolled (n = 12)	19.8	3.7–140
Paradoxical (n = 2)	77.0	14.1–140
Nonparadoxical (n = 10)	8.4	3.7–17.4
Pain controlled (n = 7)*	1.1	0.3–2.4

Note: Variance controlled vs. uncontrolled by Kruskal-Wallis analysis gave $P < 0.001$; nonparametric paired test (Kotmogovow-Sminraff) gave $P < .018$. Paradoxical vs. nonparadoxical not significant.
*n = 6 from our earlier study (Venn et al. 1990).

Table IV
Reported mean ratios of metabolites during oral administration of morphine (pain mainly controlled)

Study	Type (Number) of Patients	M3G/M6G	M3G/M6G+M
Plasma			
Venn et al. 1990	cancer (40)	5.0	4.5
McQuay et al. 1990	cancer (151)	4.8	4.2
Cerebrospinal fluid			
Venn et al. 1990	cancer (40)	6.0	0.6
Hand et al. 1987	prostatectomy (15)	6.0	0.9

were: "Use an initial dose of methadone that is one tenth of the total daily morphine dose, but not greater than 100 mg, and give this dose at intervals determined by the patient (Sawe et al. 1981), but not more frequently than three hourly. Typically, the patient requires three to eight doses per day for the first few days (3 doses per day, i.e., 8-hourly dosing, is usual), then settles on a lower fixed intake (1–4 doses per day) after one week. The steady-state total daily dose may then be divided into a twice daily regime, and future adjustments made (as in the use of MST)."

The subsequent experience of Dr. Finnigan, Good Shepherd Hospice, Chester, UK, is typical. He has so far applied the recommendations in five cases (three paradoxical, two nonparadoxical), and in all but one case the switch to methadone brought immediate pain relief. We thank him for the following two case histories.

Case history 3: Female (44), carcinoma of uterus, with lumbar and leg pain worsening on Oramorph (up to 1000 mg/day). Plasma concentrations were 3138 nmol/l M3G, 480 nmol/l M6G, and 32 nmol/l morphine (M3G/M6G+M ratio 6.1). The Oramorph administration was then stopped and replaced by methadone (100 mg t.i.d. decreasing to 60 mg b.i.d.), with total pain relief. Pain control was so good that the patient stopped taking the methadone, causing return of severe pain within 24 hours. Total pain relief was restored when methadone (60 mg b.i.d.) was retaken.

Case history 4: Female (46), carcinoma of anus, with pelvic lymph node involvement. Rectal pain, first controlled by MST (270 mg b.i.d.), rapidly escalated and became unresponsive to MST (400 mg b.i.d.). Plasma concentrations were 15,732 nmol/l M3G, 1805 nmol/l M6G, and 489 nmol/l morphine (M3G/M6G+M ratio 6.9). The MST administration was stopped and replaced by methadone (80 mg q.i.d. decreasing to 50 mg b.i.d.) with total pain relief. Accidental underdose (4 mg b.i.d.) due to prescription error, when returned to home. Severe rectal pain returned. Total pain relief on restarting correct dose.

The unsuccessful case was a male (49) with neuralgic pain in the arm (from a mesothelioma) poorly controlled by MST Continus (100 mg b.i.d.), who developed marked agitation. When transferred to methadone (30 mg t.i.d.), his agitation lifted but the pain remained poorly responsive.

Successful use of methadone is not confined to pain arising from carcinomas. A recent admission to our hospital is illustrative:

Case history 5: Male (24), acute lymphoblastic leukemia, with severe constant abdominal pain, agitation, and allodynia, worsening over 14 weeks during diamorphine administration (up to 75 mg/hr, iv.). No sampling was possible. Changed to methadone (10 mg/3 hr iv.). After 18 hours, no pain, no agitation, no allodynia.

We hope that concerns about the safety of methadone therapy (Harding-Pink 1993) do not deter clinicians from its appropriate use. The concerns arise mainly because of its long and unpredictable half-life. However, the experience of many physicians is that the drug may be used safely and successfully if care is taken in the titration of dose against pain. O'Neill and Onen (1993) comment: "The effective management of cancer pain was delayed for decades (and continues to be delayed in some areas) because of an unbalanced focus on the risks rather the benefits of opioids. We do not wish the same to be true of methadone."

An alternative strategy when uncontrolled pain of the type we have described is suspected is the use of M6G, but this is presently an expensive chemical. Use of ketamine is also indicated (Laird and Lovel 1993).

ACKNOWLEDGMENTS

We gratefully acknowledge the cooperation and help of the medical and nursing staff of many U.K. hospices, and generous grants from the Trustees of Remedi, the Liverpool General Cancer Charity Committee, and the BUPA Medical Foundation Ltd.

REFERENCES

Bowsher, D., Paradoxical pain, Br. Med. J., 306 (1993) 473–474.

Carrupt, P.-A., Testa, B., Bechalany, A., Tayer, N.E., Descas, P. and Perrissoud, D., Morphine 6-glucuronide and morphine 3- glucuronide as molecular chameleons with unexpected lipophilicity, J. Med. Chem., 34 (1991) 1272–1275.

Chen, S.R., Irvine, R.J., Somogyi, A.A. and Bochner, F., Mu receptor binding of some commonly used opioids and their metabolites, Life Sci., 48 (1991) 2165–2171.

Davis, C.L. and Turner, R., Paradoxical pain, Br. Med. J., 306 (1993) 793.

Gong, Q.-L., Hedner, J., Bjorkman, R. and Hedner, T., Morphine-3-glucuronide may functionally antagonize morphine-6-glucuronide induced antinociception and ventilatory depression in the rat, Pain, 48 (1992) 249–255.

Hanks, G.W.C., O'Neill, W.M. and Fallon, M.T., Paradoxical pain, Br. Med. J., 306 (1993) 793.

Hanna, M.H., Peat, S.J., Woodham, M., Knibb, A. and Fung, C., Analgesic efficacy and CSF pharmacokinetics of intrathecal morphine-6-glucuronide: comparison with morphine, Br. J. Anaesth., 64 (1990) 547–550.

Harding-Pink, D., Methadone: one person's maintenance dose is another's poison, Lancet, 341 (1993) 665–666.

Hardy, P.A.J., Paradoxical pain. Br. Med. J., 306 (1993) 794.

Hewett, K., Dickenson, A.H. and McQuay, H.J., Lack of effect of morphine-3-glucuronide on the spinal antinociceptive actions of morphine in the rat: an electrophysiological study, Pain, 53 (1993) 59–63.

Jacquet, Y.F., Excitatory and inhibitory effects of opiates in the rat vas deferens: a dual mechanism of opiate action, Science, 210 (1980) 95–97.

Jessop, J., Paradoxical pain, Br. Med. J., 306 (1993) 794.

Laird, D. and Lovel, T. Paradoxical pain, Lancet, 341 (1993) 241.

Morley, J.S., Miles, J.B., Wells, J.C. and Bowsher, D., Paradoxical pain, Lancet, 340 (1992) 1045.

O'Neill, W.M. and Onen, T.S., Methadone therapy, Lancet, 341 (1993) 1277–1278.

Osborne, R., Joel, S., Trew, D. and Slevin, M., Analgesic activity of morphine-6-glucuronide, Lancet, i (1988) 828.

Pasternak, G,W., Bodnar, R.J., Clark, J.A. and Inturrisi, C.E., Morphine-6-glucuronide, a potent mu agonist, Life Sci., 41, (1987) 2845–2849.

Paul, D., Standifer, K.M., Inturrisi, C.E. and Pasternak, G.W., Pharmacological characterization of morphine-6β-glucuronide, a very potent morphine metabolite, J. Pharmacol. Exp. Ther., 251 (1989) 477–483.

Portenoy, R.K., Thaler, H.T., Inturrisi, C.E., Friedlander-Klar, H. and Foley, K.M., The metabolite morphine-6-glucuronide contributes to the analgesia produced by morphine infusion in patients with pain and normal renal function, Clin. Pharmacol. Ther., 51 (1992) 422–431.

Sawe, I., Hansen, J., Ginman, C., Hartvig, P., Jakobsson, P.A., Nilsson, M.-I. and Rane, A., Patient-controlled dose regimen of methadone for chronic cancer pain, Br. Med. J., 282 (1981) 771–773.

Smith, M.T., Watt, J.A. and Cramond, T., Morphine-3-glucuronide: a potent antagonist of morphine analgesia, Life Sci., 47 (1990) 579–585.

Suzuki, N., Kalso, E. and Rosenberg, P., Intrathecal morphine-3-glucuronide does not antagonize spinal antinociception with morphine or morphine-6-glucuronide in rats, Eur. J. Pharmacol., 249 (1993) 247–250.

Twycross, R., Paradoxical pain, Br. Med. J., 306 (1993) 793.

Venn, R.F. and Michaelkiewicz, A., Fast reliable assay for morphine and its metabolites using high-performance liquid chromatography and native fluorescence detection, J. Chromatogr., 525 (1990) 379–388.

Venn, R.F., Michaelkiewicz, A., Hardy, P. and Wells, C., Concentrations of morphine, morphine metabolites and peptides in human CSF and plasma, Pain, Suppl. 5 (1990) S188.

Yaksh, T.L., Harty, G.J. and Onofrio, B.M., High doses of spinal morphine produce a nonopiate receptor-mediated hyperesthesia: clinical and theoretical implications, Anesthesiology, 64 (1986) 590–597.

Correspondence to: J.S. Morley, PhD, DSc, Pain Research Institute, Pain Relief Foundation, Rice Lane, Liverpool L9 1AE, UK. Tel: 44-51-523-1486; Fax: 44-51-521-6155.

Proceedings of the 7th World Congress on Pain,
Progress in Pain Research and Management, Vol. 2,
edited by G.F. Gebhart, D.L. Hammond, and T.S.
Jensen, IASP Press, Seattle, © 1994.

42

A Comparison of Kapanol (a New Sustained-Release Morphine Formulation), MST Continus, and Morphine Solution in Cancer Patients: Pharmacokinetic Aspects of Morphine and Morphine Metabolites

Geoffrey K. Gourlay, John L. Plummer,
David A. Cherry, and Margaret M. Onley

*Pain Management Unit, Flinders Medical Centre, Bedford Park,
South Australia, Australia*

INTRODUCTION

Potent mu receptor opioid agonist drugs and a range of adjuvant medications are administered to almost all patients with severe pain related to cancer in those countries where such medications are readily available. Indeed, the WHO analgesic ladder has been shown to provide effective pain relief using orally administered medication in approximately 80% of patients with severe pain; the majority of patients are at Step 3 of the ladder (i.e., morphine or equivalent) when they die (Grond et al. 1991).

Morphine is the preferred opioid because there are well-established guidelines for its use (governmental and literature publications); it is inexpensive; its pharmacokinetic profile shows less interpatient variability than do other potent opioids; and morphine or its metabolites have no major organ toxicities other than the accumulation of the active metabolite, morphine-6-glucuronide (M6G) in renal failure.

Traditionally, morphine was administered orally as an immediate-release solution or tablet between four and six times per 24 hours. While this regimen was effective if regular attention was given to optimizing the dose and dosage interval, it was inconvenient as patients frequently had interrupted sleep patterns caused by the necessity to take early morning doses (i.e., between 0100 to 0600 hr) to maintain pain control.

Approximately one decade ago, a controlled-release tablet formulation of morphine, MST Continus® (or MS Contin® in some countries; Napp Labs; abbreviated herein as MST) was marketed, and this preparation quickly became the formulation of choice because it overcame many of the disadvantages of the immediate-release morphine formulations. Recently, a new sustained-release morphine formulation, Kapanol® (polymer-coated pellets in a capsule; Glaxo; abbreviated herein as KAP) was developed. This chapter compares the morphine pharmacokinetic profile at steady state of the new pellet formulation, KAP, with the established controlled-release morphine tablet, MST and immediate-release morphine solution (SOLN) in cancer patients with severe pain. Further, the plasma concentration–time profile for the major morphine metabolites, morphine-3-glucuronide (M3G) and M6G also were characterized together with the influence of renal function on these metabolite levels.

METHODS

This study was approved by the Committee on Clinical Investigation (ethics committee) at Flinders Medical Centre.

PATIENTS

Fifty adult patients at Step 3 of the WHO analgesic ladder (i.e., requiring opioids for pain control), with documented pathological and/or radiological evidence of cancer, were entered into this randomized, open-label, pharmacokinetic study. Of these, 24 patients completed the three-period, crossover study at steady state. No patient withdrew due to a major complication of any of the formulations. Disease progression together with poor venous access for frequent blood sampling were the main factors leading to withdrawal. Exclusion criteria included the "standard" restrictions regarding hepatic (transaminase and bilirubin levels), renal (creatinine), hematological (WCC and platelets), and gross abnormalities in pulmonary function. Attention was paid to any factor that could influence the absorption of morphine from the gastrointestinal tract (GIT) and therefore influence the derived morphine pharmacokinetic parameters—for example, gastric or upper GIT surgery, any obstruction, or other similar factors. Radiotherapy and/or chemotherapy administered in the week preceding entry or during the study and protracted nausea and vomiting were other exclusion criteria.

LEAD-IN PHASE

For each patient, the morphine dose was optimized to provide the most favorable balance between pain relief and side effects using immediate-release morphine solution. The patient was contacted daily by telephone and also recorded the extent of pain relief and side effects into a daily diary. The prescribed morphine doses were administered at four-hour intervals starting at 1000 hr on the first day. Rescue analgesia in this phase consisted of a half dose of morphine solution as required. The minimum duration of the lead-in phase was eight days and toward the end of this phase, the 24-hour morphine dose was adjusted such that the same dose could be administered with all three formulations. Dose optimization was achieved when the 24-hour morphine dose was constant for three consecutive days, with no rescue doses.

CROSS-OVER PHASE

The sequence of formulation administration was determined by random allocation to a balanced block design. The optimized 24-hour morphine dose administered was identical (to within 1 mg) for the three formulations. The two modified-release formulations (i.e., KAP and MST) were administered at 1000 and 2200 hr while SOLN was administered at four-hour intervals in an identical manner to the lead-in phase. Rescue analgesia was dextromoramide (5 mg tablets). Patients were contacted daily by phone to ensure the medication was taken as prescribed. Blood samples were collected immediately before the 1000-hr and 2200-hr doses on day six for KAP and MST and at 0200 and 0600 hr on day seven for SOLN to verify the patient was at steady state with respect to plasma morphine trough concentrations. The patient was admitted to the Pain Management Unit on the evening of day six to ensure that the two morphine doses prior to the intense blood sampling period for pharmacokinetic analysis were administered at the correct time. An indwelling centrally situated venous catheter was placed at 0800 hr on day seven to allow for collection of the steady-state blood samples. Creatinine clearance was measured during the 12-hour dosing interval. The meal times were standardized for all patients as was the composition of the meals for each patient during the three detailed blood sampling periods during day seven for each formulation. All procedures for weeks two and three of the cross-over phase were identical to week one, with the exception of the morphine formulation.

BLOOD SAMPLING AND DRUG ANALYSIS

Hourly blood samples were collected from 1000 to 2200 hr on day seven for all three formulations. In addition, samples were collected at 30-minute intervals for two hours for the three doses at 1000-, 1400-, and 1800-hr doses for the SOLN formulation. Plasma was harvested by centrifugation and stored below –20°C until assayed. Morphine was quantitated by high-performance liquid chromatography (HPLC) with electrochemical detection (Todd et al. 1982), while M3G and M6G were measured using HPLC with UV detection (Milne et al. 1991). The lower level of quantitation was 2.5 µg/l, 50 µg/l, and 20 µg/l for morphine, M3G, and M6G, respectively. Assays were linear over the ranges, 2.5–100 µg/l, 50–2000 µg/l, and 20–500 µg/l for morphine, M3G, and M6G, respectively. The morphine metabolite concentrations were measured in the plasma samples of six patients randomly selected from the 24 evaluable patients.

STATISTICS

The following pharmacokinetic parameters were derived from the plasma morphine concentration–time curves for each morphine formulation: maximum plasma morphine concentration (Cmax), time at which Cmax occurs (Tmax), area under the plasma morphine concentration–time curve (AUC), time that the plasma morphine concentration equaled or exceeded 0.75 Cmax, and the fluctuation in plasma morphine concentrations according to the formula, Fluctuation = (Cmax – Cmin)/Css, where Cmin and Css are the minimum and average steady-state plasma morphine concentrations, respectively, during a 12-hour dosing interval. Differences between formulations for these pharmacokinetic parameters were assessed using ANOVA with treatment and sequence effects included in the analysis. Because of the small number of subjects, data relating to the morphine metabolites were compared by Friedman's test using the Wilcoxon signed-rank test for pairwise comparisons if a significant difference was found. To examine possible differences in time profiles of plasma morphine concentrations, AUC was determined for each time interval, 0–4, 4–8, and 8–12 hours, during the period of sampling. These were compared for the three formulations using a two-factor (formulation × time interval) repeated measures ANOVA. Following a significant formulation × time interval interaction, formulations were compared, pair-wise, within each time interval, using paired *t*-tests.

A *P* value of less than 0.05 was required to reject the null hypothesis.

RESULTS

The mean age and weight of the patients who enrolled in the study were 65 years (range 39–85 years) and 66 kg (range 44–110 kg), respectively. The 24-hour morphine dose during the study was 142.5 ± 75.6 mg (mean ± SD, range 40–320 mg).

Fig. 1 shows the plasma morphine concentration (μg/l) as a function of time (hours) following the 1000-hr dose on day seven for each of the three formulations in the same patient. This profile is essentially similar to the plot of mean plasma morphine concentrations for all 24 patients for the three formulations. The similar morphine concentrations in the 1000- and 2200-hr plasma samples for each formulation indicates that the patients were at steady state when these pharmacokinetic determinations were made. Further, the trough plasma concentrations measured in samples collected before the pharmacokinetic study (two doses) for each formulation provide additional evidence to support this contention (data not shown).

The plasma morphine concentration–time profile for the immediate-release SOLN formulation shows wide fluctuation in morphine concentration

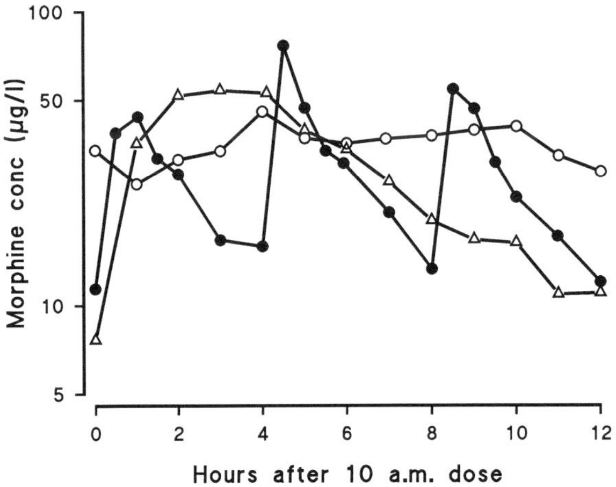

Fig. 1. Plasma morphine concentration (μg/l) as a function of time (hours) at steady state (i.e., after seven days) following the administration of the same morphine dose (120 mg per 24 hours) to an individual patient as encapsulated sustained-release pellets (KAP; open circles), as controlled-release tablets (MST; open triangles), and as immediate release solution (SOLN; filled circles). The treatments were randomized, each formulation was administered for seven days with the pharmacokinetic characterization on day seven (see Methods).

over the 12-hour sampling interval. The trough morphine concentrations prior to each dose are consistent. The profile for the MST shows a slower increase in morphine concentration after the dose relative to the SOLN, but a peak morphine concentration similar to that observed for SOLN. The actual morphine concentrations are similar for MST and SOLN at the 1000- and 2200-hr sampling times. Therefore, the fluctuations in peak and trough morphine concentrations are similar for four-hour SOLN and 12-hour MST (vide infra).

In contrast, the profile of plasma morphine concentration for KAP is quite different, showing minimal fluctuation over the dosing interval. There is a marked difference in the trough morphine concentrations for KAP relative to MST and SOLN, remembering the morphine dose was identical for each formulation.

Table I summarizes the relevant pharmacokinetic parameters of Cmax, Tmax, time that the plasma morphine concentration equaled or exceeded 0.75 Cmax, fluctuation in morphine concentration over the 12-hour dosing interval, and AUC for the three formulations in the 24 evaluable patients. The mean Cmax values (dose normalized to a nominal dose of 100 mg) were 32.2 μg/l, 42.3 μg/l, and 48.3 μg/l for KAP, MST, and SOLN, respectively. There was no significant difference between the MST and SOLN formulations, but KAP was significantly different from the other two formulations (represented as $K \neq [M = S]$ in Table I).

The mean Tmax values were 5.7 hours, 3.4 hours, and 0.7 hours for KAP, MST, and SOLN, respectively, and all three values were significantly different from each other ($K \neq M \neq S$). This finding indicates that both the solid dosage forms (i.e., KAP and MST) have modified release characteristics relative to SOLN. However, the variability in Tmax for KAP (coefficient of variation (CV = 52%) was much greater than for the other controlled-release formulation, MST (CV = 27%). This occurred because the flat plasma morphine concentration–time profile for KAP depicted in Fig. 1 was observed in many patients. In fact, the Tmax value could have easily varied by two to four hours in these patients because of the similar numerical value of many of the morphine concentrations around Tmax as indicated by the range of Tmax value for KAP (0–10 hours) relative to MST (1–5 hours) and SOLN (0.5–2 hours).

The pharmacokinetic parameter of time $\geq$ 0.75 Cmax has been proposed as an index of the control the formulation exerts over the release of the pharmacologically active agent prior to absorption. The larger the value, the flatter the release profile as can clearly be seen by comparing the different formulations in Fig. 1. It is obtained by drawing a line parallel to the x-axis at 75% of the Cmax value for each formulation and then determining the time

Table I
Pharmacokinetic parameters for three morphine formulations, Kapanol, MST Continus, and solution, at steady state in cancer patients (mean ± SD, n = 24)

	Cmax*	Tmax†	Time ≥ 0.75 Cmax‡	Fluctuation§	AUC#
Kapanol**	32.2 ± 14.9	5.7 ± 3.0	9.1 ± 2.8	60 ± 22	297.7 ± 136.5
MST Continus††	42.3 ± 17.4	3.4 ± 0.9	3.1 ± 1.3	151 ± 40	272.4 ± 104.9
Solution	48.3 ± 22.1	0.7 ± 0.4	4.4 ± 1.5	173 ± 151	267.6 ± 87.5
Significance‡‡	K ≠ (M=S)	K ≠ M ≠ S	K ≠ (M=S)	K ≠ (M=S)	K = M = S

* Cmax represents the dose normalized (to 100 mg) maximum plasma morphine concentration (µg/l) in the dosing interval, i.e., 1000–2200 hr.

† Tmax represents the time at which Cmax occurs (hour).

‡ Time ≥ 0.75 Cmax represents the time period (hour) that the plasma morphine concentration equalled or exceeded 75% of Cmax (see Results).

§ Fluctuation represents the fluctuation in plasma morphine concentration according to the formula fluctuation = (Cmax – Cmin)/Css, where Cmin and Css are the dose-normalized minimum and average steady-state plasma morphine concentration, respectively. Css = AUC/12 where 12 represents the dosing interval.

\# AUC represents the dose-normalized area under the plasma morphine concentration–time curve (µg • hr/1) from 1000–2200 hr for each formulation and was calculated using the trapezoidal rule.

** Kapanol is an encapulated pellet sustained-release morphine formulation developed and manufactured by FH Faulding & Co. Limited, Australia.

†† MST Continus is a controlled-release tablet morphine formulation manufactured by Napp Laboratories.

‡‡ Statistical differences were assessed using ANOVA with treatment and sequence effects taken into consideration and a level of significance of at least $P < 0.05$. A representation of K ≠ (M=S) means there was no significant difference between MST Continus (M) and solution (S), while Kapanol (K) was significanlty different than the other two formulations for that parameter.

that the plasma morphine concentration is at or above this line. The mean (± SD) value for the four-hour SOLN (4.4 ± 1.5 hours) was not significantly different from that for 12-hour MST (3.1 ± 1.3 hours). In contrast, the value for KAP (9.1 ± 2.8 hours) was significantly greater than for MST or SOLN.

Similarly, the fluctuation in plasma morphine concentrations over the 12-hour dosing interval for each formulation reflects the release characteristics of the different formulations, because it relates the difference in dose-normalized (to 100 mg) maximum and minimum morphine concentrations to the average steady-state concentration during the dosing interval (see Methods). There was no significant difference in the extent of fluctuation in plasma morphine concentrations between MST and SOLN, but KAP had significantly less fluctuation than did the other two formulations and was only 40% of the MST value (Table I). There was no significant difference in the dose-normalized (to 100 mg) AUC values between the three formulations, indicating that an equivalent amount of morphine was absorbed from SOLN, KAP, and MST.

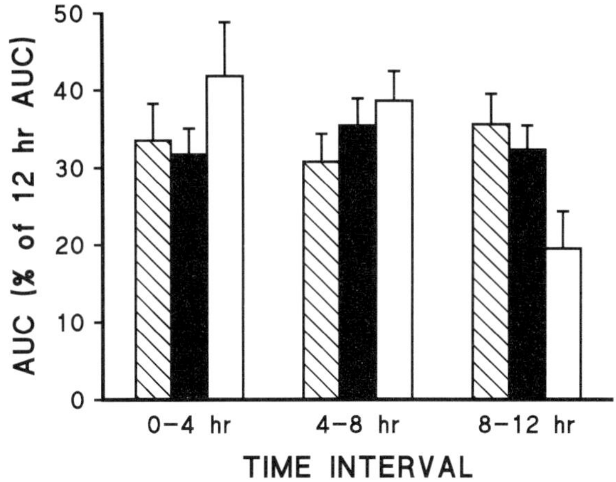

Fig. 2. AUC (% of the 12-hour AUC) as a function of time interval (i.e., 0–4, 4–8, and 8–12 hour) at steady-state for the three formulations. SOLN, KAP, and MST are represented by the slashed, solid, and open bars, respectively. The bars represent mean ± SD for the 24 patients. The AUC was calculated using the trapezoidal rule for each four-hour time interval.

When the AUC data were subdivided into four-hour time intervals (0–4, 4–8, and 8–12 hours), marked differences between the formulations became apparent (Fig. 2). We chose the four-hour time intervals because the SOLN doses were administered with this as the dosing interval. There was a highly significant ($P < 0.0001$) formulation × time interval interaction for the dose-normalized AUC values (repeated measures ANOVA), indicating marked differences between the three formulations in the time profile of plasma concentrations. The AUC for the 0–4 hour time interval for MST was significantly greater than either SOLN ($P < 0.001$) or KAP ($P < 0.0001$), but there was no difference between the latter two formulations. The AUC for the 4–8 hour time interval for SOLN was significantly less than either KAP ($P < 0.003$) or MST ($P < 0.0001$), but there was no difference between the two modified-release formulations ($P = 0.95$). Further analysis of these data indicated that while the mean ratio for either the first or third time interval (relative to the second time interval) for SOLN was 1.05 and 1.17, respectively, considerable interpatient variability existed in these ratios. The AUC for the 8–12 hour time interval for MST was significantly less for both SOLN and KAP ($P < 0.0001$).

The plasma concentrations of the two major morphine metabolites, M3G and M6G, were determined in the plasma samples from six randomly selected patients. Fig. 3 shows the plasma morphine, M3G, and M6G concentrations

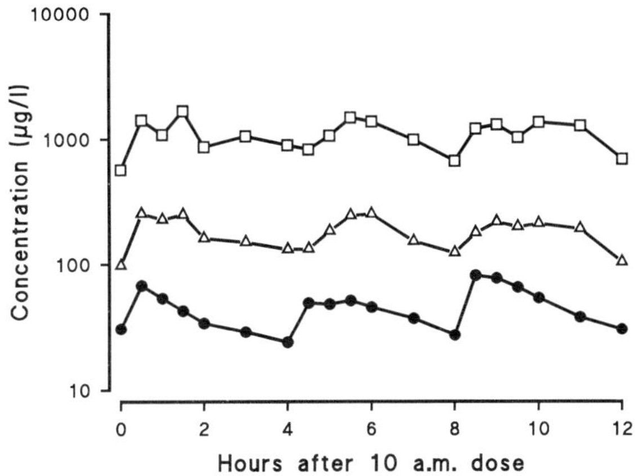

Fig. 3. Plasma morphine (filled circles), M6G (open triangles), and M3G (open squares) concentrations at steady state as a function of time (hours) after the administration of morphine as an immediate-release solution (SOLN, 23.3 mg at 1000, 1400, and 1800 hr on day seven) to an individual patient (see Methods).

(µg/l) as a function of time (hours) from 1000 to 2200 hr following the solution doses (23.3 mg at 1000, 1400, and 1800 hr, i.e., 140 mg/24 hours) at steady state in an individual patient. There was a high degree of congruence in the profiles of the plasma concentrations as a function of time for the parent drug and the two major metabolites. This high degree of congruence was also apparent for the two modified-release formulations (data not shown).

There were no significant differences in the dose-normalized AUC values for morphine, M3G, and M6G between the KAP, MST, and SOLN phases, suggesting that the extent of conversion of morphine to M3G and M6G was independent of the formulation when administered in the fasting state. There were also no significant differences between the formulations in the M6G/morphine or M3G/morphine molar ratios (Table II). For example, the mean M6G/morphine molar ratios were 4.0, 4.4, and 4.3 for KAP, MST, and SOLN, respectively, while the equivalent data for M3G/morphine ratios were 24.4, 27.1, and 25.9 respectively (Table II).

There were significant differences between the formulations in the time ≥ 0.75 Cmax values for both M6G and M3G. For example, the time ≥ 0.75 Cmax for the active metabolite M6G following KAP was significantly greater than that for SOLN, even though the mean values appear similar (Wilcoxon signed-rank test). In all 6 patients, the time ≥ 0.75 Cmax for KAP was larger than the value for SOLN. Further, the time ≥ 0.75 Cmax for M6G for SOLN

Table II
Metabolite /morphine molar ratios and time ≥ 0.75 Cmax for M6G and M3G for three morphine formulations, Kapanol, MST Continus, and solution, at steady state in cancer patients (mean ± SD, n = 6)

	M6G		M3G	
	Molar Ratio*	Time ≥0.75 Cmax†	Molar Ratio*	Time ≥ 0.75 Cmax†
Kapanol‡	4.0 ± 0.6	8.4 ± 1.9	24.4 ± 5.6	6.3 ± 3.9
MST Continus§	4.4 ± 0.9	3.8 ± 0.8	27.1 ± 5.0	2.5 ± 1.5
Solution	4.3 ± 0.8	7.3 ± 2.0	25.9 ± 4.7	7.7 ± 2.0
Significance#	K = M = S	K ≠ S ≠ M	K = M = S	S ≠ M

* Molar ratio represents either morphine metabolite /morphine molar ratio.
† Time ≥ 0.75 Cmax is the time period (hours) that the plasma morphine metabolite concentration equalled or exceeded 75% of Cmax for that metabolite for each formulation.
‡ Kapanol is an encapsulated pellet sustained-release morphine formulation developed and manufactured by FH Faulding & Co. Limited, Australia.
§ MST Continus is a controlled-release tablet morphine formulation manufactured by Napp Laboratories.
\# Statistical differences among the three formulations were assessed by Friedman's test, groups being compared pairwise by the Wilcoxon signed-rank test following a significant result. Differences were considered to be significant if P was less than 0.05. A representation of K ≠ (M=S) means there was no significant difference between MST Continus (M) and solution (S), while Kapanol (K) was significantly different than the other two formulations for that parameter.

was significantly greater than for MST. In contrast, the only difference in the time ≥ 0.75 Cmax for M3G, the inactive metabolite, was that the value for SOLN was significantly larger than for MST (Table II).

A creatinine clearance determination was made during the 12-hour steady-state pharmacokinetic aspect of the study for each formulation to investigate the relationship between the concentrations of M6G or M3G and renal function. Fig. 4 shows the M6G/morphine molar ratios as a function of creatinine clearance (ml/sec) for the three morphine formulations in all six patients with morphine metabolite determinations. There was no clear relationship between the two parameters within the range of creatinine clearance studied: i.e., 0.8–1.6 ml/sec in this study compared with the normal range of 1.5–2.0 ml/sec.

DISCUSSION

This study evaluated cancer patients with moderate to severe pain who required the prescription of morphine as part of the pharmacological regimen. The morphine dose (per 24 hours) was optimized in the lead-in phase for each

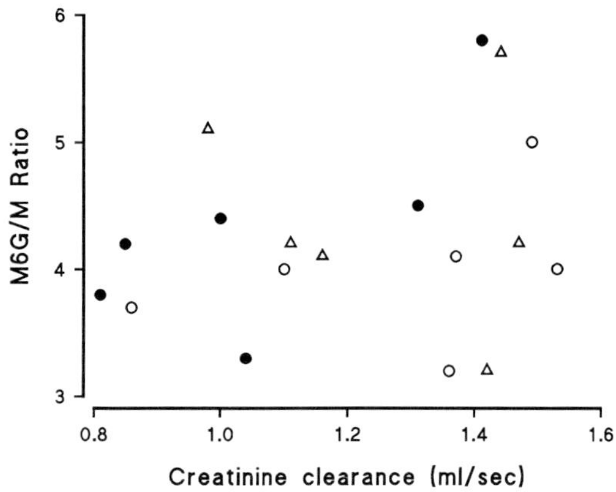

Fig. 4. M6G/morphine molar ratios as a function of creatinine clearance (ml/sec) determined during the characterization of the plasma morphine concentration–time curves following the administration of KAP (open circles), MST (open triangles), and SOLN (solid circles) for seven days for each formulation (see Methods).

patient but remained constant during the three periods of the cross-over phase, each lasting seven days. This study used an eightfold dosage range rather than the fixed-dose protocol that is frequently used in volunteer studies of an equivalent design. While other drugs, including those with analgesic activity but excluding all opioid agonists, were allowed during the study, the dose and frequency of such drugs could not be altered.

Frequent blood samples were collected to enable an accurate characterization of the plasma morphine concentration–time curve for the three formulations such that the derived pharmacokinetic parameters should realistically reflect changes that can be attributed to the formulations. In addition, validated chemical analytical techniques were used to quantitate morphine and metabolite concentrations.

Previously published pharmacokinetic parameters for SOLN (Gourlay et al. 1989; Thirlwell et al. 1989) and MST (Thirlwell et al. 1989) are almost identical to the data obtained in this study. Inspection of Fig. 1 reveals substantial differences among the three formulations, also confirmed in Table I. There were no significant differences between 12-hour MST and four-hour SOLN for any pharmacokinetic parameters except Tmax. The significantly longer Tmax, smaller Cmax, smaller fluctuations (40% of MST) in plasma morphine concentrations during the dosing interval, and almost threefold greater time ≥ 0.75 Cmax for KAP relative to MST indicate that KAP has a superior sustained-release morphine profile than does MST.

There is much debate in the literature regarding the role of the active metabolite M6G in the analgesic effect observed following morphine administration. This study demonstrated a marked congruence between either M6G or M3G plasma concentrations and morphine concentrations (Fig. 3) and the resultant derived pharmacokinetic parameters for the glucuronides. Therefore, not unexpectedly, the time ≥ 0.75 Cmax for M6G for KAP relative to MST (Table II) was similar to the equivalent values for morphine for these formulations (Table I).

Osborne and colleagues (1992) showed a direct relationship ($r = 0.81$) between M6G clearance and creatinine clearance in 20 patients with cancer pain. Two of the patients in their study had creatinine clearances of 0.3 ml/sec; a level much lower than in our patients and which is normally associated with frank renal failure. In those two patients, there was a delayed elimination of M6G with resultant increased plasma concentrations. Data from our patients suggest that modest changes in renal function, but not approaching levels associated with renal failure, do not effect M6G elimination. Prolonged sedation and other opioid side effects observed in morphine-treated patients with renal failure have been ascribed to M6G accumulation.

In conclusion, there were marked similarities in the pharmacokinetic parameters characterizing 12-hour MST and four-hour SOLN (the only exception was Tmax), while the parameters for 12-hour KAP were significantly different from MST and SOLN with the exception of AUC. This similarity would be expected as it would indicate an equivalent extent of morphine absorption from each of the formulations. However, Fig. 2 clearly shows that MST releases proportionally more morphine than KAP in the 0–4 hour time interval, equivalent amounts of morphine in the 4–8 hour time interval, but significantly less morphine in the 8–12 hour time interval (mean SD ± 8–12-hour AUC as a percentage of 0–12 hour AUC was 32.5 ± 3% for KAP and 19.5 ± 4.8% for MST). These results are consistent with the clinical finding that MST must be administered at eight-hour intervals in a percentage of patients. These findings indicate that KAP has a sustained-release profile that is superior to MST, resulting in a flat plasma morphine concentration–time profile, which will allow KAP to be administered at 12-hour intervals.

ACKNOWLEDGMENTS

The authors greatly appreciate the skilled assistance of the following PMU senior registrars: A. Beaumont, A. Russell, F. Fugere, and M. Hooper. We also happily acknowledge the generous help from the PMU nursing staff. Raelene West, Faulding Pharmaceuticals, provided constructive criticism and encouragement as well as organizing the onerous pharmaceutical industry side of the project. We thank Dr. A. Somogyi, Department of Clinical Pharmacology, University of Adelaide, for doing the assays of morphine, M3G, and M6G in plasma samples from this study.

REFERENCES

Gourlay, G.K, Plummer, J.L., Cherry, D.A., Foate, J.A. and Cousins, M.J., Influence of a high fat meal on the absorption of morphine from oral solutions, Clin. Pharmacol. Ther., 46 (1989) 463–468.

Grond, S., Zech, D., Schug, S.A., Lynch, L. and Lehmann, K.A., Validation of World Health Organisation guidelines for cancer pain relief during the last days and hours of life, J. Pain Symptom Manage., 6 (1991) 411–422.

Milne, R.W., Nation, R.L., Reynolds, G.D., Somogyi, A.A. and Van Crugten, J.T., High performqance liquid chromatographic determination of morphine and its 3- and 6-glucuronide metabolites: improvements to the method and application to stability studies, J. Chromatog., 565 (1991) 457–464.

Osborne, R., Thompson, P., Joel, S., Trew, D., Patel, N. and Slevin, M., The analgesic activity of morphine-6-glucuronide, Br. J. Clin. Pharmacol., 34 (1992) 130–138.

Thirlwell, M.P., Sloan, P.A., Maroun, J.A., Boos, G.J., Besner, J-G., Stewart, J.H. and Mount, B.M., Pharmacokinetics and clinical efficacy of oral morphine solution and controlled-release morphine tablets in cancer patients, Cancer, 63 (1989) 2275–2283.

Todd, R.D., Muldoon, S.M. and Watson, R.L., Determination of morphine in cerebrospinal fluid and plasma by high-performance liquid chromatography with electrochemical detection, J. Chromatogr., 232 (1982) 101–110.

Correspondence to: Geoffrey K. Gourlay, Pain Management Unit, Flinders Medical Centre, Bedford Park, South Australia 5042, Australia. Tel: 61-8-204-5511; Fax: 61-8-374-1758.

Part VIII

Pharmacology of Pain Control

Proceedings of the 7th World Congress on Pain,
Progress in Pain Research and Management, Vol. 2,
edited by G.F. Gebhart, D.L. Hammond, and T.S.
Jensen, IASP Press, Seattle, © 1994.

43

Effects of Intravenous Ketamine and Alfentanil on Hyperalgesia Induced by Intradermal Capsaicin

Karen M. Park, Mitchell B. Max, Elaine Robinovitz,[a] Richard H. Gracely, and Gary J. Bennett

Neurobiology and Anesthesiology Branch, National Institute of Dental Research, and the [a]Clinical Center Nursing Department; National Institutes of Health, Bethesda, MD, USA

INTRODUCTION

The phenomena produced by intradermal capsaicin have been well characterized (Simone et al. 1989; LaMotte et al. 1991). After the initial intense pain, areas of hyperalgesia and allodynia surrounding the injection site persist for several hours. Some of these symptoms are like those described by patients with nerve injury, including intense burning pain, allodynia evoked by light stroking, and hyperalgesia evoked by punctate stimuli such as a safety pin or stiff nylon filament. Psychophysical (LaMotte et al. 1991; Treede and Cole 1993; Gracely et al. 1993) and neurophysiological evidence in animals (Dougherty and Willis 1992) and humans (Torebjörk et al. 1992) suggests that the intense discharge of nociceptors initiated by capsaicin injection causes neurons in the central nervous system (CNS) to become abnormally sensitized, accounting at least in part for the allodynia and hyperalgesia. Some neuropathic pain patients also demonstrate altered central sensory processing (Campbell et al. 1988; Price et al. 1989; Gracely et al. 1992). These parallels suggest that intradermal capsaicin may be useful as a model for allodynic and hyperalgesic conditions involving the sensitization of central neurons.

The intradermal capsaicin model also has appeal because it potentially links one of the posited mechanisms of central sensitization—N-methyl-D-aspartate (NMDA) receptor activation (Dubner 1991; Wilcox 1991)—to clinically testable therapies. For example, the spinal administration of NMDA receptor antagonists in animals prevents the central sensitization produced by the peripheral injection of capsaicin (Dougherty et al. 1992; Ault and Hildebrand 1993; Nagy et al. 1993). NMDA receptor antagonists can reduce pain and hyperalgesia in neuropathic pain patients (Byas-Smith et al. 1993; Backonja et al. 1994) and in animal models of neuropathic pain (Tal and Bennett 1993; Mao et al. 1993; Yamamoto and Yaksh 1992). Thus, a similar reduction in intradermal capsaicin-induced hyperalgesia produced by NMDA receptor antagonists would further support intradermal capsaicin as a tool for testing new treatments for neuropathic pain.

We studied the NMDA receptor antagonist ketamine in an initial pharmacological study using the intradermal capsaicin model. We also examined another centrally acting drug, the μ-receptor opioid agonist alfentanil, because opioids inhibit nociceptive neurons in the CNS, reduce pain behavior in animal models of neuropathic pain (Attal et al. 1991), and reduce pain intensity in experimental pain models (Gracely 1991) and in some patients with chronic neuropathic pain (Rowbotham et al. 1991; Cherny et al. 1994; but see also Arner and Meyerson 1988).

METHODS

SUBJECTS

Twelve normal subjects participated in a randomized, double-blind, crossover study. The study was approved by the Clinical Research Institutional Review Board of the National Institute of Dental Research, and all the patients gave informed, written consent. Each subject received three treatment trials (ketamine, alfentanil, or placebo) at least 24 hours apart.

INTRADERMAL CAPSAICIN

Capsaicin (Fluka) was prepared using the method described by Simone et al. (1989). Twenty-five μl (250 μg) of capsaicin was injected using a 0.5-ml syringe fitted with a 27-gauge 3/8 inch intradermal beveled needle. All injections were made on the left volar forearm. The injection site for the first treatment trial was approximately 5 cm proximal from the wrist crease along the midline of the volar surface. The injection site and points that were 2.5 and 10 cm proximal from the injection site were marked with a felt-tip pen.

These marks were then traced onto an 8 × 11-inch acetate sheet along with markings of veins and other landmarks. We used these tracings to determine the injection site for subsequent days. Each subsequent injection was 2 cm proximal from the previous one. Movement of the injection site is necessary because capsaicin injection desensitizes primary afferents at the immediate site of injection (LaMotte et al. 1991).

ASSESSMENT OF PAIN, HYPERALGESIA, AND ALLODYNIA

For the first 10 minutes after capsaicin injection, the ongoing pain level was assessed using a 0–100 numerical scale at two-minute intervals. At 10-minute intervals thereafter, the research nurse (E.R.) carried out the following sequence of measurements:

1. Ongoing pain: 100 mm visual analog scale (VAS).
2. Area of allodynia: A cotton gauze pad was swept at a rate of 1 cm/sec toward the injection site, starting at a point approximately 10 cm away. This procedure was repeated in a pattern of eight radial spokes. With movement along each radial spoke, the subject was asked to report when the sensation became different and annoying. This process produced a plot of the area of allodynia (Simone et al. 1989).
3. Area of pinprick hyperalgesia: A standard safety pin was applied until dimpling of the skin was just visible. The subject was asked to report when the sensation became different and painful. As with the cotton gauze, the safety pin mapping produced a plot of the area of pinprick hyperalgesia.

DRUG INFUSION

Treatments with ketamine, alfentanil, or saline placebo were given from 25 to 60 minutes after capsaicin injection, and consisted of an initial intravenous bolus followed by a continuous infusion and additional boluses at the same dosage as the first, titrated as described below. The rationale for the additional bolus doses was to rapidly titrate subjects to the maximal attainable drug effect short of significant cognitive changes. Doses were adjusted proportionate to weight. Doses for a 70-kg subject were: ketamine, 5 mg bolus + 40 mg/hr infusion; alfentanil, 500 μg bolus + 4000 μg/hr infusion; or saline placebo, 1 ml + 20 ml/hr infusion. Additional bolus doses were repeated at 35, 45, and 55 minutes after capsaicin injection if the subject appeared alert, responded quickly and appropriately to questions, and gave an affirmative response to the query, "Do you feel like you could safely drive a car right now?"

The primary period of interest in each study was 0–105 minutes after capsaicin injection. Because pinprick hyperalgesia persists for many hours (LaMotte et al. 1991), the time after 105 minutes could be used to carry out a separate pilot study exploring the hypothesis that benzodiazepines reduce the transmission of nociceptive input from A-delta nerve fibers (Clavier et al. 1992). A-delta nerve fibers are the thinly myelinated fibers largely responsible for mediating pinprick-evoked sensation in normal skin (Greenspan 1991). Nine subjects who were thought to have received a placebo infusion because they had minimal side effects from 25 to 60 minutes received 1–4 mg midazolam at 145 minutes. The midazolam was titrated over five minutes until they reported drowsiness or gave a negative response to the query, "Do you feel like you could safely drive a car right now?" The benzodiazepine antagonist flumazenil, at one-tenth of the midazolam dose, was given at 165 minutes to determine whether it reversed midazolam's putative effects on pain.

ABORTED TRIALS

If the area of pinprick hyperalgesia 20 minutes after capsaicin was less than approximately 500 mm^2, no infusion was given and the subject returned on another day.

STATISTICAL ANALYSIS

For each treatment session, baseline pain, allodynia, or pinprick hyperalgesia scores were calculated as the mean of the observations at 10 and 20 minutes after capsaicin injection. Data from subsequent points were converted to percent of baseline. The primary outcome measures defined at the beginning of the study were the mean areas and intensities of pain averaged over the 30, 40, 50, and 60-minute points. Comparisons of ketamine vs. placebo and alfentanil vs. placebo were made using repeated measures analyses of variance followed by two-tailed Dunnett's tests.

RESULTS

ONGOING PAIN

Baseline value, i.e., average of the 10- and 20-minute data points, for ongoing pain was 53 ± 3 (mean ± S.E.M.) on a 100-point scale. Ongoing pain decreased during both ketamine and alfentanil infusions compared to placebo ($P < 0.01$ for both comparisons; Table I).

PINPRICK HYPERALGESIA

Baseline area of pinprick hyperalgesia was 1923 ± 82 mm^2 (mean ± S.E.M.). Saline infusion had no effect. Both ketamine and alfentanil (Table I) reduced the area of pinprick hyperalgesia by approximately one-third during the infusion ($P < 0.01$ for each drug vs. placebo).

ALLODYNIA

Baseline area of allodynia was 592 ± 133 mm^2 (mean ± S.E.M.). Allodynia was shorter-lived and showed greater variability than did pinprick hyperalgesia. Allodynia persisted for at least 20 minutes after 21/41 injections, allowing comparison of placebo to ketamine in six and alfentanil in five subjects (Table I). Alfentanil significantly reduced allodynic area during infusion ($P < 0.05$). Ketamine tended to reduce the area of allodynia, but the effect was not statistically significant. Forty-one injections were required instead of 36 (3 for each of 12 subjects) because five were aborted by the criteria noted in Methods.

MIDAZOLAM

Nine subjects (who had received placebo infusions from 25 to 60 minutes) received open-label midazolam at 145 minutes (mean dose 3.4 mg; range 1–4 mg), followed by flumazenil at 165 minutes (mean dose 0.3 mg; range 0.1–0.4 mg). The baseline area of pinprick hyperalgesia was defined as

Table I
Effect of drug infusions on hyperalgesia, allodynia, and ongoing pain

	30–60 minutes after Capsaicin (% baseline, mean ± S.E.M.)		
	Ketamine	Alfentanil	Placebo
Ongoing pain	49 ± 7	34 ± 4	75 ± 8
Pinprick hyperalgesia, area	67 ± 7	66 ± 7	101 ± 7
Allodynia to cotton gauze	31 ± 13 (n = 6)	17 ± 7 (n = 5)	62 ± 17

the average of the 125- and 140-minute time points and the drug effect was expressed a percent of baseline for the average of the 150- and 160-minute points. The pinprick hyperalgesic area did not change significantly with midazolam; the mean ± S.E.M. was 121 ± 20% of baseline ($P = 0.31$, paired t-test). Allodynia was present in only one subject at 125 minutes, obviating analysis of midazolam's effect on allodynia. The mean area of pinprick hyperalgesia at 170 and 180 minutes, just following flumazenil, was 96 ± 16% of baseline.

SIDE EFFECTS

All 12 subjects developed subjective effects with ketamine and alfentanil, as a feeling of mild intoxication was an endpoint for drug titration. One subject reported "feeling drunk" with placebo. Pruritus occurred in four subjects with alfentanil and in none with ketamine. Two subjects reported during a ketamine infusion a feeling "as though my limbs are not connected to my body," or "as though I am in a test tube."

DISCUSSION

Our results suggest promise for intradermal capsaicin as a model for testing drug therapies that might be useful in clinical pain states involving central sensitization. The model was efficient enough to detect a 30% reduction in the area of pinprick hyperalgesia in a group as small as 12 subjects. The variability of the occurrence and duration of allodynia made the model less sensitive for detecting drug effects on this sensory abnormality, however.

Both ketamine and alfentanil affect cerebral function, requiring consideration of the possible nonspecific sedative effect of these drugs on the reports of subjects. Even though the treatment design did not have a formal control for this effect, the data from the midazolam-flumazenil pilot study are relevant to this issue. In nine subjects, the midazolam given at 145 minutes after capsaicin had no significant effect on the area of pinprick hyperalgesia even though subjects were titrated to the same level of sedation as they had been with ketamine and alfentanil. Despite this result, however, we cannot fully rule out the possibility that the sedative effect of either drug caused the reduction of hyperalgesia and pain.

A-delta and C nociceptor primary afferents predominantly mediate sensation to pinprick in normal skin (Greenspan 1991). We infer that capsaicin-induced pinprick hyperalgesia is partly mediated by altered central processing rather than by peripheral afferent sensitization because: (1) Pinprick hyperalgesia was present up to 12 cm from the capsaicin injection site. Although sensitized C polymodal nociceptors (Baumann et al. 1991) and heat hyperalgesia (LaMotte et al. 1991) develop in a small ring of skin adjacent to the capsaicin intradermal bleb, neither phenomenon occurs outside this small ring, which makes up most of the area of pinprick hyperalgesia. This observation argues that sensitization of C polymodal nociceptors cannot account for pinprick hyperalgesia in the latter area. (2) Pinprick hyperalgesia lasts as long as 48 hours after capsaicin (LaMotte et al. 1991; Simone 1989), in contrast to hyperalgesia due to sensitization of primary afferents after a burn, which subsides after two hours (Meyer and Campbell 1981).

Even though we found a reduction in ongoing pain, pinprick hyperalgesia, and allodynia, the effect was only partial at drug doses that would limit daily activities. This recurring clinical limitation has been reported in chronic neuropathic pain patients treated with opioids (Arner and Meyerson 1988) and NMDA receptor antagonists (Backonja et al. 1994; Byas-Smith et al. 1993; Kristenson et al. 1992). Only if additional measures can be found to improve efficacy or reduce toxicity will NMDA receptor antagonists be able to realize the potential seen in animal models (Tal and Bennett 1993; Yamamoto and Yaksh 1992; Mao et al. 1993). Such approaches might include combining NMDA receptor antagonists and opioids, finding NMDA receptor antagonists more specific for analgesia, or infusing the drugs via the intrathecal or epidural route.

ACKNOWLEDGEMENT

The authors thank Ronald Dubner for his review of the manuscript.

REFERENCES

Arner, S. and Meyerson, B.A., Lack of analgesic effect of opioids on neuropathic and idiopathic forms of pain, Pain, 33 (1988) 11–24.

Attal, N., Chen, Y.L., Kayser, V. and Guilbaud, G., Behavioural evidence that systemic morphine may modulate a phasic pain-related behaviour in a rat model of peripheral mononeuropathy, Pain, 47 (1991) 65–70.

Ault, B. and Hildebrand, L.M., Effects of excitatory amino acid receptor antagonists on a capsaicin-evoked nociceptive reflex: a comparison with morphine, clonidine and baclofen, Pain, 52 (1993) 341–349.

Backonja, M., Arndt, G., Gombar, K.A., Check, B. and Zimmerman, M., Response of chronic neuropathic pain syndromes to ketamine: a preliminary study, Pain, 56 (1994) 51-57.

Baumann, T.K., Simone, D.A ., Shain, C.N. and LaMotte, R.H., Neurogenic hyperalgesia: the search for the primary cutaneous afferent fibers that contribute to capsaicin-induced pain and hyperalgesia, J. Neurophysiol., 66 (1991) 212–217.

Byas-Smith, M.G., Max, M.B., Gracely, R.H. and Bennett, G.J., Intravenous ketamine and alfentanil in patients with chronic causalgic pain and allodynia. In: Abstracts: 7th World Congress on Pain. IASP Press, Seattle, 1993, pp. 454–455.

Campbell, J.N. , Raja, S.N., Meyer, R.A . and MacKinnon, S.E., Myelinated afferents signal the hyperalgesia associated with nerve injury, Pain, 32 (1988) 89–94.

Cherny, N.I., Thaler, H.T., Friedlander-Klar, H., Lapin, J., Foley, K.M., Houde, R. and Portenoy, R.K., Opioid responsiveness of cancer pain syndromes caused by neuropathic or nociceptive mechanisms: a combined analysis of controlled single dose studies, Neurology, 44 (1994) 857–861.

Clavier, N., Lombard, M.-C. and Besson, J.-M., Benzodiazepines and pain: effects of midazolam on the activities of nociceptive non-specific dorsal horn neurons in the rat spinal cord, Pain, 48 (1992) 61–71

Dougherty, P.M. and Willis, W.D., Enhanced responses of spinothalamic tract neurons to excitatory amino acids accompany capsaicin-induced sensitization in the monkey, J. Neurosci., 12 (1992) 883–894.

Dougherty, P.M., Palecek, J., Paleckova, V., Sorkin, L.S. and Willis, W.D., The role of NMDA and non-NMDA excitatory amino acid receptors in the excitation of primate spinothalamic tract neurons by mechanical, chemical, thermal, and electrical stimuli, J. Neurosci., 12 (1992) 3025–3041.

Dubner, R., Neuronal plasticity and pain following peripheral tissue inflammation or nerve injury. In: M.R. Bond, J.E. Charlton and C.J. Woolf (Eds.), Proceedings of the VIth World Congress on Pain. Pain Research and Clinical Management, Vol. 4. Elsevier, Amsterdam, 1991, pp. 263–276.

Gracely, R.H., Experimental pain models. In: M.B. Max, R.K. Portenoy and E.M. Laska (Eds.), The Design of Analgesic Clinical Trials. Advances in Pain Research and Therapy, Vol. 18. Raven Press, New York, 1991, pp.33–48.

Gracely, R.H., Lynch, S.A. and Bennett, G.J., Painful neuropathy: altered central processing maintained dynamically by peripheral input, Pain, 51 (1992)175–194.

Gracely, R.H., Barcellos, S.A., Saltzman, S.J., Byas-Smith, M.G., Max, M.B. and Bennett, G.J., Ab mechano-allodynia and cold hyperalgesia following large doses of intradermal capsaicin(abstract), Society of Neuroscience, 19 (1993) 1073.

Greenspan, J.D. and McGillis, S.L.B., Stimulus features relevant to the perception of sharpness and mechanically evoked cutaneous pain. Somatosens. Mot. Res., 8 (1991) 137–147.

Kristenson, J.D., Svensson, B. and Gordh, T., Jr., The NMDA receptor antagonist CPP abolishes neurogenic "windup pain" after intrathecal administration in humans, Pain, 51 (1992) 249–253.

LaMotte, R.H., Shain, C.N., Simone, D.A. and Tsai, E.-F.P., Neurogenic hyperalgesia: psychophysical studies of underlying mechanisms, J. Neurophysiol., 66 (1991) 190–211.

LaMotte, R.H., Lundberg, L.E.R. and Torebjörk, H.E., Pain, hyperalgesia and activity in nociceptive C units in humans after intradermal injection of capsaicin, J. Physiol., 448 (1992) 749–764.

Mao, J., Price, D.D., Hayes, R.L., Lu, J., Mayer, D.J. and Frenk, H., Intrathecal treatment with dextrorphan or ketamine potently reduces pain-related behaviors in a rat model of peripheral mononeuropathy, Brain Res., 605 (1993) 164–168.

Meyer, R.A . and Campbell, J.N., Myelinated nociceptive afferents account for the hyperalgesia that follows a burn to the hand, Science, 213 (1981) 1527–1529.

Nagy, I., Maggi, C.A., Dray, A., Woolf, C.J. and Urban, L., The role of neurokinin and N-methyl-D-aspartate receptors in synaptic transmission from capsaicin-sensitive primary afferents in the rat spinal cord in vitro, Neuroscience, 52 (1993) 1029–1037.

Price, D.D., Bennett, G.J. and Rafii, A., Psychophysical observations on patients with neuropathic pain relieved by a sympathetic block, Pain, 36 (1989) 273–288.

Rowbotham, M.C., Reisner-Keller, L.A. and Fields, H.L., Both intravenous lidocaine and morphine reduce the pain of postherpetic neuralgia, Neurology, 41 (1991) 1024–1028.

Simone, D.A., Baumann, T.K. and LaMotte, R.H., Dose-dependent pain and mechanical hyperalgesia

in humans after intradermal injection of capsaicin, Pain, 38 (1989) 99–107.
Tal, M. and Bennett, G.J., Dextrorphan reliefs neuropathic heat-evoked hyperalgesia, Neurosci. Lett., 151 (1993) 107–110.
Torebjörk, H.E., Lundberg, L.E.R. and LaMotte, R.H., Central changes in processing of mechanoreceptive input in capsaicin-induced secondary hyperalgesia in humans, J. Physiol.,448 (1992) 765–780.
Treede, R.D. and Cole, J.D., Dissociated secondary hyperalgesia in a subject with a large fibre sensory neuropathy, Pain, 53 (1993) 169–174.
Wilcox, G.L., Excitatory neurotransmitters and pain. In: M.R. Bond, J.E. Charlton and C.J. Woolf (Eds.), Proceedings of the VIth World Congress on Pain. Pain Research and Clinical Management, Vol.4. Elsevier, Amsterdam, 1991, pp. 97–117.
Yamamoto, T. and Yaksh, T.L., Comparison of the antinociceptive effects of pre- and posttreatment with intrathecal morphine and MK801, an NMDA antagonist, on the formalin test in the rat, Anesthesiology, 77 (1992) 757–763.

Correspondence to: Mitchell B. Max, M.D., NIDR/NIH Pain Research Clinic, National Institutes of Health, Building 10, Room 3C-405, Bethesda, MD 20892, USA. Tel: 301-496-5483 or 6695; Fax: 301-402-4347.

Proceedings of the 7th World Congress on Pain,
Progress in Pain Research and Management, Vol. 2,
edited by G.F. Gebhart, D.L. Hammond, and T.S.
Jensen, IASP Press, Seattle, © 1994.

44

Dissociation of Analgesia and Anesthesia under Ketamine

Burkhart Bromm, Eckehard Scharein, Eberhard Kochs,[a] and Jochen Schulte am Esch[a]

Institute of Physiology and [a]Department of Anesthesia, University Hospital Eppendorf, Hamburg, Germany

INTRODUCTION

The aim of general anesthesia is the induction and maintenance of sufficient relief of pain during surgery. The action of the anesthetic, however, is unspecific: it induces loss of sensory experience, skeletomotor control, memory, and consciousness. Furthermore, it influences the autonomic nervous system, modulating cardiac and respiratory functions, blood pressure, and circulation in brain and body. In the clinical setting, these vegetative parameters are continuously recorded in order to monitor whether the depth of anesthesia is sufficient, but the question remains: Which of them reflects the degree of pain relief?

The analgesic state is defined as the absence of pain, but the loss of consciousness prohibits a report of pain. How can we be sure that the neuronal activity induced by the surgeon is not felt by the patient? This question is of special meaning since we know that most anesthetics do not inhibit nociceptive activity, i.e., they do not develop antinociceptive properties. Under most anesthetics, the nociceptive input elicited under surgery reaches central structures in the midbrain, thalamus, and cortex, as has been shown in many animal experiments (see, e.g., Willis 1985; Angel 1991).

In the past decade, the continuous recorded electroencephalogram (EEG) has been successfully used to monitor the depth of anesthesia. Information about the functional state of the brain can facilitate the individual tailoring of anesthetics (for detailed review see Schwilden and Stoeckel 1993). Furthermore,

EEG monitoring indicates cerebral risks or disturbances in the course of surgery or anesthesia (Prior 1979). Power spectral density of the spontaneous EEG gives some evidence about the vigilance level of the subject under medication (Steriade 1991). For example, it is well known that the EEG is characteristically modified in deep sleep (Berger 1938).

Evoked brain potentials are stimulus-induced changes of the spontaneous EEG. The late cognitive components elicited by pain-inducing stimuli have been shown to correlate highly with the subject's verbal report of pain (for review see Chudler and Dong 1983). These late pain-related components have therefore been used as tools for the comparative evaluation of the analgesic potency of drugs (for review see Bromm and Desmedt 1994). The method of late brain potential analysis in response to experimental pain-inducing stimuli has also been applied in the operating room to monitor the degree of analgesia under general anesthesia (Kochs et al. 1990, 1991). The appearance of pain-related components gives evidence for the cortical processing of nociceptive information, even if the subjects are unable to indicate their pain, as, for example, under general anesthesia.

This chapter summarizes results of new methods in pain measurement based on a close cooperation between anesthesiology and neurophysiology, in the laboratory as well as in the operating theater. We investigate combined measures of spontaneous and stimulus-evoked EEG in order to differentiate between specific pain-reducing components and nonspecific vigilance-reducing components of general anesthesia. In this study, the phencyclidine derivative ketamine was used because it is known to be an anesthetic with an analgesic component, but lacking respiratory depression. Therefore, low-dose ketamine (0.25 to 0.50 mg/kg) is clinically used to provide adequate analgesia for postoperative pain treatment without inducing major anesthetic effects (Austin 1976; Clements and Nimmo 1981; White et al. 1982). Ketamine induces a state of sedation, immobility, and amnesia and a marked analgesia; the duration of unconsciousness is brief (Marshall and Wollman 1985).

METHODS

Twenty healthy volunteers (11 females and 9 males, 28 ± 5 years, free of neurological or psychiatric disorders, who had not taken centrally acting drugs for at least 3 months) were randomly assigned to two groups: the placebo group received 5 ml saline iv. (n = 10); the test group received 0.5 mg/kg ketamine iv. (racemate; n = 10). The study was approved by the Institutional Ethics Committee; written informed consent was obtained.

Pain was induced experimentally by intracutaneously applied brief electrical shocks (Fig. 1, inset). A small hole is drilled through the horny layer of the skin. This way the transition resistance is reduced by a factor of 10 (Bromm and Meier 1984), and the electrical stimulus is directly fed to the most superficial terminals, the thinnest A-delta-fibers and C-fibers of the nociceptive system (Munger and Halata 1983). A stinging and burning phasic pain is elicited, very similar to a stimulation of tooth pulp and essentially different from that induced by conventional superficially applied electrical currents. Stimuli were continuously applied during the entire session, with random intensities (two- and threefold individual pain threshold) and random interstimulus intervals (between 10 and 20 s). Randomization is an essential prerequisite to minimize effects of habituation (for details see Bromm 1989).

We stimulate, for example, the afferents in the left middle finger tip and measure the stimulus-evoked changes in the EEG (Fig. 1). Cognitive components, consisting of a large negativity with a latency of 150 ms (N150) and a positivity at 250 ms (P250) can be seen after averaging over a series of stimulus repetitions. By means of principal component analysis, we were able to identify typical pain-related components in these waveforms that appear if the subject reports pain. If the subject is distracted or his or her vigilance is decreased, the late potentials are decreased as well (for details see Bromm 1989).

The EEG was continuously recorded from vertex (Cz) versus linked earlobes (A1-A2), the electro-oculogram from supra- and infraorbital leads. All electrode impedances were kept below 5 kOhm (at 12 Hz). The records were stored on analog tape (Store 7DS, Racal) and digitized off-line (200 Hz sampling rate). The system bandpass was set at 0.5 and 30 Hz. Pain-related brain potentials were calculated by averaging the 500 ms poststimulus EEG segments over 40 subsequent stimuli. Prestimulus EEG segments of 5 s duration were analyzed by computing the power in selected frequency bands (delta: 1.0–4.0 Hz; theta: 4.0–8.0 Hz; alpha: 8.0–12.0 Hz; beta: 12.0–30.0 Hz) using a fast Fourier transformation after weighting the data with a Kaiser window (40 dB side lobe suppression).

On the subjective level, pain sensation induced by the intracutaneous stimulus was rated verbally on a numerical scale ranging from 0 (no sensation) to 10 (unbearable pain). The pain threshold was given the value 4. The subjects were familiarized with the experimental setup for 30 minutes. To exclude major habituation effects, the first 10 minutes (40 stimuli) were excluded from the analysis. The subsequent 10 minutes (40 stimuli) were used to assess the baseline values and to build the first brain potential. Then either placebo or ketamine 0.5 mg/kg were given iv., and all data were recorded for another 50 minutes, resulting in five averaged brain potentials. Individual

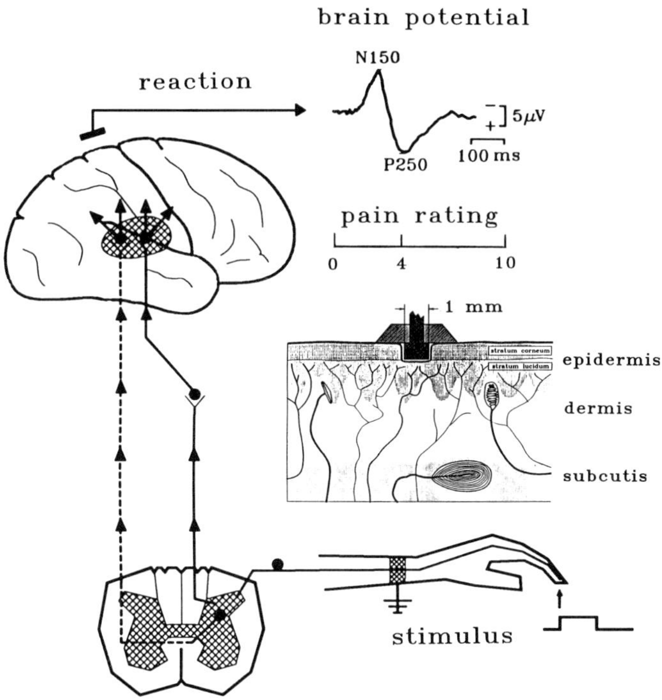

Fig. 1. The experimental pain model. Pain is induced by intracutaneously applied current pulses; by drilling a hole through the stratum corneum the electrode is directly placed in the vicinity of A-delta- and C-fibers, which belong to the nociceptive system (inset). The stimulus is applied to the left middle fingertip; it induces a sharp and stabbing painful sensation. Measured are the ratings and the brain potentials in response to each stimulus. Pain related brain potentials consist of a large vertex negativity with a maximum at 150 ms (N150), followed by a positive component (P250).

thresholds for detection and pain were determined by four series of increasing and decreasing stimulus intensities.

In the same way, the following variables were recorded simultaneously for 10 minutes before and 50 minutes after placebo or ketamine administration: heart rate (HR, beats per minute; RM300, Honeywell), mean arterial blood pressure (MAP, mm Hg; Dinamap, Critikon), end-tidal PCO_2 (P_{ETCO_2}, mm Hg; Datex, Hoyer) and arterial oxygen saturation (Sa_{O_2}, %; Nellcor 100, Draeger).

RESULTS AND DISCUSSION

Fig. 2 illustrates the effects of ketamine on one of the ten volunteers. The pain ratings in response to the intracutaneous stimuli of two- and threefold

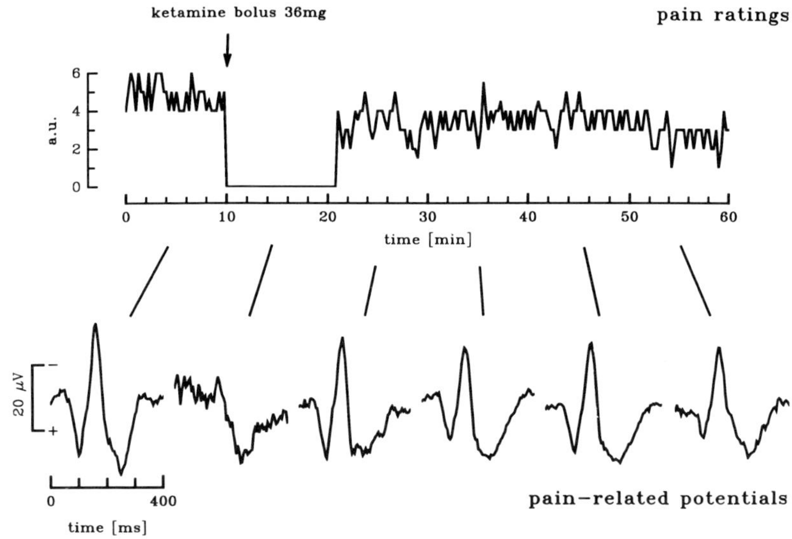

Fig. 2. Pain ratings and pain-related cerebral potentials after a bolus injection of 36 mg ketamine (single case). **Top,** the pain ratings in response to intracutaneous stimuli of two- and threefold pain threshold strength (randomly applied) are given (a.u. = arbitrary units; see Methods). Immediately after ketamine injection, a brief (11 min) state of unconsciousness occurs. Later on the pain ratings remained decreased by approximately 25%. **Bottom,** the brain potentials in response to the painful stimuli; they also are reduced by approximately 25% at the end of the period of measurement, but were still present in the state of unconsciousness.

individual pain threshold are shown in the upper graph. Because of intensity randomization, the ratings vary between 4 and 6. Before medication, the stimuli were clearly in the pain range. After injection of 0.5 mg/kg ketamine hydrochloride, the subject became unconscious within 1 to 2 minutes, and no pain ratings were available. This subject became conscious 11 minutes later, and pain ratings were again available. But these ratings in response to the same stimulus intensities were now reduced by at least 25% compared to the premedication level.

The corresponding brain potentials evoked by these stimuli in the same subject are given in Fig. 2, bottom. The initial mean peak-to-peak amplitude difference, an estimate of analgesic effects, was 46 mV. After ketamine injection it was reduced by 25% until the end of the period of measurement. This long-lasting effect of ketamine on the pain-related brain potentials corresponded well with the pain ratings. The striking result, however, was that in the beginning phase of unconsciousness, the evoked potentials did not completely disappear like the pain ratings did. In spite of unconsciousness, the antinociceptive component of the anesthetic was not sufficient; the subject might have felt pain but could not remember it.

The data of all the 10 subjects who received ketamine were similar (Fig. 3). In each subject, the pain ratings (top) and the peak-to-peak amplitude differences of the late brain potential components N150 and P250 (bottom) exhibit a comparable time course: a brief state of unconsciousness of varying duration and a long-lasting reduction of evoked brain potentials and pain ratings. Subjects under ketamine became unconscious within 65 ± 13 sec and were unresponsive for 6 ± 3 min. Furthermore, in all subjects brain potentials appeared during the state of unconsciousness, and these potentials had the same mean amplitude as those at the end of the period of measurement, for which pain ratings were again available.

Late brain potentials in response to pain-inducing stimuli reflect the subject's pain. They have therefore been used in many studies for the comparative evaluation of analgesic efficacy of drugs (Chapman et al. 1982; Buchsbaum 1984; Kobal and Raab 1986; Bromm et al. 1989; for review see Bromm and Desmedt 1994). In particular, a high correlation (r = 0.93) has

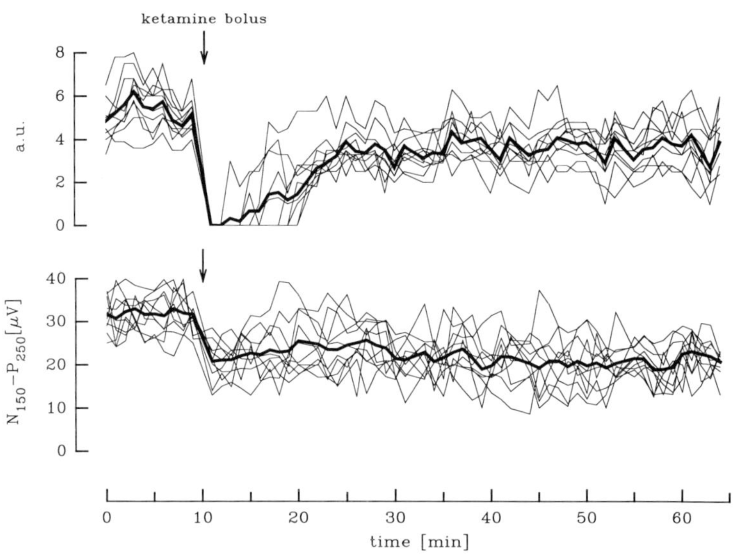

Fig. 3. Pain ratings and pain-related cerebral potentials after a bolus injection of 0.5 mg/kg ketamine. Pain ratings (**above**) and amplitude differences of the N150–P250 components (**below**) in response to the pain-inducing stimuli are given for the 10 subjects; bold lines indicate the grand means. In all subjects ketamine injection causes unconsciousness with an individually different duration (between 1 and 10 min); thereafter a long-lasting state of reduced pain sensation occurs. In contrast, in no subject did the brain potentials in response to the stimuli disappear completely. Instead they were reduced by approximately 25% during the entire period of measurement. The ketamine-induced analgesia is reflected in both pain ratings (so far as measurable) and evoked brain potentials.

been found between drug-induced pain relief and a decrease in pain-related brain potentials for narco-analgesics (Bromm et al. 1986) as well as for NSAIDs (Bromm et al. 1992). From these data we can conclude that the analgesic efficacy of 0.5 mg/kg ketamine corresponds to that of 100 mg tramadol.

The ketamine effects mentioned above were statistically significant compared to the effects in the placebo group (analysis of variance). In the placebo group, pain ratings did not change significantly over the observation period ($F_{5,45}$ = 0.38, $P[F]$ = 0.86). In contrast, in the ketamine group a significant time effect was observed ($F_{5,45}$ = 62.5, $P[F] < 0.001$). In all subjects the state of unconsciousness was brief, and pain ratings could again be recorded at most 11 minutes after ketamine administration (3.4 ± 0.3); these ratings were significantly lower than the corresponding values in the placebo group (4.9 ± 0.5).

The brain potential measured in the first 10 minutes after ketamine injection in Fig. 2 looks as if it was amplified. This is due to an alteration of the spontaneous EEG activity after ketamine application (Schwarz et al. 1974; Tatsuno et al. 1990). Fig. 4 shows the smoothed single-trial EEG spectra as grand means averaged over all subjects of the study for placebo (top) and for ketamine (bottom). The bolus injection was given after 10 minutes of baseline recordings. In the placebo group, the alpha activity remained constant over time. In contrast, ketamine administration resulted in loss of alpha activity and a fivefold increase in theta activity within the first minutes after bolus injection. Thereafter, both effects disappeared. The increased theta activity vanished within about 10 minutes, whereas the recovery of alpha activity took considerably longer. Statistical analysis revealed that the theta effect was gone within at most 20 minutes after ketamine injection, whereas alpha activity did not regain baseline values over the observation period of 50 minutes. In contrast, no ketamine effect was seen upon delta and beta activity, and no significant changes were observed in the EEG spectra of the placebo group.

The time courses of the ketamine effects on the measured cardiovascular variables for the 10 subjects are given in Fig. 5. Cerebral blood flow, blood pressure, and heart rate exhibited a marked transient increase after bolus injection of ketamine, reaching maximal values within 2 to 5 minutes. Thereafter the values slowly dropped, reaching a steady-state level after about 20 to 30 minutes. The level during the entire postmedication period—about 1 hour—was significantly higher than the premedication level . The Sa_{O_2} and P_{ETCO_2} values after drug treatment were not different from premedication values. Using analysis of variance, no significant time effect was noted in either group.

In a last step, we compared the ketamine-induced periods of unconsciousness with those of altered neurophysiological and cardiovascular parameters. The result indicates that the duration of unconsciousness in each individual

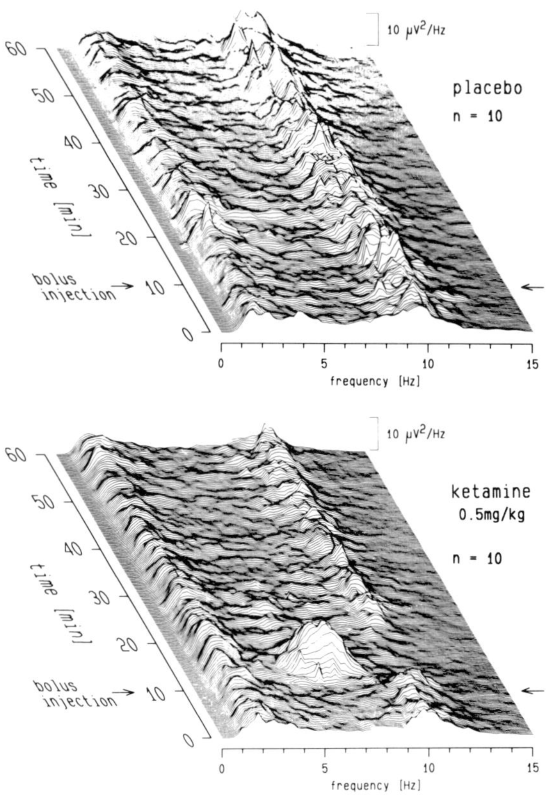

Fig. 4: Power spectra of spontaneous EEG activity after a bolus injection of 0.5 mg/kg ketamine (grand means over 10 subjects). Each prestimulus EEG segment of 5 seconds duration was subjected to Fourier transformation. Then the single trial power spectra were smoothed and averaged over all 10 subjects. Immediately after ketamine bolus injection, the alpha rhythm (8–12 Hz) is destroyed and a large increase in theta power (4–7 Hz) appears. The duration of these effects is individually different. The duration of the period of increased theta power correlates highly ($P < 0.001$) with the duration of unconsciousness.

corresponds to the period of increased theta activity in the spontaneous EEG (Fig. 6). The ketamine-induced enhancement of theta power can be used to predict the duration of the state of unconsciousness with high accuracy ($r = 0.96$). In contrast, the changes over time in the cardiovascular variables, such as blood pressure, heart rate, and cerebral blood flow, were in parallel with changes in alpha activity of the spontaneous EEG.

SUMMARY AND CONCLUSIONS

Sedative effects of general anesthesia can be assessed by frequency analysis of spontaneous EEG activity, a routine method in clinical applications (Prior 1979; Angel 1991). New experiments give evidence that the degree of pain relief under anesthesia can be monitored by the attenuation of brain potentials evoked by painful stimuli (Kochs et al. 1990, 1991). Combined analysis of

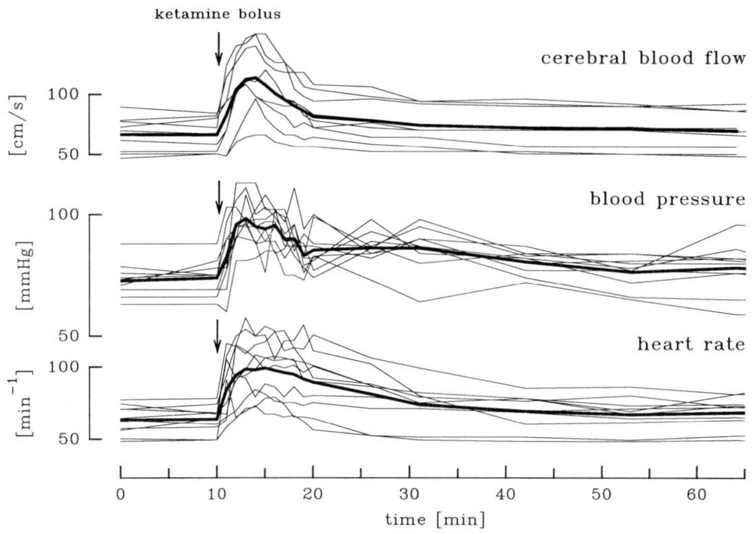

Fig. 5: Cardiovascular variables after a bolus injection of 0.5 mg/kg ketamine (10 subjects with grand mean). Cerebral blood flow, blood pressure, and heart rate after ketamine bolus injection (0.5 mg/kg) are given for the 10 subjects (bold line = mean value). In all subjects ketamine induces a transient strong activation of the cardiovascular system for a period of 10 to 15 min. Afterward a steady state of moderately enhanced activity is maintained.

spontaneous and evoked EEG allows the differentiation between analgesic and anesthetic components of general anesthesia, as demonstrated in experiments with ketamine, a so-called dissociative anesthetic that has analgesic properties but induces often unpleasant hallucinations and worrying dreams (Austin 1976; White 1982).

In spite of the relatively low dose used here (0.5 mg/kg), ketamine induced in all 10 subjects a brief period of unconsciousness (mean 6.8 $\pm$ 3.1 min), which was accompanied by a period of enhanced theta activity in the spontaneous EEG. The duration of unconsciousness corresponded well to that of increased theta activity ($r = 0.96$). Furthermore, ketamine induced an activation of the cardiovascular system (increased heart rate, blood pressure, and cerebral blood flow); all these effects lasted until the end of the period of measurement (postmedication 50 min), with a typical biphasic decay. A very similar time course was found in the ketamine-induced reduction of alpha activity.

The analgesic efficacy of ketamine 0.5 mg/kg (iv.), estimated from the attenuation of pain-induced brain potentials and pain ratings, corresponded to

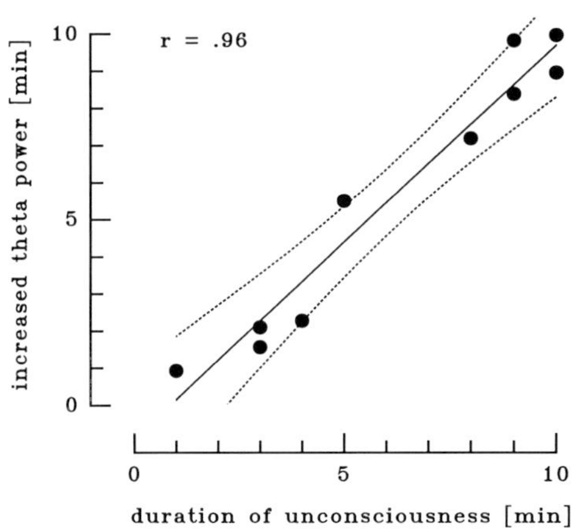

Fig. 6: Correlation between periods of unconsciousness and increased theta activity under ketamine 0.5 mg/kg (n = 10). Each point represents the results of one subject. Given are the regression line, the 95% confidence intervals, and the Pearson correlation coefficient.

that of 100 mg tramadol (p.o.). However, even during the period of unconsciousness, brain potentials could be evoked indicating the same analgesic state. In other words, ketamine anesthesia is dissociative: complete loss of consciousness, but incomplete analgesia. In anesthetized, unconscious subjects, pain-related potentials can appear if analgesia is insufficient. In particular, combined measurement of spontaneous EEG and pain-related brain potentials may be useful for the intraoperative detection of inadequate analgesia.

ACKNOWLEDGMENTS

Supported by the Deutsche Forschungsgemeinschaft (Br 310/20-1).

REFERENCES

Angel, A., Adventures in anaesthesia, Exp. Physiol., 76 (1991) 1–38.

Austin, T.R., Ketamine-hydrochloride: a potent analgesic, Br. Med. J., 2 (1976) 943–946.

Berger, H., Über das Elektroenkephalogramm des Menschen, Nova acta Leopoldina, 6 (1938) 6–173.

Bromm, B. and Desmedt, J. (Eds.), Pain and the Brain: From Nociception to Cognition, Raven Press, New York, 1994.

Bromm, B. and Meier, W., The intracutaneous stimulus: a new pain model for algesimetric studies, Meth. Find. Exp. Clin. Pharmacol., 6 (1984) 405–410.

Bromm, B. and Treede, R.D., Laser-evoked cerebral potentials in the assessment of cutaneous pain sensitivity in normal subjects and in patients, Rev. Neurol. (Paris), 147 (1991) 625–643.

Bromm, B., Forth, W., Richter, E. and Scharein, E., Effects of acetaminophen and antipyrine on non-inflammatory pain and EEG activity, Pain, 50 (1992) 213–221.

Bromm, B., Meier, W. and Scharein, E., Imipramine reduces experimental pain, Pain, 25 (1986) 245–257.
Bromm, B., Meier, W. and Scharein, E., Pre-stimulus/post-stimulus relations in EEG spectra and their modulation by an opioid and an antidepressant, Electroenceph. Clin. Neurophysiol., 73 (1989) 188–197.
Buchsbaum, M.F., Quantification of analgesic effects by evoked potentials. In: B. Bromm (Ed.), Pain Measurement in Man. Neurophysiological Correlates of Pain, Elsevier, Amsterdam, 1984, pp. 291–300.
Chapman, C.R., Colpitts, Y.M., Benedetti, C. and Butler, S., Event-related potential correlates of analgesia: comparison of fentanyl, acupunture, and nitrous oxide, Pain, 14 (1982) 327–337.
Chudler, E.H. and Dong, W.K., The assessment of pain by cerebral evoked potentials, Pain, 16 (1983) 221–244.
Clements, J.A. and Nimmo, W.S., Pharmacokinetics and analgesic effects of ketamine in man, Br. J. Anaesth., 53 (1981) 27–30.
Kobal, G. and Raab W., The effects of analgesics on pain-related somatosensory potentials, Agents Actions, Suppl., 19 (1986) 75–88.
Kochs, E., Schulte am Esch, J., Treede, R.D. and Bromm, B., Evoked cerebral responses to painful stimulation during general anesthesia. In: S. Lipton, E. Tunks and M. Zoppi (Eds.), Advances in Pain Research and Therapy, Vol. 13, Raven Press, New York, 1990, pp. 99–105.
Kochs, E., Schulte am Esch, J., Treede, R.D. and Bromm, B., Modulation of pain-related somatosensory evoked potentials by general anesthesia, Anesth. Analg., 71 (1991) 225–230.
Marshall, B.E. and Wollman, H., General anesthetics. In: A. Goodman Gilman, L.S. Goodman, T.W. Rall and F. Murad (Eds.), Goodman and Gilman's The Pharmacological Basis of Therapeutics, MacMillan, New York, 1985, pp. 276–301.
Munger, B.L. and Halata, Z., The sensory innervation of primate skin, Brain Res. Rev., 5 (1983) 45–80.
Prior, P.F., Monitoring Cerebral Function, Elsevier, Amsterdam, 1979.
Ryder, S., Way, W.L. and Trevor, A.J., Comparative pharmacology of the optical isomers of ketamine in mice, Europ. J. Pharmacol., 49 (1978) 15–23.
Schwarz, M.S., Virden, S. and Scotte, D.F., Effects of ketamine on the electroencephalograph, Anaesthesia, 29 (1974) 135–140.
Schwilden, H. and Stoeckel, H., Closed-loop feedback controlled administration of alfentanil during alfentanil–nitrous oxide anaesthesia, Br. J. Anaesth., 70 (1993) 389–393.
Steriade, M., Alertness, quiet sleep, dreaming, Cereb. Cortex, 9 (1991) 279–357.
Tatsuno, J., Kawakami, Y., Suzuki, H. and Fujita, M., Ketamine induced changes in the electroencephalogram (EEG). Investigated by two-dimensional maps. In: E.F. Domino (Ed.), Status of Ketamine in Anesthesiology, NPP Books, Ann Arbor, 1990, pp. 167–180.
White, P.F., Way, W.L. and Trevor, A.J., Ketamine: its pharmacology and therapeutic uses, Anesthesiology, 56 (1982) 119–136.
Willis, W.D., The pain system: the neural basis of nociceptive transmission in the mammalian nervous system, Pain Headache, 8 (1985) 341–346.

Correspondence to: Prof. Dr. Dr. B. Bromm, Institute of Physiology, University Hospital Eppendorf, 20246 Hamburg, Germany. Tel: 49-40-4717-3182; Fax: 49-40-4717-4920.

Proceedings of the 7th World Congress on Pain,
Progress in Pain Research and Management, Vol. 2,
edited by G.F. Gebhart, D.L. Hammond, and T.S.
Jensen, IASP Press, Seattle, © 1994.

45

Serotonergic Mechanisms of Pain Control

François Cesselin, Anne-Marie Laporte,
Marie-Christine Miquel, Sylvie Bourgoin,
and Michel Hamon

INSERM U288, Neurobiologie Cellulaire et Fonctionnelle, Faculté de Médecine Pitié-Salpêtrière, Paris, France

INTRODUCTION

That the transmission of spinal information can be modulated by supraspinal neurons located in the ventromedial medulla has been known since the nineteenth century. Initial studies focused on the role of descending inhibitory systems in the centrifugal control of motor systems and spinal reflex integration. Subsequent investigations, however, demonstrated that the transmission of sensory (particularly nociceptive) messages by afferent fibers entering the dorsal horn of the spinal cord is also under the control of descending pathways originating in the ventromedial medulla (Besson and Chaouch 1987). Within this area, the raphe obscurus and raphe pallidus nuclei, along with the paraolivary nucleus, contain neurons that project mainly onto the motoneurons of the ventral horn and the autonomic nuclei. In contrast, neurons in the nucleus raphe magnus (NRM) project predominantly to the dorsal horn, including the superficial laminae and the area around the central canal (lamina X; see Hammond 1986 for a review).

As soon as it was established that among the neurons of the midbrain and medullary raphe nuclei that project to the spinal cord, those expressing serotonin (5-hydroxytryptamine, or 5-HT) are particularly abundant (see Björklund and Skagerberg 1982 for a review), the possible role of this descending 5-HT system in the modulation of nociceptive processing became the subject of special attention. The objective of this review is to take stock of the recent data concerning the involvement of serotonergic mechanisms in the control of the first relay of nociceptive messages within the dorsal horn of the spinal cord.

THE RAPHE-SPINAL SEROTONERGIC PATHWAYS

5-HT immunoreactive neurons projecting to the dorsal horn have been visualized within the rostroventromedial medulla and caudal pons, especially in the NRM, the nucleus paragigantocellularis, and the ventral portion of the nucleus gigantocellularis (Kwiat and Basbaum 1992). Although there is a contralateral contribution, 5-HT fibers projecting to the dorsal horn are mainly located in the ipsilateral dorsolateral funiculus of the spinal cord (Bullitt and Light 1989).

The 5-HT neurons have extensive collateralization at nearly all spinal cord levels. Thus, almost 90% of the medullary 5-HT neurons can be retrogradely labeled from the lumbar spinal cord (Bowker and Abbott 1990). Moreover, many individual 5-HT neurons within the medulla project not only to the spinal cord but also to supraspinal nuclei via collateral fibers (Bowker and Abbott 1990). This is notably the case for a significant proportion of 5-HT neurons in the nucleus raphe dorsalis (NRD) that project to the medial thalamus and send collaterals to the caudal spinal trigeminal nucleus or the spinal cord as well as to the cerebral cortex, nucleus accumbens, amygdala, and/or NRM (Kazakov et al. 1993; Matsuzaki et al. 1993). In addition to the bulbospinal pathways originating in the NRM, the descending serotonergic fibers issued from NRD neurons may also contribute to some modulatory mechanisms of nociceptive transmission at the spinal level (Morgan et al. 1989).

Within the dorsal horn of the spinal cord, fibers and nerve endings specifically labeled by anti–5-HT antibodies have been identified in all laminae, with the highest densities in laminae I, II, IV, V, and X (Ruda et al. 1986). Although some targets of 5-HT terminals have been identified (spinothalamic neurons in laminae I and V, lamina IV neurons, and enkephalin immunoreactive neurons; Ruda et al. 1986), only one-fifth of all 5-HT immunoreactive profiles apparently contribute to differentiated synapses within the dorsal horn (Ridet et al. 1993).

At least at the lumbar level, 5-HT terminals appear to have an exclusive supraspinal origin, because transection of the thoracic spinal cord leads to an extensive depletion of 5-HT and the disappearance of 5-HT immunoreactivity in the lumbar segments (Oliveras et al. 1977; Ruda et al. 1986). There is some evidence for a few intrinsic 5-HT cells in restricted portions of the spinal cord in monkeys (LaMotte et al. 1982), but their contribution to the spinal 5-HT fiber plexus is likely to be small.

Although numerous studies have focused on the serotonergic pathways, this is clearly not the only system that contributes to descending projections from the bulbomesencephalon to the spinal cord. Indeed, non–5-HT cells sending axons to the dorsal horn of the spinal cord have been shown to outnumber 5-HT neurons within both the rostroventral medulla and the caudal pons (Jones and Light 1992; Kwiat and Basbaum 1992). Among non–5-HT cells, cholinergic neurons do exist as large cells, notably in the NRM. Specific GABAergic neurons also contribute to the reticulo- and raphe-spinal pathways, in addition to those which synthesize both gamma-aminobutyric adic (GABA) and 5-HT in the NRM (Jones et al. 1991). Several neuropeptides are also present in the descending projections that innervate the spinal cord. Many of these peptides (substance P, somatostatin, enkephalin, thyrotropin-releasing hormone) have been shown to be colocalized with 5-HT in the same neurons within the medullary raphe nuclei (Bowker and Abbott 1990). Cholecystokinin is also a potential non–5-HT neurotransmitter of NRM neurons projecting into the dorsal horn of the spinal cord (Mantyh and Hunt 1984). Accordingly, all effects due to the stimulation (electrical, chemical, or physiological) of NRM neurons cannot be solely attributed to the activation of descending serotonergic fibers, and early data based on this approach might well have been overinterpreted regarding, for instance, the contribution of spinal 5-HT to the analgesic action of the direct electrical stimulation of NRM neurons (Sorkin et al. 1993).

5-HT RECEPTORS IN THE DORSAL SPINAL CORD

The existence of multiple receptors for 5-HT is now well established (Humphrey et al. 1993), and very probably accounts for the great variety of 5-HT actions on various cell types both in the central nervous system (CNS) and at the periphery. The receptors can be divided into four main classes, namely 5-HT_1 (with several subclasses: 5-HT_{1A}, 5-HT_{1B}, etc.), 5-HT_2, 5-HT_3, and 5-HT_4. All but the 5-HT_3 class are G protein-coupled receptors. Another distinction concerns their respective affinities for 5-HT, as 5-HT_1 receptor subtypes are characterized by a Kd value in the nanomolar range, whereas the other three classes exhibit a Kd value in the micromolar range. However, the recent discovery of novel 5-HT receptor types with high affinity for the indolamine (for instance, the 5-HT_7; Shen et al. 1993) indicated that this property is not restricted to 5-HT_1 receptors. Among the G protein-coupled 5-HT receptors, the 5-HT_{1A}, 5-HT_{1B}, 5-HT_{1E}, and 5-HT_{1F} subtypes exert their cellular actions through the inhibition of adenylate cyclase and/or the opening of K^+ channels (Miquel and Hamon 1992). Conversely, activation of the 5-$HT_{2(A,B,C)}$ receptors results in the closure of K^+ channels and the stimulation of phospholipase C, and that of 5-HT_4 receptors produces an increase in adenylate cyclase activity, and consequently the closure of other K^+ channels (Humphrey et al. 1993). The 5-HT_3 receptor is a 5-HT–gated cation channel, whose activation triggers an increased conductance for Na^+, K^+, and Ca^{2+} ions, leading to plasma membrane depolarization in cell types expressing this receptor (Yakel et al. 1990).

All the 5-HT receptors identified to date apparently exist in all mammalian species, except the 5-HT_{1B}, which has been found only in rats and mice. In other species, this particular receptor is called 5-$HT_{1D\beta}$, to account for its different pharmacological properties as compared to those of the 5-HT_{1B} type in rodents (Humphrey et al. 1993). Indeed, the distinction among the various 5-HT receptors was first achieved through pharmacological considerations, and numerous agonists and antagonists are currently available for the identification of the specific receptor type(s) responsible for a given action of 5-HT in a particular tissue or cell.

A number of selective 5-HT receptor agonists and antagonists have been radiolabeled, and have proven to be useful for the visualization and quantification of these receptors using autoradiographic and membrane binding techniques. At the spinal level, quantitative analysis of high affinity $[^3H]$5-HT binding (5-HT_1 receptors) revealed specific binding throughout the gray matter, with the highest levels of binding sites in laminae I and II of the dorsal horn, and the lowest in lamina VII of the ventral horn (Daval et al. 1987; Marlier et al. 1991; Pubols et al. 1992). There is a relatively good correspondence between the degree of $[^3H]$5-HT specific binding and the density of 5-HT–containing fibers and terminals within the dorsal horn (Oliveras et al. 1977; Daval et al. 1987).

Both autoradiographic experiments using a selective radioligand ($[^3H]$8-OH-DPAT) and immunohistochemical studies with a specific anti–5-HT_{1A} receptor antiserum (Fig. 1) showed that 5-HT_{1A} receptors (which comprise about half of all 5-HT_1 sites in the spinal cord) are concentrated within two superficial layers in the dorsal horn (Marlier et al. 1991; Radja et al. 1991; Thor et al. 1993). Variations in 5-HT_{1A} receptor density can be observed along the rostro-caudal axis; several groups reported that 5-HT_{1A} binding sites are more numerous at the lumbar and sacral levels than at the cervical and thoracic levels (Marlier et al. 1991; Thor et al. 1993). As shown in Fig. 2, similar conclusions could be drawn from studies in humans, in which 5-HT_{1A}

$5\text{-}HT_{1A}$ RECEPTOR

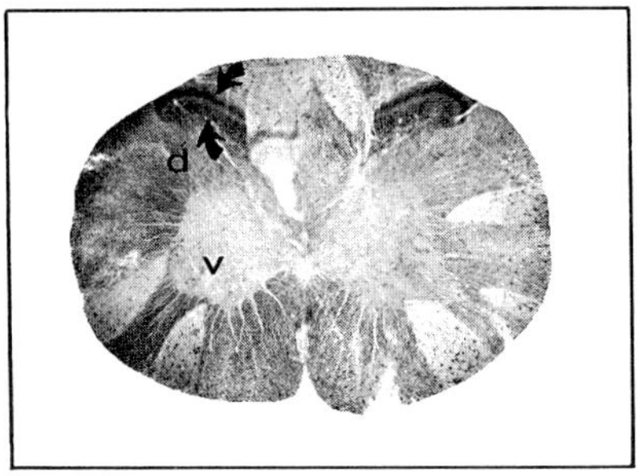

Fig. 1. Immunohistochemical labeling of $5\text{-}HT_{1A}$ receptors in the rat spinal cord. Specific anti–rat $5\text{-}HT_{1A}$ receptor antibodies (final dilution: 1/1,000; Riad et al. 1991) used with the peroxidase-antiperoxidase technique allows the visualization of $5\text{-}HT_{1A}$ receptors within two superficial layers (arrows) of the dorsal (d) horn (lamina 1 and substantia gelatinosa) at the cervical level. No $5\text{-}HT_{1A}$ receptors could be detected in the ventral (v) horn.

sites specifically labeled by [^{3}H]8-OH-DPAT almost exclusively within the superficial layers of the dorsal horn are more abundant in the lumbar cord than in cervico-thoracic segments.

Like the $5\text{-}HT_{1A}$ receptors, $5\text{-}HT_{1B}$ receptors in rats and mice and $5\text{-}HT_{1D\beta}$ receptors in humans (and other mammalian species) are concentrated within the superficial layers of the dorsal horn at the cervical, thoracic, and lumbar levels of the spinal cord (laminae I, III, and IV in the rat; Thor et al. 1993; Fig. 2). The density of $5\text{-}HT_{1B}$ sites is relatively low, however, about 35–40% that of $5\text{-}HT_{1A}$ sites all along the spinal cord (Daval et al. 1987; Thor et al. 1993). Furthermore, no clear-cut rostrocaudal gradient exists regarding the density of $5\text{-}HT_{1B}$ sites in the rat spinal cord (Thor et al. 1993).

Evidence for the presence of both $5\text{-}HT_{2A}$ and $5\text{-}HT_{2C}$ sites in the rat spinal cord has been obtained through mRNA detection (Julius et al. 1990) and receptor binding studies (Lyon et al. 1987; Marlier et al. 1991; Thor et al. 1993). In contrast to $5\text{-}HT_{1A}$ and $5\text{-}HT_{1B}$ sites, $5\text{-}HT_{2A}$ and $5\text{-}HT_{2C}$ sites are not concentrated in the superficial layers of the dorsal horn but are diffusely distributed throughout the gray matter, with some enrichment within the ventral motor neuron area in the case of $5\text{-}HT_{2A}$ receptors (Thor et al. 1993). Nevertheless, the density of $5\text{-}HT_{2A}$ sites within the rat spinal cord is very low, and several groups even concluded that binding studies with appropriate radioligands ([^{3}H]ketanserin, [^{125}I]DOI) do not allow the detection of these receptors (Blackshear et al. 1981; Leysen et al. 1982; Monroe and Smith

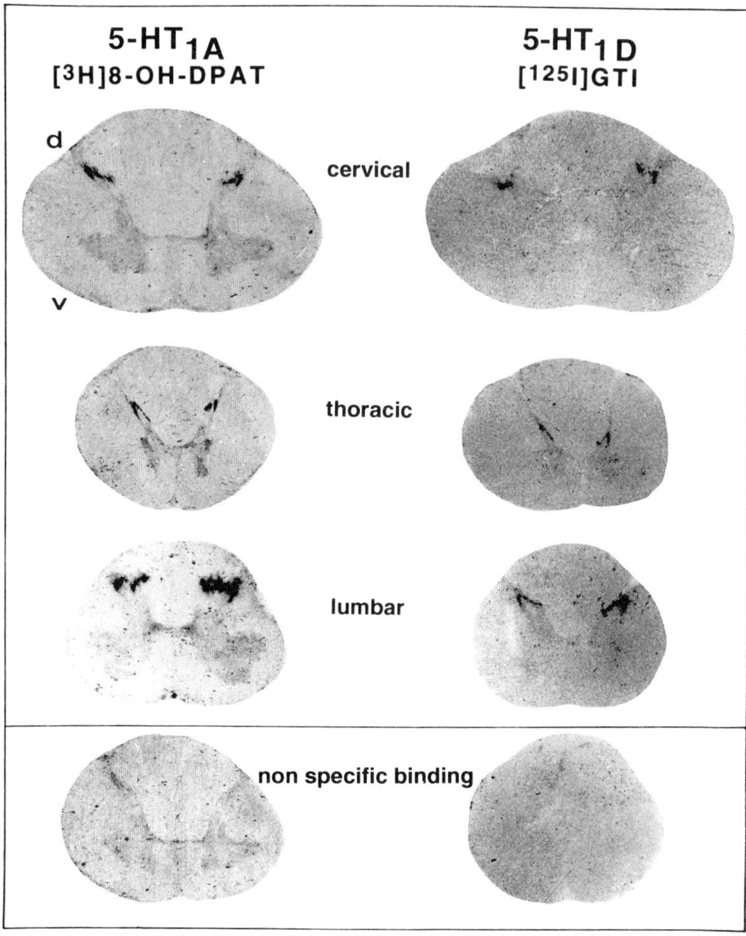

Fig. 2. Autoradiograms of sections of the human spinal cord after incubation with [^{3}H]8-OH-DPAT or [^{125}I]GTI for the specific labeling of 5-HT$_{1A}$ and 5-HT$_{1D}$ receptors, respectively. Sections at the cervical, thoracic, and lumbar levels were incubated with 1 nM [^{3}H]8-OH-DPAT or 10 pM [^{125}I]GTI, washed in appropriate buffers and water, and then exposed to ^{3}H-Hyperfilm to generate autoradiograms (see Laporte et al. 1992 for technical details). Nonspecific binding was obtained from sections at the cervical ([^{3}H]8-OH-DPAT) or lumbar ([^{125}I]GTI) level incubated with an excess (10 µM) of 5-HT. At all segments of the spinal cord, 5-HT$_{1A}$ and 5-HT$_{1D}$ receptors are concentrated within the superficial layers of the dorsal (d) horn. Only very low levels of [^{3}H]8-OH-DPAT or [^{125}I]GTI specific binding could be detected in the ventral (v) horn.

1983). Similarly, investigations in the human spinal cord showed that [^{3}H]ketanserin specific binding to 5-HT_{2A} receptors could not be found in thoracic and lumbar segments, and only a low density of such receptor sites could be labeled within the cervical cord (Laporte and Hamon, unpublished observations). In contrast, 5-HT_{2C} sites could be labeled by [^{3}H]mesulergine at all levels of the human spinal cord. Their density is 2-4 times higher in the dorsal horn than in the ventral horn all along the rostro-caudal axis. However, even in the dorsal horn, absolute values of the density (Bmax) of 5-HT_{2C} sites are only about 20% of those for 5-HT_{1A} receptors (Laporte and Hamon, unpublished observations).

It is important to keep in mind that approximately 30% of the 5-HT_1 binding sites in the rat spinal cord cannot be accounted for by 5-HT_{1A}, 5-HT_{1B}, and other identified high-affinity 5-HT receptors (Huang and Peroutka 1987; Zemlan et al. 1990). This indicates the existence of unknown sites, which have been termed 5-HT_{1S} (Zemlan et al. 1990; Zemlan and Schwab 1991; Murphy and Zemlan 1992). The 5-HT_{1S} receptors demonstrate a nanomolar affinity for 5-HT, are coupled to a GTP binding protein, and possess a unique pharmacological profile (Zemlan et al. 1990; Zemlan and Schwab 1991). They appear to be exclusively localized in the spinal cord, where their greatest density is found in the superficial laminae of the dorsal horn (Murphy and Zemlan 1992). These data strongly suggest that a specific 5-HT receptor has yet to be cloned and sequenced in the spinal cord. Its location within the key area for the transfer of nociceptive messages allows the inference that drugs acting selectively at the 5-HT_{1S} receptor might be potential pro- or antinociceptive agents with low incidence of secondary effects (in line with the probable absence of 5-HT_{1S} receptors in the brain).

The specific binding of [^{3}H]zacopride (Hamon et al. 1989) and that of an anti–5-HT_3 receptor antiserum (Fig. 3) showed that 5-HT_3 receptors are even more restricted to the superficial layers (mainly the lamina I) of the spinal cord than 5-HT_1 sites, in both the rat and the human. 5-HT_3 receptors are also highly concentrated in the nucleus of the spinal tract of the trigeminal nerve (equivalent, for the face, to the superficial layers of the dorsal horn, for the rest of the body; Waeber et al. 1988; Reynolds et al. 1991, Laporte et al. 1992).

No data are yet available regarding the possible presence of 5-HT_4 receptors in the spinal cord. However, the recent synthesis of a new selective radioligand, [^{3}H]GR 113808 (Grossman et al. 1993), should permit relevant autoradiographic investigations in the near future. Indeed, 5-HT_4 receptor agonists have been shown to exert potent antinociceptive activity through central mechanisms (Romanelli et al. 1993), and one can wonder whether they involve the first relay in the transfer of nociceptive messages, that is, the dorsal horn of the spinal cord.

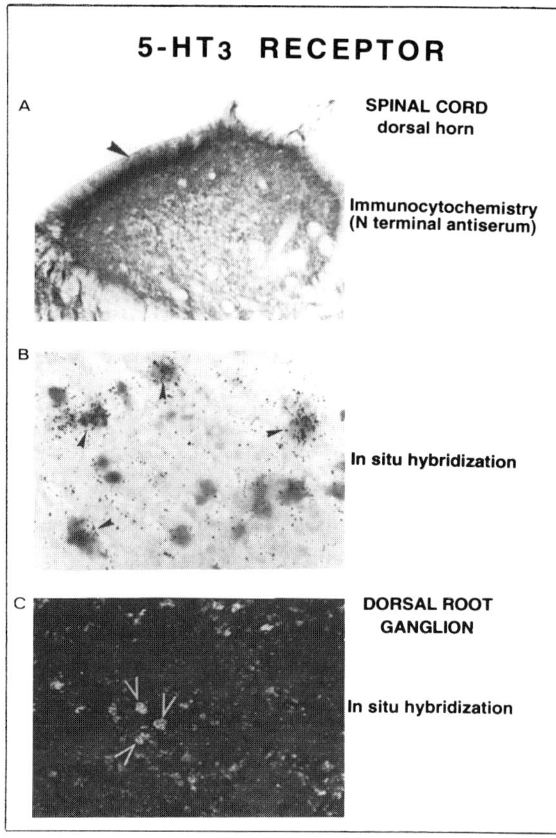

Fig. 3. Visualization of 5-HT_3 receptor protein and/or mRNA in the dorsal horn and dorsal root ganglion in rats. **A,** Immunohistochemical labeling of 5-HT_3 receptors in the cervical dorsal horn, showing the marked enrichment of these receptors in lamina 1 (arrowhead). Specific anti–5-HT_3 receptor antibodies (Turton et al. 1993) were used at a final dilution of 1:10,000 (peroxidase-antiperoxidase technique). **B,** In situ hybridization with a specific [^{35}S] labeled anti-sense riboprobe showing neurons (arrowheads) expressing the 5-HT_3 receptor mRNA in the superficial zone of the dorsal horn. **C,** Dark field photomicrograph of a section of a cervical dorsal root ganglion hybridized with the same specific anti-sense riboprobe as that used in B. Arrowheads point to cells expressing the 5-HT_3 receptor mRNA.

Because of the preferential distribution of 5-HT_{1A}, 5-HT_{1B}, and 5-HT_3 receptor binding sites in the dorsal horn, one would expect that these sites are intimately involved in the processing of sensory information. This hypothesis is somewhat sustained by data from lesion studies, which give some information about the localization of these receptors on certain spinal neuronal elements. Thus, the selective degeneration of descending serotonergic pathways in rats treated with the neurotoxin 5,7-dihydroxytryptamine (5,7-DHT) is not associated with any change in the density of 5-HT_1 binding sites in the spinal cord, indicating that these sites are probably located on postsynaptic targets of bulbo-spinal 5-HT neurons (Brown et al. 1989). Interestingly, an increased density of 5-HT_{1A} receptors has been observed after such a lesion, notably in the superficial layers of the dorsal lumbar cord (approximately 40% increase, Laporte et al., unpublished observations), leading to the suggestion that postsynaptic targets of descending serotonergic neurons adapt to the loss of 5-HT input by developing supersensitivity to 5-HT_{1A} receptor ligands. Several groups (Sawynok and Reid 1990; Eide et al. 1992) confirmed that 5,7-DHT–treated rats are supersensitive to the antinoniceptive effects of 5-HT and 5-HT_1 receptor agonists administered directly into the intrathecal space. The changes in 5-HT_{1A} receptors in these animals might, however, reflect more complex neuronal alterations than only some kind of denervation supersensitivity, because the selective lesion of descending noradrenergic systems by the alkylating agent DSP-4 [N-(2-chloroethyl)-N-ethyl-2-bromo-benzylamine, 50 mg/kg ip.] also leads to a significant enhancement in the density of 5-HT_{1A} receptors in the superficial layers of the lumbar cord in rats (Laporte et al., unpublished observations).

That the selective lesion of descending serotonergic pathways by 5,7-DHT does not reduce the density of a given receptor type is not enough to completely exclude its location at the presynaptic level. Indeed, no change in the density of spinal 5-HT_{1B} sites has been reported in 5,7-DHT–treated rats (Brown et al. 1989), in spite of the clear-cut demonstration of the existence of presynaptic 5-HT_{1B} autoreceptors on 5-HT terminals in the rat spinal cord (Brown et al. 1988; Murphy and Zemlan 1988). Accordingly, it can be concluded that the proportion of presynaptic 5-HT_{1B} autoreceptors with respect to postsynaptic 5-HT_{1B} receptors is probably very small (i.e., less than 10%). Furthermore, an increased density of the latter receptors might also occur in 5,7-DHT–treated rats, thus masking any decrease expected from the disappearance of 5-HT_{1B} autoreceptors located on serotonergic terminals. Although some behavioral studies (Archer et al. 1986, 1987; Post et al. 1986) concluded that the antinociceptive effects of intrathecally administered 5-HT and related agonists might involve some excitatory effects of these ligands on noradrenergic terminals within the dorsal horn, data from lesion studies excluded the existence of 5-HT_{1B} (and 5-HT_{1A}, see above) receptors on these terminals. Rather than a decrease, which would be expected from such a location, Laporte et al. (unpublished observations) observed a significant increase (23%) in the density of 5-HT_{1B} sites within the superficial laminae of the dorsal horn in rats whose spinal noradrenergic terminals had been lesioned by DSP-4.

It is likely that some of the 5-HT_{1A} and 5-HT_{1B} sites are on the terminals of primary afferent fibers, because degeneration of the latter due to dorsal rhizotomy (Table I) or neonatal administration of capsaicin (which preferentially destroys C-fibers) produces a 20–25% decrease in their density within the superficial layers of the dorsal horn in rats (see also Daval et al. 1987). In agreement with this conclusion, mRNAs encoding 5-HT_{1A} and 5-HT_{1B} recep-

Table I
Effect of dorsal rhizotomy on the specific labeling of 5-HT_{1A}, 5-HT_{1B}, and 5-HT_3 receptors in the dorsal horn of the rat cervical cord

	Control Rats	Rhizotomized Rats Control Side	Rhizotomized Rats Lesioned Side
5-HT_{1A} ([^{3}H]8-OH-DPAT)	25.1 ± 0.4 (74)	25.0 ± 0.4 (36)	20.3 ± 0.4* (36) −19%
5-HT_{1B} ([^{125}I]GTI)	0.89 ± 0.02 (88)	0.90 ± 0.03 (35)	0.67 ± 0.02* (35) −26%
5-HT_3 ([^{3}H]S-zacopride	28.8 ± 1.3 (56)	27.8 ± 1.2 (46)	5.6 ± 1.9* (46) −80%

Note: Unilateral dorsal rhizotomy (C_4–T_2) was performed in adult rats 10 days before death. Sections of the cervical cord were labeled with [^{3}H]8-OH-DPAT (1 nM), [^{125}I]GTI (10 pM), and [^{3}H]S-zacopride (1.2 nM) for the autoradiographic quantification of 5-HT_{1A}, 5-HT_{1B}, and 5-HT_3 receptor binding sites, respectively, within the superficial layers of the dorsal horn. Each value (± S.E.M. of the number of determinations indicated in parentheses) corresponds to the specific binding of each radioligand expressed in fmol bound per mg tissue. A significant decrease (*, $P < 0.001$) in the specific binding of each radioligand was found on the lesioned vs. the control side.

tors were recently detected in neurons of the rat dorsal root and trigeminal ganglia using in situ hybridization histochemistry (Bruinvels et al. 1992; Pompeiano et al. 1992).

The mRNA coding for 5-HT_3 receptors has also been visualized in neurons of the rat dorsal root ganglia, as well as in the dorsal horn of the spinal cord (Fig. 3; see also Tecott et al. 1993). This is congruent with the finding that dorsal rhizotomy or neonatal capsaicin treatment leads to a 50–80% decrease in the density of 5-HT_3 receptor binding sites in the superficial layers of the dorsal horn (Table I; Hamon et al. 1989; Kidd et al. 1993). There is now no doubt that a large proportion of spinal 5-HT_3 receptors are located on primary afferent fibers entering the dorsal horn of the spinal cord. Nevertheless, 5-HT_3 receptor binding sites located postsynaptically with regard to these fibers also exist within the superficial laminae of the dorsal horn (Hamon et al. 1989; Kidd et al. 1993). In situ hybridization histochemistry with a specific antisense riboprobe furthermore demonstrated that neurons expressing the 5-HT_3 receptor mRNA could be detected at this particular level of the rat spinal cord (Fig. 3).

At least three classes of 5-HT receptors, namely the 5-HT_{1A}, 5-HT_{1B} (5-$HT_{1D\beta}$ in humans), and 5-HT_3, are located on neuronal elements that participate in the transfer and/or control of nociceptive messages within the dorsal horn of the spinal cord. As discussed below, behavioral and electrophysiological data support their implication in the antinociceptive action of intrathecally administered 5-HT and related ligands in rats.

IMPLICATION OF THE RAPHE-SPINAL 5-HT PATHWAY IN THE ANTINOCICEPTIVE EFFECTS OF MORPHINE OR OF THE DIRECT ELECTRICAL STIMULATION OF BRAIN STEM SITES

The well-known inhibitory effects of direct electrical stimulation of the periaqueductal gray (PAG) on spinal noxious reflexes (Besson and Chaouch 1987) is thought to be mediated by the activation of the raphe-spinal pathway. Similarly, analgesia due to systemic morphine is believed to be partly the result of the activation of medullary neurons projecting to the spinal cord. Numerous data emphasize the contribution of 5-HT descending fibers to these processes, but it should be remembered that the descending pathways contain multiple neurotransmitters that could be released at the spinal level, with or without 5-HT, depending on the experimental conditions. This could explain, at least partly, why some of the experiments failed to reveal clearly the absolute requirement of 5-HT for the analgesic effects of central stimulation or morphine.

Earlier studies indicated that the turnover of spinal 5-HT is enhanced by the direct electrical stimulation of the NRM (Bourgoin et al. 1980), and voltametric studies have provided evidence for an increased production of 5-hydroxyindoleacetic acid (5-HIAA, the major metabolite of 5-HT) within the dorsal horn under such a treatment (Rivot et al. 1982). More recently, extracellular levels of 5-HT and 5-HIAA in the dorsal horn of the spinal cord were measured using in vivo microdialysis coupled with high-performance liquid chromatography and electrochemical detection. Thus, it could be directly demonstrated that the electrical stimulation of the NRM efficiently activates the bulbospinal serotonergic pathways (Sorkin et al. 1988). Direct electrical stimulation of the ventroposterior lateral nucleus of the thalamus also increases extracellular 5-HT concentration in the spinal cord of the monkey, presumably through an indirect activation of the raphe-spinal pathway (Sorkin et al. 1992).

Numerous pharmacological studies have shown that the analgesia as well as the inhibition of the responses of spinal dorsal horn neurons to peripheral noxious stimuli that result from chemical (by glutamate) or electrical stimulation of the PAG can be prevented—at least partially—by 5-HT depletion or intrathecal administration of 5-HT receptor antagonists (Carstens et al. 1981a; Jensen and Yaksh 1984; Paul and Phillips 1986; Liu et al. 1988). Accordingly, the release of 5-HT elicited at the spinal level by central stimulation is very probably responsible (at least in part) for the analgesic effect of this treatment.

Several lines of evidence also support the hypothesis that opioid-induced analgesia involves the activation of medullary neurons, including those containing 5-HT. In particular, the lesion of these neurons or of their terminals in the spinal cord markedly reduces the analgesic action of morphine (Yaksh et al. 1977; Proudfit 1980; Kuraishi et al. 1983; Rodriguez and Rodriguez 1989). In addition, intrathecal or systemic administration of 5-HT receptor antagonists attenuates morphine-induced analgesia (Yaksh 1979; Paul et al. 1988; Crisp et al. 1991b). The same effect has, paradoxically, been reported for the 5-HT_{1A} agonist 8-OH-DPAT (Millan and Colpaert 1991), but it is now well established that this ligand in fact reduces 5-HT neurotransmission by stimulating the somatodendritic 5-HT_{1A} autoreceptors (Hamon et al. 1988).

In spite of these well established pharmacological data, results concerning the effects of morphine on the spinal release of 5-HT are equivocal. Although previous studies concluded that morphine administration enhances the spinal release of 5-HT in awake or anesthetized animals (Yaksh and Tyce 1979; Bardon and Ruckebusch 1984), a recent investigation using in vivo microdialysis in the awake rat showed that morphine (administered either systemically or icv., even at high doses) very inconstantly modifies the release of the indolamine (Matos et al. 1992). Since behavioral analgesia was nevertheless produced in animals in which an increase in 5-HT was not observed, Matos et al. (1992) concluded that an evoked release of 5-HT in the spinal cord is not necessary for opioids to exert their analgesic action. Alternatively, it can be proposed that for some technical reason (e.g., 5-HT levels in the extracellular fluid are just at the limit of possible quantitative determination by electrochemical detectors used in microdialysis experiments), morphine-induced release of 5-HT is a regular response but cannot be detected in all animals. Indeed, as expected from such a response, the extracellular levels of 5-HIAA constantly increase as a result of morphine treatment in rats (Suzuki and Taguchi 1986; Rivot et al. 1989).

The stimulatory effect of morphine on serotonergic neurons is not limited to the descending bulbospinal pathways; evidence that the systemic administration of the opiate agonist, in a dose range producing antinociceptive effects, can evoke an increased release of 5-HT in the rat diencephalon has also been obtained (Grauer et al. 1992). Supraspinal 5-HT receptors probably also play an important role in morphine-induced antinociception. Some of these receptors could be located in the medioventral medulla. Indeed, the PAG-NRM pathway primarily contains 5-HT (Beitz 1982), and the administration of 5-HT receptor antagonists into the medioventral medulla or the PAG has been shown to reduce morphine-induced analgesia (Schul and Frenk 1991; Kiefel et al. 1992).

DOES THE DESCENDING 5-HT PATHWAY TONICALLY REDUCE NOCICEPTIVE PROCESSING AT THE SPINAL LEVEL?

Hyperalgesia consecutive to the administration of 5-HT receptor antagonists or the lesion of the raphe-spinal 5-HT system has been reported in the tail-flick and hot-plate tests (Hutson et al. 1982; Fasmer et al. 1985; Liu et al. 1988; Saito et al. 1990). In line with these observations, Rivot et al. (1987) demonstrated that 5-HT receptor antagonists increase the responsiveness of dorsal horn convergent neurons to nociceptive C-fiber stimulation. Accordingly, one can propose that 5-HT normally exerts a tonic inhibitory control on pain neurotransmission in rats.

The raphe-spinal systems also play a role in vasomotor control, however, and the decrease in tail-flick latency after the blockade of spinal 5-HT neurotransmission may well be accounted for by an increase in skin temperature occurring under this condition (Hole and Tjolsen 1993 and references therein). Furthermore, results in other tests have not confirmed the existence of a tonic inhibitory descending system (Fasmer et al. 1985). In the formalin test, hypoalgesia has even been found in mice after lesioning of the descending spinal 5-HT system with 5,6-dihydroxytryptamine (Fasmer et al. 1985; Tjolsen et al. 1991).

The problem of the existence of a tonic inhibitory control of nociception through descending serotonergic neurons is still pending. It is in fact a very difficult problem to solve because the behavioral tests that are used to assess the sensitivity to nociceptive stimuli are unavoidably stressful, and a general activation of serotonergic systems occurs under such conditions (Pei et al. 1990). Any possible tonic control by 5-HT systems may be switched over to a phasic regulatory mechanism during testing.

AT WHAT 5-HT RECEPTOR SUBTYPE(S) DOES 5-HT ACT TO MODULATE NOCICEPTION?

Depending on the dose, route of administration, species under study, and experimental procedures used to assess sensitivity to nociceptive stimuli, 5-HT may either facilitate or inhibit nociceptive transmission. The availability of selective ligands of the various 5-HT receptor subtypes made possible the identification of the receptors responsible for these various effects of the indolamine. However, the situation is still unclear, probably because all 5-HT receptors within the dorsal horn of the spinal cord are not yet known (Zemlan et al. 1990; Zemlan and Schwab 1991; Murphy and Zemlan 1992).

Numerous studies have shown that intrathecal administration of 5-HT itself produces an antinociceptive effect, as shown by an increase in tail-flick latency in mice and rats (Yaksh and Wilson 1979; Hylden and Wilcox 1983; Solomon and Gebhart 1988; Advokat 1993), which can be blocked by various 5-HT receptor antagonists injected via the same route (Yaksh and Wilson 1979; Schmauss et al. 1983; Solomon and Gebhart 1988). However, spinal 5-HT does not seem to influence pain perception in the formalin test (Abbott and Young 1988).

Evidence for the involvement of 5-HT_1, 5-HT_2, and/or 5-HT_3 receptors in the modulation of spinal nociceptive reflexes by 5-HT has been reported. Thus the antinociceptive effects of intrathecally administered 5-HT against a visceral stimulus (colorectal distension) appear to be mediated by all these receptors in the rat (Danzebrink and Gebhart 1991a). Interestingly, neither 5-HT_{1A}, 5-HT_{1B}, 5-HT_2, nor 5-HT_3 receptor agonists alone increase tail-flick latency in rats, although the increase in latency produced by 5-HT itself could be prevented by antagonists acting at any of these receptor subtypes (Crisp et al. 1991a). This suggests that concomitant stimulation of several receptor subtypes may be necessary for 5-HT to exert its antinociceptive action.

Another difficulty in identifying the various receptor subtypes responsible for the modulatory actions of 5-HT on nociception is that variable effects have been obtained with selective agonists, depending on the test used for assessing sensitivity to nociceptive stimuli. For instance, the 5-HT_{1A} receptor agonist 8-OH-DPAT was initially shown to decrease tail-flick latency when given intrathecally to rats (Solomon and Gebhart 1988; Crisp et al. 1991a). More recently, using a test adjusted for skin temperature, it was shown that neither 8-OH-DPAT nor the 5-$HT_{1A/1B}$ receptor agonist RU 24969 [5-methoxy-3-(1,2,3,6-tetrahydropyridin-4-yl)-1H-indole succinate] administered via the same route were active on tail-flick latency in rats. However, 8-OH-DPAT exhibited an antinociceptive activity in the hot-plate test (Mjellem et al. 1992). Spinal 5-HT is involved not only in nociception but also in non-nociceptive functions, such as motor control, and this may affect the response in nociceptive testing. In particular, spontaneous tail-flicks can be elicited by the systemic administration of 8-OH-DPAT, which acts on postsynaptic 5-HT_{1A} receptors at the spinal level in rats (Bervoets et al. 1993). This effect probably reflects an increased excitability of motoneurons, as demonstrated after iv. administration of this 5-HT_{1A} receptor agonist in rats (Jackson and White 1990).

Experiments in spinal rats showed that stimulation of 5-HT_{1A} and 5-HT_{1B} receptors by systemic administration of selective agonists produced opposite effects on nociceptive reflexes (Murphy and Zemlan 1990). Thus, the 5-HT_{1A} receptor agonists 8-OH-DPAT and buspirone were found to increase the receptive field area of a spinal nociceptive ventroflexion reflex after noxious levels of mechanical stimulation, whereas the 5-HT_{1B} receptor agonists m-chlorophenylpiperazine (m-CPP) and trifluoro-methylphenylpiperazine (TFMPP) produced the opposite effect. In support of antinociceptive properties of 5-HT_{1B} receptor agonists, Zemlan et al. (1988) also reported that iontophoretic application of m-CPP inhibited the glutamic acid–induced firing of dorsal horn wide-dynamic-range nociceptive units, as well as their response to noxious peripheral stimulation. El-Yassir et al. (1988) similarly found that the nonselective 5-HT_{1B} receptor agonist RU 24969 inhibited the response of wide-dynamic-range spinal units to noxious stimulation. Therefore, in contrast to 5-HT_{1A} receptor agonists, for which the situation is still unclear regarding their pro- versus antinociceptive effects (Fasmer et al. 1986; Archer et al. 1987; Eide and Tjolsen 1988), there is a general consensus on the antinociceptive influence of 5-HT_{1B} receptor stimulation at the spinal level (Alhaider and Wilcox 1993).

The involvement of 5-HT_2 receptors in the spinal antinociceptive action of 5-HT has received some support (Solomon and Gebhart 1988). In contrast, Eide and Hole (1991) concluded that the stimulation of spinal 5-HT_2 receptors facilitates the transmission of nociceptive information. Indeed, subcutaneous administration of the selective 5-HT_2 receptor antagonist, ketanserin, produces antinociception in the hot-plate and acetic acid–induced writhing tests in mice, but not in the tail-flick test. This effect could involve supraspinal 5-HT_2 receptors, however, because their stimulation may produce an inhibition of descending (including aminergic) control pathways (Barber et al. 1989; Alhaider 1991).

According to Glaum et al. (1988, 1990), spinal 5-HT_3 receptors mediate, possibly via the release of GABA (Alhaider et al. 1991), the antinociceptive effect of intrathecally administered 5-HT. The involvement of 5-HT_3 receptors in the transfer and/or control of nociception is not limited to this effect, however; the stimulation of these receptors located on peripheral sensory nerves has—in contrast—been shown to induce pain in humans (Richardson and Buchheit 1988) and produces pain-related behavior in rats (Meller et al. 1992). Thus, opposite modulations of nociception may occur through 5-HT_3 receptor stimulation, depending on the location of these receptors. Within the spinal cord, Alhaider et al. (1991) provided clear-cut evidence that only the 5-HT_3 receptors located postsynaptically with respect to primary afferent fibers mediate the antinociceptive action of 5-HT and 5-HT_3 receptor agonists. In contrast, the 5-HT_3 receptors located on the terminals of these fibers within the dorsal horn, like those on the peripheral sensory fibers, might mediate an excitatory action of 5-HT leading to the release of neuropeptides ensuring the transfer of nociceptive messages, such as substance P and calcitonin gene-related peptide (CGRP) (Saria et al. 1990). However, systemic injection of 5-HT_3 antagonists has been shown to prevent only the behavioral responses to chemical noxious stimuli but not those to mechanical or thermal noxious stimuli in rats (Sufka and Giordano 1991), suggesting that 5-HT_3 receptors on peripheral sensory fibers only participate in inflammatory pain (Eschalier et al. 1989; Giordano and Dyche 1989; Giordano and Rogers 1989).

5-HT_3 receptors are not the only receptors involved in 5-HT–dependent nociceptive processes at the periphery. 5-HT_{1A} and 5-HT_2 receptor subtypes also participate to some extent in the pain-triggering action of the indolamine (Grubb et al. 1988; Giordano and Rogers 1989; Guilbaud et al. 1989; Meller et al. 1992; Taiwo and Levine 1992). In particular, in addition to 5-HT_3 receptors, 5-HT_2 receptors have been reported to be involved in 5-HT–induced activation of nociceptive afferent fibers in inflamed tissues such as an arthritic joint (Grubb et al. 1988; Giordano and Rogers 1989).

Despite the availability of an increasing number of selective ligands of the various 5-HT receptors, it remains difficult to identify the particular subtype(s) on which 5-HT really acts to modulate nociception. It is possible that a great part of the spinal actions of 5-HT are mediated through the activation of the so-called 5-HT_{1S} receptor (Zemlan et al. 1990), and there is therefore an urgent need for a better characterization of this receptor type and development of selective agonists and antagonists. Another reason for the difficulty in identifying the receptor types responsible for 5-HT–induced modulations of nociception is linked to the fact that serotonergic systems are not isolated in the CNS but interact with many other systems, which may also participate, independently, in some modulatory mechanisms of nociception. In this context, it can be recalled that Advokat (1993) recently noted that intrathecal administration of 5-HT is antinociceptive in intact rats but promotes nociceptive responses in spinal rats. Accordingly, one can propose that the action of 5-HT in intact rats is in fact mediated by another neurotransmitter which is eliminated by spinalization.

Interactions between 5-HT and other neuroactive substances, such as substance P and adenosine, have been shown to exist at the spinal level, but much emphasis has been put on noradrenaline (NA). In particular, Archer and his coworkers reported that NA depletion resulting from the systemic or intrathecal administration of neurotoxins blocks the antinociceptive effect of intrathecally injected 5-HT in the tail-flick test, and that NA injected via the same route restores the antinociceptive effect of the potent 5-HT_1 receptor agonist 5-methoxy-N,N-dimethyltryptamine, in NA-depleted rats (Minor et al. 1985, 1988; Archer et al. 1986; Post et al. 1986). This could not be due to some toxin-induced decrease in spinal 5-HT receptor densities, because the selective lesion of the noradrenergic system by DSP-4 actually enhances the density of both 5-HT_{1A} and 5-HT_{1B} sites (Laporte et al., unpublished observations). However, if the net effect of intrathecally administered 5-HT on nociception results from a balance between a pronociceptive effect due to 5-HT_{1A} receptor stimulation and an antinociceptive effect due to 5-HT_{1B} receptor stimulation (Murphy and Zemlan 1990; Alhaider and Wilcox 1993), it is possible that the lack of analgesic action of 5-HT after NA depletion may be due to a relatively higher 5-HT_{1A} receptor-mediated effect in NA-depleted rats than in intact animals. Other mechanisms can also be proposed. Delander and Hopkins (1987) reported that intrathecally injected NA and 5-HT potentiate each other as antinociceptive agents in the tail-flick test in mice. Danzebrink and Gebhart (1991b) found that the intrathecal coadministration of the alpha-2 adrenoceptor agonist, clonidine, with 5-HT receptor agonists produces supra-additive visceral antinociception in the rat. Conversely, alpha-2 adrenoceptor blockade by yohimbine has been shown to prevent the inhibitory effect of intrathecally administered 5-HT on noxious-evoked activity of wide-dynamic-range neurons in the cat dorsal horn (Nakagawa et al. 1990). Finally, a recent report indicates that 5-methoxy-N,N-dimethyltryptamine facilitates NA release from rat spinal cord slices (Reinmann and Schneider 1993). All these observations point to a NA mediation of the antinociceptive effect of spinal 5-HT that probably involves both pre- and postsynaptic mechanisms with respect to noradrenergic terminals. Although the 5-HT receptor or receptors that interact with NA receptors (alpha-2 adrenoceptors) on the postsynaptic targets of noradrenergic terminals have not yet been identified, those responsible for the stimulatory effect of 5-HT on NA release from presynaptic noradrenergic terminals probably belong to the 5-HT_{1S} and/or 5-HT_{1C} subtypes (Sawynok and Reid 1992).

Relatively little is known about the cellular mechanisms underlying 5-HT modulation of dorsal horn activity. Local administration of the indolamine generally produces an inhibition of nociceptive neurons, although excitatory effects on deep dorsal horn neurons were also observed. 5-HT has diverse actions on frog dorsal horn neurons (depolarization, hyperpolarization, and biphasic responses), which appear to be mediated by at least three receptor subtypes: depolarization is triggered by the stimulation of 5-$HT_{2A/2C}$ receptors in some cells and by stimulation of 5-HT_3 receptors in others; hyperpolarization results from the stimulation of 5-HT_{1A} receptors (Tan and Miletic 1992). Some data suggest that 5-HT fibers may participate in axo-axonic synapses in the dorsal horn. In particular, 5-HT receptors exist on primary afferent fibers (see above), and it has been shown that iontophoretic application of 5-HT increases the threshold for antidromic activation of such fibers in the cat (Carstens et al. 1981b). Holohean et al. (1990) described both hyperpolarizations and depolarizations of frog primary afferent fibers upon local application of 5-HT. The indolamine could either decrease the amplitude of primary afferent-evoked excitatory postsynaptic potential (EPSP) or increase the electrical stimulation threshold for primary afferent-evoked action potentials, as expected of an action on the primary afferent fibers themselves (Tan and Miletic 1992). Several types of 5-HT receptors appear to mediate the effects of the indolamine on primary afferent fibers. The stimulation of 5-HT_{1A} receptors produces their hyperpolarization, whereas that of 5-HT_2 receptors has a depolarizing action (Holohean et al. 1990).

5-HT also causes a variety of membrane responses in cell bodies of primary afferent neurons (Holz et al. 1986; Morita and Katayama 1987; Tan and Miletic 1992). 5-HT_2 and 5-HT_3 receptors have been implicated in the 5-HT–induced depolarization of dorsal root ganglion (DRG) cells (Todorovic and Anderson 1990; Robertson and Bevan 1991). In contrast, 5-HT hyperpolarizes capsaicin-sensitive C-type sensory neurons in the rat DRG by activating 5-HT_{1A} receptors. (Todorovic and Anderson 1992). If this membrane response also occurs at the central terminals of C-type DRG neurons, it would be expected to produce presynaptic inhibition.

Most data, however, do not support the idea that 5-HT exerts its antinociceptive effect at the spinal level through a presynaptic control of primary afferent fibers containing substance P and/or CGRP (Pang and Vasko 1986; Go and Yaksh 1987; Bourgoin et al. 1993). As shown in Table II, among 5-HT itself, the 5-HT_{1A} receptor agonists 8-OH-DPAT and ipsapirone, the $5\text{-HT}_{1B/1D}$ receptor agonist sumatriptan (an anti-migraine drug), and the 5-HT_3 receptor agonist 2-methyl-5-HT, none significantly affected the K^+-evoked overflow of CGRP or substance P ($P > 0.05$) from rat spinal cord slices. However, the evoked release of substance P from the trigeminal nucleus of the rabbit can be reduced by 5-HT, in a methysergide-reversible manner (Yonehara et al. 1991), as expected from a possible involvement of $5\text{-HT}_{2A/2C}$ receptors. In line with the peripheral excitatory effect of 5-HT via the stimulation of 5-HT_3 receptors, it has recently been shown that the indolamine enhances the release of CGRP evoked by capsaicin from C-fibers in the rat trachea, and that this effect can be blocked by the potent 5-HT_3 receptor antagonist tropisetron (ICS 205-930) but not by 5-HT_1 or 5-HT_2 receptor

Table II
Effects of 5-HT and other ligands of 5-HT receptors on the K^+-evoked release (K_2/K_1)of CGRP and substance P from rat spinal cord slices

		CGRP	Substance P
Control		0.33 ± 0.02	0.58 ± 0.03
5-HT	0.1 μM	0.31 ± 0.06	0.52 ± 0.08
	1 μM	0.32 ± 0.04	0.57 ± 0.08
	10 μM	0.38 ± 0.03	0.54 ± 0.07
8-OH-DPAT	0.01 μM	0.36 ± 0.05	0.51 ± 0.07
	0.1 μM	0.36 ± 0.04	0.55 ± 0.07
	1 μM	0.33 ± 0.05	0.57 ± 0.09
Ipsapirone	0.01 μM	0.36 ± 0.08	0.60 ± 0.03
	0.1 μM	0.34 ± 0.06	0.64 ± 0.05
	1 μM	0.38 ± 0.04	0.56 ± 0.07
Sumatriptan	0.01 μM	0.30 ± 0.05	0.70 ± 0.06
	0.1 μM	0.31 ± 0.03	0.72 ± 0.07
	1 μM	0.30 ± 0.06	0.66 ± 0.04
	10 μM	0.33 ± 0.05	0.58 ± 0.06
2-methyl-5-HT	1 μM	0.39 ± 0.05	0.59 ± 0.07
	10 μM	0.36 ± 0.04	0.56 ± 0.05
	100 μM	0.38 ± 0.03	0.51 ± 0.08

Note: Slices of the dorsal half of the lumbar enlargement were depolarized twice (K_1, K_2) by 30 mM K^+ in the course of continuous superfusion with an artificial cerebrospinal fluid. Drugs were added to the superfusing fluid for the second K^+ pulse only, so that the ratio K_2/K_1 of the peptide overflow due to the two K^+ pulses allowed the detection of any significant drug-induced alteration of the K^+-evoked, Ca^{2+}-dependent release of CGRP and/or substance P (Bourgoin et al. 1993). Each value of the ratio K_2/K_1 is the mean ± S.E.M. of at least six independent determinations.

antagonists (Hua and Yaksh 1993). Such an excitatory effect of 5-HT_3 receptor stimulation on CGRP-containing terminals of primary afferent fibers within the dorsal horn has also been reported by Saria et al. (1990). The latter effect is probably unrelated to the modulatory action of 5-HT_3 receptor agonists on nociception at the spinal level, because Alhaider et al. (1991) convincingly showed that only the postsynaptic 5-HT_3 receptors, that is, those located downstream of (CGRP-containing) primary afferent fibers, participate in the analgesic action of intrathecally administered 5-HT.

CONCLUSION

To date, no approach, be it anatomical, biochemical, pharmacological, behavioral, or electrophysiological, has succeeded in completely defining the modulatory role of the raphe-spinal serotonergic system in the spinal processing of nociception. The involvement of the various 5-HT receptor subtypes in the spinal effects of 5-HT also remains poorly understood. Further investigations, which would also take into account the actions of 5-HT on functions other than nociception (functions able to affect nociception, or the responses to algesic tests), as well as the interactions of 5-HT with other neurotransmitter systems (especially because of the multiple transmitter nature of the raphe-spinal pathways) should be conducted for a better understanding of the physiological relevance of serotonergic mechanisms in pain control. Ideally, such studies should end with the development of specific drugs and/or appropriate therapies involving these mechanisms for the alleviation of pain.

ACKNOWLEDGMENTS

The generous gift of anti–5-HT_3 receptor antiserum by Dr. R. McKernan (Harlow, UK) is gratefully acknowledged. We are grateful to Drs. K. Kia and D. Vergé for their kind gift of the photographs in Figs. 1 and 3A. Original data reported in this review have been obtained thanks to financial support by INSERM, DRET, and Université Paris 6.

REFERENCES

Abbott, F.V. and Young, S.N., Effect of 5-hydroxytryptamine precursors on morphine analgesia in the formalin test, Pharmacol. Biochem. Behav., 31 (1988) 855–860.

Advokat, A., Intrathecal coadministration of serotonin and morphine differentially modulates the tail-flick reflex of intact and spinal rats, Pharmacol. Biochem. Behav., 45 (1993) 871–879.

Alhaider, A.A., Antinociceptive effect of ketanserin in mice: involvement of supraspinal 5-HT_2 receptors in nociceptive transmission, Brain Res., 543 (1991) 335–340.

Alhaider, A. A. and Wilcox, G.L., Differential roles of 5-hydroxytryptamine$_{1A}$ and 5-hydroxytryptamine$_{1B}$ receptor subtypes in modulating spinal nociceptive transmission in mice, J. Pharmacol. Exp. Ther., 265 (1993) 378–385.

Alhaider, A.A., Lei, S.Z. and Wilcox, G.L., Spinal 5-HT3 receptor-mediated antinociception: possible release of GABA, J. Neurosci., 11 (1991) 1881–1888.

Archer, T., Danysz, W., Jonsson, G., Minor, B.G. and Post, C., 5-methoxy-N-N-dimethyltryptamine–induced analgesia is blocked by α-adrenoreceptor antagonists in rats, Br. J. Pharmacol., 89 (1986) 293–298.

Archer, T., Arwestrõm, E., Minor, B.G., Persson, M.L., Post, C., Sundstrom, E. and Jonsson, G., (+)-8-OH-DPAT and 5-MeODMT induced analgesia is antagonized by noradrenaline depletion, Physiol. Behav., 39 (1987) 95–102.

Barber, A., Harting, J. and Wolf, H.P., Antinociceptive effects of the 5-HT_2 antagonist ritanserin in rats: evidence for an activation of descending monoaminergic pathways in the spinal cord, Neurosci. Lett., 99 (1989) 234–238.

Bardon, T. and Ruckebusch, M., Changes in 5-HIAA and 5-HT levels in lumbar CSF following morphine administration to conscious dogs, Neurosci. Lett., 49 (1984) 147–151.

Beitz, A.J., The nuclei of origin of brainstem serotonergic projections to the rodent spinal trigeminal nucleus, Neurosci. Lett., 32 (1982) 223–228.

Bervoets, K., Rivet, J.M. and Millan, M.J., 5-HT_{1A} receptors and the tail-flick response. IV. Spinally localized 5-HT_{1A} receptors postsynaptic to serotoninergic neurones mediate spontaneous tail-flicks in the rat, J. Pharmacol. Exp. Ther., 264 (1993) 95–104.
Besson, J.M. and Chaouch, A., Peripheral and spinal mechanisms of nociception, Pharmacol. Rev., 67 (1987) 67–186.
Björklund, A. and Skagerberg, G., Descending monoaminergic projection to the spinal cord. In: B. Sjölund and A. Björklund (Eds.), Brain Stem Control of Spinal Mechanisms, Elsevier, Amsterdam, 1982, pp. 55–88.
Blackshear, M.A., Steranka, L.R. and Sanders-Bush, E., Multiple serotonin receptors: regional distribution and effects of raphe lesions, Eur. J. Pharmacol., 76 (1981) 326–334.
Bourgoin, S., Oliveras, J.L., Bruxelle, J., Hamon, M. and Besson, J.M., Electrical stimulation of the nucleus raphe magnus in the rat: effects on 5-HT metabolism in the spinal cord, Brain Res., 194 (1980) 377–389.
Bourgoin, S., Pohl, M., Mauborgne, A., Benoliel, J.J., Collin, E., Hamon, M. and Cesselin, F., Monoaminergic control of the release of calcitonin gene-related peptide- and substance P–like materials from spinal cord slices, Neuropharmacology, 32 (1993) 633–640.
Bowker, R.M. and Abbott, L.C., Quantitative re-evaluation of descending serotonergic and non-serotonergic projections from the medulla of the rodent: evidence for extensive co-existence of serotonin and peptides in the same spinally projecting neurons, but not from the nucleus raphe magnus, Brain Res., 512 (1990) 15–25.
Brown, L., Amedro, J., Williams, G.M. and Smith, D., A pharmacological analysis of the rat spinal cord serotonin (5-HT) autoreceptor, Eur. J. Pharmacol., 145 (1988) 163–171.
Brown, L.M., Smith, D.L., Williams, G.M. and Smith, D.J., Alterations in serotonin binding after 5,7-dihydroxytryptamine treatment in the rat spinal cord, Neurosci. Lett., 102 (1989) 103–107.
Bruinvels, A.T., Landwehrmeyer, B., Moskowitz, M.A. and Hoyer, D., Evidence for the presence of 5-HT_{1B} receptor messenger RNA in neurons of the rat trigeminal ganglia, Eur. J. Pharmacol. Mol. Pharmacol. Sect., 227 (1992) 357–359.
Bullitt, E. and Light, A.R., Intraspinal course of descending serotoninergic pathways innervating the rodent dorsal horn and lamina X, J. Comp. Neurol., 286 (1989) 231–242.
Carstens, E., Fraunhoffer, M. and Zimmermann, M., Serotonergic mediation of descending inhibition from midbrain periaqueductal gray, but not reticular formation, of spinal nociceptive transmission in the cat, Pain, 10 (1981a) 149–167.
Carstens, E., Klumpp, D., Randic, M. and Zimmermann, M., Effect of iontophoretically applied 5-hydroxytryptamine on the excitability of single primary afferent C- and A-fibers in the cat spinal cord, Brain Res., 220 (1981b) 151–158.
Crisp, T., Stafinsky, J.L., Spanos, L.J., Uram, M., Perni, V. and Donepudi, H.B., Analgesic effects of serotonin and receptor-selective serotonin agonists in the rat spinal cord, Gen. Pharmacol., 22 (1991a) 247–251.
Crisp, T., Stafinsky, J.L., Uram, M., Perni, V.C., Weaver, M.F. and Spanos, L.J., Serotonin contributes to the spinal antinociceptive effects of morphine, Pharmacol. Biochem. Behav., 39 (1991b) 591–595.
Danzebrink, R.M. and Gebhart, G.F., Evidence that spinal 5-HT_1, 5-HT_2 and 5-HT_3 receptor subtypes modulate responses to noxious colorectal distension in the rat, Brain Res., 538 (1991a) 64–75.
Danzebrink, R.M. and Gebhart, G.F., Intrathecal coadministration of clonidine with serotonin agonists produces supra-additive visceral antinociception in the rat, Brain Res., 555 (1991b) 35–42.
Daval, G., Vergé, D., Basbaum, A.I., Bourgoin, S. and Hamon, M., Autoradiographic evidence of $serotonin_1$ binding sites on primary afferent fibres in the dorsal horn of the rat spinal cord, Neurosci. Lett., 83 (1987) 71–76.
Delander, G.E. and Hopkins, C.J., Interdependence of spinal adenosinergic, serotonergic and noradrenergic systems mediating antinociception, Neuropharmacology, 26 (1987) 1791–1794.
Eide, P.K. and Hole, K., Different role of 5-HT_{1A} and 5-HT_2 receptors in spinal cord in the control

of nociceptive responsiveness, Neuropharmacology, 30 (1991) 727–731.
Eide, P.K. and Tjolsen, A., Effects of serotonin receptor antagonists and agonists on the tail flick response in mice involve altered tail-skin temperature, Neuropharmacology, 27 (1988) 889–893.
Eide, P.K., Hole, K. and Broch, O.J., Supersensitivity to the antinociceptive effect of a 5-HT$_1$ receptor agonist after lesion of raphe-spinal serotonergic neurones, Pharmacol. Toxicol., 71 (1992) 62–64.
El-Yassir, N., Fleetwood-Walker, S.M. and Mitchell, R., Heterogeneous effects of serotonin in the dorsal horn: the involvement of 5-HT$_1$ receptor subtypes, Brain Res., 456 (1988) 147–158.
Eschalier, A., Kayser, V. and Guilbaud, G., Influence of a specific 5-HT$_3$ antagonist on carrageenan-induced hyperalgesia in rats, Pain, 36 (1989) 249–255.
Fasmer, O.B., Berge, O.G. and Hole, K., Changes in nociception after lesions of descending serotonergic pathways induced with 5,6-dihydroxytryptamine, Neuropharmacology, 24 (1985) 729–734.
Fasmer, O.B., Berge, O.G., Post, C. and Hole, K., Effects of the putative 5-HT$_{1A}$ receptor agonist 8-OH-2-(di-n-propylamino)tetralin on nociceptive sensitivity in mice, Pharmacol. Biochem. Behav., 25 (1986) 883–888.
Giordano, J. and Dyche, J., Differential analgesic actions of serotonin 5-HT$_3$ receptor antagonists in the mouse, Neuropharmacology, 28 (1989) 423–427.
Giordano, J. and Rogers, L.V., Peripherally administered serotonin 5-HT$_3$ receptor antagonists reduce inflammatory pain in rats, Eur. J. Pharmacol., 170 (1989) 83–86.
Glaum, S.R., Proudfit, H.K. and Anderson, E.G., Reversal of the antinociceptive effects of intrathecally administered serotonin in the rat by a selective 5-HT$_3$ receptor antagonist, Neurosci. Lett., 95 (1988) 313–317.
Glaum, S.R., Proudfit, H.K. and Anderson, E.G., 5-HT$_3$ receptors modulate spinal nociceptive reflexes, Brain Res., 510 (1990) 12–16.
Go, V.L.W. and Yaksh, T.L., Release of substance P from the cat spinal cord, J. Physiol. (Lond.), 391 (1987) 141–167.
Grauer, S.M., Tao, R. and Auerbach, S.B., Morphine induces an increase in extracellular serotonin in the rat diencephalon, Brain Res., 599 (1992) 277–282.
Grossman, C.J., Kilpatrick, G.J. and Bunce, K.T., Development of a radioligand binding assay for 5-HT$_4$ receptors in guinea-pig and rat brain, Br. J. Pharmacol., 109 (1993) 618–624.
Grubb, B.D., McQueen, D.S., Iggo, A., Birrell, G.J. and Dutia, M.B., A study of 5-HT receptors associated with afferent nerves located in normal and inflamed rat ankle joints, Agents Actions, 25 (1988) 216–218.
Guilbaud, G., Benoist, J.M., Eschalier, A., Gautron, M. and Kayser, V., Evidence for peripheral serotonergic mechanisms in the early sensitization after carrageenan-induced inflammation: electrophysiological studies in the ventrobasal complex of the rat thalamus using a specific antagonist of peripheral 5-HT receptors, Brain Res., 502 (1989) 187–197.
Hammond, D.L., Control systems for nociceptive afferent processing: the descending inhibitory pathways. In: T.L. Yaksh (Ed.), Spinal Afferent Processing, Plenum Press, New York, 1986, pp. 363–390.
Hamon M., Fattaccini C.M., Adrien J., Gallissot M.C., Martin P. and Gozlan H., Alterations of central serotonin and dopamine turnover in rats treated with ipsapirone and other 5-hydroxytryptamine$_{1A}$ agonists with potential anxiolytic properties, J. Pharmacol. Exp. Ther., 246 (1988) 745–752.
Hamon, M., Gallissot, M.C., Ménard, F., Gozlan, H., Bourgoin, S. and Vergé, D., 5-HT$_3$ receptor binding sites are on capsaicin-sensitive fibres in the rat spinal cord, Eur. J. Pharmacol., 164 (1989) 315–322.
Hole, K. and Tjolsen, A., The tail-flick and formalin tests in rodents: changes in skin temperature as a confounding factor, Pain, 53 (1993) 247–254.
Holohean, A.M., Hackman, J.C. and Davidoff, R. A., An in vitro study of the effects of serotonin on frog primary afferent terminals, Neurosci. Lett., 113 (1990) 175–180.
Holz, G.G., Shefner, S.A. and Anderson, E.G., Serotonin decreases the duration of action potentials recorded from tetraethylammonium-treated bullfrog dorsal root ganglion cells, J. Neurosci.,

6 (1986) 620–626.
Hua, X.Y. and Yaksh, T.L., Pharmacology of the effects of bradykinin, serotonin, and histamine on the release of calcitonin gene-related peptide from C-fiber terminals in the rat trachea, J. Neurosci., 13 (1993) 1947–1953.
Huang, J.C. and Peroutka, S.J., Identification of 5-hydroxytryptamine$_1$ binding site subtypes in rat spinal cord, Brain Res., 436 (1987) 173–176.
Humphrey, P.P.A., Hartig, P. and Hoyer, D., A proposed nomenclature for 5-HT receptors, Trends Pharmacol. Sci., 14 (1993) 233–236.
Hutson, P.H., Tricklebank, M.D. and Curzon, G., Enhancement of foot-shock-induced analgesia by spinal 5,7-dihydroxytryptamine lesions, Brain Res., 237 (1982) 367–372.
Hylden, J.L. and Wilcox, G.L., Intrathecal serotonin in mice: analgesia and inhibition of a spinal action of substance P, Life Sci., 33 (1983) 789–795.
Jackson, D.A. and White, S.R., Receptor subtypes mediating facilitation by serotonin of excitability of spinal motoneurons, Neuropharmacology, 29 (1990) 787–797.
Jensen, T.S. and Yaksh, T.L., Spinal monoamine and opiate systems partly mediate the antinociceptive effects produced by glutamate at brainstem sites, Brain Res., 321 (1984) 287–297.
Jones, B.E., Holmes, C.J., Rodriguez-Veiga, E. and Mainville, L., GABA-synthesizing neurons in the medulla: their relationship to serotonin-containing and spinally projecting neurons in the rat, J. Comp. Neurol., 313 (1991) 349–367.
Jones, S.L. and Light, A.R., Serotoninergic medullary raphespinal projection to the lumbar spinal cord in the rat: a retrograde immunohistochemical study, J. Comp. Neurol., 322 (1992) 599–610.
Julius, D., Huang, K.N., Livelli, T.J., Axel, R. and Jessell, T.M., The 5-HT$_2$ receptor defines a family of structurally distinct but functionally conserved serotonin receptors, Proc. Natl. Acad. Sci. U.S.A., 87 (1990) 928–932.
Kazakov, V.N., Kravtsov, P.Y., Krakhotnika, E.D. and Maisky, V.A., Sources of cortical, hypothalamic and spinal serotonergic projections: topical organization within the nucleus raphe dorsalis, Neuroscience, 56 (1993) 157–164.
Kidd E.J., Laporte A.M., Langlois X., Fattaccini C.-M., Doyen C., Lombard M.C., Gozlan H. and Hamon M., 5-HT$_3$ receptors in the rat central nervous system are mainly located on nerve fibres and terminals, Brain Res. 612 (1993) 289–298.
Kiefel, J.M., Cooper, M.L. and Bodnar, R.J., Serotonin receptor subtype antagonists in the medial ventral medulla inhibit mesencephalic opiate analgesia, Brain Res., 597 (1992) 331–338.
Kuraishi, Y., Harada, Y., Aratani, S., Satoh, M. and Takagi, H., Separate involvement of the spinal noradrenergic and serotonergic systems in morphine analgesia: the differences in mechanical and thermal algesic tests, Brain Res., 273 (1983) 245–252.
Kwiat, G.C. and Basbaum, A.I., The origin of brainstem noradrenergic and serotonergic projections to the spinal cord dorsal horn of the rat, Somatosens. Mot. Res., 9 (1992) 157–173.
LaMotte, C.C., Johns, D.R. and DeLanerolle, N.C., Immunohistochemical evidence of indolamine neurons in monkey spinal cord, J. Comp. Neurol., 206 (1982) 359–370.
Laporte A.M., Koscielniak T., Ponchant M., Vergé D., Hamon M. and Gozlan H., Quantitative autoradiographic mapping of 5-HT$_3$ receptors in the rat CNS using [^{125}I]iodo-zacopride and [^{3}H]zacopride as radioligands, Synapse, 10 (1992) 271–281.
Leysen, J.E., Niemegeers, C.J.E., Van Nueten, J.M. and Laduron, P.M., [^{3}H]ketanserin (R 41468), a selective ^{3}H-ligand for serotonin$_2$ receptor binding sites. Binding properties, brain distribution, and functional role, Mol. Pharmacol., 21 (1982) 301–314.
Liu, M.Y, Su, C.F. and Lin, M.T., The antinociceptive role of bulbospinal serotonergic pathway in the rat brain, Pain, 33 (1988) 123–129.
Lyon, R.A., Davis, K.H. and Titeler, M.,^{3}H-DOB labels a guanylnucleotide-sensitive state of 5-HT$_2$ receptor, J. Pharmacol. Exp. Ther., 31 (1987) 194–199.
Mantyh, P.W. and Hunt, S.P., Evidence for cholecystokinin-like immunoreactive neurons in the rat medulla oblongata which project to the spinal cord, Brain Res., 291(1984) 49–54.

Marlier, L., Teilhac, J.R., Cerruti, C. and Privat, A., Autoradiographic mapping of 5-HT_1, 5-HT_{1A}, 5-HT_{1B}, and 5-HT_2 receptors in the rat spinal cord, Brain Res., 550 (1991) 15–23.
Matos, F.F., Rollema, H., Brown, J.L. and Basbaum, A.I., Do opioids evoke the release of serotonin in the spinal cord? An in vivo microdialysis study of extracellular serotonin in the rat, Pain, 48 (1992) 439–447.
Matsuzaki, S., Takada, M., Li, Y.Q., Tokuno, H. and Mizuno, N., Serotoninergic projections from the dorsal raphe nucleus to the nucleus submedius in the rat and cat, Neuroscience, 55 (1993) 403–416.
Meller, S.T., Lewis, S.J., Brody, M.J. and Gebhart, G.F., Vagal afferent-mediated inhibition of a nociceptive reflex by iv serotonin in the rat. II. Role of 5-HT receptor subtypes, Brain Res., 585 (1992) 71–86.
Millan, M.J. and Colpaert, F.C., 5-hydroxytryptamine $(5\text{-HT})_{1A}$ receptors and the tail-flick response. II. High efficacy 5-HT_{1A} agonists attenuate morphine-induced antinociception in mice in a competitive-like manner, J. Pharmacol. Exp. Ther., 256 (1991) 983–992.
Minor, B.G., Post, C. and Archer, T., Blockade of intrathecal 5-hydroxytryptamine–induced antinociception in rats by noradrenaline depletion, Neurosci. Lett., 54 (1985) 39–44.
Minor, B.G., Persson, M.L., Post, C., Jonsson, G. and Archer, T., Intrathecal noradrenaline restores 5-methoxy-N,N-dimethyltryptamine–induced antinociception abolished by intrathecal 6-hydroxydopamine, J. Neural Trans., 72 (1988) 107–120.
Miquel M.C. and Hamon M., 5-HT_1 receptor subtypes: pharmacological heterogeneity. In: S.Z. Langer, N. Brunello and J. Mendlewicz, (Eds.), Serotonin Receptor Subtypes: Pharmacological Significance and Clinical Implications, Vol. 1, Int. Acad. Biomed. Drug Res., Karger A.G., Basel., 1992, pp.13–30.
Mjellem, N., Lund, A., Eide, P.K., Storkson, R. and Tjolsen, A., The role of 5-HT_{1A} and 5-HT_{1B} receptors in spinal transmission and in the modulation of NMDA-induced behaviour, Neuroreport, 3 (1992) 1061–1064.
Monroe, P.J. and Smith, D.J., Characterization of multiple [^{3}H]5-hydroxytryptamine binding sites in rat spinal cord tissue, J. Neurochem., 41 (1983) 349–355.
Morgan, M.M., Sohn, J.H. and Liebeskind, J.C., Stimulation of the periaqueductal gray matter inhibits nociception at the supraspinal as well as spinal level, Brain Res., 502 (1989) 61–68.
Morita, K. and Katayama, Y., 5-hydroxytryptamine effects on the soma of bullfrog primary afferent neurons, Neuroscience, 21 (1987) 1007–1018.
Murphy, R.M. and Zemlan, F.P., Selective 5-HT_{1B} agonists identify the 5-HT autoreceptor in lumbar spinal cord of rat, Neuropharmacology, 27 (1988) 37–42.
Murphy, R.M. and Zemlan, F.P., Selective serotonin1A/1B agonists differentially affect spinal nociceptive reflexes, Neurpharmacology, 29 (1990) 463–468.
Murphy, R.M. and Zemlan, F.P., Quantitative autoradiographic mapping of a novel serotonin receptor-5-HT_{1S}, Neuroreport, 3 (1992) 837–840.
Nakagawa, I., Omote, K., Kitahata, L.M., Collins, J.G. and Murata, K., Serotonergic mediation of spinal analgesia and its interaction with noradrenergic systems, Anesthesiology, 73 (1990) 474–478.
Oliveras, J.L., Bourgoin, S., Héry, F., Besson, J.M. and Hamon, M., The topographical distribution of serotoninergic terminals in the spinal cord of the cat: biochemical mapping by the combined use of microdissection and microassay procedures, Brain Res. 138 (1977) 393–406.
Pang, I.K. and Vasko, M.R., Morphine and norepinephrine but not 5-hydroxytryptamine and γ-aminobutyric acid inhibit the potassium-stimulated release of substance P from rat spinal cord slices, Brain Res., 376 (1986) 268–279.
Paul, D. and Phillips, A.G., Selective effects of pirenperone on analgesia produced by morphine or electrical stimulation at sites in the nucleus raphe magnus and the periaqueductal gray, Psychopharmacology, 88 (1986) 172–176.
Paul, D., Mana, M.J., Pfaus, J.G. and Pinel, J.P.J., Attenuation of morphine-produced analgesia by serotonin type-2 receptor blockers, pirenperone and ketanserin, Pharmacol. Biochem. Behav., 31 (1988) 641–647.

Pei, Q., Zetterström, T. and Fillenz, M., Tail pinch–induced changes in the turnover and the release of dopamine and 5-hydroxytryptamine in different brain regions of the rat, Neuroscience, 35 (1990) 133–138.

Pompeiano, M., Palacios, J.M. and Mengod, G., Distribution and cellular localization of mRNA coding for 5-HT_{1A} receptor in the rat brain: correlation with receptor binding, J. Neurosci. 12 (1992) 440–453.

Post, C., Minor, B.G., Davies, M. and Archer, T., Analgesia induced by 5-hydroxytryptamine receptor agonists is blocked or reversed by noradrenaline-depletion in rats, Brain Res., 363 (1986) 18–27.

Proudfit, H.K., Effect of raphe magnus and raphe pallidus lesions on morphine-induced analgesia and spinal cord monoamines, Pharmacol. Biochem. Behav., 13 (1980) 705–714.

Pubols, L.M., Bernau, N.A., Kane, L.A., Dawson, S.D., Burleigh, A.L. and Polans, A.S., Distribution of 5-HT_1 binding in cat spinal cord, Neurosci. Lett., 142 (1992) 111–114.

Radja, F., Laporte, A.M., Daval, G., Vergé, D., Gozlan, H. and Hamon, M., Autoradiography of serotonin receptor subtypes in the central nervous system, Neurochem. Int., 18 (1991) 1–15.

Reinmann, W. and Schneider, F., The serotonin receptor agonist 5-methoxy-N,N-dimethyltryptamine facilitates noradrenaline release from rat spinal cord slices and inhibits monoamine oxidase activity, Gen. Pharmacol., 24 (1993) 449–453.

Reynolds, D.J.M., Leslie, R.A., Grahame-Smith, D.G. and Harvey, J.M., Autoradiographic localization of 5-HT_3 receptor ligand binding in the cat brainstem, Neurochem. Int., 18 (1991) 69–73.

Riad, M., El Mestikawy, S., Vergé, D., Gozlan, H. and Hamon, M., Visualization and quantification of central 5-HT_{1A} receptors with specific antibodies, Neurochem. Int., 19 (1991) 413–423.

Richardson, B.P. and Buchheit, K.H., The pharmacology, distribution and function of 5-HT_3 receptors. In: N.N. Osborne and M. Hamon (Eds.), Neuronal Serotonin, John Wiley & Sons, Chichester, 1988, pp. 465–506.

Ridet, J.L., Rajaofetra, N., Teilhac, J.R., Geffard, M. and Privat, A., Evidence for nonsynaptic serotonergic and noradrenergic innervation of the rat dorsal horn and possible involvement of neuron-glia interactions, Neuroscience, 52 (1993) 143–157.

Rivot, J.P., Chiang, C.Y. and Besson, J.M., Increase of serotonin metabolism within the dorsal horn of the spinal cord during nucleus raphe magnus stimulation, as revealed by in vivo electrochemical detection, Brain Res., 238 (1982) 117–126.

Rivot, J.P., Calvino, B. and Besson, J.M., Is there a serotonergic tonic descending inhibition of the responses of dorsal horn convergent neurons to C-fibre inputs? Brain Res., 403 (1987) 142–146.

Rivot, J.P., Pointis, D. and Besson, J.M., A comparison of the effects of morphine on 5-HT metabolism in the periaqueductal gray, ventromedial medulla and medullary dorsal horn: in vivo electrochemical studies in freely moving rats, Brain Res., 495 (1989) 141–144.

Robertson, B. and Bevan, S., Properties of 5-$hydroxytryptamine_3$ receptor-gated currents in adult rat dorsal root ganglion neurones, Br. J. Pharmacol., 102 (1991) 272–276.

Rodriguez, F.D. and Rodriguez, R.E., Intrathecal administration of 5,6-DHT or 5,7-DHT reduces morphine and substance P-antinociceptive activity in the rat, Neuropeptides, 13 (1989) 139–146.

Romanelli, M.N., Ghelardini, C., Dei, S., Matucci, R., Mori, F., Scapecchi, S., Teodori, E., Bartolini, A., Galli, A., Giotti, A. and Gualtieri, F., Synthesis and biological activity of a series of aryltropanyl esters and amides chemically related to 1H-indole-3-carboxylic acid and endo-8-methyl-8-azabicyclo(3.2.1)oct-3-yl ester: development of a 5-HT_4 agonist endowed with potent antinociceptive activity, Arzneim. Forsch. Drug Res., 43 (1993) 913-918.

Ruda, M.A., Bennett, G.J. and Dubner, R., Neurochemistry and neural circuitry in the dorsal horn. In: P.C. Emson, M. Rossor and M. Tohyama (Eds.), Progress in Brain Research, Vol. 66, Elsevier, Amsterdam, 1986, pp. 219–268.

Saito, Y., Collins, J.G. and Iwasaki, H., Tonic 5-HT modulation of spinal dorsal horn neuron activity evoked by both noxious and non-noxious stimuli: a source of neuronal plasticity, Pain, 40 (1990) 205–219.

Saria, A., Javorsky, F., Humpel, C. and Gamse, R., 5-HT_3 receptor antagonists inhibit sensory neuropeptide release from the rat spinal cord, Neuroreport, 1 (1990) 104–106.
Sawynok, J. and Reid, A., Supersensitivity to intrathecal 5-hydroxytryptamine, but not noradrenaline, following depletion of spinal 5-hydroxytryptamine by 5,7-dihydroxytryptamine administered into various sites, Naunyn-Schmiedebergs Arch. Pharmacol., 342 (1990) 1–8.
Sawynok, J. and Reid, A., Noradrenergic mediation of spinal antinociception by 5-hydroxytryptamine: characterization of receptor subtypes, Eur. J. Pharmacol., 223 (1992) 49–56.
Schmauss, C., Hammond, D.L., Ochi, J.W. and Yaksh, T.L., Pharmacological antagonism of the antinociceptive effects of serotonin in the rat spinal cord, Eur. J. Pharmacol., 90 (1983) 349–357.
Schul, R. and Frenk, H., The role of serotonin in analgesia elicited by morphine in the periaqueductal gray matter (PAG), Brain Res., 553 (1991) 353–357.
Shen, Y., Monsma, F.J., Jr., Metcalf, M.A., Jose, P.A., Hamblin, M.W. and Sibley, D.R., Molecular cloning and expression of a 5-$hydroxytryptamine_7$ serotonin receptor subtype, J. Biol. Chem., 268 (1993) 18200–18204.
Solomon, R.E. and Gebhart, G.F., Mechanisms of effects of intrathecal serotonin on nociception and blood pressure in rats, J. Pharmacol. Exp. Ther., 245 (1988) 905–911.
Sorkin, L.S., Steinman, J.L., Hughes, M.G., Willis, W.D. and McAdoo, D.J., Microdialysis recovery of serotonin released in spinal cord dorsal horn, J. Neurosci. Meth., 23 (1988) 131–138.
Sorkin, L.S., McAdoo, D.J. and Willis, W.D., Stimulation in the ventral posterior lateral nucleus of the primate thalamus leads to release of serotonin in the lumbar spinal cord, Brain Res., 581 (1992) 307–310.
Sorkin, L.S., McAdoo, D.J. and Willis, W.D., Raphe magnus stimulation-induced antinociception in the cat is associated with release of amino acids as well as serotonin in the lumbar dorsal horn, Brain Res. 618 (1993) 95–108.
Sufka, K.J. and Giordano, J., Analgesic effects of S and R isomers of the novel 5-HT_3 receptor antagonists ADR-851 and ADR-852 in rats, Eur. J. Pharmacol., 204 (1991) 117–119.
Suzuki, Y. and Taguchi, K., In vivo voltametric studies on the effect of morphine on the serotonergic system in the cat spinal cord, Brain Res., 398 (1986) 413–418.
Taiwo, Y.O. and Levine, J.D., Serotonin is a directly-acting hyperalgesic agent in the rat, Neuroscience, 48 (1992) 485–490.
Tan, H. and Miletic, V., Diverse actions of 5-hydroxytryptamine on frog spinal dorsal horn neurons in vitro, Neuroscience, 49 (1992) 913–923.
Tecott, L.H., Maricq, A.V. and Julius, D., Nervous system distribution of the serotonin 5-HT_3 receptor mRNA, Proc. Natl. Acad. Sci. U.S.A., 90 (1993) 1430–1434.
Thor, K.B., Nickolaus, S. and Helke, C.J., Autoradiographic localization of 5-$hydroxytryptamine_{1A}$, 5-$hydroxytryptamine_{1B}$ and 5-$hydroxytryptamine_{1C/2}$ binding sites in the rat spinal cord, Neuroscience, 55 (1993) 235–252.
Tjolsen, A., Berge, O.G. and Hole, K., Lesions of bulbo-spinal serotonergic or noradrenergic pathways reduce nociception as measured by the formalin test, Acta Physiol. Scand., 142 (1991) 229–236.
Todorovic, S. and Anderson, E.G., Pharmacological characterization of 5-$hydroxytryptamine_2$ and 5-$hydroxytryptamine_3$ receptors in rat dorsal root ganglion (DRG) neurons, J. Pharmacol. Exp. Ther., 254 (1990) 109–115.
Todorovic, S. and Anderson, E.G., Serotonin preferentially hyperpolarizes capsaicin-sensitive C-type sensory neurons by activating 5-HT_{1A} receptors, Brain Res., 585 (1992) 212–218.
Turton, S., Gillard, N.P., Stephenson, F.A. and McKernan, R.M., Antibodies against the 5-HT_3-A receptor identify a 54 kDa protein affinity-purified from NCB20 cells, Mol. Neuropharmacol,. 3 (1993) 167–171.
Waeber, C., Dixon, K., Hoyer, D. and Palacios, J.M., Localization by autoradiography of neuronal 5-HT_3 receptors in the mouse CNS, Eur. J. Pharmacol., 151 (1988) 351–352.
Yakel, J.L., Shao, X.M. and Jackson, M.B., The selectivity of the channel coupled to the 5-HT_3

receptor, Brain Res. 533 (1990) 46–52.
Yaksh, T.L., Direct evidence that spinal serotonin and noradrenaline terminals mediate the spinal antinociceptive effects of morphine in the periaqueductal gray, Brain Res., 160 (1979) 180–185.
Yaksh, T.L. and Tyce, G.M., Microinjection of morphine into the periaqueductal gray evokes release of serotonin from spinal cord, Brain Res., 171 (1979) 176–181.
Yaksh, T.L. and Wilson, P.R., Spinal serotonin terminal system mediates antinociception, J. Pharmacol. Exp. Ther., 208 (1979) 446–453.
Yaksh, T.L., Plant, R.L. and Rudy, T.A., Studies on the antagonism by raphe lesions on the antinociceptive action of systemic morphine, Eur. J. Pharmacol., 41 (1977) 399–408.
Yonehara, N., Shibutani, T., Imai, Y., Ooi, Y., Sawada, T. and Inoki, R., Serotonin inhibits release of substance P evoked by tooth pulp stimulation in the trigeminal nucleus caudalis in rabbits, Neuropharmacology, 30 (1991) 5–13.
Zemlan, F.P. and Schwab, E.F., Characterization of a novel serotonin receptor subtype ($5\text{-}HT_{1S}$) in rat CNS: interaction with GTP binding protein, J. Neurochem., 57 (1991) 2092–2099.
Zemlan, F.P., Behbehani, M.M. and Murphy, R.M., Serotonin receptor subtypes and the modulation of pain transmission. In: H.L. Fields and J.M. Besson (Eds.), Progress in Brain Research, Vol. 77, Elsevier, Amsterdam, 1988, pp. 349–355.
Zemlan, F.P., Schwab, E.F., Murphy, R.M. and Behbehani, M.M., Identification of a novel $5\text{-}HT_1$ binding site in rat spinal cord, Neurochem. Int., 16 (1990) 507–513.

Correspondence to: Dr M. Hamon, INSERM U288, Neurobiologie Cellulaire et Fonctionnelle, Faculté de Médecine Pitié-Salpêtrière, 91, boulevard de l'Hôpital, 75634 Paris Cedex 13, France. Tel: 33-1-4077-9708; Fax: 33-1-4077-9790.

Proceedings of the 7th World Congress on Pain,
Progress in Pain Research and Management, Vol. 2,
edited by G.F. Gebhart, D.L. Hammond, and T.S.
Jensen, IASP Press, Seattle, © 1994.

46

NSAIDs for Cancer Pain: Meta-analysis of Efficacy

Elon Eisenberg,[a] Catherine Berkey,[b] Daniel B. Carr,[c]
Thomas C. Chalmers,[d] and Frederick Mosteller[b]

[a]Department of Neurology, Massachusetts General Hospital, [b]Technology Assessment Group, Harvard School of Public Health, and [c]Department of Anesthesia and [d]Division of Clinical Care Research, Department of Medicine, New England Medical Center, Boston, Massachusetts, USA

INTRODUCTION

The World Health Organization method for cancer pain relief (WHO 1986, 1992) recommends NSAIDs (or other nonopioid analgesics) as the sole treatment of mild to moderate pain, combined with weak opioids for moderate to severe pain, and in conjunction with strong opioids for more severe pain. Although this "WHO ladder" approach has been applied successfully by clinicians worldwide and is considered a fundamental principle of pharmacological management of cancer pain (APS 1992; Portenoy 1990; Ashburn and Lipman 1993; Inturrisi 1989; Schug et al. 1990; Ventafridda et al. 1987), there remain unresolved some basic pharmacological questions concerning use of NSAIDs. These questions include: What is the efficacy of NSAIDs in cancer pain compared to other drugs or placebo? Do NSAIDs produce dose-dependent analgesia? and Do they have a ceiling analgesic effect in patients with cancer pain? (Twycross 1983; Portenoy 1990). To address these questions, we examined the scientific evidence on efficacy of NSAIDs in the treatment of cancer-related pain by conducting a meta-analysis of data from published randomized controlled trials (RCTs). Meta-analysis refers to the application of statistical methods to integrate, and thereby to potentially increase the strength of, findings from individual studies (L'Abbe et al. 1987; Sacks et al. 1987; Thacker 1988).

METHODS

A literature search was conducted through BRS Colleague and Docline (National Library of Medicine) for 1966–1992. The search terms were *anti-inflammatory-agents, non-steroidals, neoplasms,* and *pain.* Full length reports (i.e., not simply abstracts) in the English language were selected, provided they were double-blind randomized controlled studies related to NSAID use in cancer pain in humans. References listed in these reports were reviewed and also screened for inclusion. Data regarding number of patients, type of cancer, NSAID used, number of doses (single versus multiple), analgesic efficacy, dropout rates, and global evaluation of the drugs used were extracted. Analgesic efficacy data were based on visual analogue or similar self-report scales. Pain scores used for the analyses were: (a) peak pain intensity difference (PPID)—the difference between baseline pain and the minimal pain intensity reported at any time during the postdrug observation period; (b) summed pain intensity difference (SPID)—the sum of differences between baseline pain and pain intensity at each time during postdrug observation (the area above the curve in a graph of pain intensity versus time); and (c) peak pain relief (PPAR) and total pain relief (TOPAR)—maximal and summed pain relief, respectively, during the post-drug observation period.

Scale variations required that we convert all data to percentage scales. For PPID and PPAR this transformation used the formula

$$\frac{\text{presented value (PPID or PPAR)}}{[\text{maximal value - minimal value (on scale)}]} \times 100 = \text{value in } \%$$

In the case of TOPAR and SPID, the following formula was used:

$$\frac{\text{presented values (SPID or TOPAR)}}{[\text{maximal value-minimal value (on scale)}] \times n} \times 100 = \text{value in } \%$$

where n is the number of measurements taken within the observation period. For both formulas, higher values (in %) indicate greater analgesic effects. Only comparable observation periods, six hours in the single-dose, and 10–14 days in the multiple-dose studies, were analyzed. To minimize exclusion of studies (e.g., that presented mean values without standard deviations) only mean values were used.

The n-weighted mean effect, used throughout this meta-analysis, calculates the mean effect of a treatment from several studies that vary in their sample size by weighting each study according to its relative sample size (i.e., large studies have greater weight than small ones).

We employed the DerSimonian and Laird Random Effects Model (1986) to estimate between-treatment efficacy differences. The combined estimates are presented with confidence intervals, and approximate significance is indicated at the 0.05 level.

RESULTS

Twenty-five studies met inclusion criteria (see chapter Appendix). The studies involved 1545 patients, but reported specific cancer diagnosis only in 515 (33%). Outcomes of patients with varied malignancies were not reported separately, so we could not conduct an analysis of NSAID efficacy in specific types of cancer. Baseline pain intensity was rated moderate or higher in 81% of patients in whom this measurement was reported (or 69% of all patients).

Analgesic efficacy of NSAIDs was compared to that of placebo only in single-dose studies. Better pain relief was obtained from NSAIDs than placebo in three scores (SPID, PPAR, TOPAR) based on five to six studies, and in another score (PPID) based on eight studies (Table I).

The dose-response relationship was evaluated by comparing the analgesic efficacy of 600 mg versus 1000 mg of oral aspirin, 100 versus 200 mg of oral indoprofen, and 10 versus 20 mg of im. ketorolac. Three single-dose studies allowed analysis of 157 patients (80 received low doses and 77 high doses). The two scores used, PPID and SPID, were approximately 1.3 times greater in the high-dose patients than in the low-dose patients, but the differences did not attain statistical significance (Table II).

We tested ceiling analgesic effect by comparing pain scores for recommended and supramaximal single doses of three NSAIDs: ketoprofen 100 versus 300 mg, and 75 versus 225 mg p.o.; zomepirac 100 versus 200 mg p.o.; and ketorolac 10 and 30 mg versus 90 mg im. Both doses showed similar efficacy according to all four scores used (PPID, SPID, PPAR, and TOPAR), indicating a ceiling analgesic effect (Table III).

To assess efficacy of first versus second steps on the WHO analgesic ladder, we compared the peak (PPID) and the sum (TOPAR) effects of single doses of NSAIDs alone to scores for combinations of NSAID plus weak opioid (e.g., codeine). Both scores indicated about 50% efficacy for NSAID alone or with weak opioid, i.e., no difference (Table IV).

Only two multiple-dose analgesic efficacy analyses were possible; they showed no significant differences in either PPAR or TOPAR between one NSAID and two weak opioid or weak opioid–nonopioid combination drugs

Table I
Analgesic efficacy of NSAIDs vs. placebo, single dose

Scale	Studies	Comparisons	Drugs	Patients	Effect: NSAIDs	Placebo	RD	95% Confidence Interval: Low	High
PPID	8	14	6	401/395	48%	29%	0.19	0.12	0.25*
SPID	6	12	5	289/281	31%	15%	0.16	0.08	0.22*
PPAR	5	11	5	277/269	60%	36%	0.24	0.16	0.32*
TOPAR	6	12	5	377/369	43%	26%	0.17	0.11	0.24*

Sources: PPID: Moertel 1974; Carlson 1990; Ventafridda 1974; Staquet 1989; Puglisi 1989; Pellegrini 1983; Stambaugh 1981, 1988a. SPID: Carlson 1990; Ventafridda 1974; Staquet 1989; Pellegrini 1983; Stambaugh 1981, 1988a. PPAR: Carlson 1990; Ventafridda 1974; Staquet 1989; Stambaugh 1981, 1988a. TOPAR: Moertel 1974; Carlson 1990; Ventafridda 1974; Staquet 1989; Stambaugh 1981, 1988a.

Drugs used: PPID: ketorolac, indoprofen, piprofen, ketoprofen, ASA, zomepirac. SPID: ketorolac, indoprofen, ketoprofen, ASA, zomepirac. PPAR: ketorolac, indoprofen, ketoprofen, ASA, zomepirac. TOPAR: ketorolac, indoprofen, ketoprofen, ASA, zomepirac.

RD = pooled rate difference.

* = significant at 0.05 level.

(WO/C). These analyses, however, were based on a small number of patients (20–29) in each group, and on ketorolac as the sole NSAID. The other multiple-dose analysis compared patient dropout rates during 7–10 days of administration of either NSAIDs or WO/C and showed an insignificant trend favoring NSAIDs over the WO/C drugs, with dropout rates of 27% and 30%, respectively.

DISCUSSION

Our analyses confirm the analgesic efficacy of NSAIDs for cancer pain. NSAIDs produced peak pain relief (PPAR) of 60% on average even in the face of moderate to severe baseline pain intensity. NSAIDs gave more analgesia than did placebo as measured by all pain intensity difference and relief scales—differences that were both statistically and clinically significant.

The present results are consistent with, but do not confirm, a long-suggested dose-response relationship for analgesic efficacy for NSAIDs in cancer pain (perhaps because of the small sample size per group). The comparison of recommended to supramaximal single doses, on the other hand,

Table II
Analgesic effecacy of low vs. high single doses of NSAIDs

Scale	Studies	Comparisons	Drugs	Patients	Effect: Low Dose	High Dose	RD	95% Confidence Level: Low	High
PPID	3	5	3	80/77	39%	51%	–0.12	–0.27	0.02
SPID	3	5	3	80/77	32%	40%	–0.08	–0.23	0.06

Sources: PPID and SPID: Martino 1976; Ventafridda 1974; Staquet 1989.
Drugs used: PPID and SPID: ASA, 600 vs. 1000 mg; indoprofen, 100 vs. 200 mg; ketorolac, 10 vs. 30 mg.
RD = pooled rate difference.

confirms the analgesic ceiling effect of NSAIDs; since not one of the four analgesic scores evaluated showed either a clinically (0–4%) or statistically significant difference.

With respect to the second step of the WHO analgesic ladder for cancer pain treatment, single doses of weak opioid plus NSAID combinations did not provide superior analgesic efficacy compared to NSAIDs alone. This negative result is based on a relatively large number of patients (> 450 in each treatment), assessed by several scales and given a variety of NSAIDs or combinations. Multiple-dose analyses, although based on a much smaller number of patients, further support these findings by showing that an NSAID (ketorolac in this case) has efficacy comparable to a weak opioid plus NSAID combination, and demonstrating roughly equal dropout rates in both treatment groups.

CONCLUSIONS

NSAIDs appear to reduce cancer related pain significantly more than do placebos. Further, NSAID-induced analgesia has a trend of dose-dependence up to a ceiling.

Intriguingly, the present results raise the question of whether the WHO second analgesic step is an optimal treatment protocol, or whether to proceed from NSAIDs directly to strong opioids for unrelieved pain. Although the efficacy of the WHO three-step protocol as a whole is well established, further trials to assess the importance of step 2 to the overall success of the three steps appear warranted.

Table III

Analgesic efficacy of recommended vs. supra-maximal single doses of NSAIDs

					Effect				
					Dose			95% Confidence Interval	
Scale	Studies	Comparisons	Drugs	Patients	Recommended	Supra-maximal	RD	Low	High
PPID	3	4	2	125/124	50%	48%	0.02	–0.09	0.15
SPID	5	6	3	197/196	39%	39%	0.00	–0.09	0.09
PPAR	3	4	2	133/132	65%	69%	–0.02	–0.13	0.09
TOPAR	4	5	3	173/172	48%	46%	0.02	–0.08	0.12

Drugs used:	Recommended dose:	Scale used:
Ketoprofen iv. 100 vs. 400 mg	iv. 100–300 mg	PPID, SPID
Ketoprofen p.o. 75 vs. 225 mg	p.o. 50–100 mg	SPID, PPAR, TOPAR
Ketoprofen p.o.100 vs. 300 mg	p.o. 50–100 mg	PPID, SPID, PPAR, TOPAR
Ketorolac im. 10 vs. 90 mg	im. 10–30 mg	PPID, SPID, PPAR, TOPAR
Ketorolac im. 30 vs. 90 mg	im. 10–30 mg	PPID, SPID, PPAR, TOPAR
Zomepirac p.o. 100 vs. 200 mg	p.o. 100 mg	SPID, TOPAR

Sources: PPID: Sacchetti 1984; Staquet 1989; Stambaugh 1988a. SPID: Sacchetti 1984; Staquet 1989; Stambaugh 1982, 1988a; Sunshine 1988. PPAR: Staquet 1989; Stambaugh 1988a; Sunshine 1988. TOPAR: Staquet 1989; Stambaugh 1982, 1988a; Sunshine 1988.

RD = pooled rate difference.

Table IV
Analgesic efficacy of NSAIDs vs. weak opioid or weak opioid–nonopioid combinations, single dose

					Effect				
								95% Confidence Interval	
Scale	Studies	Comparisons	Drugs	Patients	NSAID	WO/C	RD	Low	High
PPID*	6	9	5/7	471/472	49%	54%	–0.04	–0.10	0.01
TOPAR†	5	8	4/7	458/463	44%	45%	–0.01	–0.07	0.05

Sources: PPID: Moertel 1974; Carlson 1990; Estape 1990; Puglisi 1989; Stambaugh 1981, 1988a. TOPAR: Moertel 1974; Carlson 1990; Estape 1990; Stambaugh 1981, 1988a.
*Drugs used: NSAIDs: ASA, ketorolac, piprofen, ketoprofen, zomepirac.
WO/C: ASA + codeine, ASA + pentazocine, ASA + propoxyphen, acetaminophen + codeine, pentazocine, ASA + oxycodone, ASA + oxycodone + phenacetin + caffeine.
†Drugs used: NSAIDs: ASA, ketorolac, piprofen, ketoprofen, zomepirac.
WO/C: ASA + codeine, ASA + pentazocine, ASA + propoxyphen, acetaminophen + codeine, pentazocine, ASA + oxycodone, ASA + oxycodone + phenacetin + caffeine.
WO/C = weak opioid or weak opioid–nonopioid combinations.
RD = pooled rate difference.

ACKNOWLEDGMENTS

This work was supported by the Office of the Forum for Quality and Effectiveness in Health Care, Agency for Health Care Policy and Research, U.S. Department of Health and Human Services. The support was provided in connection with the development of a clinical practice guideline on cancer pain management by a panel co-chaired by Dr. Carr and Ada Jacox, RN, PhD, Independence Foundation Professor, Johns Hopkins University School of Nursing. This chapter does not necessarily represent the position of the U.S. Department of Health and Human Services. The primary literature searches were undertaken by the National Library of Medicine under the direction of Ione Auston and by Janice Ulmer, RN, PhD, and Donna Mahrenholz, RN, PhD, of the Johns Hopkins University School of Nursing. We thank Dr. Richard Kitz for continued support and encouragement. Miss Evelyn Hall provided expert secretarial assistance.

APPENDIX: Study Characteristics

Author and Year	No. of Patients	No. of Centers	Study Design	Type of Cancer	No. of Doses	Type of NSAID
Carlson 1990	75	M	P	NR	S+M	Ketorolac
Epstein 1986	75	S	P	Oropharyngeal	M	Benzyamide
Estape 1990	40	S	P	NR	S+M	Ketorolac
Ferrer-Brechner 1984	30	S	C	NR	S	Ibuprofen (combination)
Kim 1985	67	S	P	Oropharyngeal	M	Benzydamide
Levick 1988	100	M	P	NR	M	Naproxen sodium
Lomen 1986	26	S	C	Breast	M	Flubiprofen
Martino 1976	24	S	C	NR	S	Indoprofen ASA
Martino 1978	18	S	C	Mixed	S	Indoprofen Naproxen
Minotti 1989	99	S	P	Mixed	M	Diclofenac
Moertel 1974	100	S	C	NR	S	ASA
Pellegrini 1983	12	S	C	Mixed	S	Indoprofen
Puglisi 1989	45	S	P	NR	S	Piprofen
Sacchetti 1984	36	S	C	Mixed	S	Ketoprofen ASA
Stambaugh 1980	170	M	P	Mixed	M	Zomepirac
Stambaugh 1981	40	S	C	NR	S	Zomepirac
Stambaugh 1982	45	S	C	NR	S	Zomepirac
Stambaugh 1988a	160	S	P	NR	S	Ketoprofen
Stambaugh 1988b	30	S	P	NR	M	Ibuprofen (combination)
Staquet 1989	126	S	P	NR	S	Ketorolac

continued

Author and Year	No. of Patients	No. of Centers	Study Design	Type of Cancer	No. of Doses	Type of NSAID
Sunshine 1988	123	S	P	NR	S	Ketoprofen
Tonachella 1985	20	S	C	NR	M	Diclofenac
Turnbull 1986	28	S	C	Mixed	S+M	Naproxen ASA
Ventafridda 1974	24	S	C	Mixed	S	Indoprofen
Ventafridda 1990	72	S	C	NR	M	ASA Indomethacin Piprofen Diclofenac Ibuprofen Naproxen Suprofen Sulindac
Total: 25	1545	S: 21 M: 4	P: 12 C: 13	Mixed: 7 NR: 15 One organ: 3	S: 16 M: 12	

Note: C = crossover, M = multiple, P = parallel, S = single, NR = not reported

REFERENCES

American Pain Society, Principles of Analgesic Use in the Treatment of Acute Pain and Cancer Pain, American Pain Society Publications, Skokie, 1992, 41 pp.

Ashburn, M.A. and Lipman, A.G., Management of pain in the cancer patient, Anesth. Analg., 76 (1993) 402–416.

Carlson, W.R., Borrison, A.R., Harvey, B.S., Eisenberg, D.P., Nowry, A.P. and Wolin, M.E., A multiinstitutional evaluation of the analgesic efficacy and safety of Ketorolac tromethamine, acetaminophen plus codeine, and placebo in cancer pain, Pharmacotherapy, 10 (1990) 211–216.

DerSimonian, R. and Laird, N.M., Meta-analysis in clinical trials, Controlled Clin. Trials, 7 (1986) 177–188.

Epstein, J.B. and Stevenson-Moore, P., Benzydamine hydrochloride in prevention and management of pain in oral mucositis associated with radiation therapy, Oral Surg. Oral Med. Oral Pathol., 62 (1986) 145–148.

Estape, J., Vinolas, N., Gonzales, B., Ingles, F., Bofill, T., Guzman, M.C. and Tarrago, E., Ketorolac, a new non-opioid analgesic: a double-blind trial versus pentazocine in cancer pain, J. Int. Med. Res. 18 (1990) 298–304.

Ferrer-Brechner, T. and Ganz, P., Combination therapy with ibuprofen and methadone for chronic cancer pain, Am. J. Med., 77 (1984) 78–83.

Inturrisi, C.E., Management of cancer pain, Cancer, 63 (1989) 2308–2320.

Kim, J.H., Chu, F., Lakshmi, V. and Houde, R., A clinical study of benzydamine for the treatment of radiotherapy-induced mucositis of the oropharynx, Int. J. Tissue React., 7 (1985) 215–218.

L'Abbe, K.A., Detsky, A.S. and O'Rourke, K., Meta-analysis in clinical research, Ann. Int. Med., 107 (1987) 224–233.

Levick, S., Jacobs, C., Loukas, D.F., Gordon, D.H., Meyskens, F.L. and Uhm, K., Naproxen sodium in treatment of bone pain due to metastatic cancer, Pain, 35 (1988) 253–258.

Lomen, P.L., Samal, B.A., Lamborn, K.R., Sattler, L.P. and Crampton, S.L., Flubiprofen for the treatment of bone pain in patients with metastatic breast cancer, Am. J. Med. 80 (1986) 83–87.

Martino, G., Ventafridda, V., Parini, J. and Emanueli, A., A controlled study on the analgesic activity of indoprofen in patients with cancer pain. In: J.J. Bonica and D. Albe-Fessard (Eds.), Proceedings of the First World Congress on Pain. Advances in Pain Research and Therapy, Vol. 1. Raven Press, New York, 1976, pp. 573–578.

Martino, G., Emanueli, A., Mandelli, V. and Ventafridda, V., A controlled study of the analgesic effect of two non-steroidal anti-inflammatory drugs in cancer pain, Drug. Res., 28 (1978) 1657–1659.

Minotti, V., Patoia, L., Roila, F., Basurto, C., Tonato, M., Pasqualucci, V., Maresca, V. and del Favero, A., Double-blind evaluation of analgesic efficacy of orally administered diclofenac, nefopam, and acetylsalicylic acid (ASA) plus codeine in chronic cancer pain, Pain, 36 (1989) 177–183.

Moertel, C.G., Ahmann, D.L., Taylor, W.F. and Schwartau, N., Relief of pain by oral medications. A controlled evaluation of analgesic combinations, JAMA, 229 (1974) 55–59.

Pellegrini, A., Massidda, B., Pellegrini, P., Defraia, E., Usai, A., Parrinello, L., Bruni, G., Rigamonti, G. and Sacchetti, G., Effect of i.v. indoprofen on cancer pain and serum prolactin and growth hormone levels: a controlled pharmacologic study vs im. morphine and placebo, Int. J. Clin. Pharmacol. Ther. Toxicol., 21 (1983) 483–486.

Portenoy, R.K., The management of cancer pain, Compr. Ther., 16 (1990) 53–65.

Puglisi, G. and Garagiola, U., Piprofen and pentazocine in the treatment of cancer pain, Curr. Ther. Res., 45 (1989) 333–338.

Sacchetti, G., Camera, P., Rossi, A.P., Martoni, A., Bruni, G. and Pannuti, F., Injectable ketoprofen vs. acetylsalicylic acid for the relief of severe cancer pain: a double-blind crossover trial, Drug Intell. Clin. Pharm., 18 (1984) 403–406.

Sacks, H.S., Berrier, J., Reitman, D., Ancona-Berk, V.A. and Chalmers, T.C., Meta-analysis of randomized controlled trials, N. Eng. J. Med. 316 (1987) 450–455.

Schug, S.A., Zech, D. and Dorr, U., Cancer pain management according to WHO analgesic guidelines, J. Pain Symptom Manage., 5 (1990) 27–32.

Stambaugh, J.E., Tejada, F. and Trudnowski, R.J., Double-blind comparisons of zomepirac and oxycodone with APC in cancer pain, J. Clin. Pharmacol. 20 (1980) 261–270.

Stambaugh, J.E. and Sarajian, C., Analgesic efficacy of zomepirac sodium in patients with pain due to cancer, J. Clin. Pharmacol., 21 (1981) 501–507.

Stambaugh, J.E., Analgesic efficacy, safety, and acceptability of zomepirac sodium in comparison to morphine sulphate in the treatment of pain secondary to malignancy, Curr. Ther. Res., 31 (1982) 922–929.

Stambaugh, J.E. and Drew, J.A., A double-blind parallel evaluation of the efficacy and safety of a single dose of ketoprofen in cancer pain, J. Clin. Pharmacol., 28 (1988a) S34–39.

Stambaugh, J.E. and Drew, J., The combination of ibuprofen and oxycodone/acetaminophen in the treatment of chronic cancer pain, Clin. Pharmacol. Ther., 44 (1988b) 665–669.

Staquet, M.J., A double-blind study with placebo control of intramuscular ketorolac tromethadine in the treatment of cancer pain, J. Clin. Pharmacol., 28 (1989) 1031–1036.

Sunshine, A. and Olson, N.Z., Analgesic efficacy of ketoprofen in post partum, general surgery, and chronic cancer pain, J. Clin. Pharmacol., 28 (1988) S47–54.

Thacker, S.B., Meta-analysis: a quantitative approach to research integration, JAMA, 259 (1988) 1685–1689.

Tonachella, R., Gallo Curcio, C. and Grossi, E., Diclofenac sodium in cancer pain. A double-blind within patients comparison with pentazocine, Curr. Ther. Res., 37 (1985) 1130–1133.

Turnbull, R. and Hill, L.J., Naproxen versus aspirin as analgesics in advanced malignant disease, J. Palliat. Care. 1 (1986) 25–28.

Twycross, R.G. and Lack, S.A., Symptom Control in Far Advanced Cancer: Pain Relief, Pitman, London, 1983, pp. 167–189.

Ventafridda, V., Martino, G., Mandelli, V. and Emanueli, A., Indoprofen, a new analgesic and anti-inflammatory drug in cancer pain, Clin. Pharmacol. Ther. 17 (1975) 284–289.

Ventafridda, V., Tamburini, M., Caraceni, A., DeConno, F. and Naldi, F., A validation study of the WHO method for cancer pain relief, Cancer, 59 (1987) 850–856.

Ventafridda, V., De Conno, F., Panerai, A.E., Maresca, V., Monza, G.C. and Ripamonti, C., Non-steroidal anti-inflammatory drugs as the first step in cancer pain therapy: double-blind, within patient study comparing nine drugs, J. Int. Med. Res. 18 (1990) 21–29.

World Health Organization, Cancer Pain Relief, World Health Organization, Geneva, 1986.

World Health Organization Expert Committee, Cancer Pain Relief and Palliative Care, World Health Organization, Geneva, 1992.

Correspondence to: Daniel B. Carr, MD, Department of Anesthesia, New England Medical Center, 750 Washington St., Boston, MA 02111. Tel: 617-956-6044; Fax: 617-350-8384.

Proceedings of the 7th World Congress on Pain,
Progress in Pain Research and Management, Vol. 2,
edited by G.F. Gebhart, D.L. Hammond, and T.S.
Jensen, IASP Press, Seattle, © 1994.

47

Do Preemptive Treatments Provide Better Pain Control?

Henry J. McQuay

Clinical Reader in Pain Relief, University of Oxford, UK

The essence of understanding experiments . . . understanding when a thing is really known and when it is not really known.

—R.P. Feynman

INTRODUCTION

Widespread clinical interest in preemptive analgesia was triggered by an editorial (Wall 1988) that drew clinicians' attention because it linked fundamental work to clinical studies. The editorial related the findings in fundamental studies, the changes in the central nervous system that followed nociceptive stimuli and the ways in which these changes could be preempted, to clinical work in postoperative pain. Since that time the academic question has been sharpened; now we need to know whether an intervention made before the pain begins has greater analgesic effect than the same intervention (same dose, same route) made after the pain occurs. This is an active research area, and one major problem in writing this chapter is that any conclusions may be overtaken by new evidence. The aim of the chapter is to define the questions we need to ask, and, by reviewing the clinical evidence systematically, to see whether we have definitive answers.

THE BACKGROUND

Preemptive analgesia is given before the painful stimulus to prevent or reduce subsequent pain. The idea that preemptive analgesia might provide better pain control came from basic science studies. Initial observations indicated that noxious stimuli induced changes in neural function (Woolf 1983), such as hyperexcitability, in the spinal cord. Later studies suggested that analgesia given before the nociceptive stimulus began was more effective than the same dose given after the stimulus.

The hypothesis is that the preemptive analgesia prevents or reduces the development of any memory of the pain stimulus in the nervous system. Any subsequent lower analgesic requirement is a result of this prevention or reduction of the pain memory (McQuay and Dickenson 1990). This effect has generated the scientific interest in the basic mechanism and clinical interest in the potential for improving postoperative pain management.

The idea of preemptive analgesia, and the explanation, are attractive. Management of postoperative pain has rightly been criticized many times over the last 30 years. Despite the advent of increasingly high-technology approaches, it is doubtful that most patients are any better served. If preemptive analgesia worked, then these patients' pain might be reduced. Unfortunately, there are difficulties with the details of the idea and in interpreting conflicting evidence from clinical studies.

We have been slow to distinguish that preemptive treatment with one kind of analgesic intervention, for instance opioids, may not give the same answer as preemptive treatment with another, such as nonsteroidal anti-inflammatory drugs (NSAIDs). We also have been slow to distinguish between two different outcomes, that of a preemptive treatment on nociceptive pain and of a preemptive treatment on neuropathic pain.

PROBLEMS WITH THE FUNDAMENTAL EVIDENCE

Timing is one critical problem. If preemptive treatment reduces the memory of the subsequent noxious stimulus, how long does this effect last? Evidence of any preemptive effect is of great academic interest, but a short-lived effect (e.g., less than two hours) might be of little clinical relevance, particularly if the preemptive treatment carried any risk of increased morbidity. Conversely, preemptive treatments that lasted for 10 hours with minimal increase in morbidity would be of immense clinical importance. It is not easy to extrapolate from effects demonstrated in various animal models, which might last two hours, to clinical pain in humans.

A second problem is whether any preemptive effect influences acute postoperative pain (nociceptive pain) or the development of long-term sequelae such as phantom limb pain (neuropathic pain), or both. Different preemptive interventions might be required to obviate these two different problems. Positive or negative demonstrations of an effect of a particular intervention on nociceptive pain might not apply to neuropathic pain, and vice versa.

Preemptive analgesic effects have been shown in one animal model, the formalin test in which the subcutaneous injection of formalin into the paw gives rise to two peaks of nociceptive input. Interventions may be made at various times relative to the injection of formalin, and their relative efficacy may be compared. With opioids intrathecal injection of DAMGO before the formalin produced 70% greater inhibition of the C-fiber response than the same dose injected intrathecally after the formalin (Dickenson and Sullivan 1987; Dickenson 1991). With peripheral infiltrations of local anesthetic, one before and one after the formalin injection, the behavioral response to the formalin was abolished (Coderre et al. 1990). Infiltration with local anesthetic 25 minutes after the formalin made the hindpaw anesthetic but did not abolish the behavioral response. Intrathecal injection of local anesthetic before the formalin abolished the behavioral response; the same intrathecal dose five minutes after the formalin had no effect (Coderre et al. 1990). NSAIDs injected systemically or intrathecally before the formalin injection produce a reduction in the behavioral response (Coderre et al. 1990; Malmberg and Yaksh 1992); it is not clear whether the same dose of NSAID given after the formalin is less effective.

The end of the second peak of the formalin model occurs within an hour, a short time when compared with the clinical context. However, in another animal model—the development of autotomy after peripheral nerve section—longer term preemptive effects have been reported with the use of local anesthetic. The speed with which autotomy developed in response to nerve section, and the severity of the autotomy, were altered by the application of local anesthetic to the nerve fiber before the operation (Selzer et al. 1991). Preemptive use of local anesthetic delayed the onset of autotomy (42 vs. 23 days) and reduced its severity (15 vs. 41%). Similarly, 50 μg of intrathecal morphine reduced autotomy following unilateral sciatic nerve section (Puke and Wiesenfeld-Hallin 1993). These studies are perhaps more analogous to the clinical context of the development of chronic pain, and the effect of such a nerve injury is believed to be analogous to neuropathic as opposed to nociceptive pain.

From basic science then comes the idea that the same dose of an analgesic given by the same route may be more effective if given before surgery compared with after. Neither of these models operates on a time scale that is a totally convincing analogy of the clinical operative and postoperative states. The formalin model is perhaps too brief and the autotomy model too long. The formalin model involves inflammatory change, the autotomy model nerve damage. Clinical procedures may involve both inflammatory response and nerve damage. Could preemptive analgesia alter outcome in all pain contexts, or is it limited, operating for example in somatic but not visceral pain, and are the underlying mechanisms the same? Clinical demonstration of preemptive analgesia might fail if the wrong setting was chosen. The secondary issue is which is the pertinent outcome? For clinical postoperative pain the outcome is measured over hours to days. The prevention of chronic pain development requires outcome measurement over weeks, months, and perhaps years.

THE CLINICAL EVIDENCE

This chapter provides a systematic review of the evidence that an intervention given before the pain starts has greater effect than the same intervention (same dose, same route) given after the pain begins. Each of three classes of intervention—NSAIDs, local anesthetics, and opioids—is reviewed separately.

The inclusion criterion for the review was randomized controlled trials (RCTs) that addressed the question of preemptive versus the same treatment given after the pain had begun (Fig. 1). Randomized studies reduce the chance of selection bias; non-randomized studies give no such protection. Ideally, the studies should be double-blind, and double-dummy if different routes were compared in the treatment and control groups. Studies were excluded from the review if they were not RCTs or if they were RCTs that did not compare preemptive with posttreatment (Fig. 1).

Studies were identified by a MEDLINE search (Silver Platter MEDLINE version 3.0 and 3.1) for 1966 to May 1993, and by hand search. The strategy was designed to identify the maximum number of randomized and/or double-blind reports by using a combination of text words, "wild cards," and MeSH terms as described previously (Jadad and McQuay 1993). Medical journals were hand searched. They were selected from a list of the 50 journals with the highest number of reports in MEDLINE, and nine specialist journals that were not included in that list or were not indexed. The search process included volumes published between 1950 and 1992. The studies included (and excluded) are shown in Table I.

EXCLUDED STUDIES

Comparisons of Preemptive Treatment with No Treatment (± not RCT)

Several of the excluded papers (Table I) are often quoted as showing evidence of a preemptive effect. They were, however, designed to show that

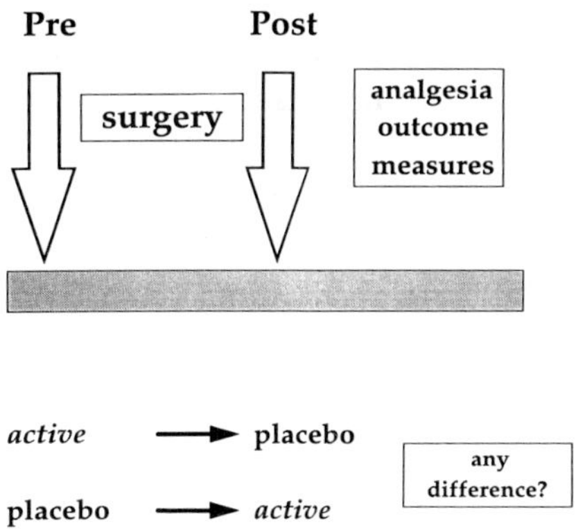

Fig. 1. Design required to show preemptive effect.

an analgesic intervention made before surgery was more effective than no intervention at all, and do not address the question of whether an analgesic intervention made before surgery is more, less, or as effective than the same intervention made after surgery. Nonetheless, the conclusion has been made that these studies produce evidence of a preemptive effect. A positive result in such designs suggests a worthwhile clinical benefit, but it is not evidence for or against a preemptive effect. Such evidence requires the control of the same intervention made after surgery (Fig. 1).

Comparisons of Preemptive Treatment with Preemptive Plus Posttreatment

These studies compared NSAID given before surgery with the same NSAID given both before and after surgery. It is not possible from these studies to answer the question of whether an analgesic intervention made before surgery is more, less, or as effective than the same intervention made after surgery.

STUDIES INCLUDED

NSAID and Paracetamol

Three RCTs with NSAIDs and one with paracetamol met the inclusion criterion. All were in oral surgery patients. Flath et al. (1987) studied four groups of 30 patients having endodontic surgery (Table II). One of these four groups had preoperative flurbiprofen and postoperative placebo. A second group had preoperative placebo and postoperative flurbiprofen. The preoperative dose was given 30 minutes before surgery and the postoperative dose 3 hours after surgery. There was no evidence of a preemptive effect on the outcome measures of categorical pain intensity and visual analogue pain intensity. The

Table I
Studies included or excluded for review

	NSAID	Local Anesthetic	Opioid
Studies included			
	Flath et al. 1987	Dahl et al. 1992	Katz et al. 1992
	Sisk et al. 1989	Pryle et al. 1993	Richmond et al. 1993
	Sisk and Grover 1990	Dierking et al. 1992	Amanor-Boadu et al. 1993
	Gustafsson et al. 1982	Rice et al. 1990	
		Gunter et al. 1990	
		Ejlersen et al. 1992	
Studies excluded			
Preemptive treatment with no postoperative comparison ± not RCT			
	Hutchison et al. 1990	Tverskoy et al. 1990	McQuay et al. 1988
	McGlew et al. 1991	Jebeles et al. 1991	Koskinen et al. 1991
	Smith and Brook 1990	Bugedo et al. 1990	
	Campbell et al. 1990	Bach et al. 1988	
		Narchi et al. 1991	
RCT but preemptive treatment plus postoperative treatment compared with postoperative only			
	Hill et al. 1987		
	Dupuis et al. 1988		
	Murphy and Medley 1993		

study had adequate sensitivity to detect a difference because one of the groups had preoperative and postoperative placebo, and the pain scores in that group were significantly higher than those in the groups that had flurbiprofen.

Sisk et al. (1989) compared diflunisal 1 g with placebo in 20 patients having third-molar extraction (Table II). The design was crossover, as shown in Fig. 1. Over eight hours, categorical pain intensity and visual analogue pain intensity scales showed no significant difference between preoperative and postoperative dosing. Sisk and Grover (1990) used a similar design to investigate naproxen 550 mg in third-molar extraction (Table II). Again, these same pain intensity scales showed no significant difference between preoperative and postoperative dosing.

Gustafsson et al. (1983) also used a two-occasion crossover design in third-molar extraction, comparing paracetamol 1 g with placebo (Table II). They used a visual analogue pain intensity scale and time to first analgesic as outcome measures and found no significant difference between preoperative and postoperative dosing.

These four studies provide a consistent answer to the question; they found

Table II
NSAID and paracetamol studies reviewed

Study	Design	No. of Patients	Procedure	Treatments	Outcome Measures	Timing preop	Timing postop	Outcome (preop vs. postop)
Flath et al. 1987	parallel	120	endodontic procedures	flurbiprofen 100 mg vs. placebo	cat PI and VASPI	15 min	3 hr	no significant difference
Sisk et al. 1989	crossover	20	third molar	diflunisal 1 g vs. placebo	cat PI and VASPI	30 min	30 min	no significant difference
Sisk and Grover 1990	crossover	36	third molar	naproxen 550 mg vs. placebo	cat PI and VASPI	30 min	30 min	no significant difference
Gustafsson et al. 1982	crossover	50	third molar	paracetamol 1 g vs. placebo	VASPI and TFA	45 min	35 min	no significant difference

Note: cat PI, categorical pain intensity scale; VASPI, visual analog pain intensity scale.

no measurable difference between the same dose given preoperatively and postoperatively. All four studies necessarily used local anesthetic; none used opioids. Thus, the balance of the evidence is that no preemptive effect was demonstrable at normal therapeutic oral doses of NSAID.

Local Anesthetic

Studies of preemptive effect with local anesthetics may be divided into trials of epidural (spinal), nerve block, and infiltration (Table III).

Epidural. Dahl et al. (1992) used a parallel group design on 32 colonic surgery patients (Table III). Epidural bolus and infusion of a local anesthetic and opioid combination was given 40 minutes before surgery for the preoperative group, and after surgery for the postoperative group (some two hours after the preoperative). There was no dummy injection. Categorical pain intensity and visual analogue pain intensity scales showed no evidence of a preemptive effect.

Pryle et al. (1993) used a similar design in 36 abdominal hysterectomy patients (Table III). Local anesthetic with adrenaline was given as a lumbar epidural bolus either 40 minutes before incision or after surgery (75 minutes after the preoperative group). The outcome measures of categorical pain intensity and visual analogue pain intensity scales, time to first use of intravenous morphine via patient controlled analgesia (PCA), and amount of intravenous morphine via PCA showed no demonstrable preemptive effect.

Table III
Local anaesthetic studies reviewed

Study	Design	No. of Patients	Procedure	Treatments	Outcome Measures	Timing pre	Timing post	Outcome (pre vs. post)
EPIDURAL								
Dahl et al. 1992	parallel group	32	major colonic surgery	epidural (T9-T12) bupivacaine and morphine	VASPI and cat PI at rest, cough and sitting up	bolus + infusion 40 min preop	bolus + infusion after surgery (still asleep)	no significant difference
Pryle et al. 1993	parallel group	36	abdominal hysterectomy	epidural (lumbar) bupivacaine and adrenaline	VASPI, cat, PI, PCA iv. morphine	40 min preincision	after surgery (still asleep)	no significant difference
Rice et al. 1990	parallel group	40	hernia, orchidopexy	caudal bupivacaine	pediatric objective score, TFA	after induction	after surgery	no significant difference
Gunter et al. 1990	parallel group	24	distal hypospadias	caudal bupivacain	TFA, analgesic needs	after induction	after surgery	no significant difference
NERVE BLOCK								
Dierking et al. 1992	parallel group	32	herniorrhaphy	inguinal field block lignocaine	VASPI and cat PI at rest, cough and moving	15 minute preop	after closure	no significant difference
IINFILTRATION								
Ejlersen et al. 1992	parallel group	37	herniorrhaphy	infiltration lignocaine	TFA, analgesic needs	5 min preincision (19 patients)	before closure (18 patients)	significantly delayed remedication time in pre group

Note: cat PI, categorical pain intensity scale; iv., intravenous; PCA, patient controlled analgesia; TFA, time to first analgesic; VASPI, visual analogue pain intensity scale.

Rice et al. (1990) compared caudal blocks pre- and postsurgery (Table III) in 40 children having outpatient surgery (mean operation time 30 minutes). An objective pain score did not show any preemptive effect. Gunter et al. (1990) used a similar design in 24 boys having hypospadias repair (Table III). The caudal block before surgery did reduce operating time and blood loss significantly compared with the same block after surgery, but there was no significant difference on the pain outcomes of time to first analgesic (TFA) or on overall analgesic consumption.

Nerve Block. Dierking et al. (1992) compared inguinal field block preoperatively and postoperatively in 32 patients having herniorrhaphy (Table III). Categorical and visual analogue pain intensity scales showed no evidence of a preemptive effect.

Infiltration. Ejlersen et al. (1992) investigated preoperative and postoperative wound infiltration in 37 herniorrhaphy patients (Table III). Using time to remedication as the outcome measure, they found a significantly longer time until remedication in patients who had the infiltration 5 minutes before incision (Fig. 2), clear evidence of a preemptive effect.

The study that did show a preemptive effect is the least subject to criticism (Ejlersen et al. 1992), but it is still balanced by five negative studies. The two pediatric studies (Rice et al. 1990; Gunter et al. 1990) both had the problem of pain scoring in children, but both showed no preemptive effect. Importantly, neither study involved the use of opioid and both therefore sought, and did not find, a preemptive effect of local anesthetic alone. It is difficult to

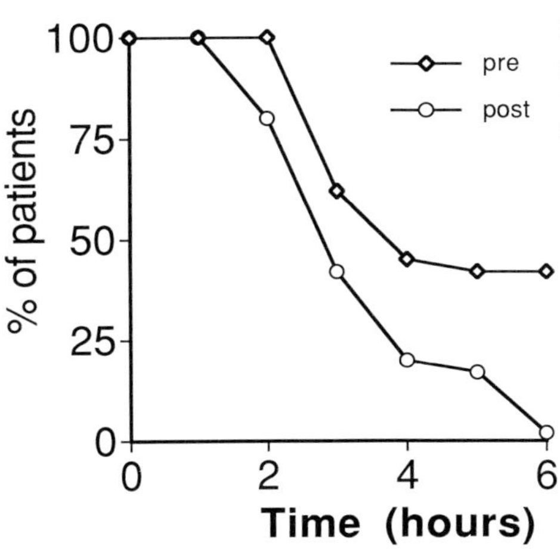

Fig. 2. Percentage of patients requiring remedication after pre- or postoperative wound infiltration with local anesthetic. (Redrawn from Ejlersen et al. 1992)

Table IV
Opioid studies reviewed

Study	Design	No. of Patients	Procedure	Treatments	Outcome Measures	Timing pre	Timing post	Outcome (pre vs. post)
EPIDURAL								
Katz et al. 1992	parallel group	30	thoracotomy	lumbar epidural fentanyl	VASPI and PCA iv. morphine	30 min infusion started 55 min pre incision	30 min infusion started 15 min after incision	significant difference (VASPI lower at 6 h and PCA morphine lower 12–24 h in pre group)
INTRAVENOUS								
Richmond et al. 1993	parallel group	76	total abdominal hysterectomy	10 mg iv. or im. morphine	VASPI and PCA iv. morphine	im. premed (16) or iv. at induction (23)	iv. at closure (21)	significant difference (PCA morphine lower to 24 h in iv. pre group at equivalent VASPI)
Amanor-Boadu et al. 1993	parallel group	41	body surface	5 mg iv. morphine	VASPI and cat PI at TFA	at induction (21)	at closure (20)	significant difference (cat PI lower at TFA in pre group)

Note: Number in parentheses are numbers of patients. Cat PI, categorical pain intensity scale; im., intramuscular; iv., intravenous; PCA, patient controlled analgesia; TFA, time to first analgesic; VASPI, visual analogue pain intensity scale.

understand why the infiltration study should have produced a positive result when the other five studies showed no preemptive effect.

In all the negative studies the local anesthetic intervention worked well, whether given before or after surgery. The power of these studies, the certitude in stating that the lack of difference is a true result, becomes a major issue. Ideally, the design in Fig. 1 could be extended to include a group that has placebo pre and placebo post. Significant difference between that placebo-placebo group and the active treatment groups would ensure that the methods were of adequate sensitivity. For the present we have a set of negative studies, without internal sensitivity checks, none of which is of adequate size to be totally convincing.

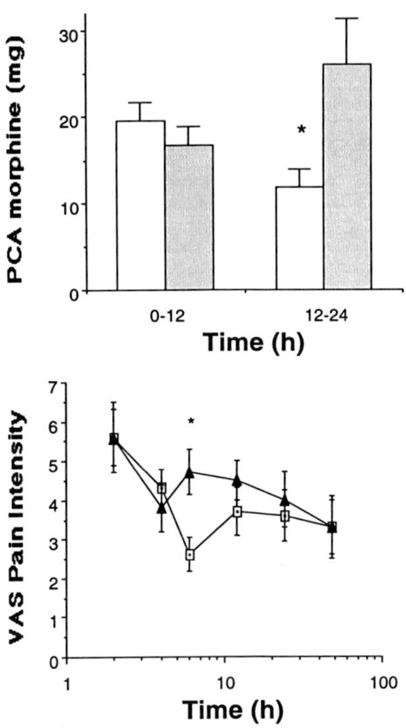

Fig. 3. **Top**: mean ± S.E.M. (mg) for preoperative (plain) and intraoperative (stippled) epidural opioid (* significant difference). **Bottom**: mean ± S.E.M. visual analogue pain intensity (cm) for preoperative (squares) and intraoperative (triangles) epidural opioid (* significant difference). (Redrawn from Katz et al. 1992)

Opioids

Three opioid studies (Table IV) conform to the design required to answer the preemptive question. Katz et al. (1992) looked at spinal opioid, while Richmond et al. (1993) and Amanor-Boadu et al. (1993) investigated the intravenous route.

Katz et al. randomized 30 thoracic patients to lumbar epidural fentanyl infusion, either preoperatively or intraoperatively (Table IV). The infusion in the postincision group was started 15 minutes after incision. Using a visual analogue pain intensity scale and PCA intravenous morphine as outcome measures, they found significantly lower visual analogue pain intensity scores at six hours in the preoperative group (with no significant difference in the PCA morphine consumption). From 12–24 hours they found significantly lower PCA morphine consumption in the preoperative group with no significant difference in the visual analogue pain intensity score (Fig. 3).

Richmond et al. (1993) randomized 76 total abdominal hysterectomy patients to 10 mg intramuscular morphine as premedication, 10 mg intravenous morphine at induction, or 10 mg intravenous morphine at closure (Table IV).

Analgesic outcome measures were visual analogue pain intensity scores and PCA intravenous morphine consumption. They found significantly lower PCA intravenous morphine consumption in the group that had received intravenous morphine at induction compared with the group that received the same dose by the same route at closure (Fig. 4).

Amanor-Boadu et al. (1993) in a similar design looked at the effect of 5 mg of intravenous morphine given at induction or at closure to 41 body-surface surgery patients (Table IV). Outcome measures were the time to first analgesic and the visual analogue pain intensity and categorical pain intensity scores at that time. Categorical pain intensity scores were significantly lower at the time of remedication in the group given morphine at induction compared with the group given morphine at closure (Fig. 5).

Each of these three studies suggests that opioids may have a preemptive effect. Unfortunately, none of the studies is perfect. The epidural study showed a significant preemptive effect at only one of the six visual analogue pain intensity scale measurement points. In the 10-mg intravenous study the PCA morphine consumption was reversed in the subsequent 24 hours (Richmond et al. 1993). In the 5-mg intravenous study only one of the two outcomes showed a significant effect. Nonetheless, we have three studies that showed a weak positive preemptive effect with opioid.

CONCLUSION

The question in the title was "Do preemptive treatments provide better pain control?" It should be answered separately for each of the three drug classes reviewed, because the answers may be different. For NSAIDs and paracetamol there are four good studies, all with no evidence of a preemptive effect. If there is a preemptive effect of NSAID it is unlikely to be seen with conventional dosing. For local anesthetics, one good infiltration study showed a preemptive effect. Five other studies, spinal and nerve block, did not show

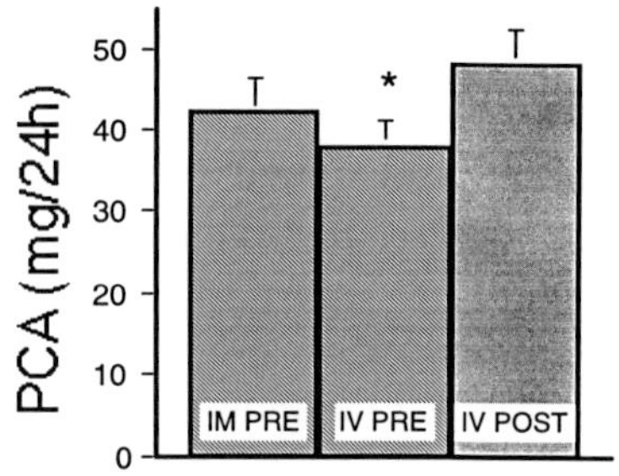

Fig. 4. PCA morphine consumption (mg/24 hours) after 10 mg intravenous morphine given as im. premed (diagonal), iv. at induction (plain), or iv. postop (stippled). Mean ± S.E.M., * significant difference iv. preemptive vs. iv. post. (Redrawn from Richmond et al. 1993)

any effect. These negative local anesthetic studies have been criticized (Katz 1993) because they were contaminated by opioid, but in two of the studies (Rice et al. 1990; Gunter et al. 1990) patients received no opioid. Perhaps a stronger criticism of these negative studies is that they lacked power.

The evidence with opioids is tantalizing but inconclusive. The evidence from fundamental studies for a preemptive effect of opioid (Dickenson and Sullivan 1987; Puke and Wiesenfeld-Hallin 1993) is also stronger than the equivalents for local anesthetic and NSAID. Inevitably, we now need studies of adequate design and size to establish whether or not there is indeed a measurable preemptive effect of opioid in humans. It does appear that the intravenous route can be used to answer the question, and that makes the studies easier to do than if the effect was only found with spinal routes. The caveat must be that the doses used in the (intrathecal) basic studies were large (up to 50 µg), and that the effect was demonstrated via the intrathecal route. This makes the human findings with relatively small intravenous doses all the more remarkable. Evidence of a preemptive effect with opioid would offer great potential benefit to patients with postoperative pain. It also would be important to know if such a preemptive effect applied to neuropathic pain (Bach et al. 1988; Puke and Wiesenfeld-Hallin 1993).

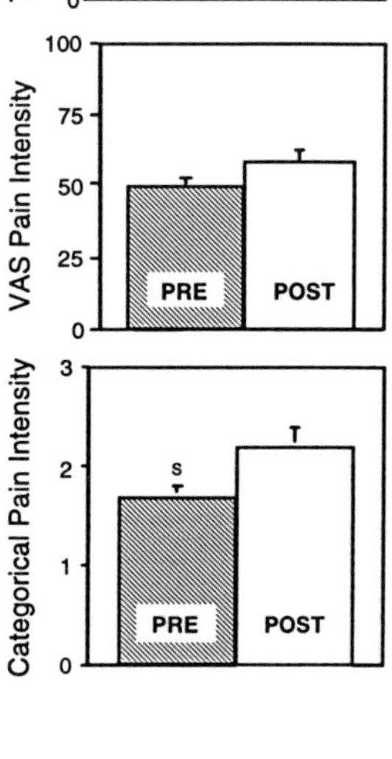

Fig. 5. Time to first analgesic (minutes; median), visual analogue pain intensity (mm; mean ± S.E.M.) and categorical pain intensity (mean ± S.E.M.) after 5 mg intravenous morphine given iv. at induction (pre) or iv. postop (post) (* significant difference preemptive vs. post). (From Amanor-Boadu et al. 1993)

REFERENCES

Amanor-Boadu, S.D., Jadad, A.R., Glynn, C.J., Jack, T.M. and McQuay, H.J., Influence of pre and postoperative morphine administration on pain after body surface surgery: a double-blind randomised controlled study. In: Abstracts: 7th World Congress on Pain, IASP Publications, Seattle, 1993, pp 538–539.

Bach, S., Noreng, M.F. and Tjellden, N.U., Phantom limb pain in amputees during the first 12 months following limb amputation, after preoperative lumbar epidural blockade, Pain, 33 (1988) 297–301.

Bugedo, G.J., Cárcamo, C.R., Mertens, R.A., Dagnino, J.A. and Muñoz, H.R., Preoperative percutaneous ilioinguinal and iliohypogastric nerve block with 0.5% bupivacaine for post-herniorrhaphy pain management in adults, Reg. Anesth., 15 (1990) 130–133.

Campbell, W.I., Kendrick, R. and Patterson, C., Intravenous diclofenac sodium. Does its administration before operation suppress postoperative pain? Anaesthesia, 45 (1990) 763–766.

Coderre, T.J., Vaccarino, A.L. and Melzack, R., Central nervous system plasticity in the tonic pain response to subcutaneous formalin injection, Brain Res., 535 (1990) 155–158.

Dahl, J.B., Hansen, B.L., Hjortsø, N.C., Erichsen, C.J., Møiniche, S. and Kehlet, H., Influence of timing on the effect of continuous extradural analgesia with bupivacaine and morphine after major abdominal surgery, Br. J. Anaesth., 69 (1992) 4–12.

Dickenson, A.H., Recent advances in the physiology and pharmacology of pain: plasticity and its implications for clinical analgesia, J. Psychopharmacol., 5 (1991) 342–351.

Dickenson, A.H. and Sullivan, A.F., Subcutaneous formalin-induced activity of dorsal horn neurones in the rat: differential response to an intrathecal opiate administered pre or post formalin, Pain, 30 (1987) 349–360.

Dierking, G.W., Dahl, J.B., Kanstrup, J., Dahl, A. and Kehlet, H., Effect of pre- vs postoperative inguinal field block on postoperative pain after herniorrhaphy, Br. J. Anaesth., 68 (1992) 344–348.

Dupuis, R., Lemay, H., Bushnelle, M.C. and Duncan, G.H., Preoperative flurbiprofen in oral surgery: a method of choice in controlling postoperative pain, Pharmacotherapy, 8 (1988) 193–200.

Ejlersen, E., Andersen, H.B., Eliasen, K. and Mogensen, T., A comparison between preincisional and postincisional lidocaine infiltration and postoperative pain, Anesth. Analg., 74 (1992) 495–498.

Flath, R.K., Hicks, M.L., Dionne, R.A. and Pelleu, G.B., Pain suppression after pulpectomy with preoperative flurbiprofen, J. Endodontics, 13 (1987) 339–347.

Gunter, J.B., Forestner, J.E. and Manley, C.B., Caudal epidural anesthesia reduces blood loss during hypospadias repair, J. Urology, 144 (1990) 517–519.

Gustafsson, I., Nystrom, E. and Quiding, H., Effect of preoperative paracetamol on pain after oral surgery, Eur. J. Clin. Pharmacol., 24 (1983) 63–65.

Hill, C.M., Carroll, M.J., Giles, A.D. and Pickvance, N., Ibuprofen given pre and post operatively for the relief of pain, Int. J. Oral Maxillofac. Surg., 16 (1987) 420–424.

Hutchison, G.L., Crofts, S.L. and Gray, I.G., Preoperative piroxicam for postoperative analgesia in dental surgery, Br. J. Anaesth., 65 (1990) 500–503.

Jadad, A.R. and McQuay, H.J., A high yield strategy to identify randomized controlled trials for systematic reviews [article], Online J. Curr. Clin. Trials [serial online], 1993 (Doc 33) (1993 Feb 27).

Jebeles, J.A., Reilly, J.S., Gutierrez, J.F., Bradley, E.L. and Kissin, I., The effect of pre-incisional infiltration of tonsils with bupivacaine on the pain following tonsillectomy under general anesthesia, Pain, 47 (1991) 305–308.

Katz, J., Preop analgesia for acute pain, Lancet, 342 (1993) 65–66.

Katz, J., Kavanagh, B.P., Sandler, A.N., Nierenberg, H., Boylan, J.F., Friedlander, M. and Shaw, M.F., Preemptive Analgesia: clinical evidence of neuroplasticity contributing to postoperative pain, Anesthesiology, 77 (1992) 439–446.

Koskinen, R., Tigerstedt, I. and Tammisto, T., The effect of peroperative alfentanil on the need for immediate postoeprative pain relief, Acta Anaesthesiol. Scand., 35, Suppl. 96 (1991) O21.

Malmberg, A.B. and Yaksh, T.L., Hyperalgesia mediated by spinal glutamate of substance P receptor blocked by spinal cyclooxygenase inhibition, Science, 257 (1992) 1276–1279.

McGlew, I.C., Angliss, D.B., Gee, G.J., Rutherford, A. and Wood, A.T., A comparison of rectal indomethacin with placebo for pain relief following spinal surgery, Anaesth. Intensive Care, 19 (1991) 40–45.

McQuay, H.J., Carroll, D. and Moore, R.A., Postoperative orthopaedic pain: the effect of opiate premedication and local anaesthetic blocks, Pain, 33 (1988) 291–295.

McQuay, H.J. and Dickenson, A.H., Implications of nervous system plasticity for pain management, Anaesthesia, 45 (1990) 101–102.

Murphy, D.F. and Medley, C., Preoperative indomethacin for pain relief after thoracotomy: comparison with postoperative indomethacin, Br. J. Anaesth., 70 (1993) 298–300.

Narchi, P., Benhamou, D. and Fernandez, H., Intraperitoneal local anaesthetics for shoulder pain after day-case laparoscopy, Lancet, 338 (1991) 291–295.

Pryle, B.J., Vanner, R.G., Enriquez, N. and Reynolds, F., Can pre-emptive lumbar epidural blockade reduce postoperative pain following lower abdominal surgery? Anaesthesia, 48 (1993) 120–123.

Puke, M.J.C. and Wiesenfeld-Hallin, Z., The differential effects of morphine and the alpha2-adrenoreceptor agonists clonidine and dexmedetomidine on the prevention and treatment of experimental neuropathic pain, Anesth. Analg., 77 (1993) 104–109.

Rice, L.J., Pudimat, M.A. and Hannalah, R.S., Timing of caudal block placement in relation to surgery does not affect duration of postoperative analgesia in paediatric ambulatory patients, Can. J. Anaesth., 37 (1990) 429–431.

Richmond, C.E., Bromley, L.M. and Woolf, C.J., Preoperative morphine pre-empts postoperative pain, Lancet, 342 (1993) 73–75.

Selzer, Z., Beilin, B.Z., Ginzburg, R., Paran, Y. and Shimko, T., The role of injury discharge in the induction of neuropathic pain behavior in rats, Pain, 46 (1991) 327–336.

Sisk, A.L. and Grover, B.J., A comparison of preoperative and postoperative naproxen sodium for suppression of postoperative pain, J. Oral Maxillofac. Surg., 48 (1990) 674–678.

Sisk, A.L., Mosley, R.O. and Martin, R.P., Comparison of preoperative and postoperative diflunisal for suppression of postoperative pain, J. Oral Maxillofac. Surg., 47 (1989) 464–468.

Smith, A.C. and Brook, I.M., Inhibition of tissue prostaglandin synthesis during third molar surgery: use of preoperative fenbufen, Br. J. Oral Maxillofac. Surg., 44 (1990) 251–253.

Tverskoy, M., Cozacov, C., Ayache, M., Bradley, E.L. and Kissin, I., Postoperative pain after inguinal herniorrhaphy with different types of anesthesia, Anesth. Analg., 70 (1990) 29–35.

Wall, P.D., The prevention of postoperative pain, Pain, 33 (1988) 289–290.

Woolf, C.J., Evidence for a central component of post-injury pain hypersensitivity, Nature, 306 (1983) 686–688.

Correspondence to: H.J. McQuay, DM, Pain Relief Unit, Churchill Hospital, Old Road, Headington, Oxford OX3 7LJ, UK. Tel: 44-865-226161; Fax: 44-865-226160.

Proceedings of the 7th World Congress on Pain,
Progress in Pain Research and Management, Vol. 2,
edited by G.F. Gebhart, D.L. Hammond, and T.S.
Jensen, IASP Press, Scattle, © 1994.

48

Lamotrigine and Analogs: A New Treatment for Chronic Pain?

Meire Nakamura-Craig and
Rhonda Lesley Follenfant

*Department of Pharmacology, Wellcome Research Laboratories,
Beckenham, Kent, UK*

INTRODUCTION

Among the different chronic pain conditions, the cause of neuropathic pain, characterized by continuing and/or episodic pain, hyperalgesia, and allodynia, is not well known and the treatment is not adequate. A recent study (Jeanmonod et al. 1993) has shown a bursting neuronal activity in the medial thalamus of patients with neurogenic pain suggesting that certain chronic pain conditions correlate with long-term neuronal changes. In the last few years, studies have suggested that excitatory amino acids, particularly glutamate acting at the NMDA receptor subtype, are involved in mechanisms that result in long-term, use-dependent changes in neuronal excitability and synaptic plasticity (Woolf 1989; Dickenson 1990). Lamotrigine (Lamictal®), a novel antiepileptic drug, is known to block sodium channels in a use-dependent manner (Cheung et al. 1992) and can inhibit glutamate release in the rat striatum (McGeer and Zhu 1990) and rat cortex (Leach et al. 1986). Our study investigated the effects of lamotrigine and a related triazine compound, BW524C79 [3,5-diamino-6-(2,3,5-trichlorophenyl)-1,2,4-triazine], in models of chronic pain in rats.

MATERIALS AND METHODS

MEASUREMENT OF PAIN THRESHOLD IN DIABETIC RATS

Following a 48-hour fast, male Wistar rats (200–250 g) were treated with streptozotocin (70 mg/kg ip.). Three to four weeks after treatment, blood glucose concentrations were measured by tail-clip sampling. Streptozotocin-treated rats with blood glucose levels of 12 mmol/l were considered diabetic. Pain threshold in the paw of normal and diabetic rats was measured by a modification of the Randall-Selitto test (1957). In this test, a constant pressure of 40 mm Hg is applied to the hind paws of rats and is discontinued when the animals withdraw the paw (reaction time, s).

MEASUREMENT OF HYPERALGESIA INDUCED BY ULTRAVIOLET RADIATION

The experiments followed ethical guidelines of the International Association for the Study of Pain (IASP) and Home Office regulations on humane use of research animals. Wistar rats (150–200 g) were exposed on one hindpaw to ultraviolet radiation (UV, intensity maximum 363 nm, 280 microwatts CM2) for 90 seconds; this exposure repeated 18 hours later (Perkins et al. 1992). Six days after the UV radiation, both paws exhibited thermal hyperalgesia evaluated by withdrawal of the paw from a focused beam of heat applied to the dorsal surface. Compounds were evaluated on day 6. In all experiments the experimenter was unaware of the group treatments during the test period.

All results are presented as means ± S.E.M. The level of statistical significance was determined with Student's *t* test for paired samples and differences with $P < 0.05$ were considered statistically significant.

RESULTS

The reaction time (seconds) to paw pressure in the streptozotocin-induced diabetic rats was significantly lower than that of nondiabetic controls (mean ± S.E.M. 13.6 ± 0.2 seconds, n = 102, compared to 26.4 ± 0.3 seconds, n = 45, $P < 0.001$). Treatment with insulin in doses that normalized the levels of blood glucose did not change the pain threshold in diabetic rats. Blood glucose concentrations were unaffected by treatment with lamotrigine or the compound BW524C79.

Lamotrigine (20 and 40 mg/kg p.o.) given to diabetic rats three weeks

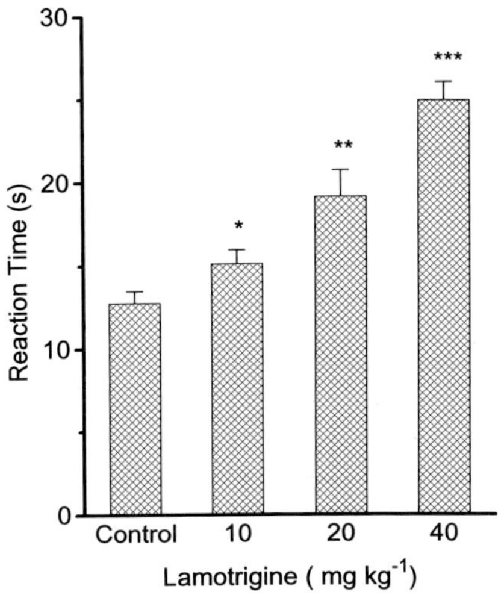

Fig. 1. Effect of lamotrigine (10–40 mg/kg p.o.) on pain threshold in diabetic rats. Lamotrigine or Celacol was given to diabetic rats three weeks after streptozotocin administration (70 mg/kg ip.). Results show the effect of lamotrigine and Celacol (control) on reaction time to paw pressure three hours after the administration. Significant difference from control (Student's *t* test, * $P < 0.05$, ** $P < 0.01$, *** $P < 0.001$, n = 8).

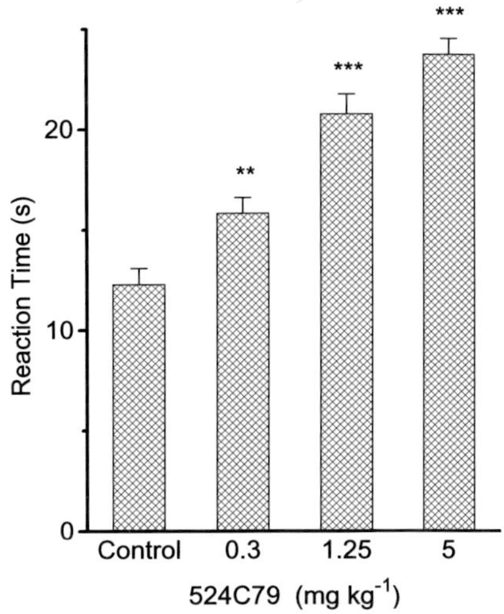

Fig. 2. Effect of compound BW524C79 (0.3–5 mg/kg)on pain threshold in diabetic rats. Compound BW524C79 or Celacol (p.o.) was given three weeks after streptozotocin treatment (70 mg/kg ip.). Results show the effect of compound BW524C79 and Celacol (control) on reaction time to paw pressure three hours after the administration. (Student's *t* test, ** $P < 0.01$, *** $P < 0.001$, n = 8).

after streptozotocin administration (70 mg/kg ip.) induced analgesia that lasted for at least five hours in the paw pressure test (Fig. 1). The lamotrigine related triazine compound BW524C79 (2.5 and 10 mg/kg p.o.) given to diabetic rats induced analgesia that lasted for at least 7 hours (Fig. 2).

To study whether lamotrigine could induce tolerance to its analgesic effect, lamotrigine (20 mg/kg p.o.) or Celacol (methyl-cellulose, lamotrigine vehicle) was given twice daily for four days to diabetic rats with low pain threshold. On day 5, the animals were treated with lamotrigine (20 mg/kg p.o.). Fig. 3 shows that the effect of this dose of lamotrigine was comparable in lamotrigine and Celacol-treated animals (four days treatment).

The application of UV radiation to the rat paw induces sustained hyperalgesia that is present from 4 to 10 days after the radiation (Perkins et al. 1992). Lamotrigine (10 and 25 mg/kg p.o.) given six days after the UV application to the hind paw of rats and one hour prior to paw flick test induced

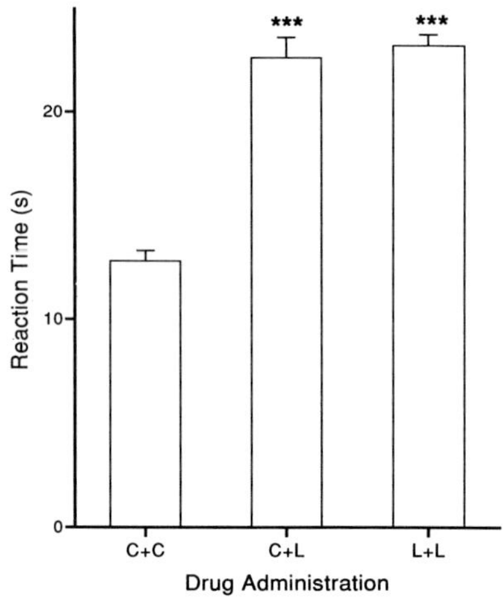

Fig. 3. Effect of chronic administration of lamotrigine on pain threshold in diabetic rats. Rats were given Celacol (C) or lamotrigine (L, 20 mg/kg p.o.) twice daily for four days. On day 5, the animals were treated with lamotrigine (20 mg/kg p.o.) or Celacol one hour before the paw pressure test. Significant difference from C+C is shown as *** $P < 0.001$ (Student's t test, n = 6).

a significant increase in the pain threshold in rats with sustained hyperalgesia (Fig. 4). Compound BW524C79 (2.5 and 10 mg/kg p.o.) also induced a significant increase in the reaction time on the paw flick test in rats that had UV radiation (Fig. 5).

DISCUSSION

Rats with streptozotocin or alloxan-induced diabetes have been used as models to study neuropathic pain as well as other complications of diabetes. In these models, nociceptive thresholds are reduced for both mechanical and thermal stimuli (Forman et al. 1986; Lee et al. 1990; Ahlgren and Levine 1993). Lamotrigine (20 and 40 mg/kg p.o.) and the related triazine, compound BW524C79 (2.5 and 10 mg/kg p.o.) significantly increased the pain threshold in rats with diabetes induced by streptozotocin.

Sustained hyperalgesia, a phenomenon that occurs after multiple injections of hyperalgesic substances into the rat paw (Nakamura-Craig and Smith 1989; Ferreira et al. 1990) or after exposure of the paw to ultraviolet radiation (Perkins et al. 1992), could be associated with some chronic pain conditions. Lamotrigine and compound BW524C79 induced significant increase of pain threshold in rats whose paw was exposed to ultraviolet radiation. These results suggest that these compounds could be used in the treatment of chronic pain conditions such as neuropathic pain and cancer with associated hyperalgesia and/or allodynia.

The development of tolerance to the analgesic effects is one of the major problems in the treatment of chronic pain conditions. Chronic administration

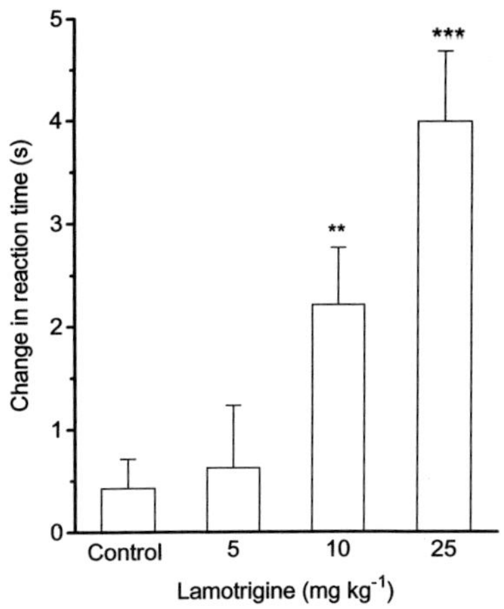

Fig. 4. Effect of lamotrigine (5–25 mg/kg p.o.) on ultraviolet-induced sustained hyperalgesia. Lamotrigine (p.o.) or Celacol (control) was given six days after the UV application to the hind paw and one hour prior to paw-flick test. Significant statistical difference from control (Student's *t* test, ** $P < 0.01$, *** $P < 0.001$, n = 8).

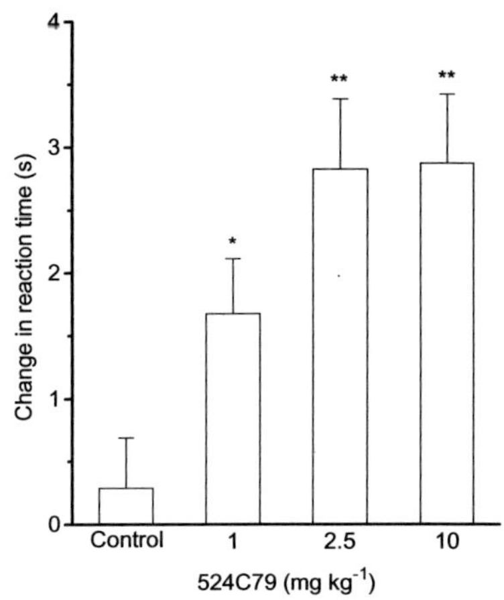

Fig. 5. Effect of compound BW524C79 (1–10 mg/kg p.o.) on ultraviolet-induced sustained hyperalgesia. Compound BW524C79 or Celacol (control) was given six days after the UV application to the hind paw and one hour prior to paw-flick test. Significant statistical difference from control (Student's *t* test, * $P < 0.05$, ** $P < 0.01$, n = 8).

of lamotrigine (20 mg/kg p.o.) twice daily for four days did not cause tolerance to the analgesic effects in diabetic rats. Thus lamotrigine and analogs could be used chronically without causing tolerance to the analgesic effects. Lamotrigine and analogs may represent a new class of analgesics for the treatment of some chronic pain conditions where hypersensitivity exists and where conventional analgesics are ineffective.

ACKNOWLEDGMENT

The authors thank Miss A. Wyatt for technical assistance in part of the experiments.

REFERENCES

Ahlgren, S.C. and Levine, J.D., Mechanical hyperalgesia in streptozotocin-diabetic rats, Neuroscience, 52 (1993) 1049–1055.

Cheung, H., Kamp, D. and Harris, E., An in vitro investigation of the action of lamotrigine on

neuronal voltage-activated sodium channels, Epilepsy Res., 13 (1992) 107–112.
Dickenson, A.H., A cure for wind up: NMDA receptor antagonists as analgesics, Trends Neurol. Sci., 11 (1990) 307–309.
Ferreira, S.H., Lorenzetti, B.B. and De Campos, D.I., Induction, blockade and restoration of a persistent hypersensitive state, Pain, 42 (1990) 365–372.
Forman, L.J., Estelow, S., Lewis, M. and Vasilenko, P., Streptozotocin diabetes alters immunoreactive of β-endorphin levels and pain perception after 8 weeks in female rats, Diabetes, 35 (1986) 1309–1313.
Jeannmonod, D., Magnin, M. and Morel, A., Thalamus and neurogenic pain: physiological, anatomical and clinical data, Neuroreport, 4 (1993) 475–478.
Leach, M.J., Marden, C.M. and Miller, A.A., Pharmacological studies on lamotrigine, a novel potential antiepileptic drug: II. Neurochemical studies on the mechanism of action, Epilepsia, 27 (1986) 490–497.
Lee, J.H., Cox, D.J., Mook, D.J. and McCarty, R.C., Effect of hyperglicemia on pain threshold in alloxan-diabetic rats, Pain, 40 (1990) 105–107.
McGeer, E.G. and Zhu, S.G., Lamotrigine protects against kainate but not ibotenate lesions in rat striatum, Neurosci. Lett., 112 (1990) 348–351.
Nakamura-Craig, M. and Smith, T.W., Substance P and peripheral inflammatory hyperalgesia, Pain, 38 (1989) 91–98.
Perkins, M.N., Patel, S., Kelly, D. and Dray, A., Persistent hyperalgesia in the rat induced by ultraviolet radiation, Abstracts from International Congress New Trends in Referred Pain and Hyperalgesia, held in Chieti, Italy, 1992, p. 79.
Woolf, C.J., Recent advances in the pathophysiology of acute pain, Br. J. Anaesth., 63 (1989) 139–146.

Correspondence to: Dr. M. Nakamura-Craig, Department of Pharmacology, Wellcome Research Laboratories, Langley Court, Beckenham, Kent BR3 3BS, England. Tel: 44-81-658-2211 ext. 25249; Fax: 44-81-663-6176.

Part IX

Headache

Proceedings of the 7th World Congress on Pain,
Progress in Pain Research and Management, Vol. 2,
edited by G.F. Gebhart, D.L. Hammond, and T.S.
Jensen, IASP Press, Seattle, © 1994.

49

Pathophysiology of Human Vascular Headache

Jes Olesen

Department of Neurology, Glostrup Hospital, University of Copenhagen, Glostrup, Denmark

INTRODUCTION

The vascular headaches in humans are migraine, cluster headache, some of the posttraumatic headaches, and headaches due to vascular diseases. To some extent they probably share pain mechanisms. Because migraine is by far the most common and best studied of these disorders, it is the focus of this chapter.

WHAT IS MIGRAINE?

This question was not easy to answer in the past. Until 1988 there was no generally agreed upon definition of migraine or subdivision of the syndrome. The most commonly used so-called definition was that of an ad hoc committee of the National Institutes of Health in America (Ad Hoc Committee 1962), a short description without specified requirements for the diagnosis. For the purpose of pathophysiological investigations in migraine. I therefore had to develop my own operational diagnostic criteria (Olesen 1978; Olesen et al. 1981a). Studies of regional cerebral blood flow (rCBF) supported the idea that migraine with aura (previously called classic migraine) and migraine without aura (previously called common migraine) were pathophysiologically different in the early phase of the attack, and such evidence played an important role in the considerations of the Headache Classification Committee of the International Headache Society, which, in 1988, published a new international headache classification with operational diagnostic criteria for all headache disorders (Headache Classification Committee 1988). The operational diagnostic criteria for the two main forms of migraine—migraine without aura and migraine with aura—are given in Table I. Basically the two conditions share the same kind of headache and associated symptoms, but migraine with aura is initiated by neurological symptoms called the aura.

Aura symptoms most typically are visual or sensory and, occasionally, also include motor and speech disturbances. They begin focally and spread out topographically to reach a maximum usually within 5–15 minutes; they usually last between 20 and 60 minutes. They often consist of positive phenomena at the edge—for example, flickering light in the visual field or pins and needles sensations in the extremities—followed by negative phenomena—for example, scotoma in the visual field or numbness in the extremities. They are fully reversible, often followed by an unexplained symptom-free interval of up to one hour before the headache develops.

PREVIOUS THEORIES OF MIGRAINE NOCICEPTION

For more than a century it has been debated whether migraine pain is neuronal or vascular. This literature has been very elegantly discussed by Schiller (1975). In the 1940s and 1950s the vascular theory became dominant, mainly because of the work of Harold G. Wolff at the New York Hospital (Wolff 1963). The arguments available at that time in favor of vascular nociception were the following: migraine pain is usually pulsating; it is associated with visible dilatation of the superficial temporal artery and measurably increased pulsations in the superficial temporal artery; it is relieved by compression of the common carotid or the superficial temporal arteries; and it is relieved by ergotamine and other vasoconstrictors such as noradrenaline. The migraine aura was thought to be caused by intracranial arterial constriction and cerebral ischemia because it reportedly could be relieved by inhalation of amyl nitrate. Migraine pain was not alleviated by saline injection into the lumbar spinal fluid, increasing intracranial pressure and thereby dampening intracranial but not extracranial pulsations. Migraine nociception was therefore thought to be primarily extracranial. Histamine-induced headache could be relieved by intrathecal saline and was therefore considered to be intracranial.

Wolff's experiments, ingenious for his time, were internationally accepted almost without question. Some of them could not easily be reproduced, however. Brazil and Friedman (1956) did not find the increased extracranial pulsations, and Hare (1966) could not reproduce the effect of amyl nitrate on the visual aura. Ergotamine has several other effects in addition to its vasoconstrictor properties, and the finding of extracranial origin of nociception was only partly reproduced by Blau and Dexter (1981) and by Drummond and Lance (1983).

Table I
Diagnostic criteria for the most important types of migraine

1.1 Migraine without aura

A. At least 5 attacks fulfilling B–D

B. Headache attacks lasting 4–72 hours (untreated or unsuccessfully treated)

C. Headache has at least two of the following characteristics:

1. Unilateral location
2. Pulsating quality
3. Moderate or severe intensity
4. Aggravation by walking stairs or similar routine physical activity

D. During headache at least one of the following:

1. Nausea and/or vomiting
2. Photophobia and phonophobia

E. At least one of the following:

1. History, physical- and neurological examinations do not suggest one of the disorders listed in groups 5–11 [not reprinted here]
2. History and/or physical- and/or neurological examinations do suggest such disorder, but it is ruled out by appropriate investigations
3. Such disorder is present, but migraine attacks do not occur for the first time in close temporal relation to the disorder

1.2 Migraine with aura

A. At least 2 attacks fulfilling B.

B. At least 3 of the following 4 characteristics:

1. One or more fully reversible aura symptoms indicating focal cerebral cortical and/or brain stem dysfunction.
2. At least one aura symptom develops gradually over more than 4 minutes or, 2 or more symptoms occur in succession.
3. No aura symptom lasts more than 60 minutes. If more than one aura symptom is present, accepted duration is proportionally increased.
4. Headache follows aura with a free interval of less than 60 minutes. (It may also begin before or simultaneously with the aura.)

C. At least one of the following:

1. History, physical- and neurological examinations do not suggest one of the disorders listed in groups 5–11 [not reprinted here].
2. History and/or physical- and/or neurological examinations do suggest such disorder, but it is ruled out by appropriate investigations.
3. Such disorder is present, but migraine attacks do not occur for the first time in close temporal relation to the disorder.

Source: Reprinted with permission from Headache Classification Committee 1988.

MIGRAINE NOCICEPTION IS NOT PRIMARILY EXTRACRANIAL

Wolff's hypothesis that migraine nociception is primarily extracranial cannot be sustained. In an extensive clinical investigation, compressing either the carotid artery or the superficial temporal artery and performing a number of maneuvers thought to primarily augment extracranial pain, Blau and Dexter (1981) concluded that migraine pain was likely to be intracranial in the majority of cases. Similar compression and clinical studies supplemented by indirect photoplethysmographic measurements of the diameter of the superficial temporal artery showed that extracranial vasculature could explain migraine pain in only a minority of patients (Drummond and Lance 1983).

Applying quantitative techniques, we have shown that focal blood flow in the subcutaneous tissues of the temporal region is normal during attacks of migraine without aura (Jensen 1987). The regulation of subcutaneous blood flow in the same area was also normal. Temporal muscle blood flow, measured by clearance of 133-Xenon injected into the temporal muscle, was normal during migraine attacks without aura when compared to measurements outside of attacks and comparing the painful side to the nonpainful side (Jensen and Olesen 1985).. Also, the regulation of temporal muscle blood flow during tonic or dynamic work was normal during migraine attacks (Jensen and Olesen 1985). Abnormalities can therefore be ruled out with a reasonable degree of certainty.

Blood flow reflects resistance of the arterioles, but it does not vary in parallel with vasomotion of the arteries. Using high-frequency ultrasound, we have recently been able to measure the absolute luminal diameter of the superficial temporal artery in migraine patients during and outside of attacks (Iversen et al. 1990). During attacks of unilateral migraine pain, there was a mild constriction of both right and left radial arteries (4%) and of the superficial temporal artery on the nonpainful side (9%). On the painful side the diameter of the superficial temporal artery was significantly larger than on the nonpainful side (9%). It was not different, however, from measurements outside of attacks. The findings were interpreted as follows: There is a (neurogenic?) dilatory effect on the pain side during unilateral migraine attacks. It is not strong enough to cause actual dilatation of the superficial temporal artery but is strong enough to compensate for a systemic arterial constriction. The latter is most likely due to pain activation of the sympathetic nervous system. In addition to the lack of absolute arterial dilatation during migraine attacks, the superficial temporal artery is not tender to palpation (Iversen et al. 1990). It therefore appears unlikely that the primary source of nociception could be extracranial arteries.

ARTERIOLAR RESPONSES AS MEASURED BY rCBF CAUSE PAIN INDIRECTLY BY TRIGGERING OTHER MECHANISMS

Skinhøj and Paulson (1969) were the first to measure regional cerebral blood flow (rCBF) during a migraine attack. As expected according to Wolff's theory, they found a focal decrease during the aura phase. Subsequently, several other casuistic reports were published (for references see Olesen 1991a). To really evaluate the chain of events spatially and topographically it was, however, necessary to employ equipment with a much better spatial resolution. Such equipment has been used by our group. Parts of our findings have recently been confirmed using the non-quantitative technique of technetium HMPAO injection and a rotating gamma camera. (For a complete discussion of the literature please see Olesen 1991b.)

Angiography triggers attacks in patients suffering from migraine with aura. This has made it possible occasionally to measure rCBF before and during the development of the migraine aura (Olesen et al. 1981b; Lauritzen et al. 1983a; Skyhøj Olsen et al. 1987; Friberg et al. 1987; Olesen et al. 1990). A complicated and probably pathognomonic series of events were shown to take place, as documented earlier (Olesen et al. 1981), and these findings have largely been confirmed and amplified in subsequent studies. The rCBF becomes reduced at the posterior pole of the hemisphere before or at the onset of the migraine aura. This reduction gradually spreads anteriorly (Fig. 1). The rate of spread was calculated by Lauritzen et al. (1983a) to be 2.2 mm/min without taking the convolutions of the cortex into account. If the convolutions are taken into account, the rate of spread is more likely around 5 mm/min, but the estimate is imprecise. Sometimes the reduced flow spreads to the whole hemisphere, but there was a tendency for the changes to stop at the central sulcus, and in some cases they spread even less. Occasionally a secondary focus in the frontal lobe was seen to spread out circularly, and Lauritzen et al. (1983a) suggested that it was in fact the spreading oligemia coming from behind which, after traversing the insular cortex, appeared in the frontal region. In the area of reduced rCBF, the autoregulation was preserved, but carbon dioxide reactivity was decreased and functional activation was impaired or abolished (Olesen et al. 1981b; Lauritzen et al. 1983b). The degree of measured rCBF reduction ranged from a few per cent to approximately 50%. As demonstrated by Skyhøj Olsen et al. (1987) and subsequently by Skyhøj Olsen and Lassen (1988), however, inherent methodological difficulties with the Xenon method imply that rCBF in low flow areas is overestimated. Skyhøj Olsen et al. (1987) suggested rCBF reduction to reach ischemic values in all migraine patients and proposed that migrainous aura symptoms could be caused by ischemia, in agreement with Wolff (1963). This seems unlikely, however, as discussed by Olesen (1991a). In several patients rCBF values are only marginally reduced, and the gradual spread of oligemia as well as the gradual spread of aura symptoms seem incompatible with vasoconstriction as the causative mechanism.

Attacks induced by angiography might not be identical to spontaneous attacks. It is now possible to record rCBF changes during spontaneous migraine attacks using 133-Xenon inhalation and a brain-dedicated SPECT system. This was first done by Lauritzen and Olesen (1984), who described studies in 10 patients having migraine with aura. In three patients rCBF was normal. In the other seven, rCBF was reduced in the posterior part of the relevant hemisphere (Fig. 2). No focal start of reduced rCBF or gradual spread was observed, probably because the patients were studied from half an hour up to several hours after onset of aura symptoms. rCBF remained depressed for one to several hours after disappearance of aura symptoms (i.e., it was reduced in several patients after headache had fully developed). Patients were studied at least three times: as soon after onset as possible, after successful treatment with ergotamine, and when free from headache for at least a week. In two patients the area of initially reduced rCBF later exhibited an increased blood flow. Andersen et al. (1988) studied this phenomenon prospectively. Reduced rCBF was indeed gradually transformed into increased blood flow after one to several hours. The swing from decreased via normal to increased rCBF was not associated with increased headache. Recently we have combined the above mentioned studies with a new series of patients studied using either intracarotid injection or inhalation of 133-Xenon (Olesen et al. 1990). We were able to establish the sequence of events in a statistically reliable fashion (Fig. 3). In some patients, rCBF is focally depressed already before the onset of aura symptoms. In others rCBF reduction and aura symptoms occur simultaneously. After the aura symptoms disappear, rCBF continues to be depressed while headache develops. At some point during the headache phase, rCBF in the focal area begins to increase, normalizes, and then becomes pathologically increased. Quite often headache disappears despite the continuation of increased rCBF. Thus, headache seems to correlate neither with low nor with high blood flow. The impression is that the cerebrovascular abnormality that causes low blood flow also, with a considerable time delay, causes the headache. Once triggered, headache persists independent from rCBF (arteriolar) changes. Increased rCBF thus seems unassociated with the headache and may be regarded as a secondary consequence of the initial flow reduction.

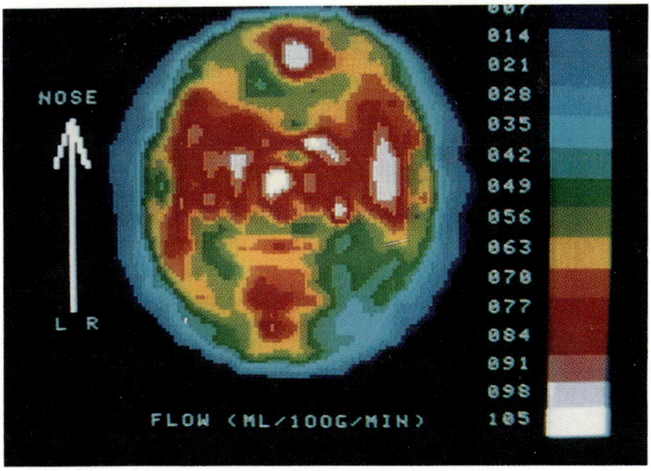

Fig. 1. Regional cerebral blood flow studied by intracarotid 133-Xenon injection and 254 external stationary detectors. Blood flow values are translated into colors: red represents high flow, yellow and green medium flow, and blue low flow. During the first measurement in the resting state (labeled FL 3), rCBF distribution is normal. Subsequently a blue area develops at the posterior pole of the brain (FL 5) and spreads anteriorly (FL 8), indicating reduced blood flow as an attack of migraine with aura develops.

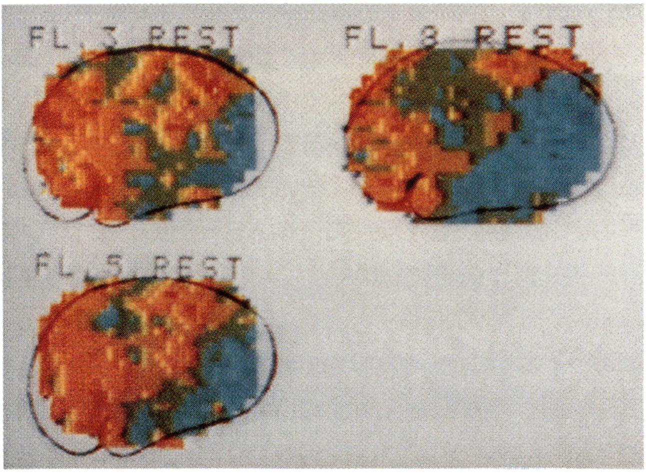

Fig. 2. 133-Xenon SPECT study of regional cerebral blood flow during a spontaneous attack of migraine with aura. Note reduced cerebral blood flow (blue and green colors) in the right occipital lobe corresponding to left homonymous visual aura symptoms.

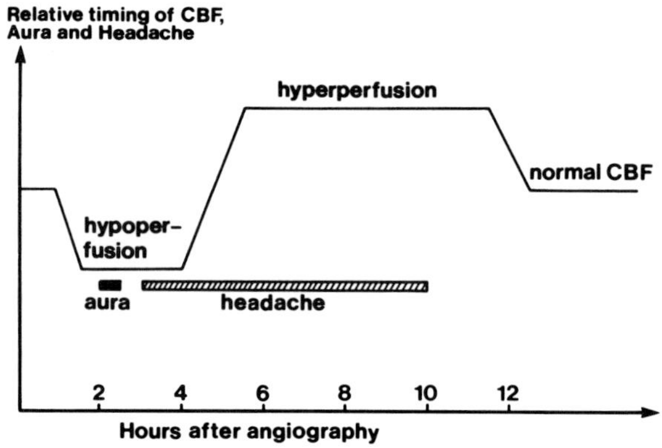

Fig. 3. Schematic drawing of the sequence of events during attacks of migraine with aura. Note the lack of correlation between blood flow changes (ordinate scale) and headache. (Reprinted with permission from Olesen et al. 1990)

SPREADING CORTICAL DEPRESSION OF LEAO MAY EXPLAIN MIGRAINE AURA SYMPTOMS AND ASSOCIATED rCBF CHANGES

The gradual spread of migrainous aura symptoms is a unique feature that led Leao to suggest that the phenomenon of cortical spreading depression (CSD), which he had previously discovered (Leao 1944), could be the underlying mechanism of migraine (Leao and Morrison 1945). Not every patient reports this spread of aura symptoms, but it is likely that inability to remember and/or to give a detailed explanation of the very complicated aura phenomena disturb clinical description (Olesen 1988). The gradual spread of rCBF reduction observed by Olesen et al. (1981) led to a revival of the idea that CSD might be operating.

Laurtizen et al. (1983a) designed a study specifically to demonstrate gradual spread of rCBF changes, and calculated a rate of spread quite similar to the rate of spread of CSD in animal experiments. Further studies by Lauritzen in animals established a number of features associated with CSD which had also been observed in human patients during migraine attacks (Lauritzen 1987). A comparison between migraine with aura and experimental CSD is given in Table II. Against this idea it has been argued that cortical spreading depression is difficult to elicit in higher animal species and that it has never been observed in humans. Bures and coworkers (1974) have clearly demonstrated the phenomenon in the human hippocampus, however, and CSD is easy to elicit in cats (Piper et al. 1991).

Table II
Comparison of migraine with aura and Leao's corical spreading depression (CSD)

	Migraine	CSD
Site of origin	primary visual cortex	high neuron density
Way of spread	contiguous, cortical	contiguous, cortical
Excitation/depression	yes	yes
Rate of spread	2–6 mm/min	2–6 mm/min
Unilateral	yes	yes
Repeated waves	yes	yes
Initial hyperemia	yes	yes
Oligemia lasting	hours	hours
Degree of oligemia	ischemic threshold	less marked?
Cerebrovascular tone instability	yes	?
Autoregulation	preserved?	preserved
CO2 reactivity	abolished?	impaired
Provocation by arteriography	yes	?

Spreading depression consists of a wave of depolarization of cortical cellular elements and presynaptic nerve terminals followed by repolarization. At the front of the wave is a burst of neuronal activity followed by electrical silence and gradual recovery of electrical activity. It is associated with a negative shift in cortical direct current (DC) potentials, a temporary but marked increase in the concentration of hydrogen and potassium ions, and a decrease in extracellular calcium (Hansen and Lauritzen 1988). Glutamate and other neurotransmitters leak from depolarized nerve terminals. Glutamate is considered instrumental in the propagation of CSD (Scheller et al. 1991) and plays an important role as a transmitter in nociceptive neural pathways (Jessell and Dodd 1989). Many of the leaking substances, such as K^+, H^+, glutamate, substance P, and CGRP, are known to sensitize sensory nerve endings which, on the cortical surface, are largely confined to perivascular spaces (Edvisson et al. 1988).

The headache cannot easily be explained, however, as the result of direct local stimulation of nociceptors caused by the wave of CSD. First of all, headache usually occurs half an hour to one hour after the onset of aura symptoms, often with a considerable free interval between the termination of aura symptoms and the onset of headache. Second, the pial surface over the convexities is not sensitive to a variety of noxious stimuli (Ray and Wolff 1940). Third, we have observed typical migraine aura symptoms and associated rCBF changes without subsequent development of migrainous headache, in keeping with the fact that, in males, migraine auras are only associated with pain in about half of the cases (Rasmussen and Olesen 1992). Spreading depression/migrainous aura therefore causes the pain of migraine via some indirect mechanism.

MIGRAINE WITHOUT AURA IS NOT TRIGGERED BY CORTICAL SPREADING DEPRESSION

Until 10 years ago it was considered that migraine without aura had the same pathophysiology as migraine with aura, just in a less severe form. Several authors suggested that the two forms of migraine were part of a continuum of headaches ranging from tension-type headache at one end of the spectrum, through migraine without aura, to migraine with aura. According to this hypothesis, rCBF changes in migraine without aura could be expected to be of the same nature as those in migraine with aura.

It is difficult to know precisely when migraine attacks without aura begin. They very often start insidiously with a headache similar to tension-type headache. Only as the headache gets worse and becomes unilateral and pulsating does the patient realize that it is a migraine attack. Negative rCBF findings could therefore be due to wrong timing. We eliminated this problem by studying migraine that could be induced quickly by drinking red wine. We measures rCBF before and after drinking red wine, and repeated the measurements until the patient developed a migraine attack (Olesen et al. 1981c). At no point in time was a focal rCBF reduction observed, however. An analysis of absolute blood flow values before and during the development of migraine showed no significant abnormalities. Lauritzen and Olesen (1984) studied 12 patients during spontaneous attacks of migraine without aura. Patients were studied from three hours until 12 hours after onset of the attack (median 7 hours). No focal areas of decreased or increased blood flow were observed, and measurements during attack were not significantly different from measurements immediately after successful treatment nor from measurements when patients had been free from migraine for a week or more.

It might be argued that we missed an early rCBF reduction, but if changes were similar to those in migraine with aura, we should at least have seen the subsequent focal rCBF increase which persists for several hours. In our most recent series of studies of migraine attacks (Olesen et al. 1990), we also failed to observe any focal or global rCBF abnormalities using 133-Xenon inhalation and SPECT or technetium HMPAO and SPECT. Again, we compared measurements during attacks to measurements outside of attacks. At present there are no rCBF findings to suggest CSD in migraine without aura. The fact that it often lasts several hours before pain reaches maximum and the lack of focal neurological symptoms are also evidence against spreading depression in this disorder.

A COMMON FINAL PATHWAY FOR PAIN IN MIGRAINE WITH AND WITHOUT AURA?

Clinical features of the painful phase of attacks with aura and of attacks without aura have recently been shown to be the same (Rasmussen and Olesen 1992). Both forms of migraine respond to prophylactic treatment with metoprolol (Kangasniemi et al. 1987). Ergot preparations are effective in the treatment of both forms of migraine according to general experience, although this has never been formally tested in a double-blind experiment. The newly developed specific 5-HT_1-like receptor agonist sumatriptan has been extensively tested in very large double-blind trials where patients have been carefully diagnosed according to the operational diagnostic criteria of the International Headache Society (Headache Classification Committee 1988). It has shown dramatic effectiveness in both forms of migraine (Glaxo 1991; Subcutaneous Sumatriptan International Study Group 1991). All evidence combined, it seems substantiated that the two forms of migraine are triggered by different mechanisms, but that mechanisms of the painful phase of the attacks are shared. Most recently we have provided evidence that dilatation of large cerebral arteries, perhaps combined with perivascular inflammation and sensitization of periarterial nociceptors, may be such a final common pathway (Friberg et al. 1991).

We measured rCBF using 133-Xenon inhalation and SPECT in 10 patients during attacks of migraine (6 with aura and 4 without aura), and simultaneously recorded middle cerebral artery blood velocity (MCAV) using transcranial doppler. We then treated patients with iv. infusion of sumatriptan (2 mg) over 10 minutes, which rapidly aborted the attacks. rCBF was measured again 30 minutes after treatment. All patients had strictly unilateral migraine pain. MCAV was initially decreased on the painful side but normalized during the 10 minutes of sumatriptan infusion. No change occurred on the nonpainful side, and no changes occurred in mean rCBF in the MCA territory. When flow and velocity of an artery only changes moderately, the relationship between flow (*rCBF*), velocity (*V*) and cross-sectional area (*A*) of an artery can be described by the equation

$$A = \frac{rCBF}{V} \cdot \mathrm{K}$$

where K is a constant.

In the study by Friberg et al. (1991), velocity was decreased and rCBF normal during the migraine attack. The cross sectional lumen of the MCA must therefore have been increased (25%); velocity normalized during 10 minutes of sumatriptan infusion in parallel with the amelioration of migraine pain, while rCBF was unchanged (Fig. 4). Therefore, the MCA was constricted by sumatriptan. This was seen both in patients with aura and in patients without aura. The superficial temporal artery showed a relative dilatation during attacks of both forms of migraine (Iversen et al. 1990).

We propose, therefore, that activation of cerebral periarterial nociceptors and simultaneous dilatation of large cerebral and possibly extracranial arteries as a result of neuropeptide release is a mechanism that can explain the pain in both migraine with aura and migraine without aura.

POSSIBLE MOLECULAR MECHANISMS OF MIGRAINE PAIN

Although the site of migraine pain has been localized to the intracranial perivascular spaces with reasonable certainty, the same cannot be said about the molecular mechanisms of migraine pain. Endogenous opioids in cerebrospinal fluid seem to be normal in migraine patients (Bach et al. 1985), and blood chemistry has not been systematically abnormal with two exceptions: there is a decrease in whole-blood 5-HT during the migraine attack (for references see Olesen and Saxena 1992), and CGRP increases in blood from the external jugular vein during migraine attack (Goadsby et al. 1990). 5-HT injected intravenously does not cause pain; local injection into the superficial temporal muscle is not painful (Jensen et al. 1990a; Olesen and Saxena 1992). However, 5-HT does aggravate bradykinin-induced pain in the temporal muscle (Jensen et al. 1990b) and may play a role as part of a cascade of biochemical changes. CGRP by contrast is not painful when injected into the superficial temporal muscle and does not seem to potentiate pain induced by other substances (Pedersen-Bjerregaard et al. 1991). Overall, the pain-inducing properties of 5-HT and CGRP are absent or very modest, and these substances are not likely to explain migraine pain.

Histamine and nitroglycerin are among the very few substances that reliably produce a headache in non–headache prone normal volunteers and/or migraine sufferers (Krabbe and Olesen 1980; Iversen et al. 1989). The mechanisms of histamine-induced headache have not been extensively evaluated, but a considerable amount of work has been done to elucidate the effects of histamine on cerebral and extracranial arteries (for references see Edvinsson et al. 1993). Most of this work, however, does not relate to the intravenous use of histamine, since it has been done either on isolated blood vessels or on pial blood vessels in situ. In both cases, the blood-brain barrier is circumvented. Histamine reaches the vessel wall from the adventitial side, which has no barrier. There is a very tight blood-brain barrier in the human cerebral

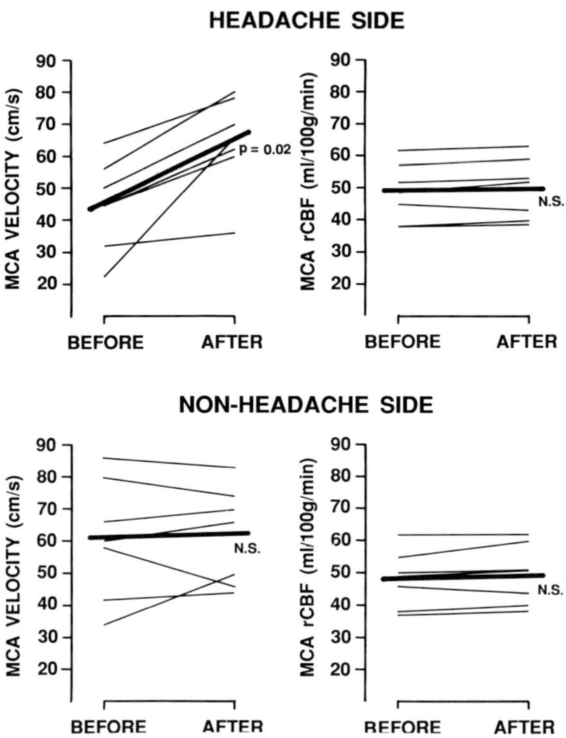

Fig. 4. Velocity in middle cerebral artery (MCA velocity) and regional cerebral blood flow in the middle cerebral artery territory (MCA rCBF) during a migraine attack and after treatment with sumatriptan 2 mg iv. On the headache side, velocity is low before treatment but normalizes, whereas rCBF stays normal. On the non-headache side, both parameters remain unchanged. This indicates that the middle cerebral artery has been dilated on the side of migraine pain and that this was normalized after sumatriptan treatment.

circulation and probably also in the resistance vessels. Thus, intravenous and even intracarotid infusion of histamine in the human does not affect cerebral blood flow, which means that cerebral arterioles have not been dilated (Krabbe and Olesen 1980). In animal experiments, histamine does increase the permeability of the blood-brain barrier when given intracarotidly, but doses of 10^{-5} M were necessary. These doses were so high that, even infused into the carotid artery, they caused severe systemic hypotension (Gross et al. 1982). Studies of isolated blood vessels have shown little effect on cerebral veins but marked effects on cerebral arteries, and considerable species difference. There are at least four different varieties of receptors (Edvinsson et al. 1993): a constrictive H_1 receptor, which is very prevalent; a dilatory H_1 receptor, which is primarily seen in primates and humans and is endothelium-dependent (Sercombe and Verrecchia 1986; Chang et al. 1988); an H_2 receptor, which is dilatory and non-endothelium-dependent; and an H_3 receptor, which is presynaptically located on nerve fibers and the effect of which has not been studied in primate blood vessels. In humans, the endothelial dilatory H_1 receptor is the most interesting. In all likelihood it works via release of endothelial-derived relaxing factor (Toda et al. 1990)—i.e., the effect of histamine on the endothelial dilatory H_1 receptor in humans is probably mediated via nitric oxide (NO). It is of the greatest interest that migraine sufferers respond to histamine infusion with much stronger headache than do migraine-free controls (Krabbe and Olesen 1980). In fact, as seen in Table III, a threshold dose may be defined at which controls experience no headache but the majority of migraine sufferers do.

Nitric oxide has rapidly been established in recent years as a ubiquitous and extremely important messenger molecule. Researchers have demonstrated the presences of its synthesizing enzyme, nitric oxide synthase, in the endothelium of cerebral blood vessels and in perivascular nerve fibers originating primarily from the parasympathetic nerve system (Nozaki et al. 1993). The physiological and pathophysiological role of these nerve fibers have not been established. Nitroglycerin has been shown to act almost exclusively as a prodrug for NO (Rand 1992). It easily penetrates the blood-brain barrier because of its high lipid solubility, and it is converted to NO in the smooth muscle cells of the blood vessels by mechanisms that are not fully elucidated. In the smooth muscle cells, NO stimulates soluble guanylate cyclase, increasing cyclic GMP and thereby resulting in vasodilatation. Whether NO from muscle cells may diffuse into perivascular nerve terminals and what effect it has in these nerve terminals is so far uncertain. It is also uncertain whether nitroglycerin donates NO in the endothelium or directly in the perivascular nerve fibers.

The effect of nitroglycerin on cerebrovascular responses and headache in normal volunteers has recently been extensively characterized. Nitroglycerin induces dilatation of cerebral arteries and extracranial as well as extremity arteries but does not change cerebral blood flow, indicating either that it acts predominantly on the arteries or that any effect on arterioles is counteracted by other mechanisms in vivo (Dahl et al. 1990; Holm et al. 1990). Nitroglycerin has a strong effect on veins and increases cerebral blood volume (Edvinsson et al. 1993, Holm et al. 1990). In normal volunteers, steady-state intravenous infusion of nitroglycerin results in a steady-state headache after approximately 10 minutes. The headache is maintained at a relatively constant level for up to several hours if the infusion continues (Iversen et al. 1989, Iversen et al. 1993). After discontinuation of the infusion, headache rapidly disappears, as expected from the very short half-life of nitroglycerin in plasma. The headache in normal volunteers is mild to medium, pulsating, bifronto-temporal, and sometimes associated with nausea and/or photophobia and/or phonophobia. Thus it only occasionally fulfills migraine diagnostic criteria, although both clinically and pathophysiologically the two types of headache strongly

Table III
Headache characteristics, blood pressure, and pulse rate during iv. histamine

Diagnosis	Dose (µg/kg/min)	Headache (number of patients) None	Pressing	Pulsating +	++	+++	BP	Pulse Rate
Normals (N = 13)	Baseline	13	0	0	0	0	130/80	66
	0.16	12	1	0	0	0	125/78	67
	0.33	10	3	0	0	0	125/75	75**
	0.66	9	4	0	0	0	120*/67**	87**
Muscle contraction headache (N = 10)	Baseline	4	6	0	0	0	137/84	79
	0.16	2	6	3	0	0	142/86	82
	0.33	1	4	5	0	0	133/78	86*
	0.66	1	4	4	1	0	133/73	91**
Common migraine (N = 25)	Baseline	16	9	0	0	0	131/81	76
	0.16	6	10	9	0	0	127**/79	86*
	0.33	2	2	11	8	2	122**/74**	89**
	0.66	1	0	2	9	13	120**/70**	97**

Source: Reprinted with permission from Krebbe and Olesen 1980.
*P < 0.05.
**P < 0.01.

resemble each other. It has been shown that N-acetylcysteine, a donor of SH-groups, augments both arterial responses and headache intensity when used as a pretreatment before nitroglycerin (Iversen 1992). Dose-response relationships between nitroglycerin and headache have been delineated, and a ceiling effect has been documented around a dose of 0.5 µg/kg per minute. A similar ceiling effect pertains to arterial dilatation. The percentage dilatation of the superficial temporal artery is significantly higher than the percentage dilatation of the radial artery, and N-acetylcysteine augments the response of the superficial temporal artery more than that of the radial artery. Although nitroglycerin affects blood vessels throughout the body, there is thus evidence of increased sensitivity and differing modulatory mechanisms in the cranial as compared to systemic arteries. This illuminates the fact that nitroglycerin, and therefore nitric oxide (NO) causes headache, but no pain in the rest of the body.

Sicuteri et al. (1987) reported that migraine patients are more sensitive to nitroglycerin than are non-migraineurs. This study, however, was not done with a degree of scientific rigor sufficient to meet current standards. We therefore studied 17 patients suffering from migraine without aura according to the diagnostic criteria of the International Headache Society (Headache

Classification Committee 1988), 9 patients with episodic tension-type headache according to the same headache classification, and 17 age- and sex-matched healthy control subjects with no history of migraine (Olesen et al. 1993). The investigator did not know the diagnosis of the experimental subjects, and the subjects did not know the main aim of the investigation (which was to analyze whether migraine patients were more sensitive to nitroglycerin and therefore to NO than normal controls or sufferers of tension-type headache). The investigation could thus be regarded as double-blind. Nitroglycerin 0.015, 0.03, 0.25, and 0.50 μg/kg per minute was infused intravenously in a staircase fashion, each dose for 15 minutes by a volume-directed pump. Clinical characteristics necessary to classify the headaches according to criteria for migraine of the International Headache Society were recorded every 5 minutes. Headache intensity was scored on a 0–10 scale, and pulse rate and blood pressure were recorded every 2 minutes throughout all infusions and during 60 minutes after the end of the last infusion. The velocity in the middle cerebral artery was determined repeatedly using transcranial doppler. Patients also answered a questionnaire about headache during the 24 hours following the study.

Total headache experienced during all doses and the post-infusion period differed significantly among migraineurs, tension-type sufferers, and controls, with migraineurs having the highest value ($P < 0.001$, Kruskal Wallis; Fig. 5). At lesser doses, more migraine patients than controls and tension-type headache patients developed headache. At the greater doses, migraine patients as well as patients with tension-type headache and headache-free control subjects developed headache. However, at the greater doses, the median steady-state headache intensity was higher in the migraine group (5, range 1–10) compared with headache-free controls (2, range 1–5). The time profile of headache changes is shown in Fig. 6. There is little difference between groups at the lesser doses but clear differences at greater doses. After end of the infusion, headache rapidly disappeared in the control subjects. Some tension-type headache patients retained a mild headache after half an hour, but migraineurs had significantly more headache in the post-infusion period ($P < 0.002$; Kruskal Wallis). In addition to the greater intensity of headache in migraine patients, headache also fulfilled diagnostic criteria for migraine without aura more often than in the other groups. The biggest difference between the groups was seen during the subsequent 24 hours, when 11 of 17 migraineurs had headaches fulfilling the IHS criteria for migraine without aura, but only one tension-type headache patient and none of the controls had such migraine attacks ($P < 0.001$; Kruskal Wallis). This large difference occurred despite the fact that 14 of the migraine patients, but only one tension-type headache patient and no controls, took antimigraine treatment.

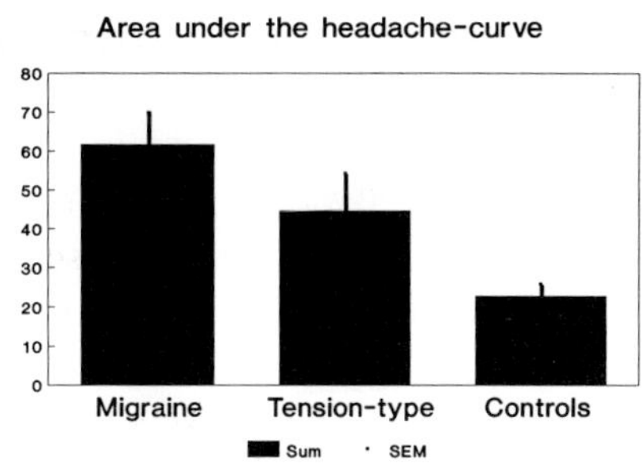

Fig. 5. Total headache experienced by migraine sufferers, tension-type headache sufferers, and headache-free controls during infusion of four ascending doses of intravenous nitroglycerin. Migraine sufferers (who were not having a migraine attack at the time of the study) had more headache than tension-type headache sufferers and considerably more than headache-free controls.

This nitroglycerin supersensitivity in migraine patients regarding the development of migraine-like headache was not just a subjective phenomenon. Transcranial doppler measurements showed that there was a significant difference between groups with regard to middle cerebral artery dilatation at the higher doses, migraine subjects displaying the most marked response. Thus, supersensitivity to nitroglycerin in migraine sufferers as demonstrated by increased headache response is paralleled by increased dilatation of the middle cerebral artery and probably by increased dilatation of the entire pial arterial vascular bed. Whether the middle meningeal artery and the extracranial arteries and/or perivascular sensory nerve endings are also supersensitive remains to be shown. The localization of this response to the pial arteries corresponds nicely to the previous conclusion from cerebral blood flow studies that migraine pain in all likelihood originates from pial perivascular sensory nerve endings.

CONCLUSION

Studies during the past decade have extensively characterized specific changes of regional cerebral blood flow during migraine attacks. In migraine with aura, reduced blood flow in the occipital region gradually spreads forward and is associated with preserved autoregulation, abolished CO_2 reactivity, and decreased response to functional activation. Cortical spreading depression is considered to be the underlying mechanism. Cerebral blood flow is normal, however, during attacks of migraine without aura. Pain in both

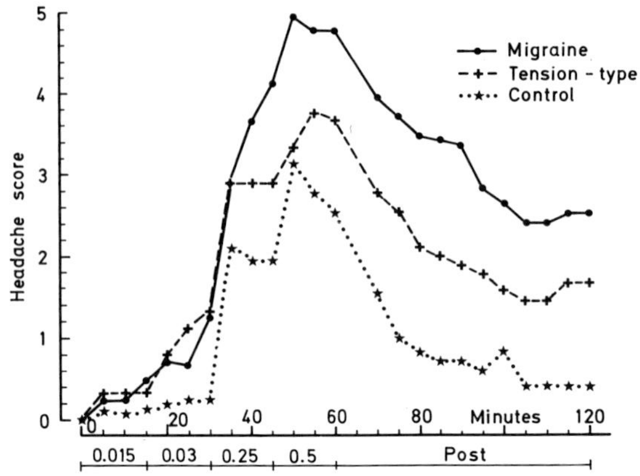

Fig. 6. Headache scores in the course of intravenous infusion of four ascending doses of nitroglycerin (doses and times indicated below the x-axis). Headache was scored on a 0–10 scale at 2 min intervals. With the two higher doses, migraine sufferers had significantly more headache than normal controls, with tension-type headache sufferers being intermediate. Headache also remained longer after the infusion in migraineurs and actually worsened during the post-infusion period (not shown).

forms of migraine probably originates from periarterial nerve plexus, with cerebral arteries being dilated on the side of pain relative to the nonpainful side.

It may be concluded from the studies of nitroglycerin that NO directly causes a headache, fulfilling migraine criteria in most migraine sufferers, and that this starts a chain reaction leading to a migraine attack that continues several hours after nitroglycerin/NO has been completely eliminated. The dilatory response of the middle cerebral artery to nitroglycerin is increased, and migraine sufferers experience more severe headache than controls. These findings lead to the conclusion that NO is likely to be significantly involved in the generation of spontaneous migraine attacks.

Studies of the interaction among NO, neuropeptides, and monoamines in and around the cerebral arteries constitute an interesting future avenue of headache research.

REFERENCES

Ad Hoc Committee on the Classification of Headache, Classification of headache, JAMA, 179 (1962) 717–718.

Andersen, A.R., Friberg, L., Olsen, T.S. and Olesen, J., SPECT demonstration of delayed hyperemia following hypoperfusion in classic migraine, Arch. Neurol., 45 (1988) 154–159.

Bach, F., Jensen, K., Blegvad, N., Fenger, M., Jordal, R. and Olesen, J., Beta-endorphin and ACTH

in plasma during attacks of common and classic migraine, Cephalalgia, 5 (1985) 177–182.
Blau, J.N. and Dexter, S.L., The site of pain origin during migraine attacks, Cephalalgia, 1 (1981) 143–147.
Brazil, P. and Friedman, A.P., Craniovascular studies in headache. A report and analysis of pulse volume tracings, Neurology, 6 (1956) 96–102.
Bures, J., Buresova, O. and Krivanek, J., The Mechanism and Applications of Leao's Spreading Depression of Electroencephalographic Activity, Academic Press, New York, 1974.
Chang, J.Y., Hardebo, J.E. and Owman, C., Differential vasomotor action of noradrenaline, serotonin and histamine in isolated basilar artery from rat and guinea-pig, Acta Physiol. Scand., 132 (1988) 91–102.
Dahl, A., Russell, D., Nyberg-Hansen, R. and Rootwelt, K., Cluster headache: transcranial doppler ultrasound and rCBF studies, Cephalalgia, 10 (1990) 87–94.
Drummond, P.D. and Lance, J.W., Extracranial vascular changes and the source of pain in migraine headache, Ann. Neurol., 13 (1983) 32–37.
Edvinsson, L., McKenzie, E.T., McCulloch, J. and Uddman, R., Nerve supply and receptor mechanisms in intra- and extracerebral blood vessels. In: J. Olesen and L. Edvinsson (Eds.), Basic Mechanisms of Headache, Elsevier, Amsterdam, 1988, pp. 129–144.
Edvinsson, L., McKenzie, E.T. and McCullogh, J., Cerebral Blood Flow and Metabolism, Raven Press, New York, 1993.
Friberg, L., Skyhøj Olsen, T., Roland, P.E. and Lassen, N.A., Focal ischemia caused by instability of cerebrovascular tone during attacks of hemiplegic migraine, Brain, 110 (1987) 917–934.
Friberg, L., Olesen, J., Iversen, H.K. and Sperling, B., Migraine pain associated with middle cerebral dilatation: reversal by sumatriptan, Lancet, 338 (1991) 13–17.
Glaxo, Sumatriptan: from molecule to man, Eur. Neurol., 31 (1991) 277–344.
Goadsby, P.J., Edvinsson, L. and Ekman, R., Vasoactive peptide release in the extracerebral circulation of humans during migraine headache, Ann. Neurol., 28 (1990) 183–187.
Gross, P.M., Teasdale, G.M., Graham, D.I., Angerson, W.J. and Harper, A.M., Intra-arterial histamine increases blood-brain transport in rats, Am. J. Physiol., 243 (1982) H307–H317.
Hansen, A.J. and Lauritzen, M., Spreading depression of leao. In: J. Olesen and L. Edvinsson (Eds.), Basic Mechanisms of Headache, Elsevier, Amsterdam, 1988, pp. 99–107.
Hare, E.H., Personal observations on the spectral march of migraine, J. Neurol. Sci., 3 (1966) 259–264.
Headache Classification Committee of the International Headache Society (Jes Olesen, chairman), Classification and diagnostic criteria for headache disorders, cranial neuralgias and facial pain, Cephalalgia, 8, Suppl 7 (1988) 1–96.
Holm, S., Friberg, L., Iversen, H.K. and Lassen, N.A., Dual energy brain SPECT: methods and applications. In: H.A.E. Schmidt and J. Chambion (Eds.), Nuclear Medicine. Quantitative Analysis in Imaging and Function. Schattauer, Stuttgart and New York, 1990, pp. 11–13.
Iversen, H.K., N-acetylcysteine potentiates nitroglycerin induced headache and dilatation of cranial but not extremity arteries, Clin. Pharmacol. Ther., 52 (1992) 125–133.
Iversen, H.K., Olesen, J. and Tfelt-Hansen, P., Intravenous nitroglycerin as an experimental model of vascular headache: basic characteristics, Pain, 38 (1989) 17–24.
Iversen, H.K., Nielsen, T.H., Olesen, J. and Tfelt-Hansen, P., Arterial responses during migraine headache, Lancet, 336 (1990) 837–839.
Iversen, H.K., Nielsen, T.H., Tfelt-Hansen, P. and Olesen, J., Lack of tolerance of headache and radial artery diameter during a 7 hour intravenous infusion of nitroglycerin, Eur. J. Clin. Pharmacol., 44 (1993) 47–50.
Jensen, K., Subcutaneous blood flow in the temporal region of migraine patients, Acta Neurol. Scand., 75 (1987) 310–318.
Jensen, K. and Olesen, J., Temporal muscle blood flow in common migraine, Acta Neurol. Scand., 72 (1985) 561–570.
Jensen, K., Tuxen, C., Pedersen-Bjergaard, U., Jansen I., Edvinsson, L. and Olesen, J., Pain and tenderness in human temporal muscle induced by bradykinin and 5-hydroxytryptamine,

Peptides, 11 (1990a) 1127–1132.

Jensen, K., Tuxen, C., Pedersen-Bjergaard, U., Jansen I., Edvinsson, L. and Olesen, J., Pain, wheal and flare in human forearm skin induced by bradykinin and 5-hydroxytryptamine, Peptides, 11 (1990b) 1133–1138.

Jessell, T.M. and Dodd, J., Functional chemistry of primary afferent neurons. In: P.D. Wall and R. Melzack (Eds.), Textbook of Pain, 2nd ed., Churchill Livingstone, London, 1989, pp. 84–85.

Kangasniemi, P., Andersen, A.R., Andersson, P.G., Gilhus, N.E., Hedman, C., Hultgren, M., Vilming, S. and Olesen, J., Classic migraine: effective prophylaxis with metoprolol, Cephalalgia, 7 (1987) 231–238.

Krabbe, A.Æ. and Olesen, J., Headache provocation by continuous intravenous infusion of histamine. Clinical results and receptor mechanisms, Pain, 8 (1980) 253–259.

Lauritzen, M., Cerebral blood flow in migraine and cortical spreading depression, Acta Neurol. Scand., 76, Suppl. 113 (1987) 1–40.

Lauritzen, M. and Olesen, J., Regional cerebral blood flow during migraine attacks by Xenon-133 inhalation and emission tomography, Brain, 107 (1984) 447–461.

Lauritzen, M., Skyhøj Olsen T., Lassen, N.A. and Paulson, O.B., The changes of regional cerebral blood flow during the course of classical migraine attacks, Ann. Neurol., 13 (1983a) 633–641.

Lauritzen, M., Skyhøj Olsen T., Lassen, N.A. and Paulson, O.B., The regulation of regional cerebral blood flow during and between migraine attacks, Ann. Neurol., 14 (1983b) 569–572.

Leao, A.A.P., Spreading depression of activity in cerebral cortex, J. Neurophysiol., 7 (1944) 359–390.

Leao, A.A.P. and Morrison, R.S., Propagation of spreading cortical depression, J. Neurophysiol., 8 (1945) 33–45.

Nozaki, K., Moskowitz, M.A., Maynard, K., Koketsa, V., Dawson, T.M., Bredt, S. and Snyder, S.H., Possible origins and distribution of immunoreactive nitric oxide synthetase-containing nerve fibres in cerebral arteries, J. Cereb. Blood Flow Metab., 13 (1993) 70–79.

Olesen, J., Some clinical features of the acute migraine attack. An analysis of 750 patients, Headache, 18 (1978) 268–271.

Olesen, J., Pathophysiological implications of migraine aura symptomatology. In: J. Olesen and L. Edvinsson (Eds.), Basic Mechanisms of Headache, Elsevier, Amsterdam, 1988, pp. 353–363.

Olesen, J., Cerebral and extracranial circulatory disturbances in migraine: pathophysiological implications, Cerebrovasc. Brain Metab. Rev., 3 (1991a) 1–28.

Olesen, J., (Ed.) Migraine and other headaches: the vascular mechanisms, Raven Press, New York, 1991b.

Olesen, J. and Saxena, P.R. (Eds.), 5-hydroxytryptamine Mechanisms in Primary Headaches, Raven Press, New York, 1992, pp. 1–362.

Olesen, J., Krabbe, A.Æ. and Tfelt-Hansen, P., Methodological aspects of prophylactic drug trials in migraine, Cephalalgia, 1 (1981a) 127–141.

Olesen, J., Larsen, B. and Lauritzen, M., Focal hyperemia followed by spreading oligemia and impaired activation of rCBF in classic migraine, Ann. Neurol., 9 (1981b) 344–352.

Olesen, J., Tfelt-Hansen, P., Henriksen, L. and Larsen, B., The common migraine attack may not be initiated by cerebral ischemia, Lancet, 2 (1981c) 438–440.

Olesen, J., Friberg, L., Olsen, T.S., Iversen, H.K., Lassen, N.A., Andersen, A.R. and Karle, A., Timing and topography of cerebral blood flow, aura and headache during migraine attacks, Ann. Neurol., 28 (1990) 791–798.

Olesen, J., Iversen, H.K. and Thomsen, L.L., Nitric oxide supersensitivity: a possible molecular mechanism of migraine pain, Neuroreport 4 (1993), 1027–1030.

Pedersen-Bjergaard, U., Nielsen, L.B., Jensen, K., Edvinsson, L., Jansen, I. and Olesen, J., Calcitonin gene-related peptide, neurokinin A and Substance P: effects on nociception and neurogenic inflammation in human skin and temporal muscle, Peptides, 12 (1991) 333–337.

Piper, R.D., Lambert, G.A. and Duckworth, J.W., Cortical blood flow changes during spreading depression in cats, Am. J. Physiol., 261 (1991) 96–102.

Rand, M.J., Nitrergic transmission: nitric oxide as a mediator of non-adrenergic, non-cholinergic

neuro-effector transmission, Clin. Exp. Pharmacol. Physiol., 19 (1992) 147–169.
Rasmussen, B.K. and Olesen, J., Migraine with aura and migraine without aura: an epidemiological study, Cephalalgia, 12 (1992) 221–228.
Ray, B.S. and Wolff, H.G., Experimental studies in headache, Arch. Surg., 41 (1940) 813–856.
Scheller, D., Heister, U., Dengler, K. and Tegtmeir, F., Extracellular changes of aspartate and glutamate during generation and during propagation of cortical spreading depression in rats. In: J. Olesen (Ed.), Migraine and Other Headaches: The Vascular Mechanisms, Raven Press, New York, 1991, pp. 161–165.
Schiller, F., The migraine tradition, Bull. Hist. Med., 49 (1975) 1–19.
Sercombe, R. and Verrecchia, C., Role of vascular endothelium in modulating cerebrovascular effects of neurotransmitters. In: C. Owman and J. Hardebo (Eds.), Neural Regulation of Brain Circulation, Elsevier, Amsterdam, 1986, pp. 27–42.
Sicuteri, F., Del Bene, E., Poggioni, M. and Bonnazzi, A., Unmasking latent dysnociception in healthy subjects, Headache, 27 (1987) 180–185.
Skinhøj, E. and Paulson, O.B., Regional cerebral blood flow in internal carotid distribution during migraine attack, BMJ, 3 (1969) 569–570.
Skyhøj Olsen, T. and Lassen, N.A., Blood flow and vascular reactivity during attacks of classic migraine: limitations of the Xe-133 intraarterial technique, Headache, 29 (1988) 15–20.
Skyhøj Olsen, T., Friberg, L. and Lassen, N.A., Ischemia may be the primary cause of the neurological deficits in classic migraine, Arch. Neurol., 44 (1987) 156–161.
The Subcutaneous Sumatriptan International Study Group, Treatment of migraine attacks with sumatriptan, N. Engl. J. Med., 325 (1991) 316–321.
Toda, N., Mechanism underlying responses to histamine of isolated monkey and human cerebral arteries, Am. J. Physiol., 258 (1990) H311–H317.
Wolff, H.G., Headache and Other Head Pain, 2nd ed., Oxford University Press, New York, 1963.

Correspondence to: Jes Olesen, MD, PhD, Department of Neurology, Glostrup Hospital, University of Copenhagen, DK-2600 Glostrup, Denmark. Tel: 45-43-96-43-33; Fax: 45-43-42-35-70.

Proceedings of the 7th World Congress on Pain,
Progress in Pain Research and Management, Vol. 2,
edited by G.F. Gebhart, D.L. Hammond, and T.S.
Jensen, IASP Press, Seattle, © 1994.

50

Drug Mechanisms in Acute Migraine

Michael A. Moskowitz

*Stroke Research Laboratory, Neurology and Neurosurgery Services,
Departments of Neurology and Surgery, Harvard Medical School,
Massachusetts General Hospital, Boston, Massachusetts, USA*

INTRODUCTION

Sumatriptan is the first antimigraine medication to exhibit receptor-selective properties. Sumatriptan binds with nanomolar affinities to 5-HT_{1B}, 5-HT_{1D} and 5-HT_{1F} receptor subtypes and is inactive at receptor sites for norepinephrine, dopamine, gamma-aminobutyric acid (GABA), glutamate, and other 5-hydroxytryptophan receptor types (5-$HT_{2,3,4}$). In clinical trials to date, sumatriptan has shown significant success for acute treatment (Moskowitz and Cutrer 1993) and encouraging results in cluster headaches as well.

Sumatriptan has become a useful tool for probing basic mechanisms in migraine and for deciphering its molecular pharmacology. Although Humphrey and colleagues developed sumatriptan for its ability to constrict vascular smooth muscle, recent studies indicate that the most relevant actions of sumatriptan may well be neurogenic and involve prejunctional 5-HT_{1D} receptors expressed on trigeminovascular neurons. Receptor activation is coupled to blockade of neuropeptide release, neurogenic inflammation, and neural transmission.

Traditional vascular models of migraine lack experimental validation and are inconsistent with emerging clinical data—despite 60 years of intense research. Moreover, models based entirely on the contraction or relaxation of vascular smooth muscle have overlooked potentially important interactions between the trigeminal nerve and its target, the meningeal blood vessel wall. For these reasons, this chapter will focus briefly on the relevance of neurogenic mechanisms to the pathophysiology and treatment of migraine. Readers are referred to more detailed reviews and original publications for a more complete description of the trigeminovascular system and its importance to migraine headache (Moskowitz 1992; Moskowitz 199la,b; Moskowitz and Cutrer 1994).

THE VASCULAR THEORY

The vascular theory of migraine states that vasodilation is a necessary and sufficient cause of migraine headache. Several lines of evidence cast doubt on this theory. First, Harold Wolff's observation of exaggerated temporal artery pulsations during migraines is based upon tenuous data (Blau 1978), and has not been confirmed by others (Heyck 1956). Second, the extracranial vessels studied by Wolff do not appear to possess the receptor that mediates the therapeutic effect of drugs (e.g., ergot alkaloids or sumatriptan) known to be effective in treating the condition (Buzzi and Moskowitz 1990; Humphrey et al. 1990; Buzzi et al. 1992). Third, there is no consistent relationship between vessel caliber, cerebral blood flow, and headache (Andersen et al. 1988). Transcranial Doppler studies involving more than 120 patients in seven studies did not reveal consistent differences in vessel caliber between pain-free episodes and migraine attacks (Zwetsloot et al. 1991). When changes did occur, they did not always correspond to the side of the headache or neurological aura. Fourth, histamine injection into the carotid arteries of humans causes headache when injected into the intracranial but not the extracranial circulation (Northfield, 1938). Fifth, doubling of cerebral blood flow by papaverine injection or CO_2 inhalation does not cause headache (Olesen and Paulson 1971; Olesen et al. 1971).

Headache following the administration of vasodilators, such as nitrates, has been used to support the importance of a vascular cause. However, cluster headache provoked in such a manner does not develop during peak vasodilatation, but during the waning period (Dahl et al. 1989, 1990). Wei and co-workers (1992) have determined that the mechanism of dilatation by nitroglycerin and sodium nitroprusside in the cat is via the activation of perivascular sensory nerves, with subsequent release of calcitonin gene-related peptide (CGRP). This in turn relaxes vascular smooth muscle via activation of the soluble form of guanylate cyclase. If this mechanism is also true for other species, it is highly likely that it is not the vasodilatation per se that causes headache in response to nitroglycerin, but the activation of trigeminal perivascular sensory afferent nerves.

After sensitization of primary afferent axons by the neurogenic inflammatory process, hemodynamic events in arteries and veins take on greater importance to the headache (Fig. 1). In this instance, changes in venous pressure

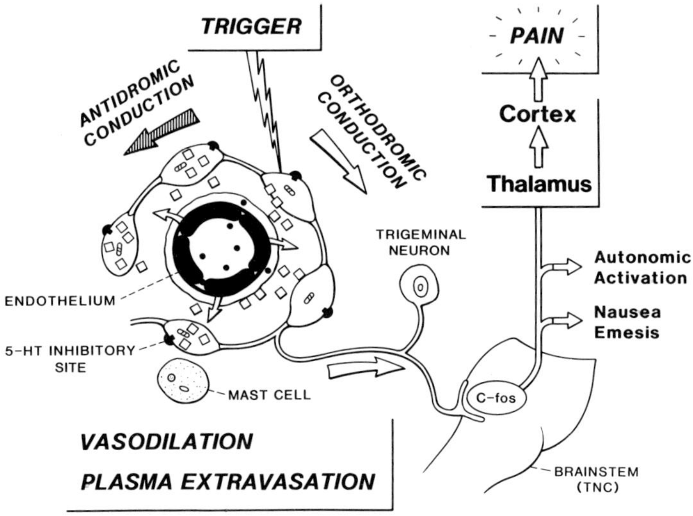

Fig. 1. Antinociceptive site for the binding of sumatriptan and ergot alkaloids in vascular headaches. Triggers for headache activate perivascular trigeminal axons, which release vasoactive neuropeptides to promote neurogenic inflammation (vasodilation, plasma extravasation, mast cell degranulation). The inflammatory response spreads to adjacent tissues via ortho- and antidromic conduction along trigeminovascular fibers and transmits nociceptive information toward the trigeminal nucleus caudalis and higher brain centers for the registration of pain. (Modified with permission from Moskowitz 1992)

and transluminal pressure (events that otherwise might be nonnoxious) may be sufficient to activate trigeminovascular neurons, thereby imparting the pulsating quality to the headache and its exaggeration with Valsalva maneuvers. These stimuli, in the absence of sensitization, would not otherwise cause pain.

NEUROGENIC MECHANISMS

Lewis (1937) proposed the term *nocifensor system* to identify the role of neurogenic inflammation as a potent endogenous defense in the early phase of tissue damage. As in other tissues, neurogenic inflammation in the dura involves the release of the vasodilator neuropeptide substance P (SP) (Lembeck 1953) and neurokinin A (NKA) (Saria et al. 1985). Substance P is the most important of the stored neuropeptides. (In fact, antagonists to the substance P receptor [NK_1 antagonists] potently block neurogenic inflammation within the meninges.) Although CGRP is a potent vasodilator, it does not cause plasma extravasation in dura mater or extracranial tissues innervated by the trigeminal nerve (Markowitz et al. 1987). Neurotransmitter release elicited by electrical trigeminal stimulation results in vasodilatation, platelet aggregation, mast cell degranulation, and an increase in vascular permeability (Markowitz et al. 1987). Systemic administration of the tachykinins mimics some of these changes as well. Leakage occurs primarily in postcapillary venules, as demonstrated by HRP light and electron microscopy studies (Dimitriadou et al. 1992). Electrical stimulation of the rat trigeminal ganglion induces neurogenic plasma extravasation and mast cell degranulation within ipsilateral dura mater. Both are abolished by neonatal capsaicin pretreatment to destroy unmyelinated sensory afferent neurons (Markowitz et al. 1987; Dimitriadou et al. 1991), as are the endothelial vesicular changes (Buzzi et al. 1990).

The close correspondence between the spectrum of drugs effective in both migraine patients and the model establish the relevance of this model to the pathophysiology and treatment of migraine. The dosage requirements for the effects of sumatriptan in both, and the ability of treatment both pre- as well as poststimulation to block the neurogenic response (Huang et al. 1993) also are relevant. The efficacy in this model of nonsteroidal anti-inflammatory drugs (Buzzi et al. 1989) and ketorolac tromethamine (unpublished) plus chronic steroid treatment also establishes the relevance of the pharmacology to the human condition.

THE 5-HT$_{1B/D}$ RECEPTOR

The mammalian peripheral and central nervous system express multiple 5-HT receptors and subtypes of which 5-HT$_{1B}$ and 5-HT$_{1D}$ receptors appear most relevant to the treatment of acute migraine and cluster headaches (Peroutka 1991). 5-HT$_{1D}$ and 5-HT$_{1B}$ are pharmacologically distinct, homologous receptor subtypes belonging to the 5-HT$_1$ receptor family, which includes at least five receptor subtypes, 5-HT$_{1A}$, 5-HT$_{1B}$, 5-HT$_{1D}$, 5-HT$_{1E}$, and 5-HT$_{1F}$ (Peroutka 1990; Branchek et al. 1991). 5-HT$_{1B/D}$ receptors belong to the ever-expanding family of receptor proteins possessing seven transmembrane-spanning segments that are coupled to G-proteins. 5-HT$_{1B/D}$ receptors are often prejunctional or presynaptic in location and inhibit neurotransmitter release, perhaps through activation and opening of potassium channels.

Recently, the genes for both 5-HT$_{1D}$ and 5-HT$_{1B}$ receptor subtypes were cloned, sequenced, and identified in mammalian tissues (Hamlin and Metcalf 1991; Maroteaux et al. 1992; Demshyshyn et al. 1992; Jin et al. 1992; Voigt et al. 1992). Two forms of the human 5-HT$_{1D}$ receptor gene were defined and designated as 5-HT$_{1D\alpha}$ and 5-HT$_{1D\beta}$, the latter exhibiting significant sequence homology to the 5-HT$_{1B}$ receptor protein (Hartig et al. 1992). 5-HT$_{1D\alpha}$ and 5-HT$_{1D\beta}$ are encoded by genes located on chromosomes 6 and 1, respectively

(Jin et al. 1992). The two receptor subtypes exhibit similar binding affinities but possess only 60% amino acid sequence homology. Available pharmacological evidence suggests that the 5-HT_{1D} subtype predominates in the peripheral and central nervous systems of most species including human and guinea pig, whereas 5-HT_{1B} predominates in rats, mice, and hamsters (Hartig et al. 1992). The rat 5-HT_{1B} gene differs from the human $5\text{-HT}_{1D\beta}$ (or human 5-HT_{1B}) by a single amino acid substitution in transmembrane domain 7. Despite the close sequence homology between the rat 5-HT_{1B} and human $5\text{-HT}_{1D\beta}$ receptor proteins, their binding affinities are distinctly different.

A receptor subtype closely related to $5\text{-HT}_{1B}/5\text{-HT}_{1D}$ is expressed on peptide-containing trigeminovascular axons within dura mater but is not present on extracranial cephalic vascular tissues also innervated by the trigeminal nerve (Saito et al. 1988; Buzzi and Moskowitz 1990; Buzzi et al. 1991a). The 5-HT_{1D} receptor subtype does not appear to be expressed by sympathetic nerves innervating dura mater (Buzzi et al. 1991b). The receptor subtype responsible for blockade of plasma protein extravasation in dura mater is species dependent (Matsubara et al. 1991). In the rat, blockade of neurogenic extravasation occurs following the administration of CP-93,129, a compound virtually selective for the 5-HT_{1B} receptor subtype. CP-93,129 (which binds only with micromolar affinity to the 5-HT_{1D} receptor subtype) is inactive in the guinea pig extravasation model (Matsubara et al. 1991).

As noted, the drugs exhibiting the greatest potency in blocking neurogenic plasma protein extravasation are those 5-HT_1 agonists exhibiting nanomolar binding affinities to the $5\text{-HT}_{1B/D}$ receptor subtype in membranes prepared from brain. We suspect that an additional as yet unidentified subtype of the 5-HT_1 receptor might mediate the response. Consistent with this formulation, we observed in the dural extravasation model pharmacological differences from the predicted effects of drugs acting at a known 5-HT_1 receptor subtype(s): (l) the very high potency of the nonselective agonist, 5-carboxamidotryptamine (5-CT) was greater than expected; (2) the effects of 5-CT were not blocked by metergoline, a 5-HT_1 receptor antagonist; (3) metergoline only partially inhibited the action of sumatriptan; (4) pretreatment with methiothepin, a 5-HT_1 receptor antagonist, did not affect inhibition by sumatriptan; (5) the putative antagonists promote plasma extravasation when administered alone; and (6) serotonin itself is inactive in this model (Buzzi et al. 1991b).

The newest subtype of the 5-HT_1 receptor series has been designated 5-HT_{1F} (Adham et al. 1993). The 5-HT_{1F} subtype is encoded by a distinct gene and like the 5-HT_{1D} receptor subtype, binds sumatriptan with high (nM) affinity. The 5-HT_{1F} receptor subtype binds 5-carboxamidotryptamine with low affinity. Because 5-carboxamidotryptamine blocks neurogenic plasma extravasation with greatest potency among the drugs we have tested to date, the relevance of the 5-HT_{1F} receptor subtype to the treatment of migraine requires further study. Moreover, whether the 5-HT_{1F} receptor subtype is expressed by vascular smooth muscle or trigeminovascular neurons remains to be determined.

Several lines of pharmacologic evidence support the existence of prejunctional inhibitory 5-$HT_{1B/D}$ receptors on sensory nerve fibers. First, administration of ergot alkaloids and sumatriptan in therapeutically relevant doses blocks the neurogenically-mediated plasma protein leakage that follows either electrical stimulation of the trigeminal ganglion or capsaicin administration (Saito et al. 1988; Buzzi and Moskowitz 1990). However, plasma protein extravasation induced directly by SP or NKA administration is unaffected by these agents (vasoconstriction alone cannot account for the ergot action because extravasation is not abolished by the vasoconstrictors angiotensin or phenylephrine (Saito et al. 1988; Dimitriadou et al. 1992). Second, sumatriptan and dihydroergotamine attenuate the concomitant increase in plasma CGRP content within the superior sagittal sinus (Buzzi et al. 1990). Furthermore, serum CGRP levels are reduced in humans who have received sumatriptan (Goadsby and Edvinsson 1991). Third, sumatriptan and ergot alkaloids reduce the ultrastructural changes in endothelium, platelets, and mast cells, which result from trigeminal sensory nerve fiber stimulation (Buzzi et al. 1992). A receptor site for acute antimigraine drugs like sumatriptan is postulated to reside outside the blood-brain barrier (BBB) because sumatriptan penetrates into the brain very poorly, and there is no evidence that the BBB is disrupted in migraine.

Molecular biological techniques recently were used to localize the 5-$HT_{1B/D}$ receptor within trigeminovascular neurons. Using polymerase chain reaction (PCR) technology, Rebeck et al. amplified a single oligonucleotide sequence homologous to 5-$HT_{1D\alpha}$ (85%) and 5-HT_{1B} receptor (74%) mRNA within guinea pig trigeminal ganglion. Using reverse transcriptase-PCR and specific probes complementary to either the 5-$HT_{1D\alpha}$ or 5-$HT_{1D\beta}$ gene, Rebeck and his colleagues could amplify only the 5-$HT_{1D\alpha}$ message, thereby suggesting selective expression of this gene. Rebeck's findings complement Bruinvels' results using in situ hybridization documenting the existence of the receptor mRNA in trigeminal ganglion neurons (Bruinvels et al. 1992). Using probes complementary to codons encoding the amino acid residues 249–264, hybridization signals were observed in perikaryons in all three divisions of the rat trigeminal ganglion. By contrast, specific 5-$HT_{1B/D}$ binding sites were not found within the ganglia when in vitro receptor autoradiography was performed using ^{125}I-GTI. The pharmacological and molecular data together suggest that

5-HT_{IB} receptor proteins are transported primarily to the nerve terminals of the trigeminovascular fibers within the meninges. The data appear to rule out the trigeminal ganglia itself as a binding site for the antimigraine drugs such as sumatriptan and dihydroergotamine.

Rebeck's recent data suggest that the alpha subtype of the 5-HT_{ID} receptor is expressed selectively by trigeminovascular neurons (Rebeck et al. 1994). These findings take on greater importance based on Hamel's recent publication showing that the 5-$HT_{ID\beta}$ receptor subtype is selectively expressed by the pial arteriolar vascular smooth muscle (Hamel et al. 1993). Hamel found a stronger correlation between the constrictor potency of 5-HT_{ID} ligands on pial vessels and the binding affinity of these same compounds to the cloned and expressed 5-$HT_{ID\beta}$ (than 5-$HT_{ID\alpha}$) receptor subtype. Furthermore, she observed a strong hybridizing signal on northern blots to mRNA prepared from vascular smooth muscle using probes selective for 5-$HT_{ID\beta}$, no hybridizing signal was detected using probes for the 5-$HT_{ID\alpha}$ subtype. Confirmation of both findings would raise the possibility of designing drugs that bind selectively to the prejunctional receptor to avoid vasoconstriction of pial and contraction in other vascular beds (e.g., coronary vessels). Developing second-generation drugs with selective prejunctional binding has the potential to circumvent some of the untoward effects of both sumatriptan and the ergot alkaloids in patients with angina pectoris and hypertension.

CONCLUSION

Migraine can be treated by serotonin receptor agonists that couple to prejunctional 5-$HT_{IB/D}$ receptors on unmyelinated perivascular sensory nerves to block activity in the trigeminovascular system. We propose that the vasodilatation that may accompany migraine is not the source of headache, but reflects neuropeptide release from perivascular sensory nerves as a consequence of activation of trigeminal pathways, and neurogenic inflammation. Rather than causing the headache, vasodilatation may develop as a consequence of sensory nerve activation. This supposition, however, does not rule out that vasoconstriction could, in some secondary way, also contribute to headache relief. It has been hypothesized that vasoconstriction will alter the geometry of perivascular axons and, by so doing, may modify their electrophysiologic properties (Moskowitz 1991b). However, the existing clinical data addressing the merits of an additional mechanism based on vasoconstriction are far from definitive and, for the most part, have not provided convincing results to support a primary vascular mechanism of drug action.

Recent data examining the expression of c-*fos* antigen within superficial laminae of trigeminal nucleus caudalis following noxious meningeal stimulation confirm the important neurogenic actions of the ergot alkaloids and sumatriptan in models of meningovascular pain (Nozaki et al. 1992a,b; Moskowitz et al. 1993).

ACKNOWLEDGMENT

This work was supported by the National Institute of Neurological Disorders and Stroke (NINDS) grant NS 21558.

REFERENCES

Adham, N.H.-T., Kao, L.E., Schechter, L.E., Bard, J., Olsen, M., Urguhart, D., Durkin, M., Hartig, P.R., Weinshank, L. and Brancek, T., Cloning of another human serotonin receptor (5-HT_{1F}): a fifth 5-HT_1 receptor subtype coupled to inhibition of adenylate cyclase, Proc. Natl. Acad. Sci. USA, 90 (1993) 408–412.

Andersen, A.R., Friberg, L., Olsen, T.S. and Olesen, J., Delayed hyperemia following hypoperfusion in classic migraine, Arch. Neurol., 45 (1988) 154–159.

Blau, J.N., Migraine: a vasomotor instability of the meningeal circulation, Lancet, 2 (1978) 1136–1139.

Branchek, T., Zgombick, J., Macchi, M., Hartig, P. and Weinshank, R., Cloning and expression of a human 5-HT_{1D} receptor. In: J.R. Fozard and P.R. Saxena (Eds.), Serontonin Molecular Biology, Receptors and Functional Effects, Birkhauser Verlag, Basel, Switzerland, 1991, pp. 21–32.

Bruinvels, A.T., Landwehrmeyer, B., Moskowitz, M.A. and Hoyer, D., Autoradiographical evidence for the presence of serotonin 5-HT_{1B} messenger RNA in neurons of the rat trigeminal ganglia, Eur. J. Pharmacol., 227 (1992) 357–359.

Buzzi, M.G. and Moskowitz, M.A., The antimigraine drug, sumatriptan (GR43175), selectively blocks neurogenic plasma extravasation from blood vessels in dura mater, Br. J. Pharmacol., 99 (1990) 202–206.

Buzzi, M.G., Sakas, D.E. and Moskowitz, M.A., Indomethacin and acetylsalicylic acid block neurogenic plasma protein extravasation in rat dura mater, Eur. J. Pharmacol., 165 (1989) 251–258.

Buzzi, M.G., Dimitriadou, V., Theoharides, T.C. and Moskowitz, M.A., Morphological effects of electrical trigeminal ganglion stimulation (ETG) on intra- and extracranial vessels, Soc. Neurosci., 16 (1990) 160.

Buzzi, M.G., Carter, B., Shimizu, T., Heath, H., III and Moskowitz, M.A., Dihydroergotamine and sumatriptan attenuate levels of CGRP in plasma in rat superior sagittal sinus during electrical stimulation of the trigeminal ganglion, Neuropharmacology, 30 (1991a) 1193–1200.

Buzzi, M.G., Moskowitz, M.A., Peroutka, S.J. and Byun, B., Further characterization of the putative 5-HT receptor which mediates blockade of neurogenic plasma extravasation in rat dura mater, Br. J. Pharmacol., 103 (1991b) 1421–1428.

Buzzi, M.G., Dimitriadou, V., Theoharides, T.C. and Moskowitz, M.A., 5-hydroxytriptamine receptor agonists for the abortive treatment of vascular headaches block mast cell, endothelial and platelet activation within the rat dura mater after trigeminal stimulation, Brain Res., 583 (1992) 137–149.

Dahl, A., Russell, D., Nyberg-Hansen, R. and Rootwelt, K., Effect of nitroglycerin on cerebral

circulation measured by transcranial Doppler and SPECT, Stroke, 20 (1989) 1733–1736.
Dahl, E., Russell, D., Nyberg-Hansen, R. and Rootwelt, K., Cluster headache: transcranial Doppler ultrasound and rCBF studies, Cephalgia, 10 (1990) 87–94.
Demshyshyn, L., Sunahara, R.K., Miller, K., Teitler, M., Hoffman, B.J., Kennedy, J.L., Seeman, P., Van Tol, H.H. and Niznik, H.B., A human serotonin ID receptor variant ($5HT_{1\beta}$) encoded by an intronless gene on chromosome 6, Proc. Natl. Acad. Sci. USA, 89 (1992) 5522–5526.
Dimitriadou, V., Buzzi, M.G., Moskowitz, M.A. and Theoharides, T.C., Trigeminal sensory fiber stimulation induces morphological changes reflecting secretion in rat dura mater mast cells, Neurosci., 44 (1991) 97–112.
Dimitriadou, V., Buzzi, M.G., Theoharides, T.C. and Moskowitz, M.A., Ultrastructural evidence for neurogenically mediated changes in blood vessels of the rat dura mater and tongue following antidromic trigeminal stimulation, Neurosci., 48 (1992) 187–203.
Goadsby, P.J. and Edvinsson, L., Sumatriptan reverses the changes in calcitonin gene-related peptide seen in the headache phase of migraine, Cephalgia, 11, Suppl. 11 (1991) 3.
Hamel, E., Fan, E., Linville, D., Ting, V., Villemure, J.-G. and Chia, S.-S., Expression of mRNA for the serotonin 5-hydroxytryptamine$_{1D\beta}$ receptor subtype in human and bovine cerebral arteries, Mol. Pharmacol., 44 (1993) 242–246.
Hamlin, M.W. and Metcalf, M.A., Primary structure and functional characterization of a human 5-HT_{1D} type serotonin receptor, Mol. Pharmacol., 40 (1991) 143–148.
Hartig, P.R., Branchek, T.A. and Weinsank, R.L., A subfamily of 5-HT_{1D} receptor genes, Trends Pharmacol. Sci., 13 (1992) 152–159.
Heyck, H., Neue Beitrage zur Kl inik und Pathogenese der Migraine, Georg Thieme Verlag, Berlin, 1956, p. 29.
Huang, Z., Byun, B.J., Matsubara, T. and Moskowitz, M.A, Time-dependent blockade of neurogenic plasma extravasation in dura mater by 5-$HT_{1B/D}$ agonists and endopeptidase 24,11, Br. J. Pharmacol., 108 (1993) 331–335.
Humphrey, P.P.A., Feniuk, W., Perren, M.J., Berseford, I.J.M. and Skingle, M., Serotonin and migraine. In: P.M. Whitaker-Azmitia and S.J. Peroutka (Eds.), The Neuropharmacology of Serotonin, Ann. NY Acad. Sci., 600 (1990) 587–600.
Jin, H., Oksenberg, D., Ashkenazi, A., Peroutka, S.J., Duncan, A., Rozmahel, R., Yang, Y., Mengod, G., Palaxios, U.M. and Dowd, B.F., Characterization of the human 5-hydroxytrytpamine$_{1B}$ receptor, J. Biol. Chem., 267 (1992) 5735–5738.
Lembeck, F., Zur fragen der zentralen ubertragung afferenter Impulse. III. Mitteilung. Das Vorkommen und die Bedeutung der Substanz P in den dorsal en wurzeln des Ruckenmarks, Naunyn-Schmiedeberg's Arch. Exp. Pathol. Pharmakol., 219 (1953) 197–213.
Lewis, T., The nocifensor system of nerves and its reactions, Br. Med. J., 194 (1937) 431–435.
Markowitz, S., Saito, K. and Moskowitz, M.A., Neurogenically mediated leakage of plasma protein occurs from blood vessels in dura mater but not brain, J. Neurosci., 7 (1987) 4129–4136.
Maroteaux, L., Saudou, F., Amlaidy, N., Boscert, U., Plassat, J.L. and Hen, R., Mouse 5-HT_{1B} serotonin receptor: cloning, functional expression, and localization in motor control centers, Proc. Natl. Acad. Sci. USA, 89 (1992) 3020–3024.
Matsubara, T., Moskowitz, M.A. and Byun, B., CP-93,129, a potent and selective 5-HT_{1B} receptor agonist blocks neurogenic plasma extravasation within rat but not guinea pig dura mater, Br. J. Pharmacol., 104 (1991) 3–4.
Moskowitz, M.A., The visceral organ brain: implications for the pathophysiology of vascular head pain, Neurology, 41 (1991a) 182–186.
Moskowitz, M.A., Interpreting vessel diameter changes in vascular headaches, Cephalalgia, 12 (1991b) 5–7.
Moskowitz, M.A., Neurogenic versus vascular mechanisms of sumatriptan and ergot alkaloids in migraine, Trends Pharmacol. Sci., 13 (1992) 307–311.
Moskowitz, M.A. and Cutrer, F.M., Sumatriptan:a receptor-targeted treatment for migraine, Ann. Rev. Med., 44 (1993) 145–154.
Moskowitz, M.A. and Cutrer, F.M., Possible importance of neurogenic inflammation within the

meninges to migraine headaches. In: H.L. Fields and J.C. Liebeskind (Eds.), Pharmacological Approaches to the Treatment of Chronic Pain: New Concepts and Critical Issues. Progress in Pain Research and Management, Vol. 1. IASP Press, Seattle, 1994, pp. 43–49.

Moskowitz, M.A., Nozaki, K. and Kraig, R.P., Neocortical spreading depression provokes the expression of c-fos protein-like immunoreactivityq within trigeminal nucleus caudalis via trigeminovascular mechanisms, J. Neurosci., 13 (1993) 1167–1177.

Northfield, D.W.C., Some observations on headache, Brain, 61 (1938) 133–162.

Nozaki, K., Boccalini, P. and Moskowitz, M.A., Expression of c-fos-like immunoreactivity in brainstem after meningeal irritation by blood in the subarachnoid space, Neuroscience, 49 (1992a) 669–680.

Nozaki, K., Moskowitz, M.A. and Boccalini, P., CP-93,129, sumatriptan, dihydroergotamine block c-fos expression within rat trigeminal nucleus caudalis caused by chemical stimulation of the meninges, Br. J. Pharmacol., 106 (1992b) 409–415.

Olesen, J. and Paulson, O.B., The effect of intra-arterial papaverine on the regional cerebral blood flow in patients with stroke or intracranial tumor, Stroke, 2 (1971) 148–159.

Olesen, J., Paulson, O.B. and Lassen, L.A., Regional cerebral blood flow in man determined by the initial slope of the clearance of intra-arterially injected 133Xe, Stroke, 2 (1971) 519–540.

Peroutka, S.J., Sumatriptan in acute migraine: pharmacology and review of world experience, Headache, 30, Suppl. 2 (1990) 554–560.

Peroutka, S.J., Serotonin receptor subtypes and neuropsychiatric diseases: focus on 5-HT1D and 5-HT 3 receptor agents, Pharmacol. Rev., 43 (1991) 579–586.

Rebeck, G.W., Maynard, K.I., Hyman, B.T. and Moskowitz, M.A., Selective 5-$HT_{1D\alpha}$ receptor gene expression in trigeminal ganglia: implications for antimigraine drug development, Proc. Natl. Acad. Sci. USA (1994), in press.

Saito, K., Markowitz, S. and Moskowitz, M.A., Ergot alkaloids block neurogenic extravasation in dura mater: Proposed action in vascular headaches, Ann. Neurol., 24 (1988) 732–737.

Saria, A., Gamse, R., Lundberg, J.M., Hokfelt, T., Theodorsson-Norheim, E., Petermann, J. and Fischer, J.A., Co-existence of tachykinins and calcitonin gene-related peptide in sensory nerves in relatin to neurogenic inflammation. In: R. Hakanson and F. Sundler (Eds.), Tachykinin Antagonists, Elsevier, Amsterdam, 1985.

Voigt, M.M., Laurie, D.J., Seeburg, P.H. and Bach, A., Molecular cloning and characterization of rat brain cDNA encoding a 5-hydroxytryptamine1B receptor, EMBO J, 10 (1992) 4017–4023.

Wei, E.P., Moskowitz, M.A., Boccalini, P. and Kontos, H.A., Calcitonin gene-related peptide mediates nitroglycerin and sodium nitroprusside–induced vasodilatation in feline cerebral arterioles, Circ. Res., 70 (1992) 1313–1319.

Zwetsloot, C.P., Caekebeke, J.F.V., Jansen, J.C., Odink, J. and Ferrari, M.D., Blood flow velocity changes in migraine attacks: a transcranial Doppler study, Cephalgia, 11 (1991) 8103–8107.

Correspondence to: Michael A. Moskowitz, MD, Stroke Research Laboratory, Massachusetts General Hospital, Boston, MA 02114, USA. Tel: 617-726-8442; Fax: 617-726-2547.

Part X

Central Pain

Proceedings of the 7th World Congress on Pain,
Progress in Pain Research and Management, Vol. 2,
edited by G.F. Gebhart, D.L. Hammond, and T.S.
Jensen, IASP Press, Seattle, © 1994.

51

A Thalamic Concept of Neurogenic Pain

Daniel Jeanmonod, Michel Magnin, and Anne Morel

Laboratory of Functional Neurosurgery, Neurosurgical Clinic,
University Hospital, Zürich, Switzerland

INTRODUCTION

Chronic neurogenic pain remains today a significant problem, at the clinical as well as at anatomo-physiological levels. It is caused by a lesion along somatosensory pathways, from nerve to cortex (Déjerine and Roussy 1906; Head and Holmes 1911; Pagni 1989; Tasker and Dostrovsky 1989; Tasker et al. 1991) and is characterized by thermal (burning, cold), exteroceptive (electrical, tingling, pins and needles), and proprioceptive (crushing, tearing) dysesthesias. It can be steady, intermittent, or evoked by external stimuli (thermal, tactile, and proprioceptive allodynia, hyperalgesia). In humans as well as in an animal model, neurogenic pain was correlated with abnormal spontaneous activities at different levels of the somatosensory system, i.e., dorsal horn, thalamus and somatosensory (SI) cortex (Loeser et al. 1968; Modesti and Waszak 1975; Albe-Fessard et al. 1985; Jeanmonod et al. 1989; Lenz et al. 1989; Lenz 1991a,b; Albe-Fessard and Rampin 1991; Rinaldi et al. 1991).

The medial thalamotomy was among the first stereotactic operations against neurogenic pain. From the beginning and in contrast to most other destructive surgeries, it was recognized as a procedure with a low complication rate and no risk for the development of iatrogenic neurogenic pain. It was shown to bring a selective relief to all pain localizations, without producing somatosensory deficits (Hécaen et al. 1949; Fairman 1967; Richardson 1967; Sano 1977; Hitchcock and Teixeira 1981; Laitinen 1988; Gybels and Sweet 1989; Tasker 1989). Although cases with total and stable relief were published, recurrence of the original pain, partial or complete, was too frequent. Lesions in the dorsal root entry zone (Sindou and Daher 1988; Sindou et al. 1990) and chronic stimulation of the dorsal column and of the ventroposterior (VP) nucleus of the thalamus (Levy et al. 1988; Gybels and Sweet 1989) have nowadays taken the forefront of the surgical treatment of neurogenic pain, but a definitive treatment, with any technique, is still lacking.

In 1911, Head and Holmes proposed, in the pathogenesis of central neurogenic pain, the causal significance of an "essential thalamic centre," localized medially to the lesion in the VP and submitted to the decreased inhibitory influence of a thalamo-cortico-thalamic loop. Albe-Fessard and coworkers (1985) and Tasker and Dostrovsky (1989) emphasized the appearance of marked alterations of the responses to stimulation in the medial thalamus of patients with neurogenic pain. Experimental and clinical data reported by Cesaro et al. (1986, 1991) gave support to an imbalanced interplay between medial and lateral thalamic areas through the thalamic reticular nucleus with a postulated disinhibition, and thus hyperactivity, of the medial thalamus. Sano had already proposed in 1977 the generation of abnormal impulses in VP and their amplification in a reverberating circuit between lateral and medial thalamic nuclei. In contrast to these hypotheses based on disinhibition and hyperactivity, recent unit recordings in the lateral (Lenz et al. 1989) and the medial (Jeanmonod et al. 1993) thalamus revealed the presence of overinhibition in both structures. The aim of our work has thus been to develop a comprehensive concept of neurogenic pain integrating these data.

METHODS

PATIENT POPULATION

The medial thalamotomy, with its necessary peroperative physiological controls, was approved by the University Hospital ethics committee, and proposed to 69 fully informed patients suffering from chronic therapy-resistant peripheral or central neurogenic pain. Pain taxonomy follows propositions of Lindblom (1993) and Tasker and Dostrovsky (1989). Detailed pre- and postoperative neurologic examinations and the preoperative completion of a pain questionnaire were carried out. Pain was assessed pre- and postoperatively using: (1) three to seven visual analogue scale (VAS) determinations of pain intensity, (2) the patient's estimation in percent of the global postoperative improvement, (3) activities of daily living, and (4) pain drug intake. The age of the patients at the time of the thalamotomy ranged between 19 and 84 years, with a mean of 56 years. The dates of injury and pain onset were known in 40 patients, and 60% of them presented a delay in pain onset ranging between 2 weeks and 2 years. The duration of the pain syndrome, i.e., the time between pain onset and thalamotomy, varied between 2 months and 23 years, with a mean of 6 years. Fifty-four patients had peripheral nerve and/or dorsal root lesions (Fig. 1). Among them, 10 had lesions in the trigeminal area, 4 a postherpetic neuralgia, and 8 an amputation. These peripheral lesions covered among them the face, the head and neck, the upper and lower limb, the thoracoabdominal, and the perineal areas. Seven patients had a plexus avulsion. Among central lesions, 12 were in the spinal cord, 4 in the brain stem, 3 in the thalamus, and 5 in the parietal cortex (Fig. 1). This list amounts to 85 causal lesions, because in some patients there was more than one. Forty-one patients (59%) had pure peripheral (nerve and/or root) lesions, 15 (22%) pure central lesions, and 13 (19%) mixed peripheral and central lesions. In 11 patients, the neurogenic pain syndrome resulted from cancer, and they underwent surgery before the minimum one year of pain duration required for patients with normal life expectancies. Resistance to therapy was documented for all patients with proper antiepileptic and thymoleptic treatments, and often with trials of physiotherapy, transcutaneous electrical nerve stimulation, and local blocks. Nineteen dorsal column and thalamic stimulations and 12 interruptive surgeries had been performed before thalamotomy. The mean of the highest preoperative pain intensity values on the VAS was 85. Preoperative somatosensory deficits were present in 91% of the patients; the remaining patients had no deficits clinically visible but had neurological or anamnestic evidence of former, compensated somatosensory damage.

As shown in Fig. 2, steady pain was present in 92% of the patients prior to surgery, intermittent pain in 72%, and evoked pain in 51%. Steady pain alone was present in 21%, intermittent pain alone in 7%, and the three pain types together in 43% of the patients. As shown in Fig. 3, thermal pain qualities were observed preoperatively in 76%, exteroceptive in 86%, and proprioceptive in 92% of the patients. Pain qualities were rarely seen alone (8%); the most frequent association was the combination of the three, seen in 62% of the patients.

STEREOTACTIC AND RECORDING TECHNIQUES

Operations took place under local anesthesia in 69 fully awake patients. Each thalamotomy session included the exploration of one to two medial thalamic targets, so that a total of 159 penetrations were performed during 104 operative sessions. A stereotactic frame (Cosman Roberts Wells, Radionics, Burlington, Mass.) compatible with magnetic resonance (MR) was used. Stereotactic MR pictures were taken to localize the medial thalamic targets using an adaptation of a CT technique (Jeanmonod and Thomas 1989). The

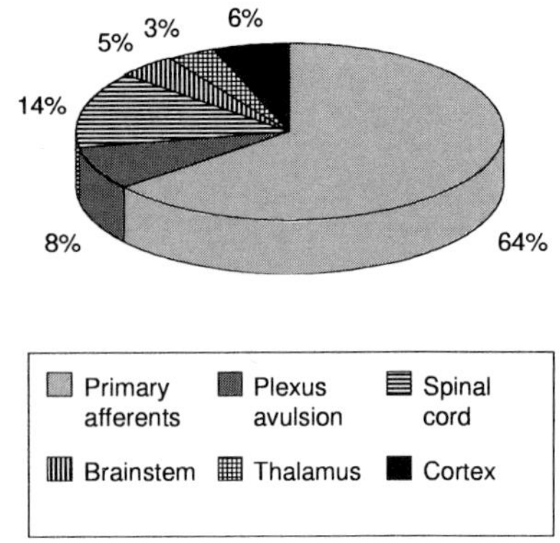

Fig. 1. Distribution of lesion localizations in our patient population with neurogenic pain. The large majority of these lesions concern the primary afferents, i.e., the peripheral nerve and/or the nerve root. Plexus avulsions which involve an additional spinal cord injury are displayed separately. The total number of lesions amounts to 85 because in some patients there was more than one lesion.

electrode reached the computer-calculated thalamic target through a prefrontal approach, under impedance monitoring. All targets, in general two per operation, were localized in the central lateral (CL), parafascicular (Pf), limitans (Li), oral and medial pulvinar (PuO and PuM), posterior thalamic complex (PO), center median (CM), and midline nuclei. Targets chosen were primarily contralateral or, if necessary (11 patients), ipsilateral to pain localization. Unit recordings were obtained using tungsten microelectrodes with an impedance between 0.5 and 1 megohm. Unit responses were searched with a protocol including tests of motor voluntary function and tactile, nociceptive, and proprioceptive stimuli. Quantitative analysis of the data was done off-line using the software Discovery (Brainwave, Broomfield) to produce interspike interval histograms and autocorrelation histograms. At the end of the recording session, the macroelectrode replaced the microelectrode in the common guide tube and a stimulation session was performed analyzing somesthetic, motor, and psychic manifestations. Neurophysiological data guided the location of radiofrequency thermolesions (volume 40–160 mm^3). All patients underwent a postoperative (2–6 months) three-dimensional MR examination to determine the lesion location.

Target positions, lesion reconstructions, and unit localizations were projected on our stereotactic atlas of the human thalamus.

RESULTS

UNIT RECORDINGS

A total of 972 thalamic units were analyzed from 99 penetrations. Only two units (0.2%) responded to tactile and nociceptive stimuli with large and

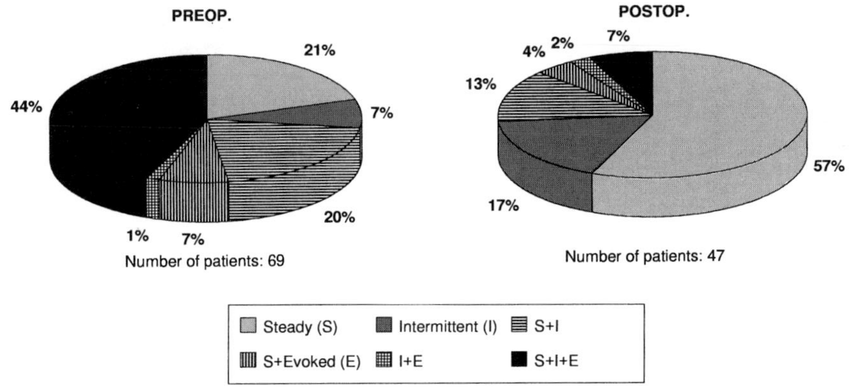

Fig. 2. Pre- versus postoperative pain type distribution. Note the large increase in the steady component to the detriment of the combination S + I + E when pain remains postoperatively. Difference in pre- and postoperative patient numbers corresponds to the 14 patients showing a complete relief and 8 patients with known global postoperative improvement but no data on pain types.

bilateral receptive fields. Of the 970 unresponsive units, 45% had sporadic spontaneous activities, and 55% showed bursting activities, random in 291 (30%) and rhythmic in 240 (25%). When analyzed with interspike interval and autocorrelation histograms, rhythmic bursting units were characterized by interburst intervals between 200 and 300 msec, corresponding to a frequency between 3 and 5 Hz (Fig. 4). Random bursting units showed a more or less marked rhythmic tendency toward these frequencies. The first spike of each burst was often of higher amplitude, and interspike intervals within a burst increased with each successive interval (from 2 to 8 msec). The shorter the first interspike interval in a burst, the greater the number (3 to 10) of spikes within this burst (Fig. 5). All these characteristics are recognized as hallmarks of low-threshold calcium spike (LTS) bursts (Steriade et al. 1990).

The anatomical distribution of the bursting units (localization error ± 1 mm) showed a clustering in and around CL, as illustrated at three thalamic levels in Fig. 6.

CLINICAL RESULTS

Follow-ups ranged from 2 weeks to 4 years (mean: 13 months). Fig. 7 gives the distribution of patients in different relief categories after the medial thalamotomy. 67% experienced a 50–100% improvement, and 20% of them complete relief. A 50–100% improvement was found in 71% of patients with peripheral neurogenic pain, in 60% of the patients with central pain, and in

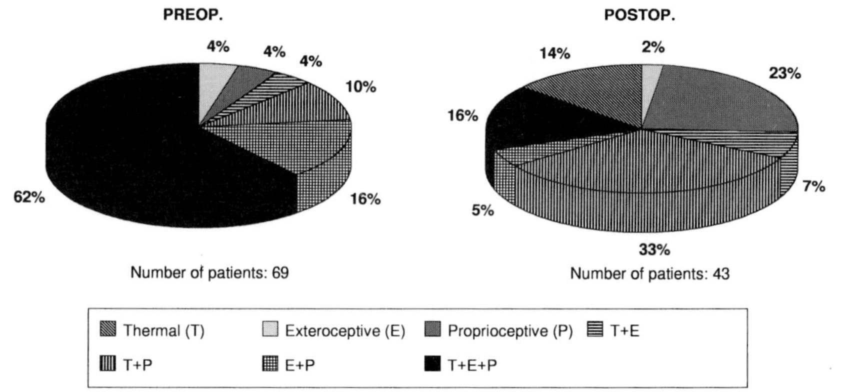

Fig. 3. Pre- versus postoperative pain quality distribution. An isolated thermal component is present only with pain recurrence and, together with the proprioceptive quality, alone or in combination, represents the major postoperative trait. Difference in pre- and postoperative patient numbers corresponds to the 14 patients showing a complete relief and 12 patients with known global postoperative improvement but no data on pain qualities.

62% of patients with pain of mixed central and peripheral origin. The mean of the highest postoperative pain intensity values on the VAS was 49 (compared with 85 preoperatively). Significant decrease or even elimination of consumption of specific drugs (antiepileptics and thymoleptics) was observed in 54% of patients. Significant improvement up to normalization of the activities of daily living was observed in 45% of patients. The majority of the patients (91%) showed no postoperative somatosensory—including pain—deficits. A postoperative improvement of the somatosensory examination was even seen in 47% of patients. Accidental lateral expansion of the lesion (bleeding, edema, or ischemia) into VP or the lateral spinothalamic tract produced in six patients (9%) slight to moderate somatosensory deficits, completely reversible in three of them. In only one patient, a lasting change of the pain qualities and an extension of its localization indicated iatrogenic pain production, fortunately without global worsening. In four of the six patients with acute somatosensory deficits, reversible motor, oculomotor, and pupillary symptoms, as well as fatigability were observed. Somatosensory outcome data are presented in Fig. 8. One additional patient had an anterior thalamic vasospasm with lasting verbal mnestic deficits, representing the unique serious complication of the whole series.

The pain types and qualities that were resistant to the thalamotomy were studied postoperatively (Figs. 2 and 3). Steady pain remained present in 81% of the patients with partial relief, intermittent pain in 39%, and evoked pain in 13%. Fifty-seven percent of the patients reported a persisting isolated steady

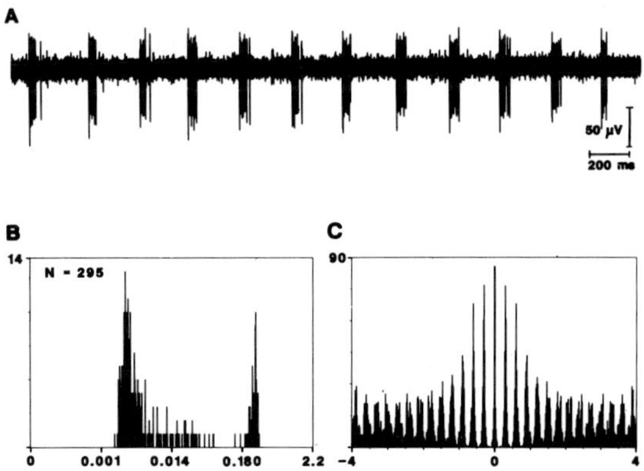

Fig. 4. **A,** Typical example of a rhythmic bursting unit recorded in the CL of a patient suffering from central neurogenic pain. **B,** Bimodal distribution (inter- and intraburst) as shown by an interspike interval histogram of the same unit (N: number of intervals analyzed; ordinate: number of intervals; abscissa: logarithmic time scale in sec; bin size: 0.02 msec). **C,** Corresponding autocorrelogram showing the stability of this bursting activity (ordinate: number of spikes; abscissa: time scale in sec; bin size: 16 msec).

pain. Proprioceptive pain qualities remained in 77% of the patients with partial relief, thermal ones in 70%, and exteroceptive ones in 30%. Isolated proprioceptive pain qualities were present in 23%, and coupled thermal and proprioceptive in 33% of the patients. Steady pain with proprioceptive and thermal qualities is thus clearly the pain profile that so far is the most resistant to medial thalamotomy.

The lesions centered in CL, where most bursting units were found, revealed themselves to be the most efficient (Figs. 9 and 10). Next, in descending order of efficiency, came Pf, PO, PuO, and PuM nuclei. Results after lesions in CM and midline nuclei were the least efficient, so these targets were progressively abandoned.

DISCUSSION

UNIT ACTIVITIES

One characteristic of the vast majority (99.8%) of our medial thalamic units is their lack of responsiveness to somatosensory stimulation, in contrast to the large and often bilateral receptive fields reported in animals (Guilbaud et al. 1984; Willis 1985) and humans (Ishijima et al. 1975; Sano 1977). This unresponsiveness bears a strong relation to neurogenic pain, since the only two responsive units of our series were found in one patient with cancer-related nociceptive and neurogenic pain in the CL contralateral to the nociceptive pain component.

In addition to their unresponsiveness, half of the units show a striking bursting activity, rhythmic in 25% and random in 30%. Rhythmic activities with a similar bursting frequency (3–5 Hz) have been found in animals in slow wave sleep but never in wakefulness (Steriade and Deschenes 1984; Steriade et al. 1990). This indicates a clear state-dependent abnormality, because all our patients were fully awake during the operation. The random bursting units can also be considered as abnormal, for two reasons. First, similar activities were observed in awake cats (Steriade et al. 1990), but displayed a tendency toward much higher frequencies (20–40 Hz) than those recorded here (3–5 Hz). Second, these random bursting cells were found only in a restricted dorso-lateral area of CL, whereas we discovered them widely distributed throughout the posterior half of CL. Even more relevant to the

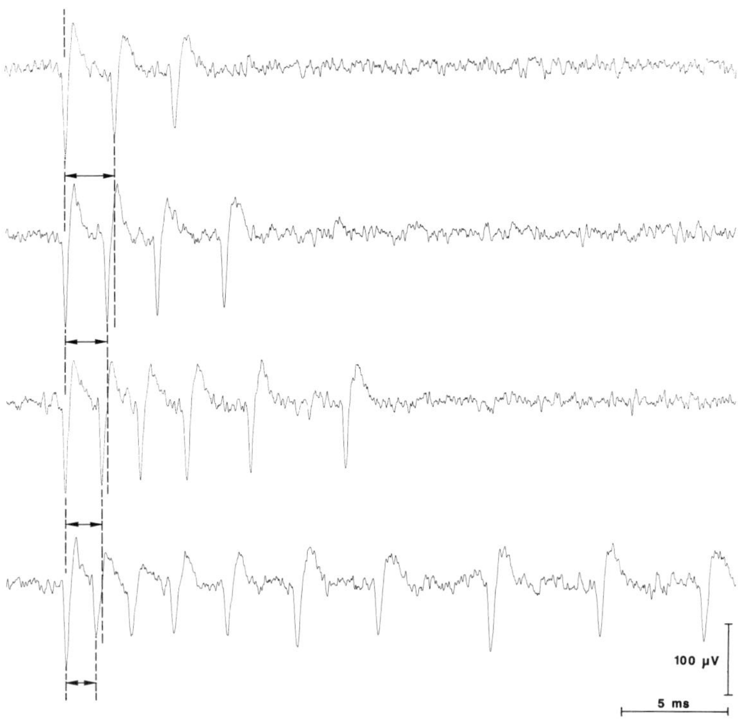

Fig. 5. Example of four bursts of a rhythmic bursting unit.

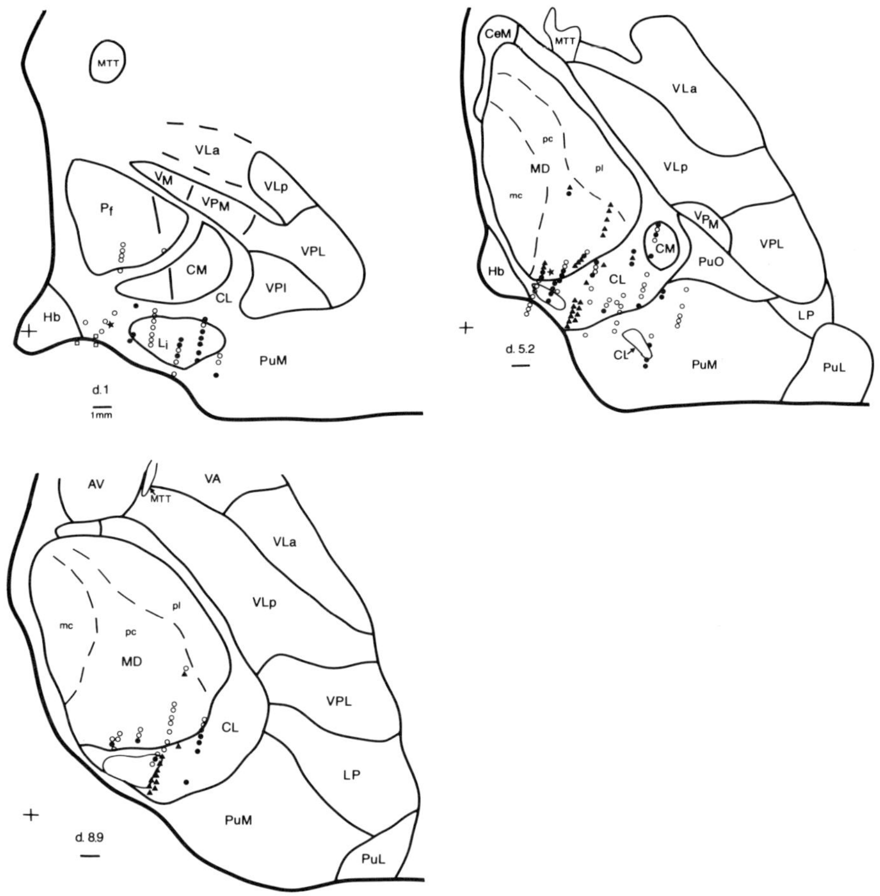

Fig. 6. Anatomical localization of a representative sample of recorded cells on three horizontal sections of our atlas of the human thalamus, at levels 1, 5.2, and 8.9 mm dorsal to the intercommissural plane. Posterior commissure level is indicated by a cross in the lower left of each section. Open square: pretectal; star: responsive; open circle: sporadic; black dot: random bursting; black triangle: rhythmic bursting units. AV: anterior ventral; CeM: central medial CL: central lateral; CM: center median; Hb: habenula; Li: limitans; LP: lateral posterior; MD: mediodorsal (pl: paralamellar, pc: parvocellular, mc: magnocellular); MTT: mamillothalamic tract; Pf: parafascicular; PuL, PuM, and PuO: lateral, medial, and oral pulvinar; R: reticularis thalami VA: ventral anterior; VLa: ventral lateral anterior; VLp: ventral lateral posterior; VPI: ventral posterior inferior VPL: ventral posterior lateral; VPM: ventral posterior medial; VM: ventral medial.

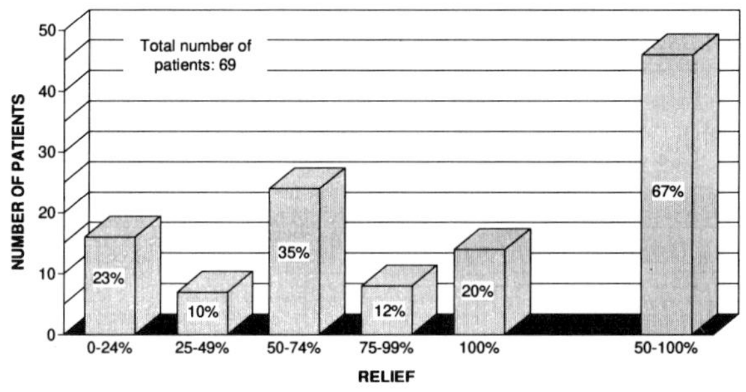

Fig. 7. Distribution of the number of patients with respect to the percentage of relief obtained after medial thalamotomy. Results corresponding to a worthwhile to complete relief (50–100%) are represented by the rightmost bar. Values on each bar indicates the percentage of the total population of patients in each class.

situation of patients with lesions in the somatosensory system, thalamic bursting activities were also described in the animal after cortical (Curro Dossi et al. 1992) or thalamic reticular (Steriade et al. 1990) experimental lesions.

The above-mentioned bursting activities observed experimentally and those presented in this chapter in humans (see Results) have the same characteristics, i.e., those of LTS bursts, known to result from an overinhibition of relay thalamic cells (Steriade et al. 1990). Such LTS bursts were also found in VP of patients with neurogenic pain by Lenz et al. (1989, 1990). They were concentrated in and around the part of VP which was deafferented, i.e., centered on the pain area. Studies in the rat using a rhizotomy model (Albe-Fessard and Rampin 1991) have also demonstrated the presence of rhythmic activities in both VP and CL.

The rest of our sampled units displayed unresponsive sporadic activities. Many of them exhibited occasional LTS bursts, suggesting that they are under a more limited inhibitory influence than cells showing random or rhythmic bursts. Such an interpretation is supported by data from Steriade et al. (1990), who showed the occurrence of isolated spikes after a moderate hyperpolarization and of LTS bursts after a stronger hyperpolarization of thalamic relay cells. This suggests a continuum of increasingly inhibited thalamic neurons.

A THALAMIC CONCEPT OF NEUROGENIC PAIN

Fig. 11 highlights the anatomical and physiological central elements of our concept: (a) CL, VP, and nucleus reticularis thalami (RT) are interconnected by reciprocal reticulothalamic and thalamoreticular pathways, (b) The reticulothalamic connection is inhibitory (GABAergic), and (c) CL has more

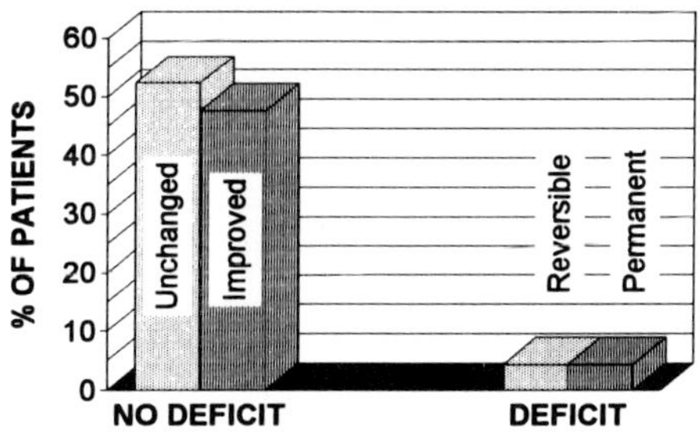

Fig. 8. The postoperative somatosensory status. The sum of the 4 columns is greater than 100% because some patients had both an improvement on a body part and a temporary deficit on another part.

diffuse and multiple connections with the spinal cord and cortex than VP (Albe-Fessard et al. 1985; Jones 1985; Willis 1985; Hodge 1990; Steriade et al. 1990; Craig 1991; Bentivoglio et al. 1993).

There is evidence that neurogenic pain typically arises after a lesion of the lateral spinothalamic system with a relative sparing of the medial spinothalamic, spinoreticular, and spinomesencephalic systems (Gybels and Sweet 1989; Pagni 1989). Such a lesion—as well as any lesion along the somatosensory pathways—deprives VP more extensively of its excitatory inputs than CL (Fig. 11.1). A self-limiting down-regulation of the VP-RT-VP loop should ensue. CL, however, with its spared excitatory afferents and decreased inhibitory reticular input, is in a position to overactivate RT, leading to an inappropriate inhibition of VP (Fig. 11.2). In this condition, VP cells produce LTS bursts. The next steps are the overactivation of RT by these VP bursts and the resulting overinhibition of CL, which in turn initiates LTS bursts (Fig. 11.3). These CL bursts further overactivate RT, which then overinhibits VP, thus closing a vicious circle (Fig. 11.3). This vicious circle can be broken by (1) the destruction of VP at the cost of marked deficits (Mauguière and Desmedt 1988) and with the risk, if parts of it are spared, of reactivating or even increasing the physiopathology; (2) the stimulation of VP, counteracting its overinhibition, but limited by topographic, temporal, and technical factors; or (3) the lesion of CL and other medial thalamic nuclei, with no decrease of remaining somatosensory functions and no risk of producing neurogenic pain.

The idea of a disturbed balance between medial and lateral thalamic areas at the source of neurogenic pain dates back to the beginning of this century (Head and Holmes 1911). Along the years many hypotheses have been proposed (Albe-Fessard et al. 1985; Pagni 1989; Tasker and Dostrovsky 1989; Cesaro et al. 1991) which postulated a hyperactivation, or a loss of inhibition, at the thalamic level, although the origin of the neurogenic pain phenomenon was soon recognized as the suppression of excitatory inputs to the thalamus.

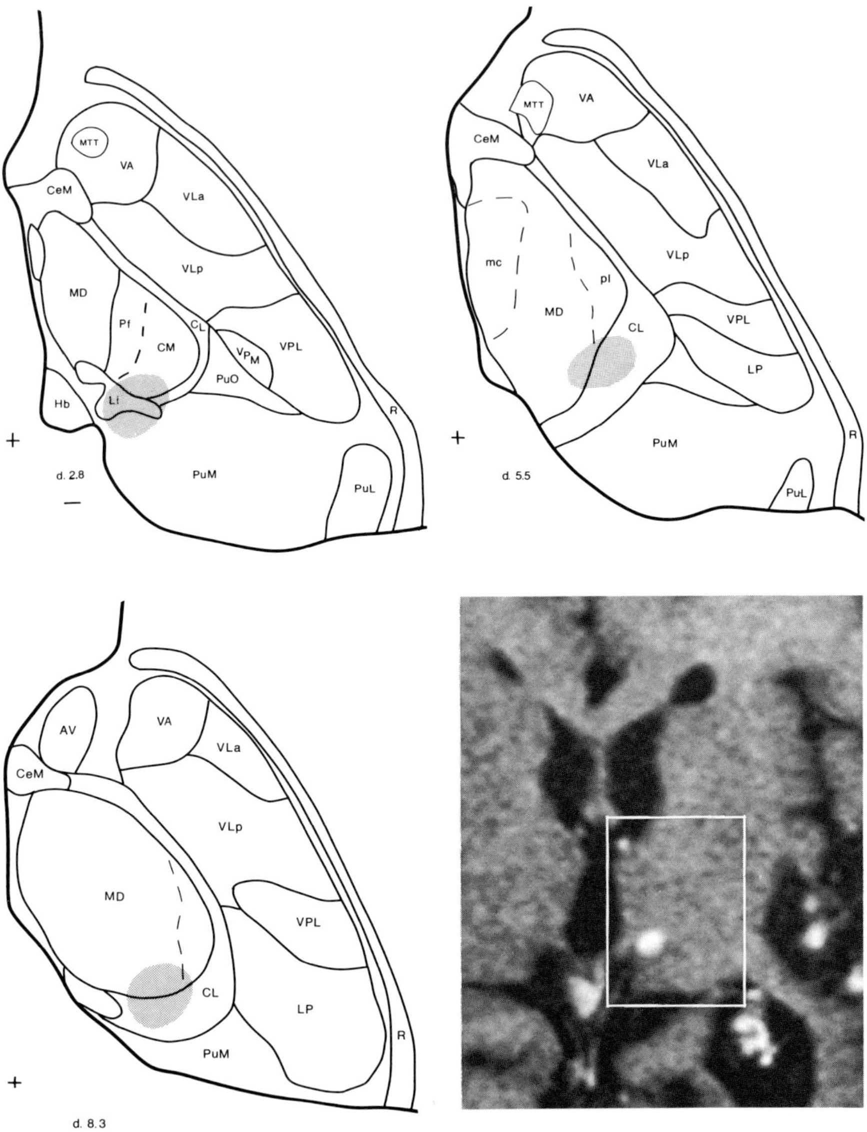

Fig. 9. Anatomical reconstructions of a lesion made in the thalamus of a patient suffering from central neurogenic pain. The projection of the lesion on three horizontal sections of our atlas (2.8, 5.5, and 8.3 mm above the intercommissural plane) shows its localization in the caudal part of the central lateral (CL) nucleus. Scale bar: 1 mm. Posterior commissure level is indicated by a cross in the lower left of each section. Anatomical abbreviations as in Fig. 6. Lower right: MR picture of the lesion; the white rectangle shows the localization of the upper left atlas reconstruction.

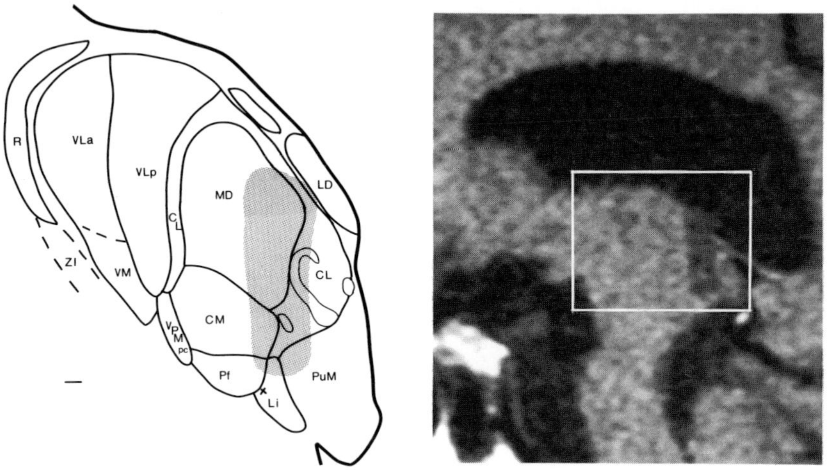

Fig. 10. Anatomical reconstruction and MR picture of a lesion made in a patient suffering from neurogenic pain of peripheral origin. The lesion is projected on a parasagittal plane 7 mm lateral to the midline. LD: lateral dorsal; VPMpc: ventral posterior medial, parvocellular; ZI: zona incerta. Other abbreviations as in Fig. 6. Scale bar: 1 mm. White rectangle on MR picture corresponds to the localization of the left atlas reconstruction. Posterior commissure level is indicated by a cross over nucleus limitans (Li).

Our concept, integrating the presence of LTS bursts in both the medial (this work; see also Jeanmonod et al. 1993) and lateral (Lenz et al. 1989) thalamus, resolves the paradox of a hyperactivity induced by a loss of excitation. This hyperactivity reaches cortical areas devoted to pain perception, resulting in the somatosensory hallucination called neurogenic pain. The unexpected improvement of the somatosensory examination, observed in 47% of our patients after thalamotomy in addition to pain relief, may find an explanation in the liberation of cortical integrations, which were impaired by the thalamic bursting discharges.

CLINICAL RESULTS

The present study confirms that the medial thalamotomy brings a selective relief of neurogenic pain, be it central or peripheral, at all body localizations, without risk, except accidental, of iatrogenic neurogenic pain or somatosensory deficits. The obtained 67% of patients experiencing worthwhile to complete pain relief stands among the best results reported for all techniques. Applying also the medial thalamotomy, Sano (1977) and Laitinen (1988) published very similar, and Hitchcock and Teixeira (1981) and Young et al. (1993) even better results, but on smaller series. From a review of the litera-

Fig. 11. Thalamic concept of neurogenic pain. Upper diagram shows the significant structures and excitatory (+) or inhibitory (–) connections involved in neurogenic pain. CL: central lateral nucleus; RF: reticular formation; RT: reticularis thalami; SCDH: spinal cord, dorsal horn; VP: ventral posterior nucleus. Lower three diagrams illustrate the temporal sequence of events that lead to neurogenic pain after a lesion of the lateral spinothalamic tract (broken arrow). For details see text. Open arrows with headings Ca^{2+} indicate LTS bursting activity. The breadth of all other arrows represents the decrease or increase of activity relative to the normal situation shown in the upper diagram.

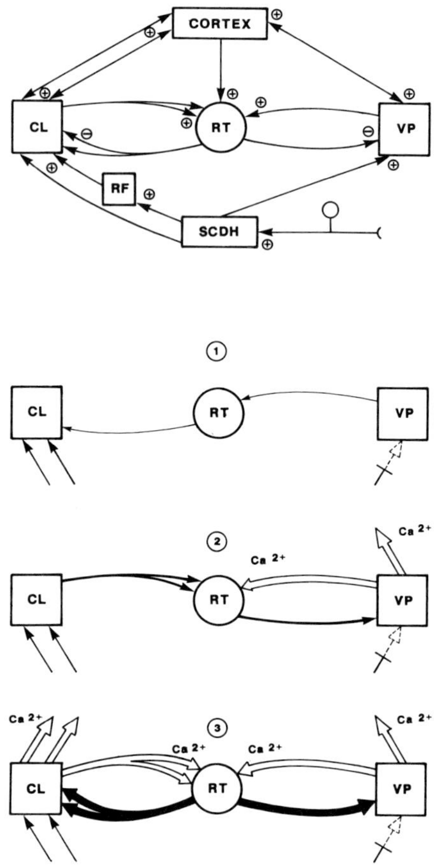

ture, results of VP stimulation and dorsal column stimulation can be averaged to 47 and 43%, respectively (Levy et al. 1988; Gybels and Sweet 1989; North et al. 1993). These results, however, have been obtained against peripheral neurogenic pain, and both procedures have shown much more limited or no effect against central pain syndromes. Even motor cortex stimulation (Tsubokawa et al. 1993), recently claimed to bring relief to central (but not paraplegia) pain, showed only 45% satisfactory results. To compare adequately results of stimulation with results of the medial thalamotomy, it is necessary to consider together neurogenic pain patients who received only a temporary—unsatisfactory—stimulation test and those who underwent permanent implantation. In general, quoted percentages of success are based only on the latter patients, and are thus too optimistic, for they do not consider patients having shown immediate resistance to stimulation.

The fact that central neurogenic pain is more difficult to control than peripheral neurogenic pain could be due to a direct anatomical deafferentation of VP with loss of presynaptic endings. The potential short-distance collateral sprouting of new reticulothalamic synapses on VP deafferented cells could increase the control of RT on these cells, thus promoting their overinhibition when the physiopathology develops.

The analysis of our data indicates the separation of neurogenic pain in two forms on the basis of their response to medial thalamotomy (see also Tasker et al. 1992): a phasic one with intermittent and evoked exteroceptive characteristics, and a tonic one with steady proprioceptive and thermal characteristics. The phasic form, being more easily controlled, would be preponderantly linked to physiopathology in CL. The tonic form, more resistant, could be related to a broader and/or bilateral extension of the physiopathology in the medial thalamus, including Pf, PuO, PuM or PO. Improvements of our results can thus reasonably be expected, because many patients have had so far only a unilateral thalamotomy limited to CL. In 11 patients with unilateral pain source and localization, a complementary ipsilateral thalamotomy has indeed brought further relief, in agreement with the presence of ipsilateral as well as contralateral bursting activities, as observed in the rat rhizotomy model (Albe-Fessard and Rampin 1991). Further improvements are also possible thanks to an optimization of lesion placement in CL, a complex three-dimensional shell-like structure, and a progressive exploration of the other neighboring medial thalamic nuclei.

The good to excellent results of the medial thalamotomy on the phasic form of neurogenic pain could result not only from a more limited and well recognized localization of the physiopathology in CL, but also from more fluctuating and thus more fragile levels of overinhibition. In patients with intermittent pain without steady component, recordings were made only during pain-free periods, and never showed a large amount of LTS bursts, as can be the case in patients with steady pain. A plausible hypothesis, then, is that a further recruitment of the already active but subclinical physiopathology arises at the time of the pain attack.

The effectiveness of the medial thalamotomy against evoked pain in both peripheral and central pain situations puts an accent on central, thalamic mechanisms, at variance with current studies concentrated on the periphery and spinal cord (Willis 1992). Peripheral inputs to normally afferented neighboring parts of VP can, through a VP-RT-VP diverging loop, increase the hyperpolarization of the deafferented VP cells and thus increase temporarily the symptomatology (Roberts et al. 1992). This hypothesis requires neighbor relationship in VP, which is in accordance with the clinical observation that evoked pain is typically present in partially deafferented body parts. The medial thalamotomy efficiently relieves evoked pain through a suppression of the overactivation of RT by CL (Fig. 11) and a consequent decrease of the efficacy of the VP-RT-VP afferent inhibition loop.

Our data also support a role of the thalamus in the mechanisms of peripheral neurogenic pain, which have so far mostly been attributed to primary afferent fibers and dorsal horn neurons. Indeed, some of the most impressive results in this series were obtained in peripheral neurogenic pain situations, particularly lumbosacral root lesions after disc surgeries. These positive results can be explained by the relatively easy control of a thalamic imbalance resulting from a limited peripheral deafferentation.

Animal models of compressive peripheral neurogenic (or neuropathic) pain are currently being extensively studied (Munger et al. 1992; Guilbaud et al. 1993). Most if not all of these studies are performed in the acute postlesion period, and not at longer term. They show lowered threshold to stimuli and broadened receptive fields in thalamus and cortex (Guilbaud et al. 1992). These characteristics and their opiate dependence bring them close to nociceptive models (Guilbaud et al. 1984). Recordings in the medial thalamus are lacking in the neuropathic model, and no LTS bursts have been described until now in VP. It could well be that the acute neuropathic models have mixed nociceptive and neurogenic properties, and correspond only for parts of their physiopathology to the pure chronic neurogenic pain situation seen in patients coming to surgery after months to years of therapy-resistant pain. Some evidence indeed does speak in favor of a separation between acute and chronic neurogenic pain syndromes. In the rhizotomy model, Albe-Fessard and collaborators demonstrated an early but temporary physiopathology at the dorsal horn level, and the emergence, after two months, of stable rhythmic thalamic and cortical activities that correlated with an ongoing or re-emerging and then long-lasting pain behavior (Lombard et al. 1979; Albe-Fessard and Lombard 1983; Albe-Fessard et al. 1985; Albe-Fessard and Rampin 1991). Clinical studies show the possibility of spontaneous regression of neurogenic pain during the first year of symptomatology (Friedman and Nashold 1985; Jensen and Rasmussen 1989), a phenomenon that is also observed in the animal neuropathic model (Guilbaud et al. 1993). Thus, neurogenic pain mechanisms, triggered rather frequently after a somatosensory insult, may show a spontaneous tendency to normalize over time. Patients with a chronic syndrome may have a somatosensory system unable to restabilize itself, thus entertaining a long term physiopathology. In this sense, no present animal model corresponds to the human syndrome. In surgical practice, it is necessary to consider the possibility of spontaneous regression during the first year of pain, and that only relief obtained after longer periods of pain can firmly be considered as resulting from the surgical treatment.

Clinical and experimental evidence indicates a role of the medial thalamus in mechanisms of attention (Heilman et al. 1985). The fact that lesions in CL in neurogenic pain patients do not produce attentional (or other) deficits suggests that this structure is no longer functional. This is supported by the unresponsiveness of the recorded units to somatosensory stimuli known to activate CL normally, and implies a redistribution of its function to other areas through extensive plastic reorganizations (Kaas 1991).

A striking characteristic of chronic neurogenic pain in humans is the frequent, sometimes overwhelming influence of emotional factors, which often pose difficult differential diagnostic questions. The existence of numerous direct thalamo-cortical and cortico-thalamic, including cortico-reticular, connections of all mesocortical (cingular, orbitofrontal, insular, parahippocampal, temporopolar) areas offers an anatomical explanation for this emotional influence on thalamic neurogenic pain mechanisms (Akert and Hartmann-von Monakow 1980; Mufson and Mesulam 1984; Moran et al. 1987; Vogt et al. 1987; Witter et al. 1989; Morecraft et al. 1992; Sadikot et al. 1992; Bentivoglio et al. 1993). A strong activation of the cortical excitatory input to RT can indeed result in an increase of inhibition of thalamic neurons, with a consequent increase in symptomatology. The reverse scenario can also be proposed, with an influence of the thalamic physiopathology on the function of the emotional mesocortical areas. We think that these direct reciprocal influences explain the frequent clinical observations that patients with neurogenic pain (in contrast to many with psychogenic pain) typically recognize an emotional dependence of the pain, and that such patients describe clear-cut emotional problems, mainly anxio-depressive. In these conditions, it seems clear that strong negative emotional inputs like fear, frustration, despair, and sadness can enhance postoperatively a thalamic imbalance which in fact is only weak, and thus a symptomatology that could otherwise wear off to insignificance. This demonstrates the necessity of adequate and thorough postoperative psychotherapeutic support. Most if not all our patients with absence of relief after medial thalamotomy display emotional problems. Long-lasting and rigidly patterned emotional, mnestic, and attentional mechanisms can be thought to be at work at the mesocortical level, more or less difficult to overcome. Because these patients fulfilled all clinical criteria for neurogenic pain and presented with the typical thalamic overinhibition described above, they were maintained in this neurogenic pain patient group.

ACKNOWLEDGMENTS

We thank Prof. M. G. Yasargil and Prof. K. Akert for their support; Dr. B. Schurch for her collaboration; S. Hess, H. Rayvadera, S. Richter, P. Roth, and V. Streit for technical assistance; Dr. Huisman, Dr. Schefer, H. Bosshard, J. Dodd, M. Petrovic, and D. Sokman for clinical assistance; and V. Cucci for secretarial help. The study was supported by grants from the University Hospital Zürich and the University of Zürich, and by a grant (31-36330.92) from the Schweizerischer Nationalfonds zur Förderung der wissenschaftlichen Forschung.

REFERENCES

Akert, K. and Hartmann-von Monakow, K., Relationships of precentral premotor and prefrontal cortex to the mediodorsal and intralaminar nuclei of the monkey thalamus, Acta Neurobiol. Exp., 40 (1980) 7–25.

Albe-Fessard, D., Berkley, K.J., Kruger, L., Ralston, H.J. and Willis, W.D., Jr., Diencephalic mechanisms of pain sensation, Brain Res. Rev., 9 (1985) 217–296.

Albe-Fessard, D. and Lombard, M.C., Use of an animal model to evaluate the origin of and protection against deafferentation pain. In: J. J. Bonica, U. Lindblom and A. Iggo (Eds), Proceedings of the Third World Congress on Pain. Advances in Pain Research and Therapy, Vol. 5. Raven Press, New York, 1983, pp. 691–700.

Albe-Fessard, D. and Rampin, O., Neurophysiological studies in rats deafferented by dorsal root sections. In: B.S. Nashold Jr. and J. Ovelmen-Levitt (Eds.), Deafferentation Pain Syndromes: Pathophysiology and Treatment, Raven Press, New York, 1991, pp. 125–139.

Bentivoglio, M., Kultas-Ilinsky, K. and Ilinski, I., Limbic thalamus: structure, intrinsic organization, and connections. In: B.A. Vogt and M. Gabriel (Eds.), Neurobiology of Cingulate Cortex and Limbic Thalamus, Birkhäuser, Boston, 1993, pp. 71–122.

Cesaro, P., Amsallem, B., Pollin, B., Nguyen-Legros, J. and Moretti, J.L., Organisation des noyaux médians et intralaminaires du thalamus: hypothèses sur leur rôle dans la survenue de certaines douleurs centrales, Rev. Neurol., 142 (1986) 297–302.

Cesaro, P., Mann, M.W., Moretti, J.L., Defer, G., Roualdès, B., Nguyen, J.P. and Degos, J.D., Central pain and thalamic hyperactivity: a single photon emission computerized tomographic study, Pain, 47 (1991) 329–336.

Craig, A.D., Supraspinal pathways and mechanisms relevant to central pain. In: K.L. Casey (Ed.), Pain and Central Nervous System Disease: The Central Pain Syndromes, Raven Press, New York, 1991, pp. 157–170.

Curro Dossi, R., Nunez, A. and Steriade, M., Electrophysiology of a slow (0.5–4 Hz) intrinsic oscillation of cat thalamocortical neurones in vivo, J. Physiol., 447 (1992) 215–234.

Dejerine, J. and Roussy, G., Le syndrome thalamique, Rev. Neurol., 14 (1906) 521–532.

Fairman D., Unilateral thalamic tractotomy for the relief of bilateral pain in malignant tumors, Confin. Neurol., 29 (1967) 146–152.

Friedman, A.H. and Nashold, B.S., Jr., Postherpetic neuralgia. In: R.H. Wilkins and S.S. Rengachary (Eds.), Neurosurgery, McGraw-Hill, New York, 1985, pp. 2367–2371.

Guilbaud, G., Benoist, J.M., Levante, A., Gautron, M. and Willer, J.C., Primary somatosensory cortex in rats with pain-related behaviours due to a peripheral mononeuropathy after moderate ligation of one sciatic nerve: neuronal responsitivity to somatic stimulation, Exp. Brain Res., 92 (1992) 227–245.

Guilbaud, G., Gautron, M., Jazat, F., Ratinahirana, H., Hassig, R. and Hauw, J.J., Time course of degeneration and regeneration of myelinated nerve fibres following chronic loose ligatures of the rat sciatic nerve: can nerve lesions be linked to the abnormal pain-related behaviours? Pain, 53 (1993) 147–158.

Guilbaud, G., Peschanski, M. and Besson J.-M., Experimental data related to nociception and pain at the supraspinal level. In: P.D. Wall and R. Melzack (Eds.), Textbook of Pain, Churchill Livingstone, Edinburgh, 1984, pp. 141–149.

Gybels, J.M. and Sweet, W.H., Neurosurgical Treatment of Persistent Pain, Karger, Basel, 1989, 442 pp.

Head, H. and Holmes, G., Sensory disturbances from cerebral lesions, Brain, 34 (1911) 102–254.

Hécaen, H., Talairach, J., David, M. and Dell, M.B., Coagulations limitées du thalamus dans les algies du syndrome thalamique, Rev. Neurol., 81 (1949) 917–931.

Heilman, K., Watson, R.T. and Valenstein, E., Neglect and related disorders. In: K.M. Heilman and E. Valenstein (Eds.), Clinical Neuropsychology, Oxford University Press, New York, 1985, pp. 243–293.

Hitchcock, E.R. and Teixeira, M.J., A comparison of results from center-median and basal thalamotomies for pain, Surg. Neurol., 15 (1981) 341–351.

Hodge, C.J., Jr., and Apkarian, A.V., The spinothalamic tract, Crit. Rev. Neurobiol., 5 (1990) 369–397.

Ishijima, B., Yoshimasu, N., Fukushima, T., Hori, T., Sekino, H. and Sano, K., Nociceptive neurons in the human thalamus, Confin. Neurol., 37 (1975) 99–106.

Jeanmonod, D., Magnin, M. and Morel, A., Thalamus and neurogenic pain: physiological, anatomical and clinical data, Neuroreport, 4 (1993) 475–478.

Jeanmonod, D., Sindou M., Magnin, M. and Boudet M. Intra-operative unit recordings in the human dorsal horn with a simplified floating microelectrode, Electroencephalogr. Clin. Neurophysiol., 72 (1989) 450–454.

Jeanmonod, D. and Thomas, D.G.T., Application of CT-directed stereotaxy in the determination of functional neurosurgical targets in the diencephalon and cerebral hemisphere, Brit. J. Neurosurg., 3 (1989) 337–342.

Jensen, T.S. and Rasmussen, P., Phantom pain and related phenomena after amputation. In: P.D. Wall and R. Melzack (Eds.), Textbook of Pain, 2nd ed., Churchill Livinstone, Edinburgh, 1989, pp. 508–521.

Jones, E.G., The Thalamus, Plenum Press, New York, 1985, 935 pp.

Kaas, J.H., Plasticity of sensory and motor maps in adult mammals, Ann. Rev. Neurosci., 14 (1991) 137–167.

Laitinen, L.V., Mesencephalotomy and thalamotomy for chronic pain. In: L.D. Lunsford (Ed.), Modern Stereotactic Neurosurgery, Nijhoff, Boston, 1988, pp. 269–276.

Lenz, F.A., Evidence that thalamus is involved in the generation of sensory abnormalities observed in human central pain syndromes. In: B.S. Nashold Jr. and J. Ovelmen-Levitt (Eds.), Deafferentation Pain Syndromes: Pathophysiology and Treatment, Raven Press, New York, 1991a, pp. 141–150.

Lenz, F.A., The thalamus and central pain syndromes: human and animal studies. In: K.L. Casey (Ed.), Pain and Central Nervous System Disease: The Central Pain Syndromes, Raven Press, New York, 1991b, pp. 171–182.

Lenz, F.A., Kwan, H.C., Dostrovsky, J.O. and Tasker, R.R., Characteristics of the bursting pattern of action potentials that occurs in the thalamus of patients with central pain, Brain Res., 496 (1989) 357–360.

Lenz, F.A., Kwan, H.C., Martin, R., Tasker, R.R. and Dostrovsky, J.O., Characteristics of spontaneous neuronal activity at different locations in ventrocaudal thalamus of patients with central pain following spinal cord transsection, Pain, Suppl. 5, (1990) S493.

Levy, R.M., Lamb, S. and Adams, J.E., Deep brain stimulation for chronic pain: long-term results and complications. In: L.D. Lunsford (Ed.), Modern Stereotactic Neurosurgery, Nijhoff, Boston, 1988, pp. 395–406.

Lindblom, U., Pathophysiological pain taxonomy for clinical use. In: Abstracts: 7th World Congress on Pain, IASP Publications, Seattle, 1993, p. 189.
Loeser, J.D., Ward, A.A., Jr., and White, L.E., Jr., Chronic deafferentation of human spinal cord neurons, Neurosurg., 29 (1968) 48–50.
Lombard M.C., Nashold, B.S., Jr., and Pelissier, T., Thalamic recordings in rats with hyperalgesia. In: J.J. Bonica, J.C. Liebeskind and D. Albe-Fessard (Eds.). Proceedings of the Second World Congress on Pain. Advances in Pain Research and Therapy, Vol. 3. Raven Press, New York, 1979 pp. 767–772.
Mauguière, F. and Desmedt, J.E., Thalamic pain syndrome of Dejérine-Roussy: Differentiation of four subtypes assisted by somatosensory evoked potentials data, Arch. Neurol., 45. (1988) 1312–1320.
Modesti, L.M. and Waszak, M., Firing pattern of cells in human thalamus during dorsal column stimulation, Appl. Neurophysiol., 38 (1975) 251–258.
Moran, M.A., Mufson, E.J. and Mesulam, M.M., Neural inputs into the temporopolar cortex of the rhesus monkey, J. Comp. Neurol., 256 (1987) 88–103.
Morecraft, R.J., Geula, C. and Mesulam, M.-M., Cytoarchitecture and neural afferents of orbitofrontal cortex in the brain of the monkey, J. Comp. Neurol., 323 (1992) 341–358.
Mufson, E.J. and Mesulam, M.M., Thalamic connections of the insula in the rhesus monkey and comments on the paralimbic connectivity of the medial pulvinar nucleus, J. Comp. Neurol., 227 (1984) 109–122.
Munger, B.L., Bennett, G.J. and Kajander, K.C., An experimental painful peripheral neuropathy due to nerve constriction, Exp. Neurol., 118 (1992) 204–214.
North, R.B., Kidd, D.H., Zahurak, M., James, C.S. and Long, D.M., Spinal cord stimulation for chronic, intractable pain: experience over two decades, Neurosurg., 32 (1993) 384–395.
Pagni, C.A., Central pain due to spinal cord and brain stem damage. In: P.D. Wall and R. Melzack (Eds.), Textbook of Pain, 2nd ed., Churchill Livingstone, Edinburgh, 1989, pp. 634–655.
Richardson, D.E., Thalamotomy for intractable pain, Confin. Neurol., 29 (1967) 139–145.
Rinaldi, P.C., Young, R.F., Albe-Fessard, D. and Chodakiewitz, J., Spontaneous neuronal hyperactivity in the medial and intralaminar thalamic nuclei of patients with deafferentation pain, J. Neurosurg., 74 (1991) 415–421.
Roberts, W.A., Eaton, S.A. and Salt, T.E., Widely distributed GABA-mediated afferent inhibition processes within the ventrobasal thalamus of rat and their possible relevance to pathological pain states and somatotopic plasticity, Exp. Brain Res., 89 (1992) 363–372.
Sadikot, A.F., Parent, A. and François, C., Efferent connections of the centromedian and parafascicular thalamic nuclei in the squirrel monkey: a PHA-L study of subcortical projections, J. Comp. Neurol., 315 (1992) 137–159.
Sano K., Intralaminar thalamotomy (thalamolaminotomy) and postero-medial hypothalamotomy in the treatment of intractable pain, Prog. Neurol. Surg., 8 (1977) 50–103.
Sindou, M. and Daher, A., Spinal cord ablation procedures for pain. In: R. Dubner, G.F. Gebhart and M.R. Bond (Eds.), Proceedings. of the Vth World Congress on Pain. Pain Research and Clinical Management, Vol. 3. Elsevier, Amsterdam, 1988, pp. 477–495.
Sindou, M., Jeanmonod, D. and Mertens, P., Ablative neurosurgical procedures for the treatment of chronic pain, Neurophysiol. Clin., 20 (1990) 399–423.
Steriade, M. and Deschenes, M., The thalamus as a neuronal oscillator, Brain Res. Rev., 8 (1984) 1–63.
Steriade, M., Jones, E.G. and Llinas, R.R., Thalamic Oscillations and Signaling, Wiley, New York, 1990, 431 pp.
Tasker, R.R., Stereotactic surgery. In: P.D. Wall and R. Melzack (Eds.), Textbook of Pain, Churchill Livingstone, 2nd ed., Edinburgh, 1989, pp. 840–855.
Tasker, R.R., DeCarvalho, G.T.C. and Dolan, E.J., Intractable pain of spinal cord origin: clinical features and implications for surgery, J. Neurosurg., 77 (1992) 373–378.
Tasker, R.R., DeCarvalho, G. and Dostrovsky, J.O., The history of central pain syndromes, with observations concerning pathophysiology and treatment. In: K.L. Casey (Ed.), Pain and

Central Nervous System Disease: The Central Pain Syndromes, Raven Press, New York, 1991, pp. 31–58.

Tasker, R.R. and Dostrovsky, J.O., Deafferentation and central pain. In: P.D. Wall and R. Melzack (Eds.), Textbook of Pain, 2nd ed., Churchill Livingstone, Edinburgh, 1989, pp. 154–174.

Tsubokawa, T., Katayama, Y., Yamamoto, T., Hirayama, T. and Koyama, S., Chronic motor cortex stimulation in patients with thalamic pain, J. Neurosurg., 78 (1993) 393–401.

Vogt, B.A., Pandya, D.N. and Rosene, D.L., Cingulate cortex of the rhesus monkey: cytoarchitecture and thalamic afferents, J. Comp. Neurol., 262 (1987) 256–270.

Willis, W., Hyperalgesia and Allodynia, Raven Press, New York, 1992, 400 pp.

Willis, W.D., The Pain System, Karger, Basel, 1985, 346 pp.

Witter, M.P., Groenewegen, H.J., Lopes da Silva, F.H. and Lohman, A.H.M., Functional organization of the extrinsic and intrinsic circuitry of the parahippocampal region, Prog. Neurobiol., 33 (1989) 161–253.

Young, R.F., Rand, R.W., Jacques, D.S. and Copcutt, B., Stereotactic medial thalamotomy with the Leksell Gamma Knife for treatment of chronic pain. In: Abstracts: 7th World Congress on Pain, IASP Publications, Seattle, 1993, p. 570.

Correspondence to: Daniel Jeanmonod, Laboratory of Functional Neurosurgery, Neurosurgical Clinic, University Hospital, Rämistrasse 100, 8091 Zürich, Switzerland. Tel: 41-1-255-2684; Fax: 41-1-255-4505.

Proceedings of the 7th World Congress on Pain,
Progress in Pain Research and Management, Vol. 2,
edited by G.F. Gebhart, D.L. Hammond, and T.S.
Jensen, IASP Press, Seattle, © 1994.

52

The Clinical Characteristics and Sensory Abnormalities of Patients with Central Pain Caused by Multiple Sclerosis

Anders Österberg,[a] Jörgen Boivie,[a] Helen Holmgren,[b] Karl-Åke Thuomas,[c] and Ingegerd Johansson[c]

Departments of [a]Neurology, [b]Clinical Neurophysiology, and [c]Radiology, University Hospital, Linköping, Sweden

INTRODUCTION

Pain has not been considered important in multiple sclerosis (MS). This attitude is evident in both textbooks and neurology journals. The notion is incorrect, as shown in studies from Clifford et al. (1984) and Moulin et al. (1988), and in our study. These studies show that pain is in fact a major problem for a large proportion of MS patients. This incorrect notion has led to a lack of interest in pain in MS over the years. However, two pain conditions in MS are well known among neurologists, namely trigeminal neuralgia and painful tonic seizures, but these account for only a minor proportion of all pain in MS.

The most recent prevalence study found that 48% of all MS patients had a chronic pain syndrome (Moulin et al. 1988). Several different pain syndromes were recognized, but analysis of the pain did not aim at a thorough differentiation among nociceptive, peripheral neuropathic, and central pain. Each of these three may occur, and it is quite possible, for instance, that those patients who have paresis and spasticity may have nociceptive pain due to these dysfunctions.

We attempted to identify the various pain components, with special emphasis on central pain, which is defined as pain caused by a lesion or dysfunction in the central nervous system (CNS). In most patients with MS it is not possible to show the localization of the individual lesion causing a particular symptom, not even with the best available techniques, including advanced magnetic resonance imaging (MRI), but diagnosis of the disease often can be made with certainty. In the search for the mechanisms of central pain it would be useful to know the location of the lesion, but another, and perhaps more interesting approach, is to identify the functional abnormalities that accompany the condition. Previous studies of central pain indicate that the only neurological dysfunctions that accompany central pain are abnormalities in somatic sensibility (Boivie 1994; Boivie et al. 1989). The leading hypothesis regarding the kind of lesions that cause central pain states that it only occurs in patients who have lesions affecting the spino-thalamo-cortical pathways serving pain and temperature sensibility (Boivie 1994). Because one of the aims of our study was to elucidate the mechanisms of central pain in MS, one of the major parts of the project has been to analyze the sensory abnormalities in detail to see if the hypothesis holds true for central pain in MS.

This chapter reports the results from the analysis of the first 255 patients. It concerns the incidence of pain, the characteristics of the central pain, and the sensory abnormalities in the patients with central pain.

PATIENTS AND METHODS

The basis for this study is a group of 439 patients with the diagnosis of MS from the patient register at our neurology department. They were all sent a questionnaire asking if they had experienced pain or sensory symptoms currently or previously during the course of the disease. The patients were asked to describe the character and location of the pain, to indicate the location on a pain diagram, and to report all forms of pain. All patients admitting to pain were interviewed and examined at the outpatient clinic.

Eighty-three percent of the patients responded (366 patients); the results are based on the evaluation of 255. Table I gives demographic data on the patients. Four patients could not be analyzed because of dementia, psychiatric illness, and other reasons preventing an adequate pain history.

The diagnosis of central pain is based partly on exclusion, partly on specific criteria. The most important determinants of this diagnosis are the following:

- Negative outcome of a thorough examination of the painful region to find signs of nociceptive pain. Normal blood and other laboratory tests to exclude general or regional non-neurological disease. Pure back pain was not considered to be central pain even if the examination failed to demonstrate a cause in musculoskeletal structures.

- Negative outcome of a thorough neurological examination to find possible signs of peripheral neuropathy or rhizopathy, indicating the possibility of peripheral neurogenic pain.
- Normal neurography, or abnormal results from neurography, but the pain does not conform with known forms of peripheral neurogenic pain.
- Vascular and tension headache are not included in central pain.
- No signs of psychiatric disease.
- Pain with a regional distribution compatible with a CNS lesion.
- Pain arising from muscle spasm or other forms of spasticity are included in central pain.
- Quantitative analysis of sensory abnormalities (Fruhstorfer et al. 1976).

The examination of sensibility was done using conventional clinical and quantitative methods. The clinical examination included the following tests: touch by strokes of cotton wool, cold by applying the round surface of a tuning fork at room temperature (area 3.9 cm^2), and pinprick using a pin.

In the quantitative examination of sensibility, we analyzed vibration, touch, warmth, cold, cold pain, and heat pain. Thresholds to vibration were measured with a Vibrameter (Somedic AB, Sweden; Goldberg et al. 1979). The threshold amplitude in µm was measured with a constant probe pressure at a vibration frequency of 100 Hz. We recorded the mean of three consecutive readings on each side of the body.

We measured the threshold for touch by applying graded punctate stimuli to the skin using a set of 15 nylon filaments of varying bending pressures (von Frey's hairs). The series of filaments represents stimuli from 10 mg to 300 g. The weakest stimulus that the patient identified more than 50% of the time was recorded as the perception threshold.

We used a Thermotest apparatus to quantitatively assess sensibility for non-noxious and noxious (cold pain, heat pain) temperatures. With this tech-

Table I
Age, duration of MS, and pain duration of 40 patients with central pain (29 women/11 men)

	Age (years)	Disease Duration (years)	Pain Duration (years)
Range	34–79	4–42	1–40
Mean	52	20	14

nique the stimuli are given via a 25 × 50-mm plate that is fixed to the skin. The plate consists of 36 peltier elements that can be heated or cooled in a controlled manner. The difference limen was used as the threshold for innoxious temperature (Fruhstorfer et al. 1976).

The following regions were examined: vibrametry—second metacarpal, first metatarsal; von Frey's for touch—cheek, pulp of index finger, dorsum of the foot; thermotest—cheek, thenar eminence, dorsum of the foot; pinprick, cotton wool, cold surface of a tuning fork—cheek, dorsum of the hand, dorsum of the foot.

RESULTS

Table I gives information about how long the patients had had MS and how long they had suffered pain. About one-third of the patients (14) reported pain throughout the course of the disease, and one patient had pain before the onset of other MS symptoms. We list here the pain categories of 164 MS patients (of 255 evaluated). Numbers of patients are given, with percentage in parentheses.

Nociceptive Pain	107 (42)	Neurogenic Pain	57 (22)
Tension headache	23 (9)	Central MS pain	40 (16)
Migraine	9 (3)	Trigeminal neuralgia	13 (5)
Other type of headache	23 (9)	Postherpetic neuralgia	1
Neck and back pain	34 (13)	Central poststroke pain	1
Joint pain	12 (5)	Nerve root pain	2
Muscle pain	8 (3)	Peripheral nerve entrapment	1

Nociceptive pain including headache was reported by 42%, whereas the prevalence of all pain was 64%. Four patients had neurogenic pain that was judged not related to their MS: one patient had right-sided central poststroke hemipain; two had nerve root pain; and one had pain that was part of a carpal tunnel syndrome. Twenty-two per cent had central pain. Trigeminal neuralgia is included because in MS this pain condition is caused by a lesion in the CNS; it occurred in 5% of the patients during the course of the disease. The rest (16%) had more traditional forms of central pain. Seven of these patients were unable to come to the outpatient clinic because of long traveling distances (three patients), lack of interest (three), and recent stroke episode (one).

The location and the quality of the pain of 40 MS patients with central pain are listed below. The pain was largely confined to the lower extremities. Most patients experienced two or three pain locations and two to four pain qualities.

Pain Location	%
Lower extremities	88
Upper extremities	18
Trunk	5

Pain Quality	%
Burning	58
Aching	55
Pricking	32
Stabbing	25
Squeezing	25
Cutting	19
Other	45

One of the questions asked was if central pain was accompanied by other neurological symptoms. The prevalences of the most common MS symptoms in the patients with central pain (N = 33) are: ataxia, 37%; paresis, 51%; sensory abnormalities, 98%; and bladder dysfunction, 55%. It is evident that central pain is only associated with sensory symptoms.

The most important results from the examination of somatic sensibility are given in Tables II (clinical examination) and III (quantitative examination). When we analyzed the results from each patient we found that all patients except two had abnormal sensibility to temperature and/or pain. One of these also had normal sensibility to vibration and touch.

Many patients were abnormal for all four submodalities that were examined (touch, vibration, innoxious temperature, and pain), but the submodalities were not affected to the same degree. The abnormalities were more pronounced regarding the sensibility to temperature and pain than to touch and vibration. In the quantitative sensory tests (QST) the thresholds to temperature were severely abnormal in 76%, whereas the corresponding figures for touch and vibration were 17% and 59%, respectively.

Central pain is often accompanied by allodynia, hyperalgesia, paresthesias, and dysesthesias. In this study none had paresthesias or allodynia, only one had hyperalgesia for cold and pinprick, whereas three to six patients had dysesthesias for touch, cold, and pinprick.

DISCUSSION

Our results support the notion that pain is common in patients with MS. Our figure for the prevalence of pain (i.e., 64%) is in the same order of magnitude as the prevalence found by Moulin et al. (1988) About one-third is central pain, i.e., caused by a demyelinating lesion in the brain or spinal cord. Apart from the cases with trigeminal neuralgia, it is not possible to draw any conclusion about the location of the lesions that produce the pain. It is reasonable to suppose that the lesions that cause the trigeminal neuralgia are located in the lower brainstem, either in the nerve as it passes to the trigeminal nuclei

Table II
Results from clinical examinations of somatic sensibility at the site of pain in 33 MS patients with central pain

	Touch		Cold		Pinprick	
Clinical Finding	No.	(%)	No.	(%)	No.	(%)
0 (normal)	10	(30)	10	(30)	14	(43)
1 (hypoesthesia)	14	(43)	13	(39)	11	(33)
2 (total loss of sensibility)	5	(15)	6	(18)	4	(12)
3 (hyperesthesia)	—	—	—	—	1	(3)
4 (dysesthesia)	3	(9)	3	(9)	2	(6)
1/4 (hypoesthesia & dysesthesia)	1	(3)	2	(6)	1	(3)

or in the nuclei. Demyelinating lesions have been demonstrated in postmortem preparations in the intrabulbar portion of the nerve in four patients with trigeminal neuralgia and MS (Jensen et al. 1982).

In patients with other forms of central pain, we can only speculate about the location of the lesions responsible for the development of central pain because disseminated lesions are commonly found in both the brain and the spinal cord in MRI examinations. According to traditional thinking, CNS symptoms that affect both legs or both sides below a spinal level are caused by lesions in the spinal cord, and it is reasonable to suspect that many of the lesions that lead to bilateral leg pain, which is common, are spinal.

Central pain in MS can have many different characteristics; thus, it is impossible to describe a pathognomonic clinical picture for this pain condition, but some features are more common than others. The most common syndrome is one of constant burning and aching pain in the legs. Stabbing, squeezing, cutting, and smarting pains are also rather frequent. In MS-associated trigeminal neuralgia the pain characteristics are rather homogeneous and similar to those found in idiopathic tic douloureux.

Our results show that the only symptoms and signs that regularly accompany central pain in MS are sensory abnormalities, whereas only about half of the patients had paresis at the time of clinical examination and less than two-thirds had ataxia. These results are similar to those found in patients with central pain following stroke (Leijon et al. 1989).

In the detailed analysis of the sensory abnormalities we found that the sensibility to temperature and pain is more severely affected than the sensibility to vibration and touch. Thus, all patients except two had abnormal temperature and pain sensibility, and the degree of abnormality also was more

Table III
Results from quantitative examination of sensibility at the site of pain in 29 MS patients with central pain temperature includes noxious and non-noxious temperature

Sensibility Rating	Touch No.	Touch (%)	Vibration No.	Vibration (%)	Temperature No.	Temperature (%)
0 (normal)	11	(38)	6	(21)	4	(14)
1 (mild)	9	(31)	3	(10)	2	(7)
2 (moderate)	4	(14)	3	(10)	1	(3)
3 (severe)	3	(10)	10	(35)	7	(24)
4 (total loss of sensibility)	2	(7)	7	(24)	15	(52)

pronounced in these submodalities. Surprisingly, central pain in MS is not accompanied to any great extent by allodynia, hyperalgesia, paresthesias, or dysesthesias.

In textbooks, sensory abnormalities in MS usually have been ascribed to lesions in the spinal dorsal columns. Our results indicate that lesions affecting the spinothalamic pathways are also common in MS, because they show that many patients with MS have abnormal temperature and pain sensibility. This conclusion also has relevance in discussions regarding the mechanisms of central pain in MS, because one of the aims of our study was to test the hypothesis that it only occurs in patients with lesions affecting the spinothalamic pathways. This hypothesis has been tested in patients with central poststroke pain (Boivie et al. 1989). Results from studies of this condition and other conditions (Boivie 1994) support this notion.

Furthermore, almost all our patients had signs of spinothalamic pathway dysfunctions (i.e., abnormalities in temperature and pain sensibility), whereas it was more common to find that patients with central pain had normal tactile and vibration sensibility, indicating normal dorsal column medial lemniscal pathways. Thus, we concluded that our results provide further support for the hypothesis that central pain only occurs in patients with lesions affecting the spinothalamic pathways, although admittedly they do not show conclusively that the hypothesis is correct.

In the first half of this century it was commonly thought that the crucial lesion for the occurrence of central pain was a lesion affecting the dorsal column medial lemniscal pathways (Foerster 1927). It now appears that such a lesion is probably not necessary for the development of central pain. It may not even affect the character of the pain, but it does, of course, affect the character of the sensory abnormality.

SUMMARY

We present the results from investigations of 255 patients with multiple sclerosis (MS) with regard to the presence of pain and its characteristics. Sixty-four percent experienced pain, and 22% (40 patients) had central pain. Of the latter patients, 5% had trigeminal neuralgia and 16% had central pain of other kinds. The most common location was in the lower extremities, the site for about 85% of the patients with central pain. Many different pain qualities were reported, with burning, aching, and pricking the most common.

All patients with central pain, except one, had sensory abnormalities, which were dominated by abnormal temperature and pain sensibility, whereas tactile and vibration sensibility were less frequently and less severely affected. From these findings we concluded that the results support the hypothesis that central pain only occurs in patients with lesions affecting the spinothalamic pathways.

REFERENCES

Boivie, J., Central pain. In: P.D. Wall and R. Melzack (Eds.), Textbook of Pain, 3rd ed., Churchill Livingstone, Edinburgh, 1994.

Boivie, J., Leijon, G. and Johansson, I., Central post-stroke pain: a study of mechanisms through analyses of the sensory abnormalities, Pain, 37 (1989) 173–185.

Clifford, D.B. and Trotter, J.L., Pain in multiple sclerosis, Arch. Neurol., 41 (1984) 1270–1272.

Foerster, O., Die Leitungsbahnen des Schmerzgefühls und die chirurgische Behandlung der schmerzzustande, Urban und Schwarzenberg, Berlin, 1927.

Fruhstorfer, H., Lindblom, U. and Schmidt, W.G., Method for quantitative estimation of thermal thresholds in patients, J. Neurol. Neurosurg. Psychiatry, 39 (1976) 1071–1075.

Goldberg, J.M. and Lindblom, U., Standardized method of determining vibratory perception thresholds for diagnosis and screening in neurological investigation, J. Neurol. Neurosurg. Psychiatry, 42 (1979) 793–803.

Jensen, T.S., Rasmussen, P. and Reske-Nielsen, E., Association of trigeminal neuralgia with multiple sclerosis: clinical and pathological features, Acta Neurol. Scand., 65 (1982) 182–189.

Leijon, G. and Boivie, J., Central post-stroke pain: a controlled trial of amitriptyline and carbamazepine, Pain, 36 (1989) 27–36.

Moulin, D.E., Foley, K.M. and Ebers, G.C., Pain syndromes in multiple sclerosis, Neurology, 38 (1988) 1830–1834.

Correspondence to: Dr. Anders Österberg, Department of Neurology, University Hospital, S-581 85 Linköping, Sweden. Tel: 46-13-22-20-00; Fax: 46-13-22-44-38.

Part XI

Nociceptive Processing

Proceedings of the 7th World Congress on Pain,
Progress in Pain Research and Management, Vol. 2,
edited by G.F. Gebhart, D.L. Hammond, and T.S.
Jensen, IASP Press, Seattle, © 1994.

53

Parabrachial Projections to the Forebrain Rostral to the Amygdala Studied with the PHA-L Method in the Rat

Jean-François Bernard, Marie Aldén,
and Jean-Marie Besson

*Unité de Recherches de Physiopharmacologie du Système Nerveux and EPHE,
INSERM U 161, Paris, France*

INTRODUCTION

The pontine parabrachial (pPB) area is a group of cells that surrounds the brachium conjunctivum (bc) in the dorsolateral pons up to the mesencephalon, where it continues into the mesencephalic parabrachial (mPB) area. The pPB area is implicated in gustatory functions and in a large number of autonomic processes (see references in Bernard et al. 1993). More recently it has also been implicated in nociceptive processes. Several authors (see references in Light et al. 1992) have found that a portion of this area receives a marked input from neurons located in lamina I of the spinal and medullary dorsal horns, which are driven by noxious stimuli. In addition, a large proportion of neurons backfired from the central nucleus of the amygdala (Ce) and located in the external pPB (pPBe) area (i.e., external lateral [pPBel] and external medial [pPBem] subnuclei of the pPB area) respond specifically to noxious stimuli, as do numerous neurons in the Ce (Bernard and Besson 1990; Bernard et al. 1992). These nociceptive responses are depressed by intravenous (iv.) morphine in a dose-dependent and naloxone reversible fashion in both the pPBe and the Ce (Huang et al. 1993a,b).

We found that the dense projection of the pPB area onto the Ce includes three sets of connections (Bernard et al. 1993). In the present investigation, a follow-up of the former, we used a very sensitive and selective anterograde axonal marker, *Phaseolus vulgaris* leucoagglutinin (PHA-L) (Gerfen and Sawchenko 1984), injected into very restricted sites in the pPB area, to determine projections from subregions of the pPB to the bed nucleus of the stria terminalis (BST) and neighboring regions.

METHODS

Iontophoretic applications of a 10% solution of PHA-L were made in the pPB area in 85 rats. Following a postoperative survival time of two weeks, the animals were re-anesthetized and perfused, the brain was removed, and 50-μm-thick coronal sections were cut on a freezing microtome. The sections were incubated overnight in the primary anti serum (1/2000) goat anti-PHA-L (Vector), then one hour in the secondary anti serum (1/200 goat anti-IgG Vector), and then one hour in the avidin-biotin-HRP complex solution (kit Vector). One group of sections was processed only with 3,3'-diaminobenzidine (DAB, Sigma). The two other groups were processed with DAB enhanced with nickel. One of the latter series was counterstained with neutral red. The delineation and nomenclature of this region was adopted from the relevant literature (Fulwiler and Saper 1984; Paxinos and Watson 1986; Moga et al. 1989; see also Fig. 14 in Bernard et al. 1993).

RESULTS

Results are based on 78 experiments, in which the PHA-L injection sites were located in (n = 53), or around (control experiments, n = 25), the pPB area. Taken together, these injections covered almost all of the pPB subnuclei. It must be remembered that in the earlier study (Bernard et al. 1993), a topographical organization of the pPB projections to the Ce was discovered. Interestingly, a close correlation between the pPB-Ce and the pPB-BST connections was observed in the present study.

- The first pPB area (corresponding to injection sites in Fig. 1A), which projected very densely onto the medial subdivision of the Ce (CeM; Bernard et al. 1993), also projected strongly onto the lateral division of the BST (BSTL) and the Ce-BSTL continuum (see below), exhibiting a rather diffuse labeling (Fig. 2B).
- The second pPB area (corresponding to injection sites in Fig. 2A), which projected very densely to the lateral subdivision of the Ce (CeL; Bernard et al. 1993), had concentrated projections to the dorsal lateral subnucleus

of the BST (BSTdl; Fig. 2B). Furthermore, a subgroup of these injections projected onto the preoptic hypothalamus (Fig. 2B).

- The third pPB area (corresponding to injection sites in Fig. 3A), which projected very densely onto the lateral capsular subdivision of the Ce (CeLC; Bernard et al. 1993), resulted in no or weak labeling in the BST.

PROJECTIONS OF THE FIRST pPB AREA

This pPB area corresponds to the injection sites of experiments (Fig. 1A, gray and black), which covered the whole medial subnucleus (pPBm), the waist area (pPBwa), and part of the ventral lateral subnucleus (pPBvl) of the pPB area and the more medial portion of the pPBem. In this experimental series, the pattern of labeling was quite similar in the ipsilateral CeM (Fig. 1C) as to the region investigated. Experiment 13, illustrated in Fig. 1, was chosen to represent the group. The injection in this experiment (Fig. 1A, black) was almost exclusively located in the pPBm. In the forebrain region investigated, the two major areas of termination were the ipsilateral BST and Ce-BSTL continuum.

In the ipsilateral BST, a medium to high density of labeled terminals was seen throughout the rostro-caudal extent of the BSTL division (except for the juxtacapsular subnucleus, [BSTjxc])—i.e., in the BSTdl, the posterior lateral (BSTpl), the anterior lateral (BSTal), and the ventral lateral (BSTvl) subnuclei of the BST (Fig. 1B). The labeling covered the whole area in a diffuse manner, although lower density of labeling was seen in the BSTdl. In the medial division of the BST (BSTM), labeling was of lower density in the ventral medial subnuclei (BSTvm; Fig. 1B) and was almost absent in the other subnuclei.

The Ce-BSTL continuum is an indefinite region that extends roughly from the rostral pole of the Ce up to the BSTL division. It includes the dorsal portion of the substantia innominata (SI) and the ventral portion of the globus pallidus (GPv), the fundus striatum (FStr) and the substriatal area (SStr). In this region we discovered both numerous fibers of passage (which appeared to be directed towards the BST) and a medium to high density of terminals. The density of labeled terminals, at maximum in the caudal parts, diminished progressively towards the more rostral parts (Fig. 1B1).

We also found a medium density of labeled terminals on the ipsilateral side, in the caudal portion of the agranular insular cortex (AI) and the magnocellular preoptic nucleus (Fig. 1B). Throughout the area studied, the labeling was clearly lower on the contralateral side.

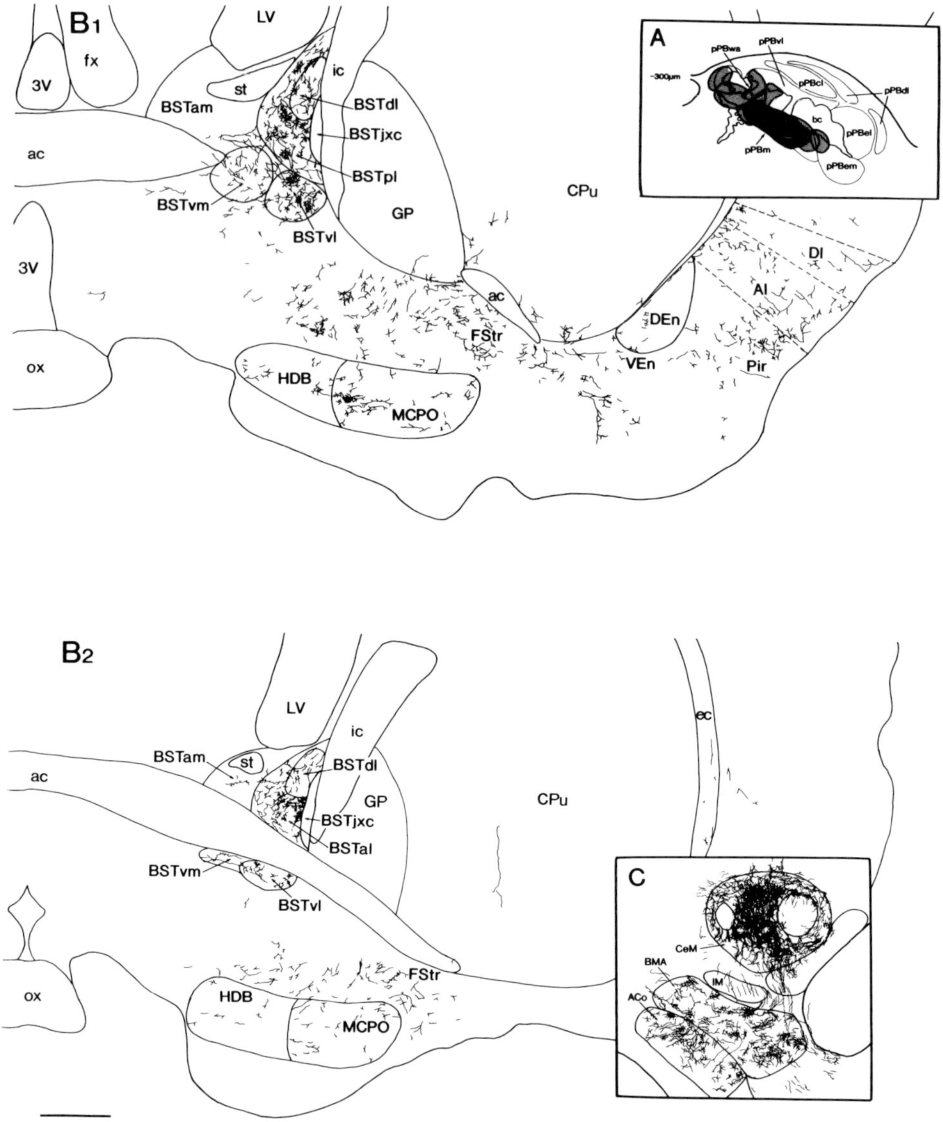

Fig. 1. *Experiment 13:* camera lucida drawings of coronal sections (from caudal to rostral), illustrating the extent of labeled terminals in tne BSTL division (**B1 and B2**) and in the CeM (**C**), following an injection (black) in the pPBm (**A**). The other injection sites of this first group correspond to areas filled with gray (**A**). Distance (caudal direction) of the sections throughout the pPB with the coronal plan where the inferior colliculus merges with the pons is indicated in –µm. The distance between two successive coronal sections is 300 µm. Scale is 500 µm. For abbreviations, see Appendix.

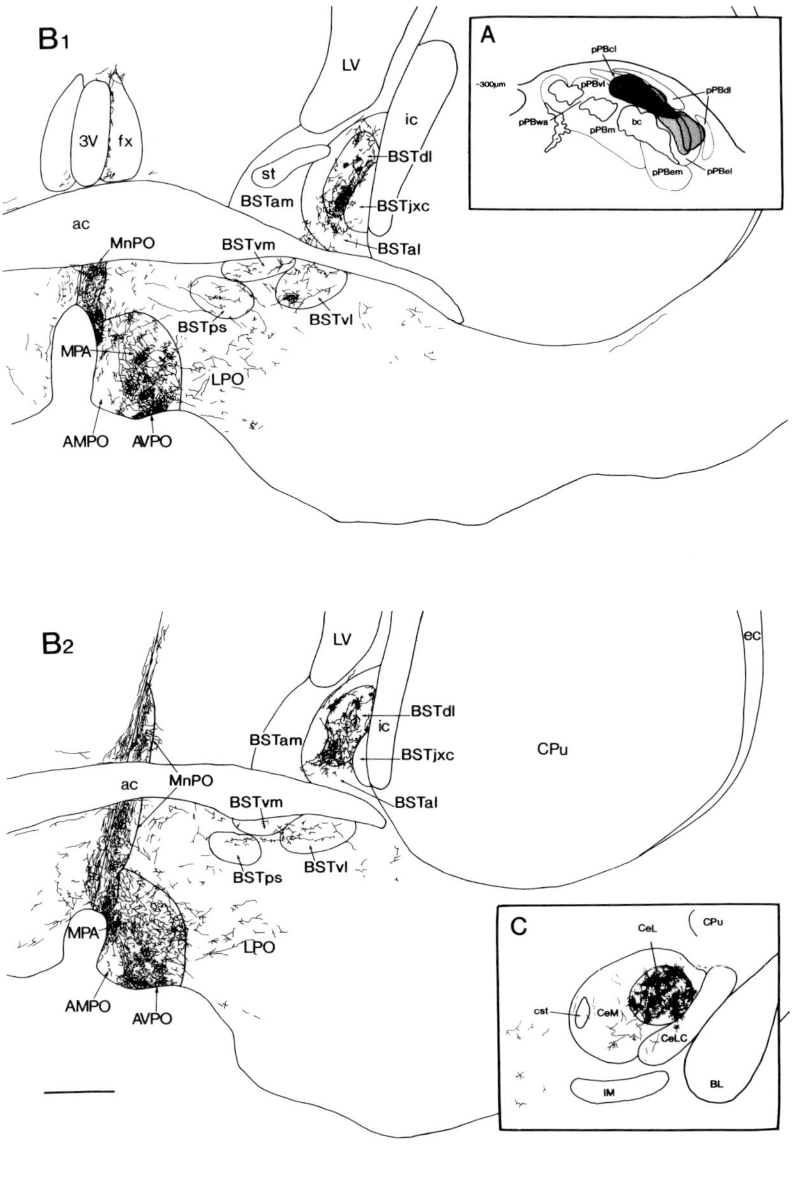

Fig. 2. *Experiment 27:* distribution of terminal fibers in the BSTdl, the preoptic hypothalamus nuclei (**B1** and **B2**), and in the CeL (**C**), following an injection (black) in the pPBcl (**A**). The other injection sites of this second group correspond to areas filled with gray (**A**). Note that the two lateral sites (in gray) exhibited similar (even if stronger) projection in the BST and the CeL, but on the contrary of the medial sites (represented by case 27), they do not project onto the preoptic hypothalamus. For further information see Results and Fig. 1; for abbreviations see Appendix.

PROJECTIONS OF THE SECOND pPB AREA

This pPB area corresponds to the injection sites (Fig. 2A, gray and black) that covered the central lateral subnucleus (pPBcl; medial subgroup) and the outer portion of the pPBel (lateral subgroup). All these experiments produced a similar pattern of labeling in the ipsilateral CeM (Fig. 2C) and in the ipsilateral BSTL division.

The two injection sites of the medial subgroup (in the pPBcl; Fig. 2A, gray and black) represented by experiments 27 (Fig. 2A, black) projected into the ipsilateral BSTL division and the hypothalamus. (1) In the ipsilateral BSTL division, we found that a very high density of labeled terminals were concentrated in the BSTdl (Fig. 2B). Contrasting with this dense labeling, a low to medium density of terminals covered the adjacent BSTpl, the BSTal, and the BSTvl subnuclei (Fig. 2B). Furthermore, a low to medium density of terminals was found in the caudal portion of the BSTM division; only a few or no labeled fibers were present in the rostral portion of the BSTM division (i.e., the anterior medial subnucleus of BST [BSTam] and the BSTvm, Fig. 2B). (2) In the preoptic hypothalamus, a high density of labeled terminals was observed both in the whole median preoptic nucleus (MnPO) and in the ipsilateral medial preoptic area (MPA), mainly in the anteroventral preoptic nucleus (AVPO) and the periventricular nucleus (Pe; Fig. 2B) but not in the anterior medial preoptic nucleus (AMPO). On the contralateral side the labeling, present exclusively in the BSTdl, was weak.

The two injection sites in the lateral subgroup (in the pPBel; Fig. 2A, gray) projected more densely onto the ipsilateral BSTdl than did those in the medial subgroup but, in contrast, they did not, or only weakly, project onto the preoptic hypothalamus.

PROJECTIONS OF THE THIRD pPB AREA

This pPB area corresponds to the injection sites that covered the dorsal lateral subnucleus of the pPB area (pPBdl), the inner portion of the pPBel and the pPBem (Fig. 3A, gray and black). All these injections, represented by injection 31 (Fig. 3A, black), produced a dense labeling in the ipsilateral CeLC (Fig. 3C) and projected weakly or not at all onto the BST and the preoptic hypothalamus (Fig. 3B). Furthermore, the injection sites in the pPBem and the caudal pPBel, which projected onto the rostral portion of the CeLC, gave rise to significant, although not dense, labeling in the ipsilateral nucleus of the horizontal limb of the diagonal band (HDB).

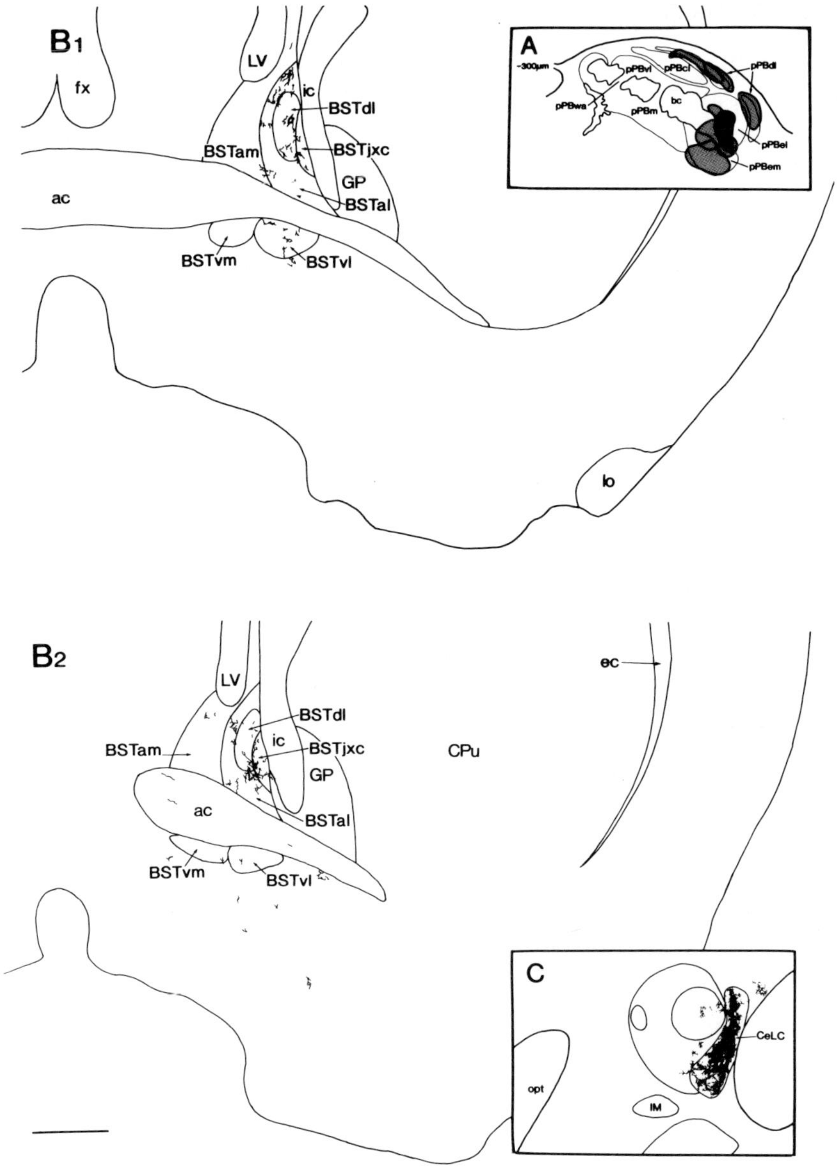

Fig. 3. *Experiment 31:* very weak labeling in the BST (**B1** and **B2**) and strong labeling in the CeLC (**C**) as the result of an injection (black) in the inner portion of the pPBel (**A**). The other injection sites of this third group correspond to areas filled with gray (**A**). For further information see Fig. 1; for abbreviations see Appendix.

CONTROL EXPERIMENTS

When sites were in mPB area without spread into the pPB area, we observed no projection to the BSTL division. It must be pointed out that in most of the mesencephalic injections, a medium to very high density of labeled terminals was found in the medial amygdaloid nucleus, in the BSTM division, and in other regions of the hypothalamus (primarily the ventromedial and retrochiasmatic nuclei).

DISCUSSION

COMPARISON WITH DATA IN THE LITERATURE

Concerning the BST, the present data are in general agreement with the studies carried out by Saper and Loewy (1980), Weller and Smith (1982), and Fulwiler and Saper (1984), but a precise comparison is difficult because earlier observations were built on experimental cases with relatively large injections. Moga et al. (1990) carried out a detailed retrograde study, and we found, as they did, that the pPBm, pPBwa, pPBvl, and especially the pPBel projected to the BSTL. On the other hand, unlike the Moga study, we did not see any significant projections from the mPB to the BSTL. Finally, we observed an additional and important projection from the pPBcl onto the BSTdl. With regard to the hypothalamus, we, like Saper and Levisohn (1983), Lind and Swanson (1984), Simerly and Swanson (1986), and Moga et al. (1990), found a heavy projection from the pPBcl to the MnPO. We also demonstrated that the pPBcl not only projects onto the MnPO but also densely projects onto neighboring hypothalamic nuclei (i.e., the Pe and the AVPO).

CORRELATION TO AMYGDALOID PATHWAYS

Considering the present results, the organization of the pPB projection onto the Ce (Bernard et al. 1993) and the Ce projection onto the BST (Sun et al. 1991) suggest the existence of: (1) a pPB(m)-CeM-BSTL indirect pathway that accompanies the direct pPB(m)-BSTL pathway and (2) a pPB(l)-CeL-BSTdl indirect pathway that accompanies the direct pPB(l)-BSTdl pathway. The pPB-CeLC pathway described earlier had no equivalent in the present study.

FUNCTIONAL IMPLICATIONS

1. On the basis of the role of the pPB(m) region in the learning of taste aversion (Ivanova and Bures 1990; Flynn et al. 1991), as well as the projections from the BSTL division to the lateral hypothalamus and the autonomic regions of the brainstem (de Olmos et al. 1985), the pPB(m)-BSTL diffuse pathway could be implicated in both motivational and autonomic responses related to taste in a manner similar to the pPB(m)-CeM pathway (see discussion in Bernard et al. 1993).
2. The pPB(l)-BSTdl concentrated pathway would primarily act in the processing of autonomic and visceral messages, as suggested for the pPB(l)-CeL pathway (Bernard et al. 1993). As suggested by the studies implicating the BST in stress behavior (Henke 1984; Casada and Dafny 1991) and the parabrachial area in analgesia (de Salles et al. 1985), this pathway could play an important role in what is called stress-produced analgesia.
3. The pPB(l)-MnPO could be partly a collateral pathway of the pPB(l)-BSTdl and might, more precisely, be implicated in osmotic and volemic regulation as suggest by anatomical data (Saper and Levisohn 1983; Simerly and Swanson 1986) and physiological data (O'Neill and Brody 1987; McAllen et al. 1990) on the MnPO.

ACKNOWLEDGMENTS

We thank Dr. A.H. Dickenson for advice in the preparation of the manuscript and J. Carroue for histological help. This study was supported by l'Institut National de la Santé et de la Recherche Médicale (INSERM), and by an Unrestricted Pain Research Award from the Bristol-Myers Squibb Co.

APPENDIX: Abbreviations Used in Figs. 1–3

ac	anterior commissure
Aco	anterior cortical amygdaloid nucleus
AI	agranular insular cortex
AMPO	anterior medial preoptic nucleus
AVPO	anteroventral preoptic nucleus
bc	brachum conjunctivum
BL	basolateral amygdaloid nucleus

BMA	basomedial ant. amygdaloid nucleus
BST	bed nucleus of stria terminalis
1) BSTL	lateral division of the BST
BSTal	anterior lateral subnucleus of BST
BSTdl	dorsal lateral subnucleus of BST
BSTjxc	juxtacapsulars subnucleus of BST
BSTpl	posterior lateral subnucleus of BST
BSTvl	ventral lateral subnucleus of BST
2) BSTM	medial division of the BST
BSTam	anterior medial subnucleus of BST
BSTps	parastrial subnucleus of BST
BSTvm	ventral medial subnucleus of BST
Ce	central nucleus of the amygdala
CeL	lateral subdivision of the Ce
CeLC	lateral capsular subdivision of the Ce
CeM	medial subdivision of the Ce
CPu	caudate putamen
cst	commisural stria terminalis
DEn	dorsal endopiriform nucleus
DI	dysgranular insular cortex
ec	external capsule
Fstr	fundus striati
fx	fornix
GP	globus pallidus
HDB	nu. horizontal limb diagonal band
ic	internal capsule
IM	intercalated amygdaloid nucleus
LPO	lateral preoptic area
LV	lateral ventricle
MCPO	magnocellular preoptic nucleus
MnPO	median preoptic nucleus
MPA	medial preoptic area
opt	optic tract
ox	optic chiasm
pPB	pontine parabrachial area
pPBcl	central lateral subnucleus of pPB
pPBdl	dorsal lateral subnucleus of pPB
pPBel	external lateral subnucleus of pPB
pPBem	external medial subnucleus of pPB
pPBm	medial subnucleus of pPB
pPBvl	ventral, lateral subnucleus of pPB
pPBwa	waist area of the pPB
Pir	piriform cortex
st	stria terminalis
VEn	ventral endopiriform nucleus
3V	3rd ventricle

REFERENCES

Bernard, J.F. and Besson, J.M., The spino (trigemino) pontoamygdaloid pathway: electrophysiological evidence for an involvement in pain processes, J. Neurophysiol., 63 (1990) 473–489.

Bernard, J.F., Huang, G.F. and Besson, J.M., Nucleus centralis of the amygdala and the globus pallidus ventralis: electrophysiological evidence for an involvement in pain processes, J. Neurophysiol., 68 (1992) 551–569.

Bernard, J.F., Aldén, M. and Besson, J.M., The organization of the efferent projections from the pontine parabrachial area to the amygdaloid complex: A *Phaseolus vulgaris* leucoagglutinin (PHA-L) study in the rat, J. Comp. Neurol., 329 (1993) 201–229.

Casada, J.H. and Dafny, N., Restraint and stimulation of bed nucleus of the stria terminalis produce similar stress-like behaviors, Brain Res. Bull., 27 (1991) 207–212.

de Olmos, J., Alheid, G.F. and Beltramino, C.A., Amygdala. In: G. Paxinos (Ed.), The Rat Nervous System: Forebrain and Midbrain, Vol. 1, Academic Press, Sydney, 1985, pp. 223–334.

de Salles, A.A.F., Katayama, V., Becker, D.P. and Hayes, R.L., Pain suppression induced by electrical stimulation of the pontine parabrachial region, J. Neurosurg., 62 (1985) 397–407.

Flynn, F.W., Schulkin, J., Grill, H.J. and Norgren, R., Central gustatory lesions: effects on sodium appetite, taste aversion learning and feeding behaviors, Behav. Neurosci., 105 (1991) 944–954.

Fulwiler, C.E. and Saper, C.B., Subnuclear organization of the efferent connections of the parabrachial nucleus in the rat, Brain Res. Rev., 7 (1984) 229–259.

Gerfen, C.R. and Sawchenko, P.E., An anterograde neuroanatomical tracing method that shows the detailed morphology of neurons, their axons and terminals: immunohistochemical localization of an axonally transported plant lectin, *Phaseolus Vulgaris* leucoagglutinin (PHA-L), Brain Res., 290 (1984) 219–238.

Henke, P.G., The bed nucleus of the stria terminalis and immobilization stress: unit activity, escape behaviour and gastric pathology in rats, Behav. Brain Res., 11 (1984) 35–45.

Huang, G.F., Besson, J.M. and Bernard, J.F., Morphine depresses the transmission of noxious messages in the spino (trigemino)-ponto-amygdaloid pathway, Eur. J. Pharmacol., 230 (1993a) 279–284.

Huang, G.F., Besson, J.M. and Bernard, J.F., Intravenous morphine depresses the transmission of noxious messages to the nucleus centralis of the amygdala, Eur. J. Pharmacol., 236 (1993b) 449–456.

Ivanova, S.F. and Bures, J., Acquisition of conditioned taste aversion in rats is prevented by tetrodoxin blockade of a small midbrain region centered around the parabrachial nuclei, Physiol. Behav., 48 (1990) 543–549.

Light, A.R., The initial processing of pain and its descending control: spinal and trigeminal systems. In: P.L. Gildenberg (Ed.), Pain and Headache, Vol. 12, Karger, Basel, 1992, 306 pp.

Lind, R.W. and Swanson, L.W., Evidence for corticotropin releasing factor and leu-enkephalin in the neural projections from the lateral parabrachial nucleus to the median preoptic nucleus: a retrograde transport, immunohistochemical double labelling study in the rat, Brain Res., 321 (1984) 217–224.

McAllen, R.M., Pennington, G.L. and McKinley, M.J., Osmoresponsive units in sheep median preoptic nucleus, Am. J. Physiol., 259 (1990) R593–R600.

Moga, M.M., Saper, C.B. and Gray, T.S., Bed nucleus of the stria terminalis: cytoarchitecture, immunohistochemistry and projection to the parabrachial nucleus in the rat, J. Comp. Neurol., 283 (1989) 315–332.

Moga, M.M., Herbert, H., Hurley, K.M., Yasui, Y., Gray, T.S. and Saper, C.B., Organization of cortical, basal forebrain and hypothalamic afferents to the parabrachial nucleus in the rat, J. Comp. Neurol., 295 (1990) 624–661.

O'Neill, T.P. and Brody, M.J., Role for the median preoptic nucleus in centrally evoked pressor responses, Am. J. Physiol., 252 (1987) R1165–R1172.

Paxinos, G. and Watson, C., The Rat Brain in Stereotaxic Coordinates, Academic Press, Sydney, 1986.

Saper, C.B. and Loewy, A.D., Efferent connections of the parabrachial nucleus in the rat, Brain Res., 197 (1980) 291–317.

Saper, C.B. and Levisohn, D., Afferent connections of the median preoptic nucleus in the rat: anatomical evidence for a cardiovascular integrative mechanism in the anteroventral third ventricular (AV3V) region, Brain Res., 288 (1983) 21–31.

Simerly, R.B. and Swanson, L.W., The organization of neural inputs to the medial preoptic nucleus of the rat, J. Comp. Neurol., 246 (1986) 312–342.

Sun, N., Roberts, L. and Cassell, M.D., Rat central amygdaloid nucleus projections to the bed nucleus of the stria terminalis, Brain Res. Bull., 27 (1991) 651–662.

Weller, K.L. and Smith, D.A., Afferent connections to the bed nucleus of the stria terminalis, Brain Res., 232 (1982) 255–270.

Correspondence to: Dr Jean-François Bernard, INSERM U161, 2 rue d'Alésia, F-75014 Paris, France. Tel: 33-1-45-89-36-62; Fax: 33-1-45-88-13-04.

Proceedings of the 7th World Congress on Pain,
Progress in Pain Research and Management, Vol. 2,
edited by G.F. Gebhart, D.L. Hammond, and T.S.
Jensen, IASP Press, Seattle, © 1994.

54

Morphology of Primary Somatosensory Cortical Neurons Responsive to Noxious Stimulation of the Trigeminal Regions

Rhyuji Sumino,[a] Yoshiyuki Tsuboi,[a] Junichi Yagi,[a]
Hiroyoshi Nakanishi,[b] Masahiro Kondo,[a]
and Koichi Iwata[a]

[a]Department of Physiology, School of Dentistry, and [b]Department of Anesthesiology, School of Medicine, Nihon University, Tokyo, Japan

INTRODUCTION

Previous studies have revealed that many neurons in the primary somatosensory cortex (SI) are responsive to noxious thermal and mechanical stimulation of the facial skin (Chudler et al. 1990; Chudler et al. 1986; Iwata et al. 1987, 1990; Kenshalo et al. 1988; Kenshalo and Isensee 1983a,b; Lund and Sessle 1974; Tsuboi et al. 1993). Such neurons have been classified into two different types: WDR (wide dynamic range) neurons give increasing spike discharges with an increase in mechanical stimulus intensity, and NS (noxious-specific) neurons respond exclusively to noxious mechanical stimulation. However, no reports have described the morphology of nociceptive neurons in the SI cortex. Our study focused on neurons responsive to noxious stimulation of intraoral structures and attempted to clarify their morphology.

MATERIALS AND METHODS

We performed experiments on 28 young adult cats weighing 3.0–3.5 kg. The animals were initially anesthetized with ketamine-HCl (50 mg/kg). During surgery, the anesthesia was maintained with a mixture of halothane and oxygen. Gas anesthesia was discontinued after surgery, and the depth of anesthesia was maintained throughout the experiment with α-chloralose (60 mg/kg). During recording sessions, the animals were immobilized with pancuronium bromide (1 mg/kg per hour, iv.) and ventilated artificially. Before application of noxious stimulus to the facial skin and intraoral mucosa, the depth of anesthesia was judged by miosis. When the animal's pupil responded to light presentation, additional α-chloralose (20 mg/kg) was intravenously injected. Expired CO_2 concentration was monitored and maintained between 3 and 4%. Rectal temperature was maintained between 37° and 39°C by a thermostatically controlled heating pad.

A craniotomy was performed to expose the cerebral cortex over the coronal gyrus. Glass micropipette electrodes filled with a solution of neurobiotin (Vector Lab.) with 0.5 M KCl in PBS (pH 8.0) for intracellular recording were then advanced through the cortex, and cellular activity was evoked by touching various intraoral structures. Each cell was tested for its response to mechanical and thermal stimuli in the receptive fields. When a neuronal discharge in response to innocuous mechanical stimulation of the receptive fields was obtained, neurons were tested for their responsiveness to thermal stimulation of their receptive fields. A thermal probe was placed in the area of the receptive field most sensitive to innocuous mechanical stimulation. Mechanical stimuli included touching the receptive field with brushes (touch), application of a glass rod (pressure), and application of an arterial clip (pinch). Thermal stimuli consisted of temperatures ranging between 40 and 58°C for each stimulation (duration: 10–30 seconds). We classified neurons based on the type of afferent convergence from orofacial cutaneous, mucosal, and periodontal structures. Low-threshold mechanoreceptive (LTM) neurons responded to light touch or pressure of the skin, mucosa, or tooth. WDR neurons responded to innocuous and to noxious mechanical or heat stimulation of the skin or mucosa. NS neurons responded to noxious mechanical and heat stimulation of the skin or mucosa.

When intracellular potentials were recorded, neuronal activities were fed into a tape recorder (bandwidth DC to 20 kHz) for subsequent analysis of signals. After identification of nociceptive neurons, intracellular injection was done through the neurobiotin-filled electrodes with a depolarizing pulse (3–5 nA, 300 ms duration, 2 cycles per second) for 2–10 minutes. The injection was stopped when a resting potential was no longer observed. The cellular responses were monitored every other minute to ensure the cell's identity. Following injection, the animals were allowed to survive for 6–10 hours and then were deeply anesthetized with pentobarbital sodium. They were perfused transcardially with 500 ml of phosphate-buffered saline (PBS; pH 7.4) followed by 4% paraformaldehyde in 0.1 M phosphate buffer. The brain was

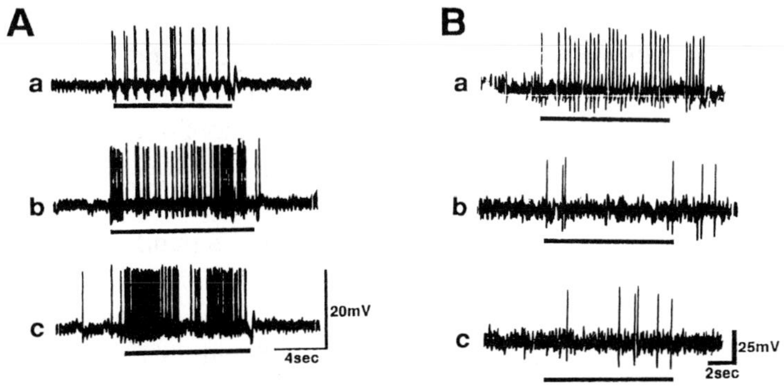

Fig. 1. Sample intracellular recordings of WDR (**A**) and LTM (**B**) neurons from the SI. **a:** responses to gentle brushing of the receptive fields, **b:** responses to pressure stimulation of the receptive fields, **c:** responses to pinching of the receptive fields. Scale bars indicate the duration of each stimulus.

removed and placed in cold fixative for four days and then transferred to cold phosphate-buffered 30% sucrose for 48 hours. Serial sections 50-μm thick were cut along the path of electrode penetration. The sections were incubated in peroxidase-conjugated avidin-biotin complex (1:100; ABC: Vecta Labs). We used 3,3'-diaminobenzidine-tetra HCl (DAB; Sigma), nickel ammonium sulfate (0.2 mg/100 ml), and 30% hydrogen peroxide (30 μl/100 ml) in Tris-buffered saline (0.05 M, pH 7.4) to develop the ABC reaction product, producing a distinctive black chromogen. Every section was counterstained with thionin. The morphology of each stained neuron was reconstructed by a camera lucida tube-equipped microscope (× 400 magnification).

RESULTS AND DISCUSSION

Intracellular potentials from 59 neurons were successfully recorded, and the neurons were injected, recovered, and reconstructed. Eleven neurons were classified as WDR neurons, and located in laminae III–V of area 3b and 47 were classified as LTM neurons. We found no nociceptive-specific neurons in the SI. Fig. 1 illustrates sample intracellular recordings of WDR and LTM neurons responsive to mechanical stimulation of the facial skin. The WDR neuron showed a graded response to an increase of stimulus intensity (Fig. 1A). Following gentle brushing of the receptive field, LTM neurons showed clear neuronal discharges but did not increase in firing frequency in response to pressure and noxious pinch stimuli. We classified WDR and LTM neurons on the basis of their response properties following mechanical stimulation of the receptive field, as illustrated in Fig. 1.

Six WDR neurons were located in lamina III, four in lamina IV, and one in lamina V, of area 3b, according to the cytoarchitectonic criteria of Hassler

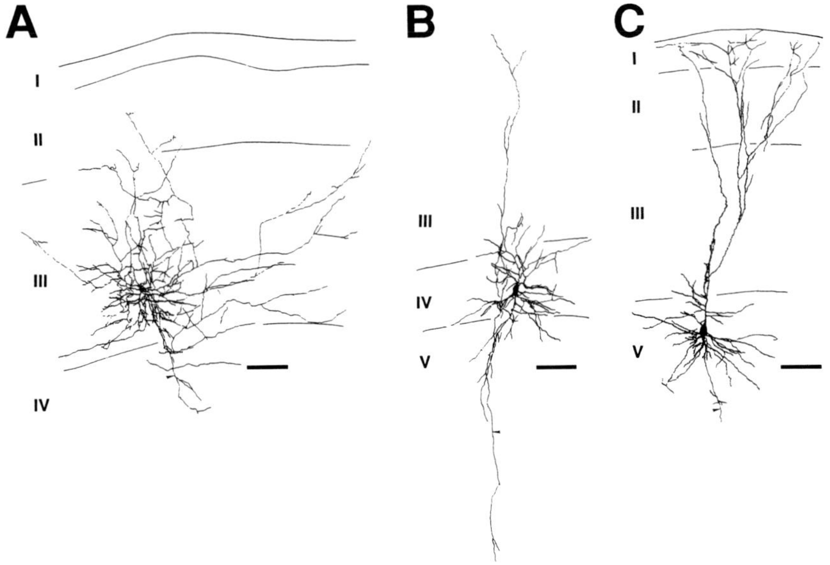

Fig. 2. Sample reconstructions of typical WDR neurons in each lamina. **A,** lamina III WDR neuron, **B,** lamina IV WDR neuron, **C,** lamina V WDR neuron. Scale bars indicate 100 μm.

and Muhs-Clement (1964). Two types of lamina III WDR neurons were identified. One type was classified as stellate cells, having oval somata with many dendrites and axon collaterals. The other type was typical pyramidal cells with pyramidal somata and thick apical dendrites with many spines. Figs. 2 and 3 show sample reconstructions of typical WDR and LTM neurons in each lamina. The lamina III stellate WDR neuron had a round soma and spiny dendrites (Fig. 2A). We did not find axons going deep into the subcortical regions, and some axon collaterals ran through lamina III. However, these collaterals did not extend far from the soma. An interesting morphological characteristic of WDR neurons was the distribution pattern of their dendrites. As shown in Fig. 2A, the dendrites of the lamina III WDR neurons were distributed mainly around the area of the soma, and a small number of apical dendrites extended up to the superficial laminae. Lamina III pyramidal WDR and LTM neurons had similar morphological properties: typical pyramidal somata and thick apical dendrites with many spines (Fig. 3A). The lamina IV WDR neurons generally had bipolar somata with dendrites spreading around the soma and axons running deep into the white matter (Fig. 1B). Lamina IV WDR neurons were similar morphologically to LTM neurons. Basically, lamina IV WDR and LTM neurons had dendrites running around the soma, expanding to only a limited extent like those of lamina III WDR neurons and having many varicosities on their dendritic trees. We successfully recorded and in-

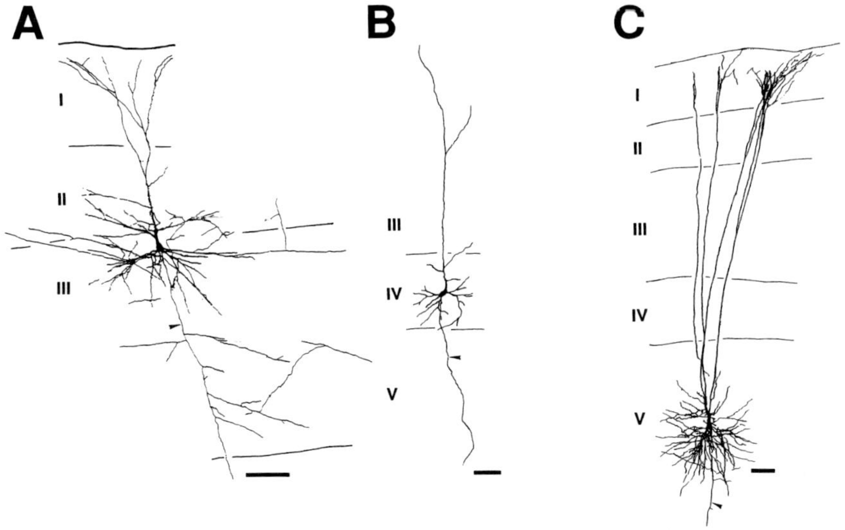

Fig. 3. Sample reconstructions of typical LTM neurons in each lamina. **A,** lamina III LTM neuron, **B,** lamina IV LTM neuron, **C,** lamina V LTM neuron. Scale bars indicate 100 μm.

jected only one WDR neuron from lamina V. The lamina V WDR and LTM neurons had similar morphological characteristics, with large somata and thick apical dendrites with many spines. Table I compares the detailed morphological properties of WDR and LTM neurons. Lamina III WDR neurons (mean ± S.E.M., 153.9 ± 37.5 μm^2, n = 6) had smaller somata than did those of lamina III LTM neurons (275.9 ± 39.2 μm^2, n=16) ($P < 0.05$), whereas no significant difference was evident between in lamina IV LTM and WDR neurons. The former (2.6 ± 0.5, n = 6) had a smaller number of basal dendrites than did those of lamina III LTM neurons (4.2 ± 0.4, n = 15) ($P < 0.05$), whereas lamina IV WDR neurons (6.5 ± 1.3, n = 4) had more basal dendrites than did lamina IV LTM neurons (2.5 ± 0.4, n = 7) ($P < 0.05$). Lamina IV WDR neurons had small oval somata, many dendrites, and axon collaterals. The one example of lamina V WDR neurons recorded in our study had larger somata, apical dendrites, and more spines than those in other laminae. We found no significant differences between LTM and WDR neurons in the diameter of apical dendrites and the number of spines.

In sum, the present data showed that nociceptive neurons in SI had some different morphological characteristics compared with those of LTM neurons: (1) WDR neurons had smaller somata and fewer spines and basal dendrites than did LTM neurons. Yamamoto and colleagues (1988, 1990) reported that SI neurons responsive to electrical stimulation of the superficial radial nerve were classified as pyramidal and nonpyramidal. The morphological properties

Table I
Incidence of wide dynamic range (WDR) and low-threshold mechanoreceptive (LTM) neurons in the SI

Lamina		Area of Somata (μm^2)	Diameter of Apical Dendrites (μm)	Number of Spines (per 50 μm of apical dendrites)	Number of Basal Dendrites
III	WDR (n = 5)	153.9 ± 37.5	2.8 ± 0.9	5.3 ± 5.3	2.6 ± 0.5
	LTM (n = 15)	275.9 ± 39.2	3.5 ± 0.4	9.2 ± 4.4	4.2 ± 0.4
IV	WDR (n = 4)	227.4 ± 14.5	2.9 ± 0.2	0	6.5 ± 1.3
	LTM (n = 7)	208.9 ± 35.7	2.5 ± 0.4	2.7 ± 1.8	2.6 ± 0.4
V	WDR (n = 1)	599.7	3.5	20	3
	LTM (n = 9)	603.2 ± 129.4	3.8 ± 0.5	6.1 ± 4.9	5.1 ± 0.6

of nonpyramidal neurons were quite similar to those of nociceptive neurons shown in our study. Previous anatomical studies (Landry et al. 1981, 1987; Yamamoto et al. 1990) have shown that the majority of laminae III and IV somatosensory cortical neurons receive direct inputs from the thalamus. In our study, almost all the WDR neurons were recorded from laminae III and IV. Furthermore, our data showed that laminae III and IV WDR neurons had axons projecting only a short distance away from the soma, which were distributed mainly around each nociceptive neuron. These findings suggest that laminae III and IV WDR neurons receive nociceptive inputs via thalamic relay neurons and relay the nociceptive sensory information to the vicinity of the soma.

ACKNOWLEDGMENTS

This study was supported by the Sato Foundation of Nihon University and in part by a Grant-in-Aid for Scientific Research (67232665) from the Japanese Ministry of Education, Science, and Culture.

REFERENCES

Chudler, E.H., Dong, W.K. and Kawakami, Y., Cortical nociceptive responses and behavioral correlates in the monkey, Brain Res., 397 (1986) 47–60.

Chudler, E.H., Anton, F., Dubner, R. and Kenshalo, D.R., Jr., Responses of nociceptive neurons in monkeys and pain sensation in humans elicited by noxious thermal stimulation: effect of interstimulus interval, J. Neurophysiol., 63 (1990) 559–59.

Hassler, R. and Muhs-Clement, K., Architectonisher Aufbar des sensomotorishen Cortex der Katze, J. Hirnforsch., 6 (1964) 377–420.

Iwata, K., Itoga, H., Muramatsu, H., Toda, K. and Sumino, R., Responses of bradykinin sensitive

tooth-pulp driven neurons in cat cerebral cortex, Exp. Brain Res., 66 (1987) 435–439.
Iwata, K., Tsuboi, Y., Muramatsu, H. and Sumino, R., Distribution and response properties of cat SI neurons responsive to changes in tooth temperature, J. Neurophysiol., 64 (1990) 822–834.
Kenshalo, D.R., JR. and Isensee, O., Effects of noxious stimuli on primate SI cortical neurons. In: J. Bonica, U. Lindblom and A. Iggo (Eds.), Proceedings of the Third World Congress on Pain. Advances in Pain Research and Therapy, Vol. 5. Raven Press, New York, 1983a, pp.139–145.
Kenshalo, D.R., Jr. and Isensee, O., Responses of primate SI cortical neurons to noxious stimuli, J. Neurophysiol., 50 (1983b) 1479–1496.
Kenshalo, D.R., Jr., Chudler, E.H., Anton, F. and Dubner, R., SI nociceptive neurons participate in the encoding process by which monkeys perceive the intensity of noxious thermal stimulation, Brain Res., 454 (1988) 378–382.
Landry, P. and Deschenes, M., Intracortical arborizations and receptive fields of identified ventrobasal thalamocortical afferents to the primary somatic sensory cortex in the cat, J. Comp. Neurol., 199 (1981) 345–371.
Landry, P., Diadori, P., Leclerc, S. and Dykes. R.W., Morphological and electrophysiological characteristics of somatosensory thalamocortical axons studied with intra-axonal staining and recording in the cat, Exp. Brain Res., 65 (1987) 317–330.
Lund, J.P. and Sessle, B.J., Oral-facial and jaw muscle afferent projections to neurons in cat frontal cortex, Exp. Neurol., 45 (1974) 324–331.
Tsuboi, Y., Iwata, K., Muramatsu, H., Yagi, J., Inomata, Y. and Sumino, R., Response properties of primary somatosensory cortical neurons responsive to cold stimulation of the facial skin and oral mucous membrane, Brain Res., 613 (1993) 193–202.
Yamamoto, T., Kisimoto, Y., Yoshikawa, H. and Oka, H., Cortical laminar distribution of rat thalamic ventrolateral fibers demonstrated by the PHL-L anterograde labeling method, Neurosci. Res., 9 (1990) 148–154.
Yamamoto, T., Samejima, A. and Oka, H., Short latency activation of local circuit neurons in the cat somatosensory cortex, Brain Res., 461 (1988) 199–203.
Yamamoto, T., Samejima, A. and Oka, H., The mode of synaptic activation of pyramidal neurons in the cat primary somatosensory cortex: an intracellular HRP study, Exp. Brain Res., 80 (1990) 12–22.

Correspondence to: Koichi Iwata, DDS, PhD, Department of Physiology, School of Dentistry, Nihon University, Kanda-surugadai, Chiyoda-ku, Tokyo 101, Japan. Tel: 81-3-3219-8122; Fax: 81-3-3219-8311.

Proceedings of the 7th World Congress on Pain,
Progress in Pain Research and Management, Vol. 2,
edited by G.F. Gebhart, D.L. Hammond, and T.S.
Jensen, IASP Press, Seattle, © 1994.

55

Reduction in the Size of Tactile Hypesthesia and Allodynia Closely Associated with Pain Relief in Patients with Chronic Pain

Katsuyuki Moriwaki, Osafumi Yuge, Kengo Nishioka, Takao Yamanoue, and Masakazu Nakao

Department of Anesthesiology and Critical Care Medicine, Hiroshima University School of Medicine, Hiroshima, Japan

INTRODUCTION

Pain is "an unpleasant sensory and emotional experience associated with actual or potential tissue damage, or described in terms of such damage," and thus, "pain is always subjective" (Merskey 1979, 1986). All indicators of the magnitude of pain such as visual analogue scales (VAS), verbal rating scores, and picture face scales (Rogers 1981) are subjective. A more objective indicator of pain, if such exists, is extremely helpful for evaluating a patient's pain.

In the last two decades, a growing body of evidence has indicated that the altered central processing in dorsal horn neurons plays a crucial role in the initiation and maintenance of painful conditions (Woolf 1983, 1991; Woolf and Thompson 1991; Dubner 1991). This altered central processing is thought to cause not only spontaneous pain but also cutaneous sensory abnormalities (Lindblom and Verrillo 1979; Dubner 1992). The magnitude of acute pain increased in association with the increasing area of mechanical hyperalgesia in a dose-dependent manner after injection of capsaicin in human subjects (Simone et al. 1989). Thus, the size of abnormal cutaneous sensibility may be also closely associated with the magnitude of spontaneous pain in patients with chronic pain. If this is true, we can estimate the change of a patient's magnitude of pain in a more objective manner. Our study investigated whether the size of tactile sensory abnormalities correlates with the magnitude of spontaneous pain in patients with chronic pain. We also studied the characteristics of tactile sensory abnormalities.

METHODS

We studied 42 patients (29 men, 13 women) who had chronic pain with tactile sensory abnormality at first visit to the pain clinic in Hiroshima University Hospital. All subjects fulfilled the criteria of chronic pain defined by Bonica (Bonica 1990). The patients' age ranged from 25 to 79 years, with an average of 55.5 years (SD=13.4). Table I summarizes the diagnoses of the painful conditions and tactile sensory abnormalities in each group. The patients were treated with sympathetic ganglion blocks or somatic nerve blocks or both, depending on the diagnosis. Nonsteroidal anti-inflammatory drugs (NSAIDs) and antidepressants also were prescribed if indicated. Table I summarizes nerve blocks and medications used for treatments in each diagnosis

Tactile sensory abnormalities were examined by using a soft writing brush. The areas of tactile hypesthesia and allodynia were delineated on the patient's skin and recorded before and after each treatment. Outcomes were classified into four grades according to relief of spontaneous pain measured by percent decrease of VAS (Table II). Statistical analysis was performed using chi-square test or Fisher's exact test. A P value less than 0.05 was considered statistically significant.

RESULTS

FINDINGS OF ABNORMAL TACTILE SENSIBILITIES AT FIRST VISIT

Before treatments, 17 patients had tactile hypesthesia without allodynia and 25 patients had both tactile hypesthesia and allodynia (Table I). The allodynic area was surrounded by an area of tactile hypesthesia in all patients with allodynia except one who had postherpetic neuralgia with severe allodynia. The area of tactile hypesthesia was reported by patients as an area of slight numbness, where "something like a very thin layer exists between the skin and the brush." The touch sensation in the area of tactile hypesthesia was usually felt with an intensity of 0.8 to 0.4 of the normal touch sensation. Degrees of both tactile hypesthesia and allodynia were lighter at the outer part and greater at the inner part in each area. The degree of hypesthesia was

Table I
Diagnoses, initial tactile sensory abnormalities, and treatments

Diagnosis	Number of Patients	Tactile Sensory Abnormality		Treatments		
		H	HA	Nerve Blocks	NSAIDs	Antidepressant
Postherpetic neuralgia	11	(0)	(11)	Trigger point injection (9) SGB (5) Epidural block (3) Spinal root block (2) Gasserian ganglion block (1)	(7)	(8)
Postoperative neuralgia	9	(2)	(7)	Trigger point injection (6) Epidural block (6) Intercostal nerve blocks (3) SGB (1)	(7)	(3)
RSD and causalgia	8	(3)	(5)	Epidural block (8) LSGB (7) ThSGB (1) Trigger point injection (2) SGB (1)	(8)	(6)
Atypical facial pain	4	(4)	(0)	SGB (4)	(2)	(0)
Cervical radiculopathy	2	(1)	(1)	SGB (2)	(2)	(1)
Other types of neuritis or neuropathy (5), myofascicular pain syndrome (1), temporomandibular arthrosis (1), or glossopharyngeal neuralgia (1)	8	(7)	(1)	SGB (5) LSGB (1) Trigger point injection (2) Temporo mandibular joint injection (1) Epidural block (1)	(2)	(3)

Note: Numbers in parentheses indicate number of patients. H, presence of tactile hypesthesia; HA, presence of both allodynia and tactile hypesthesia; SGB, stellate ganglion block; LSGB, lumbar sympathetic ganglion block.

Table II
Definition of outcome grades

Outcome Grade	% Relief of Spontaneous Pain (% decrease of VAS)
Excellent	> 75 %
Good	51–75 %
Fair	26–50 %
Poor	< 25 %

greatest at the area adjacent to the territory of allodynia. The area of allodynia or tactile hypesthesia often spread out of the territory of the affected peripheral nerve(s). The patterns and intensity distributions of these tactile sensory abnormalities were easily determined in patients with diagnoses other than postherpetic neuralgia. In patients with postherpetic neuralgia, the patterns and intensity distributions were somewhat complex and scattered; basically, the allodynic area was surrounded by tactile hypesthesia, which was the same as in patients with other diagnoses.

THE PATTERN OF IMPROVEMENT OF TACTILE SENSORY ABNORMALITIES

Summing up the observations made during the course of treatments in 42 patients, the improvement of sensory abnormalities appeared in the following stages: stage I—reduction in the size of allodynia and tactile hypesthesia; stage II—disappearance of allodynia; stage III—reduction in the size of the remaining tactile hypesthesia; and stage IV—disappearance of tactile hypesthesia. A schematic drawing of the improvement of sensory abnormalities is presented in Fig. 1. The following case report illustrates the typical pattern of improvement of tactile sensory abnormalities in a patient with postoperative neuralgia.

A Case Report

A 54-year-old man had long-standing low back pain since childhood. He had been treated with hemodialysis since 1978 because of chronic renal failure. To relieve the low back pain caused by renal stones in the nonfunctioning kidney, he underwent a left nephrectomy in July 1986 and a right nephrectomy in September 1990. After the second operation, in addition to his right low back pain, the patient developed a constant dull pain in his right flank extending into the right inguinal region with sharp pain radiating to the right femoral

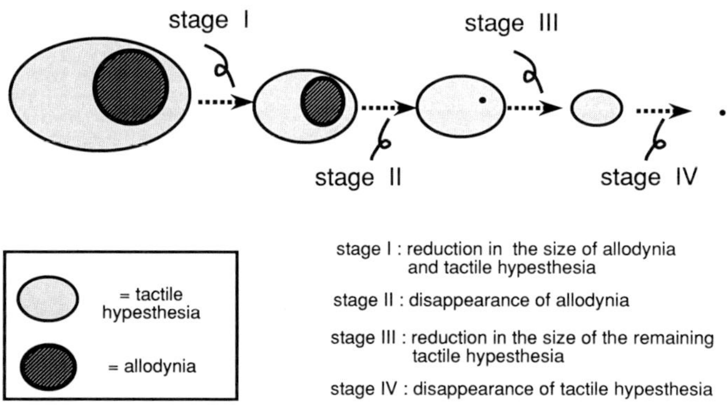

Fig. 1. Stages of improvement of cutaneous sensory abnormality.

region. The patient was referred to our pain clinic in November 1990. According to the findings of physical examinations and X-ray of the lumbosacral vertebrae, we diagnosed two diseases related to his pain—postoperative neuralgia and facet arthropathy of right L3/4. Postoperative neuralgia in his right flank was the suspected cause of his major complaint of ongoing pain. Tactile sensory abnormalities are shown in Fig. 2A. Allodynia and tactile hypesthesia surrounded the allodynic area. He received 4 ml of bupivacaine with or without triamcinolone diacetate 10 mg injected to the painful points in the postoperative scar (trigger point injection) 10 times during the subsequent two months. Facet block and epidural block also were applied several times for the treatment of facet pain and low back pain after confirmation of normal bleeding time. The areas of allodynia and tactile hypesthesia were reduced significantly after three days of treatments (Fig. 2B, stage I improvement). Following two more days of treatments, the allodynic area disappeared (Fig. 2C, stage II improvement). After two months of treatments, small area of tactile hypesthesia remained just caudal to the scar (Fig. 2D, stage III improvement). The spontaneous, constant pain of the flank to the femoral region related to the postoperative neuralgia was relieved by 70% (good outcome grade; Table II).

RELATION BETWEEN OUTCOME GRADES (RELIEF OF SPONTANEOUS PAIN) AND IMPROVEMENT OF THE ABNORMAL TACTILE SENSIBILITY

Table III summarizes the numbers of patients in each outcome grade who reached one of the four improvement stages (Fig. 1). In patients with both tactile hypesthesia and allodynia (Table IIIA), reduction in the size of tactile hypesthesia and allodynia (stage I) was observed in all patients with excellent, good, and fair outcome grades. With one exception, reduction in the size of

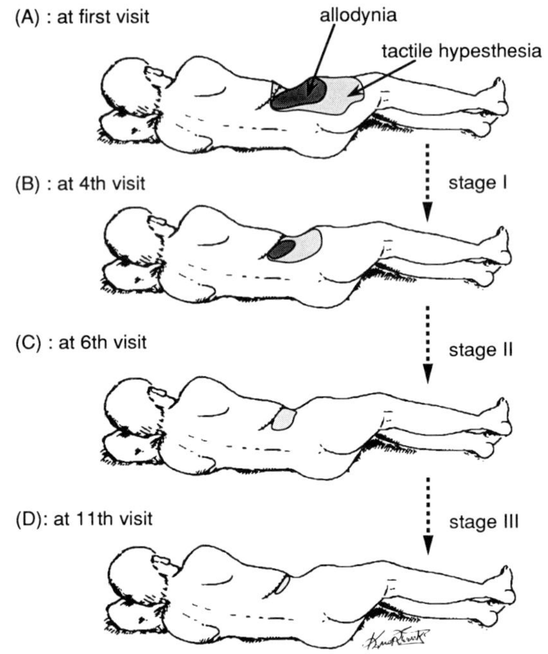

Fig 2. Improvement of abnormal tactile sensibility in a case of postoperative neuralgia.

sensory abnormalities was not observed in patients showing poor pain relief. The incidence of positive reduction in the size of allodynia and tactile hypesthesia was significantly higher in patients with good to fair outcome grades than that in patients with poor outcome grade ($P < 0.0001$). The incidence of disappearance of allodynia (stage II) and reduction in the size of remaining tactile hypesthesia (stage III) was significantly higher in patients with excellent to good outcome grades than in patients with fair to poor outcome grades ($P < 0.001$, $P < 0.01$, respectively). Tactile hypesthesia (stage IV) disappeared in one patient with excellent outcome. In patients with tactile hypesthesia without allodynia (Table IIIB), the incidence of reduction in the size of tactile hypesthesia (stage III) was significantly higher in patients with excellent to fair outcome grades than in patients with poor outcome grades ($P < 0.05$). Tactile hypesthesia disappeared in three patients with excellent and good outcome grades.

RELATION BETWEEN THE TEMPORARY EFFECT OF NERVE BLOCK ON THE TACTILE SENSORY ABNORMALITIES AND LONG-TERM OUTCOME WITH TREATMENTS

Temporary reduction in the size of tactile hypesthesia and allodynia occurred within 15 minutes after nerve blocks in all patients with excellent to

Table III
Improvement of abnormal tactile sensibility in relation to outcome grade

Outcome Grade	Stage I	Stage II	Stage III	Stage IV
A. In Patients with Allodynia and Tactile Hypesthesia: number and (percentage)				
Excellent (n = 2)	2 (100)	2 (100)	2 (100)	1 (50)
Good (n = 9)	9 (100)	8 (89)	6 (67)	0 (0)
Fair (n = 8)	8 (100)	1 (13)	1 (13)	0 (0)
Poor (n = 6)	1 (17)	1 (17)	1 (17)	0 (0)
B. In Patients with Tactile Hypesthesia without Allodynia: number and (percentage)				
Excellent (n = 2)	—	—	2 (100)	2 (100)
Good (n = 7)	—	—	7 (100)	1 (14)
Fair (n = 6)	—	—	5 (83)	0 (0)
Poor (n = 2)	—	—	0 (0)	0 (0)

fair outcome grades and in some patients with poor outcome grades. The temporary effect lasted for several days or weeks, while in others the effect lasted only a few hours. Regardless of the length of improvement of tactile sensory abnormalities, the spontaneous pain was significantly decreased during this time.

The relation between long-term outcomes and temporary improvement of tactile sensory abnormalities are schematically shown in Fig. 3. In patients with excellent or good outcome grades, spontaneous pain relief was associated with gradual improvements of the tactile sensory abnormalities (Fig. 3A). However, long-term follow-up with repetition of the effective nerve blocks, which were followed by positive temporary reduction in the size(s) of abnormal tactile sensibilities, revealed that gradual improvement of the tactile hypesthesia and allodynia rarely occurred in patients with poor outcome grades (Fig. 3B). Six of eight patients with RSD or a causalgia type of pain showed this type of refractoriness to the treatments. All patients who did not show any temporary improvement at the tactile sensory abnormalities belonged to the poor outcome grade (Fig. 3C).

DISCUSSION

Allodynia and tactile hypesthesia have been reported as two distinct cutaneous tactile sensory abnormalities in patients with neuralgia. Lindblom and

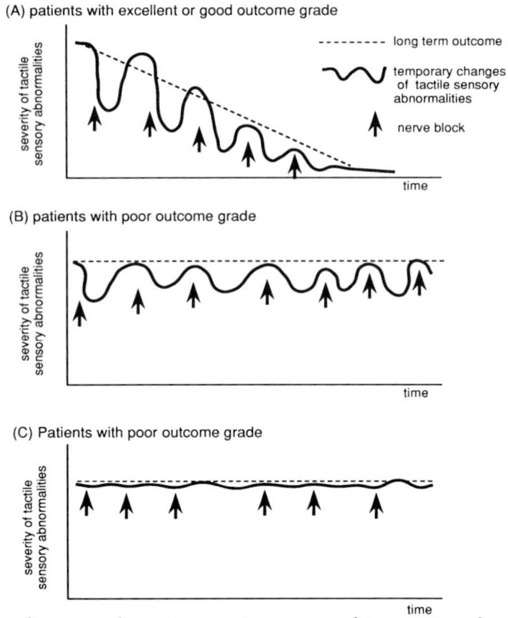

Fig. 3. The relation between long-term outcomes and temporary improvement of tactile sensory abnormalities.

Verrillo made an early important observation concerning allodynia and tactile hypesthesia. They described that the painful area was numb (i.e., hypesthetic) in all patients, but that touch was unpleasant or painful (i.e., allodynia), at least in certain patches. Recently, Rowbotham reported that their patients with postherpetic neuralgia fell into two major groups: one group with prominent allodynia and another without (Rowbotham et al. 1989). Although not always, they observed that allodynia occasionally was present in the area with the greatest sensory deficit. These notions together with our findings reported in the present study indicate that tactile sensory abnormalities in patients with chronic pain can basically be classified into two types: (1) tactile hypesthesia with allodynia where the allodynic area is surrounded by tactile hypesthesia, and (2) tactile hypesthesia without allodynia.

In our study, we observed that the tactile sensory abnormalities improved in parallel with spontaneous pain relief in certain chronic pain patients. In 1960, Nathan reported that measures which relieve pain and local tenderness, including measures that block some of the afferent fibers from the area, also may improve "the perception of stimuli," namely hypesthesia (Nathan 1960). This kind of improvement of tactile sensory abnormalities, which include not only hypesthesia but also allodynia, has been reported recently in many clinical studies involving sympathetic nerve block (Loh et al. 1978; Price et al.

1989), local anesthetic block (Arnér et al. 1990; Gracely et al. 1992), intravenous administration of lidocaine (Marchettini et al. 1992), and administration of an NMDA-receptor antagonist (Kristensen et al. 1992). The transient reversal of these tactile sensory abnormalities strongly suggests that the reversible allodynia and tactile hypesthesia are not caused by organic changes of peripheral nerves, rather they reflect the plastic changes in central perceptions. This agrees with the early notion made by Lindblom and Verrillo (1979) that both "hypoesthesia" and "painful tactile dysesthesia," (now called allodynia) may occur by central mechanisms. On the contrary, it is presumed that fixed areas of tactile sensory abnormalities, which are refractory to any treatment in patients with poor outcome grade, reflect either organic changes or loss of plasticity in peripheral and/or central nervous systems; i.e., deafferentation or lesions of dorsal horn neurons.

The temporary improvement of tactile sensory abnormalities itself, however, does not necessarily indicate excellent or good long-term outcomes, although the long-term good outcome can not be expected without the temporary improvement of the tactile sensory abnormalities. Gradual improvements of the tactile sensory abnormalities found by several sequential examinations during the course of repetitive treatments seem to be important (Fig. 3).

One of the most intriguing results of the present study is the four stages of improvement of the tactile sensory abnormalities observed in association with pain relief (Fig. 1). Some of these stages already have been reported fragmentarily. For example, Loh and Nathan (1978) reported that when the hyperpathia and hyperesthesia disappeared following a sympathetic block, the patient sometimes became aware of a diminution of sensibility, a numbness. This finding may correspond to stage II improvement of cutaneous sensory abnormalities in our study. The point is that the four stages occur sequentially in association with relief of spontaneous pain by repetitive therapeutic interventions. Thus, with careful sequential examinations and determinations of the changing pattern of these tactile sensory abnormalities, it becomes possible to evaluate patients' ongoing pain in a more objective manner.

What are the pathophysiological mechanisms of the four sequential stages of improvement of the tactile sensory abnormalities in association with pain relief in our study? We have a growing body of evidence that the peripheral nerve injury causes dynamic pathophysiological and anatomical changes in dorsal horn neurons (Devor et al. 1978; Woolf 1983; Sugimoto et al. 1987; Woolf 1991; Wolf and Thompson 1991), of which some may give us the clue to solve the problem. An important question is how does expansion of receptive fields of nociceptive neurons lead to hyperalgesia? Dubner proposed one hypothesis that "expanded receptive fields will lead to a greater number of neurons activated by a stimulus applied to a hyperalgesic zone than the same stimulus applied to a normal zone. The increase in neuronal activity may ultimately be perceived as more intense pain" (Dubner 1992). According to this hypothesis, reduction in the size of allodynia could be elucidated reversely by reduction in the size of receptive fields of dorsal horn neurons. The concept that cutaneous tactile sensory abnormalities are caused by the altered central processing of dorsal horn neurons through their changes of receptive fields seems to be extremely attractive for understanding the distribution and improvement patterns of abnormal tactile sensibilities. To prove the concept, at least two fields of investigations are mandatory. One is to investigate the character of receptive fields to tactile stimulation. The other is to establish a mathematical model elucidating the cutaneous tactile sensory abnormalities by the changes of receptive fields of dorsal horn neurons based on precise anatomical and physiological findings of the neuronal network. The essential part of the former investigations has already been reported by Hillmann and Wall (1969). They recognized three distinct zones as the receptive fields of lamina 5 cells in decerebrate cats (Fig. 4). The receptive fields of a single lamina 5 cell to tactile stimuli (touching and brushing) can be divided into two distinct zones. One is the excitatory zone, where the tactile stimulus causes excitation of the cell. The other is the inhibitory zone, where the same stimulus causes inhibition of the cell. The excitatory zone is surrounded by the inhibitory zone. They reported that both zones expanded (Fig. 4 SP) when the descending inhibitory fibers were blocked at the cephalad site by cooling. We would like to point out that there may be a correspondence of the distribution pattern of allodynia and tactile hypesthesia in our patients to that of excitatory and inhibitory zones in the receptive fields of lamina 5 of the decerebrate cats. We speculate that the change of these excitatory and inhibitory zones in the recep-

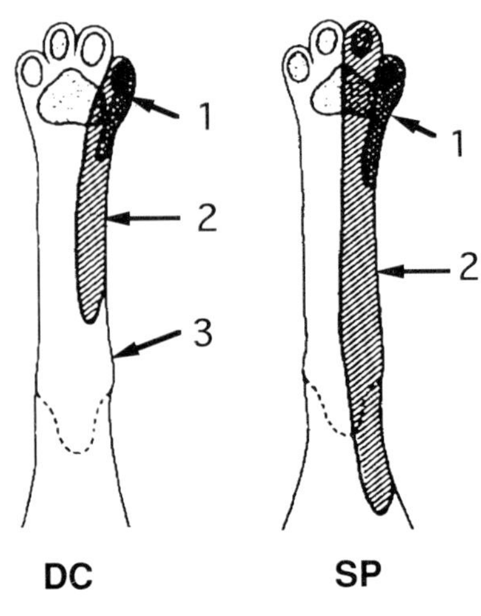

Fig. 4. Receptive fields of a single neuron in the lamina 5. **DC**: the receptive field in the decerebrate cat. *Zone 1*, the cell responded to brush, touch, and crushing of the skin. *Zone 2*, brushing inhibited the cell while pressure and pinch excited it. *Zone 3*, brush, touch, and pressure inhibited the cell but did not excite it. **SP**: the receptive field of the same cell after the lower thoracic spinal cord had been blocked by cooling. Zones 1 and 2 had expanded. Zone 3 had disappeared. (Reproduced from Hillman and Wall 1969)

tive field of dorsal horn neurons, which are influenced by descending inhibitory systems, play extremely important roles for the occurrence of both tactile hypesthesia and allodynia and their improvement in association with relief of pain by therapeutic interventions.

In conclusion, we have reported the pattern of improvement of tactile sensory abnormalities and the positive relation between such improvement of tactile sensory abnormality and relief of spontaneous pain. Sequential examinations of the tactile hypesthesia and allodynia can be helpful for evaluating the magnitude of pain in a more objective manner in patients with these sensory abnormalities.

REFERENCES

Arnér, S., Lindblom, U., Meyerson, B.A. and Molander, C., Prolonged relief of neuralgia after regional anesthetic blocks: a call for further experimental and systematic clinical studies, Pain, 43 (1990) 287–297.

Bonica, J.J., Definition and taxonomy of pain. In: J.J. Bonica (Ed.), The Management of Pain, 2nd ed., Lea & Febiger, Philadelphia, 1990, pp. 19.

Devor, M. and Wall, P.D., Reorganization of spinal cord sensory map after peripheral nerve injury, Nature, 276 (1978) 75–76.

Dubner, R., Neuronal plasticity and pain following peripheral tissue inflammation or nerve injury. In: M.R. Bond, J.E. Charlton and C.J. Woolf, (Eds.), Proc. VIth World Congress on Pain, Pain Research and Clinical Management, Vol. 5, Elsevier, Amsterdam, 1991, pp. 263–276.

Dubner, R., Hyperalgesia and expanded receptive fields, Pain, 48 (1992) 3–4.

Gracely, R.H., Lynch, S.A. and Bennett, G.J., Painful neuropathy: altered central processing maintained dynamically by peripheral input, Pain, (1992) 175–194.

Hillman, P. and Wall, P.D., Inhibitory and excitatory factors influencing the receptive fields of lamina 5 spinal cord cells, Exp. Brain Res., 9 (1969) 284–306.

Kristensen, J.D., Svensson, B. and Gordh, T. Jr., The NMDA-receptor antagonist CPP abolishes neurogenic 'wind-up pain' after intrathecal administration in humans, Pain, 51 (1992) 249–253.

Loh, L. and Nathan, P.W., Painful peripheral states and sympathetic blocks, J. Neurol. Neurosurg. Psychiat., 41 (1978) 664–671.

Lindblom, U. and Verrillo, R.T., Sensory functions in chronic neuralgia, J. Neurol. Neurol. Neurosurg. Psychiat., 42 (1979) 422–435.

Marchettini, P., Lacerenza, M., Marangoni, C., Pellegata, G., Sotgiu, M.L. and Smirne, S., Lidocaine test in neuralgia, Pain, 48 (1992) 377–382.

Merskey, H., Pain terms: a list with definitions and notes on usage. Recommended by the IASP Subcommittee on Taxonomy, Pain, 6 (1979) 249–252.

Merskey, H., Classification of chronic pain: description of chronic pain syndromes and definitions of pain terms, Pain, Suppl. 3 (1986) S215–S221.

Nathan, P.W., Improvement in cutaneous sensibility associated with relief of pain, J. Neurol. Neurol. Neurosurg. Psychiat., 23 (1960) 202–206.

Price, D.D., Bennett, G.J. and Rafii, A., Psychophysical observations on patients with neuropathic pain relieved by a sympathetic block, Pain, 36 (1989) 273–288.

Rogers, AG., The assessment of pain and pain relief in children with cancer, Pain, 11(Suppl) (1981) S11.

Rowbotham, M.C. and Fields, H.L., Post-herpetic neuralgia: the relation of pain complaint,

sensory disturbance, and skin temperature, Pain, 39 (1989) 129–144.
Simone, D.A., Baumann, T.K and LaMotte, R.H., Dose-dependent pain and mechanical hyperalgesia in humans after intradermal injection of capsaicin, Pain, 38 (1989) 99–107.
Sugimoto, T., Takemura, M., Sakai, A. and Ishimaru, M., Rapid transneuronal destruction following peripheral nerve transection in the medullary dorsal horn in enhanced by strychnine, picrotoxin and bicuculline, Pain, 30 (1987) 385–393.
Woolf, C.J., Evidence for a central component of post-injury pain hypersensitivity, Nature, 306 (1983) 686–688.
Woolf, C.J., Central mechanisms of acute pain. In: M.R. Bond, J.E. Charlton and C.J. Woolf (Eds.), Proceedings of the VIth World Congress on Pain. Pain Research and Clinical Management, Vol. 5. Elsevier, Amsterdam, 1991, pp. 25–34.
Woolf, C.J. and Thompson, S.W.N., The induction and maintenance of central sensitization is dependent on N-methyl-D-aspartic acid receptor activation: implications for the treatment of post-injury pain hypersensitivity states, Pain, 44 (1991) 293–299.

Correspondence to: K. Moriwaki, MD, PhD, Department of Anesthesiology and Critical Care Medicine, Hiroshima University School of Medicine, Kasumi 1-2-3 Minami-ku, Hiroshima 734, Japan. Tel: 81-82-257-5267; Fax: 81-82-256-6815.

Proceedings of the 7th World Congress on Pain,
Progress in Pain Research and Management, Vol. 2,
edited by G.F. Gebhart, D.L. Hammond, and T.S.
Jensen, IASP Press, Seattle, © 1994.

56

Sensory Descriptors from Touch to Pressure-Pain and Experimental Variables: A Psychophysiological Study in Human on Pressure-Pain Threshold

Gilles J. Lavigne,[a] Marc Thu Thon,[a] Pierre Rompré,[a]
Gary H. Duncan,[a] and Jean-Paul Goulet[b]

[a]*Faculté de Médecine Dentaire and Centre de Recherche en Sciences Neurologiques, Université de Montréal, and* [b] *Université Laval, Québec, Canada*

INTRODUCTION

The measurement of pressure pain thresholds (PPT) with a pressure algometer is a diagnostic procedure used to assess a variety of muscle pain syndromes (Fisher 1987a,b). Although several studies have shown that this procedure is reasonably reliable in the hands of trained researchers (Jensen et al. 1986; Reeves et al. 1986; Schiffman et al. 1988; List et al. 1989, 1990; Ohrbach and Gale 1989), its use in clinical situations may, nevertheless, be compromised by a number of methodological variables. In the interest of establishing a more rigorous method for studying the relationship between pressure stimulation and pain perception, we have developed and tested an electronically driven algometer (EDA) that we believe should aid both the researcher and the clinician in standardizing the assessment of muscle pain.

Our efforts to improve two procedural aspects of muscle pain assessment had two primary goals: (1) to give better stimulus control than is presently possible with the commonly employed hand-held algometer, and (2) to standardize and automate recording of the subject's responses to the pressure stimulation. In addition to assessing stimulus-delivery and data-acquisition techniques, we have conducted several studies comparing psychophysical data regarding the perception of pressure-induced pain with those involving the more commonly used heat-induced pain in order to further validate the use of pressure as an experimental pain stimulus. Finally, the EDA was used to assess how pressure-pain thresholds (PPT) are influenced by distraction and muscle contraction, variables that could influence both within- and between-subject comparisons of muscle pains.

This chapter thus summarizes the results of six experiments that:

1. compare PPT values determined using the EDA with those determined with a standard hand-held spring-loaded algometer;
2. compare subject- and experimenter-controlled response paradigms on PPT;
3. investigate the stimulus-response characteristics of innocuous and noxious pressure stimuli using visual analog scales (VAS) of pain intensity and unpleasantness;
4. assess the effects of pressure duration on pain intensity and unpleasantness ratings;
5. investigate the relationship between pressure magnitude and choice of sensory verbal descriptors; and
6. assess the effects of distraction and muscle contradiction on PPT.

METHODS

Forty-five asymptomatic men [mean age 25.7 ±. 0.8 (range 18–40); mean body weight 70.2 ± 1.1 kg (range 58–85 kg)] participated in these experiments (19 subjects participated in two experiments). All signed a university-approved consent form. An electronically driven algometer (EDA), designed and built in our laboratory, was used in all experiments along with, for experiment one, a spring-loaded, hand-held algometer (Pain Diagnostics and Thermography Co., NY, USA). Both instruments had a tip surface of 1 cm^2. PPT and subjective ratings of muscle pressure stimuli were determined over the jaw masseteric and/or arm brachioradialis muscles by a trained examiner using a standardized protocol. The patient sat in a dental chair to which the EDA was fixed to a frame that restrained the head or the arm with foam pads to prevent any motion while pressure was applied over selected sites. All tests were randomized and repeated six times in each experimental protocol; to avoid habituation and/or sensitization, no site was tested more frequently than once every five minutes.

In experiment 1, PPT values were estimated over the masseter muscle with a hand-held algometer and the EDA. With the EDA used in the fixed mode, pressure was increased at a constant rate of 0.5 kg/cm^2 per second; with the hand-held algometer, the investigator was trained to approximate the same rate of stimulus application. The tests were terminated at the first report of pain by a signal cue to the investigator who then turned off the EDA or stopped applying the manual pressure with the hand-held algometer.

For experiment 2, the EDA was employed in a fixed position to compare PPTs over the masseter muscle obtained using subject- and experimenter-controlled response paradigms. Thresholds were determined either by the subject's pressing a button to turn off the EDA at the first sensation of pain, or by the experimenter's termination of EDA stimulation when the subject signaled that pain threshold was reached.

In experiment 3, the stimulus-response characteristics associated with sensation evoked by muscle pressure were evaluated using the EDA to deliver stimuli between 0.5 and 3.0 kg/cm^2, at 0.5 kg/cm^2 per second increments, randomly presented to the right and left jaw masseteric and arm brachioradialis muscles. Following each stimulus period, subjects rated pain intensity and unpleasantness on a 100-mm visual analogue scale (VAS).

In experiment 4, which assessed the effects of stimulus duration, the desired pressure was reached at a rate of 1 kg/cm^2 per second and then was sustained for a total test duration of one, two, or three seconds at 1.0 kg/cm^2 and two and three seconds at 2 kg/cm^2. All the tests were performed in random order, on both muscles. Subjected rated pain as in experiment 3.

During experiment 5, subjects used sensory verbal descriptors (Table I) to characterize the magnitude of pressure stimuli ranging from 0.5 to 3.0 kg/cm^2, at 0.5 kg/cm^2 per second increments. Following each stimulus, delivered randomly on the jaw masseteric muscle, subjects chose the most appropriate word from the list of seven French sensory verbal descriptors.

Finally, experiment 6 used the EDA to assess the influence of muscle contraction and distraction on PPTs. Reports of PPT during a rest condition were compare with those obtained while the subject maintained a constant level of contraction (50% of maximum) in the muscle being tested. Tests involving the masseter muscle employed an electromyographic biofeedback system (Myotrac, Thought Technology, Montréal, Canada) to monitor muscle contraction, while those involving the brachioradialis muscle used a hand-grip dynamometer (Stoeling-Smedley Dynamometer, USA). The distraction task consisted of reading a difficult text.

Statistical analyses employed MANOVA for repeated measures with C-Matrix sample contrasts when appropriate (Sysat software, IL, USA). Simple regressions were used to estimate the correlation. A significance level of

Table I
Sensory verbal descriptors used for
PPT evaluation (in French)

Pressure	Pain
Touch (toucher)	Light (légère)
Light (légère)	Moderate (modérée)
Moderate (modérée)	Strong (forte)
Strong (forte)	

$P < 0.05$ was used. Sample sizes were estimated, similarly to Jensen et al. (1986), for each experiment with an alpha of 0.05 and a power of 0.80.

RESULTS

Experiment 1: Comparison of PPTs obtained using the EDA and hand-held algometer: The mean PPT was 33% less when pain was evoked using the EDA, compared with that evoked using a spring-loaded, hand-held algometer (Fig. 1). Although this difference was significant, (F[1,7] - 32.3; $P = 0.001$), measurements using the EDA were not more precise as seen by the variance attributed to the two stimulation methods (S.E.M. = 0.13 and 0.14, respectively).

Experiment 2: Comparison of subject- and experimenter-controlled response paradigms on PPT: Compared with that observed in the experimenter-controlled tests, the mean PPT was 11% less when the subjects themselves terminated the test by pressing the push-button (Fig. 2). Although this effect was statistically significant (F[1,9] = 7.8; $P = 0.02$), the threshold was shifted without reducing the variability of the measurement (S.E.M. = 0.2, for both cases).

Experiment 3: Stimulus-response characteristics derived using the EDA: For both muscles tested (Fig. 3A and B), VAS ratings of pain intensity (Int) and unpleasantness (Unp) were a linear function of stimulus magnitude (F[1,7] = 52.9; $P < 0.001$ and $r^2 = 0.98$ and 0.96 for masseteric INT and UNP ratings; F[1,9] = 29.4; $P < 0.001$ and $r^2 = 0.98$ for both brachioradialis ratings). VAS ratings for pain intensity were always higher than those of unpleasantness, although this difference was not significant for the brachioradialis (F[1,9] = 1.; $P = 0.24$); significant differences were noted for the masseters muscle (F[1,7]: 9.8; $P < 0.05$) at 1.0 and 1.5 kg/cm^2.

Experiment 4: Effect of stimulus duration on VAS pain ratings: Fig. 4A illustrates that stimulus durations of one, two, or three seconds did not significantly influence the ratings of either pain intensity or of unpleasantness evoked

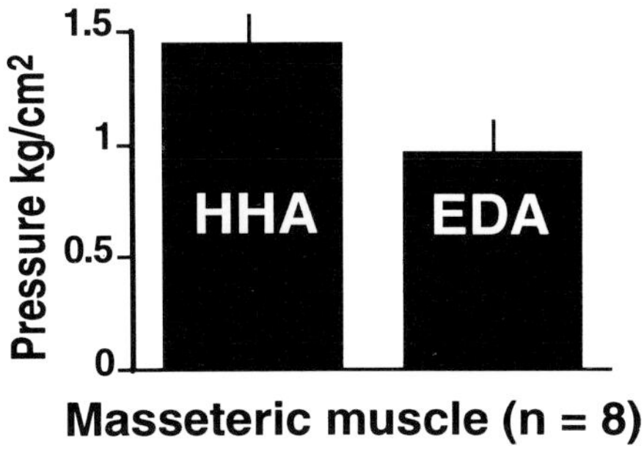

Fig. 1. Difference in PPT using a manually driven HHA (hand-held algometer) or the EDA (electronically driven algometer) fixed to a frame. The investigator terminated pressure application. No difference was noted between right and left masseteric muscles ($F[1,7] = 2.7$; $P = 0.14$); consequently, data were pooled.

by a stimulus pressure of 1 kg/cm^2 ($F[2,14] = 2.3$; $P = 0.13$ for masseters and $F[2,14] = 0.39$; $P = 0.67$ for brachioradialis). Similar results were observed for stimulus durations of two and three seconds applied to a pressure of 2 kg/cm^2 (Fig. 4B). These data indicate that the duration of the stimulus does not explain the linear relationship between stimulus magnitude and pain ratings observed in experiment 3.

Experiment 5: Sensory verbal descriptors chosen to characterize pressure stimuli: Interestingly, although all levels of pressure stimuli had been rated as unpleasant or painful on the pain VAS (Fig. 3), all subjects chose words in the innocuous pressure range for the 0.5 kg/cm^2 stimuli (Fig. 5 and Table II). Similarly, only 6% of the subjects reported light pain sensations for a pressure stimulation of 1.0 kg/cm^2. For the 3.0 kg/cm^2 stimulus, 22% reported a sensation of strong pressure while 78% chose descriptors indicating light to strong pain.

Experiment 6: Influence of distraction and muscle contraction on PPT: Shifting the focus of attention with the distraction task, as used in this study, had no significant effect on PPT. The statistical analyses, however, revealed that muscle contraction did influence the PPT values of both the masseteric and brachioradialis muscles ($F[2,18] = 9.6$; $P < 0.01$ and $F[2,18] = 9.0$; $P < 0.01$ respectively (Fig. 6). Simple contrast analysis further showed a significant increase of at least 36% in PPT when subjects maintained voluntary contraction of approximately 50% of their maximum capacity.

DISCUSSION

Our experiments have shown that an electronically-driven algometer (EDA) and subject-controlled response paradigm minimize the apparent thresholds determined for pressure pain; however, they had no influence on the variation of the measures. In addition, these studies support the validity of pressure-pain

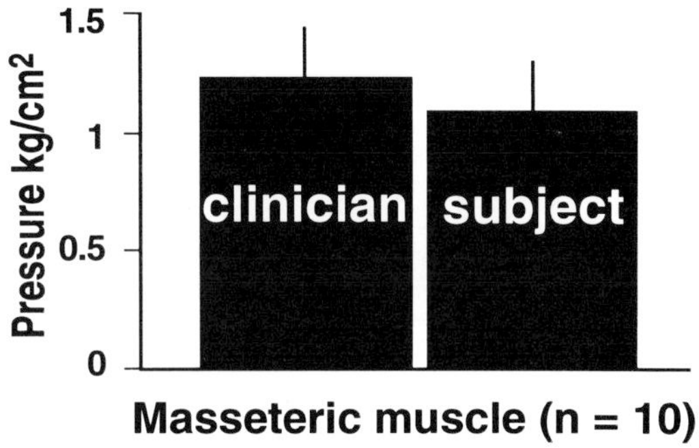

Fig. 2. Difference in PPT when the investigator or the subject stopped the test. The EDA was used over the masseteric muscle.

measurements by demonstrating a linear relationship between the strength of the pressure stimuli applied and the subjects' visual analog and verbal responses, an effect that was shown to be independent of the duration of the stimulation. And, most importantly, we observed a substantial effect of muscle contraction on the determination of PPT.

Lower PPT values were obtained when recorded with the EDA instead of the hand-held algometer (HHA). The difference could probably be explained by the manually controlled rate of pressure application required by the HHA and/or by the additional reaction time needed to interrupt the pressure application. To terminate the stimulus using the HHA, the experimenter must move an arm and/or the upper body; in comparison, use of the EDA requires only that the experimenter lift a finger switch that instantly allows removal of the stimulus. However, because both systems exhibit similar precision characteristics (with almost identical S.E.M.), the HHA may be preferred in some clinical environments because of its smaller size and simplicity. Users must then be aware that the resulting PPT will fall in a higher range of values than that reported with most automated systems.

In using a subject-controlled response paradigm, PPT values also were lower than the ones observed under experimenter-controlled conditions. These higher measurements were not surprising and probably reflect the longer latency resulting from time elapsed between the subject's cue signal and the reaction time of the investigator. In a previous study, Jensen (1990) used a similar subject-controlled system to assess PPT, but gave no rationale and no data in favor of such a system. As in Jensen's study, our data do not show any reduction in the variability of the subject-controlled measurements—the S.E.M. is identical with both technics. Although neither approach seems better in terms of accuracy, elimination of the investigator's reaction time would, in principle, increase the validity of repeated PPT measurements. An obvious conclusion from these two experiments is that PPT data recorded with

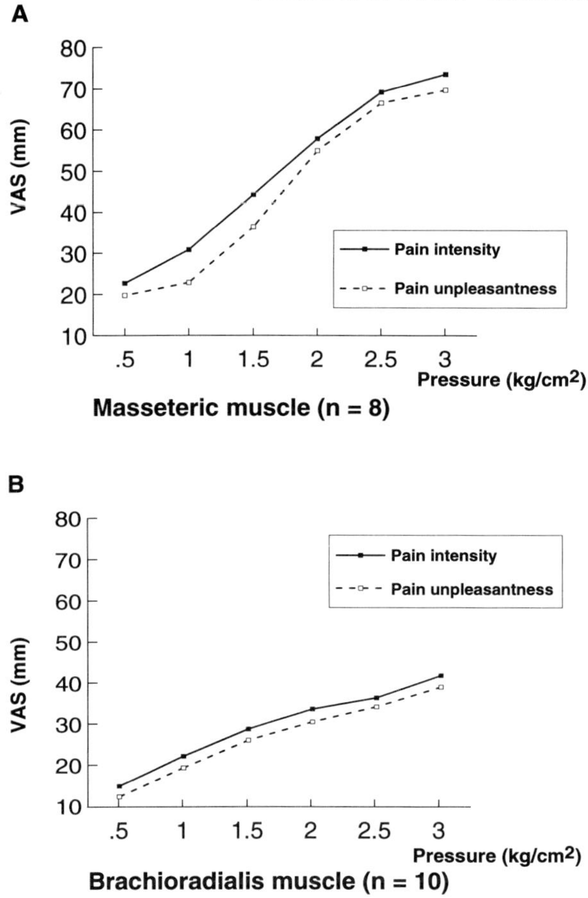

Fig. 3. Stimulus-response characteristics of pressure algometer. **A,** data of jaw masseteric muscles; **B,** data of arm brachioradialis.

algometers using different drive modalities or interruption paradigms should be compared with caution.

Jensen (1990) has suggested a linear relationship between pain and pressure stimulus magnitude, but did not present supportive data. To our knowledge, we are the first to report data showing linear relations between VAS pain reports and pressure magnitude for both jaw and arm muscles. Interestingly, this relationship was similar to that observed for thermal pain (Duncan et al. 1989). Moreover, for stimuli between 0.5 and 3.0 kg/cm^2, subjects clearly discriminate pressure differences of 0.5 kg/cm^2. Furthermore, the results of experiment 4 indicate that the linear stimulus-response relationship was not due to the longer duration of the larger stimulus because increasing the duration of 1 or 2 kg/cm^2 had no significant effect on pressure-pain ratings. We conducted our experiment with normal, young subjects; we do not know whether this degree of discriminative ability applies to muscle-pain patients.

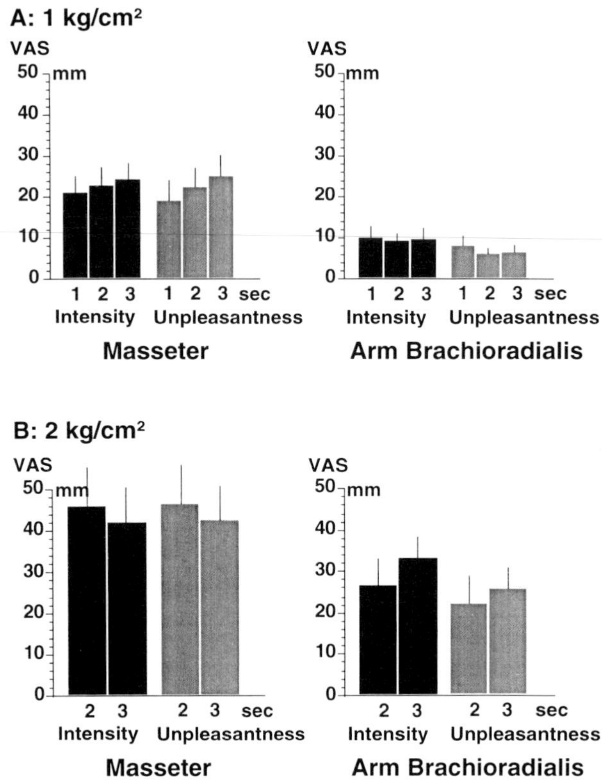

Fig. 4. Effect of stimulus duration (1 to 3 sec) on VAS ratings for a stimulus magnitude of 1 (**A**) and 2 (**B**) kg/cm^2 for both masseter and brachioradialis muscles (n = 8).

Although pain was reported on the VAS for every level of pressure presented, parallel reports of sensory verbal descriptor responses suggest that low pressure (0.5 kg/cm^2) stimuli evoked no pain sensation at all. This apparent evaluation of perceived pain at low stimulus levels may reflect the subjects' tendency to make some small response on the VAS; however, it is unknown if this represents the "prepain sensation" (Handwerker and Kobal 1993). At the other extreme, it appears that even though all subjects rated high scores on the VAS for 3.0 kg, only 78% used pain verbal descriptive words for this level of stimulation, while 22% reported only strong pressure; these findings suggest some discrepancy between the sensory VAS reports and the selection of a descriptive word.

The distraction task used in our study, reading a text, had no significant effect on PPT. Our results differ from those of others for two possible reasons: differences in the attentional manipulation and in the nature of the stimulus. For example, Miron et al. (1989) observed that active participation of the subjects in a detection task involving a different sensory modality decreased their ratings of noxious thermal stimuli. Interestingly, another presentation at

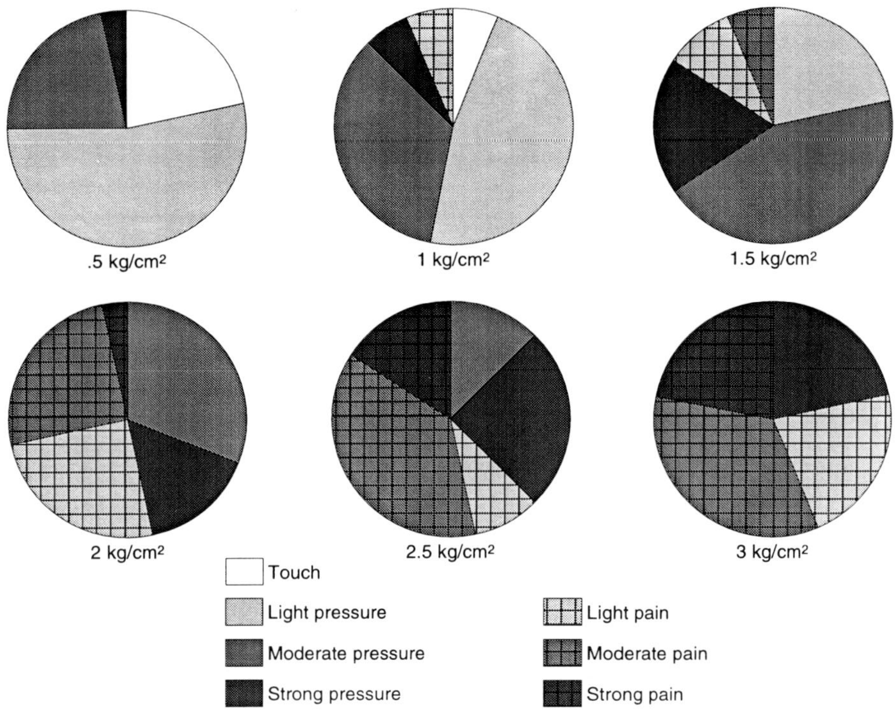

Fig. 5. Sensory verbal descriptors chosen to characterize pressure of different magnitudes. Same subjects as for experiments 3 and 4. Data are presented in %; Table II gives the raw values.

Table II
Sensory verbal descriptors chosen to characterize pressure at different magnitudes (raw data in %)

Pressure (kg)	Touch	Light Pressure	Moderate Pressure	Strong Pressure	Light Pain	Moderate Pain	Strong Pain
0.5	22	53	22	3	0	0	0
1	6	47	34	6	6	0	0
1.5	0	22	44	19	9	6	0
2	0	0	31	16	25	25	3
2.5	0	0	12	25	9	38	16
3	0	0	0	22	22	34	22

Note: These data are presented graphically in Fig. 5.

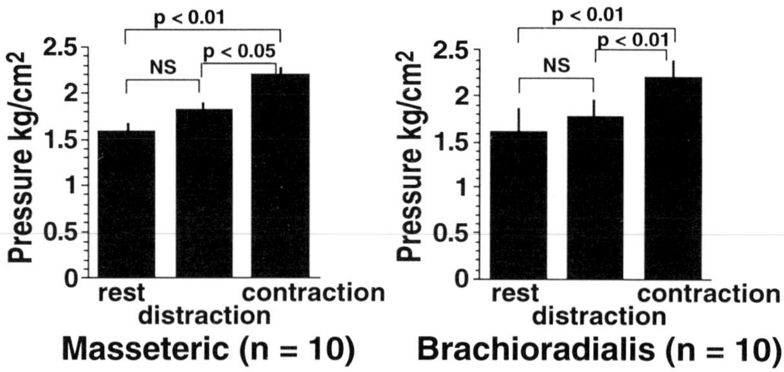

Fig. 6. Influences of distraction and muscle contraction on PPT for both muscles. The *P* values are for simple contrast analysis.

this World Congress reported that reading a novel was associated with a great variability of the threshold and amplitude of the nociceptive reflex RIII (Docekal et al. 1993). The different attentional effects observed in these studies could be due to different levels of arousal associated with protective mechanisms evoked by thermal, electric, and pressure stimuli. The possible effects of the attentional and stimulus-related variables on the determination of pain thresholds need further study.

One of the most important observations of our study is that moderate muscle contraction significantly elevates the apparent PPT. Similarly, Kosek and Ekholm (1993) reported comparable observations in asymptomatic subjects using a lower level of voluntary contraction (30%). A recent study from McMillan and Lawson (in press) reports similar findings, showing that PPT measured over the temporalis muscle increased in a linear fashion when subjects clenched their teeth with increasing force. From a clinical perspective, these findings are important because the level of muscle contraction during the examination procedure of a subject could vary for numerous reasons. This point is supported by our recent study of patients with torticollis, a dystonia associated with muscle pain. Without control of the level of muscle contraction, these patients had the same PPT, both at trapezius or sternocleidomastoid muscles, as did their matched controls. However, a reevaluation of the PPT in controls while they contracted their neck muscles revealed higher PPT than those observed in torticollis patients (Lavigne et al. 1992). The level of muscle contraction thus is an important parameter and needs to be standardized when estimating PPT. This factor is even more important when we compare contralateral muscles in a patient; the PPT could be even more variable due to different level of muscle activity.

ACKNOWLEDGMENTS

The authors thank L. TenBokum for his research skills in electrotechnics; F. Guitard and L. Noce for the experiments; C. Manzini for the graphics; A. Tremblay for manuscript preparation; and A. Lobbezo-Scholte for reviewing this chapter. The research was supported by the Fonds de la recherche en santé du Québec and the Canadian MRC.

REFERENCES

Docekal, P., Convers, P., Peyron, R., Laurent, B., Michel, D., Nociceptive reflex R III and subjective evaluation of pain: the influence of the repeated stimulation and of the distracting effect of the selective attention. In: Abstracts: 7th World Congress on Pain, IASP Publications, Seattle, 1993, p. 156

Duncan, G.H., Bushnell, M.C., Lavigne, G.J., Comparison of verbal and visual analogous scales for measuring the intensity and unpleasantness of experimental pain, Pain, 37 (1989) 295–303.

Fischer, A.A., Pressure algometry over normal muscles. Standard values, validity and reproducibility of pressure threshold, Pain, 30 (1987a) 115–126.

Fischer, A.A., Pressure threshold measurement for diagnosis of myofascial pain and the evaluation of treatment results, Clin. J. Pain, 2 (1987b), 207–214.

Handwerker, H.O. and Kobal, G., Psychophysiology of experimentally induced pain, Physiol. Rev., 73, 3 (1993) 639–671.

Jensen, K., Quantification of tenderness by palpation and use of pressure algometers. In: J.R. Friction and E. A. Awad (Eds.), Myofascial Pain and Fibromyalgia, Advances in Pain Research and Therapy, Vol. 17. Raven Press, New York, 1990, pp. 165–181.

Jensen, K., Andersen, H.O., Olesen, J. and Lindblom, U., Pressure-pain threshold in human temporal region: evaluation of a new pressure algometer, Pain, 25 (1986) 313–323.

Kosek, E. and Eckholm, J., Modulation of pressure pain thresholds during and following isometric contraction. In: Abstracts: 7th World Congress on Pain, IASP Publications, Seattle, 1993, p. 153.

Lavigne, G.J., Rémillard, G., Thu Thon, M., Guitard, F., Rompré, P.H. and Montplaisir, J., Spasmodic torticollis and sleep: a controlled study, Sleep Res., 21 (1992) abstract 226.

List, T., Helkimo, M. and Falk, G., Reliability and validity of a pressure threshold meter in recording tenderness in the masseter muscle and the anterior temporalis muscle, J. Craniomand. Pract., 7, 3 (1989) 223–229.

List, T., Helkimo, M., Karlsson, R., Influence of pressure rates on the reliability of a pressure threshold meter, J. Craniomand Disord. Facial Oral Pain, 5 (1991), 173–178.

McMillan, A.S. and Lawson, E.T., Effect of tooth clenching and jaw opening on pressure-pain thresholds in the human jaw muscles, J. Orofacial Pain, (in press).

Miron, D., Duncan, G.H., Bushnell, M.C., Effects of attention of the intensity and unpleasantness of thermal pain, Pain, 39 (1989) 345–352.

Ohrbach, R. and Gale, E.N., Pressure pain threshold, clinical assessment, and differential diagnosis: reliability and validity in patients with myogenic pain, Pain, 39, (1989) 157–169.

Reeves, J.L., Jaeger, B., Graff-Radford, S.B., Reliability of the pressure algometer as a measure of myofacial trigger point sensitivity, Pain, 24, (1986) 313–321.

Schiffman, E., Fricton, J., Haley, D. and Tylka, D., A pressure algometer for myofascial pain syndrome: reliability and validity testing. In: R. Dubner, G.F. Gebhart and M.R. Bond (Eds.), Proceedings of the Vth World Congress on Pain. Pain Research and Clinical Managment, Vol. 3. Elsevier, Amsterdam, 1988, pp. 407–413.

Correspondence to: Gilles J. Lavigne, Faculté de médecine dentaire, Université de Montréal, C.P. 6128, Centre Ville, Montréal, Québec H3C 3J7, Canada. Tel: 514-343-2310; Fax: 514-343-2233.

Proceedings of the 7th World Congress on Pain,
Progress in Pain Research and Management, Vol. 2,
edited by G.F. Gebhart, D.L. Hammond, and T.S.
Jensen, IASP Press, Seattle, © 1994.

57

The Somatotopic Organization of Nociceptor-Induced Vascular Response Pattern Reflects Central Nociceptive Processing in Humans

Walter Magerl,[a,c] Martin Koltzenburg,[b,c]
Dirk Meyer-Jürgens,[c] and Hermann O. Handwerker[c]

[a]Institut für Physiologie und Pathophysiologie, Universität Mainz, Germany;
[b]Neurologische Klinik, Universität Würzburg, Germany;
and [c]Institut für Physiologie und Biokybernetik, Universität Erlangen-Nürnberg, Erlangen, Germany

INTRODUCTION

There is a long and elaborate tradition of reflex measurement in pain research, sustained by the assumption that protective reflex responses are intimately linked to nociception in order to counteract factual or potential damages to an organism. In Sherrington's words, "Pain is the psychical adjunct to protective reflexes" (Sherrington 1900). In the past, however, research has mainly concentrated on the analysis of skeletomotor withdrawal reflexes, notably tail flick, paw flick or head flick (D'Amour and Smith 1941; Randall and Selitto 1957; Hargreaves et al. 1988).

We know from everyday experience that painful events may also lead to strong excitation of autonomic effector systems, but careful examination of autonomic responses has yielded conflicting results in many of the parameters. Rapid adaptation and proneness to habituation were reported to be associated with autonomic response, which seemingly precludes their use as robust output parameters for pain assessment. Consequently, these parameters have attracted less attention as tools for the investigation of the sensory-discriminative dimension of nociception, and it has been suggested that autonomic responses may perhaps primarily reflect the emotional-affective rather than sensory-discriminative dimension of the pain experience (Chapman et al. 1985). However, we have recently been able to show in human volunteers that a distinct component of sustained vasoconstrictor reflexes may adapt very slowly and be almost devoid of habituation (Magerl et al. 1990b). These reflexes also readily reflect intensity and discrimination of painful stimuli (Magerl et al. 1990b; Nakagawa et al. 1993).

Here we present evidence that the sustained nociception-related vascular reflex component, but not arousal responses, exhibits differentially a specific, somatotopically organized pattern. This is reminiscent of a nociceptor-driven autonomic response pattern in animals and suggests that the sustained vascular reflex pattern reflects the spinal segmental processing of nociceptive afferent inputs.

METHODS

Experiments were conducted to determine the temporal and spatial pattern of somatosensory-induced autonomic reflexes in human volunteers, comparing the perception of sustained-type noxious stimulation with the pattern of skin vascular responses.

EXPERIMENT 1: NOXIOUS INPUT AND AUTONOMIC OUTPUT AT DIFFERENT SEGMENTAL LEVELS

Twenty-two young male volunteers (age: 22–30, mean: 26 years) participated in the experiment, which consisted of repetitive painful squeezing of the interdigital skin for 2 minutes using feedback-controlled forceps (8 N with a stylus of 6 mm diameter; for details see Magerl et al. 1990b) or painful electrical stimulation of tooth pulp of vital incisors for 2 minutes. The tooth was isolated against the oral cavity by a rubber foil. The labial surface of the incisor was then carefully cleansed both mechanically and chemically with a 3% solution of hydrogen peroxide. A rubber foam chamber containing an Ag/AgCl-plate electrode was glued to the labial incisor surface. The closed chamber was injected with electrolyte gel and sealed with cyanoacrylate. The active electrode had an area of 16 mm^2, and a larger reference electrode (300 mm^2) was placed inside the oral cavity. The impedance of the pair of electrodes was checked before and after the experimental session (range: 400–700 kΩ, mean: 590 kΩ) to exclude current leakage at the dental surface and to certify current passage through the pulp. Electrical pain thresholds ranged from 14 to 44 μA (mean: 30 μA). During the experimental sessions, dental pulp was stimulated at twice individual pain threshold (2 ms pulse width at 15 Hz for 2 min). Squeeze stimuli were alternated with electrical stimulation of tooth pulp in 10-minute intervals (4 stimuli each). Skin vascular reflexes of the ipsilateral thumb and head (cheek and earlobe) were measured by laser Doppler flowmetry (LDF; Periflux Pf2B, Perimed, Stockholm, Sweden). Arterial blood pressure and heart rate were monitored continuously at the contralateral middle finger using a noninvasive cuff method (FINAPRES, Ohmeda, Zürich, Switzerland).

EXPERIMENT 2: NOXIOUS INPUT AND AUTONOMIC OUTPUT WITHIN A SEGMENTAL LEVEL

Noxious chemical stimulation was used to excite selectively skin nociceptors. A cotton pad was soaked in 500 µl of pure mustard oil (allylisothiocyanate, Merck, Darmstadt) and placed into a closed chamber glued to the ventral forearm in 12 subjects (9 men, 3 women, 24–50 years) for 10 minutes to elicit burning pain (stimulated skin area: 5 cm^2). After 10 minutes, the remaining mustard oil was removed with soft cotton pads. The stimulation was repeated on the contralateral arm in 10 of the 12 subjects after several weeks. Histamine (1% aqueous solution of histamine dihydrochloride, Serva, Heidelberg) was iontophoresed from the chamber with a constant current of 330 µA for 10 minutes (total charge transferred: 200 mC) in 10 of the 12 subjects to elicit itch (for details see Magerl and Handwerker 1988, Magerl et al. 1990a). The autonomic reflex responses were assessed under thermoneutral conditions (24 ± 0.5 °C) in the palms of both hands by computer-aided infrared thermography (AGEMA 870) operating at 2–5 µm wavelength (thermal infrared; sensitivity: 0.1 °C). Thermograms were taken at 30-second intervals and analyzed off-line by densitometry.

In experiments 1 and 2, the subjects rated their sensations of either pain or itch at 10-second intervals on an electronic visual analogue scale (VAS).

The experiments were approved by the ethics committee of the medical faculty of the University of Erlangen-Nürnberg, and subjects were freely consenting volunteers according to the declaration of Helsinki.

RESULTS

ROSTRO-CAUDAL ORGANIZATION OF VASCULAR REFLEXES TO NOXIOUS INPUT

We adjusted the stimulation of the skin and dental pulp to produce comparable magnitudes of pain sensation on average, as determined in pilot experiments. The average pain ratings throughout the 2-minute stimulation period were therefore of almost equal magnitude (43.0 ± 2.6 for squeeze stimuli vs. 41.4 ± 2.0% of VAS for pulp stimuli, $P > 0.50$, *t* test).

Painful stimulation of either type led to a typical sequence of vascular responses in both body regions. Using the nomenclature introduced by Sokolov (1963), we will refer to "digital responses" for responses in the thumb and to "cephalic responses" for responses in the skin of the head.

We observed vasodilation in the skin of the cheek and earlobe. Responses in the cheek and earlobe were qualitatively and quantitatively identical. The structure of these cephalic vasodilatation reflexes were characterized by

- rapid rise of cutaneous blood flow following stimulus onset, which readily adapted within the first minute of stimulation, and
- vasodilatation of similar time course but smaller amplitude following the end of stimulation (Fig. 1A).

In contrast, vasoconstrictor reflexes were registered in the thumb and consisted of

- a rapid "on-response" phase with steeply rising and steeply declining flanks, followed by
- a tonic vasoconstrictor response lasting for the remaining stimulus time. During this time segment, vasoconstriction adapted very slowly and was followed by
- a rapid "off-response" phase following the end of 2 minutes of stimulation, similar to the initial phasic response (Fig. 1B).

We analyzed separately the different components of the vascular responses for their dependence on stimulus type and region (hand vs. tooth pulp) and region of blood-flow recording (head vs. digits) by a two-way analysis of variance (ANOVA). Vascular responses in the head and digits were qualitatively different at every time during and shortly after stimulation. In the thumb, we observed vasoconstriction, whereas vasodilatation prevailed in the skin of the head. The difference was highly significant (ANOVA, $P << 0.0001$ each; Table I). The early- and late-phase reflex components were differentially affected by the different sites of stimulus application. The amplitudes and latencies of the phasic immediate responses following switching on or off of the stimulus ("on" and "off" components) were almost identical, and neither depended on the type or region of stimulus application (ANOVA, $P > 0.60$ each). In contrast, the late tonic reflex component (the nociceptor-specific component) was markedly influenced by the different stimulus sites (ANOVA, $P < 0.0001$; Table I). Even within each LDF recording site, the response

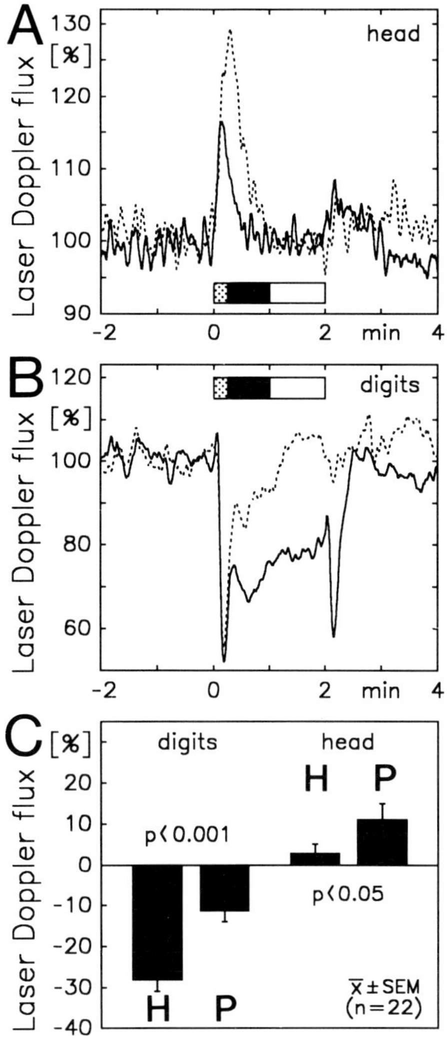

Fig. 1. Average vascular responses to painful stimulation of the hand or tooth pulp. **A:** Vasodilatation in the skin of the head (cheeks and earlobes), which appears to be enhanced and prolonged after painful electrical stimulation of the tooth pulp (dashed line) compared to painful squeezing of the skin of the hand (continuous line). **B:** Vasoconstriction develops in the skin of the digits (thumbs). A sustained late-phase component (> 15 s) is enhanced after painful squeezing the skin of the hand compared to painful tooth pulp stimulation. The duration of the stimuli (2 min) is marked by the horizontal bar in A and B. The stippled segment corresponds to the phase, which was operationally defined as the early reflex phase (1–15 s). The black segment corresponds to the period, which was defined as the late ("nociceptor-related") reflex phase (>15 s). **C:** Analysis of the late-phase component of vascular reflexes in the head and digits following painful squeeze stimuli at the hand (H) and painful electrical pulp stimuli (P) (mean ± SEM). The reflexes in both skin areas are significantly more intense after close (homotopic) as compared to remote (heterotopic) painful stimuli.

magnitudes were significantly different depending on the stimulus type. The slowly adapting digital vasoconstriction during painful squeezing of the interdigital skin averaged –28.20 ± 2.70% compared to –11.50 ± 2.55% after painful pulp stimulation ($P < 0.001$, *t* test). The late phase of the cephalic vasodilatation after pulp stimulation was on average 11.12 ± 3.80% compared to 2.99 ± 2.14% after painful squeezing ($P < 0.05$, *t* test; Fig. 1C). The latter difference is probably caused by a late second shoulder which is present in the vasodilatation following tooth pulp stimulation but not following squeezing of interdigital skin (Fig. 1A). Thus only the late reflex component was largely determined by the spatial relationship of stimulation and LDF recording site.

Table I
Two-way ANOVA on the components of the vascular reflexes elicited by painful stimuli (F values and statistical significance)

Factor	On Component	Nociceptor-Specific Component	Off Component
Stimulation site*	0.17 (n.s.)	16.62 (P < 0.0001)	0.00 (n.s.)
LDF site†	167.17 (P < 0.0001)	78.00 (P < 0.0001)	27.83 (P < 0.0001)
Stimulation site × LDF site interaction	0.46 (n.s.)	1.98 (n.s.)	2.14 (n.s.)

*Body region where stimuli were applied.
†Body region where vascular reflexes were obtained by laser Doppler flowmetry.
n.s. = not significant.

In general, there appeared to be a parallel shift of response magnitudes between head and hand areas of blood flow recording by approximately 10–15%, such that the local cutaneous LDF responses at each recording site were significantly more pronounced when induced by painful stimulation of a spatially close (homotopic) than by stimulation of a remote (heterotopic) area. The phasic on- and off-responses were totally independent of the stimulation site, however, suggesting that they may reflect a non-nociceptive arousal or startle response.

Painful stimulation of either type induced slight cardiovascular changes characterized by a pressor response (approximately 6%) and heart rate deceleration (approximately –3%). There were no differences between stimulus types regarding the amplitude and time course in heart rate and blood pressure.

BILATERAL ORGANIZATION OF VASCULAR REFLEXES TO NOXIOUS INPUT

Histamine and mustard oil, which are known to excite overlapping subsets of human cutaneous nociceptors (Handwerker et al. 1991), resulted in sensations of different qualities. Application of mustard oil elicited a strong sensation of burning pain that outlasted stimulation time (10 min) by more than an hour. Histamine iontophoresis led to an equally fast rising sensation of itch that peaked early, after 2–3 minutes. Itch sensation declined much faster than burning pain and was essentially gone after 30 minutes (Fig. 2A).

Upon stimulation, an immediate cooling of the palmar skin developed in all of the histamine (10/10) and almost all of the mustard oil (21/22) experiments. A thermographic specimen record is shown for mustard oil in Fig. 3. The time course of the skin cooling largely matched the time course of the

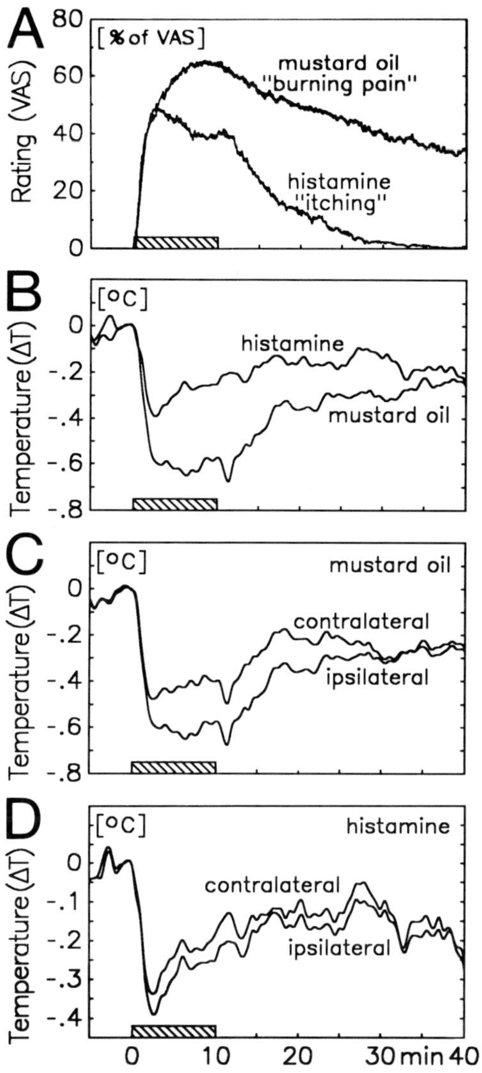

Fig. 2. Temporal relationship of nociceptor-induced sensations (pain or itch) and the palmar cooling reflex. **A:** Pain and itch sensation increase rapidly after stimulus onset. After 2–3 minutes, the time courses of the VAS rating magnitudes differ. Histamine-induced itching diminishes slightly even during ongoing stimulation, and more rapidly after the end of histamine iontophoresis. Mustard oil–induced burning pain increases progressively during stimulation and wanes slowly after wiping the mustard oil from the skin surface. **B:** The time course of the palmar cooling reflexes mirror the VAS ratings during and after stimulation. At 20–30 min after stimulation, the relationship becomes unstable, presumably because of overlapping thermoregulatory changes. **C** and **D:** Similar time courses are observed in the ipsilateral and contralateral palm after induction of burning pain by mustard oil (**C**) and itch sensation by histamine iontophoresis (**D**), but the response magnitude is generally smaller contralateral to the stimulated side. The duration of stimulus delivery (10 min) is marked by a hatched bar at the bottom of each figure.

pain or itch rating with respect to onset, peak, plateau, and decline during and after stimulation (Fig. 2B). Quantitative differences between histamine- and mustard oil–induced cooling responses generally corresponded to quantitative differences in the respective percept, that is, higher magnitude of pain and reflexes after mustard oil vs. lower magnitude of itch and reflexes after histamine. Reflex magnitudes thus fit into the same kind of response pattern predicted by the corresponding ratings of pain or itch magnitude ($r = 0.49$, $P < 0.005$).

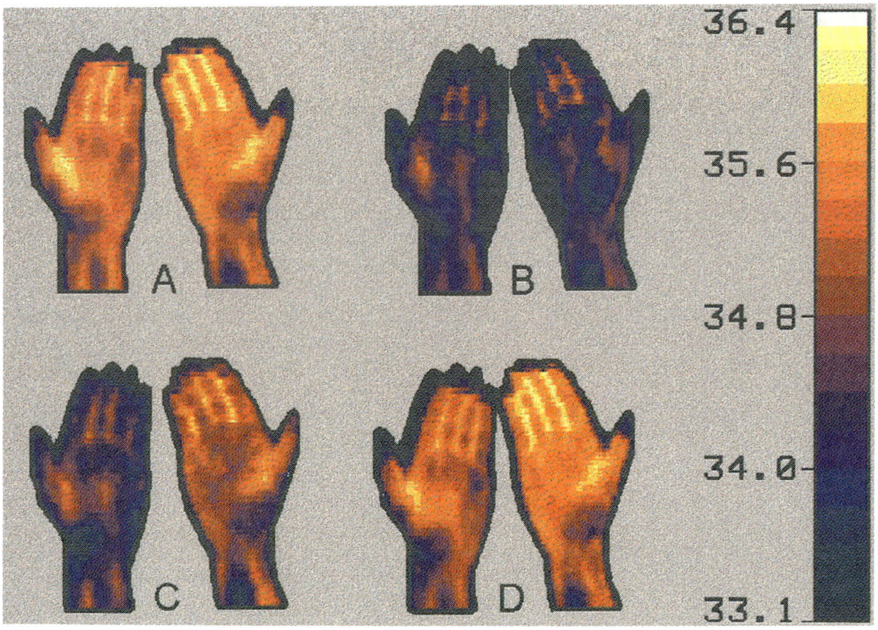

Fig. 3. A specimen thermographic record of the palmar cooling pattern following topical mustard oil stimulation of the left ventral forearm. The skin surface temperatures are shown in false color codes (see color code panel at right). **A:** Baseline, **B:** 2 minutes after stimulation, **C:** 10 minutes after stimulation, **D:** 30 minutes after stimulation. This typical temporal sequence of responses illustrates the symmetry of palmar skin temperatures prior to noxious stimulation (**A**). Skin cooling is induced by the painful stimulus, and thermal asymmetry between palms develops. A more intense cooling is seen ipsilateral to the side of stimulus application (**B** and **C**). Recovery of the skin temperature and restoration of the thermal balance emerges when the perception of burning pain fades (**D**).

Reflexes may be homogeneously induced by both nociceptive submodalities, irrespective of their different qualities, and may be maintained for prolonged periods in parallel to the subjective perceptions.

The cooling reflexes were qualitatively similar but quantitatively different on both sides of the body. They were consistently smaller contralateral to the site of stimulus application both after mustard oil (20 of 22 cases; Fig. 2C) and after histamine (7 of 10 cases) (Fig. 2D). The reverse was never observed. The difference developed immediately upon onset of stimulation and was statistically significant for the time of stimulus application and for 20 minutes after mustard oil and 5 minutes after histamine. The magnitude of ipsilateral and contralateral reflex responses was highly correlated at any time ($r > 0.85$, typically 0.95). The proportion of contralateral attenuation was rather constant (27 % on average) and correlated to ipsilateral and contralateral reflex magnitudes ($r = 0.64$). Additionally, the degree of asymmetry was fairly reproducible between both trials employing mustard oil ($r = 0.65$), and also when comparing histamine with mustard oil experiments ($r = 0.58$; $P < 0.05$ each).

DISCUSSION

Protective reflex responses are commonly believed to be intimately linked with nociception. Consequently, the precise operational definition of such reflex outputs has been a topic of major concern in pain research. Such definition has been achieved for skeletal muscle reflexes, which are now the most common measures of nociceptive processing in animal experiments (for a survey on human nociceptive reflexes, see Willer 1984). In humans, a close relation has been demonstrated between the nociceptive component of the electrically evoked flexion reflex (RIII component) and the magnitude of painful stimuli as well as with the magnitude of pain sensations, although the relation of the RIII component to pain threshold is under debate (Bromm and Treede 1980; Willer 1977). Pain and flexion reflexes can be modified in parallel by stress and pharmacological intervention (Bromm and Seide 1982; Willer 1977).

In contrast, a reliable relationship has usually been denied for pain and autonomic reflexes, usually galvanic skin response. Occasionally a linear relationship has been found, but thresholds for changes in skin resistance and pain diverged (Bromm and Treede 1980). We have demonstrated, using sustained painful squeezing of the skin, that a late component of vasoconstrictor reflexes parallels pain perception (Magerl et al. 1990b). The present data extend these observations and indicate that a sustained sympathetic vascular reflex component is linked to nociception. We have shown previously that this tonic reflex activation is slow-adapting and is exceptionally resistant to habituation. Even reflex increment that parallels hyperalgesia has been found upon stimulus repetition (Magerl et al. 1990b; Magerl, Beck, Gall, Schmitz, and Handwerker, unpublished data).

Sustained nociceptive inputs seem to be essential to elicit this late reflex component. This corroborates early studies in anesthetized cats, which have shown that sympathetic reflexes are efficiently induced by stimulation of the peripheral nerves at C-fiber strength. However, single shocks were rather ineffective, whereas stimulus repetition at intervals of fewer than 8 seconds led to continuous reflex buildup (Schmidt and Weller 1970), which parallels the phenomenon of action potential windup in dorsal horn cells (Mendell and Wall 1965). This may explain why earlier studies of autonomic reflexes in humans, which used brief pain stimuli, failed to show nociceptive-specific autonomic reflex responses.

We have tentatively proposed that the particular nociception-related reflex component may be primarily organized at spinal rather than supraspinal levels (Magerl et al. 1990b). To examine this hypothesis, we used data from electrophysiological investigations of lumbar and thoracic white rami in the cat. Studies have shown that after electrical or natural stimulation of primary afferents, there is evidence for functionally independent autonomic reflex circuits organized at the spinal cord level. Importantly, it has also been demonstrated that only nociceptor-driven discharges in white rami of spinal origin (short-loop spinal group IV potentials) exhibit a distinct reflex topography, while long-loop reflexes relayed through the brainstem do not. The spread of spinal group IV potentials was restricted to the same and neighboring spinal segments (Beacham and Perl 1964; Coote et al. 1969; Sato and Schmidt 1971; Sato 1973; for review see Sato and Schmidt 1973). Such reflex topography has generally been confirmed at the level of single postganglionic fiber recordings in anaesthetized cats (Horeyseck and Jänig 1974; Jänig and Spilok 1978; Jänig and Kümmel 1981). Based on these electrophysiological grounds, the existence of independent spinal sympathetic functional units has been proposed, as the keyboard on which the primary afferent and descending supraspinal systems play (Jänig 1985, 1986). Our results in awake humans are analogous to electrophysiological recordings from animals after noxious stimulation and extend the concept of a somatosympathetic reflex topography driven exclusively by nociceptor input. The measurement of vascular reflexes induced by nociceptor stimulation and accompanied by perceptions of pain or itch disclosed that they match the time course of sensation. They are most prominent when the stimulation is exerted to a segmentally nearby area (homotopic stimulation) and significantly diminished when the stimulation affects a remote area, either far outside a segment or even contralateral within the same segment (heterotopic stimulation). This has been demonstrated in the rostro-caudal axis of the body directly by blood flow measurements (LDF) and indirectly by infrared thermography as a side-to-side asymmetry. The latter result has also been confirmed by LDF blood flow measurement (Magerl, Zimmermann, and Handwerker, unpublished data).

Interestingly, the reflex topography relates not only to the digital vasoconstrictor reflex, but also to the cephalic vasodilatation. The latter can not be explained in our experiments by the rather small amplitude blood pressure changes and are certainly not passive blood flow enhancements. The mechanism of cephalic vasodilatation is not yet fully understood. In animal experiments (cat) it has been found that presumed vasoconstrictor neurons projecting into the cervical sympathetic trunk were inhibited during noxious stimulation, which may result in passive vasodilatation (Boczek-Funke et al. 1992). Active parasympathetic vasodilatation has been found in the mandibular region of the cat face (Izumi and Karita 1992). Parasympathetic vasodilatation may be mediated by vasoactive intestinal polypeptide (VIP) in the cat and guinea pig (Goadsby and MacDonald 1985; Gibbons 1990). Neither mechanism has so far been demonstrated in humans. Vasodilatation in the human face may instead be sympathetic; it is absent in the respective facial areas in patients with unilateral lesions of the sympathetic pathways (Drummond and Lance 1987) and is abolished by acute blockade of respective sympathetic ganglia (Drummond and Finch 1989). Recent correlative microneurographic studies in the human supraorbital nerve also suggest that there is active sympathetic vasodilatation in the forehead (Nordin 1990).

Regionally organized sympathetic activity has also been demonstrated in deep tissue. Sympathetic efferents, presumably muscle vasoconstrictors, were specifically inhibited in the working muscle, and bilateral discharge synchrony in corresponding muscle nerves was increasingly lost, but sympathetic outflow to the neighboring agonists or antagonists was unaffected (Wallin et al. 1992). Interestingly, inhibition of muscle vasoconstrictor activity directed specifically to the working muscle and uncoupling of bilateral sympathetic outflow occur at contraction levels sufficient to excite nociceptive muscle afferents (Kniffki et al. 1978; Mitchell and Schmidt 1983). We do not at all exclude the contribution of supraspinal loop reflexes or more indirect contributions of higher brain centers, for example, the limbic system, to the overall magnitude of the vascular reflexes, but in the light of animal physiology we infer that in humans there may also be a quantitatively important direct contribution of spinal circuits to nociception-induced autonomic vascular reflexes. Alternatively, a somatotopic organization of brain stem reflexes or even more complex interactions between excitatory and inhibitory spinal and supraspinal centers may be conceived to explain the reflex topography, but this possibility lacks experimental support.

We do not know yet whether the nociception-related reflexes and their regional specificity have a bearing on clinical pain states. Thermal asymmetries are frequently present in neuropathic painful conditions in animals (Bennett and Ochoa 1991; Wakisaka et al. 1991) and humans (Blumberg 1989; Bonica 1992). Temperature asymmetry in trigeminal neuralgia has been shown to fade upon pain relief and reappear upon reappearance of the pain (Hampf et al. 1990). The present findings invite speculation that such changes are not causally related to the pathophysiology of the pain syndrome, but are mere epiphenomenal sequels of a regionally restricted nociceptive input.

CONCLUSIONS

1. Sustained painful stimulation of the skin and teeth induces strong sympathetic vascular reflexes in the skin of humans.
2. The vascular responses are differentially organized in the head (vasodilatation) and digits (vasoconstriction).
3. Cutaneous sympathetic vascular responses involve rapidly fading nonspecific on- and off-components, probably reflecting arousal and a tonic, slowly adapting somatosympathetic reflex component, reflecting to a large extent the nociceptive input .
4. The nociceptive-specific reflex component can be sustained and matches the time course of pain and itch perception.
5. The nonspecific arousal components are independent of the site of stimulus application.
6. In contrast, both along and across the neuraxis, the nociceptive sympathetic reflexes are somatotopically organized and depend strongly on the segmental level of nociceptive input. As a rule, close (homotopic) stimulation is more effective than remote (heterotopic) stimulation.
7. Previous failure to identify autonomic responses as valid measures of nociceptive input may be the result of inadequate experimentation rather than genuine lack of correlation.

REFERENCES

Beacham, W.S. and Perl, E.R., Background and reflex discharge of sympathetic preganglionic neurones in the spinal cat, J. Physiol., 173 (1964) 400–416.

Bennett, G.J. and Ochoa, J.L., Thermographic observations on rats with experimental neuropathic pain, Pain, 45 (1991) 61–67.

Blumberg, H., Griesser, H.J. and Hornyak, M.E., Mechanisms and role of peripheral blood flow dysregulation in pain sensation and edema in reflex sympathetic dystrophy. In: M. Stanton-Hicks, W. Jänig and R.A. Boas (Eds.), Reflex Sympathetic Dystrophy, Kluwer Academic Publishers, Boston, 1989, pp. 101–112.

Boczek-Funcke, A., Dembowsky, K., Häbler, H.-J., Jänig, W., McAllen, R.M. and Michaelis, M., Classification of preganglionic neurones projecting into the cat cervical sympathetic trunk, J. Physiol., 453 (1992) 319–339.

Bonica, J.J., Causalgia and other sympathetic reflex dystrophies. In: J.J. Bonica (Ed.), The Management of Pain, Lea and Febiger, Philadelphia, 1992, pp. 220–243.

Bromm, B. and Seide, K., The influence of tilidine and prazepam on withdrawal reflex, skin reaction and pain rating in man, Pain, 12 (1982) 247–258.

Bromm, B. and Treede, R.D., Withdrawal reflex, skin resistance and pain rating due to electrical stimuli in man, Pain, 9 (1980) 339–354.

Chapman, C.R., Casey, K.L., Dubner, R., Foley, K.M., Gracely, R.H. and Reading, A.E., Pain measurement: an overview, Pain, 22 (1985) 1–31.

Coote, J.H., Downman, C.B.B. and Weber, W.V., Reflex discharges into thoracic white rami elicited by somatic and visceral afferent excitation, J. Physiol., 202 (1969) 147–159.

D'Amour, F.E. and Smith, D., A method for determining loss of pain sensation, J. Pharmacol. Exp. Ther., 72 (1941) 74–79.

Drummond, P.D. and Finch, P.M., Reflex control of facial flushing during body heating in man, Brain, 112 (1989) 1351–1358.

Drummond, P.D. and Lance, J.W., Facial flushing and sweating mediated by the sympathetic nervous system, Brain, 110 (1987) 793–803.

Gibbins, I.L, Target-related pattern of co-existence of neuropeptide Y, vasoactive intestinal peptide, enkephalin and substance P in cranial parasympathetic neurons innervating the facial skin and exocrine glands of guinea pigs, Neuroscience, 38 (1992) 541–560.

Goadsby, P.J. and MacDonald, G.J., Extracranial vasodilatation mediated by vasoactive intestinal polypeptide (VIP), Brain Res., 329 (1985) 285–288.

Hampf, G., Bowsher, D., Wells, C. and Miles, J., Sensory and autonomic measurements in idiopathic trigeminal neuralgia before and after radiofrequency thermocoagulation: differentiation from some other causes of facial pain, Pain, 40 (1990) 241–248.

Handwerker, H.O., Forster, C. and Kirchhoff, C., Discharge patterns of human C-fibres induced by itching and burning stimuli, J. Neurophysiol., 66 (1991) 307–317.

Hargreaves, K.M., Dubner, R., Brown, F., Flores, C. and Joris, J., A new and sensitive method for measuring thermal nociception in cutaneous hyperalgesia, Pain, 32 (1988) 77–88.

Horeyseck, G. and Jänig, W., Reflexes in postganglionic fibers within skin and muscle nerves after noxious stimulation of skin, Exp. Brain Res., 20 (1974) 125–134.

Izumi, H. and Karita, K., Selective excitation of parasympathetic nerve fibers to elicit the vasodilatation in cat lip, J. Auton. Nerv. Syst., 37 (1992) 99–108.

Jänig, W., Organization of the lumbar sympathetic outflow to skeletal muscle and skin of the cat hindlimb and tail, Rev. Physiol. Biochem. Pharmacol., 102 (1985) 119–213.

Jänig, W., Spinal cord integration of visceral sensory systems and sympathetic nervous system reflexes. In: F. Cervero und J.F.B. Morrison (Eds.), Visceral sensation. Progress in Brain Research, Vol. 67. Elsevier, Amsterdam, 1986, pp. 255–277.

Jänig, W. and Kümmel, H., Organization of the sympathetic innervation supplying the hairless skin of the cat's paw, J. Auton. Nerv. Syst., 3 (1981) 215–230.

Jänig, W. and Spilok, H., Functional organization of the sympathetic innervation supplying the hairless skin of the hindpaws in chronic spinal cats, Pflügers Arch., 377 (1978) 25–31.

Kniffki, K.-D., Mense, S. and Schmidt, R.F., Responses of group IV afferent units from skeletal muscle to stretch, contraction and chemical stimulation, Exp. Brain Res., 31 (1978) 511–522.

Magerl, W. and Handwerker, H.O., A reliable model of experimental itching by iontophoresis of histamine. In: R. Dubner, G.F. Gebhart and M.R. Bond (Eds.), Proceedings of the Vth World Congress on Pain. Pain Research and Clinical Management, Vol.3. Elsevier, Amsterdam, 1988, pp. 536–540.

Magerl, W., Westerman, R.A., Möhner, B. and Handwerker, H.O., Properties of transdermal histamine iontophoresis: differential effects of season, gender and body region, J. Invest. Dermatol., 94 (1990a) 347–352.

Magerl, W., Geldner, G., and Handwerker, H.O., Pain and vascular reflexes in man elicited by prolonged noxious mechano-stimulation, Pain, 43 (1990b) 219–225.

Mendell, L.M. and Wall, P.D., Responses of single dorsal cord cells to peripheral cutaneous unmyelinated fibres, Nature, 206 (1965) 97–99.

Mitchell, J.H. and Schmidt, R.F., Cardiovascular reflex control by afferent fibers from skeletal muscle receptors. In: J.T. Shepherd and F.M. Abboud (Eds.), Handbook of Physiology, Section 2: The Cardiovascular System, Vol. III. Peripheral circulation and organ blood flow, Part 2. American Physiological Society, Bethesda, Md., 1983, pp. 623–658.

Nakagawa, H., Omori, M., Fujiwara, A., Hosokawa T. and Tanaka, Y., Quantitative measurement

of pain is possible by the analysis of skin blood flow using laser-Doppler flow meter. In: Abstracts: 7th World Congress on Pain, IASP Publications, Seattle, 1993, p. 349.
Nordin, M., Sympathetic discharges in the human supraorbital nerve and their relation to sudo- and vasomotor responses, J. Physiol., 423 (1990) 241–255.
Randall, L.O. and Selitto, J.J., A method for measurements of analgesic activity on inflamed tissue, Arch. Int. Pharmacodyn., 111, 409–419 (1957).
Sato, A., Spinal and medullary reflex components of the somato-sympathetic reflex discharges evoked by stimulation of the Group IV somatic afferents, Brain Res., 51 (1973) 307–318.
Sato, A. and Schmidt, R.F., Spinal and supraspinal components of the reflex discharges into the lumbar and thoracic white rami, J. Physiol., 212 (1971) 839–850.
Sato, A. and Schmidt, R.F., Somatosympathetic reflexes. Afferent fibers, central pathways, discharge characteristics, Physiol. Rev., 53 (1973) 916–947.
Schmidt, R.F. and Weller E., Reflex activity in the cervical and lumbar sympathetic trunk induced by unmyelinated somatic afferents, Brain Res., 24 (1970) 207–218.
Sherrington, C.S., Cutaneous sensations. In: E.A. Schäfer (Ed.), Textbook of Physiology, Vol.2, Pentland, London, 1900, pp. 920–1001.
Sokolov, E.N., Perception and the Conditioned Reflex, Pergamon Press, Oxford 1963, 309 pp.
Wakisaka, S., Kajander, K.C. and Bennett, G.J., Abnormal skin temperature and abnormal sympathetic vasomotor innervation in an experimental painful peripheral neuropathy, Pain, 46 (1991) 299–313.
Wallin, B.G., Burke, D., Gandevia, S.C., Coherence between the sympathetic drives to relaxed and contracting muscles of different limbs of human subjects, J. Physiol., 455 (1992) 219–233.
Willer, J.C., Comparative study of perceived pain and nociceptive flexion reflex, Pain, 3 (1977) 69–80.
Willer, J.C., Nociceptive flexion reflex as a physiological correlate of pain sensation in humans. In: B. Bromm (Ed.), Pain Measurement in Man. Neurophysiological Correlates of Pain. Elsevier, Amsterdam, 1984, pp. 87–110.

Correspondence to: Dr. Walter Magerl, Institut für Physiologie und Pathophysiologie, Universität Mainz, Saarstr. 21, D-55099 Mainz, Germany. Tel: 49-6131-395218; Fax: 49-6131-395902.

Proceedings of the 7th World Congress on Pain,
Progress in Pain Research and Management, Vol. 2,
edited by G.F. Gebhart, D.L. Hammond, and T.S.
Jensen, IASP Press, Seattle, © 1994.

58

Similarity of Threshold Temperatures for First Pain Sensation, Laser-Evoked Potentials, and Nociceptor Activation

Rolf-Detlef Treede,[a] Richard A. Meyer,[b]
and Ronald P. Lesser[c]

[a]*Institute of Physiology and Pathophysiology, Johannes Gutenberg University, Mainz, Germany, and Departments of* [b]*Neurosurgery and* [c]*Neurology, Johns Hopkins University, Baltimore, Maryland, USA*

INTRODUCTION

Several studies have compared primary afferent nociceptor discharges in humans and monkeys with human psychophysical measurements of pain (Raja et al. 1988). Other studies have compared human psychophysics with human evoked potentials (Bromm and Treede 1991). However, the vastly different heat stimuli used in these studies make comparisons difficult. We thus conducted a study comparing all three parameters, using the same radiant heat stimulator.

Fig. 1 illustrates examples of the typical heat stimuli used in these types of experiments, giving the time course for temperature changes at the skin surface and at the dermal-epidermal junction (50 µm). Laser stimuli for evoked-potential studies are usually energy-controlled (Fig. 1, left). The risetime of skin temperature is approximately equal to the stimulus duration, followed by passive cooling. Base temperature is not controlled and hence may vary between subjects; as a typical value, 30°C was chosen. The adequate stimulus for heat pain sensation is elevated skin temperature, so most neurophysiological and psychophysical studies use temperature-controlled stimuli on top of a controlled base temperature (Fig. 1, right). The high base temperature of

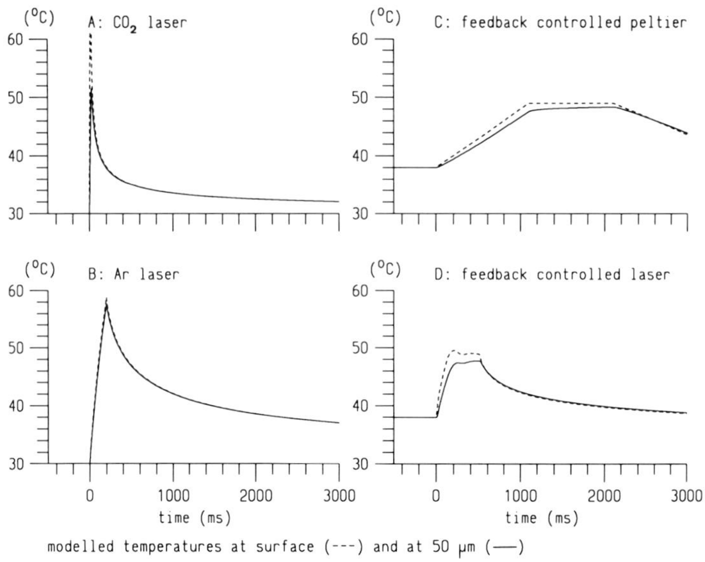

Fig. 1. Various types of heat stimuli that are used in evoked potential studies (left) or primary afferent studies (right). Modeled temperature changes at the skin surface (dashed line) and at the dermal-epidermal interface (solid line), thermal diffusivity alpha = 0.0015 cm^2/s, volumetric heat capacity ρc = 1.0 cgs units. **A:** CO_2 laser radiant heat pulse of pain threshold intensity (10 W, 20 ms, 5 mm); reflectivity 0.0078, absorption coefficient 950 cm^{-1} (Bromm and Treede 1983). **B:** Argon laser radiant heat pulse of pain threshold intensity (1.25 W, 200 ms, 3 mm); reflectivity 0.37, absorption coefficient 65 cm^{-1} (Arendt-Nielsen and Bjerring 1988, Van Gemert et al. 1982). **C:** Heat pulse from a fast Peltier stimulator (10°C/s) can elicit nociceptor activity and painful sensations; risetime is too slow for evoked-potential studies. **D:** Feedback-controlled CO_2 laser stimulator can also apply controlled temperature changes. Risetimes are comparable to those of the Argon laser.

35–38°C is used to saturate the activity of low-threshold warm sensitive afferents (LaMotte and Campbell 1978).

Contact heat stimulators are much too slow to elicit the synchronous response needed to allow stimulus-locked EEG-averaging for evoked potentials (e.g., 10°C/s in Fig. 1C). Although temperature risetime in most laser evoked-potential studies has been on the order of tens of milliseconds (Fig. 1A), there are several papers on Argon laser evoked potentials, which use a risetime of 200 ms (Fig. 1B). This risetime is within reach of the fastest temperature-controlled stimulator, the laser stimulator at the Johns Hopkins School of Medicine (Fig. 1D, Meyer et al. 1976). This stimulator has been used for several comparative studies of human psychophysics and peripheral afferent activity in the monkey (e.g., LaMotte and Campbell 1978; Meyer and

Campbell 1981). In our study, we used this laser stimulator to compare human psychophysics, monkey neurophysiology, and human evoked potentials.

METHODS

A CO_2-laser stimulator under radiometer feedback control delivered step increases in temperature to the skin (150 ms risetime). The 0.5-second duration stimuli ranged from 42°C to 50°C (in 2°C increments, with a 38°C base) and were presented to the dorsum of the left hand in a randomized sequence every 15 seconds with the constraint that each stimulus was presented 10 times in a given run. Each stimulus was delivered to a different site on the dorsum of the hand to avoid stimulus interaction (LaMotte and Campbell, 1978). After a 30-minute interval, a second run of heat stimuli was given to the same skin area.

The EEG was recorded from three midline electrode positions (Fz, Cz, Pz according to the 10–20 system) vs. left earlobe reference (bandpass 0.1–30 Hz) and digitized at 200 per second. The vertical EOG was recorded with the same filter settings; contaminated trials were discarded. Averaged laser evoked potentials (LEPs) were calculated off-line. In addition, subjective ratings were collected after each stimulus. Subjects were instructed to categorize the stimulus as not detected, detected, or pricking pain. For this purpose, a tone was presented three seconds after each stimulus, prompting the subjects to give a rating. Seven subjects participated in these studies that were approved by the Johns Hopkins Committee on Clinical Investigations.

Recordings from single nociceptive afferents were made in monkeys that were anesthetized with pentobarbital. Standard teased-fiber techniques were used for recording from the following nerves: superficial radial ($n = 19$), medial antebrachial cutaneous ($n = 7$), saphenous ($n = 8$), sural ($n = 1$), and superficial peroneal ($n = 1$). A-delta nociceptors were initially identified with distal electrical nerve stimulation and then characterized with mechanical and heat stimuli at the receptive field (Meyer et al. 1991). Heat stimuli were delivered with the same stimulator as in the combined psychophysical and evoked-potential study. Base temperature was also 38°C, but the stimulus duration was one second. We report only results from type II AMHs in this chapter. AMHs were classified as type II based on their fast response to a 53°C, 30-second stimulus given after the threshold determination. Type I AMHs, in contrast, respond to this heat stimulus with several seconds delay and a slowly increasing discharge (cf. Treede et al. 1991). The data on CMHs are from a previous study (Treede et al. 1990).

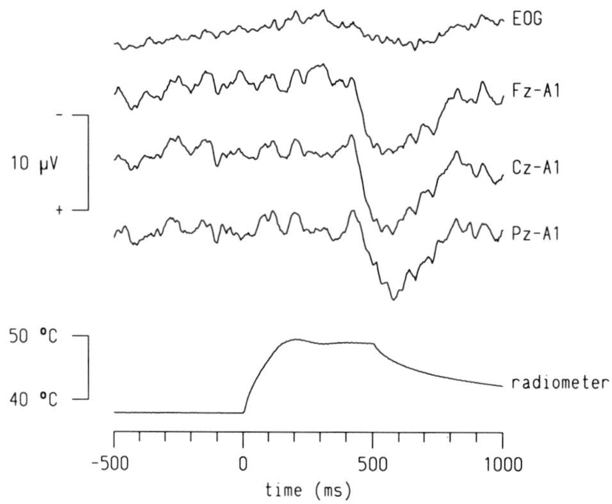

Fig. 2. Averaged laser evoked potential in one subject; 47 artifact-free sweeps. Stimulus intensity was 49°C, delivered with a risetime of 150 ms from a base temperature of 38°C and maintained for 500 ms. The evoked response occurred before the end of the stimulus and was maximal at the vertex.

RESULTS

In the first three subjects, the stimulus temperature was kept constant within a run. Fig. 2 shows an example of an averaged evoked potential (47 artifact-free sweeps) in one subject in response to a 49°C stimulus. As with other late LEPs, the potential was maximal at the vertex. It consisted of a negativity at 420 ms and a positivity at 575 ms with 10.5 µV peak-to-peak amplitude. The temperature waveform recorded by the radiometer is shown on the bottom. The risetime to the target temperature of 49°C was about 150 ms. In contrast, the risetime of skin temperature with the usual energy-controlled laser is about equal to the pulse duration of 20 ms (Fig. 1A). If the risetime of the temperature is relevant for the LEP latency, a difference of about 130 ms to previous studies would be expected. If the end of the stimulus is relevant, the difference should be 480 ms.

The late LEP as a function of stimulus temperature was studied in four subjects using stimulus temperatures that ranged from 42–50°C in 2°C increments. Each subject participated in two runs separated by 30 minutes and each run consisted of 50 stimulus trials (i.e., 10 trials of each temperature in a randomized order). The resulting grand mean waveforms recorded at the vertex are shown in Fig. 3. At 42–46°C, only deflections similar to those in the prestimulus EEG occurred. At 48 and 50°C, the LEP could be detected visu-

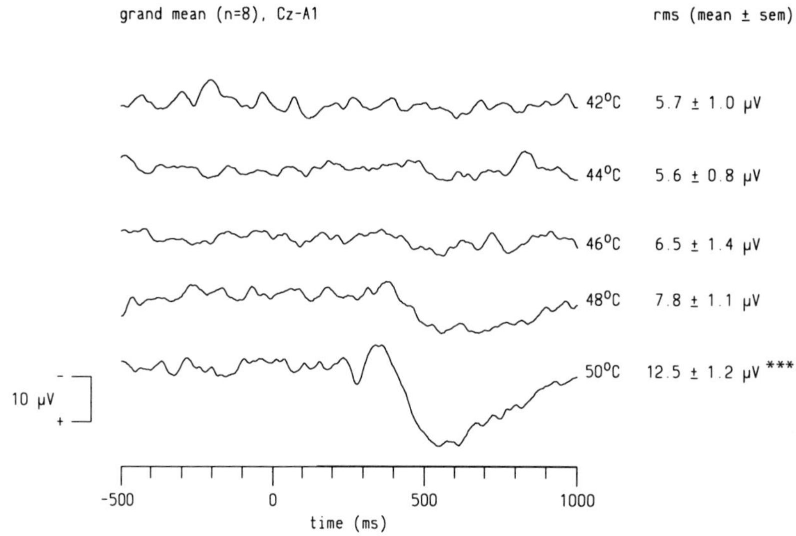

Fig. 3. Laser evoked potential as a function of stimulus intensity; grand means over eight runs; recording from vertex versus left earlobe. An evoked potential can be seen for 48° and 50°C. The RMS amplitude in a window from 150 to 1000 ms was significant for 50°C.

ally. At 50°C, the average peak latency for the negativity and the positivity was 346 ms and 595 ms, respectively (Table I). These latencies were 100–200 ms longer than those recorded with brief laser pulses that have 20 ms temperature risetime (Treede et al. 1988).

Fig. 4 can be used to compare the results from the electrophysiological, psychophysical, and evoked-potential studies. As there is no established statistical method to test for the presence of an evoked potential, we tried a simple measure, the root mean square (RMS) amplitude from 150 to 1000 ms. In Fig. 4B, the RMS values of the vertex potential are plotted as a function of stimulus temperature. The mean RMS value for 50°C was significantly higher than for all other intensities ($P \leq 0.001$ versus 42–46°C; $P \leq 0.05$ versus 48°C). Although the LEP was detectable visually also for 48°C, the RMS amplitude values were only significant for 50°C.

The results from the psychophysical ratings of the stimuli in the evoked-potential runs are presented in Fig. 4C. The mean percentage of stimuli that was detected (open circles) or perceived as pricking pain (filled circles) was plotted as a function of stimulus temperature. At 46°C, the subjects detected virtually all stimuli. The percentage of stimuli that was rated as pricking pain was significantly higher for 48–50°C stimuli than for 42–44°C stimuli ($P \leq 0.001$), and marginally higher for 46° than for 42–44° ($P \approx 0.05$). The threshold for pricking pain was 47.1 ± 2°C (mean ± SD), whereas the detec-

Table I
Evoked potentials following temperature-controlled or energy-controlled CO2 laser stimuli

	150 ms Risetime, 50°C			20 ms Duration, 15 W*		
	mean	SD	n	mean	SD	n
Vertex negativity (ms)	346	42	8	244	21	22
Vertex positivity (ms)	595	85	8	384	31	22
Amplitude (μV pp)	30.7	9.9	8	23.2	8.5	23

* Data from Treede et al. 1988; intensities were 1.5 times the individual pain threshold, which was 10.6 ± 4.1 W (mean and standard deviation).

tion threshold was near 42°C. These data indicate that the LEP appeared only with stimulus intensities above pricking pain threshold.

The receptive fields of high-threshold A-fiber nociceptors were located with an electrical search technique (Meyer et al. 1991). Of the 39 fibers studied in the monkey hand, 16 responded with a short latency and a phasic response to an intense (53°C, 30-second) heat stimulus and were therefore classified as type II AMHs (Treede et al. 1991). The mean response latency (from stimulus onset to generation of the first action potential at the receptive field) was 220 ms. The peak discharge occurred on the average 470 ms after stimulus onset, followed by rapid adaptation. Eleven of the 16 type II AMHs had a mechanical threshold above 5 bar; these fibers would not normally be found with mechanical search techniques and are referred to as mechanically insensitive afferents (Meyer et al. 1991). Their mean conduction velocity of 12 m per second corresponds well to previous estimates from evoked potentials. The cumulative heat threshold distribution of the type II AMHs is given in Fig. 4A. The threshold temperature for these AMHs was 47.3 ± 2.7 °C. The threshold distribution of type II AMHs matched the evoked potential data, whereas that of CMHs did not.

DISCUSSION

Our study showed that step increases in skin temperature, generated by a feedback-controlled CO_2 laser, have a risetime that is fast enough to study laser evoked potentials (LEPs). The risetime of skin temperature was about 150 ms, whereas the risetime with the usual energy-controlled CO_2 laser pulse is about 20 ms. If the risetime of skin temperature is relevant for the LEP latency, a difference of about 130 ms to previous studies would be expected.

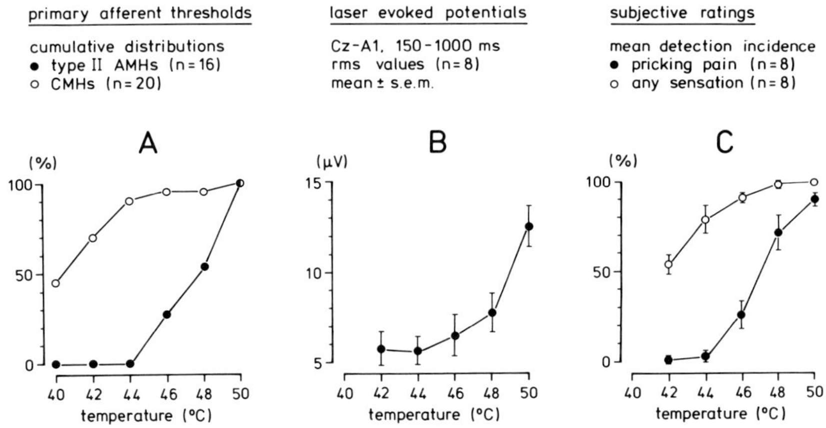

Fig. 4. Stimulus response functions for monkey primary afferent, human evoked potential, and human psychophysical data. **A:** Nociceptor recruitment was plotted as the percentage of fibers that had a threshold less than or equal to the value on the abscissa. **B:** Evoked-potential amplitude was quantified as root mean square value within a window from 150 to 1000 ms after stimulus onset. **C:** Subjective ratings were plotted as percentage of stimuli detected (open circles) or rated as pricking pain (filled circles).

latency, a difference of about 130 ms to previous studies would be expected. Compared with our own data (Treede et al. 1988), we found a 100-ms difference for the negativity and 200-ms difference for the positivity. These data suggest that the risetime of a temperature stimulus, not the duration of the plateau, is important for triggering an evoked potential. This finding is also consistent with data of evoked potentials following Argon laser pulses of 200 ms duration (Arendt-Nielsen and Bjerring 1988), which have 420-ms peak latency for the negativity. The vertex negativity thus always appears about 200 ms after the temperature peak.

We had the unique opportunity to compare the stimulus-response curve of LEPs with the recruitment of nociceptive afferents. At 48°C, where the LEP was first visually detected in the averaged waveforms, more than 50% of the type II AMHs were activated, and more than 50% of the stimuli were perceived as pricking pain. For a statistically significant LEP (i.e., at 50°C), these percentages had to be above 90%. These data indicate that the LEP appeared only with stimulus intensities above pricking pain threshold and depended upon activation of type II AMHs. The rapid adaptation of type II AMHs to a sustained heat stimulus may explain why only the temperature risetime is important for LEP latencies.

A large percentage of stimuli were detected at temperatures below 48°C;

thus, detection of brief heat pulses cannot depend upon activation of type II AMHs. The recruitment of CMHs matched, however, the percentage of stimuli detected. Although these nonpainful stimuli were described as hot by the subjects, it is likely that they were mediated by nociceptors, because sensitive thermoreceptors should have been saturated by the 38°C base temperature (LaMotte and Campbell 1978).

Evidently, CMHs can play no role for the late LEPs because of their slow conduction velocity leading to an arrival of the afferent volley at the spinal cord no earlier than 700 ms (Treede et al. 1991). Also, more than 90% of CMHs were already recruited at intensities that did not elicit a late LEP. In earlier studies with nerve blocks, C-fiber activity has been related to the occurrence of ultralate LEPs with peak latencies beyond 1000 ms (Bromm and Treede 1987). Stimuli of 44–46°C may be suitable for studying ultralate potentials, because these intensities already recruit more than 90% of CMHs, but less than one-third of the AMHs. We have seen ultralate potentials at these intermediate temperatures on several occasions, but are not yet able to demonstrate their presence statistically, perhaps because our mathematical methods are not sensitive enough. Other techniques such as spectral analysis of evoked potentials may be necessary (e.g., Bromm et al. 1989).

CONCLUSIONS

Stepped increases in skin temperature above pricking pain threshold are able to produce an evoked potential in human subjects. The latency of this potential is related to the risetime of skin temperature, not to the total stimulus duration. Pricking pain and late laser-evoked potentials are likely to be mediated by type II AMHs. Detection of brief heat pulses, however, depends upon activation of CMHs rather than type II AMHs.

ACKNOWLEDGMENTS:

This work was supported by a travel grant from the Möller foundation (RDT) and by the NIH (NS-14447). We appreciate the technical assistance of T.V. Hartke and P. Poon.

REFERENCES

Arendt-Nielsen, L. and Bjerring, P., Selective averaging of argon laser induced pre-pain and pain related cortical responses, J. Neurosci. Methods, 24 (1988) 117–123.

Bromm, B. and Treede, R.D., CO_2 laser radiant heat pulses activate C nociceptors in man, Pflügers Arch., 399 (1983) 155–156.
Bromm, B. and Treede, R.D., Human cerebral potentials evoked by CO_2 laser stimuli causing pain, Exp. Brain Res., 67 (1987) 153–162.
Bromm, B. and Treede, R.D., Laser evoked cerebral potentials in the assessment of cutaneous pain sensitivity in normal subjects and in patients, Révue Neurologique, 147 (1991) 625–643.
Bromm, B., Meier, W. and Scharein, E., Pre-stimulus/post-stimulus relations in EEG spectra and their modulations by an opioid and an antidepressant, Electroenceph. Clin. Neurophysiol., 73 (1989) 188–197.
LaMotte, R.H. and Campbell, J.N., Comparison of responses of warm and nociceptive C-fiber afferents in monkey with human judgements of thermal pain, J. Neurophysiol., 41 (1978) 509–528.
Meyer, R.A. and Campbell, J.N., Myelinated nociceptive afferents account for the hyperalgesia that follows a burn to the hand, Science, 213 (1981) 1527–1529.
Meyer, R.A., Walker, R.E. and Mountcastle, V.B., A laser stimulator for the study of cutaneous thermal pain sensation, IEEE Trans. Biomed. Eng., 23 (1976) 54–60.
Meyer, R.A., Davis, K.D., Cohen, R.H., Treede, R.D. and Campbell, J.N., Mechanically insensitive afferents (MIAs) in cutaneous nerves of monkey, Brain Res., 561 (1991) 252–261.
Raja, S.N., Meyer, R.A. and Campbell, J.N., Peripheral mechanisms of somatic pain, Anesthesiology, 68 (1988) 571–590.
Treede, R.D., Kief, S., Hölzer, T. and Bromm, B., Late somatosensory evoked cerebral potentials in response to cutaneous heat stimuli, Electroenceph. Clin. Neurophysiol., 70 (1988) 429–441.
Treede, R.D., Meyer, R.A. and Campbell, J.N., Comparison of heat and mechanical receptive fields of cutaneous C-fiber nociceptors in monkey, J. Neurophysiol., 64 (1990) 1502–1513.
Treede, R.D., Meyer, R.A. and Campbell, J.N., Classification of primate A-fiber nociceptors according to their heat response properties, Pflüger's Archiv., Suppl. 418 (1991) R42.
Van Gemert, M.J.C., De Kleijn, W.J.A. and Hulsbergen-Hennings, J.P., Temperature behaviour of a model port-wine stain during argon laser coagulation, Phys. Med. Biol., 27 (1982) 1089–1104.

Correspondence to: Prof. Dr.med. Rolf-Detlef Treede, Institute of Physiology and Pathophysiology, Johannes Gutenberg University, Saarstr. 21, D-55099 Mainz, Germany. Tel: 49-6131-39-5715; Fax: 49-6131-39-5902.

Part XII

Pain and Age

Proceedings of the 7th World Congress on Pain,
Progress in Pain Research and Management, Vol. 2,
edited by G.F. Gebhart, D.L. Hammond, and T.S.
Jensen, IASP Press, Seattle, © 1994.

59

Pain, Affect, and Cognition in Children: 1. The Influence of Affective State on Pain in Children

Robert Johnson,[a] Susan H. Spence,[b]
G. David Champion,[c] and John B. Ziegler[c]

[a]*Department of Psychology, University of Sydney, New South Wales, Australia,* [b]*Department of Psychology, University of Queensland, Queensland, Australia, and* [c]*The Prince of Wales Children's Hospital, Randwick, New South Wales, Australia.*

INTRODUCTION

Insufficient research has been conducted into the cognitive and affective components of pain (Erskine et al. 1990; Jamison et al. 1993), particularly for children (Lander et al. 1992). This chapter examines the relationship between pain and affect in children. It is important to identify factors that have the potential to exacerbate or remediate the experience of pain in children. Children are particularly susceptible to environmental influences that may impact their affective state. The risk of negative emotional influence is especially likely in the unfamiliar surroundings of a hospital to which they have been admitted for surgery.

In our study we defined the term *affect* as mood, emotion, or feeling state, along a bipolar dimension ranging from negative affect to positive affect, or sad to happy mood. We distinguish between the concept of affect and pain-specific affect, which is a subset of a person's overall affective state and operates as a unipolar dimension ranging from neutral to negative. The association between the experience of pain and negative affect is well established and it is commonly assumed that the direction of causality is unilateral, with the aversive experience of pain leading to negative affect. There is some suggestion in the clinical literature, however, that the causal direction may be reciprocal in adults. Some longitudinal studies have suggested that negative emotional states such as depression may serve to exacerbate the intensity of pain experience (e.g., Leino and Magni 1993). Other studies have found that pain severity tends to predict future depression (Rudy et al. 1988; Brown 1990). Thus, it appears that the relationship between affect and pain is a complex one with reciprocal influences operating.

We investigated whether an increase in negative affect produces an increase in the intensity of pain experienced and conversely whether an increase in positive affect produces a reduction in pain intensity. We studied children who experienced pain following a minor surgical procedure and experimentally manipulated mood to examine the impact upon perceived pain.

METHOD

SUBJECTS

The subjects consisted of 45 children, 8 to 12 years of age (mean 9.71 years), who were admitted to The Prince of Wales Children's Hospital for minor surgery, such as tonsillectomy and/or adenoidectomy. There were 23 females and 22 males.

ASSESSMENT OF PAIN AND AFFECT

Pain was measured with a Visual Analog Scale (VAS), an 18 by 4-cm plastic card with a 15-cm red-colored wedge, measuring from 1 cm to 3 cm in width. The intensity of redness of the wedge increased with the increasing width of the wedge. Additionally, at the narrow end were the words NO PAIN and at the wide end were the words MOST PAIN. A sliding cursor could be moved to any position on the wedge. On the reverse of the scale were graduations from 1 to 10 corresponding to the length of the wedge. (This VAS was designed by P.A. McGrath and her colleagues and given to participants at the Second International Symposium on Pediatric Pain, Montreal, Canada, 1991). The subjects were asked to position the cursor at the point on the wedge that corresponded to their pain. A numerical rating was then obtained from the reverse of the scale. VAS-derived numerical estimates are reliable and valid measures of acute, recurrent, and chronic pain in children aged 5 to 16 years (McGrath 1990, 1991).

We assessed affective state using a scale consisting of seven basic schematic drawings of faces positioned in a horizontal row and identical in every respect except the mouth. The expressions of the mouths varied from a downturn, depicting sadness, in the extreme left drawing, through to an upturn, depicting a smile, in the extreme right drawing. Under each drawing, from left to right respectively, were the words Very Sad, Sad, A little Sad, Neutral, A little Happy, Happy, and Very Happy. The original scale was developed by Buck (1975) and used to measure self-reported affective state in children aged from 5 to 6 years. Forgas et al. (1988) modified it to a seven-point scale for research with older children, and successfully used it with 8- to 10-year-olds in a study employing a similar mood manipulation technique to that of our study.

STUDY PROCEDURE

Subsequent to consent and preceding the operation, we administered the State-Trait Anxiety Inventory for Children (STAIC; Spielberger et al. 1973) and the Children's Depression Inventory (CDI; Kovacs 1981) to all subjects. No further contact was made with subjects until a minimum of three hours after surgery. At this time, we assessed baseline measures of self-reported pain on a scale of zero (no pain) to 10 (most pain), and affective state on a scale of one (very sad) to seven (very happy).

Fifteen subjects were assigned to each of three conditions, positive affect, negative affect, and neutral (control), by stratified random sampling on the basis of their baseline pain and affect scores. The groups also were matched as closely as possible for age and gender. We then manipulated the affective state of subjects by showing them age-appropriate video clips of the required affective valence. That is, subjects assigned to the positive affect condition saw a happy video clip, subjects assigned to the negative affect condition saw a sad video clip, and subjects assigned to the neutral condition saw a clip that was neither happy nor sad. We obtained these video clips from Eliot Brenner and Peter Salovey at Yale University, who developed them specifically for the induction of affective states in children. They consisted of five- to six-minute excerpts from movies entitled *Pee Wee's Big Adventure, The Bear,* and *Turner and Hooch.*

Compared with other methods of mood manipulation, such as manipulated task performance feedback, hypnosis, and the Velten technique (which uses self-referent statements; Velten 1968), the video observation method used in this study has several advantages. It is a highly familiar medium to children; it does not require a select population such as hypnotizable subjects; it produces strong and predictable positive and negative affective states; and the videos can be shown with minimal interruption to the subject's environment.

In our study the video clips were shown at the subject's bedside on a television monitor with a 51-cm (20-in) screen. The audio was played through headphones to minimize external distraction. Immediately following video observation, we again assessed pain and affective state.

RESULTS

The STAIC and CDI scores were consistent with normative data (Spielberger et al. 1973; Spence and Kennedy 1989), and analysis of variance (ANOVA) indicated homogeneity across experimental groups on each scale. Table I shows the age, gender, and baseline affect and pain scores for each experimental group.

Analysis of the pain and affect data consisted of comparisons of pre- and post-video self-reported pain and affect levels between groups, and changes in pre- to post-video ratings of pain and affect by subjects within each group. As shown in Table I, the mean group affect ratings prior to mood manipulation ranged from 4.33 to 4.53. The ANOVA revealed no significant difference between groups in affect ratings prior to mood manipulation ($F[2, 42] = 0.08$, $P = 0.921$). Following mood manipulation, the affect rating of the neutral (control) group remained almost the same, at 4.67 (SD = 1.05), while that of the positive affect group increased to 5.93 (SD = 0.70), and the negative group decreased to 2.53 (SD = 0.99). ANOVA performed on these data showed that after mood manipulation all group differences were highly significant ($F[2, 42] = 51.67$, $P < 0.001$). This finding confirms that the experimental procedure was effective in producing the desired manipulation in mood.

These results were confirmed by repeated measures analysis of each subject's affect score before and after mood manipulation. Paired *t* tests showed that there was no significant change in the affect ratings of subjects in the neutral group, but highly significant changes for subjects in both the positive affect group ($t[14] = -6.81$, $P < 0.001$) and the negative affect group ($t[14] = 6.12$, $P < 0.001$).

The pain ratings were subjected to the same statistical tests as the affect data. Prior to mood manipulation the mean pain ratings for each group were almost the same, ranging from 2.42 to 2.51 (Table I). No significant difference between groups was found with the ANOVA ($F[2,42] = 0.02$, $P = 0.982$). After mood manipulation the neutral group's mean pain rating remained almost the same, at 2.29 (SD = 1.14), whereas the negative affect group's rating increased to 3.18 (SD = 1.39), and the positive affect group's rating decreased to 1.62 (SD = 1.27). The difference between the positive affect and negative affect groups, for the post-manipulation pain ratings, was highly significant ($F[2, 42] = 5.72$, $P = 0.006$).

Table I
The baseline characteristics of each experimental group

	Positive Affect Group	Negative Affect Group	Neutral Group
Mean age (years)	9.73 (SD = 1.62)	9.80 (SD = 1.42)	9.60 (SD = 1.50)
Gender (female/male)	8/7	7/8	8/7
Mean affect rating	4.33 (SD = 1.35)	4.47 (SD = 1.36)	4.53 (SD = 1.41)
Mean pain rating	2.51 (SD = 1.40)	2.42 (SD = 1.11)	2.44 (SD = 1.58)

The repeated measures analysis of each subject's pain score before and after mood manipulation confirmed these results. Paired *t* tests showed that there was no significant change in the pain ratings of subjects in the neutral group, but a significant increase in the pain ratings of subjects in the negative affect group ($t[14] = -2.87$, $P = 0.012$) and significant decrease in the pain ratings of subjects in the positive affect group ($t[14] = 4.88$, $P < 0.001$). Fig. 1 summarizes the results for mean pain scores for each group before and after mood manipulation.

Finally, correlations of the pain and affect data revealed a strong inverse relationship such that higher affect scores corresponded with lower pain scores, and higher pain scores corresponded with lower affect scores. The Pearson product-moment correlations between pain and affect ratings were –0.73 before mood change and –0.65 following mood change.

DISCUSSION

Our study found a strong correlation between current affective state and self-reported pain intensity. The results also support the direction of causality hypothesis, that changes in affective state produced significant alterations in the level of pain experienced by children.

The analysis of affect ratings made before and after video observation showed the effectiveness of the mood manipulation technique in bringing about the desired changes in the affective state of the children. The affective state of subjects who observed the neutral material did not change. However, as designed, the affective state of subjects assigned to the positive affect condition became more positive, while the affective state of subjects assigned to the negative affect condition became more negative.

Corresponding ratings of pain intensity clearly supported the hypotheses that when the affective state of children in pain becomes more negative, they will report increased pain, and when their affective state becomes more posi-

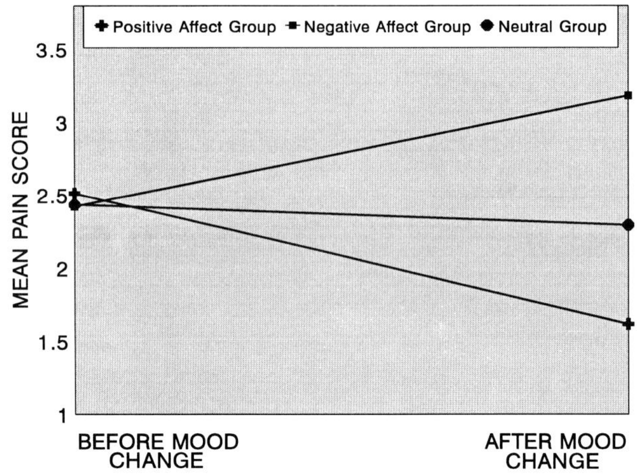

Fig. 1. The mean pain scores for each experimental group before and after mood change.

tive, they will report decreased pain. Homogeneity of the STAIC and CDI scores across the groups indicated that these effects could not be attributed to pre-existing conditions of anxiety or depression.

These findings have theoretical and practical implications. From a theoretical perspective the results strongly suggest that the relationship between affect and pain is not a unidirectional one in which the experience of pain produces negative affect. Rather, it appears that the relationship is bidirectional, and that changes in affect may produce alterations in the intensity of perceived pain. From a practical perspective, many children have to undergo painful and aversive medical procedures, and it is desirable to ensure that they experience as little pain as possible. The experience of such procedures is likely to generate negative emotional states, over and above the impact of pain. For example, separation from parents, an unfamiliar environment, and inability to take part in interesting activities all may serve to generate negative affect. Such negative emotional states are likely to increase the intensity of postoperative pain experienced. Wherever possible, attempts should be made to enhance mood postoperatively to reduce postoperative pain levels.

ACKNOWLEDGMENTS

This research was conducted as partial fulfillment of the requirements for the Ph.D. degree by Robert Johnson and was supervised by Associate Professor Susan H. Spence. Financial support was provided by a scholarship from Johnson & Johnson Australia Pty. Limited.

REFERENCES

Brown, G.K., A causal analysis of chronic pain and depression, J. Ab. Psych., 99, (1990), 127–137.

Buck, R., Nonverbal communication of affect in children, J. Pers. Soc. Psychol., 31 (1975) 644–653.

Erskine, A., Morley, S. and Pearce, S., Memory for pain: a review, Pain, 41 (1990) 255–265.

Forgas, J. P., Burnham, D. K. and Trimboli, C., Mood, memory and social judgments in children, J. Pers. Soc. Psychol., 54 (1988) 697–703.

Jamison, R. N., Pearce, S., Morley, S., Reeves, J. L., Graber, L. M. and Lander, J., Memory and pain, Topical Seminar at VIIth World Congress on Pain, Paris, France, 22–29 August, 1993.

Kovacs, M., Rating scales to assess depression in school age children, Acta Paedopsychiatr., 46 (1981) 305–315.

Lander, J., Hodgins, M. and Fowler-Kerry, S., Children's pain predictions and memories, Behav. Res. Ther., 30 (1992) 117–124.

Leino, P., & Magni, G., Depressive and distress symptoms as predictors of low back pain, neck-shoulder pain and other musculoskeletal morbidity: a 10 year follow-up of metal industry employees, Pain, 53, (1993) 163–169.

McGrath, P. A., Pain in children: Nature, assessment, and treatment, Guilford Press, New York, 1990.

McGrath, P. A., Versatile pain measures for children, Paper presented at the Second International Symposium on Pediatric Pain, Montreal, Canada, April 24–27, 1991.

Rudy, T.E., Kerns, R.D., and Turk, D.C., Chronic pain and depression: towards a cognitive-behavioural mediation model, Pain, 35, (1988), 129–140.

Spence, S. H. and Kennedy, E., Australian data for the Children's Action Tendency Scale, the Children's Depression Inventory and Fear Survey Schedule for Children-Revised, Aust. Ed. Dev. Psychol., 6 (1989) 16–21.

Spielberger, C. D., Edwards, C. D., Lushene, R. E., Montuori, J. and Platzek, D., Preliminary test manual for the state-trait anxiety inventory for children, Consulting Psychologists Press, Palo Alto, 1973.

Velten, E., Jr., A laboratory task for induction of mood states, Behav. Res. Ther., 6 (1968) 473–482.

Correspondence to: Robert Johnson, PhD, 3 Norton Street, Kingsford, NSW 2032, Australia. Tel: 61-2-398-8323.

Proceedings of the 7th World Congress on Pain,
Progress in Pain Research and Management, Vol. 2,
edited by G.F. Gebhart, D.L. Hammond, and T.S.
Jensen, IASP Press, Seattle, © 1994.

60

Pain, Affect, and Cognition in Children: 2. Recall Bias Associated with Pain

Robert Johnson[a] and Susan H. Spence[b]

[a]Department of Psychology, University of Sydney, New South Wales, Australia, and [b]Department of Psychology, University of Queensland, Queensland, Australia

INTRODUCTION

There is now considerable evidence that specific emotional states are associated with bias in the cognitive processing of material relating to that emotional state (MacLeod and Mathews, 1991). This mood congruency effect has been demonstrated consistently in studies of affect and cognition (Isen et al. 1978; Bower et al. 1981; Nasby and Yando 1982), particularly for the recall of affectively laden material. Given that the experience of pain has much in common with negative affect states, it was hypothesized that subjects in pain would show a similar type of cognitive bias with respect to material related to their pain state. Thus, subjects who experience pain should recall a greater number of words associated with pain than subjects who are not experiencing pain. Indeed, a study by Pearce et al. (1990) found that chronic pain patients recalled more pain words and less neutral words than did controls. It is unclear, however, whether this effect was a pain-congruent recall effect or a demonstration of a well-learned vocabulary salient to the chronic pain patients' environment. In other words, is it frequent contact with an environment related to pain stimuli (such as hospital contact) that produces the effect or the experience of pain? Additionally, it was important to demonstrate that any recall bias for pain-related material was not simply due to higher levels of negative mood among those who experience pain. Furthermore, we needed to determine whether cognitive bias in recall for pain-related words only occurs when subjects are in pain (including acute pain), or whether it is the long-term experience of pain that creates this cognitive bias effect irrespective of current pain levels.

Our study examined recall bias for pain-related material in children in four experimental groups: acute postoperative pain, chronic pain, no-pain but in hospital, and no-pain outside of the hospital environment. The use of these groups allowed us to examine the influences of pain chronicity, environment, and pain experience (pain vs. no pain). To further separate environmental bias from pain bias in information processing, the experimental tasks included both pain-related and pain-descriptive words. This distinction was necessary because a related study found that bias in the recall of pain-related information was not related to differences in pain intensity if that information was composed only of descriptions of the pain environment (e.g., nurse, doctor, operation). Instead, just as cognitive bias in recall for affect-laden material is associated with prevailing mood state, we hypothesized that recall bias in children experiencing pain would be found for pain-descriptor material (e.g., ache, throbbing) rather than words associated with the pain environment (e.g., doctor, operation). Furthermore, we expected that such bias would not be found for children who have high levels of contact with the hospital environment but who do not experience pain. Finally, we hypothesized that cognitive bias in the recall of pain descriptive words would be related to the level of pain experienced rather than to negative affect states such as depression.

METHOD

SUBJECTS

The subjects consisted of 120 children aged 8 to 12 years, divided equally into four experimental groups: (1) an acute postoperative pain group consisting of children admitted to hospital for minor surgery such as tonsillectomy and appendectomy; (2) a chronic pain group consisting of children, mostly with juvenile arthritis, who had been experiencing pain for at least six months; (3) a no-pain group of children admitted to hospital for nonpainful procedures and observations; and (4) a no-pain group from outside of the hospital environment consisting of school children from a similar catchment area as that of the hospital. These last children were tested in the school and are referred to as the no-pain school group.

MEASURES

Assessment of Pain and Affect

At the commencement and conclusion of the experimental task, pain and affect ratings were elicited from all subjects. Pain was measured with a Visual Analog Scale (VAS) that consisted of an 18 by 4-cm plastic card on which was a 15-cm red-colored wedge, measuring from 1 cm to 3 cm in width. The intensity of redness of the wedge increased with the increasing width of the wedge. Additionally, at the narrow end were the words NO PAIN and at the wide end were the words MOST PAIN. A sliding cursor could be moved to any position on the wedge. On the reverse of the scale were graduations from 1 to 10 corresponding to the length of the wedge. (This VAS was designed by P.A. McGrath and her colleagues and given to participants at the Second International Symposium on Pediatric Pain, Montreal, Canada, 1991). Subjects were required to position the cursor at the point on the wedge that corresponded to their pain. A numerical rating was then obtained from the reverse of the scale. VAS-derived numerical estimates are reliable and valid measures of acute, recurrent, and chronic pain in children aged 5 to 16 years (McGrath, 1990, 1991).

Affective state was assessed using a scale consisting of seven basic schematic drawings of faces positioned in a horizontal row and identical in every respect except for the mouth. The expressions of the mouths varied from a downturn, depicting sadness, in the extreme left drawing, to an upturn, depicting a smile, in the extreme right drawing. Under each drawing, from left to right respectively, were the words Very Sad, Sad, A little Sad, Neutral, A little Happy, Happy, and Very Happy. The original scale was developed by Buck (1975) and used to measure self-reported affective state in children aged 5 to 6 years. The scale was modified by Forgas et al. (1988) to a seven-point scale for research with older children.

Recall Task

The recall task demanded that subjects attempt to recall and verbalize as many words as possible immediately after hearing a list of 30 words and again five minutes after hearing the list. The word list consisted of six pain descriptors obtained from the sensory group of the McGill Pain Questionnaire (Melzack 1982, 1987); six pain-related words that were salient within the hospital environment and had been used in related studies; six affectively negative words; six neutral words; and six filler words. The negative words, neutral words, and some filler words were obtained from previous research on affect and cognition (Isen et al. 1978; Clark et al. 1983; Teasdale and Russell 1983; Clark and Teasdale 1985; Williams and Broadbent 1986). The words were matched for frequency of usage and length, across categories. Within categories, no synonyms, antonyms, rhyming words, or words beginning with the same letter were used. Words that were hard to pronounce also were excluded. The filler words were positioned at the beginning and end of the word list to minimize the effects of primacy and recency on the recall of the other words. Within these constraints, all words were presented in a fixed randomized order.

RESULTS

The mean age of subjects was approximately 10.5 years. There was no significant difference in age between the groups. The gender ratio within each group varied from 2:1 males to females in the acute pain group to 1:1 in the chronic pain group; however, the results showed no gender-related effects.

There was no significant difference in the pain scores of the acute pain and chronic pain groups before or after the recall task. The difference between the pain groups and the no-pain groups on the pain rating measure was significant ($F[3, 116] = 68.15$, $P < 0.001$). All group mean affect ratings were similar across groups at a mean score of approximately five, and there was no significant difference between groups. The pain and affect scores were significantly correlated for the pain groups. The Pearson product-moment correlations ranged from –0.32 to –0.49, indicating a strong inverse relationship between pain and affect such that higher pain ratings correspond with lower affect ratings and vice versa.

Comparison of the scores at immediate recall showed no significant difference in the total recall of words across groups, with group means ranging from 7.1 words to 7.6 words. The comparison of recall data did, however, reveal significant differences between groups in the recall of specific word types. Fig. 1 shows the mean number of words recalled in each word category by each experimental group at immediate recall. The pattern of results at delayed recall mirrored those at immediate recall and will not be discussed in this chapter.

DIFFERENCES BETWEEN GROUPS FOR PAIN DESCRIPTOR WORDS

The acute pain group and the chronic pain group recalled significantly more pain-descriptor words (means of 1.7 and 1.8 words, respectively) than

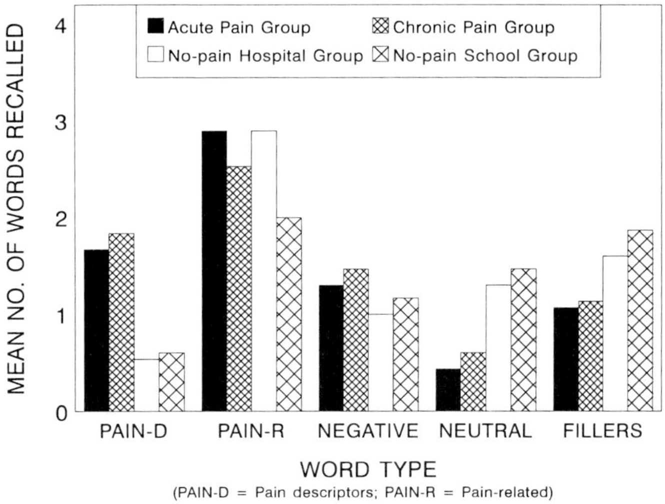

Fig. 1. The mean number of words recalled in each word category by each experimental group at immediate recall.

did the no-pain hospital group (mean = 0.5 words) and the no-pain school group (mean = 0.6 words) ($F[3, 116] = 24.34$, $P < 0.001$).

DIFFERENCES BETWEEN GROUPS FOR PAIN-RELATED WORDS

Significantly more pain-related words were recalled by the acute pain group (mean = 2.9 words) and the no-pain hospital group (mean = 2.9 words) than by the no-pain school group (mean = 2.0 words) ($F[3, 116] = 4.47$, $P = 0.005$). Fig. 1 shows that the chronic pain group also recalled more pain-related words than did the no-pain school group (mean = 2.5 words at immediate recall); however, this effect just failed to reach statistical significance.

DIFFERENCES BETWEEN GROUPS FOR NEGATIVE, NEUTRAL, AND FILLER WORDS

Significantly more neutral words were recalled by the no-pain hospital group (mean = 1.3 words) and the no-pain school group (mean = 1.5 words) than by the acute pain group (mean = 0.4 words) and chronic pain group (mean = 0.6 words). This is the inverse of the pain descriptor effect and may indicate that the bias of the pain groups toward recall of pain-descriptor words leaves less recall capacity for neutral words. In addition, the no-pain school group recalled more filler words than did the acute pain group, and the same explanation may apply. There was no significant difference in the recall of negative words across groups.

RELATIONSHIP BETWEEN CURRENT PAIN LEVELS AND RECALL

To test the hypothesis that greater pain results in the recall of more pain-descriptive words than does less pain, all pain subjects (i.e., acute and chronic) were divided into two groups, low pain and high pain, on the basis of a median split of their pain scores. Fig. 2 shows the mean word recall for each word type by group.

High- and low-pain groups were compared using analysis of covariance, taking affect as a covariate to ensure that differences between groups could not be explained by different levels of affective state. As hypothesized, subjects in the high-pain group recalled more pain descriptors (mean = 2.1 words) than did subjects in the low-pain group (mean = 1.4 words) ($F[1, 57] = 8.77$, $P = 0.004$). No significant differences were found between groups for recall of other word types.

DISCUSSION

The results from the analysis of the recall task data showed two major effects. First, the pain groups recalled significantly more pain descriptors than did the no-pain groups. That is, there was a positive recall bias of pain-descriptive words by subjects in the pain groups compared with those in the no-pain groups. Even those children who were in hospital, yet did not experience pain, did not show an elevation in recall of pain descriptor words. This finding indicates that the effect was specific to the experience of pain rather than to the hospital environment. Additional results showed that the subjects who were experiencing greater pain recalled more pain-descriptive words than did the subjects with less severe pain. Thus, the recall bias of pain-descriptive words appears to be progressive with increasing pain, rather than a simple off-on effect.

Second, the acute pain group, the no-pain hospital group, and the chronic pain group recalled more pain-related words than did the no-pain school group. The critical variable was the subject's environment. All acute pain and no-pain hospital subjects were tested in the hospital environment; the no-pain school subjects were not. Approximately half of the chronic pain subjects were tested in the hospital, the other half outside. Thus, the results of the study suggest that recall bias for pain-related information occurs in hospitalized children, irrespective of their prevailing pain state. This finding is perhaps not

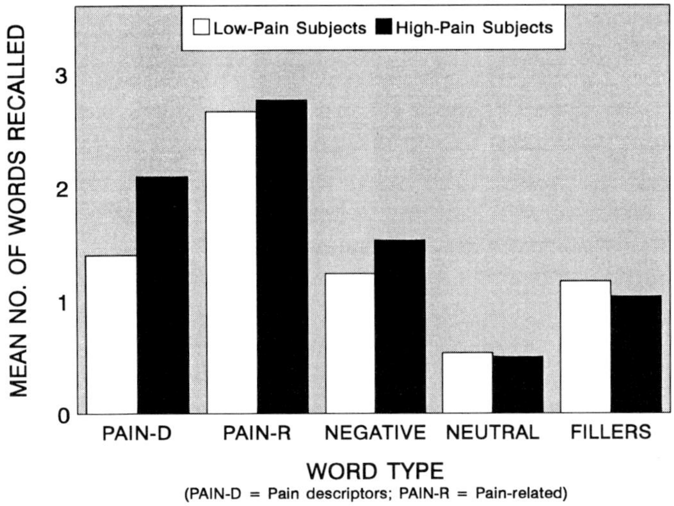

Fig. 2. The mean number of words recalled in each word category by low-pain and high-pain groups.

surprising given that pain-related words are strongly associated with the hospital environment (e.g., doctor, operation) and are likely to have high salience to children who are in hospital whether or not they experience pain. Only the pain descriptor words were proposed to have specific relevance to the experience of pain (e.g., ache, throbbing).

In summary, the study found that the experience of pain produced a bias in the recall of material associated with the state of pain. This effect increased as the level of pain increased, and was not attributable to the negative affective state associated with being in pain. Furthermore, the effect was not explained by association with the physical environment in which the pain was experienced (e.g., the hospital). Nevertheless, the subject's environment evidently facilitated the recall of information. Material relating to the physical environment associated with pain (pain-related words) was recalled better by children who were in hospital, regardless of whether they were experiencing pain. It appears that aspects of the hospital environment become highly salient to children and influence subsequent information processing of stimuli associated with that environment, thereby producing a bias in retrieval from memory.

Overall, the results confirmed the proposed bias in recall for pain-descriptor material in association with the experience of pain. Thus, pain appears to have a similar influence to other forms of negative affective state, such as depression, for which bias in recall from memory has previously been demonstrated.

ACKNOWLEDGMENTS

This research was conducted as partial fulfillment of the requirements for the Ph.D. degree by Robert Johnson and was supervised by Associate Professor Susan H. Spence. Financial support was provided by a scholarship from Johnson & Johnson Australia Pty. Limited. Special thanks are due to Dr. G. David Champion and Dr. John B. Ziegler of The Prince of Wales Children's Hospital, where all inpatient subjects were recruited.

REFERENCES

Bower, G. H., Gilligan, S. G. and Montiero, K. P., Selectivity of learning caused by affective states, J. Exp. Psychol. Gen., 110 (1981) 451-473.

Buck, R., Nonverbal communication of affect in children, J. Pers. Soc. Psychol., 31 (1975) 644-653.

Clark, D. M., Teasdale, J. D., Broadbent, D. E. and Martin, M., Effect of mood on lexical decisions, Bull. Psychonomic Soc., 21 (1983) 175-178.

Clark, D. M. and Teasdale, J. D., Constraints on the effects of mood on memory, J. Pers. Soc. Psychol., 48 (1985) 1595-1608.

Forgas, J. P., Burnham, D. K. and Trimboli, C., Mood, memory and social judgments in children, J. Pers. Soc. Psychol., 54 (1988) 697-703.

Isen, A. M., Shalker, T. E., Clark, M. and Karp, L., Affect, accessibility of material in memory, and behaviour: A cognitive loop?, J. Pers. Soc. Psychol., 36 (1978) 1-12.

MacLeod, C. and Mathews, A. M., Cognitive-experimental approaches to the emotional disorders. In P. R. Martin (Ed.), Handbook of behavior therapy and psychological science. Pergamon Press, New York, 1991, pp. 116-150.

McGrath, P. A., Pain in children: Nature, assessment, and treatment, Guilford Press, New York, 1990.

McGrath, P. A., Versatile pain measures for children, Paper presented at the Second International Symposium on Pediatric Pain, Montreal, Canada, April 24-27, 1991.

Melzack, R., The McGill Pain Questionnaire: Major properties and scoring methods, Pain, 11 (1982) 275-299.

Melzack, R., The short-form McGill Pain Questionnaire, Pain, 30 (1987) 191-197.

Nasby, W. and Yando, R., Selective encoding and retrieval of affectively valent information: Two cognitive consequences of children's mood states, J. Pers. Soc. Psychol., 43 (1982) 1244-1253.

Pearce, S. A., Isherwood, S., Hrouda, D., Richardson, P. H., Erskine, A. and Skinner, J., Memory and pain: tests of mood congruity and state dependent learning in experimentally induced and clinical pain, Pain, 43 (1990) 187-193.

Teasdale, J. D. and Russell, M. L., Differential effects of induced mood on the recall of positive, negative and neutral words, Br. J. Clin. Psychol., 22 (1983) 163-171.

Williams, J. M. G. and Broadbent, K., Distraction by emotional stimuli: Use of a Stroop task with suicide attempters, Br. J. Clin. Psychol., 25 (1986) 101-110.

Correspondence to: Robert Johnson, PhD, 3 Norton Street, Kingsford, NSW 2032, Australia. Tel: 61-2-398-8323.

Proceedings of the 7th World Congress on Pain,
Progress in Pain Research and Management, Vol. 2,
edited by G.F. Gebhart, D.L. Hammond, and T.S.
Jensen, IASP Press, Seattle, © 1994.

61

Factors Contributing to the Properties of the Cutaneous Withdrawal Reflex in Human Neonates

Katharine Andrews and Maria Fitzgerald

Department of Anatomy and Developmental Biology,
University College London, UK

INTRODUCTION

In view of the recent increase of interest in the study of human neonatal responses to painful stimuli, it is clear that more information is required concerning the development of human somatosensory function in general. An understanding of the functional development of the somatosensory system and its responses to both noxious and non-noxious stimuli is essential if we are to reach conclusions about neonates' experiences of pain. The increased numbers of preterm neonates surviving and undergoing traumatic procedures make it an important field of study (Craig et al. 1993; Fitzgerald 1991).

One measure of somatosensory function that seems relatively unaffected by factors such as hunger or stress is the cutaneous withdrawal reflex threshold. It has already yielded useful information on somatosensory development (Fitzgerald et al. 1988, 1989; Andrews and Fitzgerald 1994). The threshold of the nociceptive flexor reflex in the adult has been demonstrated to be a sensitive measure of spinal cord excitability, and nociceptive activity of the kind generated postoperatively or in intensive care can lower the threshold of the reflex, indicating a hyperalgesic response (Woolf and Wall 1986; Woolf 1983, 1984). Despite its low threshold in the neonate, the cutaneous withdrawal reflex also appears to be a useful measure of such central excitability, as demonstrated by the fall in its threshold in the presence of injury (Fitzgerald et al. 1989).

The questions addressed here are:

1. What are the special features of the developing withdrawal reflex that can add to our knowledge of the developing somatosensory system?
2. What are the relative contributions of the sensory and motor components of the reflex arc that result in the features observed in the developing withdrawal reflex?

METHODS

The properties of the cutaneous withdrawal reflex in 29 female and 21 male infants were tested using calibrated von Frey hairs. Each infant was tested between one and four times, and a total of 108 tests were performed. The weights of the hairs ranged from 0.08 to 12.6 g. The infants were tested only when they were being disturbed for some other reason, such as an eight-hourly "all-care" procedure. They were tested either in the prone position or on their side, and were either quietly awake or lightly asleep when tested. Each test took approximately 20 minutes and was performed on one leg only.

The initial threshold for the withdrawal reflex was determined by applying a von Frey hair perpendicularly on the plantar surface of the foot toward the outer aspect of the heel. A very fine hair was used to begin with, and working upward in force, the initial threshold was considered to have been reached when a clear, brisk withdrawal of the foot away from the stimulus was obtained.

Repeated innocuous stimuli were applied immediately after establishing initial threshold. In exactly the same place on the foot, the von Frey hair two steps above threshold (3.4 times more weight applied) was applied in the same way, at 10-second intervals 10 times. The response was noted after each stimulation. The threshold following repeated stimuli was then determined starting with the von Frey hair at one grade of intensity below that used to obtain the initial threshold.

In order to define the receptive field for the withdrawal reflex, 11 points on the lower leg along distal-proximal lines were tested, beginning on the plantar surface of the foot with the grade of von Frey hair used to evoke initial threshold. Where possible, the thigh and buttock were also tested.

A contralateral stimulus was applied by gently holding and stroking the contralateral foot while stimulating the ipsilateral foot with the grade of von Frey hair used for the initial threshold. The infant was always left for a few minutes following the last experiment before this test was performed. The foot was stimulated three times without holding the contralateral foot, then there was a five-minute waiting period before the ipsilateral foot was tested three times more, this time while the other foot was being held and stroked.

More recently, preliminary surface EMG recordings of withdrawal responses to von Frey hair stimulation have been made from flexor and extensor muscles of the lower limb, particularly biceps femoris and quadriceps femoris, using standard silver/silver chloride electrodes (5 mm in diameter with centers separated by 15 mm). Electrode impedances were measured and maintained below 2 kOhms. Single sweeps were recorded and saved using a Sapphire 2M EMG unit (Medelec Ltd., UK).

Prior approval for the study was obtained from the Ethics Committee at University College Hospital, and written parental consent was obtained for each infant.

RESULTS

INITIAL THRESHOLD

In both preterm and full-term human neonates, the cutaneous withdrawal reflex is evoked with low intensity mechanical stimuli to the foot (Fitzgerald et al. 1988, 1989) and has a much lower threshold than the nociceptive flexion reflex in the adult (RIII; Hugon 1973). This result was confirmed here. The threshold of the withdrawal reflex in the neonate rises with increasing postconceptional (PC) age (Fitzgerald et al. 1988) and is therefore an interesting index of somatosensory development (Fig. 1). Neonatal rats demonstrate similar low threshold reflex withdrawal responses following cutaneous stimulation observed by behavioral methods (Fitzgerald et al. 1988), and on direct recording from flexor motor axons (Fitzgerald and Gibson 1984).

REPEATED STIMULATION

Another feature of the cutaneous withdrawal reflex in neonatal rats and in human infants below 30–35 weeks PC age is the sensitization that occurs with repeated innocuous stimulation (Fitzgerald et al. 1988). Here this was studied in more detail by looking at the drop in threshold as well as the number of responses to repeated stimulation. The effect in the human neonate is not as profound as in the neonatal rat.

Above approximately 37 weeks PC age, habituation to repeated innocuous stimulation occurs, characterized by a decrease in the number of re-

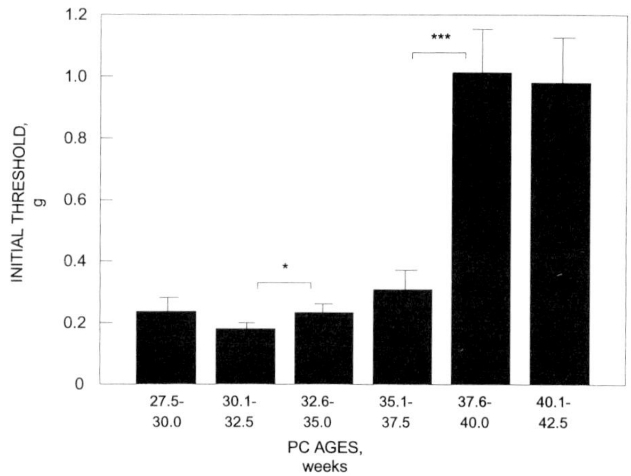

Fig. 1. Postconceptional (PC) age versus initial threshold, in infants without leg injury. Error bars denote S.E.M. Stars denote levels of significance of differences in threshold between age bands (* $P < 0.05$; *** $P < 0.001$). (Reproduced with permission from Andrews and Fitzgerald 1994)

sponses and no drop in threshold on repeated stimulation (Fitzgerald et al. 1988; see Fig 2). This is more akin to the habituation of withdrawal reflex responses seen in adults following repeated stimulation at regular intervals (Dimitrijevic and Nathan 1970; Dimitrijevic et al. 1972; Wickelgren 1967a,b), although Hugon (1973) has reported sensitization occurring in adults, but only in response to noxious stimulation. The point of interest here is that, in the human neonate, *non-noxious* stimulation produces sensitization.

RECEPTIVE FIELDS

The receptive field for the withdrawal reflex in the human neonate occupies the same area as that of the flexor reflex in the adult cat and rat, extending from the toes to the top of the thigh and buttock (Sherrington 1910; Woolf and Swett 1984; Andrews and Fitzgerald 1994). In the human neonate, as in the adult cat (Sherrington 1910) and rat (Woolf and Swett 1984), there is also a graded distribution of thresholds within the receptive field, with a "hotspot" of maximum sensitivity on the plantar surface of the foot and a decrease in sensitivity progressing up the leg toward the knee (Andrews and Fitzgerald 1994; see Fig. 3). However, there is far more uniformity of threshold within the receptive field in the younger neonates (below 35 weeks PC age), and overall, the thresholds within the receptive field are lower in this age group.

CONTRALATERAL STIMULATION

Despite the preceding phenomena, which are indicative of a higher level of excitability in the neonatal spinal cord, there is evidence that segmental

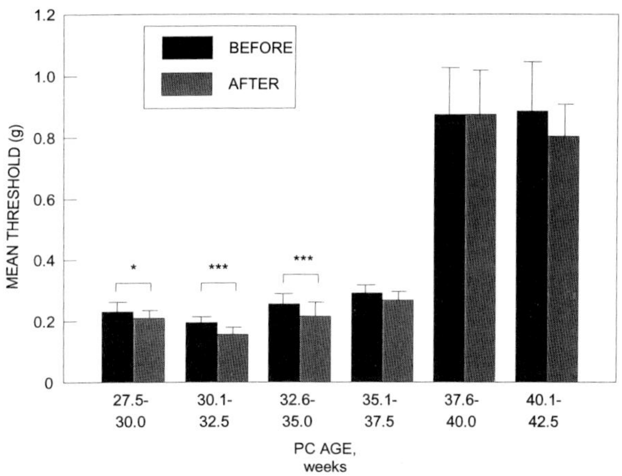

Fig. 2. Effect of repeated stimulation on threshold. Error bars denote S.E.M. Stars denote levels of significance of differences in threshold before and after repeated stimulation within age bands (* $P < 0.05$; *** $P < 0.001$). (Reproduced with permission from Andrews and Fitzgerald 1994)

inhibitory mechanisms are well established. The withdrawal reflex in the human neonate is clearly inhibited by non-noxious contralateral stimulation, even in infants as young as 27.5 weeks PC age (Andrews and Fitzgerald 1994). The responses are similar across all PC ages up to full-term (see Fig. 4). Contralateral inhibition has been clearly observed in spinal adult rats, in response to both noxious stimuli involving A-delta- and C-fibers, and non-noxious stimuli involving A-beta-fibers (Fitzgerald 1982). The former type of inhibition appears to be more powerful in the adult (Fitzgerald 1982), but this seems not to be the case in the neonate (Andrews and Fitzgerald 1994).

EMG RECORDINGS

Surface EMG recordings, which have been so useful in the study of other reflexes in neonates (Mayer and Mosser 1969; Vecchierini-Blineau and Guiheneuc 1981; Issler and Stephens 1983; Myklebust et al. 1986; O'Sullivan et al. 1991), provide a quantitative measure of the withdrawal reflex. Fig. 5 shows a preliminary surface EMG recording from biceps femoris and its antagonist, quadriceps femoris, of a withdrawal response to a mechanical stimulus. Initial findings suggest that the radiation of reflex responses to antagonistic muscles seen in other neonatal studies (Bergstrom et al. 1962; Issler and Stephens 1983; Myklebust et al. 1986; O'Sullivan et al. 1991) does not occur to the same degree in the cutaneous withdrawal reflex when non-noxious mechanical stimuli are applied (Fig. 5). Further detailed EMG studies are being undertaken to determine the latency, duration, and magnitude of the withdrawal reflex in the neonate, in response to both noxious and non-noxious stimulation, and under a variety of clinical conditions.

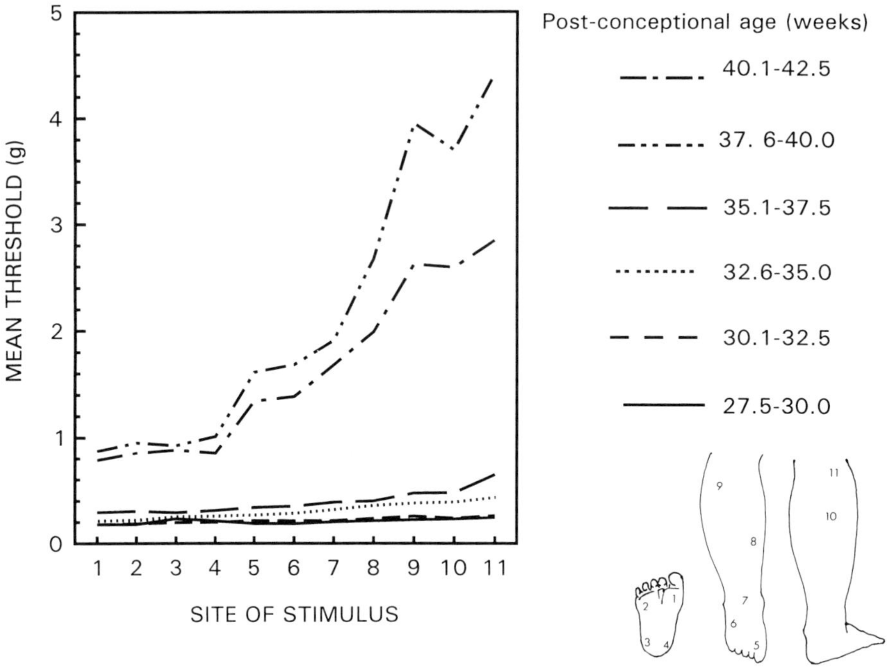

Fig. 3. Effect of increasing PC age and site of stimulus on threshold. Error bars are not inserted as the S.E.M.s are so small. The numbers marked on the abscissa correspond to the sites of stimulation shown on the leg. (Modified with permission from Andrews and Fitzgerald 1994)

DISCUSSION

There has been much discussion about the relative contributions of changes in sensory versus motor excitability to the developmental changes seen in the cutaneous withdrawal reflex in the neonate, and its usefulness as an index of somatosensory processing, particularly in response to noxious stimuli. We take the opportunity here to examine this issue.

Immature motor neurons are more easily excitable than those in the adult (Kellerth et al. 1971; Fulton and Walton 1986; Kudo and Yamada 1987), and this is thought to underlie the large amplitude of motor reflex responses in the neonate (Thomas and Lambert 1960; Mayer and Mosser 1973; Myklebust et al. 1986; O'Sullivan et al. 1991). Also, lesions of the pyramidal tract in adults result in increased reflex excitability (Kugelberg et al. 1960; Dimitrijevic 1973; Jenner and Stephens 1982), so the lack of functional development of

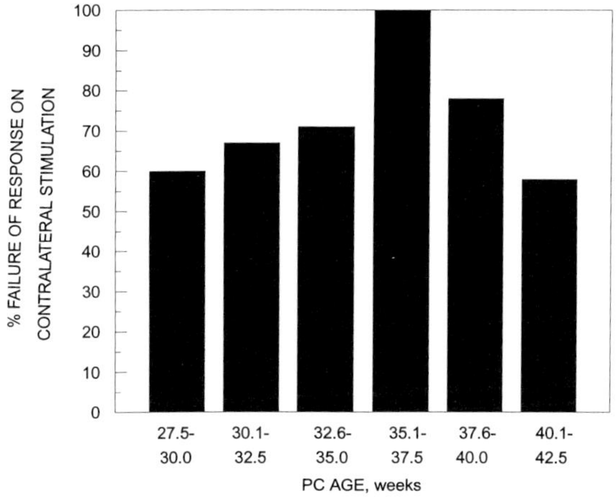

Fig. 4. Effect of a contralateral stimulus on ipsilateral response to stimulation. Percentages of tests that showed a decrease in the number of responses on contralateral stimulation.

this tract in neonates may be responsible for their augmented motor reflexes (Issler and Stephens 1983; Leonard et al. 1991). In contrast to this, however, Mayer and Mosser (1973) found that both the H:M ratio (an index of motor neuron excitability) and the F response (antidromic excitation of motor neurons) are the same in human newborns as in adults. This suggests that increased motor neuron excitability does not play a major role in the augmented reflex responses seen in neonates. Furthermore, motor units in awake unrestrained newborn rats are surprisingly inactive (Navarrete and Vrbova 1983). In addition, proprioceptive excitation is relatively weak at a time when flexion responses to skin stimulation are exaggerated, and excitatory skin areas are largest in the newborn being gradually restricted during development (Ekholm 1967). The increased excitability of motor neurons found in some studies is therefore likely to be a part of a general increased neuronal excitability in the immature spinal cord due to higher input resistance (Fulton and Walton 1986) and lack of descending inhibition (Issler and Stephens 1983). It does not explain the differential increased responsiveness to cutaneous versus muscle inputs (Ekholm 1967).

The most striking effects of sensory excitability unique to the cutaneous withdrawal reflex are seen in responses to repeated noxious and non-noxious skin stimuli, both of which result in sensitization in preterm infants below 32–34 weeks PC age (Fitzgerald et al. 1988, 1989; Andrews and Fitzgerald 1994). The stretch reflex, although highly synchronized in the neonate and therefore large in amplitude, does not sensitize (Myklebust et al. 1986). Similar changes are seen in the flexion reflex in the adult as a result of long-term injury (Woolf 1983, 1984) and reflect changes in central excitability of inter-

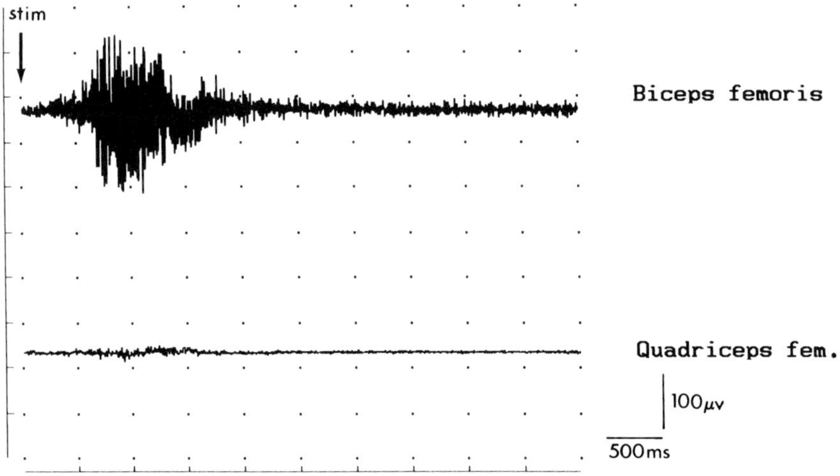

Fig. 5. Surface EMG recording (single sweep) from biceps femoris and quadriceps femoris of a withdrawal response to a non-noxious mechanical stimulus. The EMG burst in biceps is not accompanied by a corresponding large burst in quadriceps. Vertical calibration 100 μV, sweep speed 5 sec. Arrow indicates time of stimulus.

neurons in the spinal cord (Woolf 1992; Woolf and Wiesenfeld-Hallin 1986). These processes may also occur in the neonate, albeit against a general background of increased neuronal excitability due to immaturity.

CONCLUSION

Despite the undeniable contributions of general neuronal immaturity to the features of the cutaneous withdrawal reflex in the neonate, the specific changes in responses to cutaneous stimuli seen over 27 to 42 weeks PC age indicate that this reflex is a useful tool in the study of somatosensory processing in the neonate. Progress will undoubtedly be enhanced by the continued use of EMG studies using mechanical stimuli, through which we hope to gain an accurate picture of the responses of neonates to the type of stimuli they encounter every day while receiving intensive care, which are not like the electrical stimuli used in the experimental situation. The end result of these studies must be to increase our understanding of neonatal responses to inputs resulting from intensive care, and thus to begin to find ways of preventing the kinds of long-term changes in the nervous system that would be so detrimental to their subsequent development.

ACKNOWLEDGMENTS

We thank the Wellcome Trust for financial support, and Alan Ainsworth for technical advice and for making the von Frey hairs. We also thank the staff of the Neonatal Unit at University College Hospital, particularly Osmund Reynolds, for their help and cooperation in this study. Last, we thank the parents of all the babies who were included in the study for their consent and cooperation.

REFERENCES

Andrews, K.A. and Fitzgerald, M., The cutaneous withdrawal reflex in human neonates: sensitization, receptive fields, and the effects of contralateral stimulation, Pain, 56 (1994) 95–102.

Bergstrom, R.M., Hellstrom, P.-E. and Stenberg, D., Studies in reflex irradiation in the foetal guinea-pig, Ann. Chir. Gynaec. Fenn., 51 (1962) 171–178.

Craig, K.D., Whitfield, M.F., Grunau, R.V.E., Linton, J. and Hadjistavropoulos, H.D., Pain in the preterm neonate: behavioural and physiological indices, Pain, 52 (1993) 287–299.

Dimitrijevic, M.R., Withdrawal reflexes. In: J.E. Desmedt (Ed.), New Developments in Electromyography and Clinical Neurophysiology, Vol. 3, Karger, Basel, 1973, pp. 744–750.

Dimitrijevic, M.R. and Nathan, P.W., Studies of spasticity in man. 4. Changes in flexion reflex with repetitive cutaneous stimulation in spinal man, Brain, 93 (1970) 743–768.

Dimitrijevic, M.R., Faganel, J., Gregoric, M., Nathan, P.W. and Trontelj, J.K., Habituation: effects of regular and stochastic stimulation, J. Neurol. Neurosurg. Psych., 35 (1972) 234–242.

Ekholm, J., Postnatal changes in cutaneous reflexes and in the discharge pattern of cutaneous and articular sense organs, Acta Physiol. Scand., Suppl., 297 (1967) 1–130.

Fitzgerald, M., The contralateral input to the dorsal horn of the spinal cord in the decerebrate spinal rat, Brain Res., 236 (1982) 275–287.

Fitzgerald, M., The developmental neurobiology of pain. In: M.R. Bond, J.E. Charlton and C.J. Woolf (Eds.), Proceedings of the VIth World Congress on Pain, Elsevier, Amsterdam, 1991, 253–261.

Fitzgerald, M. and Gibson, S., The postnatal physiological and neurochemical development of peripheral sensory C fibres, Neurosci., 13 (1984) 933–944.

Fitzgerald, M., Millard, C. and McIntosh, N., Cutaneous hypersensitivity following peripheral tissue damage in newborn infants and its reversal with topical anaesthesia, Pain, 39 (1989) 31–36.

Fitzgerald, M., Shaw, A. and McIntosh, N., The postnatal development of the cutaneous flexor reflex: comparative study of preterm infants and newborn rat pups, Dev. Med. Child Neurol., 30 (1988) 520–526.

Fulton, B.P. and Walton, K., Electrophysiological properties of neonatal rat motoneurons studied in vitro, J. Physiol., 370 (1986) 651–678.

Hugon, M., Exteroceptive reflexes to stimulation of the sural nerve in normal man. In: J.E. Desmedt (Ed.), New Developments in Electromyography and Clinical Neurophysiology, Vol. 3, Karger, Basel, 1973, 713–729.

Issler, H. and Stephens, J.A., The maturation of cutaneous reflexes studied in the upper limb in man, J. Physiol., 335 (1983) 643–654.

Jenner, J.R. and Stephens, J.A., Cutaneous reflex responses and their central nervous pathways studied in man, J. Physiol., 333 (1982) 405–419.

Kellerth, J., Mellstrom, A. and Skoglund, S., Postnatal excitability changes of kitten motoneurones, Acta Physiol. Scand., 83 (1971) 31–41.

Kudo, N. and Yamada, T., Morphological and physiological studies of development of the monosynaptic reflex pathway in the rat lumbar spinal cord, J. Physiol., 389 (1987) 441–459.
Kugelberg, E., Eklund, K. and Grimby, L., An electromyographic study of the nociceptive reflexes of the lower limb. Mechanism of the plantar responses, Brain Res., 83 (1960) 394–410.
Leonard, C.T., Hirschfeld, H. and Forssberg, H., The development of independent walking in children with cerebral palsy, Dev. Med. Child Neurol., 33 (1991) 567–577.
Mayer, R.F. and Mosser, R.S., Excitability of motoneurones in infants, Neurology, 19 (1969) 932–945.
Mayer, R.F. and Mosser, R.S., Maturation of human reflexes. In: New Developments in Electromyography and Clinical Neurophysiology, Vol. 3, Karger, Basel, 1973, 294–307.
Myklebust, B.M., Gottlieb, G.L. and Argawal, G.C., Stretch reflexes of the normal infant, Dev. Med. Child Neurol., 28 (1986) 440–449.
Navarrete, R. and Vrbova, G., Changes of activity patterns in slow and fast muscles during postnatal development, Dev. Brain Res., 8 (1983) 11–19.
O'Sullivan, M.C., Eyre, J.A. and Miller, S., Radiation of phasic stretch reflex in biceps brachii to muscles of the arm in man and its restriction during development, J. Physiol., 439 (1991) 529–543.
Sherrington, C.S., Flexion reflex of the limb, crossed extension reflex, and reflex stepping and standing, J. Physiol., 40 (1910) 28–121.
Thomas, J.E. and Lambert, E.H., Ulnar nerve conduction velocity and H-reflex in infants and children, J. Appl. Physiol., 15 (1960) 1–9.
Vecchierini-Blineau, M.F. and Guiheneuc, P., Excitability of the monosynaptic reflex pathway in the child from birth to four years of age, J. Neurol. Neurosurg. Psych., 44 (1981) 309–314.
Wickelgren, B.G., Habituation of spinal motoneurons, J. Neurophysiol., 30 (1967a) 1404–1423.
Wickelgren, B.G., Habituation of spinal interneurons, J. Neurophysiol., 30 (1967b) 1424–1438.
Woolf, C.J., Evidence for a central component of post-injury pain hypersensitivity, Nature, 306 (1983) 686–688.
Woolf, C.J., Long term alterations in the excitability of the flexion reflex produced by peripheral tissue injury in the chronic decerebrate rat, Pain, 18 (1984) 325–343.
Woolf, C.J., Excitability changes in central neurons following peripheral damage: role of central sensitization in the pathogenesis of pain. In: W.D. Willis (Ed.), Hyperalgesia and Allodynia, Raven Press, New York, 1992, 221–243.
Woolf, C.J. and Swett, J., The cutaneous contribution to the hamstring flexor reflex in the rat: an electrophysiological and anatomical study, Brain Res., 303 (1984) 299–312.
Woolf, C.J. and Wall, P.D., The relative effectiveness of C primary afferent fibres of different origins in evoking a prolonged facilitation of the flexor reflex in the rat, J. Neurosci., 6 (1986) 1433–1443.
Woolf, C.J. and Wiesenfeld-Hallin, Z., Substance P and calcitonin gene-related peptide synergistically modulate the gain of the nociceptive flexor withdrawal reflex in the rat, Neurosci. Lett., 66 (1986) 226–230.

Correspondence to: Mrs. Katharine Andrews, Department of Anatomy and Developmental Biology, University College London, Gower Street, London WC1E 6BT. Tel: 44-71-380-7376; Fax: 44-71-383-0929.

Proceedings of the 7th World Congress on Pain,
Progress in Pain Research and Management, Vol. 2,
edited by G.F. Gebhart, D.L. Hammond, and T.S.
Jensen, IASP Press, Seattle, © 1994.

62

Comparison of Chronic Pain Experience Between Young and Elderly Patients

Trevor M. Corran, Stephen J. Gibson,
Michael J. Farrell, and Robert D. Helme

National Research Institute of Gerontology and Geriatric Medicine,
Parkville, Australia

INTRODUCTION

The effect of age has received little attention in the pain literature (Harkins and Price 1992; Melding 1991). From the limited number of published studies comparing the pain experience across the age spectrum, it would appear that similarities are more remarkable than differences (Sorkin et al. 1990). In the earliest of the published studies Middaugh et al. (1988) looked at the differences between two small groups of patients with mean ages of 62.4 years (range 55–78, n = 17) and 38.5 years (range 29–48, n = 20). They found minor differences, with more physical impairments in the older group. A gender effect, with women tending to report more pain and a higher use of health services, was present at all ages. Sorkin et al. (1990), in a study that used the West Haven–Yale Multidimensional Pain Inventory, compared two groups with mean ages of 72.5 years (SD = 6.6, n = 26) and 27.7 years (SD = 4.8, n =26). They identified no differences between these groups other than a greater number of abnormal physical findings among the older group.

The evidence from these cross-sectional studies must be interpreted circumspectly (Middaugh et al. 1988; Sorkin et al. 1990). Harkins (1988) has noted that very few of the elderly are treated in general pain management clinics, despite an apparent age-related increase in the prevalence of chronic pain. This factor may have contributed to additional sources of selection bias for the elderly portion of the sample in those studies cited above. Moreover, the sample numbers were small and the very old (greater than 80 years) were either absent or underrepresented. The psychometric instruments employed in these studies had not been validated for use with older persons, yet this issue may be important when examining age differences (Helme et al. 1989a; Corran et al. 1991; Gibson et al. in press). As a result, the conclusion that age is not a significant factor in the pain experience may be somewhat premature.

Another important consideration when examining the chronic pain experience of older adults concerns the issue of age differences in the use of coping strategies and in the ability to cope with the negative consequences of persistent pain. There is some evidence that older persons are more accepting of pain as a normal consequence of aging (Harkins et al. 1984; Helme et al. 1992), which might be expected to influence the choice and use of coping strategies. Sorkin et al. (1990) showed that older chronic pain patients displayed a lower ratio in the use of cognitive to physical coping skills than did their younger counterparts. Keefe and Williams (1990) examined coping strategies in four groups of 22 patients with mean ages of 28.77 (SD = 2.29), 39.86 (SD = 3.66), 59.09 (SD = 1.88), and 72.05 (SD = 5.46) years, using the Coping Strategies Questionnaire. In contrast to Sorkin et al. (1990), they reported no significant difference in the frequency of use of coping strategies, although there was a strong trend for the elderly adults to use more praying and hoping. Keefe and Williams (1990) also examined the relationship between coping strategies and the level of adjustment using this sample, which did include chronic pain patients of advanced age. Consistent with previous studies of young adults (Jensen et al. 1991), the use of catastrophizing as a strategy was found to be maladaptive, leading to higher levels of pain, depression, and psychological distress. While these findings support the notion of similar relationships between coping and measures of adjustment across the age spectrum, no attempt was made to examine these relationships within each age group.

Our study examined the chronic pain experience and the use of coping strategies in young, middle-aged, old, and very old patients suffering from chronic pain. We explored the question of whether older people differ in the absolute levels of suffering and the reported use of coping strategies and looked for differences in the relationships between coping skills and levels of pain, mood disturbance, and disability.

METHOD

SUBJECTS

We collected data from patients consecutively assessed at entry to two multidisciplinary pain clinics—the North West Hospital Pain Clinic and the

Caulfield Pain Clinic in Melbourne, Australia. The North West Clinic manages pain predominantly in the elderly and contributed data from 179 subjects with a mean age of 71.37 years (range 39–92) collected over 26 months between March 1991 and May 1993. The Caulfield Clinic caters mainly to younger adults. This portion of the sample consisted of 171 subjects with a mean age of 42.52 years (range 18–83) who attended the clinic between March 1992 and May 1993. All subjects were divided by age into four groups irrespective of the clinic they attended.

PROCEDURE

Subjects were assessed in their homes before attending the clinic, and then were screened for eligibility by a physician. Patients were not included in the study if the physician concluded further assessment by team members was not appropriate, if English was not their first language, if they showed signs of dementia as assessed by an Abbreviated Mental Test Score of less than 8 (Hodkinson 1972), or if the patient had a visual or physical impairment that would prevent them from completing the pen and paper psychometric instruments. A more complete description of these procedures may be found in Helme et al. (1989b).

MEASURES

Demographic information was recorded for each patient on age, gender, marital status, and months in pain. Pain was assessed using the McGill Pain Questionnaire (MPQ; Melzack 1975). This instrument consists of four classes of word descriptors: sensory, affective, evaluative, and miscellaneous that are used by patients to specify subjective pain experience. This study employed the sensory (PRIS) and affective (PRIA) dimensions. Previous experience with the MPQ has supported its use with older persons (Corran et al. 1991). The two clinics used different depression scales. The Caulfield Pain Clinic used the self-rating depression scale (SRDS; Zung 1965), while the North West Clinic had adopted the Geriatric Depression Scale (GDS; Yesavage et al. 1983). Scores were not used in parametric analysis. Cutoffs of 50 (Zung 1974) and 11 (Yesavage et al. 1983) were used for the SRDS and the GDS, respectively, as an indicator of depression. Anxiety was measured using the state version of the Spielberger State/Trait Anxiety Inventory (STAI; Spielberger 1983). The Sickness Impact Profile (SIP; Gilson et al. 1975) was selected as a measure of disability and adapted for use with chronic pain patients. This behaviorally based measure consists of 14 subscales of sickness-related dysfunction and has been previously validated for use with the elderly (Fletcher et al. 1992). These subscales can be collated into two areas of sickness impact involving psychosocial (PSYCSOC) and physical (PHYS) function. Our study used these two global measures. The final measure was the Coping Strategies Questionnaire (CSQ) developed by Rosenthiel and Keefe (1983). This instrument assesses the coping strategies used by the patient to deal with pain. The questionnaire consists of seven classes of coping strategies (i.e., ignoring sensations, diverting attention, praying and hoping, increased behavioral activity, reinterpreting sensation, catastrophizing, and coping self-statements), as well as two effectiveness ratings—ability to decrease pain (ADP) and control over pain (COP). The CSQ has been successfully administered to older subjects in the past (Keefe and Williams 1990).

RESULTS

The original sample for this study comprised 350 patients. Seventy-four patients had missing data on one or more of the dependent variables, leaving a total of 276 patients for the multivariate analyses and 297 patients for univariate analyses.

Given that the data were collected from two multidisciplinary pain management centers, we conducted an initial analysis to examine possible differences in patient ratings of the chronic pain experience between the clinics. Patient scores on the PRIS, PRIA, STAI, PHYS, PSYCSOC, ADP, and COP were analyzed conjointly using MANOVA with age as a covariate. The findings indicated no significant differences between the clinics on the scores from the psychometric questionnaires after matching for age.

Patients were divided into four groups on the basis of age: 18–39, 40–59, 60–79, and greater than 80 years. Table I provides descriptive information concerning the numbers in each group, the mean age, sex, marital status, and duration of pain. A chi-square analysis for differences between age groups revealed that the proportion of women patients was significantly higher in the older groups, $\chi^2 = 16.5$, $P = .001$, as was the proportion of widowed/divorced versus married or single patients, $\chi^2 = 102.6$, $P < .0001$. Table I shows that these differences were most noticeable between the youngest and oldest age cohorts. It also shows that all patients had been suffering from pain for an extended period. However, ANOVA indicated a significant difference between age groups, $F_{(3,227)} = 3.85$, $P = .01$. Post-hoc Newman Keuls pairwise comparisons demonstrated that patients aged 40–60 reported a significantly longer duration of pain than did patients aged 18–40 or greater than 80 years.

To examine possible age-related differences in the chronic pain experience, self-report measures of PRIS, PRIA, STAI, PSYCSOC, PHYS, COP, and ADP were entered into a MANOVA. Due to significant differences in the

Table I
Demographic information for sample by age group

	Age Group			
	18–39	40–59	60–79	80+
Number	57	77	121	42
Mean age, years (S.E.M.)	31.4 (0.7)	49.5 (0.6)	70.4 (0.5)	84.6 (0.4)
Gender, number (%)				
Men	30 (53)	30 (39)	40 (32)	5 (12)
Women	27 (47)	47 (61)	87 (68)	37 (88)
Marital status, number (%)				
Single	26 (45)	14 (18)	11 (9)	4 (10)
Married	25 (44)	45 (58)	63 (52)	8 (20)
Divorced/widowed	6 (11)	18 (24)	47 (39)	30 (70)
Mean duration of pain, months (S.E.M.)	46.8 (7.5)	83.4 (10.6)	67.8 (8.0)	35.9 (5.5)

proportion of women and the duration of pain between age groups, both age and gender were entered as factors, while duration of pain was entered as a covariate in the analysis. Depression scores were not included in this analysis because the two clinics used different screening instruments. Scores on the depression scales were converted to dichotomous data (i.e., depressed vs. nondepressed) and analyzed separately.

The MANOVA revealed a highly significant effect of age, $F_{(21,720)} = 4.28$, $P < .0001$, with no difference between the genders and no significant interaction effect. In addition, duration of pain was not a significant covariate with patient scores on measures of pain, mood, and disability. A post-hoc univariate analysis was then conducted for each of the dependent variables using one-way ANOVA with Newman Keuls pairwise comparisons. The results from this analysis indicate that STAI, $F_{(3,356)} = 11.6$, $P < .0001$, PHYS, $F_{(3,284)} = 11.1$, $P < .0001$ and PSYCSOC, $F_{(3,284)} = 3.29$, $P = .0215$ differed, with the two older age groups reporting less anxiety (Fig. 1) and psychosocial impact (Fig. 2), but a greater pain impact on physical activity (Fig. 2). The sensory and affective dimensions of pain, ADP and COP (Fig. 3; Table II), were not significantly different between the four age groups. A chi-square analysis of the proportion of patients suffering from depression also indicated no difference between age groups (Fig. 1).

To examine the issue of whether patients in the four age cohorts differed in the frequency of use of pain coping strategies, we conducted a MANOVA of the scores on the seven subscales of the CSQ. In common with the first analysis, age and gender were entered as factors, while duration of pain was entered as a covariate. The findings indicate a significant effect for age,

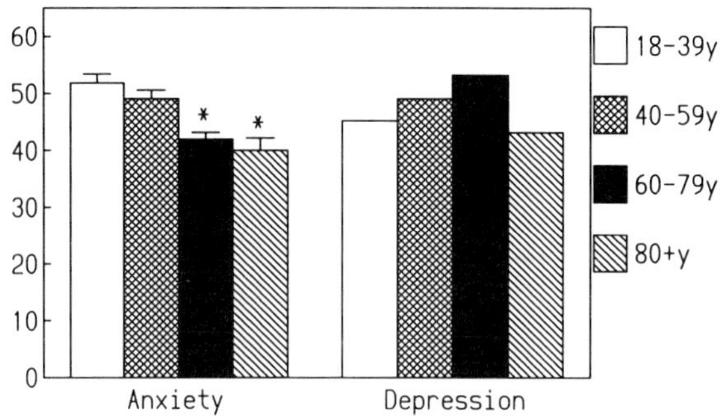

Fig 1. The histograms on the left present mean values and S.E.M. for the State Trait Anxiety Index (STAI) for each of the four age groups. The histograms on the right correspond to the number of persons in each group that exceeded the cutoff score for mild depression on either the Geriatric Depression Scale or the Self-Rating Depression Scale. The two older groups had significantly lower scores on the STAI than did the younger two groups, $P < 0.0001$.

$F_{(21,789)} = 1.95$, $P = .007$, with no difference between the genders, no age by sex interaction, and no significant effect for duration of pain as a covariate with each of the coping subscales. A post-hoc analysis using one-way ANOVA with Newman Keuls pairwise comparisons revealed that patients in the two oldest groups were significantly less likely to use ignoring sensation as a strategy when compared to the young, $F_{(3,298)} = 5.63$, $P = .0009$, and were more likely to use praying and hoping, $F_{(3,298)} = 3.97$, $P = .0085$ (Table II). All other subscales were used with similar frequency in the four age groups (Table II).

We conducted further analysis to examine age-related differences in the effectiveness of various coping strategies. Twelve stepwise multiple-regression analyses were performed using the seven subscales of the CSQ as independent variables and the psychometric measures of PRIS, PRIA, STAI, SRDS, GDS, PHYS, and PSYCSOC as the separate dependent variables. To increase the sample size and thereby increase the reliability of this analysis, patients were combined into two age groups (18–59, greater than 60 years of age). Scores from the depression scales were treated as continuous variables for this analysis. Table III provides a summary of the multiple-regression analyses using coping strategies to predict scores on pain, mood, and disability in patients aged less than 60 years, while Table IV provides a summary of the complementary analyses conducted in patients 60 years and older.

Of the seven coping subscales, catastrophizing was the most important predictor of pain, mood, and disability scores in both young and elderly chronic

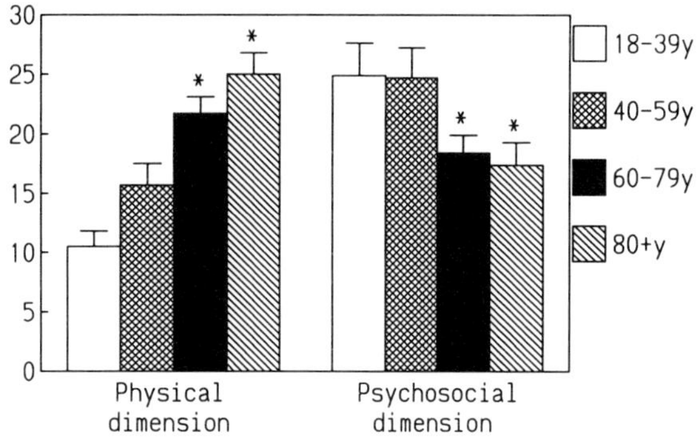

Fig. 2. This graph presents mean values and S.E.M. for both dimensions of the Sickness Impact Profile. Each histogram corresponds to one of four age groups. The histograms on the left and right relate to the physical and psychosocial dimensions of the Sickness Impact Profile, respectively. The two older groups reported more dysfunction on the physical dimension (* $P < 0.0001$) and less dysfunction on the psychosocial dimension (* $P = 0.02$) than did the two younger groups.

pain patients. An examination of the beta weight values indicates that this strategy was maladaptive; that is, patients who frequently engaged in catastrophizing reported higher levels of anxiety, depression, a greater impact of pain on physical and psychosocial function, as well as higher scores on the affective dimension of pain. The only notable departure from this general pattern involved scores on the sensory dimension of pain. Once again, catastrophizing was the most important predictor in young adults, accounting for approximately 10% of the variation in sensory pain ratings, while in older adults, an increased use of diverting attention was most related to increased sensory pain, accounting for 4% of the variance in this measure.

The types of coping strategies entered on the second and subsequent steps of the multiple regression analyses revealed some subtle but consistent age-related differences (Tables III, IV). In the elderly cohort the use of coping self-statements featured prominently as a positive influence on self-reported levels of depression, anxiety, physical, and psychosocial function. This was not the case for younger patients. Instead, ignoring pain sensations appeared to be the most important positive strategy adopted by the young and was associated with lower levels of anxiety and depression. Conversely, the frequent use of reinterpreting pain sensation was related to higher reports of pain (both sensory and affective dimensions) and higher scores on the SRDS in the young, but with exception of psychosocial disability, this maladaptive strategy did not occur in the elderly.

DISCUSSION

Contrary to previously published studies, our results support the existence of subtle differences in the experience of young and old patients with chronic pain. Demographic variables, for the most part, reflected the process of aging in the community at large. The older subjects were more likely to be female and widowed. The difference in duration of pain was counterintuitive. Older persons, who would be expected to have had pain of longer duration, actually experienced it for less time than did the young adult cohort. Referral patterns might have influenced this finding (Harkins 1988). None of these variables, nor the effect of different pain clinics, were significant factors in distinguishing differences on the psychometric measures. Age alone consistently identified differences in the chronic pain experience. It is of interest, however, that these differences occurred between persons aged less than 60 years and those in their seventh decade and beyond. Octo- and nonagenarians, a purportedly vulnerable group, appeared to suffer no more or less impact of chronic pain than did the 60- to 79-year-old cohort.

The age-related differences in the two dimensions of the SIP were in opposite directions with psychosocial effects less apparent in the older groups and physical effects less apparent in the young. Variations also were found in the reported levels of suffering. While all groups reported a similar prevalence of depressive symptoms, the two older groups had lower levels of anxiety. There was no age difference in self-reported ability to control or decrease pain. In keeping with the trend identified by Keefe and Williams (1990), older subjects more frequently employed praying and hoping. In addition, the strategy of ignoring pain was more prevalent in the young. However, the four age groups showed no discernible difference in pain reports.

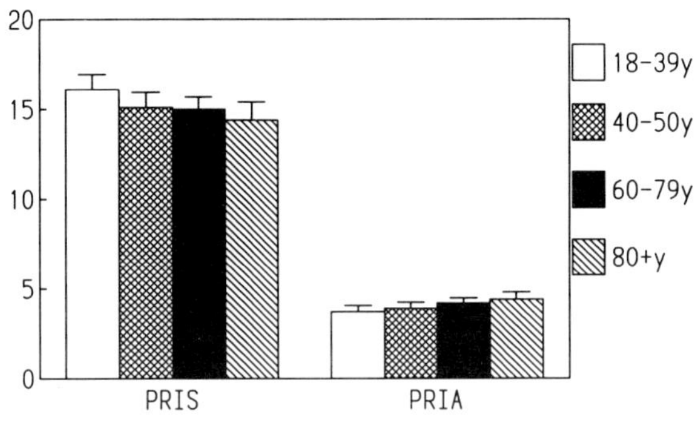

Fig. 3. This graph represents mean scores and S.E.M. for the sensory (PRIS) and affective (PRIA) dimensions of the McGill Pain Questionnaire (MPQ) for each of four age groups. The PRIS scores are on the left and the PRIA on the right. No two groups had significantly different scores.

Elderly patients tend to be more physically impaired, and their responses on the SIP may reflect an interaction between the effects of chronic pain and the increased comorbidity expected with age. The respective coping strategies employed by the two age groups do not appear to explain differences on the measures of anxiety and psychosocial functioning. Differences in anxiety levels might reflect an age-related change that occurs irrespective of the presence of pain. A previous study using the Profile of Mood States Questionnaire has noted that older, active community-dwelling subjects report less mood disturbance by up to one standard deviation when compared to younger subjects (Helme et al. 1992). The reasons for the difference in the psychosocial dimension of the SIP are less apparent. Perhaps older persons, who potentially suffer from a range of maladies and lack of social resources, are less inclined to ascribe disabilities in the psychosocial area to pain alone.

There is a selection bias for pain clinics, and the frequent use of maladaptive strategies is likely to characterize those who are referred to such treatment programs. Consequently, it is not unexpected that catastrophizing predicted significant proportions of the variance in almost all of the components of the pain experience regardless of age. The one exception was the sensory dimension of the MPQ. In the older group, diverting attention was the most important predictor, although it accounted for little of the variance in sensory pain ratings. Similarly, although catastrophizing was related to sensory pain in the young, the proportion of variance explained by this strategy was lower than for any other aspect of the pain experience. Clearly, other factors are contrib-

Table II
Mean values (± S.E.M.) for each of the subscales of the coping strategies questionnaire for the four age groups

	Age Group			
	18–39	40–59	60–79	80+
Reinterpreting pain	6.3 (0.9)	6.3 (0.8)	5.1 (0.6)	5.0 (0.9)
Catastrophizing	17.5 (1.1)	17.6 (1.1)	16.2 (0.8)	15.6 (1.5)
Increased behavioral activities	14.1 (0.9)	17.3 (0.9)	15.8 (0.6)	16.2 (1.5)
Diverting attention	12.1 (0.9)	14.0 (0.8)	13.0 (0.7)	11.7 (1.4)
Ignoring pain*	12.4 (1.0)	11.9 (0.8)	9.0 (0.7)	8.2 (0.9)
Praying and hoping*	14.6 (1.0)	16.3 (1.2)	18.3 (0.7)	20.2 (1.4)
Self-coping statements	19.1 (1.0)	20.3 (0.8)	18.7 (0.7)	19.3 (1.0)
Ability to decrease pain	2.1 (0.2)	2.0 (0.2)	1.9 (0.2)	1.6 (0.2)
Control over pain	2.1 (0.2)	2.3 (0.2)	2.3 (0.2)	1.9 (0.3)

* The older two groups had significantly higher scores on praying and hoping (P = 0.0085) and lower scores on ignoring pain (P = 0.0009).

Table III
Stepwise multiple-regression analyses using coping strategies to predict scores on pain, mood, and disability in subjects aged less than 60 years (N = 133)

	Multiple R	Beta Weight	Change in R^2	P value
MPQ–Sensory Rating				
Catastrophizing	.3105	.3458	.0964	.0001
Reinterpretation	.3664	.1976	.0559	.0195
MPQ–Affective Rating				
Catastrophizing	.4501	.4909	.2026	.0000
Reinterpretation	.5029	.2281	.0528	.0039
Zung–Depression				
Catastrophizing	.5498	.4881	.3023	.0000
Ignoring sensation	.5758	–.2633	.0260	.0052
Reinterpretation	.5961	.1750	.0203	.0487
Speilberger–Anxiety				
Catastrophizing	.4637	.4053	.2150	.0000
Ignoring sensation	.4991	–.1938	.0354	.0173
SIP–Physical Impact				
Catastrophizing	.3947	.3984	.1558	.0000
Diverting attention	.4558	.2279	.0611	.0100
SIP–Psychosocial Impact				
Catastrophizing	.4406	.4405	.1941	.0000

uting to variations in the report of sensory pain. It is possible, therefore, that treatment directed toward the adoption of more adaptive coping strategies may have less impact on reports on the sensory dimension of pain than on other aspects of suffering. This finding is consistent with those of Puder (1988), who observed that cognitive-behavioral therapy had little effect on pain intensity irrespective of age despite an association with improvement on other outcomes.

Other subtle differences could be discerned among the coping strategies used by the two age groups. There was an absolute difference in the level of praying and hoping between the groups, although this strategy does not have an important impact on their pain experience. The difference in absolute frequency of use is most likely due to a cohort effect. Young subjects more often ignored pain, which constituted an adaptive strategy. Older persons received benefit from the use of coping self-statements. Reinterpreting the pain and diverting attention had negative consequences for the younger and older subjects, respectively. Given that the frequency of use of coping self-statements was similar across the groups, this approach only appears to benefit older persons. The age differences in the level of ignoring pain have implications

Table IV
Stepwise multiple-regression analyses using coping strategies to predict scores on pain, mood, and disability in subjects aged greater than 60 years (N = 164)

	Multiple R	Beta Weight	Change in R^2	P value
MPQ–Sensory Rating				
Diverting attention	.2004	.2004	.0401	.0092
MPQ–Affective Rating				
Catastrophizing	.3432	.3432	.1175	.0000
GDS–Depression				
Catastrophizing	.5217	.4631	.2722	.0000
Self-coping statements	.5966	–.2951	.0749	.0000
Speilberger–Anxiety				
Catastrophizing	.5503	.4874	.3028	.0000
Self-coping statements	.6502	–.3519	.0999	.0000
SIP–Physical Impact				
Catastrophizing	.3361	.2398	.1129	.0024
Diverting attention	.3711	.2439	.0350	.0027
Self-coping statements	.4272	–.2309	.0561	.0043
SIP–Psychosocial Impact				
Catastrophizing	.3981	.3318	.1585	.0000
Self-coping statements	.4451	–.2587	.0470	.0008
Reinterpretation	.4798	.1879	.0347	.0126

for treatment. Are older persons unaware of the potential utility of this approach?

Clearly there are factors, other than ways of coping, that influence the chronic pain experience in both young and old. For example, it might be anticipated that factors such as social, family, and community support, diagnosis, and even activity itself might have differing influences on pain in patients across the age spectrum. Regardless of these unexplored domains, there are significant differences in pain and its sequelae between groups defined by age in this sample. The methods used in this study have not uncovered the reasons for these differences, and future studies will need to consider these issues.

ACKNOWLEDGMENTS

Preparation of this study was aided by a grant to Prof. R.D. Helme and Dr. S.J. Gibson from the Victorian Health Promotion Foundation. The authors gratefully acknowledge the work of the staff at the two clinics who were involved in collecting data for this study.

REFERENCES

Corran, T.M, Helme, R.D. and Gibson, S.J., An assessment of psychometric instruments used in a geriatric outpatient pain clinic, Australian Psychologist, 26 (1991) 121–131.

Fletcher, A.E., Dickinson, E.J. and Philp, I., Audit measures: quality of life measures for everyday use with elderly patients, Age Ageing, 12 (1992) 142–150.

Gibson, S.J., Katz, B., Corran, T.M., Farrell, M.J. and Helme, R.D., Pain in older persons, Disabil. Rehabil., (1994) in press.

Gilson, B.S., Gilson, J.S., Bergner, M., Bobbitt, R.A., Kressel, S., Pollard, W.E. and Vesselago, M., The Sickness Impact Profile: development of an outcome measure of health care, Am. J. Public Health, 65 (1975) 1304–1310.

Harkins, S.W. Pain in the elderly. In: R. Dubner, G.F. Gebhart and M.R. Bond (Eds.), Proceedings of the Vth World Congress on Pain. Pain Research and Clinical Management, Vol. 3. Elsevier, Amsterdam, 1988, pp. 355–367.

Harkins, S.W. and Price, D.D., Assessment of pain in the elderly. In: R. Melzack and D.C. Turk (Eds.), Handbook of Pain Assessment, Guilford Publications, New York, 1992, pp. 315–331.

Harkins, S.W., Kwentus, J. and Price, D.D., Pain and the elderly. In: C. Benedetti, C.R. Chapman and G. Moricca (Eds.), Recent Advances in the Management of Pain, Vol. 7, Raven Press, New York, 1984, pp. 103–122.

Helme, R.D., Katz, B., Gibson, S. and Corran, T.M., Can psychometric tools be used to analyse pain in a geriatric population? Clin. Exp. Neurol., 26 (1989a) 113–117.

Helme, R.D., Katz, B., Neufeld, M., Lachal, S., Herbert, J. and Corran, T., The establishment of a geriatric pain clinic: a preliminary report of the first 100 patients, Australian Journal on Ageing, 8 (1989b) 27–30.

Helme, R.D., Corran, T.M. and Gibson, S.J., Pain in the elderly, Proc. Aust. Assoc. Gerontol., 27 (1992) 22–26.

Hodkinson H.M., Mental Test Score, Age Ageing, 1 (1972) 233–238.

Jensen, M.P., Turner, J.A., Romano, J.M. and Karoly, P., Coping with chronic pain: a critical review of the literature, Pain, 47 (1991) 249–283.

Keefe, F.J. and Williams, D.A., A comparison of coping strategies in chronic pain patients in different age groups, J. Gerontol., 45 (1990) 161–165.

Melding, P., Is there such a thing as geriatric pain? Pain, 46 (1991) 119–121.

Melzack, R., The McGill Pain Questionnaire: major properties and scoring method, Pain, 1 (1975) 277–299.

Middaugh, S.J., Levin, R.B., Kee, W.G., Barchiesi, F.D. and Roberts, J.M., Chronic pain: its treatment in geriatric and younger patients, Arch. Phys. Med. Rehabil., 69 (1988) 1021–1026.

Puder, R.S., Age analysis of cognitive-behavioural group therapy for chronic pain outpatients, Psychol. Ageing, 3 (1988) 204–207.

Rosensthiel, A.K. and Keefe, F.J., The use of coping strategies in chronic low back pain patients: relationship to patient characteristics and current adjustment, Pain, 17 (1983) 38–44.

Sorkin, B.A., Rudy, T.E., Hanlon, R.B., Turk, D.C. and Steig, R.L., Chronic pain in old and young patients: differences appear less important than similarities, J. Gerontol., 45 (1990) 64–68.

Spielberger, C. D., Manual for the state-trait anxiety inventory. Consulting Psychologists Press, Palo Alto, 1983.

Yesavage, J.A., Brink, T.L., Rose, T.L., Lum,O., Huang, V., Adey, M. and Leirer, V.O., Development and validation of a geriatric depression screening scale: a preliminary report, J. Psych. Res., 17 (1983) 37–49.

Zung, W.W.K., A self-rating depression scale, Arch. Gen. Psychiatry, 12 (1965) 63–70.

Zung, W., The measurement of affects: depression and anxiety. In: P. Pichot (Ed.), Psychological Measurements in Psychopharmacology, Modern Problems of Psychopharmacology, Modern Problems of Pharmacopsychiatry, Vol. 7, Karger, Paris, 1974.

Correspondence to: Trevor M. Corran, MAP'sS, National Research Institute of Gerontology and Geriatric Medicine, North West Hospital, Poplar Road, Parkville, Victoria 3052, Australia. Tel: 61-3-389-7148; Fax: 6-13-387-4030.

Index

B

F

U

V